Critical Care Nursing: Synergy for Optimal Outcomes

Roberta Kaplow, RN, PhD, CCNS, CCRN, AOCNS

Clinical Nurse Specialist
DeKalb Medical Center
Decatur, GA

Sonya R. Hardin, RN, PhD, CCRN, APRN-BC

Associate Professor
School of Nursing
University of North Carolina at Charlotte
Charlotte, NC

JONES AND BARTLETT PUBLISHERS

Sudbury, Massachusetts

BOSTON   TORONTO   LONDON   SINGAPORE

World Headquarters

Jones and Bartlett Publishers	Jones and Bartlett Publishers	Jones and Bartlett Publishers
40 Tall Pine Drive	Canada	International
Sudbury, MA 01776	6339 Ormindale Way	Barb House, Barb Mews
978-443-5000	Mississauga, Ontario	London W6 7PA
info@jbpub.com	L5V 1J2	UK
www.jbpub.com	CANADA	

Jones and Bartlett's books and products are available through most bookstores and online booksellers. To contact Jones and Bartlett Publishers directly, call 800-832-0034, fax 978-443-8000, or visit our website, www.jbpub.com.

Substantial discounts on bulk quantities of Jones and Bartlett's publications are available to corporations, professional associations, and other qualified organizations. For details and specific discount information, contact the special sales department at Jones and Bartlett via the above contact information or send an email to specialsales@jbpub.com.

The authors, editor, and publisher have made every effort to provide accurate information. However, they are not responsible for errors, omissions, or for any outcomes related to the use of the contents of this book and take no responsibility for the use of the products and procedures described. Treatments and side effects described in this book may not be applicable to all people; likewise, some people may require a dose or experience a side effect that is not described herein. Drugs and medical devices are discussed that may have limited availability or are controlled by the Food and Drug Administration (FDA) for use only in a research study or clinical trial. Research, clinical practice, and government regulations often change the accepted standard in this field. When consideration is being given to use of any drug in the clinical setting, the health care provider or reader is responsible for determining FDA status of the drug, reading the package insert, and reviewing prescribing information for the most up-to-date recommendations on dose, precautions, and contraindications, and determining the appropriate usage for the product. This is especially important in the case of drugs that are new or seldom used.

Production Credits

Executive Editor: Kevin Sullivan
Acquisitions Editor: Emily Ekle
Associate Editor: Amy Sibley
Editorial Assistant: Lisa Gordon
Production Director: Amy Rose
Production Editor: Tracey Chapman
Marketing Manager: Katrina Gosek
Marketing Associate: Rebecca Wasley
Manufacturing and Inventory Coordinator: Amy Bacus
Composition: Auburn Associates, Inc.
Cover Design: Kristin E. Ohlin
Cover Image: © Photos.com
Printing and Binding: Malloy, Inc.
Cover Printing: Malloy, Inc.

Library of Congress Cataloging-in-Publication Data

Kaplow, Roberta.
   Critical care nursing : synergy for optimal outcomes / Roberta Kaplow, Sonya R. Hardin.
      p. ; cm.
   Includes bibliographical references and index.
   ISBN-13: 978-0-7637-3863-1 (casebound)
   ISBN-10: 0-7637-3863-8
   1. Intensive care nursing—Case studies. I. Hardin, Sonya R. II. Title.
   [DNLM: 1. Critical Care—methods—Case Reports. 2. Nursing Care—methods—Case Reports. WY 154 K17c 2007]
   RT120.I5K37 2007
   616.02'8—dc22
                           2006017424
6048

Printed in the United States of America
11 10 09 08 07   10 9 8 7 6 5 4 3 2

Dedication

This book is dedicated to Jack, Eleanor, Susan, Peter, James, Bria, Grace, Emily, Lucie, Teddy, and Princess.

The editors would like to recognize and thank James Perron for his contributions as an illustrator for this text.

The editors would also like to thank the American Association of Critical-Care Nurses for taking the initiative to develop the Synergy Model and for the years of moving practice forward through the identification of patient characteristics matched with nurse competencies to optimize patient outcomes.

The editors would like to recognize Kevin Sullivan of Jones and Bartlett for his insight into recognizing the value in publishing a critical care nursing text that utilizes the AACN Synergy Model. His patience during the process of writing this text is commendable.

Contents

Preface   xvii

Introduction   xix

Contributors   xxi

Reviewers   xxv

About the Authors   xxvii

Part I   Introduction   1

Chapter 1   Implementation of the Synergy Model in Critical Care   3
             Kevin D. Reed, Melanie Cline, and Karlene M. Kerfoot
             Overview of the Synergy Model   3
             Application of the Model: Patient Characteristics   4
             Application of the Model: Nurse Characteristics   8
             Summary   10

Part II   Caring Practices   13

Chapter 2   Family-Focused Care   15
             Fay Wright
             Definition of Family-Focused Care   15
             Definition of Family   16
             The Effect of Critical Illness on the Family   17
             Implementing Family-Focused Care   17
             Summary   22

Chapter 3   Creating a Healing Environment in the ICU   27
             Renee Rubert, L. Dianne Long, and Melissa L. Hutchinson
             Ancient Perspective   27
             Psychological and Physiological Connection of the Healing Phenomenon   28
             Physical Environment   28
             Healing Measures   33
             Recommendations for Creating a Healing Environment   35
             Summary   36

Chapter 4   Pain Issues in the ICU   41
       Celine Gélinas
       Definition and Types of Pain   41
       Physiology of Pain   42
       Pain Assessment in the Critically Ill Patient   43
       Pharmacological Management of Pain in the Critically Ill Patient   45
       Nonpharmacological Methods for Pain Management in the Critically Ill Patient   47
       Summary   48

Chapter 5   Sleep Disturbances in the ICU   53
       Catherine Vena
       Overview of Normal Sleep   53
       Sleep in the ICU   55
       Factors Contributing to Disturbed Sleep in the ICU   57
       Interventions to Improve Sleep in the ICU   60
       Summary   62

Chapter 6   Infections in the ICU   67
       Janet Eagan
       Patient Risk Factors for Infection   67
       Modes of Transmission   68
       Antibiotic-Resistant Infections in Critically Ill Adults   69
       Common Infections in the ICU   69
       Infection Control and Prevention   71
       Patient Outcomes   71
       Summary   71

Part III   Response to Diversity   75

Chapter 7   Gerontological Issues in Critical Care   77
       Diane J. Mick
       Predicting Outcomes for Elders Following Critical Illness   78
       Pathophysiology and Aging   79
       Summary   86

Chapter 8   Cultural Issues in Critical Illness   95
       Renee Twibell, Debra Siela, and Terri L. Townsend
       Cultural Concepts   96
       Cultural Assessment   97
       Cultural Factors in Planning Care   97
       Evaluating Cultural Care   104
       Summary   104

Chapter 9   Complementary Therapies in the ICU   109
       Michael Neville
       Therapeutic Touch   110
       Music Therapy   111
       Prayer and Spirituality   111
       Herbs   112
       Patient Outcomes   113
       Summary   113

Part IV	Clinical Judgment	117
	CARDIOVASCULAR	119
Chapter 10	Cardiac Anatomy and Physiology and Assessment	121
	Deborah Becker	
	The Cardiovascular System	121
	Dysrhythmia Interpretation	125
	Cardiac Assessment	132
	Summary	137
Chapter 11	Hemodynamic Monitoring	139
	Kim Blount	
	Physiologic Basics of Hemodynamic Monitoring	140
	Physical Assessment	146
	Troubleshooting Systems	151
	Clinical Inquiry and Decision Making	154
	Summary	155
Chapter 12	Coronary Artery Disease	159
	Barbara Hutton Borghardt	
	The Coronary Arteries	159
	Pathophysiology of Coronary Artery Disease (CAD)	159
	Risk Factors	161
	Markers of Inflammation	163
	Blood Supply and Demand	163
	Treatment of Chronic Stable Angina and Suspected or Known CAD	165
	Patient Outcomes	167
	Summary	167
Chapter 13	Hypertension	171
	James R. Steele and Sonya R. Hardin	
	Pathophysiology	171
	Urgent and Emergent Hypertension	173
	Nursing Management	174
	Nursing Management Based on Medical Diagnosis	175
	Patient Education	177
	Patient Outcomes	178
	Summary	178
Chapter 14	Acute Coronary Syndrome	181
	Barbara Hutton Borghardt	
	Unstable Angina	181
	Myocardial Infarction	181
	Assessment of the Patient	182
	Diagnostic Tests	183
	Complications of Myocardial Ischemia and Infarction	187
	Treatment of Acute Coronary Syndrome	188
	Interventions of the Critical Care Cardiac Patient	191
	Patient Outcomes	193
	Summary	193
Chapter 15	Heart Failure	197
	Sara Paul and Kismet D. Rasmusson	
	Pathophysiology	197
	Patient History and Physical Exam	198

Pharmacologic Treatment   199
Nonpharmacologic Treatment   203
Patient and Family Education   204
Patient Outcomes   204
Summary   204

Chapter 16   Cardiac Assist Devices   209
        Shannon L. DeLuca, Dana F. Kay, and Cathy Clark
VAD Basics   209
Care of the Patient with a VAD   216
Implantable Hemodynamic Monitoring Systems   218
Pacemakers   218
Implantable Cardioverter-Defibrillators   223
Patient Outcomes   224
Summary   224

Chapter 17   Cardiac Surgery and Heart Transplant   229
        Mary Zellinger
Preoperative Workup   229
Preoperative Education   230
The Day of Surgery   230
Operating Room   230
Immediate Postoperative Assessment   233
Immediate Postoperative Monitoring   233
Open Chest Resuscitation   236
Weaning from Mechanical Ventilation   236
Beyond the Immediate Postoperative Period   237
Preparation for Discharge   238
Cardiac Transplantation   238
Ventricular Assist Devices   239
Patient Outcomes   240
Summary   240

Chapter 18   Shock   243
        Eric S. Wolak, Ernest J. Grant, and Sonya R. Hardin
Creating a Foundation   243
Classifications of Shock Syndromes   245
Hypovolemic Shock   246
Cardiogenic Shock   247
Obstructive Shock   249
Distributive Shock   250
Stages of Shock   251
System Progression and Management   253
Managing the Patient with Shock   254
Nursing Management of Shock   255
Patient Outcomes   255
Summary   255

Chapter 19   Vascular Disorders   261
        Rebecca Long
Abdominal Aortic Aneurysm   261
Arterial Occlusion and Venous Occlusion   263
Compartment Syndrome   265
Patient Outcomes   266
Summary   266

	RESPIRATORY	269
Chapter 20	Respiratory Anatomy, Physiology, and Assessment	271
	Stephen Parkman	
	Anatomy of the Respiratory System	271
	Assessment of the Respiratory System	278
	Summary	280
Chapter 21	Respiratory Monitoring	283
	Dianna Levine	
	SpO_2 Monitoring (Saturation of Peripheral O_2)	284
	Arterial Blood Gas Monitoring	284
	pH	286
	$PaCO_2$	286
	HCO_3	287
	Compensation	287
	Base Excess	287
	$EtCO_2$ Monitoring	288
	Patient Outcomes	289
	Summary	289
Chapter 22	Select Respiratory Disorders, Airway Adjuncts, and Noninvasive Ventilation	293
	Leslie P. Golden, Roberta Kaplow, and Dianne Earnhardt	
	Vascular Causes of Respiratory Failure: Ventilation/Perfusion Mismatch (Deadspace)	293
	Restrictive Lung Disease: Ventilation/Perfusion Mismatch (Shunt)	294
	Obstructive Causes of Respiratory Failure	298
	Airway Adjuncts	299
	Noninvasive Ventilation	301
	Patient Outcomes	302
	Summary	303
Chapter 23	Mechanical Ventilation	307
	Suzanne M. Burns	
	Concepts of Positive-Pressure Ventilation	307
	Ventilator Parameters and Modes	308
	Nursing Management of the Patient on Mechanical Ventilation	311
	Weaning from the Ventilator	314
	Patient Outcomes	316
	Summary	316
Chapter 24	Common Respiratory Disorders	321
	Michael W. Day	
	Influenza	321
	Pneumonia	322
	Tuberculosis	325
	Asthma	327
	Chronic Obstructive Pulmonary Disease	330
	Patient Outcomes	333
	Summary	333
Chapter 25	Acute Respiratory Distress Syndrome	337
	Kelly Brennan-Paddock and M. Dave Hanson	
	Definition and Etiology	337
	Pathophysiology	338
	Clinical Manifestations	339
	Medical Management	339

Complications and Nursing Interventions   341
Patient Outcomes   343
Summary   343

NEUROLOGY   347

Chapter 26   Neurologic Anatomy, Physiology, and Assessment   349
              Joyce King
              Overview of Neurologic Anatomy and Physiology   350
              The Central Nervous System   351
              The Peripheral Nervous System   353
              Neurological Assessment   354
              Summary   357

Chapter 27   Multimodal Neurological Monitoring   359
              Daiwai M. Olson
              The Physical Neurological Examination   359
              Invasive Brain Monitoring   360
              Noninvasive Brain Monitoring   366
              Patient Outcomes   368
              Summary   368

Chapter 28   Common Neurologic Disorders   375
              Krista M. Garner
              Managing Elevated Intracranial Pressure   375
              Common Neurologic Disorders and Evidence-based Interventions   377
              Patient Outcomes   383
              Summary   383

Chapter 29   Neurologic Injuries   387
              Kelly Nadeau
              Pathophysiology   387
              Intracranial Pressure and Cerebral Perfusion Pressure   388
              Head Injuries   388
              Spinal Cord Injuries   390
              Vertebral Fractures   390
              Patient Outcomes   392
              Summary   392

Chapter 30   Cerebrovascular Disorders   395
              Susan Yeager
              Arteriovenous Malformations   395
              Cerebral Aneurysms   399
              Patient Outcomes   406
              Summary   406

GASTROINTESTINAL   411

Chapter 31   Gastrointestinal Anatomy, Physiology, and Assessment   413
              Joyce King
              Basic Digestive Processes   413
              Regulation of the Digestive Tract   414
              Components of the Digestive System   414
              Assessment of the Gastrointestinal System   416
              Physical Assessment   417
              Summary   419

Chapter 32   Gastrointestinal Interventions   421
              Pat Ostergaard and Roberta Kaplow
              Gastric Lavage   421
              Endoscopic Procedures   422
              Surgical Procedures   424
              Liver Biopsy   425
              Paracentesis   426
              Patient Outcomes   427
              Summary   427

Chapter 33   Nutrition Concepts for Clinical Practice in the Critically Ill Adult   431
              Linda DeStefano
              Review of the Literature   431
              Starvation Versus Stress Hypermetabolism   431
              Best Practices   432
              Practical Information for Optimal Delivery: Parenteral Nutrition   434
              Practical Information for Optimal Delivery: Enteral Nutrition   434
              Management and Safety Issues Related to Enteral Feeding   437
              Patient Outcomes   438
              Summary   439

Chapter 34   Gastrointestinal Bleeding   443
              Celeste Smith
              Etiology   444
              Assessment   444
              Diagnostic Testing   444
              Medical Management   445
              Nursing Management   447
              Patient Outcomes   447
              Summary   447

Chapter 35   Hepatic Failure   453
              Marian S. Altman
              Etiology   453
              Pathophysiology and Clinical Manifestations   454
              Other Sequelae of Hepatic Failure   457
              Patient Outcomes   461
              Summary   461

Chapter 36   Hepatitis   465
              Marian S. Altman
              Pathophysiology   465
              Etiology   466
              Hepatitis A   466
              Hepatitis B   467
              Hepatitis D   468
              Hepatitis C   469
              Hepatitis E   470
              Patient Outcomes   471
              Summary   471

Chapter 37   Pancreatitis   475
              Kelly Brewer
              Etiology and Incidence   475
              Clinical Presentation   476

Predicting Severity of Acute Pancreatitis   477
Systemic Complications   477
Local Complications   478
Metabolic Complications   478
Patient Care Management   478
Surgical Management in Acute Pancreatitis   478
Summary of Key Research   478
Challenges for the Nursing Student/Faculty   478
Patient Outcomes   480
Summary   481

ENDOCRINE   485

Chapter 38   Endocrine Anatomy, Physiology, and Assessment   487
              Linda L. Steele
              Anatomy and Physiology of the Endocrine System   487
              Assessment of the Endocrine System   490
              Disorders of the Endocrine System   491
              Summary   491

Chapter 39   Thyroid Disorders   497
              Cynthia V. Brown
              Normal Thyroid Function   497
              Thyroid Storm   498
              Myxedema Coma   499
              Euthyroid Sick Syndrome   500
              Patient Outcomes   500
              Summary   500

Chapter 40   Adrenal Disorders   503
              Donnie Jester
              Functional Anatomy and Physiology of the Adrenal Glands   503
              Significant Adrenal Disorders   504
              Patient Outcomes   508
              Summary   508

Chapter 41   Pituitary Disorders   511
              Christopher A. Vreeland
              Anatomy and Physiology   511
              Disorders of the Pituitary   513
              Management of Pituitary Disorders   514
              Patient Outcomes   515
              Summary   515

Chapter 42   Diabetic Emergencies   519
              Sarah B. Freeman
              Pathophysiology   519
              Hypoglycemia   520
              Hyperglycemic Emergencies   522
              Treatment   524
              Prevention   526
              Patient Outcomes   528
              Summary   529

RENAL   533

Chapter 43   Renal Anatomy, Physiology, and Assessment   535
              Pat Ostergaard and Roberta Kaplow
              Anatomy of the Renal System   535
              Physiology of the Renal System   536
              Assessment of the Renal System   538
              Assessment of the Renal System in the ICU   540
              Summary   540

Chapter 44   Acute Renal Failure   543
              Carol Isaac MacKusick
              Renal Failure   543
              Clinical Staging of Acute Renal Failure   546
              Key Research   548
              Patient Outcomes   548
              Summary   549

Chapter 45   Interventions for the Renal System   553
              Carol Isaac MacKusick
              Renal Replacement Therapies   553
              Principles of Dialysis   554
              Hemodialysis   555
              Peritoneal Dialysis   558
              Continuous Renal Replacement Therapy   559
              Dialysis of Drugs   560
              Key Research   561
              Patient Outcomes   561
              Summary   561

Chapter 46   End-Stage Renal Disease and Renal Transplantation   565
              Carol Isaac MacKusick
              Chronic Kidney Disease Staging   565
              The Acutely Ill ESRD Patient   566
              Renal Transplantation   568
              Patient and Family Teaching   569
              Key Research   570
              Patient Outcomes   570
              Summary   570

HEMATOLOGY   575

Chapter 47   Oncologic Emergencies   577
              Jennifer S. Webster
              Cardiac Tamponade   577
              Hypercalcemia   578
              Superior Vena Cava Syndrome   580
              Syndrome of Inappropriate Antidiuretic Hormone Secretion   581
              Tumor Lysis Syndrome   582
              Spinal Cord Compression   583
              Patient Outcomes   584
              Summary   584

Chapter 48   Human Immunodeficiency Virus and Acquired Immune
    Deficiency Syndrome   589
    Dianne Weyer
    Transmission   589
    HIV/AIDS and the Immune System   590
    Laboratory Tests   591
    Treatment   592
    Patient Outcomes   593
    Summary   593

Chapter 49   Thrombocytopenia   597
    Hildy Schell
    Platelets and Normal Hemostasis   597
    Platelet Disorders   597
    Clinical Presentation of Thrombocytopenia   598
    Evaluation and Diagnosis   599
    Treatment and Management   600
    Patient Outcomes   601
    Summary   601

Chapter 50   Disseminated Intravascular Coagulation   605
    Jan Teal
    Etiologic Factors   605
    Acute Versus Chronic DIC   605
    Coagulation   606
    Pathophysiology   608
    Diagnosis   608
    Treatment   610
    Systemic Assessment and Support   611
    Detection of DIC   613
    Patient Outcomes   613
    Summary   613

Part V   Systems Thinking   617

Chapter 51   Systemic Inflammatory Response Syndrome and Sepsis   619
    Mary Fran Tracy
    Definitions   619
    Pathophysiology   620
    Nursing Assessments   621
    Interventions   623
    Prevention of Infection   626
    Patient and Family Education and Communication   626
    Patient Outcomes   626
    Summary   626

Chapter 52   Burns   629
    Frank Costello
    Burn Assessment   629
    Burn Management   630
    Patient Outcomes   638
    Summary   638

Chapter 53   Managing the Transition from the Hospital   641
             Evelyn Koenig
             Transitional Planning as Collaborative Practice   642
             Aspects of Transitional Planning and the Nursing Role   642
             Screening   644
             Patient Outcomes   646
             Summary   646

Part VI   Collaboration   649

Chapter 54   Recovery of the Postanesthesia Patient   651
             Teresa Dozier
             Overview of Anesthetic Agents and Adjuncts   651
             Moderate Sedation/MAC   656
             Initial Postoperative Care   657
             Management of Postoperative Complications   659
             Patient Outcomes   663
             Summary   664

Chapter 55   Trauma   667
             Andy Betz, Sally Betz, and Kelly Nadeau
             Trauma Systems   667
             Phases of Trauma Care   668
             Trauma and Mechanism of Injury   668
             Physiology of Trauma and Injury   668
             Trauma Assessment   669
             Head Injury   672
             Spine Trauma   672
             Abdominal Trauma   674
             Thoracic Trauma   675
             Orthopedic Trauma   678
             ICU Considerations   678
             Patient Outcomes   680
             Summary   680

Chapter 56   Drug Overdose and Poisonings   685
             Michael Neville and Roberta Kaplow
             Acetaminophen   685
             Amphetamine and Methamphetamine   686
             Barbiturates   687
             Benzodiazepines   688
             Carbon Monoxide   688
             Cocaine   689
             Cyanide   690
             Methanol   691
             Opiates   692
             Salicylates   693
             Tricyclic Antidepressants   694
             Initial Nursing Management   695
             Patient Outcomes   695
             Summary   696

Chapter 57   Management of the Critically Ill Bariatric Patient   705
                    Catherine Head
              Indications for Bariatric Surgery   705
              Types of Bariatric Surgery   705
              Complications of Bariatric Surgery   707
              Management of the Bariatric Surgery Patient in the ICU   708
              Patient Outcomes   712
              Summary   712

Part VII   Advocacy and Moral Agency   717

Chapter 58   Bioethical Issues Concerning Death in the ICU   719
                    Shirlien Metersky
              Advance Directives   719
              Ethical Dilemmas   722
              Professional Misconceptions in Management of EOLC   723
              Summary   724

Chapter 59   Organ Donation   727
                    Jesse Scruggs, Kenneth E. Wood, and Alista "Cozzie" Watkins
              Contraindications for Donorship   727
              Brain Death Physiology   728
              Medical Management   728
              Care of the Organ Recipient   733
              Patient Outcomes   735
              Summary   735

Chapter 60   Palliative Care and End-of-Life Care in the ICU   739
                    Donna Arena and Roberta Kaplow
              Goals of Palliative Care   739
              The ICU Environment   740
              End-of-Life Care   740
              Advance Directives   741
              Symptoms and Management at the End of Life   741
              Barriers to Implementing Palliative Care in the ICU   743
              The Shift from Curative to Comfort Care   743
              Patient Outcomes   744
              Summary   744

Index   749

Preface

The purpose of this text is to create a foundation for nursing students, nurses involved in a critical care internship, or nurses already in practice who are new to the care of acute and critically ill adult patients regardless of the setting where the care is being delivered. We, the authors, also recognize that critically ill patients are being cared for outside the walls of the ICU and there are no boundaries for the setting of a critically ill patient. The book will also serve as a resource for staff seeking review in the fundamentals of critical care nursing.

This text is different from other critical care nursing texts. Like other books, it provides a foundation for care of acute and critically ill patients as well as a review of anatomy, physiology, and a system assessment. In this book, however, those chapters focused on disease entities include an application of the American Association of Critical-Care Nurses's (AACN) Synergy Model for patient care as the framework for providing nursing care.

The AACN Synergy Model is described in detail in the first chapter. According to the Synergy Model, patients who are acutely or critically ill will have variable levels of eight characteristics. The majority of patients, when admitted to the ICU, are highly complex and vulnerable—which are two of the patient characteristics. In addition, a patient may be unstable, unpredictable, and have low levels of resiliency and ability to participate in care and decision-making, depending on their acuity. The nurse caring for the patient and family brings eight competencies of his/her own to the healthcare situation. The book is divided into sections based on nurse competencies described in the model.

The primary characteristic emphasized throughout the text is clinical judgment, as this is consistent with what is stressed in academic settings and orientation programs. Inherent in caring for patients is a nurse's responsibility to facilitate learning about a disease process, treatment options, and resources available for the patient, family, and staff. Therefore, the "facilitator of learning" competency is woven throughout each of the chapters related to clinical conditions. This ought not detract from the significance of competency in the other characteristics in optimizing patient outcomes. These other characteristics are described in relation to the disease entities on the Web site associated with this text at: *http://nursing.jbpub.com/criticalcare.*

The assumptions of the AACN Synergy Model are incorporated throughout the book as patients are understood as biological, psychological, social, and spiritual entities who present at various levels of altered states of health. Patients are described within the eight patient characteristics of the model which are interrelated. The nurse–patient relationships fall within the context of the patient, family, and community. The nursing competencies of the Synergy Model should be developed, enhanced, and evaluated based on the needs of the patient. The goal of nursing is to restore a patient to an optimal level of wellness. Death can be an acceptable outcome, if the goal of nursing care is to move a patient toward a peaceful death or toward the organ donation process.

The authors and editors of this text have gone to great lengths to provide the reader with patient management strategies based on the most recent evidence. Each of the content areas includes a case study with associated critical thinking questions and some potential optimal patient outcomes, as well as Internet resources to encourage further exploration or provide ideas for further research. Each case study is analyzed based on the Synergy Model to emphasize its application to critically ill patients. (At the end of the chapters are online resources that were correct at the time the book went to press.)

In addition to these Web links, individuals are encouraged to review the authors' first book on the Synergy Model, *Synergy for Clinical Excellence: The AACN Synergy Model for Patient Care,* also published by Jones and Bartlett. This book provides the basics to understanding the Synergy Model and assigned readings can help the student to integrate the model into practice. Readers can also visit the AACN Certification Corporation homepage: *http://www.certcorp.org.* This site provides access to many articles that have been published on the Synergy Model, which will facilitate the student's use of this text book.

Caring for acute and critically ill patients and their families is a privilege. Nurses have the opportunity to promote optimal outcomes during one of the most vulnerable times in patients' lives. It is our hope that this text helps nurses achieve these optimal outcomes, however they are defined by the patient and family.

Roberta Kaplow and Sonya R. Hardin

Introduction

Congratulations on choosing *Critical Care Nursing: Synergy for Optimal Outcomes!* While this text covers core clinical content, it is unique in its incorporation of a nursing model and direct focus on patient outcomes. Jones & Bartlett Publishers is proud to bring you this exciting new book in such an important field. Below you'll find a brief overview of the key features of this text, including the complete companion Web site at *http://nursing.jbpub.com/criticalcare*. Faculty should note that this Web site takes the place of a costly CD-ROM or student workbook and is free to students. Read on to learn more about the structure of the book and about the features of the text and Web site. We hope you enjoy the book!

Organization

Critical Care Nursing: Synergy for Optimal Outcomes is organized around the American Association of Critical-Care Nurses's Synergy Model for Patient Care. The main sections of the book correspond with the nurse competencies described in this nursing model. The first part of the book defines the Synergy Model and how it functions as a framework for this textbook. The remaining parts focus on nurse competencies of the Synergy Model. Part II, "Caring Practices," describes issues specific to the critical care nursing environment—family-focused care, healing environments, and issues of pain, sleep, and infection. Part III addresses response to diversity—gerontological and cultural issues, as well as complementary and alternative therapies in the ICU. The clinical section of the book, Part IV, is entitled "Clinical Judgment," and focuses on clinical judgement and addresses the different systems that critical care nurses will work with most:

- Cardiovascular
- Respiratory
- Neurologic
- Gastrointestinal
- Renal
- Hematology

Clinical Judgement section begins with the anatomy, physiology, and assessment involved with that particular body system, and go on to cover monitoring, interventions, and specific diseases, disorders, and syndromes. Part V moves on to systems thinking for particular topics such as SIRS and sepsis, burns, transitioning from the hospital, recovery from anesthesia, trauma, overdoses and poisonings, and management of the bariatric patient. Part VI is a collaboration and addresses complex clients that require highly integrated interdisplinary care. The final unit, Part VII, delves into the challenging, yet incredibly important topics of bioethics, organ donation, and palliative care.

Every chapter includes the following features:

- **Learning Objectives**—found at the beginning of the chapter, these bullet points outline the knowledge readers will have gained once they've completed this chapter
- **Summary**—a brief paragraph recapping the key points of information
- **Case Study**—a detailed description of a particular patient or situation
- **Critical Thinking Questions**—questions to answer in response to the case study, designed specifically to encourage critical thinking and utilization of The Synergy Model
- **Online Resources**—a list of Web sites and URLs for finding additional information on the Internet

With an attractive two-color interior design, many anatomical illustrations, as well as essential points pulled out in boxes and tables, readers will find each chapter easy to navigate with key information highlighted for both quick reference and extended study.

Special Features

A variety of special features have been created to enhance this textbook and help readers fully utilize the Synergy Model concepts.

- **Optimal Patient Outcomes,** a key component of the Synergy Model, list the best possible results of effective critical care nursing.
- **Key Terms** list and define the most essential words and phrases.
- **Using the Synergy Model to Develop a Plan of Care** helps apply the Synergy Model to the specific patient situations found in the case studies and asks the reader to create a care plan.
- **Clinical Practice Guidelines** are specific strategies for guiding care and relate to different types of therapies and pharmacologic responses.
- **Critical Thinking Questions** are found throughout the text to help students process and expand upon the material they are reading and absorbing.
- **Patient and Family Education** boxes contain detailed instructions for passing on to patients and their family members for specific disease entities.
- **Drug Tables** list the most current drugs used for treating specific conditions, their dosages, and their effective ranges.
- **Diagnostic Tests** present the recommended tests, possible findings, and what diagnosis accompanies those findings.

Ancillary Package

A full companion Web site has been designed to accompany *Critical Care Nursing: Synergy for Optimal Outcomes,* found at http://nursing.jbpub.com/criticalcare. The special features here are designed to help complement and expand upon concepts found here in the main text and through typical classroom instruction. Designed to be as simple, yet as useful as possible, the features on the Web site can be accessed either by chapter number or by type of feature (i.e. Flash Cards or Web Links).

Instructors

Instructors will have access to the student resources on the Web site (below), and will also have access to the following secure resources that are designed to make teaching easier:

- **PowerPoint™** Slides to accompany each chapter and aid in classroom presentation of materials.
- **Lecture Outlines** to help guide and focus your lectures and discussions.
- **Critical Thinking Answers** to the questions found after each case study in the book. Assign the Critical Thinking Questions as homework or for small group work within the class!
- **Multiple-Choice Testbank**—over 600 multiple choice questions for use in giving exams, quizzes, and homework.

Students

The student features can be used to enhance individual study time or can be assigned by the instructor as homework. They include the following:

- The **Interactive Anatomy Review** displays an anatomical illustration and asks the student to identify certain components.
- **Animated Flash Cards** give a definition and ask for the key term—the student types in the answer.
- The **Interactive Online Glossary** allows students to search for key terms and their definitions alphabetically or by chapter.
- **Interactive Crosswords** function as real crossword puzzles—except the answers are made up of critical care nursing terms.
- **Matching and Fill-in-the-Blank Quizzes** test the students' knowledge of the key terms.
- **Web Links** contain all of the Web resources listed in each chapter of the book for easy clicking and linking!
- The **Synergy Aspects** lay out the eight patient characteristics of the Synergy Model and apply them to each of the Case Studies found within the text.
- **Audio Scenarios** provide sound clips of various patient scenarios and then ask questions regarding those clips for the student to answer.
- **Skills in Action** and **Interactive Simulations** are short video clips demonstrating different maneuvers or positions that nurses must sometimes perform.
- **Interactive Simulations** are interactive illustrations and photographs showing the mechanics of different body systems or maneuvers.
- **Assessment in Action** presents a brief scenario, and asks various questions about what the nurse in such a situation would do.

Contributors

Marian S. Altman, MS, RN, CCRN, ANP
Clinical Nurse Specialist
CCU Virginia Commonwealth University Health System
Richmond, VA

Donna Arena, PhD, RN
Palliative Care Clinical Nurse Specialist
Emory University Hospital
Atlanta, GA

Deborah Becker, MSN, RN, CRNP, BC
Program Director
Adult Acute Care Nurse Practitioner Program
University of Pennsylvania School of Nursing
Philadelphia, PA

Andy Betz, MS, RN, ANP
Nurse Practitioner, Trauma
Grant Medical Center
Columbus, OH

Sally Betz, MS, RN
Trauma Program Director
Ohio State University Medical Center
Columbus, OH

Kim Blount, MSN, RN, CCRN
Cardiovascular Clinical Nurse Specialist
Carolinas Medical Center
Adjunct Faculty, UNC Charlotte College of Nursing
Charlotte, NC

Barbara K. Hutton Borghardt, MSN, RN, CCRN
Clinical Nurse IV, Intensive Care Unit
Memorial Sloan Kettering Cancer Center
New York, NY

Kelly Brennan-Paddock, BSN, RN
Registered Nurse Associate Partner
Cardiovascular Critical Care Unit
Clarian Health Partners, Methodist Hospital
Indianapolis, IN

Kelly Brewer, MSN, RN
Instructor
Nell Hodgson Woodruff School of Nursing
Emory University
Atlanta, GA

Cynthia V. Brown, MN, RN, ANP, CDE
Adult Nurse Practitioner
Southeastern Endocrine and Diabetes
Roswell, GA

Suzanne M. Burns, MSN, RN, RRT, ACNP, CCRN,
   FAAN, FCCN, FAANP
Professor of Nursing, Acute and Specialty Care
APN 2, Medicine/MICU
School of Nursing
University of Virginia Health System
Charlottesville, VA

Cathy Clark, RN, MSN, FNP-C
Family Nurse Practitioner
Women's Health Clinic
West Jefferson, NC

Melanie Cline, MSN, RN
Director of Clinical Operations
Pediatric Specialty Care Center
Riley Hospital
Clarian Health Partners
Indianapolis, IN

Frank Costello, BA, RN, BSN, LMSW, CCRN
Nurse Clinician
The New York-Presbyterian Weill Cornell Burn Center
Independent Lecturer/Consultant in Burn, Trauma,
    Emergency and Critical Care Nursing (Adult/Pediatrics)
New York, NY

Michael W. Day, MSN, RN, CCRN
Trauma Nurse Coordinator
Sacred Heart Medical Center
Spokane, WA

Shannon L. DeLuca, BSN, RN, CCTC
Cardiac Transplant and Ventricular Assist Device Coordinator
Carolinas Medical Center
Charlotte, NC

Linda DeStefano, MSN, RN, CCRN, NP, FCCM
Cardiopulmonary CNS
Critical Care Services
MemorialCare
Saddleback Memorial Medical Center
Laguna Hills, CA

Teresa Dozier, RN, CPAN
Department Head
Perioperative Services and Pain Clinic
DeKalb Medical Center
Decatur, GA

Janet Eagan, BS, RN, MPH, CIC
Infection Control Manager
Memorial Sloan-Kettering Cancer Center
New York, NY

Dianne Earnhardt, RN, CRNA
Nurse Anesthetist
Carolinas Healthcare
Charlotte, NC

Sarah B. Freeman, PhD, RN, ARNP, FAANP
Betty Tigner Turner Clinical Professor
Nell Hodgson Woodruff School of Nursing
Emory University
Atlanta, GA

Krista M. Garner, MSN, RN, ACNP
Nurse Practitioner
Emory University Hospital
Neuroscience Critical Care
Atlanta, GA

Celine Gélinas, PhD, RN
Postdoctoral Trainee
School of Nursing
McGill University
Montreal, Quebec

Leslie P. Golden, MSN, RN, CRNA
Assistant Director, Clinical Education
Carolinas Healthcare System
Nurse Anesthesia Program/UNCC
Charlotte, NC

Ernest J. Grant, MSN, RN
Nursing Education Clinician II
Burn Outreach
N.C. Jaycee Burn Center
UNC Hospitals
Chapel Hill, NC

M. Dave Hanson, MSN, RN, CCRN, CNS
Clinical Nurse Specialist
Cardiovascular Critical Care Unit
Clarian Health Partners, Methodist Hospital
Indianapolis, IN

Sonya R. Hardin, PhD, RN, CCRN, APRN-BC
Associate Professor
University of North Carolina at Charlotte
Charlotte, NC

Catherine Head, RN, MSN, ANP-BC
Clinical Coordinator Bariatric Program
Carolinas Laparoscopic Advanced Surgery Program
Carolinas Medical Center
Charlotte, NC

Melissa L. Hutchinson, MN, RN, CCRN, CWCN
Clinical Nurse Specialist MICU/CCU
VA Puget Sound Health Care System
Seattle, WA

Donnie Jester, MSN, RN, FNP
Family Nurse Practitioner
Southeastern Endocrine and Diabetes
Roswell, GA

Roberta Kaplow, PhD, RN, CCNS, CCRN, AOCNS
Clinical Nurse Specialist
DeKalb Medical Center
Decatur, GA

Dana F. Kay, BSN, RN, CCTC
Cardiology Outcomes Manager
Carolinas Medical Center
Charlotte, NC

Karlene M. Kerfoot, PhD, RN, CNAA, FAAN
Senior Vice President for Nursing and Patient Care Services
    and Chief Nurse Executive
Clarian Health Partners
Indianapolis, IN

Joyce King, PhD, RN, CNM, MN
Assistant Professor
Nell Hodgson Woodruff School of Nursing
Emory University
Atlanta, GA

Evelyn Koenig, MSW, LCSW, ACM
Manager, Oncology Care Management
Grady Memorial Hospital
Atlanta, GA

Dianna Levine, MSN, RN, CCRN, BC
Instructor, Nursing Education
Maimonides Medical Center
Brooklyn, NY

L. Dianne Long, MN, RN, C
Clinical Coordinator, DDS
VA Puget Sound Healthcare System
Seattle, WA

Rebecca Long, MS, RN, CCRN, CMSRN
Academic Administrator/Clinical Nurse Specialist
VA Healthcare System San Diego/San Diego State University
San Diego, CA

Carol MacKusick, MSN, RN, CNN
Assistant Professor
Gordon College
Barnesville, GA

Shirlien Metersky, MSN, RN, CCRN
Heart Service Line Educator
Grant/Riverside Methodist Hospitals
OhioHealth
Columbus, OH

Diane J. Mick, PhD, RN, CCNS, GNP, FNAP
Associate Professor
University of Delaware School of Nursing
Newark, DE

Kelly Nadeau, MN, RN, CCRN
Trauma Nurse Coordinator
DeKalb Medical Center
Decatur, GA

Michael Neville, PharmD
Associate Clinical Professor
Nell Hodgson Woodruff School of Nursing
Emory University
Clinical Pharmacist
Emory University Hospital
Atlanta, GA

Daiwai M. Olson, PhD(c), RN, CCRN
Critical Care Nurse, Neuro Care Unit
Duke University Hospital
Durham, NC

Pat Ostergaard, MSN, RN
Clinical Nurse Educator
Duke University Hospital
Durham, NC

Stephen Parkman, BS, RRT
Respiratory Care Supervisor
DeKalb Medical Center
Decatur, GA

Sara Paul, MSN, RN, FNP
Director, Heart Function Clinic
Western Piedmont Heart Centers
Hickory, NC

James R. Perron, PE
Medical Illustrator
Hickory, NC

Kismet D. Rasmusson, MS, RN, BC, FNP
Heart Failure Prevention and Treatment Program
Program Development Team
LDS Hospital and Intermountain Health Care
Salt Lake City, UT

Kevin D. Reed, MSN, RN, CNA
Director of Clinical Operations
Neuroscience/Critical Care
Clarian Health Partners
Franklin, IN

Renee Rubert, MN, RN, CCRN
Clinical Nurse Manager
4 East Medical Telemetry
VA Puget Sound Healthcare System
Seattle, WA

Hildy Schell, MS, RN, CCRN, CCNS
Clinical Nurse Specialist, Adult Critical Care UCSF Medical
    Center Assistant Clinical Professor
UCSF School of Nursing
San Francisco, CA

Jesse Scruggs, MD
Fellow, Pulmonary and Critical Care Medicine
University of Wisconsin Hospital and Clinics
Madison, WI

Debra Siela, DNSc, RN, CCNS, APRN, BC, CCRN, RRT
Assistant Professor
School of Nursing, Ball State University
Clinical Nurse Specialist
Intensive Care Unit, Ball Memorial Hospital
Muncie, IN

Celeste Smith, BSN, RN, CCRN
ICU Staff Nurse
Memorial Hermann Hospital Systems
Katy, TX

James R. Steele, MSN, RN, ANP-C
Clinical Instructor
East Carolina University School of Nursing
Greenville, NC

Linda L. Steele, PhD, RN, APRN, ANP-BC
Associate Professor
East Carolina University School of Nursing
Greenville, NC

Jan Teal, MSN, RN, BC, CCRN
Staff Educator
High Point Regional Health System
High Point, NC

Terri L. Townsend, MA, RN, BC, CVN-II, FACCN
Instructor, Critical Care, Educational Services, Ball
  Memorial Hospital
Clinical Faculty, School of Nursing, Ball State University
Muncie, IN

Mary Fran Tracy, PhD, RN, CCRN, CCNS, FAAN
Critical Care Clinical Nurse Specialist
Fairview University Medical Center
Minneapolis, MN

Renee Twibell, DNS, RN
Associate Professor, School of Nursing
Ball State University
Faculty Associate, Administration and Research
Ball Memorial Hospital
Muncie, IN

Catherine Vena, PhD, RN
Postdoctoral Fellow
Nell Hodgson Woodruff School of Nursing
Emory University
Atlanta, GA

Christopher A. Vreeland, MSN, RN, FNP
Family Nurse Practitioner
Southeastern Endocrine and Diabetes
Roswell, GA

Alista "Cozzie" Watkins, BS, RN, CPTC
Inhouse Organ Recovery Specialist
Lifeshare of the Carolinas
Charlotte, NC

Jennifer S. Webster, MN, RN, APRN, BC, AOCN
Clinical Nurse Specialist/Nurse Practitioner
Georgia Cancer Specialists
Tucker, GA

Dianne Weyer, MS, RN, CFNP
Clinical Instructor
Department of Family and Preventive Medicine
Emory University
Atlanta, GA

Eric S. Wolak, BSN, RN, CCRN
Critical Care Clinical Nurse Education Specialist
Department of Nursing Practice, Education and Research
University of North Carolina Hospitals
Chapel Hill, NC

Kenneth E. Wood, DO
Director, Critical Care Medicine and Respiratory Care
The Trauma and Life Support Center
University of Wisconsin Hospital and Clinics
Section of Pulmonary and Critical Care Medicine
Madison, WI

Fay Wright, MS, RN, NP, BC
Clinical Instructor
Northern Westchester Hospital
Mt. Kisco, NY

Susan Yeager, MS, RN, CCRN, EMT
Neuroscience Nurse Practitioner
Riverside Methodist Hospital
Columbus, OH

Mary Zellinger, MN, RN, ANP, CCRN
Clinical Nurse Specialist Cardiac Surgery
Emory University Hospital
Atlanta, GA

Reviewers

Diane Brown, MSN, RN, CCRN
The University of Akron
College of Nursing

Louise Cook, RN, MSN, CCRN
The University of Akron
College of Nursing

Judy Crewell, MSN, RN
Assistant Professor of Nursing
Regis University
Per Diem Staff Nurse
Exempla Lutheran Medical Center

Susan Hurst, RN, MSN, CCRN, CNRN
Clinician Nurse Specialist
Critical Care Services
Banner Health

Roni Kearns, RN, MN
Nursing Instructor
Eastern Arizona College

Lynn Kelso, MSN, RN, APRN, FCCM
Assistant Professor of Nursing
University of Kentucky

Debbie McDonough, RN, MSN
Assistant Professor Department of Baccalaureate Nursing
Alcorn State University

Katherine Plitnick, RN, PhD, CCRN
Assistant Professor
Georgia Baptist College of Nursing
Mercer University

Debbie Pool, MS, CCRN
Instructor
Department of Nursing
Glendale Community College

Lynn Simko, PhD, RN, CCRN
Associate Professor
School of Nursing
Duquesne University

Barbara Stevenson, BSN, MS
Lecturer
School of Nursing
Washburn University

Diane White, PhD, RN, CCRN
Assistant Professor, GBCN
Mercer University

Gail Weybright, RN, MSN, CS, CCRN
Associate Professor of Nursing
Goshen College
Staff Nurse ICU
Goshen General Hospital

About the Authors

Roberta Kaplow, PhD, RN, CCNS, CCRN, AOCNS has been a critical care nurse for the past 27 years. She is currently the Clinical Nurse Specialist at DeKalb Medical Center in Decatur, GA. She also teaches online graduate nursing research and evidence-based practice courses for Excelsior College. She received her Bachelor of Science in Nursing degree from Long Island University and her Master of Arts in Nursing and Ph.D. from New York University. She has held a variety of clinical, education, and advanced practice roles. In these positions, she has strived to create an environment that promotes evidence-based practice. Dr. Kaplow has also served as a clinical professor and director of an oncology Master's program. She is the first nurse nationwide to receive Distinguished Cancer Scholar recognition by the Georgia Cancer Coalition. As an advanced practice nurse, Dr. Kaplow collaborates with the multidisciplinary team to promote optimal outcomes for the patient and family. She is the author of numerous articles and book chapters on a variety of critical care and oncology topics. She serves on the editorial board of *Applied Nursing Research* and is a peer reviewer of research manuscripts.

Dr. Kaplow has been a member of the American Association of Critical-Care Nurses for 27 years. She is certified as a CCRN and CCNS through that organization. She is serving on the Board of Directors of AACN and is a past and current director on the AACN Certification Corporation. She is also nationally recognized for her work with the AACN Synergy Model and is co-editor of the *Synergy for Clinical Excellence: AACN Synergy Model.*

Sonya R. Hardin, RN, PhD, CCRN, APRN-BC has been a critical care nurse for the past 25 years. She is certified by the American Association of Critical-Care Nurses as a CCRN and by the American Nurses Credentialing Center as a Medical-Surgical Clinical Nurse Specialist. She received her BSN and MSN from the University of NC at Charlotte, an MBA/MHA from Pfeiffer University, and a PhD from the University of Colorado Health Sciences Center. Post Doctoral work has been completed through the University of Madison Wisconsin on Hermeneutical Phenomenology and a Post-Doctoral Fellowship was completed in 2006 on Interventions for Chronic Illness through the University of NC at Chapel Hill.

As an Associate Professor in the School of Nursing at UNC Charlotte in Charlotte, NC, her teaching responsibilities include content in the graduate and undergraduate programs. Her area of expertise includes acute and critical care of chronically ill patients with a specific interest in the management of chronic heart failure. She is known nationally for her work on the AACN Synergy Model and has co-authored the first book on the *Synergy for Clinical Excellence: AACN Synergy Model.* In 2002, Dr. Hardin was chosen as a Hartford Scholar and then in 2005 attended the NIA Summer Institute for emerging researchers. She has been active locally and nationally in numerous organizations such as a former member of the Board of Directors of the AACN Certification Corporation, President of the Mu Alpha chapter of Sigma Theta Tau and board member of the local American Heart Association. She is on the review panel for the journal *Gerontological Nursing* and is Co-Editor of *Visions: The Journal of Rogerian Nursing Science.* She maintains her clinical practice by working perdiem at Davis Regional Medical Center in Statesville, NC.

Introduction

PART I

CHAPTER 1

Implementation of the Synergy Model in Critical Care

Kevin D. Reed   Melanie Cline   Karlene M. Kerfoot

LEARNING OBJECTIVES

Upon completion of this chapter, the reader will be able to:

1. Briefly state the purpose of the AACN Synergy Model in the delivery of care to acute and critically ill patients.

2. Define the eight patient characteristics a patient brings to a healthcare situation.

3. Define the eight nurse competencies needed for optimal patient outcomes.

4. Apply the Synergy Model to clinical examples.

5. Design a plan of care based on the Synergy Model to ensure optimal patient outcomes

The American Association of Critical-Care Nurses' (AACN's) Synergy Model for Patient Care has become widely accepted as a viable model for professional nursing in the 21st century. Since 1996, when the AACN Certification Corporation commissioned a think tank to conceptualize certified nursing practice, the model has been applied in both the nursing service and academic arenas. It has evolved into a practical and relevant means to enhance the articulation of nursing practice in diverse clinical practice settings. In its application, the Synergy Model brings both the work of nurses and the model to life (Curley, 2004) (see **Figure 1-1**).

The Synergy Model can be applied in various ways to foster the development of nurse competencies and to ensure an optimal match to the individual needs of patients. In the broad realm of nurse competencies, the model's concepts provide a unifying framework for the development of nursing job descriptions, peer review evaluations, and a career path trajectory. From this work, a curriculum for professional development can be envisioned and created to realize the potential for the professional nurse as a knowledge performer. The model can facilitate the evolution of a common language for nurses in identifying and communicating the needs of patients. A common language provides a structure for the development of methodologies that characterize patients and their needs, including nurse-to-nurse communication, documentation tools, and an acuity classification system.

Conceptual models are important because they illuminate what is essential or relevant to a discipline (Curley, 2004). The AACN Synergy Model for Patient Care clearly identifies the work of nurses as being based on their relationships to patients and their families. It provides a viable means for delineating the role of professional nurses in directly affecting the outcomes of patients and ultimately the overall success of healthcare organizations.

OVERVIEW OF THE SYNERGY MODEL

The beauty of the Synergy Model lies in its simplicity: It identifies the patient as the central focus, describing the patient's needs and the skills required of the nurse to best meet those needs (Curley, 1998). It is an extremely powerful tool to define the relationship between nurses and their competencies and the characteristics or needs of patients.

FIGURE 1-1 The AACN Synergy Model for Patient Care

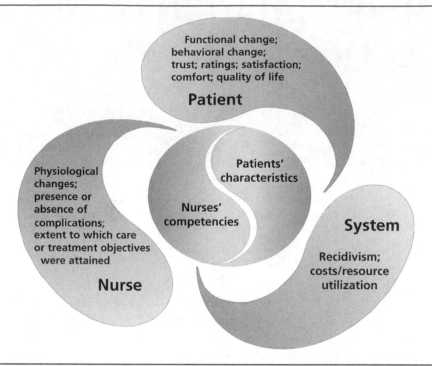

Source: From "Patient-Nurse Synergy: Optimizing Patients' Outcomes" by Martha A.Q. Curley, RN, PhD, CCRN, *American Journal of Critical Care,* January 1998, Volume 7, No. 1, Page 69.

The model describes eight patient characteristics and eight nurse competencies that constitute the practice of professional nursing (see **Tables 1-1 and 1-2**). It also provides a framework for outcome evaluation for the patient, the nurse, and the system. The basic premise of the model is that patient needs drive nurse skill sets; when nurse skills are matched to the needs of the patient, synergy occurs and patient outcomes are optimized (Curley). The model is relevant in all practice settings.

The eight patient characteristics span a continuum of health to illness: resiliency, vulnerability, stability, complexity, resource availability, participation in care, participation in decision making, and predictability. Patient outcomes include patient satisfaction with care, levels of trust, patient behavior and knowledge, patient functional change, and quality of life.

The model also defines eight dimensions of nursing practice: clinical judgment, advocacy/moral agency, caring practices, collaboration, systems thinking, response to diversity, facilitator of learning, and clinical inquiry. Nurse outcomes include the extent to which care objectives are met, management of physiological changes, and the presence or absence of preventable complications.

The third component of the model is the healthcare environment or system. The system acts as a facilitator or conduit to support patient needs and has the power to nurture the professional practice environment of the nurse. Successful outcomes for the patient and the nurse are dependent on the characteristics present in the healthcare system and the nurse's ability to create and support those system characteristics. Successful outcomes for both the patient and the nurse thus directly affect the success of the entire healthcare system. True synergy can be achieved only when all three components work synergistically to support the patient. The essential system characteristics include a patient-centered care philosophy, shared leadership, a learning environment, nurse–physician collaborative practice, and resources to support evidence-based practice, outcome evaluation, and patient safety. Outcomes viewed from the system's perspective include recidivism (i.e., repeat admissions), healthcare costs, and resource utilization (Curley, 1998).

APPLICATION OF THE MODEL: PATIENT CHARACTERISTICS

The Synergy Model presents an opportunity to build a common language for nurses in their efforts to sufficiently describe patients' needs, thus enabling the appropriate match to the competencies of the nurse. Utilizing the eight characteristics of

TABLE 1-1 The Patient Characteristics of the Synergy Model

Resiliency: The capacity to return to a restorative level of functioning using compensatory/coping mechanisms; the ability to bounce back quickly after an insult.

Level 1: Minimally resilient. Unable to mount a response; failure of compensatory/coping mechanisms; minimal reserves; brittle.

Level 3: Moderately resilient. Able to mount a moderate response; able to initiate some degree of compensation; moderate reserves.

Level 5: Highly resilient. Able to mount and maintain a response; intact compensatory/coping mechanisms; strong reserves; endurance.

Vulnerability: Susceptibility to actual or potential stressors that may adversely affect patient outcomes.

Level 1: Highly vulnerable. Susceptible; unprotected, fragile.

Level 3: Moderately vulnerable. Somewhat susceptible; somewhat protected.

Level 5: Minimally vulnerable. Safe; out of the woods; protected, not fragile.

Stability: The ability to maintain a steady-state equilibrium.

Level 1: Minimally stable. Labile; unstable; unresponsive to therapies; high risk of death.

Level 3: Moderately stable. Able to maintain a steady state for a limited period of time; some responsiveness to therapies.

Level 5: Highly stable. Constant; responsive to therapies; low risk of death.

Complexity: The intricate entanglement of two or more systems (e.g., body, family, therapies).

Level 1: Highly complex. Intricate; complex patient/family dynamics; ambiguous/vague; atypical presentation.

Level 3: Moderately complex. Moderately involved patient/family dynamics.

Level 5: Minimally complex. Straightforward; routine patient/family dynamics; simple/clear cut; typical presentation.

Resource availability: Extent of resources (e.g., technical, fiscal, personal, psychological, and social) that the patient/family/community bring to the situation.

Level 1: Few resources. Necessary knowledge and skills not available; necessary financial support not available; minimal personal/psychological supportive resources; few social systems resources.

Level 3: Moderate resources. Limited knowledge and skills available; limited financial support available; limited personal/psychological supportive resources; limited social systems resources.

Level 5: Many resources. Extensive knowledge and skills available and accessible; financial resources readily available; strong personal/psychological supportive resources; strong social systems resources.

Participation in care: Extent to which the patient/family engage in aspects of care.

Level 1: No participation. Patient and family unable or unwilling to participate in care.

Level 3: Moderate level of participation. Patient and family need assistance in care.

Level 5: Full participation. Patient and family fully able to participate in care.

Participation in decision making: Extent to which the patient/family engage in decision making.

Level 1: No participation. Patient and family have no capacity for decision making; require surrogacy.

Level 3: Moderate level of participation. Patient and family have limited capacity; seek input/advice from others in decision making.

Level 5: Full participation. Patient and family have capacity, and make decision for self.

Predictability: A characteristic that allows one to expect a certain course of events or course of illness.

Level 1: Not predictable. Uncertain; uncommon patient population/illness; unusual or unexpected course; does not follow critical pathway, or no critical pathway developed.

Level 3: Moderately predictable. Wavering; occasionally noted patient population/illness.

Level 5: Highly predictable. Certain; common patient population/illness; usual and expected course; follows critical pathway.

Source: www.certcorp.org/certcorp/certcorp.nsf/vwdoc/SynModel?opendocument

patients embedded in the Synergy Model, patient needs can be identified along a continuum of illness based on the assessment parameters of resiliency, vulnerability, stability, complexity, resource availability, participation in care, participation in decision making, and predictability. At any point, patients may fluctuate in their positions along these eight continuums, which can change within minutes (Curley, 1998). Assessing patients' needs along these eight continuums enhances the development of nurse communication via nurse-to-nurse reports, documentation systems, and articulation of patient acuity.

In the past, nurse-to-nurse communication in reporting the needs of patients has been felt to be inadequate and incomplete due to the limited amount of time allocated for this activity. Most recently, these types of communications have been identified as contributing to confusion and error (AACN, 2005). To provide adequate information between caregivers and across practice settings, nurses must first have in-depth knowledge of their patients and families. It is only by knowing patients that nurses become able to provide care respective of their

TABLE 1-2 The Nurse Competencies of the Synergy Model

Clinical judgment: Clinical reasoning, which includes clinical decision making, critical thinking, and a global grasp of the situation, coupled with nursing skills acquired through a process of integrating formal and informal experiential knowledge and evidence-based guidelines.

Level 1: Collects basic-level data; follows algorithms, decision trees, and protocols with all populations and is uncomfortable deviating from them; matches formal knowledge with clinical events to make decisions; questions the limits of one's ability to make clinical decisions and delegates the decision making to other clinicians; includes extraneous detail.

Level 3: Collects and interprets complex patient data; makes clinical judgments based on an immediate grasp of the whole picture for common or routine patient populations; recognizes patterns and trends that may predict the direction of illness; recognizes limits and seeks appropriate help; focuses on key elements of case while sorting out extraneous details.

Level 5: Synthesizes and interprets multiple, sometimes conflicting, sources of data; makes judgments based on an immediate grasp of the whole picture, unless working with new patient populations; uses past experiences to anticipate problems; helps patient and family see the "big picture;" recognizes the limits of clinical judgment and seeks multidisciplinary collaboration and consultation with comfort; recognizes and responds to the dynamic situation.

Advocacy and moral agency: Working on another's behalf and representing the concerns of the patient/family and nursing staff; serving as a moral agent in identifying and helping to resolve ethical and clinical concerns within and outside the clinical setting.

Level 1: Works on behalf of patient; self-assesses personal values; aware of ethical conflicts/issues that may surface in clinical setting; makes ethical/moral decisions based on rules; represents patient when patient cannot represent self; aware of patient's rights.

Level 3: Works on behalf of patient and family; considers patient values and incorporates them in care, even when differing from personal values; supports colleagues in ethical and clinical issues; moral decision making can deviate from rules; demonstrates give-and-take with patient's family, allowing them to speak for/represent themselves when possible; aware of patient and family rights.

Level 5: Works on behalf of patient, family, and community; advocates from patient/family perspective, whether similar to or different from personal values; advocates ethical conflict and issues from patient/family perspective; suspends rules—patient and family drive moral decision making; empowers the patient and family to speak for/represent themselves; achieves mutuality within patient–professional relationships.

Caring practices: Nursing activities that create a compassionate, supportive, and therapeutic environment for patients and staff, with the aim of promoting comfort and healing and preventing unnecessary suffering. Includes, but is not limited to, vigilance, engagement, and responsiveness of caregivers, including family and healthcare personnel.

Level 1: Focuses on the usual and customary needs of the patient; no anticipation of future needs; bases care on standards and protocols; maintains a safe physical environment; acknowledges death as a potential outcome.

Level 3: Responds to subtle patient and family changes; engages with the patient as a unique person in a compassionate manner; recognizes and tailors caring practices to the individuality of patient and family; domesticates the patient's and family's environment; recognizes that death may be an acceptable outcome.

Level 5: Has astute awareness and anticipates patient and family changes and needs; is fully engaged with and senses how to stand alongside the patient, family, and community; caring practices follow the patient and family lead; anticipates hazards and avoids them, and promotes safety throughout the patient's and family's transitions along the healthcare continuum; orchestrates the process that ensures the patient's and family's comfort and concerns surrounding issues of death and dying are met.

Collaboration: Working with others (e.g., patients, families, healthcare providers) in a way that promotes/encourages each person's contributions toward achieving optimal/realistic patient/family goals. Involves intra- and interdisciplinary work with colleagues and community.

Level 1: Willing to be taught, coached, and/or mentored; participates in team meetings and discussions regarding patient care and/or practice issues; open to various team members' contributions.

Level 3: Seeks opportunities to be taught, coached, and/or mentored; elicits others' advice and perspectives; initiates and participates in team meetings and discussions regarding patient care and/or practice issues; recognizes and suggests various team members' participation.

Level 5: Seeks opportunities to teach, coach, and mentor, and to be taught, coached, and mentored; facilitates active involvement and complementary contributions of others in team meetings and discussions regarding patient care and/or practice issues; involves/recruits diverse resources when appropriate to optimize patient outcomes.

Systems Thinking: Body of knowledge and tools that allow the nurse to manage whatever environmental and system resources exist for the patient/family and staff, within or across healthcare and non-healthcare systems.

Level 1: Uses a limited array of strategies; limited outlook—sees the pieces or components; does not recognize negotiation as an alternative; sees patient and family within the isolated environment of the unit; sees self as key resource.

Level 3: Develops strategies based on the needs and strengths of the patient/family; able to make connections within components; sees opportunity to negotiate but may not have strategies; developing a view of the patient/family transition process; recognizes how to obtain resources beyond self.

Level 5: Develops, integrates, and applies a variety of strategies that are driven by the needs and strengths of the patient/family; global or holistic outlook—sees the whole rather than the pieces; knows when and how to negotiate and navigate through the system on behalf of patients and families; anticipates needs of patients and families as they move through the healthcare system; utilizes untapped and alternative resources as necessary.

Response to diversity: The sensitivity to recognize, appreciate, and incorporate differences into the provision of care. Differences may include, but are not limited to, cultural differences, spiritual beliefs, gender, race, ethnicity, lifestyle, socioeconomic status, age, and values.

Level 1: Assesses cultural diversity; provides care based on own belief system; learns the culture of the healthcare environment.

Level 3: Inquires about cultural differences and considers their impact on care; accommodates personal and professional differences in the plan of care; helps the patient/family understand the culture of the healthcare system.

Level 5: Responds to, anticipates, and integrates cultural differences into patient/family care; appreciates and incorporates differences, including alternative therapies, into care; tailors healthcare culture, to the extent possible, to meet the diverse needs and strengths of the patient/family.

Facilitator of learning: The ability to facilitate learning for patients/families, nursing staff, other members of the healthcare team, and the community. Includes both formal and informal facilitation of learning.

Level 1: Follows planned educational programs; sees patient/family education as a separate task from delivery of care; provides data without seeking to assess the patient's readiness for or understanding information; has limited knowledge of the totality of the educational needs; focuses on the nurse's perspective; sees the patient as a passive recipient.

Level 3: Adapts planned educational programs; begins to recognize and integrate different ways of teaching into delivery of care; incorporates the patient's understanding into practice; sees the overlapping of educational plans from different healthcare providers' perspectives; begins to see the patient as having input into goals; begins to see individualism.

Level 5: Creatively modifies or develops patient/family education programs; integrates patient/family education throughout delivery of care; evaluates the patient's understanding by observing behavior changes related to learning; is able to collaborate and incorporate all healthcare providers' and educational plans into the patient/family educational program; sets patient-driven goals for education; sees the patient/family as having choices and consequences that are negotiated in relation to education.

Clinical inquiry: The ongoing process of questioning and evaluating practice and providing informed practice. Creating practice changes through research utilization and experiential learning.

Level 1: Follows standards and guidelines; implements clinical changes and research-based practices developed by others; recognizes the need for further learning to improve patient care; recognizes obvious changing patient situation (e.g., deterioration, crisis); needs and seeks help to identify patient problem.

Level 3: Questions appropriateness of policies and guidelines; questions current practice; seeks advice, resources, or information to improve patient care; begins to compare and contrast possible alternatives.

Level 5: Improves, deviates from, or individualizes standards and guidelines for particular patient situations or populations; questions and/or evaluates current practice based on patients' responses, review of the literature, research, and education/learning; acquires knowledge and skills needed to address questions arising in practice and improve patient care. (The domains of clinical judgment and clinical inquiry converge at the expert level; they cannot be separated.)

Source: www.certcorp.org/certcorp/certcorp.nsf/vwdoc/SynModel?opendocument

needs and in the context in which they become manifested. The Synergy Model framework provides a means of organizing subjective and objective data about patients so that their needs are consistently identified and continuity of care is maintained throughout the episode of illness.

The following example helps to understand the Synergy Model application in nurse-to-nurse communication. Daniel is a 42-year-old male with chronic diabetes who is in severe cardiogenic shock, following his third acute myocardial infarction. Upon reviewing his case, Daniel can be described as highly complex, unstable, unpredictable, vulnerable, and resilient, with a family that has been an active part of his care and decision making. Having been ill for some time, his resource availability has become inadequate. Incorporating the holistic view of the patient into nurse-to-nurse communication, including shift report, postoperative review, multidisciplinary rounding, and discharge planning ensures a common language and comprehensive understanding of the trajectory of illness. It also serves to clearly identify the patient's needs and assists in developing a plan of care, including identification of the competencies of individual nurses that would best match the patient's needs.

Once a common language is identified and utilized, patient documentation systems can be aligned around the eight patient characteristics as well. The traditional approaches to documentation, including the body systems and head-to-toe methods, do not allow for an adequate synthesis of the data points to characterize patients and families in advanced healthcare situations. The Synergy Model framework provides a method to understand patient needs from a broad perspective, incorporating data and qualitative information into the overall portrait of the patient. Whether they are manual or electronic, care maps, pathways, flow sheets, patient education documents, and discharge planning records can all be designed according to the needs of patients as outlined in the model. Assigning data points and other information to the categories of patient needs helps to differentiate the overall needs of the patient and enables the development of a patient acuity scoring structure.

Acuity Systems

Many healthcare systems use acuity systems as a mechanism to guide decision making related to staffing a unit. Typically, acuity systems assign numbers or categories to patients that correspond with the amount of tasks required for the care of the patient. This method of basing staffing decisions on the number of tasks required does not take into account the vulnerability or complexity of the patient with multisystem problems whom the nurse encounters in the intensive care unit (ICU).

Nurses must advocate for changing systems in such a manner as to create acuity systems that provide a holistic approach toward evaluating the needs of the patient. An acuity system based on the Synergy Model, for example, affords the system an opportunity to classify patients based on their characteristics versus the number of tasks performed during a shift.

Classifying and scoring patient acuity according to the patient characteristics of the model also requires that data and other information about patients be ranked according to the resources required to meet the patient's needs. For example, the vulnerability of a patient could be scored as a 1, 3, or 5. A score of 1 would indicate the patient had a low level of vulnerability; a score of 3 would indicate a moderate level of vulnerability; a score of 5 would indicate a high level of vulnerability.

The following example simplifies the process of assigning acuity to a patient. Sarah is a 22-year-old female undergoing an appendectomy following an episode of acute appendicitis. Her vital signs—including temperature, respiratory rate, heart rate, and blood pressure—are needed every four hours and have been stable. Sarah requires fluids, antibiotic therapy, and frequent pain assessment. She has been stable in the post-anesthesia care unit and is being prepared for transfer to the surgical unit. Her parents are assisting in her care and have adequate resource availability. In this scenario, an expert nurse could rank the patient's needs on a scale of 1, 3, or 5 based on the patient characteristics defined in the Synergy Model. The results might look similar to this: resiliency, 3; vulnerability, 3; stability, 3; complexity, 1; resource availability, 5; participation in care, 5; participation in decision making, 5; and predictability, 5. By ranking the patient's needs according to the patient characteristics, a comprehensive view of the patient becomes clear. In this case, the patient might be described as stable and resilient, with a highly predictable course of illness. She is moderately vulnerable to physiologic and environmental stressors. The patient and the family are fully engaged in participating and making decisions about the plan of care, and adequate resources are available to support them.

APPLICATION OF THE MODEL: NURSE CHARACTERISTICS

The work of nurses is also well articulated by the Synergy Model framework and leads to the ability to capitalize on individual strengths of nurses and to match those strengths to what is required by the patient. It has long been established that nursing practice can be plotted along a continuum based on levels of expertise. The work of Benner (1984) describes this continuum as being characterized by stages moving from novice to expert. The Synergy Model incorporates the idea that nursing knowledge and skills are unique to the professional practice of each individual nurse (AACN Certification Corporation, 2003; Muenzen, Greenberg, & Pirro, 2004). It emphasizes the ability to clearly differentiate various levels of expertise, including competent, proficient, and expert clinical practice and leadership (Kerfoot & Cox, 2005). Although the Synergy Model has been theoretically validated, its use in practice continues to evolve. The application of the model in the care of patients and their families presents many promising opportunities (Edwards, 1999).

The eight nurse characteristics of the Synergy Model provide a comprehensive and contemporary view of the work of nurses (Curley, 1998). These characteristics can serve as a conceptual framework for roles that distinguish levels of nursing practice for the purpose of professional development and career advancement. In the past, many career advancement programs (career ladders) have focused on the completion of tasks as the basis for moving from one level to the next. By contrast, the eight nurse characteristics of the Synergy Model provide a framework that enables a career advancement program to be constructed based on progressive levels of expertise in caring, clinical practices, and leadership.

The development of job descriptions based on the nurse characteristics of the Synergy Model serves as a blueprint for defining nursing practice and competencies that link to the needs of patients and their families (Hardin & Kaplow, 2005). Each of the eight nurse characteristics of the Synergy Model allows for categorization of essential elements of competent, proficient, and expert nursing practice. Performance standards can then be developed that are strongly linked to patient, nurse, and system outcomes. **Table 1-3** provides an example showing how three characteristics of the Synergy Model are useful for job description development (Czerwinski, Blastic, & Rice, 1999).

A job description can be developed by using the Synergy Model and three levels of performance: levels 1, 3, and 5. Each level of performance is associated with specific activities that are observed in the nurse. Such an application can be useful in evaluating nurses and in conducting annual performance reviews. These performance standards provide the nurse with clear expectations in an ICU setting and allow practice to be guided by the Synergy Model.

Educating Nurses

The Synergy Model provides a functional approach to educational programming and development that transcends customary approaches to nursing education and broadens the ability to respond to the needs of patients and their families. The model can help nursing students develop a plan of care for each patient. Utilizing the eight patient characteristics, the nurse can identify both subjective and objective data needed to choose evidence-based interventions for the patient. **Table 1-4** depicts a form that students can use in developing a plan of care. This form can be used to gather data, define individualized and standardized patient interventions, and identify optimal patient and family outcomes. Outcomes should focus on patient satisfaction, levels of trust, patient behavior, patient knowledge, patient function, and quality of life. The form can also be used to facilitate nurse-to-nurse communication during a change of shift (Hardin, 2004).

Nurses should evaluate patient needs in relation to a set of nursing characteristics for optimal outcomes to be obtained. For example, patients who have high levels of vulnerability, low levels of resiliency, and low levels of stability, and who are highly complex and highly unpredictable, would require an expert nurse overseeing their care. Competent nurses should

TABLE 1-3 Performance Standards Applied to Selected Nurse Characteristics

Nurse Characteristic	Level 1 Performance Standard	Level 3 Performance Standard	Level 5 Performance Standard
Clinical judgment	Utilizes policies, procedures, and protocols to make clinical practice decisions.	Incorporates multiple sources of assessment data in making clinical practice decisions.	Recognizes ultra-subtle changes in patients and acts to prevent adverse outcomes.
Caring practices	Develops professional and trusting relationships that facilitate patient/family coping.	Seeks various types of consultation to assist with patient/family coping.	Understands patterns in patient/family coping and proactively seeks consultation from the multiprofessional team. Provides evidence-based interventions in the management of coping.
Collaboration	Communicates patient/family needs to the multidisciplinary team.	Clearly delineates the expertise of individuals within the multiprofessional team and provides timely consultation.	Recognizes individualized needs of patients/families and proactively seeks expert consultation.

TABLE 1-4 Using the Synergy Model to Develop a Plan of Care

Patient Characteristics	Subjective and Objective Data	Evidence-Based Intervention(s)	Outcomes
Resiliency			
Vulnerability			
Stability			
Complexity			
Resource Availability			
Participation in care			
Participation in decision making			
Predictability			

be mentored by these experts when patient characteristics indicate that the patient status warrants an expert's care.

SUMMARY

The Synergy Model can be utilized as a framework for practice. Its eight patient characteristics and eight nurse competencies provide healthcare providers with an approach designed to logically formulate a plan of care, evaluate nurses' competency, and identify patient acuity to ensure adequate staffing. Furthermore, the model has served as a foundation when healthcare facilities sought to transform professional practice. The following case study describes the use of the model in a system-wide integration across a number of hospitals.

The power of the Synergy Model is reflected in the richness of the relationship between individual nurse and patient and the infinite variety of the combinations of nurses' contri-

butions to individual patient situations in all practice settings. Supported by the power of technology and the electronic medical record, this model has promise for evaluating specific nursing interventions within each of the dimensions of practice and their relationship to specific patient outcomes. This electronic support will catapult nursing practice into a future in which nurses evaluate the outcomes of their practice in real time and systematically study the results of individual and group practices on patient outcomes at the individual, unit, and system levels.

The Synergy Model is extremely effective in articulating the important role that professional nursing plays in the healthcare system and, when facilitated by the organization, defines the impact professional nursing can have not only on patient outcomes, but also on organizational transformation and success.

CASE STUDY

Organizational Exemplar: Clarian Health Partners, Indianapolis, IN

The Synergy Model for Patient Care is the framework for the Clarian Health Professional Practice model that has been implemented across this multihospital system in all clinical settings. The three major tenets of the model—the nurse, the patient, and the system—have served as a road map for the development and implementation of a revolutionary approach to patient care and professional nursing. Patient centrality is the hallmark of the Synergy Model, with patient needs driving the skills required in the nurse and in the physical environment to attain optimal patient outcomes.

Application of the Synergy Model at Clarian Health Partners

The Clarian Health model was implemented in 2003, as a result of a unique partnership with AACN. Utilizing the nurse characteristics of the model, a career advancement program was designed to differentiate practice and delineate three levels of practice and compensation. A promotional process to differentiate clinical expertise and level of contribution as the criteria for promotion was established. Foundational support for the career advancement program included a realignment of all nursing job documents as well as the development of a performance appraisal system based on the job documents. A unique compensation program was developed to acknowledge the value of advanced skill sets and the contributions that nurses make to patients, unit goals, and system outcomes. A curriculum to enable multidimensional practice and advancing skill sets was pursued, which eventually evolved into a set of core synergy classes. A career advancement board of review, whose primary purpose was to protect the integrity of the program, was established to guide the promotional process. Finally, the professional practice environment was permeated with the Synergy Model by using a shared leadership philosophy, allowing synergy and the model to thrive and supporting the staff in learning the model.

Implementation

We began our implementation on what we deemed the "nurse side" of the model. To fully develop and implement the model, we initially focused on creating a career advancement program. Our nursing staff identified the need for a professional practice environment that would reward and recognize nurses' contributions to patient care. The Synergy Model naturally delineates patient needs along on a continuum and nurses' skill sets from low to high to match those patient needs.

This delineation lent itself to the development of a differentiated practice model that defined three levels of practice: Associate Partner, Partner, and Senior Partner. The Associate Partner is a competent practitioner, the Partner is a proficient practitioner, and the Senior Partner is an expert practitioner. In addition to level of practice, the scope of responsibility for each classification was established and leveled: The Associate Partner's primary focus is the patient, the Partner focuses on unit outcomes, and the Senior Partner is accountable for patient population and system outcomes.

The design work for the model began with eight full-day sessions and included nurses from all levels of the organization and every practice setting, as well as internal experts on the nurse characteristic being analyzed. Behavioral expectations were developed, leveled, and subsequently went through an extensive review process, with more than 750 nurses providing feedback on the content for understandability, fit within the dimension, and appropriate leveling. Behaviors within each dimension were designated as primary or secondary so as to provide a developmental plan and stretch within the job documents. Primary behaviors must be met prior to application for promotion to demonstrate capacity for the work. The secondary behaviors within each document must be demonstrated within six months of promotion.

Upon completion of the behaviors, criterion measures were developed for each behavior. Criterion measures are concrete examples of how nurses can demonstrate competency. The criterion measures were reviewed, and consensus was reached that they represented equivalent practice across inpatient, outpatient, and procedural settings. This process established inter-rater reliability for the job documents, so that practice could be evaluated across all areas of practice.

Phase II of the Clarian Health model is currently under development. It will include operational definitions of the patient characteristics described in the model to quantify and measure the presence or absence of each of the characteristics; development of an ongoing assessment tool, and evidence-based interventions that will be embedded in the electronic medical record; and the development of a care delivery model that matches the patient with the nurse most qualified to meet the needs of that patient and supports the nurse–patient relationship. Phase III of the Clarian Health model is envisioned to result in the creation of a mature model, having a substantial influence on patient, nurse, and system outcomes.

CRITICAL THINKING QUESTIONS

1. Write a case example from the clinical setting highlighting one patient characteristic. Explain how this characteristic was observed through subjective and objective data.

2. Utilize the form in Table 1-4 to write up a plan of care for one client in the clinical setting.

3. Write a case example from the clinical setting. Rate the patient as a level 1, 3, or 5 on each patient characteristic. Identify the level of nurse characteristics needed in the care of this patient.

4. Take one patient outcome for a patient and list evidence-based interventions found in a literature review for this patient.

Online Resources

AACN Synergy Model for Patient Care: www.certcorp.org

Excellence in Nursing Knowledge, Issue 1: www.nursingknowledge.org

REFERENCES

AACN Certification Corporation. (2003). *The AACN Synergy Model for patient care.* Retrieved June 29, 2005, from www.aacn.org

American Association of Critical-Care Nurses. *Healthy work environment standards.* Retrieved August 15, 2005, from www.aacn.org

Benner, P. A. (1984). *From novice to expert.* Menlo Park, CA: Addison-Wesley.

Curley, M. A. Q. (1998). Patient–nurse synergy: Optimizing patient outcomes. *American Journal of Critical Care, 7*(1), 64–72.

Curley, M. A. Q. (2004). The state of synergy. *Excellence in Nursing Knowledge, 1*(1), 2–10.

Czerwinski, S., Blastic, L., & Rice, B. (1999). The Synergy Model: Building a career advancement program. *Critical Care Nurse, 19*(4), 72–77.

Edwards, D. F. (1999). The Synergy Model: Linking needs to nurse competencies. *Critical Care Nurse, 9*(1), 88–90, 97–99.

Hardin, S. R. (2004). Synergy and the undergraduate. *Excellence in Nursing Knowledge, 1*(1), 2–10.

Hardin, S. R., & Kaplow, R. (2005). *Synergy for clinical excellence: The AACN Synergy Model for patient care.* Sudbury, MA: Jones and Bartlett.

Kerfoot, K. M., & Cox, M. (2005). The Synergy Model: The ultimate mentoring model. *Critical Care Nursing Clinics of North America, 17,* 109–112.

Muenzen, P. M., Greenberg, S., & Pirro, K. A. (2004). *Final report of a comprehensive study of critical care nursing practice.* Retrieved on June 29, 2005, from www.aacn.org

Caring Practices

PART II

Family-Focused Care

Fay Wright

LEARNING OBJECTIVES

Upon completion of this chapter, the reader will be able to:

1. Identify the components of family-focused care.

2. Examine the need of families of acutely ill patients.

3. Discuss family-focused care from patient, family, and healthcare provider perspectives.

4. Integrate current knowledge of family-focused care into critical care nursing practice.

5. Analyze strategies to successfully implement family-focused care.

6. List optimal patient outcomes that may be achieved through evidence-based family-focused care.

When an individual family member is hospitalized with a critical illness, change inevitably occurs within the family system. As the family adapts to a member's illness and approaches care decisions, the nurse's role is to facilitate the changes in the family's role, function, and adaptation. Family-focused care takes patient care to the next level. This approach considers patient needs to be a priority, but it maintains familial bonds and helps the family continue to support the patient as part of the family system.

DEFINITION OF FAMILY-FOCUSED CARE

Family-focused care is a method of care delivery that recognizes and respects the pivotal role of the family. It views the patient and family as a complete entity, while supporting families in their natural caregiving roles and ensuring family collaboration and choice in treatment decisions affecting patients. By its very nature, family-focused care opens up the care delivery system to include support and communication with families. Family-focused care involves developing and individualizing interventions such as visitation, communication, family involvement in caregiving activities, patient/family education, and counseling. The key elements of family-focused care present a philosophy of care that, when incorporated into practice, recognizes the uniqueness of each patient and family. By incorporating the elements of family-focused care into professional nursing practice, interventions can be developed that facilitate patient and family coping (see **Table 2-1**).

Family-focused care is imperative for quality patient care in today's healthcare environment. Patients and families are taking control of their health to ensure they receive the best care possible. Shortened length of hospital stays, families assuming direct caregiver roles, and increased involvement during the patient's hospitalization are all trends that require family-focused care. The publicity surrounding the Institute of Medicine's report on errors in patient care (2000), television shows that detail aspects of medical care, the nursing shortage, and the potential for medical errors likewise amplify the need for families to be actively involved in understanding the patient's care and advocating for the best practice.

TABLE 2-1 Key Elements of Family-Focused Care

Recognizing that the family is the constant in the patient's life while the service systems and personnel within those systems fluctuate

Being aware of family strengths and individuality and having respect for different methods of coping

Encouraging and facilitating family-to-family support and networking

Sharing complete and unbiased information about the patient's care with family members on a continuing basis in a supportive manner

Designing accessible healthcare delivery systems that are flexible, culturally competent and responsive to family needs

Source: Shelton & Stepanek, 1994.

The American Hospital Association's *Patient Care Partnership* document (2005) mandates a decision-making partnership between the healthcare system and the patient, thus facilitating patients' efforts to determine their own future. This partnership also highlights the responsibilities of the healthcare system to fully communicate treatment options and the plan of care.

In a discussion with critical care nurses about the changes in their practice, the primary concern identified was the growing lack of trust between nurses, patients, and families (Dracup & Bryan-Brown, 2002). This concern has grown to the point that the Joint Commission on Accreditation of Healthcare Organizations (JCAHO) has developed standards to address the growing liability related to medical errors.

In JCAHO's 2005 publication *Healthcare at the Crossroads: Strategies for Improving the Medical Liability System and Preventing Patient Injury*, one of the recommendations for preventing liability in case of medical errors is to promote open communication between practitioners, patients, and families. Open communication is a hallmark of family-focused care. Family-focused care increases the communication between patients, families, and healthcare professionals, building trust between all parties. When open communication exists, there is less confusion and frustration for all participants involved in patient care.

Imagine that your parent is having coronary artery bypass surgery (CABG). The surgeon has told you that the surgery is complete and that your parent will be admitted to the intensive care unit (ICU). You are directed to the ICU waiting room, where a nurse provides you with more information about how your

parent is doing and when you can visit. When you arrive at the waiting room, you call into the ICU on the phone outside the door—but no one answers. You call again. When you get a response, you are told to wait and informed that someone will get in touch with you soon, but no specific time frame is given. You do not know if your parent is in the ICU, what your parent's condition is, or when you will be able to visit. How do you feel?

If you are like most family members, you will become increasingly anxious and afraid. The uncertainty of not knowing what is happening or when you can see your parent becomes overwhelming, and you continue to call the ICU and seek information. With your constant calling, the ICU staff become frustrated that they cannot complete their work because of the interruptions from the "difficult family." This creates a situation where both the family and the staff are frustrated, anxious about communication and distrustful of each other.

How different this situation would be if upon arrival to the ICU family waiting room, the initial call is answered and a nurse comes out, makes introductions, and gives you an overview of what will happen to your parent upon arrival to the ICU and how the monitoring will occur, and states that within 45 minutes you will be allowed to visit with your parent. Forty-five minutes later the nurse brings you in to visit. While at the bedside, the nurse explains the tubes and machines and encourages you to touch and talk with your parent. The nurse explains how you and your family can support your parent. In this scenario, trust would develop. While you would still feel concern for your parent's well-being, you would have a sense of being informed and part of the care—an active participant in the healing process for your parent. When nurses are empathetic and open to interacting with patients and families, they connect and communicate in such a way as to promote trust and form positive relationships.

DEFINITION OF FAMILY

To practice family-focused care, one must first identify the family. The family is the basic unit of care. The family is who the patient identifies as important and significant and who influences the care and well-being of the patient. The traditional definition of a two-parent, nuclear family, while still present, is not the only way to define families. According to the U.S. Census Bureau (2000), one-third of U.S. families include members who are not biologically or legally related. Single-parent families are increasing, and 35% of all U.S. children live with step-parents or grandparents at some point in their lives. The number of same-sex partners who are starting families is also increasing. In our society, there are an increasing number of elderly who live alone. Redefining the way we describe the family is essential to providing family-focused care for critically ill patients.

THE EFFECT OF CRITICAL ILLNESS ON THE FAMILY

Critical illness of a family member creates a crisis and a sense of disequilibrium within the family system. Established roles and functions are disrupted (Hepworth, Hendrickson, & Lopez, 1994). The crisis of critical illness disrupts the family's usual methods of adapting to stress. Basic emotional and physical needs may not be met and new needs may develop (Hepworth et al.).

Molter (1979) published a seminal research report that identified the needs of critically ill patients' families. Using the Critical Care Family Needs Inventory (CCFNI), she interviewed the families of critically ill patients to determine their needs related to the critical illness of a family member in the ICU. The top ten needs are listed in **Table 2-2**.

The CCFNI has been used in many research studies, and its results have been replicated and validated (Wasser et al., 2001). The identified needs can be generalized to the critical care family population. The CCFNI needs can be grouped into five common themes (**Table 2-3**), which most ICU family members experience. These themes help families support the critically ill patient, help nurses develop interventions to facilitate family understanding of the patient's illness, and assist families coping with the crisis.

Families will individually express needs based on their resources, coping methods, values, and attitudes about critical illness and health care. Evaluation and incorporation of families' individual responses into the plan of care are essential to implement family-focused care. The family's needs provide a base from which to get started. When the family understands

TABLE 2-2 Critical Care Family Needs

To have questions answered honestly
To know specific facts regarding what is wrong with the patient and his or her progress
To know the prognosis/outcome/chance of recovery
To be called at home about changes
To receive information once a day
To receive information and understandable explanations
To believe the hospital personnel care about the patient
To have hope
To know exactly what/why things are being done to the patient
To have reassurance that the best possible care is being given to the patient

Source: Molter, 1979.

TABLE 2-3 Critical Care Family Need Themes

To receive assurance
To remain near the patient
To receive information
To be comfortable
To have support available

Source: Leske, 2002.

the patient's illness and treatment options, they are able to participate in decision making and provide emotional support to the patient. Involved families have time to process the impact of the illness on the family system. They are also able to observe care that is provided and to determine if and when it is time to withhold care.

IMPLEMENTING FAMILY-FOCUSED CARE

Early assessment and communication between the nurse and the family will identify the level of intervention necessary to support the family. Needs serve as building blocks for meeting the goal of helping the patient and family maximize their health and coping during the patient's critical illness. The complexity of each situation is distinct and requires an individualized plan of care. The earlier the healthcare team develops an effective relationship with clear communication, the more coordinated and effective care will be (Tracy & Ceronsky, 2001).

Recognize That the Family Is the Constant in the Patient's Life

Before, during, and after the critical illness, the family is a part of the patient's life. Families are not mere visitors, but rather an integral part of the patient's world and support system. The nurse is the visitor in the family system and has a transient relationship in helping the family seek balance and maintain its bonds.

Recognition of these facts immediately suggests a number of nursing interventions. Ask patients who is important to them and who they want at the bedside. If the patient can not communicate, ask the family member who appears closest to the patient, who should be at the bedside.

Early relational work between the nurse and the family will facilitate communication throughout the patient's critical illness (Leske, 2002). Talking with families about the plan of care, daily changes, and the patient's progress is easier if a consistent caregiver has established trust and open communication. Johnson and colleagues (1998) reported that families experienced enhanced satisfaction when the patient had the same nurse care for them for two consecutive days.

It is important to be consistent with the plan of care and communication. For example, if you have discussed that chest x-rays are performed daily but on one day the x-ray is deferred due to a system or a clinical issue, an explanation may be warranted. If family members expect a chest x-ray and it is not performed, they may assume something is wrong with the patient if the change is not communicated. Communicating honestly and simply about changes in the plan of care will decrease family anxiety.

Families Need to Be Near the Patient

In a family-focused care ICU, flexible visiting hours allow the family and staff to reach a mutual understanding about the length and timing of visits and the visitors permitted. Families are encouraged to be at the bedside, showing sensitivity for patient needs, activity level in the unit, and their own need for positive health. Talking with families before they enter the unit, thereby explaining unit routine and patient care needs, allows them to understand what is occurring at the bedside. Strict, rigid visiting policies with access being granted based on rule rather than assessment of patient needs, nursing care demands, and unit activities sets up a conflictual relationship between the patient, family, and staff. The ICU should establish practice guidelines for family visiting that incorporate patient and family needs for proximity, maintain family relationships, and allow the family to support the patient (Kirchhoff, Pugh, Calame, & Reynolds, 1993). Research demonstrates that flexible, inclusive, and open visiting that is responsive to patient, family, and care needs is beneficial to all parties (Titler, 1998). Flexible visitation involves assessing family, patient, and unit needs and preferences in order to develop guidelines and an individualized plan that frames the frequency, time, or length of visits. The visitation plan is routinely evaluated to determine if it is responsive to individual patient and family needs. The following clinical example illustrates the communication process that takes place when establishing a flexible visitation plan.

Alexander is admitted for an acute myocardial infarction. He is married with six children, all of whom live more than one hour away from the hospital. The nurse meets with Alexander's wife Katie at his bedside. Alexander is alert, yet groggy. During the nurse's initial interaction with Katie, she asks when Katie would like to visit. Katie informs the nurse that she needs to be with Alexander and has never slept away from him in their 35 years of marriage. The nurse explains the ICU environment, the noise of machines, and routine of care. The nurse also discusses the need for Katie to take care of herself so she can support Alexander.

Alexander holds Katie's hand and states that, while he doesn't want her to get tired, he would like her to stay with him as much as possible. Together, Alexander, Katie, and the nurse decide that Katie will stay at the bedside for as long as she would like, with the expectation that she will leave to eat and take a break every few hours. The nurse and Katie also discuss that when the children arrive, they will come into the room but no more than three people will be at the bedside at any given time because of space limitations. The nurse explains the need to call the unit secretary before walking into the unit as protocol for security. The nurse also discusses the need for Alexander to rest and states that the plan will be reevaluated based on how Alexander's care proceeds.

For the first 24 hours, Katie leaves only to go to the bathroom and eat a short meal. As the children arrive, Katie explains the visiting process. The children organize themselves and move in and out of the unit, visiting their father. The next night Katie leaves to go to a nearby hotel with her son. Katie felt comfortable with Alexander's progress and care but knew that she was tired. The nurse supported Katie's decision and assured her that she could call or return at any time.

This example illustrates the process of communication and assessment that occurs when a professional nurse develops a visiting plan as part of the patient's plan of care. The family participated in the planning process. As they developed comfort with the patient's status and care, they were able to reevaluate the plan and adapt it to continue to meet their needs.

Through conversations with the family, flexible visitation plans may be developed. These plans may limit the number of visitors at the bedside and may put some restrictions on when family may visit. It is common practice to limit visitation during shift report. The time limits often become a non-issue when family-focused care is implemented, as the family becomes integral to the patient's care.

Some critical care nurses anecdotally report adverse patient responses to visiting, such as increased ventricular ectopy, intracranial pressure, and stress and anxiety. Clinical research does not support these reports, however. Routine nurse–patient interactions are as stressful as family interactions but have no harmful effects on patient blood pressure, ventricular ectopy, or intracranial pressure (Fuller & Foster, 1982; Hepworth et al., 1994). Initial adverse patient responses will diminish if the family is allowed to remain at the bedside and does not have limited access to the patient.

Schulte et al. (1993) studied the relationship between heart rate and ectopy in a cardiac care unit with restricted and flexible visitation. These researchers found no significant difference in the number of premature ventricular contractions or premature arterial contractions with flexible visitation when compared with restricted visitation. The patients with flexible visitation experienced lower heart rates and appeared more relaxed than the patients whose families were restricted from visiting. (See the American Association of Critical-Care Nurses' (AACN) protocol for practice for annotated bibliographies of these studies.)

When patients were asked about family visitation, patients reported that visiting is "a nonstressful experience because visitors offered moderate levels of reassurance, comfort, and calming" (Gonzalez, Carroll, Elliott, Fitzgerald, & Vallent, 2004). Family visitors explained clinical care information to patients and provided information to assist the nurse in understanding the patients.

If a patient requests to see a child family member or a child wishes to see the patient, that request should be honored. Developmentally appropriate education about the patient's illness and the ICU environment prepares the child to visit. Emotional support before, during, and after the visit enables the patient and child to maintain a bond and may help the child deal with the critical illness of an adult family member (Nicholson et al., 1993).

If the family is defined as whoever is significant to the patient, then the patient's beloved pet must be included in a family-focused care ICU. Pet visitation, when properly planned and monitored, can address the loneliness, isolation, and lack of emotional support that some critically ill patients face (Giulano, Bloniasz, & Bell, 1999).

Be Aware of Family Strengths and Have Respect for Different Methods of Coping

Every family has different strengths and supports. Yet research has shown that initially family members respond similarly to the crisis of critical illness regardless of their age, gender, or relationship to the patient, and the severity of the illness (Leske, 1992; Leske & Jiricka, 1998). Before the onset of a critical illness, the family is inevitably coping with the daily stresses of work, school, and finances. When a life-threatening change occurs, the family must respond. The amount of stress and the success of the family's coping prior to the critical illness affect how they will manage the new stress created by critical illness (Leske, 2003). Families with more extensive resources and coping skills will more effectively adapt to the crisis of the critical illness. If their strengths do not compensate for the new demands faced, the family will become unbalanced and their adaptation will decrease. Research has shown that problem-solving communication is a significant family strength influencing family adaptation (Leske, 2003). Nursing interventions that help mobilize family strengths and meet identified family needs promote the adaptation of families of critically ill patients.

Families Need Information

Family members will ask questions, take notes, and bring research from the Internet to discuss with the healthcare team. It is important to not assume that the family member is trying to document mistakes but rather is keeping track of what transpires and what is said. The critical care nurse should assess the knowledge that the family has and needs. The family should be encouraged to take notes and write down their questions, and their need to understand should be clearly acknowledged. Have the family identify a family spokesperson who will make sure all members remain informed. Notebooks help the family organize and gather information in a setting with a large amount of new and ever-changing information. Repeated questions are not really directed to understanding how the ventilator works or what the electrocardiogram (ECG) pattern is but rather represent a plea to understand the patient's condition and to develop some sense of control. Honest, thoughtful answers will help this inquisitive person as well as disseminate information throughout the family.

Occasionally, a family member may also be a healthcare professional. Assessment of the family member's level of knowledge and expertise should be made and can serve as a foundation for further information. One should not assume the presence of knowledge or understanding of the patient's condition.

Families Need Assurance

Family members may ask a lot of questions, want to chat about providers' lives outside the ICU, and get to know the nurse and the unit. Family members are looking for answers and assurance that the patient is receiving the best possible care. With greater understanding, their ability to support the patient grows.

One study found that having family members with high levels of optimism was strongly correlated with greater satisfaction with needs being met and feelings of affiliation with both physicians and nurses (Auerbach et al., 2005). To build on this family strength, nurses may communicate positive changes and encourage family members to participate in the patient's care.

Families Need to Be Comfortable

It is important to accept a family member's expression of feelings and to develop comfort with crying and emotionality. Assessment of the effect of crying on the patient should be made. If the patient becomes upset when the family member cries, the family should be moved away from the bedside. If it doesn't affect the patient, expression of emotion can be allowed to continue in the patient's view.

Some families are more effective than others in supporting their ill family member at the bedside. Some family members' coping behaviors may lead a novice nurse to label them as dysfunctional, needy, or difficult. Chesla and Stannard (1997) discuss the effect of labeling family behaviors. Once labels were assigned and communicated from shift to shift, the family began to take on more negative behaviors. When family behaviors were discussed in a descriptive manner, the increase in "negative behaviors" was not identified and a decrease in dysfunction was noted. However, the goal with family-focused care is not to fix any dysfunctional family dynamics. Nurses can acknowledge any perceived dysfunction and communicate with the family to focus on the common goal of patient recovery. Family members arguing at the bedside may affect the stress levels of the patient and of the ICU as a whole. The arguing family requires refocusing back on the patient, moving any heated discussions away from the bedside and developing plans of visitation and communication that keep the heated discussions away from patient care areas. Building relationships with the family early during the critical illness and clearly communicating behavioral expectations decrease and prevent behaviors that interfere with the patient's health and well-being.

Share Complete and Unbiased Information about Patient's Care with Family Members on a Continuing Basis in a Supportive Manner

The clarity of the information discussed with families as well as the attitude of the healthcare provider are important in determining the family's ability to understand the information (Jurkovich, Pierce, Pananen, & Rivara, 2000). Communication must be meaningful to the family. Understandable language that is not filled with medical jargon is essential. Think about getting a report on the first day of your first clinical rotation. How much did you understand? Did you understand what an IV, CVP, ABG, or pulse ox was? Listen to the way you communicate with families. Use simple terms to explain patient care procedures (see **Table 2-4**).

A structured plan of calling the patient's family daily (Medland & Ferrans, 1998), giving informational booklets (Henneman, McKenzie, & Dewa, 1992) about the ICU, holding orientation meetings (Chavez & Faber, 1987), and providing educational videotapes has been found to help meet the information needs of critically ill patients' families.

During initial interactions as well as in daily communication, the nurse should share specific information with the family (**Table 2-5**). This important information includes vital signs, level of consciousness, status through the night, changes in condition, and plans for the day. It is important to determine

TABLE 2-4 Communication Principles for Family Understanding

Use analogies.
Draw pictures.
Use words, not letters.
Rephrase.
Reframe.
Repeat.

what additional information is important to the family. Determine how the family thinks the patient is doing when providing these updates.

Information families receive so that they can make care decisions is often inadequate or lacking. Effective communication with the staff is the best antidote for uncertainty among the patient's family members (Kirchhoff & Beckstrand, 2000). After more than two decades of research evaluating the needs and satisfaction of families of ICU patients, it is clear that improved communication, enhanced support systems, and a friendlier environment decrease frustration and promote feelings of satisfaction. From the research, several themes and principles have become apparent, which formed the basis of the Critical Care Family Assistance Program (CCFAP) (Lederer, Goode, & Dowling, 2005). Started by the Chest Foundation, a philanthropic arm of the American College of Chest Physicians, in collaboration with the Eli Lilly and Company Foundation, the CCFAP study "supports the delivery of a family assistance program model that has the potential to significantly alter the critical care environment for ICU patients and their families" (Lederer, Goode, & Dowling, p. 65S). The study's dual purposes are "determining the efficacy of the model as a replicable model in a variety of hospital ICU environments and assessing the impact of the model on family satisfaction with the care and treatment of their loved ones in critical care units" (Lederer, Goode, & Dowling, p. 65S).

The CCFAP study is now in its third year. Preliminary data reveal an improvement in communication between the families and various members of the ICU team, increased ratings regarding family involvement in decision-making processes, and decreased stress levels for family members. It was concluded that the CCFAP has been successful in meeting the needs of families of ICU patients (information, flexible visiting policies, and assurance that the patient is receiving the best care). There was no significant difference in the families' perception of quality of care as provided by the ICU team members. In contrast,

TABLE 2-5 Example of a Family Assessment and Information Checklist

Initial Interaction

1. Introduce yourself, including your credentials.
2. Ask what the family member's relationship to the patient is.
3. Explain the ICU family-focused policy: "Families are important to us and you are welcome!"
4. Discuss the patient's current status and the nursing care routines.
5. Explain the visiting guidelines (e.g., times determined by family needs, three at the bedside at a given time, calling before entering the unit from the waiting room phone). Children may visit after meeting with the nurse.
6. Identify the family members who will be visiting. Chart the names and times each will be visiting.
7. Discuss appointing a family spokesperson to coordinate communication with other family members.
8. Give the family the unit phone number. Discuss coordinating calls. Ask who will be calling and chart these names on a flow sheet.
9. Distribute the family information book. Point out important information.
10. Follow up with any questions or concerns.

Follow-up Visits

1. Introduce yourself and give your credentials. If you don't already know, find out who the visitors are and if they have visited before.
2. Discuss the patient's current status and the nursing care routines.
3. Determine whether they have any questions or concerns.
4. Ask if they would like to speak with a physician or other team member.
5. Assess interest in participating in care activities (e.g., mouth care, foot rub, ice chips).
6. Ask how they are doing. Are they eating? Sleeping?

Sources: Henneman, McKenzie, & Dewa, 1992; Wright, 2000.

the ratings for this variable were high prior to the implementation of the study (Dowling & Wang, 2005).

Several implications have been drawn from the available data. First, "healthcare organizations have a responsibility to foster an environment that protects the physical and emotional health of severely stressed family members who assemble in their facilities to participate in the treatment of a loved one." Second, "nothing is as effective in meeting and promoting satisfaction, not only with the families but also with the hospital staff, as improved and consistent communication. All members of the staff must be able to depend on every other team mem-

ber to be faithful to communication responsibilities" (Dowling, Vender, Guilianelli, & Wang, 2005, p. 92S).

Design Accessible Healthcare Delivery Systems That Are Flexible, Culturally Competent, and Responsive to Family Needs

Family-focused care requires that all members of the healthcare team support the philosophy of care. Teaching the principles of family-focused care to unit secretaries, security, volunteers, housekeepers, and aides can be enormously helpful and effective in providing family support. "For example, instead of being viewed as 'gatekeepers,' unit secretaries should function as liaisons between patients' families and nursing staff, assisting in relaying information and helping support family-centered decisions" (Henneman & Cardin, 2002, p. 15). In a family-focused care ICU, the patient and family members are considered integral members of the healthcare team, taking part in daily rounds as active participants (Uhlig, Brown, Nason, Camelio, & Kendall, 2002). Hospital volunteers, when trained by ICU nurses, can provide nonmedical information, comfort, and support to families of critically ill patients (Appleyard, Gavaghan, Gonzalez, Ananian, & Tyrell, 2000).

Support groups can strengthen the family's understanding of ICU care as well as provide an informal network of other families who are experiencing the crisis of critical illness (Halm, 1991).

Participation in patient care in the ICU has been associated with enhanced family satisfaction (Wasser et al., 2001). Assisting with care can maintain family bonding and promote togetherness. Patient comfort and healing are also enhanced (Azoulay et al., 2003). Nurses should explore the family's preferences for participating in patient care on an ongoing basis. The family may want to participate in a minor way (e.g., passing an alcohol wipe or other piece of equipment) or a major way (e.g., assisting with bathing, turning, range of motion, or mouth care).

It is important to be aware of the diversity of patients and their families. Culture affects the individual's view of time, space, family structure, illness, health, and death, all of which color the family's interaction with the healthcare team (Wright, Cohen, & Caroselli, 1997).

Families Need Support

Family needs can often be met with basic nursing interventions, such as giving information, providing reassurance, and offering a flexible visiting schedule. Other families may need more support from colleagues in social services or spiritual care.

With appropriate resources and preparation, families can be present during most procedures, including resuscitation.

Family presence during care procedures, including resuscitation, enhances the family's ability to trust that all care measures have been implemented, understand that curative measures may no longer work, and realize that end-of-life decisions need to be made (Jones & Buttery, 1981).

Meyers et al. (2000) found that 100% of family members who stayed during resuscitation would do it again if the same situation occurred. They experienced many benefits related to their presence (**Table 2-6**). The family members understood the need for appropriate behavior during the resuscitation and felt that their presence helped them deal with the patient's status and that they provided comfort to the patient during the resuscitation.

Nurses have the power to control important end-of-life memories for the families of dying patients through communication and support of families throughout the critical illness, including end-of-life care (Lewandowski, 1994).

Nurses can help ensure attainment of optimal patient outcomes such as those listed in **Box 2-1** through the use of evidence-based interventions.

SUMMARY

Critical illness is a journey for both the patient and the family. In a family-focused care unit, the family receives navigation information that enables them to proceed on the journey of critical illness with the patient, so all parties can move together through the critical illness. Family care skills are part of becoming an expert nurse (Benner, Tanner, & Chesla, 1996).

Life-saving interventions and family interactions become much more rewarding when the work focuses on a patient instead of the accomplishment of a procedure or task. Studies have shown that where work is meaningful, critical care nurses'

> **Box 2-1**
> # Optimal Patient Outcomes
>
> - Increased collaboration between RN and family members
> - Increased communication between RN and family members
> - Increased patient and family education
> - Increased family trust
> - Implementation of open/unrestricted family visitation
> - Family participating in planning and providing care

job satisfaction increases and stress is reduced (Stechmiller & Yarandi, 1992).

One of the greatest professional satisfactions is talking with family members and teaching them about the techniques and care procedures that are being performed. Education facilitates the family's understanding of care the patient is receiving. Families who have interactions with nurses who practice family-focused care express how impressed they are with nurses' knowledge, compassion, and caring (Wright, 2000).

When the nurse develops a relationship with the family, the family develops trust with healthcare providers, which in turn decreases their stress and anxiety (Leske, 2002). Families also feel more comfortable leaving the bedside and getting rest and food when they have a trusting relationship with the ICU staff (Wright, 2000). Critical care nurses have the unique privilege of working with families during an exceptionally stressful hospitalization. Being open to the family allows the nurse to make a difference during one of the most challenging times in the life of a patient and family.

TABLE 2-6 Benefits to Family Members Who Are Present during Invasive Procedures and Resuscitation

- Relief from wondering about what was happening to the patient
- Visual and verbal knowledge of the patient's care and condition
- Provision of comfort and protection to a loved one who was in pain, vulnerable, or defenseless
- Patient/family connectedness and bonding maintained
- Opportunity for closure
- Spiritual experience

Source: Meyers et al., 2000.

CASE STUDY 1

Janet is an 83-year-old woman who was admitted to the ICU with a hemorrhagic stroke. Janet has been married to Bert for 66 years. They live independently in their own home. Janet's blood pressure is 160/100, her heart rate is 120 with 3 to 6 PVCs/minute, she is breathing with the assistance of a ventilator, and she requires sedation because she is trying to pull out her endotracheal tube and intravenous (IV) lines. Janet is agitated, confused, and restless despite the IV sedation. The visiting hours in the ICU are hourly for ten minutes. Bert sits in the family waiting room until he is able to visit.

When he is allowed in to visit, he goes to Janet's side, kisses her, and talks with her about their life together and his desire for her to return home. While he is there, Janet appears to relax; her heart rate is 110 with a decrease in PVCs, and her blood pressure decreases to 140/88 without any change in medications. Bert also appears more relaxed. When the nurse announces the end of visiting time, Bert begins to cry and asks the nurse to let him stay with his wife. He is told that it is not the policy and that Janet will get more rest if he leaves the room.

CRITICAL THINKING QUESTIONS

1. What caring practices could a nurse implement in a family-focused care environment that would address Bert's concerns?
2. Design an informational poster for staff about family-focused care.
3. Discuss the evidence-based literature that supports family visitation.
4. How will you implement your role as a facilitator of learning for this patient or staff?
5. How would you modify a plan of care for patients of diverse backgrounds who request to stay at the bedside in an ICU?
6. What patient care outcomes would you expect with family-focused care?

CASE STUDY 2

Evan is a seven-year-old boy whose mother is in the ICU. He is having difficulty sleeping and needs to visit his mother. Evan's father discusses his concern for his son as well as his belief that his wife would feel better if she saw Evan. In the discussion with Evan's father, the nurse explains that the unit has a family-focused care policy and that Evan may visit his mother after the nurse explains to him what equipment he will see and what his mother will look like with an endotracheal tube and IV lines in her arms. The nurse also explains how the unit will sound and smell.

Ater talking with the nurse, Evan went in, hugged his mother, and talked with her. His mother opened her eyes and looked at him. The nurse and his father answered questions and helped Evan sit on the bed so his mother could hold his hand. He cried because his mother could not speak to him but she smiled and he felt better. That night, Evan slept through the night for the first time since his mother was admitted to the ICU.

CRITICAL THINKING QUESTIONS

1. Describe the bedside environment and noises in the ICU in terms that a non-healthcare provider can understand.
2. Given that Evan wants to be with his mother, how would you approach this situation in a family-focused care unit?
3. Explain how the Synergy Model can help to ensure that the family has the appropriate nursing care to ensure optimal outcomes. Use the grid provided below to analyze the case. Determine whether the nurse displayed each characteristic and what actions would demonstrate competency in each characteristic.

	Nurse Characteristics	Qualities Displayed by the Nurse in the Case	Actions the Nurse Can Take to Demonstrate the Characteristic
SYNERGY MODEL	Clinical judgment		
	Advocacy/moral agency		
	Caring practices		
	Collaboration		
	Systems thinking		
	Response to diversity		
	Facilitator of learning		
	Clinical inquiry		

Online Resources

American Association of Critical-Care Nurses (2001). *For Those Who Wait: A Guide to Critical Care for Patients, Families and Friends.* Aliso Viejo, CA: American Association of Critical-Care Nurses. This information booklet for families reviews critical environment information and provides a helpful glossary of medical terms. http://www.aacn.org; go to AACN Ethics Website—Family-Centered Care.

Diagrams and definitions about the care in a critical care unit: http://www.icu-usa.com

CASE STUDY ARTICLES THAT ILLUSTRATE SUCCESSFUL FAMILY-FOCUSED CARE PRACTICE

Leske, J. S. (1998). *Creating a Healing Environment—Family Needs and Interventions in the Acute Care Environment [Protocols for Practice].* Aliso Viejo, CA: American Association of Critical-Care Nurses.

Titler, M., & Drahozal, R. (1998). *Creating a Healing Environment—Family Pet Visiting, Animal-Assisted Activities and Animal-Assisted Therapy in Critical Care [Protocols for Practice].* Aliso Viejo, CA: American Association of Critical-Care Nurses.

Society of Critical Care Medicine. (2002). *Patient and Family Resources: ICU Issues and Answers Brochures.* Chicago, IL: Society of Critical Care Medicine.

- "Common Problems of Critical Illness" addresses conditions that may bring a loved one into the ICU or that may develop while in the unit.
- "What Are My Choices Regarding Life Support?" deals with the decisions patients and families face regarding specific forms of life support.

- "Participating in Care: What Questions Should I Ask?" guides family members on how to interact most effectively with ICU team members.
- "Taking Care of Yourself While a Loved One Is in the ICU" stresses the importance of self-care while supporting a loved one in the ICU.
- "Why Do ICU Patients Look and Act That Way?" provides an illustrated guide to equipment and procedures that will affect the loved one's appearance in the ICU.
- "Helpful Hospital Safety Tips" lists ways you can work with your healthcare team to make your journey fast, easy, and, above all, safe.
- "When Your Child Is Admitted to the Intensive Care Unit" is every family's guide to understanding what is happening to their child in the pediatric intensive care unit.

- "Making Decisions When Your Child Is Very Sick" is a guide to help family and friends understand what difficult decisions need to be made when a child is in the ICU.

ONLINE ACTIVITIES

1. Provide websites with instructions for activities to enhance student learning, as appropriate.
2. Take a patient's diagnosis from a clinical experience and explore the information and links at http://www.icu-usa.com.
3. From a family member's perspective, discuss the information's effectiveness if an educational brochure.

REFERENCES

American Hospital Association. The patient care partnership: Understanding expectations, rights responsibilities. Retrieved July 12, 2005, from http://www.aha.org/aha/ptcommunication/partnership/index

Appleyard, M. E., Gavaghan, S. R., Gonzalez, C., Ananian, L., & Tyrell, R. (2000). Nurse-coached interventions for families of patients in critical care units. *Critical Care Nurse, 20*(6), 40–48.

Auerbach, S. M., Kiesler, D. J., Wartella, J., Rausch, S., Ward, K. R., & Ivatury, R. (2005). Optimism, satisfaction with needs met, interpersonal perceptions of the healthcare team, and emotional distress in patients' family members during critical care hospitalization. *American Journal of Critical Care, 14*, 202–210.

Azoulay, E., Pouchard, F., Chevret, S., Arich, C., Brivet, F., Brun, F., et al. (2003). Family participation in care to the critically ill: Opinions of families and staff. *Intensive Care Medicine, 29*, 1498–1504.

Benner, P., Tanner, C., & Chesla, C. (1996). *Expertise in nursing practice.* New York: Springer.

Chavez, C. W., & Faber, L. (1987). Effect of an education-orientation program on family members who visit their significant other in the intensive care unit. *Heart & Lung, 16*(1), 92–99.

Chesla, C. A., & Stannard, D. (1997). Breakdown in the nursing care of families in the ICU. *American Journal of Critical Care, 6*(1), 64–71.

Dowling, J., Vender, J., Guilianelli, S., & Wang, B. (2005). A model of family-centered care and satisfaction predictors: The Critical Care Family Assistance Program. *Chest, 128*(Suppl. 3), 815–925.

Dowling, J., & Wang, B. (2005). Impact on family satisfaction: The Critical Care Family Assistance Program. *Chest, 128*(Suppl. 3), 765–805.

Dracup, K., & Bryan-Brown, C. (2002). On notebooks and trust. *American Journal of Critical Care, 11*(2), 96–98.

Fuller, B. F., & Foster, G. M. (1982). The effects of family/friend visits vs. staff interaction on stress/arousal of surgical intensive care patients. *Heart & Lung, 11*, 457–463.

Giulano, K. K., Bloniasz, E., & Bell, J. (1999). Implementation of a pet visitation program in critical care. *Critical Care Nurse, 19*(3), 43–50.

Gonzalez, C. E., Carroll, D. L., Elliott, J. S., Fitzgerald, P. A., & Vallent, H. J. (2004). Visiting preferences of patients in the intensive care unit and in a complex care medical unit. *American Journal of Critical Care, 13*(3), 194–198.

Halm, M. A. (1991). Strategies for developing a family support group. *Focus on Critical Care, 71*, 600–702.

Henneman, E. A., & Cardin, S. (2002). Family-centered critical care: A practical approach to making it happen. *Critical Care Nurse, 22*, 12–19.

Henneman, E. A., McKenzie, J. B., & Dewa, C. S. (1992). An evaluation of interventions for meeting the needs of families of critically ill patients. *American Journal of Critical Care, 1*(3), 85–93.

Hepworth, J. T., Hendrickson, S. G., & Lopez, J. (1994). Time series analysis of physiological response during ICU visitation. *Western Journal of Nursing Research, 16*(6), 704–717.

Institute of Medicine. (2000). *To err is human: Building a safer health system.* Washington, DC: National Academy Press.

Johnson, D., Wilson, M., Cavanaugh, B., Bryden, C., Gudmundson, D., & Moodley, O. (1998). Measuring the ability to meet family needs in an intensive care unit. *Critical Care Medicine, 26*(2), 266–271.

Joint Commission on Accreditation of Healthcare Organizations. (2005). *Healthcare at the crossroads: Strategies for improving the medical liability system and preventing patient injury.* Oakbrook Terrace, IL: JCAHO.

Jones, W. H., & Buttery, M. (1981). Sudden death: Survivors' perceptions of their emergency department experience. *Journal of Emergency Nursing, 7*(1), 14–17.

Jurkovich, G. J., Pierce, B., Pananen, L., & Rivara, F. P. (2000). Giving bad news: The family perspective. *Journal of Trauma, 48*, 865–870.

Kirchhoff, K. T., & Beckstrand, R. L. (2000). Critical care nurses' perceptions of obstacles and helpful behaviors in providing end-of-life care to dying patients. *American Journal of Critical Care, 9*(2), 96–105.

Kirchhoff, K. T., Pugh, E., Calame, R. M., & Reynolds, N. (1993). Nurses' beliefs and attitudes toward visiting in adult critical care settings. *American Journal of Critical Care, 2*(3), 238–245.

Lederer, M. A., Goode. T., & Dowling, J. (2005). Origins and development: The Critical Care Family Assistance Program. *Chest, 128*(Suppl. 3), 65S–75S.

Leske, J. S. (1992). Needs of adult family members after critical illness. *Critical Care Nursing Clinics of North America, 4*, 587–596.

Leske, J. S. (2002). Interventions to decrease family anxiety. *Critical Care Nurse, 2*(6), 61–65.

Leske, J. S. (2003). Comparison of family stresses, strengths, and outcomes after trauma and surgery. *AACN Clinical Issues in Critical Care, 14*(1), 33–41.

Leske, J. S., & Jiricka, M. K. (1998). Impact of family demands and family strengths and capabilities on family well-being and adaptation after critical injury. *American Journal of Critical Care, 7*, 383–392.

Lewandowski, L. A. (1994) Nursing grand rounds: The power to shape memories, critical care nurses, and family visiting. *Journal of Cardiovascular Nursing, 9*(1), 54–60.

Medland, J. J., & Ferrans, C. E. (1998). Effectiveness of a structured communication program for family members of patients in an ICU. *American Journal of Critical Care, 7*(1), 24–29.

Meyers, T. A., Eichhorn, D. J., Guzzetta, C. E., Clark, A. P., Klein, J. D., Taliaferro, E., et al. (2000). Family presence during invasive procedures and resuscitation: The experience of family members, nurses and physicians. *American Journal of Nursing, 100*(2), 32–44.

Molter, N. (1979). Needs of relatives of critically ill patients: A descriptive study. *Heart & Lung, 8,* 332–339.

Nicholson, A. C., Titler, M., Montgomery, L. A., Kleiber, C., Craft, M. J., Halm, M., et al. (1993). Effects of child visitation in adult critical care units: A pilot study. *Heart & Lung, 22*(1), 36–45.

Schulte, D. A., Burrell, L. O., Gueldner, S. H., Bramlett, M. H., Fuszard, B., Stone, S. K., et al. (1993). Pilot study of the relationship between heart rate and ectopy and unrestricted visiting hours in the coronary care unit. *American Journal of Critical Care, 2*(2), 134–136.

Shelton, T. L., & Stepanek, J. S. (1994). *Family-centered care for children needing specialized health and development services.* Washington, DC: Association for the Care of Children's Health.

Stechmiller, J. K., & Yarandi, H. N. (1992). Job satisfaction among critical care nurses. *American Journal of Critical Care, 1*(3), 37–44.

Titler, M. (1998). *Creating a healing environment—Family visitation and partnership in the critical care unit [Protocols for Practice].* Aliso Viejo, CA: American Association of Critical-Care Nurses.

Tracy, M. F., & Ceronsky, C. (2001). Creating a collaborative environment to care for complex patients and families. *AACN Clinical Issues, 12*(3), 383–400.

Uhlig, P. N., Brown, J., Nason, A. K., Camelio, A., & Kendall, E. (2002). System innovation: Concord Hospital. *Journal of Quality Improvement, 28*(12), 666–672.

United States Census Bureau. (2000). Retrieved September 18, 2005, from www.census.gov

Wasser, T., Pasquale, M. A., Matchett, S. C., Bryan, Y., & Pasquale, M. (2001). Establishing reliability and validity of the critical care family satisfaction survey. *Critical Care Medicine, 29,* 192–196.

Wright, F. (2000). Unpublished interviews with families of critically ill families. Newark, NJ.

Wright, F., Cohen, S., & Caroselli, C. (1997). How culture affects ethical decision making. *Critical Care Nursing Clinics of North America, 9*(1), 63–69.

CHAPTER 3

Creating a Healing Environment in the ICU

Renee Rubert   L. Dianne Long   Melissa L. Hutchinson

LEARNING OBJECTIVES

Upon completion of this chapter, the reader will be able to:

1. Describe the issues associated with the critical care environment and optimal patient outcomes.

2. Discuss strategies that can facilitate healing environments for the critically ill patient.

3. Discuss the philosophy of family visitation policies in intensive care units.

4. Explain healing modalities that can be integrated into nursing interventions.

5. List optimal patient outcomes that may be achieved through creation of an evidence-based healing ICU environment.

While a nurse or nursing unit can possess impeccable critical care skills and knowledge, those are not the only factors that influence patient recovery. This chapter focuses on the intensive care environment, examining how it can influence physiologic measures and the holistic needs of the patient and family. Other modalities (e.g., spirituality and prayer) that may enhance a healing environment for the patient are described in Chapter 9.

Many designs of critical care units provide a cold and sterile environment in which specialized care is received. This design fails to humanize the experience for the critical care patient and family. The term "critical care unit" invokes images of very ill patients surrounded by the latest in biomedical equipment, monitoring devices, and code carts. These images alone can raise feelings of anxiety and levels of stress in patients and families alike. The lack of foresight in designing critical care programs that encompass a pleasing physical design, integrate family presence, and offer complementary therapies leaves critical care patients and their families with less than an optimal environment in which to heal.

The concept of environmental influences on healing has been known since Florence Nightingale (1970), a nursing leader, cared for soldiers of the Crimean War. New generations of critical care units are being designed to promote healing in a humanistic manner that can meet the holistic needs of patients and their families.

ANCIENT PERSPECTIVE

The interaction between humans and the different environments in which they are placed has long been known. More than 2000 years ago, the ancient Roman physician Galen recognized the healing aspect that an environment could provide. He understood the consequences of unclean conditions; thanks to his health philosophy, he had the highest survival rate among all physicians who treated the gladiators (Pearcy, 1985). Florence Nightingale was also famed for her focus on sanitation and other aspects of the environment that contribute to the health and healing of the patients. She was not only a leader in improving sanitation and ventilation, but was also instrumental in bringing forth the body-and-mind connection. She understood that the environment played a central role in a patient's healing of body and mind. Nightingale went on to influence the healthcare environment by varying the patient's visual perspective, utilizing color and natural light more effectively, and eliminating excessive noise. This early nursing leader was passionate about the nurse's role to create a milieu that would give a patient the best opportunity to heal.

Until recently, the primary strategies employed in the design of critical care units were based on the medical needs of the patients and the convenience of the provider; the architectural designs were mainly utilitarian and family visits were restricted. The utilitarian designs of the past created an ambience that dehumanized the patient's experience. Recent studies have supported Nightingale's practices from a century ago; the environment plays a significant role in the overall healthcare experience and healing process. Historically patients were placed in an open ward in beds that lined the walls. This design allowed for many patients to receive nursing care from a minimal number of nursing staff. Lack of privacy and exposure to repulsive sights and odors were some of the detractors of this type of design (Fontaine, Briggs, & Pope-Smith, 2001).

Intensive care units (ICUs) lacked aesthetic appeal and had a sterile ambience, with little visual interest being incorporated into their design. Even today, with the many advancements that have been attained in biomedical equipment and monitoring in critical care units, the same issues considered by Nightingale of air quality, color, light, view, and noise are still of concern.

Stepping into the 21st century and utilizing Nightingale's concept, today's healing environment encompasses a patient-centered approach including a pleasing physical setting and a supportive organizational culture (Malkin, 2003). There is a resurgence of interest by healthcare designers and providers in, and a demand by patients and families for, healthcare facilities that incorporate the ambience of healing into the architecture, artwork, and philosophy. Stichler (2001), in her review of related research, reports that patients experience positive outcomes when the environment incorporates natural light, elements of nature, peaceful colors, soothing sounds, pleasant views, and an overall pleasing aesthetic essence.

PSYCHOLOGICAL AND PHYSIOLOGICAL CONNECTION OF THE HEALING PHENOMENON

Psychoneuroimmunology refers to the physiologic response of the body to psychological and environmental stressors (Starkweather, Witek-Janusek, & Mathews, 2005). This stress response is initiated by the hypothalamus releasing corticotrophin-releasing factor (CRF). The CRF stimulates the pituitary gland to release a number of stress hormones, such as adrenocorticotropic hormone (ACTH). This hormone, in turn, stimulates the release of cortisol from the adrenal cortex and the release of aldosterone from the adrenal medulla. Cortisol, a glucocorticoid, stimulates the release of glucose from glycogen in the liver.

Aldosterone, a mineralocorticoid, acts to retain sodium and water. Both of these hormones cause an increased blood pressure in the ICU patient (Lusk & Lash, 2005). Furthermore, cortisol depresses phagocytosis, which can affect healing.

Psychoneuroimmunology research demonstrates that emotions influence immunological functioning and that too much stress has a negative impact on the functioning of the body's immune system. Recent research suggests that the immune system can be enhanced or suppressed by external stimuli and that the brain reacts to external stimuli at an unconscious level (Malkin, 2003). The physiological affects of stress negatively affect patients' ability to heal. Creating physical environments that support families' and patients' psychological well-being, by contrast, can produce a positive impact on therapeutic outcomes, reduce stressors, and improve staff performance and morale (Lusk & Lash, 2005).

Information received through our five senses evokes physiological and emotional responses of anxiety or serenity (Mazer, 2002). Creating a healing environment within the chaos of a critical care setting might sound daunting, but the potential benefits are well worth the effort.

PHYSICAL ENVIRONMENT
Environmental Noise

> Unnecessary noise, or noise that creates an expectation in the mind, is that which hurts a patient . . . . Such unnecessary noises undoubtedly induced or aggravated delirium in many cases. (Nightingale, 1970, p. 25)

Noise is one of the most insidious environmental stressors found in the hospital environment. In the critical care unit, where patients require more frequent and more intensive monitoring, noise can be the most pervasive stressor. On any ward, noxious noises can include the hum of medical equipment; bubbling of chest tubes; staff conversations; pagers and intercom systems; ringing of telephones; opening and closing of doors, cabinets, and supply carts; and even the clattering sounds from the wheels of a passing cart. The critical care unit, with the advent of new technologies and increased monitoring equipment, adds even more auditory stimuli—the buzzing and beeping of alarms and strange noises that the specialized monitoring equipment can produce (Petterson, 2000). These unfamiliar and unexpected noises can startle anyone, but especially a patient already stressed from a physiological strain. A constant barrage of unexpected noises has physiological manifestations as well, such as interrupted sleep. (Sleep disturbances in the ICU are discussed in Chapter 5.) It is not surprising that noise is one of the most frequently cited complaints from critical care patients and their families (Stein-Parbury & McKinley, 2000).

Not only does the chaotic environment of a critical care setting induce stress, but it can also affect patients' perception of sleep quality. Topf, Bookman, and Arand's (1996) study of critical care sounds found that individuals who were subjected to critical care sounds perceived their sleep quality less positively than individuals who roomed in quieter environments. Topf and Thompson (2001) found that the hospital environmental noises negatively influenced the quality of sleep by interacting with patients' other stressors and that noise-induced stress is very subjective, noting that what is stressful to one individual may be comforting to another.

Designing a critical care environment that supports a healing atmosphere by reducing ambient noises takes into consideration many design elements, such as flooring, ceiling material, and doors and nursing station placement (Mazer, 2002). Mazer recommends utilizing sound absorbent carpeting, acoustic ceilings, and floor tiles in heavy-traffic areas. Petterson (2000) suggests creating mini-workstations throughout the unit to reduce noise from conversations by dispersing staff away from a central station, where escalating voices can often be heard over the basal sound level of the unit.

Other design proposals include small bedside televisions with a pillow speaker or headphones (Kahn et al., 1998), earplugs or noise-canceling headsets, or therapeutic sounds either through small machines or a centralized "music" station. Even simple actions such as closing the patient's door and having single-occupancy rooms can provide relief (Topf & Thompson, 2001). Attention should also be given to noises that can be significantly reduced through judicious equipment purchases, such as purchasing delivery carts with rubber wheels, because they are quieter (Mazer, 2002).

Biomedical testing of patient care equipment for noise impact and development of maintenance programs that review quieter operation of equipment and machinery are also recommended to decrease noise levels (Mazer, 2002). A study of noise in a neonatal intensive care unit (ICU) showed that even modest modifications reduced noise by 50% (Walsh-Sukys, Reitenbach, Hudson-Bar, & DePompei, 2001). Modification of the unit included installation of acoustical material in monitor bays, carpet that was installed in high-traffic areas, weather stripping that was added to doors and drawers, metal trashcans that were replaced by rubber cans, and covers that were placed over incubators. Other research suggests that reducing noise levels can influence patient outcomes in other ways, such as nurses being less likely to make errors when they are less distracted by extraneous noise (Mazer, 2005).

When designing a new ICU from "scratch," engineers can utilize the abundance of research and knowledge for implementing an aesthetically pleasing and healing environment. Because many ICUs that are in operation today were originally designed for ease of cleaning and convenience of staff, the characteristics that make up a healing environment were not considered. To redesign an active ward in a logical manner, it is important first to assess the current noise pollution and then to develop an auditory environmental standard. Mazer (2005) recommends evaluating the decibel level at different locations and different times of the day. Kahn et al. (1998) propose formulating and implementing an official policy that addresses noise standards and leads to the continued reduction of ambient noise in the ICU.

Petterson (2000) conducted a survey of the medical critical care staffs' perception of noise levels at Henry Ford Hospital and compared the results with baseline decibel readings on the medical ICU. Although the decibel reading and staffs' perception of noise were found to be correlated, staff members were unaware of the types and times of noise. Kahn et al. (1998) measured the noise level in two ICUs. They found a peak noise level of 80 decibels and almost 50% of noxious noise generated in the ICU was created by human behavior.

Given that human behavior is one of the greatest contributors to offensive sound, the generation of unnecessary noise can be abated with modification of staffs' behavior. Most important is the education of nursing and medical staff on the effects of their behaviors on the noise level and pollution in the critical care unit (Kahn et al., 1998). Creating a culture among the staff that fosters a healing environment includes encouraging behaviors that decrease unnecessary noise, such as keeping hallway conversations low, especially at night; avoiding over-the-bed conversations; turning pagers to vibrate; avoiding the use of overhead paging; turning off unused biomedical equipment; and modifying or repairing unnecessarily loud equipment (Petterson, 2000). Along with facilitating staff behaviors that decrease unnecessary and noxious noises, therapeutic sounds can be introduced, such as music, heartbeat sounds (especially in the neonatal ICU), pleasant sounds from nature like ocean waves and rain showers, or even "white noise" that lightly stimulates the hearing receptors, making other background noises less obvious.

Environmental Light

> Second to their need for fresh air is their need for light . . . it is not only light but direct sunlight . . . the usefulness of light in treating the disease is all important. (Nightingale, 1970, pp. 47–48)

Light, like sound, can have both positive and negative influences on the human body and mind. All living things need light to exist, and light contrasted with darkness guides the tempo of the body's 24-hour circadian rhythm. Providing natural light or full-spectrum light is the best choice. One study involving school children and the effects of standard cool-white fluorescent lighting and full-spectrum light showed that the children in the classroom with full-spectrum lighting had academic and behavioral improvement one month after installation of this lighting. The report also stated that classrooms with the cool-white fluorescent lighting had more children with hyperactivity, irritability, fatigue, and attention problems. Furthermore, full-spectrum light produces less reaction to cortisol and ACTH stress hormones. Full-spectrum light is best derived from natural daylight and can be achieved through windows, skylights, and atriums; however, full-spectrum lighting fixtures are a reasonable alternative if natural daylight is not available (Mazer, 2002; Starkweather et al., 2005).

Light has healing properties, and light therapy has been instituted as part of the treatment plans of many diseases. Many forms of light exist, and a variety of therapies that use light are being studied. Photodynamic therapy is being tested at the Baylor Research Foundation in the treatment of viruses, and light therapy is being used to treat seasonal affective disorder and insomnia (Starkweather et al., 2005). Ulrich and Zimring (2004) report that climate and sunlight not only direct circadian rhythms, but can also influence a patient's length of stay. One study of unipolar and bipolar disorder patients demonstrated a decreased length of stay of 3.67 days when patients were assigned a brighter room.

The critical care unit is typically bright and devoid of full-spectrum light, instead featuring primarily harsh artificial lighting. Many ICUs are designed without windows or the patient's bed is positioned in such a manner that it does not allow a view of the window. Artificial lighting is predominately fluorescent and produces visual fatigue and headaches (Fontaine et al., 2001). Although light is a vital element of a healing environment, continuous light disrupts the natural circadian cycle and contributes to drops in melatonin levels. If the light is intense, the person can even experience a total cessation of melatonin production. Melatonin, a hormone that is released in response to darkness, is produced in the pineal gland in the eye. Even small doses of light can disrupt its production. Melatonin helps facilitate sleep, and decreased levels can cause impairment in sleep patterns, which can then lead to delirium in critically ill patients (Fontaine et al.). Without the influences of day and night, the human body's natural circadian rhythms are disturbed, which can result in disorientation, delirium, or even ICU psychosis, which may lengthen or jeopardize a patient's recovery (Starkweather et al., 2005). Studies have shown that decreasing noise and turning the lights down decrease patients' anxiety, which with other factors decreases the incidence of delirium.

Many critical care clinicians fear that reduced light will compromise patient care, but that view has not been supported by the research. One study on reducing light and sound in neonatal ICUs by Walsh-Sukys and colleagues (2001) found that modest changes, such as turning off fluorescent lights, covering incubators, and installing low-level patient-centered lighting, did not adversely affect patient safety but did increase staff satisfaction. When selecting lighting options in critical care units, a variety of characteristics must be considered: technical lighting needs, soft lighting for relaxing, and night lighting, as well as the location, intensity, and controllability of the lighting. Available lighting options are nearly endless, thanks to changing technology, miniaturization of components and systems, and the wide variety of lighting choices available. Meeting the lighting needs of patients and caregivers is not the difficult challenge it has been in the past.

Color in the Environment

> Little as we know about the way in which [we are] affected by form, by color, and by light, we do know this—that they all have an actual physical effect . . . People say the effect is only on the mind. It is no such thing. The effect is on the body, too . . . Variety of form and brilliancy of color in the objects presented to patients are actual means of recovery. (Nightingale, 1970, pp. 33–34)

The relationship between light and color dictates that neither can exist without the other. In fact, light and color enhance each other's life and energy. There are seven colors in the visible spectrum of light: red, orange, yellow, green, blue, indigo, and violet; all of these colors are present in visible light.

The energy of color is derived from light, and that energy evokes both psychological and physiological responses in the body (Starkweather et al., 2005). The response of the body and mind to color is influenced by cortical activation, the autonomic nervous system, and hormone activation. Color evokes emotional responses that produce feelings of serenity or agitation that can aggravate or alleviate stress (see **Table 3-1** for the human's responses to color). Color can also affect an individual's emotional state, inducing cheerfulness, agitation, or calmness (Starkweather et al.). Nightingale reportedly used brilliantly colored flowers as a therapy for recovery. Over the centuries, various cultures have used color for its healing powers. Ancient Egyptians designed chambers to produce a ray of prism light used for healing the sick. In Indian culture, each color is assigned to various energy centers of the body. Color has electromagnetic energy that can influence healing in similar ways to sunlight. The field of chromotherapy uses color as a therapeutic tool in the treatment of various disorders (Fontaine et al., 2001). Science is in the beginning stage of investigating color's healing nature. Color by design can be used to supplement the existing light in patient rooms and contribute to the healing milieu.

TABLE 3-1 Human Response to Color

Color	Common Association	Nature Symbol
Red	High energy, passion, excitement raised blood pressure	Earth
Orange	Emotional expression, warmth	Sunset
Yellow	Optimism, clarity, intellect, mood enhancement, excitement, aging	Sun
Green	Healing, nurturing, unconditional love	Growth
Blue	Relaxation, serenity, loyalty, calming, healing	Sky and ocean
Indigo	Meditation, spirituality	Sunset
Violet	Spirituality, stress reducer, feeling of inner calmness	Violet flower

Sources: Friedrich, 1999; Naughton, 2003.

The Society of Critical Care Medicine recommends using calming colors that promote rest in critical care units (Fontaine et al., 2001). Blues, greens, and violet are appropriate, because they have healing and calming influences and are stress-reducing colors. Reds, orange, and yellow colors should be avoided, because they induce excitement, increase blood pressure, and can cause fatigue (Starkweather et al., 2005). Many studies have concluded that cool colors have a tendency to calm, whereas warm colors excite. As another technique for using color in the environment, Stichler (2001) suggests creating painted ceilings for patients to view while they are lying in bed.

Environmental Landscape

That they [patients] should be able, without raising themselves or turning in bed, to see out a window from their beds, to see sky and sunlight at least, if you can show them nothing else, I assert to be, if not of the very first importance for recovery, at least something very near to it. (Nightingale, 1970, p. 48)

Staring at the same four walls can have just as deleterious a consequence on a patient's recovery as the chaotic environment produced in the critical care environment. Creating a healing milieu in the critical care environment necessitates that clear consideration be given to the design of the environmental landscape as well as the feelings and emotions of the individual enmeshed in that environment. A revolutionary study by Ulrich (1984) found that postsurgical patients recovered more quickly when exposed to a window view than did those without this view, suggesting that changing the

healthcare landscape reduces stress and has a positive effect on medical outcomes, including speed of recovery, and reductions in length of stay and cost.

Turner (2001) cites Ernesto Machado's experience during his father's hospitalization in a cancer care center. Machado spent many hours in a windowless waiting area, where he was appalled by the water-stained ceiling and the lack of a pleasant view. This experience inspired him to develop a product that would simulate a window view. This "virtual window" for healthcare facilities actually looks like a window. It can be installed in the wall or ceiling and brings the healing power of water and nature into the stressful hospital environment.

Air Quality

The first essential to the patient, without which all the rest that you can do for him is nothing . . . keep the air he breathes as pure as the external air. (Nightingale, 1970, p. 8)

The human sense of smell is inexorably linked with the environments in which people live. The information received through the senses evokes physiological responses and feelings. Scents stimulate the olfactory system and can trigger an immediate response (Buckle, 2001). The sense of smell is more intertwined in the memory and emotions than any of the other senses (Chu & Downes, 2000). Indeed, the sheer thought of a smell can trigger a memory or reaction (Buckle). The sense of smell stimulates reactions and actions at both subconscious and conscious levels.

The effect of an odor triggering memories embedded deep within the human mind and spirit is known as the Proust phenomenon. The phenomenon is named after the French author, who eloquently described how the smell of tea-soaked cake lifted him from a gloomy frame of mind to the pleasant state of happy childhood feelings (Chu & Downes, 2000). Buckle goes on to state not only that perception of odor evokes memories of happiness and sadness, but also that specific odors can alert us to the danger of fire, stimulate our appetite, and arouse our desire for the opposite sex. Another example of the Proust effect is the unbounded role the sense of smell plays in bonding between a new mother and her infant. New mothers unconsciously nuzzle their infants, breathing in their babies' smell, which helps in sealing the mother–baby bond (Buckle, 2001). In turn, newborns use their sense of smell to find the mother's breast. In the past, healthcare providers used their sense of smell to assist in diagnosing different illnesses. *Pseudomonas aeruginosa* bacteria, for example, smells like a musty wine cellar; typhoid smells like baking bread (Mazer, 2005).

The sense of smell plays a significant role in how humans perceive and react to environments in which they are placed. The basic medicinal smells of a hospital environment evoke strong reactions without even considering the potential for additional noxious odors. Just the "hospital smell" can produce anxiety and increase heart rate and respiration, let alone the reactions to the smell of blood, vomit, feces, and infections.

Controlling the many and varied stress-producing smells in the critical care setting can be a daunting task. One key is designing critical care units to provide good air quality and ventilation as well as single private rooms that assist in eliminating the variety of odors a roommate may emit (Malkin, 2003). Other suggestions include removing offensive odors from the immediate environment as quickly as possible and providing other, more pleasant odors to supercede the noxious ones, such as vanilla, lavender, and mint. **Table 3-2** describes additional effects of aromatherapy.

Liberalizing Family Visitation

In addition to the effects of the physical environment on a healing environment in the critical care setting, social support is a key element of the social milieu. Social support includes emotional and instrumental support provided by family and friends that is influential in a critical care patient's recovery (Tullmann & Dracup, 2000). Family should be considered crucial members of the healthcare team, because the family can provide the patient with the emotional support needed for recovery (Fontaine, Briggs, & Pope-Smith, 2001). Lack of a social network and inadequate social support are associated with a decrease of an individual's overall well-being (Tullmann & Dracup).

Liberalizing family visitation for the critically ill is an emerging concept in providing a holistic approach to healing. Historically, hospitals had restrictive visiting policies limiting family visits. Over time, many hospital floors have liberalized visiting policies. Nevertheless, many ICUs maintain restrictive visiting policies (Berwick & Kotagal, 2004). Rationales cited for such strict visiting policies in the critical care environment, though not supported by research, focus on concerns about increased physiological stress for the patients, interference with patient care, and mental fatigue of the family.

The concern that visits from family increase physiological stress in the critically ill is unfounded; in fact, empirical literature demonstrates just the opposite effect (Berwick & Kotagal, 2004). Whereas nursing visits frequently increase physiological

TABLE 3-2 Aromatherapy

Essential Oil	Properties
Chamomile	Promotes relaxation and calming
Lemon balm	Reduces anxiety and depression
Orange blossom	Reduces anxiety and depression
Sweet orange	Used for relaxation during induction of anesthesia and post-anesthesia recovery
Mandarin	Reduces stress
Rose	Reduces stress
Sweet marjoram	Reduces stress
Lavender	Promotes peaceful mood and a sense of calm
	Promotes healing of wounds and cell rejuvenation
	Aids in relief of insomnia
	Antiseptic
	Stimulates the immune system
Geranium	Reduces stress and promotes healing
Eucalyptus	Promotes healing of slow-healing wounds
Sandalwood	Promotes healing of wounds
Tea tree	Promotes healing of wounds
	Antiseptic
	Stimulates the immune system
Jasmine and rosemary	Psychologically stimulating
	Increase beta waves and alertness
Peppermint	Relieves upset stomach and headache
	Psychologically stimulating

Sources: Avis, 1999; Buckle, 2001; Flemming, 2000; Ro, Ha, Kim, & Yeom, 2002.

parameters, patients are often calmer and demonstrate decreases in blood pressure, pulse, and intracranial pressure with family visits (Berwick & Kotagal). Open visiting hours may not be appropriate for all patients, of course, and there may be times when families may be asked to leave or the unit is closed, such as during procedures or emergencies (Berwick & Kotagal).

Family presence during procedures and emergencies is now being advocated. Family members can provide the spiritual and emotional support to patients in an unfamiliar situation, and they can help give meaning and understanding of the experience of illness for the patient. Allowing the patient to control his or her own visiting hours is imperative to a healing environment (Berwick & Kotagal, 2004).

What Patients and Families Need and Want

When embarking on creating a healing environment through physical design and cultural change, it is imperative to investigate how patients and families perceive their critical care experiences. It is equally important to research what causes stress for patients and families and which stressors of a critical care experience patients and families need reduced to feel safe and secure during their stay. Patients need to feel that they have some sense of control over the environment so as to reduce their stress. Empowering patients by giving them control over temperature, lighting, privacy, visitation, and the type and volume of music decreases stress and improves healing. Rollins (2004) reports that patients were more satisfied with their care, slept better, had lower blood pressure, and were less likely to be readmitted when hospitals took measures to reduce the hospital environmental stressors.

HEALING MEASURES

Therapeutic Sounds/Music Therapy

In addition to designing critical care units and rooms to create an atmosphere that is conducive to healing, there are other healing measures to consider. Therapeutic sound is one example, demonstrating that not all sounds affect patients negatively (Chlan, 2000). In fact, some sounds can sooth and calm. Certain rhythmic patterns of music have anxiolytic effects on human psychophysiology (Chlan). Music therapy, which is classified as a noninvasive nursing intervention, is used as an adjunct to medical therapies. Music, when used as relaxation therapy, has an even rhythm that duplicates the normal pulse beat of humans, is nonsyncopated, and is lyric free. Music as therapy can be used to harmonize with or to bring back in sync the body's own rhythms.

Entrainment occurs when two elements become synchronized with one another and vibrate at the same sound frequency. Entrainment with relaxing music and the body's rhythms induces a decrease in pulse rate, respiratory rate, metabolic rate, oxygen consumption, and blood pressure (Chlan, 2000).

Studies support the effect of entrainment in the critical care population. Chlan (2000) studied the effects of music on mechanically ventilated patient in the ICU. Although there were many uncontrolled variables and the study was small, Chlan revealed that heart rate, respiratory rate, and anxiety level could be positively influenced by adjunctive music therapy. In a 2001 study of mechanically ventilated Chinese patients and the efficacy of music therapy in decreasing anxiety, Wong, Lopeez-Nahas, and Molassiotis (2001) could not replicate the decreased physiological responses found in Chlan's (2000) report. Their inability to replicate results could be related to the small sample size in both studies. Incorporation of music therapy into the plan of care can also decrease a patient's perception of pain. A study at a Swedish hospital of 60 female patients undergoing gynecological laparoscopic surgery revealed that patients required less pain medication with music therapy (Ikonomidou,

Rehnstrom, & Naesh, 2004). Further discussion of the effects of music therapy appears in Chapter 9.

A complement to traditional music therapy is the use of psychoacoustic therapy as a noninvasive nursing intervention. Psychoacoustic therapy comprises harmonies of therapeutic tones (Stichler, 2001). Sounds of nature—such as birds, water, rain, and waves—integrated with soft classical music can also reduce the anxiety of family and visitors in critical care waiting areas. Whether therapeutic sounds are utilized as a therapy to synchronize body rhythms or to provide a distraction, they can be a meaningful stimulus that can alleviate boredom and produce harmony (Chlan, 2000). When employing music as a nursing intervention, it is important to recognize that not all music can produce an anxiolytic effect. Listening to music evokes emotions and feelings that are rooted in an individual's past experiences and personal preferences. More often than not, soothing and calm music produces the desired anxiolytic results (Wong et al., 2001). When providing music listening as a therapy, the patient's cultural, geographic, economic, religious, and educational characteristics and—most importantly—reaction to the therapy must be considered. It is essential to give the patient a sense of control and respect his or her personal music preferences—for example, by having family bring in CDs—when feasible to optimize music therapy.

Art for Healing

Thoughtful art is another healing measure that can introduce light, color, and nature into an environment. Artwork in the ICU has not been considered an important element of the essence of a healing environment until recently. Naughton (2003) notes that a trigger effect is produced when art enhances the body-and-mind connection. Appropriate therapeutic art evokes positive thoughts, which increases the feeling of wellness. Many hospitals have artwork in the corridors and entrances; however, artwork has been frequently neglected or placed haphazardly in patients' rooms (Naughton). In the past, art was not considered an important element to the design of the critical care patient room. However, as the conscious design of critical care patient rooms has moved toward the creation of a healing environment, artwork, light, and color have been recognized as integral elements.

Artwork in patient rooms should produce a restful, calm feeling for patients and families. Some hospitals have art programs that can be changed at will by the patients as well as patient artwork. A peaceful nature scene is superlative in inducing feelings of calm and safety (Stichler, 2001). Roger Ulrich, director of the Center for Health System and Design in the College of Architecture at Texas A & M University, pioneered the innovative field of evidence-based design. Ulrich, Linden, and Etinge (1993), in their landmark study on the effect of nature and abstract pictures on patients recovering from open-heart surgery, found that patients who viewed nature scenes had decreased lengths of stay, had lower blood pressure readings, and required less pain medication. These researchers also suggested that patients who viewed artwork of a brick wall instead of nature recovered more slowly. Clearly, not all art has a positive influence on patients' healing and stress reduction.

Friedrich (1999) suggests that art for therapeutic purposes should be positive and should depict identifiable images; these images include caring human faces, people displaying gestures of nurturing, and calming sunny nature scenes with green vegetation instead of brown or orange landscapes. Specifically, patient rooms absent of a window view can benefit from artwork that depicts the essence of nature, color, and light (Stichler, 2001). Artwork that depicts chaotic impressions, ambiguity, and abstract pictures should be avoided, because these forms may make the patient feel more ill than if no art is present.

Aromatherapy

Another healing measure that employs one of the human senses for healing is aromatherapy. The sense of smell can be harnessed to induce a healing atmosphere within the body, mind, and spirit. Aromatherapy and the use of essential oils for healing ailments have been practiced for many centuries. Clinical aromatherapy is the therapeutic use of essential oils to promote relaxation and healing (Buckle, 2001). Pleasant fragrances and essential oils can elevate mood, alleviate symptoms of stress, and perhaps help in healing difficult wounds and ulcers of diabetic patients. Nurses have been involved in the enhancement of caring for patients with aromatherapy and touch since the beginning of nursing. Nightingale used essential oils to anoint the foreheads of those wounded during the Crimean War (Buckle). Aromatherapy was one of six complementary therapies instituted at Columbia-Presbyterian Medical Center's Complementary Care Center to enhance the patient's healing experience (Whitworth, Burkhardt, & Oz, 1998).

In the 1940s, there was a renaissance of the practice of aromatherapy, after a French chemist used the essential oil of lavender to avoid an inevitable amputation of his arm once gas gangrene set in after a severe burn. Essential oils were used during the Indo-China War to heal wounds when antibiotics were not available. In the last decade, alternative and complementary therapies have been added to the arsenal of allopathic treatment modalities (Buckle, 2001).

Each essential oil has a distinct fragrance and chemistry that induce a variety of physiological and psychological responses that affect relaxation, healing, and general well-being. Essential oils are inhaled or diluted and applied to the skin through lotions/bath oils, colognes, compresses, and mists. Most essential oils are not safe for ingestion, with the exception of peppermint (Wheeler-Robins, 1999). Essential oils are derived from aromatic plants through a process of steam distillation or cold compression (Buckle, 2001). Lavender is the most popular essential oil and is widely available. It requires 150 pounds of lavender—compared to 3000 pounds of rose—to produce just an ounce of essential oil (Wheeler-Robins).

Many studies suggest that essential oils and aromatherapy are plausible alternatives for complementary treatments for asthma, skin disorders, and wounds as well as for inducing relaxation and relieving anxiety. However, safety and efficacy are the two major concerns when considering the integration of clinical aromatherapy as an adjunct to traditional nursing practice. Another issue is the scarcity of rigorously designed research studies on the efficacy of clinical aromatherapy. The evidence thus far suggests that the use of aromatherapy has relatively few side effects; however, a few studies report contact dermatitis, cellulitis, stomatitis, or burning at the site of application (Wheeler-Robins, 1999). According to Wheeler-Robins (1999), some of these reported side effects are conditions that are purported to receive relief with aromatherapy. Avis (1999) reports other adverse effects of aromatherapy, such as headaches, tinnitus, vertigo, nausea, and even epilepsy in patients with familial history. Therefore, caution should be instituted when incorporating aromatherapy into the treatment plans of patients with these conditions, as well as in patients with allergies, atopic skin, or sensitive skin (Wheeler-Robins). One sensible precaution may be to determine whether the aromatherapy can be applied directly to the skin or whether it should be diluted. Aromatherapy should be individualized and carefully assessed for effect. Wheeler-Robins recommended that individuals receive appropriate training before engaging in the art of aromatherapy.

Another issue to consider is the length of use, as the olfactory neurons become sensitized to the scent, so that, over time, less concentration is required to detect the scent (Avis, 1999). Consequently, Avis discourages using a particular essential oil for more than three weeks because continuous use diminishes the effects of aromatherapy and increases the risk of side effects. Avis goes on to recommend against the capricious use of essential oils in vaporizers on nursing units, because this therapy will affect all present on the ward, including nurses, physicians, and visitors.

Ro, Ha, Kim, and Yeom's (2002) study demonstrated that the use of aromatherapy led to a notable decrease in pruritus scores on patients undergoing hemodialysis. In the study, neither the control group nor the experimental group showed significant changes in skin pH. However, the experimental group demonstrated improved hydration of the stratum coreum. These researchers' Complementary Care Center uses complementary modalities such as aromatherapy to provide a holistic approach toward treatment of cardiac surgery patients, which encompasses the body, mind, and spirit. Garbee and Beare (2001) described aromatherapy as one possible complementary therapy in postoperative pain control. Flemming (2000) reported evidence that aromatherapy massage provides patients with a transient reduction in anxiety. Because the use of aromatherapy and other complementary modalities have become increasingly popular as an adjunct to the traditional allopathic medicine modalities, these measures are filtering in to the critical care setting (Fontaine, Briggs, & Pope-Smith, 2001).

The Benefits of a Healing Environment

Incorporating elements that produce a healing environment is not only good for patients, but also a good business strategy for healthcare providers to sustain or gain a competitive edge (Naughton, 2003). The cultivation of a healing environment improves the healing experience for patients and families while simultaneously boosting the bottom line for healthcare providers by decreasing length of stays, improving patient outcomes, increasing family and staff satisfaction, decreasing staff turnover, and attracting new patients and competent staff.

A healing environment can still be created in areas where the environment cannot be physically changed or modified.

Critical care nurses and other personnel can make an environment toxic or healing based on their behavior. A nurse's attitude toward patients and others influences the overall environment in the ICU (Almost, 2006). Shattell, Hogan, and Thomas (2005) demonstrated that day-to-day human-to-human contact made patients feel more secure with their surroundings and environment. Human-to-human contact refers to being present and engaged with the patient and family.

RECOMMENDATIONS FOR CREATING A HEALING ENVIRONMENT

The ICU setting has the potential to afford patients the best possible opportunity to heal if key stress-reducing elements are incorporated into its physical design. Such elements may reduce noise, offer privacy, add full-spectrum lighting, and assimilate color. As well as considering the physical design, a critical program that integrates the family and other healing measures is essential to the milieu of a healing environment. Key elements that reduce stress and provide the patient with a sense of some control are listed in **Box 3-1**. **Table 3-3** compares the traditional and healing environments in the critical care environment.

Box 3-1
Strategies for Promoting a Healing Environment in the ICU

Physical Environment
- Reduce environmental stress caused by noise, offensive light, and odor
- Establish an official policy on noise standards and evaluate noise levels
- Use a mini-workstation to disperse staff
- Use sound-absorbent materials such as acoustical ceilings and carpeting in high-traffic areas
- Construct single rooms with televisions with headphones
- Test equipment for noise impact and implement a maintenance program
- Use natural light when possible
- Provide full-spectrum light
- Provide periods of low light for sleep
- Position the patient to appreciate the view
- Utilize calming color schemes such as blues, greens, and violet
- Incorporate nature and artwork

Social Environment
- Create a family friendly program

- Include the family in the plan of care
- Establish a liberal visiting policy
- Offer options to give the patient control over temperature, lighting, music, visitors, and privacy
- Design the area to accommodate families

Healing Measures
- Therapeutic music
- Psychoacoustic therapy
- Nature sounds
- Therapeutic artwork
- Aromatherapy

Other Concepts
- Pet therapy
- Performing arts
- Hypnosis
- Prayer and guided imagery
- Therapeutic touch
- Yoga and reki
- Unit and organizational culture
- Architectural design

Source: Stichler, 2001.

TABLE 3-3 The Critical Care Environment

Traditional	Healing
Physical Environment	
Designs are utilitarian/sterile ambiance	Incorporates color and architectural interest
Lack visual interest or esthetic appeal	Designs are based on patient's needs
Noisy and chaotic	Designed to limit noise with carpet and acoustical tiles
Limits natural light or window view	Full-spectrum lighting
	Incorporates natural light
Limits privacy and family presence	Private rooms and family welcoming
Limits patient's control	Offers option to give patient control over light, temperature, and visiting
Restrictive visiting policy	Liberalized visiting policy
Social Environment	
Passive role for patient and family	Holistic with active involvement of patient and family
Healing Measures	
Allopathic	Integrates complementary therapy
Symptomatic treatment	Incorporates body, mind, and spirit
Lacks connection between patient's experience and treatment plan	Connects patient's experience and treatment through music, art, and aromatherapy

Sources: Kahn et al., 1998; Berwick & Kotagal, 2004; Petterson, 2000; Stichler, 2001.

Nurses can help ensure attainment of optimal patient outcomes such as those listed in **Box 3-2** through the use of evidence-based interventions.

SUMMARY

A mounting body of research suggests that humanizing the environment in which medical and nursing care is provided improves healing and the healing process for patients, families, and providers. Meeting the challenges of reducing environmental stressors in the critical care unit will potentially avert the adverse effects of being a patient in the ICU and reduce staff stress.

Box 3-2
Optimal Patient Outcomes

- Decreased environmental noise
- Increased air quality
- Implementation of open/unrestricted family visitation
- Physical comfort in expected range
- Decreased signs and symptoms of stress

CASE STUDY

A 56-year-old homeless male was admitted to a large Veterans Administration teaching hospital with chest pain and possible myocardial ischemia during the early hours of the morning. The patient states that he has been living on the streets for several years and has no family. He denies taking any routine medication, but admits having chest pain on occasion. The patient was transferred from the emergency department (ED) to the critical care unit (CCU) and then taken to the cardiac catheterization lab later that day for evaluation of coronary artery disease. He was determined to have multivessel disease, which necessitated an immediate coronary artery bypass graft (CABG). The patient underwent a four-vessel bypass and was transferred to postoperative care in the 18-bed ICU and placed in a 2-bed ICU bay. Over the course of the first two postoperative days, the following assessment is made by the nurse:

Postoperative day 1: The patient did well and was extubated early in the morning. During the day he appeared to be anxious at times but overall he was alert, oriented, and cooperative with care. During the night, he had higher pain levels and appeared increasingly restless. He stated his restlessness was probably due to his unfamiliar surroundings and the strange noises of the busy unit.

Postoperative day 2: During the morning nurse's assessment, it was discovered that the patient consumed approximately one pint of vodka each day (there was no notation of alcohol consumption on the ED note or admission assessment). In reviewing the previous shift's assessment and care, the nurse noted that the patient's pain had been difficult to control throughout the night. Additionally, the other patient in his two-bed ICU bay suffered a code and expired after an extended resuscitation attempt, adding to his agitation.

The nurse noted the following major problems:

- Alcohol dependence with late identification (post-op)
- Pain management issues
- Anxiety
- Overstimulation throughout the patient's hospital stay
- Minimal change in lighting due to increased activity overnight
- Loud unit noises
- Hospital and unit odors

CRITICAL THINKING QUESTIONS

1. What is the top priority for this patient now?
2. What activities could help improve his recovery and aid in decreasing his anxiety level?
3. What strategies should the nurse implement to provide a healing environment for the patient?
4. Use the Synergy Model to develop a plan of care for this patient. The grid is provided to help you organize your thinking to include all patient characteristics.

Synergy Model to Develop a Plan of Care

	Patient Characteristics	Subjective and Objective Data	Evidence-based Interventions	Outcomes
SYNERGY MODEL	Resiliency			
	Vulnerability			
	Stability			
	Complexity			
	Resource Availability			
	Participation in Care			
	Participation in Decision Making			
	Predictability			

Online Resources

Institute for Healthcare Improvement, Patient Centered Care, and the Planetree Model:
www.ihi.org

Guideline for ICU Design:
www.sccm.org/professional_resources/guidelines/table_of_contents/documents/ICU_design.pdf

Healing by Design:
www.muhc-healing.mcgill.ga/english/speakers/hamilton_pl.html

The Pebble Project:
http://www.healthdesign.org/research/pebble/

Agency for Healthcare Research and Quality (AHRQ)
The Effect of Health Care Working Conditions on Patient Safety. Evidence Report/Technology Assessment: Number 74. AHRQ Publication No. 03-E024, 2003:
http://www.ahrq.gov/clinic/epcsums/worksum.htm

Smith J., & Crawford, L.
Report of findings from the practice and professional issues survey Spring 2003. *National Council of State Boards of Nursing,* 2004 (15):
http://www.ncsbn.org/pdfs/RB15_SO3PPI_ESforWeb.pdf

REFERENCES

Almost, J. (2006). Conflict within nursing work environments: Concept analysis. *Journal of Advanced Nursing, 53*(4), 444–453.

Avis, A. (1999). Aromatherapy in practice. *Nursing Standards, 13*(24), 14–15.

Berwick, D., & Kotagal, M. (2004). Restricted visiting hours in ICUs: Time to change. *Journal of the American Medical Association, 292*(6), 736–737.

Buckle, J. (2001). Aromatherapy and diabetes. *Diabetes Spectrum, 14*(3), 124–126.

Chlan, L. (2000). Music therapy as a nursing intervention for patients supported by mechanical ventilation. *AACN Clinical Issues Advanced Practice in Acute Critical Care, 11*(1), 128–138.

Chu, S., & Downes, J. (2000). Odor-evoked autobiographical memories: Psychological investigations of Proustian phenomena. *Chemical Senses, 29*, 111–116.

Flemming, K. (2000). Review: Aromatherapy massage is associated with small, transient reductions on anxiety. *British Medical Journal, 3*(4), 118–120.

Fontaine, K., Briggs, L., & Pope-Smith, B. (2001). Designing humanistic critical environments. *Critical Care Nursing Quarterly, 24*(3), 21–34.

Friedrich, M. (1999). The arts of healing. *Journal of the American Medical Association, 281*(19), 1779–1781.

Garbce, D., & Beare, P. (2001). Creating a positive surgical experience for patients. *Association of periOperative Registered Nurses Journal, 74*(3), 333–337.

Ikonomidou, E., Rehnstrom, A., & Naesh, O. (2004). Effect of music on vital signs and postoperative pain. *Association of periOperative Registered Nurses Journal, 80*(2), 269–278.

Kahn, D. M., Cook, T. E., Carlisle, C. C., Nelson, D. L., Kramer, N. R., & Millman, R. P. (1998). Identification and modification of environmental noise in an ICU setting. *Chest, 114*(2), 535–561.

Lusk, B., & Lash, A. A. (2005). The stress response, psychoneuroimmunology, and stress among ICU patients. *Dimensions of Critical Care Nursing, 24*(2), 25–31.

Malkin, J. (2003). The business case for creating a healing environment. *Business Briefing: Hospital Engineering and Facilities Management,* 1–5.

Mazer, S. (2002). Sound advice. *Health Facilities Management, 15*(5), 24–27.

Mazer, S. (2005). *Sense.* Retrieved from http://www.healinghealth.com/default.php

Naughton, C. (2003). Prescription: Art. *Contract, 45*(9), 84–86.

Nightingale, F. (1970). *Notes on nursing.* United Kingdom: Brandon/Systems Press.

Pearcy, L. (1985). Galen: A biographical sketch. Retrieved April 30, 2005, from http://course.edasu.edu/horan/ced522readings/galen/dreams/galenbio.htm

Petterson, M. (2000). Reduced noise levels in ICU promote rest and healing. *Critical Care Nurse, 20*(5), 104.

Ro, Y., Ha, H., Kim, C., & Yeom, H. (2002). The effects of aromatherapy on pruritus in patients undergoing hemodialysis. *Dermatology Nursing, 14*(4), 231–234.

Rollins, J. (2004). Evidence-based hospital design improves health care outcomes for patient and families. *Pediatric Nursing, 30*(4), 338–342.

Shattell, M., Hogan, B., & Thomas, S. P. (2005). It's the people that make the environment good or bad: The patient's experience of the acute care hospital environment. *AACN Clinical Issues, 16*(2), 159–169.

Starkweather, A., Witek-Janusek, L., & Mathews, H. L. (2005). Applying the psychoneuroimmunology framework to nursing research. *Journal of Neuroscience Nursing, 37*(1), 56–62.

Stein-Parbury, J., & McKinley, S. (2000). Patients' experience of being in the intensive care unit: A select literature review. *American Journal of Critical Care, 9*(1), 20–27.

Stichler, J. (2001). Creating healing environments in critical care units. *Critical Care Nursing Quarterly, 24*(3), 1–20.

Topf, M., Bookman, M., & Arand, D. (1996). Effects of critical care unit noise on the subjective quality of sleep. *Journal of Advanced Nursing, 24*, 545–551.

Topf, M., & Thompson, S. (2001). Interactive relationship between hospital patients' noise-induced stress and other stress with sleep. *Heart & Lung, 30*(4), 237–242.

Tullmann, D., & Dracup, K. (2000). Creating a healing environment for the elders. *AACN Clinical Issues, 11*(1), 34–50.

Turner, M. (2001). Virtual windows brighten rooms without a view. *Houston Business Journal.* Retrieved February 22, 2005, from http://houston.bizjournals.com/houston/stories/2001/9/24/focus1html?

Ulrich, R. (1984). View through a window may influence recovery from surgery. *Science, 224*(4647), 420–421.

Ulrich, R., Linden, O., & Etinge, J. (1993). Effects of exposure to nature and abstract pictures on patients recovering from open heart surgery. *Psychophysiology, 30*, 37–43.

Ulrich, R., & Zimring, C. (2004). The role of the physical environment in the hospital of the 21st century: Once-in-a-lifetime opportunity. Report to the Center of Health Design for designing the 21st Century Hospital Project. Retrieved February 22, 2005, from http://www.healthdesign.org/research/reports/pdfs/role_physical_env.pdf

Walsh-Sukys, M., Reitenbach, A., Hudson Bar, D., & DePompei, P. (2001). Reducing light and sound in the neonatal intensive care unit: An evaluation of patient safety, staff satisfaction and costs. *Journal of Perinatology, 21,* 230–235.

Wheeler-Robins, J. L. (1999). The science and art of aromatherapy. *Journal of Holistic Nursing, 17*(1), 9–16.

Whitworth, J., Burkhardt, A., & Oz, M. (1998). Complementary therapy and cardiac surgery. *Journal of Cardiovascular Nursing, 12*(4), 87–94.

Wong, H. L., Lopcez-Nahas, V., & Molassiotis, A. (2001). Effect of music therapy on anxiety in ventilator-dependent patients. *Heart & Lung, 30*(5), 376–387.

Pain Issues in the ICU

Celine Gélinas

Pain is a predominant stressor in critically ill patients (Stanik-Hutt, 2003; van de Leur et al., 2004), and it is not unusual for the intensity of this pain to be described as moderate to severe (Puntillo et al., 2001; Stanik-Hutt, Soeken, Fontaine, & Gift, 2001). Many sources of pain have been identified in critical care settings, such as the patient's illness or trauma, invasive equipment, and nursing and medical interventions (Kwekkeboom & Herr, 2001; van de Leur et al.). Pain management in the intensive care unit (ICU) poses a challenge given that patients often lack sleep (which can increase pain perception), exhibit delirium, have multisystem failure, and are unable to communicate their needs due to invasive and complex treatment modalities.

Because pain is a major problem in the ICU, its detection is a priority. To detect pain, it must be adequately assessed. Unfortunately, in the ICU, many factors alter verbal communication with patients, making pain assessment more complex. Based on the definition and physiology of pain, this chapter discusses several methods for pain assessment in critically ill patients. It then addresses pain management, because proper pain relief represents an important goal in critically ill patients.

DEFINITION AND TYPES OF PAIN

Pain is defined as an unpleasant sensory and emotional experience associated with actual or potential tissue damage or is described in terms of such damage (International Association for the Study of Pain [IASP], 1979). Essentially, pain is recognized as a subjective and multidimensional experience (Loeser & Cousins, 1990; Melzack & Casey, 1968; Melzack & Wall, 1965). Its subjective characteristic implies that pain is whatever the experiencing person says it is, and that pain exists whenever he or she says it does (McCaffery, 1979). Its multidimensional characteristics include five components (McGuire, 1992; Melzack, 1999):

- Sensory: the perception of many characteristics of pain (e.g., intensity, location, quality)
- Affective: negative emotions (e.g., anxiety, fear) associated with the experience of pain
- Cognitive: the meaning of pain by the person who experiences it
- Behavioral: the strategies used by the person to express, avoid, or control pain
- Physiological: nociception and the stress response

Under this traditional definition of pain, self-reporting is considered the most reliable and valid measure for pain identification. But what happens to critically ill patients who are unable to communicate their self-report of pain? Some authors (Anand & Craig, 1996) have proposed an alternative definition for nonverbal patients. They suggest that the behavioral alterations caused by pain are valuable forms of self-report and should be considered as alternative measures of pain. With this approach, pain assessment must be designed to conform to the patient's communication capabilities.

Many factors may alter the patient's level of consciousness in the critical care unit, such as acute disease, head trauma, and use of sedative agents. Even if it is usual to provide care for unconscious patients in the ICU, these patients remain a dilemma for clinicians. A fundamental question must be answered to support pain assessment and management in these patients: Can unconscious patients have pain? (See **Box 4-1**.)

Pain can be classified according to its duration or its onset (McCaffery & Pasero, 1999). Based on its duration, pain can be either acute or chronic. Acute pain is short lasting and implies

---

Box 4-1

Critical Thinking Question: Can Unconscious Patients Have Pain?

Pain perception is known to rely on cortical response (Dunckley et al., 2005). Based on this fact, it is believed that the patient without higher cortical function has no perception of pain (Halloran & Pohlman, 1995). Conversely, the inability to interpret the noxious message as a painful signal does not negate the transmission of pain (Laureys, 2005). Payen et al. (2001) and Gélinas et al. (2006) demonstrated that behavioral indicators can be observed in reaction to a nociceptive procedure in critically ill unconscious patients. Experts recommend assuming that unconscious patients may have pain and treating them the same way that conscious patients would be treated when they are exposed to sources of pain (Bushnell, 1997). According to studies and experts' recommendations, the ICU nurse can serve as an advocate for the patient and family and participate with the multidisciplinary team to formulate a pain management plan for the unconscious patient.

---

tissue damage that is usually generated by an identifiable cause. Acute pain lasts for the duration of the healing process, which is about 30 days. Chronic pain persists for more than 3 to 6 months following the healing process.

Depending on its characteristics, pain can be either nociceptive or neuropathic (McCaffery & Pasero, 1999; see **Figure 4-1**). Nociceptive pain refers to the nociception mechanism and can be somatic or visceral. Somatic pain involves the skin, muscles, joints, and bones; visceral pain involves organs such as the heart, stomach, and liver. Neuropathic pain is described as an abnormal sensory process caused by nerve damage following an injury, surgery, or disease. It can involve the peripheral (e.g., neuropathy) or the central (e.g., phantom pain, stroke) nervous system.

PHYSIOLOGY OF PAIN

Nociception

Nociception refers to the mechanism of pain and engages the sensory, emotional, and cognitive processing areas of the brain (Charlton, 2005). Four processes are involved in nociception: transduction, transmission, perception, and modulation (McCaffery & Pasero, 1999). Transduction refers to the mechanical (e.g., surgical incision), thermal (e.g., burn), or chemical (e.g., toxic substance) stimuli that damage tissues. These stimuli, which are also called stressors, stimulate the release of excitatory neurotransmitters, which in turn stimulate peripheral nociceptive receptors and thus serve to initiate nociceptive transmission. The noxious signal travels through the dorsal root ganglion of the spinal cord and through the spinothalamic tract into the sensory cortex for the perception of pain. Once the signal is processed, modulation begins with the release of endogenous opioids, which inhibit, through the descending pathways, the transmission of the noxious pain sensation in the spinal cord and produce analgesia. **Table 4-1** lists indicators for pain assessment generated by nociception.

Stress Response

Besides nociception, the pain mechanism involves the stress response. In the presence of pain, an obvious stressor, the sympathetic nervous system (SNS) is activated and stress hormones (epinephrine and norepinephrine) are released. Physiological signs may be observed in association with the stress response: increased blood pressure (BP), heart rate (HR), respiratory rate (RR), perspiration, pallor, and pupil dilation (Milbrandt & Ely, 2005). Many of these physiological signs have been associated with acute pain in critical care (Gélinas, 2004; Payen et al., 2001; Puntillo et al., 1997).

FIGURE 4-1 Nociceptive versus Neuropathic Pain

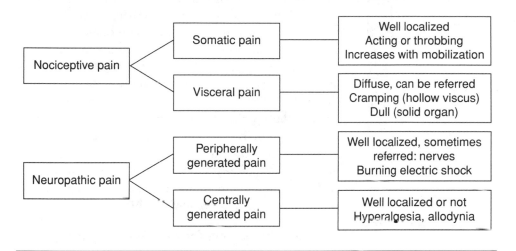

Source: Adapted from McCaffery, M., & Pasero, C. (1999). *Pain: Clinical manual* (2nd ed., p. 19). St. Louis, MO: Mosby Inc.

PAIN ASSESSMENT IN THE CRITICALLY ILL PATIENT

Pain assessment is an important part of the quality of care (Gordon et al., 2005). Because of his or her frequent presence at the patient's bedside, the ICU nurse plays a unique and im-

portant role in pain assessment and management, in collaboration with the patient, family, and multidisciplinary team. **Box 4-2** describes the information to be gathered for a complete pain assessment.

The Patient's Self-report of Pain

Pain is first recognized as a subjective experience. The patient's self-report of pain therefore represents the most reliable and valid measure of pain and must be obtained as often as possible (Kwekkeboom & Herr, 2001; Pasero, 2003; Ste-Marie, 2002). Mechanical ventilation should not be a barrier for ICU nurses to document patients' self-reports of pain. Many intubated patients can use pain scales by pointing to them (Puntillo et al., 2001) and should be encouraged to do so. Before concluding that a patient is unable to self-report, it is recommended that the nurse make three attempts to ask the patient about pain (Kwekkeboom & Herr). Sufficient time should be allowed for the patient to respond with each attempt.

On admission or in the presence of a new pain, a complete pain interview must be done. It can be obtained by questioning the patient using the mnemonic PQRSTU (Jarvis, 2004):

- P (provocative/palliative): What causes pain? What makes pain worse? Better?
- Q (quality): What does the pain feel like (e.g., throbbing, burning, cramping?)
- R (region/radiation): Where is the pain? Does it spread anywhere?
- S (severity/signs and symptoms): How intense is the pain on a scale from 0 (no pain) to 10 (worst possible pain)? Do you feel any other discomforts? (The ICU nurse also observes the patient for signs associated with pain.)
- T (timing): When did the pain first occur? How long did it last? How often did it occur?
- U (understand): What do you think it means? (The patient who had a similar experience before or is suffering from a chronic pain problem knows himself or herself well.)

Pain is considered the fifth vital sign (Lynch, 2001; Wild, 2001), and it must be assessed regularly. Pain intensity repre-

TABLE 4-1 Nociception and Indicators for Pain Assessment

Nociception	Indicators for Pain Assessment	Physiological Links
Transduction	Sources of pain Turning is the most painful procedure for critically ill adult patients (Puntillo et al., 2001)	Represent the stimuli that initiate the transduction process
Transmission	Muscular rigidity of chest wall	Reflex activity through the spinal cord
Perception	Patient's self-report of pain	Pain signal is processed by the sensory cortex of parietal lobe
	Behaviors (e.g., facial expressions, body movements)	Result from pain fiber projections to the motor cortex of the frontal lobe

Box 4-2

Steps for Complete Pain Assessment

1. Identify the sources of pain (e.g., admission diagnosis, invasive equipment, nursing and medical interventions) such as chest tube removal, turning and positioning, and suctioning.
2. Obtain the patient's self-report of pain whenever possible.
   - On admission or in the presence of new pain: PQRSTU.
   - Pain intensity (using a validated scale) as an ongoing assessment during hospitalization. If this measure is difficult to obtain, simply ask patients if they have pain (yes or no).
3. Observe behavioral and physiological indicators that may be associated with pain.
4. Always conduct pain assessments before and after an intervention for pain.

use for elderly patients because it reminds them of a thermometer (Herr & Mobily, 1991).

However, because of the patient's change in communication, a lack of concentration secondary to sedation therapies, and the life/death immediacy of most actions in the critical care environment, pain assessment may be difficult to complete. Kwekkeboom and Herr (2001) recommend asking whether the patient has pain by using a simple "yes or no" question, thereby allowing the patient to answer verbally, by head nodding, or by other signs. This way, it is easier for intubated patients to communicate with clinicians because they cannot express themselves verbally. In addition, pain intensity and location are important information for the initial assessment of pain (Gélinas et al., 2005; Puntillo, 2001).

Observable Indicators for Pain Assessment

Besides patients' self-reports of pain, the ICU nurse can rely on observation of behavioral and physiological indicators that may be associated with pain and that are part of a complete pain assessment (Gélinas, 2006). These should not be substituted for a self-report as long as the patient is able to communicate in any way. When the patient is unable to communicate, however, these indicators become unique information for pain assessment (Aslan, Badir, & Selimen, 2003;

sents the minimal information that the nurse should document during the patient's hospitalization once the pain problem is known and described (via PQRSTU). Many pain intensity scales are available (see **Figure 4-2**). In addition, visual analog scales, numeric and descriptive pain intensity scales have been used with critically ill patients, whether they were intubated or not (Mateo & Krenzischek, 1992; Puntillo, 1994; Puntillo et al., 1997; Puntillo et al., 2001; Puntillo & Weiss, 1994; Webb & Kennedy, 1994). Pain intensity scales, including faces, were preferred by adults in acute care settings (Carey et al., 1997; Stuppy, 1998). The use of a tool must take into account the patient's preference. A vertical pain intensity scale seems to be easier to

FIGURE 4-2 Pain Intensity Scales: (a) 0 to 10 numeric scale, (b) visual analog scale, (c) descriptive scale, and (d) Faces Pain Scale—Revised

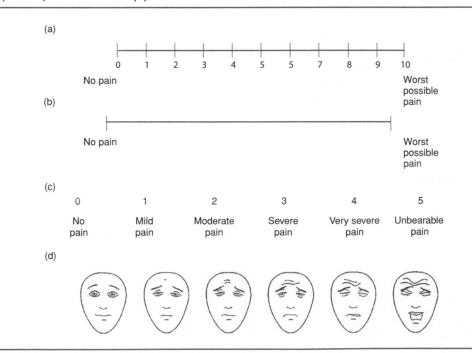

Source: Hicks, C. L., von Baeyer, C. L., Spafford, P. A., van Korlaar, I., & Goodenough, B. (2001). The Faces Pain Scale–Revised: Toward a common metric in pediatric pain measurement. Figure 1-Bottom, p. 176. *Pain,* 93, 173–183.

Gélinas, Fortier, Viens, Fillion, & Puntillo, 2004; Gélinas, Fillion, Puntillo, Viens, & Fortier, 2006; Kwekkeboom & Herr, 2001). **Table 4-2** lists behavioral and physiological indicators that may be associated with pain. Some of these indicators have been supported with empirical data from studies of critical care or postanesthesia care unit (PACU) adult patients (Gélinas et al., 2006; Mateo & Krenzischek, 1992; Payen et al., 2001; Puntillo et al., 1997; Webb & Kennedy, 1994).

Some of these observable indicators were included in tools developed and validated for clinical use in critical care: the PACU Behavioral Pain Rating Scale (PACUBPRS) (Mateo & Krenzischek, 1992), the Pain Assessment and Intervention Notation (PAIN) (Puntillo et al., 1997; Puntillo et al., 2002), the Behavioral Pain Scale (BPS) (Payen et al., 2001) and the Critical-Care Pain Observation Tool (CPOT) (Gélinas et al., 2006). Although these tools show some limitations, they may help support pain assessment in the ICU, especially in nonverbal patients. Research is still needed to improve the use of observable indicators for pain assessment in critically ill patients. The ICU nurse must also be aware that behavioral and physiological indicators are not specific to pain. They can indicate other problems, such as anxiety and discomfort (Bergbom-Engberg & Haljamõe, 1989; Carroll, et al., 1999;

Frazier et al., 2002), or can be influenced by different pharmacologic therapies.

The critical care nurse should also take into account observations from the family. Indeed, the family knows the patient best and can inform the nurse about behaviors or change in behaviors that might be related to pain (Aslan, Badir, & Selimen, 2003; Gélinas et al., 2006; JCAHO, 2001; Pasero, 2003; Puntillo, 2001).

PHARMACOLOGICAL MANAGEMENT OF PAIN IN THE CRITICALLY ILL PATIENT

The pharmacological management of pain takes many forms and is widely used in the ICU. Pain medications can be classified into three main categories: opioid agonists, nonopioids, and adjuvants. Pain can be managed using a combination of the available agents, and the nurse must consider the type of pain and the patient response to the therapy when administering such agents. The mechanisms of action of these different agents in accordance with nociception, their therapeutic uses, and their side effects are described in **Table 4-3**. Clinical practice guidelines for pain management in the critically ill adult have also been proposed (Jacobi et al., 2002; see **Box 4-3**).

TABLE 4-2 Potential Behavioral and Physiological Indicators for Pain Assessment

Behavioral Indicators		Physiological Indicators	
Facial expression	Frowning, brow lowering, orbit tightening, eyes tightly closed, levator contraction, grimacing, teeth clenched, mouth opened, teary, flushing, biting endotracheal tube (intubated patients)	Vital signs (heart rate, blood pressure, respiratory rate)	Increase or decrease
Body movements	Immobile, slow/cautious movements, trying to reach or touching the pain site or tubes, rubbing the pain site, seeking attention through movements, bracing, restlessness	SpO$_2$	Decrease
Muscle tension	Rigid, tense, stiff, splinting	End-tidal CO$_2$	Increase or decrease
Compliance with the ventilator (intubated patients)	Coughing, turning the alarms on, fighting the ventilator	Perspiration	General
Sounds or vocalizations	Groaning, moaning, sighing, sobbing, grunting	Pallor / Pupil	Skin / Dilation

Note: An absence of these indicators does not mean the absence of pain (Puntillo et al., 1997).
Sources: Gélinas, 2006; Puntillo et al., 1997.

TABLE 4-3 Pharmacological Agents Used for the Management of Pain

Analgesic Category	Mechanism of Action	Nociception	Therapeutic Uses	Side Effects
Opioid agonists (e.g., morphine, fentanyl, hydromorphone, codeine, meperidine)	Bind to μ-opioid receptors in the central nervous system (CNS) to: 1. Inhibit the release of excitatory neurotransmitters (substance P) at the dorsal root ganglion of the spinal cord (transmission) 2. Activate descending inhibitory pathways (modulation) 3. Alter limbic system activity (perception)	Transmission Perception Modulation	All types of pain Moderate to severe pain	Sedation Confusion Respiratory depression Nausea and vomiting Constipation Pruritus (itching) Urinary retention
Nonopioid: acetaminophen	Inhibit prostaglandin synthesis in the CNS	Perception	Nociceptive, acute and chronic pain Mild pain	None if recommended dosage is used (≤ 4000 mg/day) Hepatic toxicity in patients suffering from hepatic failure or alcohol abuse (recommended dosage ≤ 2400 mg/day)
Nonopioid: anti-inflammatory agents (NSAIDs) COX-1 and -2 (e.g., aspirin, ibuprofen, naprosyn, ketorolac) COX-2 (e.g., celecoxib, rofecoxib)	Inhibit the enzyme cyclooxygenase (COX-1 and COX-2), which blocks prostaglandin synthesis	Transduction Perception	Acute and chronic pain associated with the inflammatory process	COX-1 and -2 Gastrointestinal effects Bleeding (by suppressing platelet aggregation) Renal failure COX-2 Not recommended in some patients because of the risk of developing cardiovascular disease (long-term use)
Adjuvants: local and systemic anesthetics (e.g., lidocaine, bupivacaine)	Block sodium channels and inhibit the generation of abnormal impulses (local) or suppress aberrant electrical activity in structures associated with pain (systemic)	Transduction (local) Transmission (systemic)	Acute pain (procedural or postoperative pain), neuropathic and chronic pain	Allergic reaction (topical agent, such as EMLA)® Parenteral routes (e.g., IV, epidural): • CNS toxicity (dizziness, drowsiness, tremors) • Cardiovascular effects (arrhythmias)
Adjuvants: antidepressants (e.g., amitriptyline, paroxetine, venlafaxine)	Block the reuptake of serotonin and norepinephrine in the CNS, which increases the activity of endogenous opioids (modulation process)	Modulation	Neuropathic pain, chronic pain related to cancer or other pain problems (e.g., headaches, lumbago)	Sedation Hypotension Anticholinergic effects (dry mouth, blurred vision, photophobia, constipation, urinary retention, tachycardia)
Adjuvants: anticonvulsants (e.g., carbamazepine, gabapentin, phenytoin)	Possible mechanism: block sodium channels and inhibit the generation of abnormal impulses	Transduction	Neuropathic pain	Sedation Dizziness Ataxia Nausea and vomiting

Sources: JCAHO, 2001; Lehne, 2004; McCaffery & Pasero, 1999; Melzack & Wall, 2003.

Box 4-3

Clinical Practice Guidelines for Pain Management in the Critically Ill Adult Patient

1. A pain management plan should be established for every critically ill patient and communicated to all caregivers.
2. Fentanyl, hydromorphone, and morphine are the recommended agents for the IV route.
3. To provide consistent analgesia, scheduled opioid doses or a continuous infusion is preferred over an "as needed" regimen.
4. Fentanyl is preferred for a rapid onset of analgesia.
5. Fentanyl or hydromorphone is preferred in hemodynamic unstable or renal failure patients.
6. Because of their longer duration of effect, morphine or hydromorphone is preferred for intermittent therapy.
7. Nonsteroidal anti-inflammatory drugs (NSAIDs) or acetaminophen may be used as adjuncts to opioids in some patients.
8. Ketorolac should not be used for more than five days and should be monitored for the development of renal failure or gastrointestinal bleeding.

Source: Jacobi et al., 2002.

Equianalgesia

Morphine is the standard for the conversion of opioids. The goal of equianalgesia is to provide equal analgesic effects with a new agent when opioid replacement is required. Prescribed dosages must take into account the patient's age (e.g., infants and elderly patients will usually receive lower dosages of opioids than adult patients) and the patient's health condition (e.g., pain severity, diseases affecting the pharmacokinetics of opioids). The ICU nurse must know and practice equianalgesia to administer the correct dosages of opioids to critically ill patients. All critical care units need to have a chart available for easy referral.

NONPHARMACOLOGICAL METHODS FOR PAIN MANAGEMENT IN THE CRITICALLY ILL PATIENT

Numerous nonpharmacological methods of pain management appear in the literature (Garbee & Beare, 2001; McCaffery & Pasero, 1999; Menefee & Monti, 2005; National Guideline Clearinghouse, 2006). These methods may modify nociception in different ways and enhance the pharmacological management of the patient's pain. Application of heat or cold, massage, and transcutaneous electrical nerve stimulator (TENS) activate the transmission process by stimulating the nonpain fibers. Other techniques such as patient teaching, relaxation, distraction, guided imagery, and music therapy involve the cortical interpretation of pain, and may reduce pain by modifying the perception and the modulation process

of nociception. However, little research (Houston & Jesurum, 1999; Miller & Perry, 1990) has shown that relaxation techniques and music therapy are effective in reducing pain in critically ill patients who are undergoing chest tube removal or with postoperative pain. Music therapy is pleasing to patients, helping them distract themselves or relax (Broscious, 1999). Research is still needed to document the effect of nonpharmacological methods of pain management in the critically ill. The ICU nurse is encouraged to include such methods in the patient's pain management plan because they represent appropriate nursing interventions. Use of selected nonpharmacologic therapies is discussed further in Chapter 9.

Nurses can help ensure attainment of optimal patient outcomes such as those listed in **Box 4-4** through the use of evidence-based interventions.

Box 4-4

Optimal Patient Outcomes

- Physical comfort in expected range
- Reported satisfaction with symptom and pain control
- Reported physical and psychological well-being

SUMMARY

Pain is a very complex phenomenon, especially in critically ill patients. To be accurately managed, it must first be adequately assessed. Pain assessment is a vital part of critical care nursing practice. The physiology of pain allows us to identify indicators that can be used for complete pain assessment. Besides the patient's self-report, which is the most reliable and valid measure of pain, behavioral and physiological indicators represent alternative measures of pain assessment in critical care for uncommunicative patients.

The critical care nurse plays an important role in pain assessment and management. The nurse must accurately assess the patient's pain to participate, along with the multidisciplinary team, in the development of the patient's pain management plan. To do so, the critical care nurse must know about the various pain therapies available and should consider including nursing interventions to achieve proper pain relief.

CASE STUDY

V.R., a 28-year-old man, had a car accident and was admitted to the ICU. He had severe head trauma and multiple bruises. He is unconscious with a Glasgow Coma Score of 7/15. V.R. is very agitated. He moves his legs and arms spontaneously even if he has restraints. V.R. is receiving a continuous infusion of morphine (10 mg/hour). He is fighting the ventilator (the alarms are often activated) and has a rigid posture. These are his vital signs:

BP 145/90
HR 110/min
RR 30/min
SpO_2 92%

During the first 24 hours, the nurse gathers more information about the patient. He is not married but does have a supportive mother and father. V.R. is a computer programer for a local Internet company and has a degree in computer science. He has been dating a girl who has visited once with his mother. At 12 hours post-injury, V.R. has an ICP of 23. The patient remains on the ventilator and now has a Glasgow Coma Score of 8/15. CT scan shows slight diffuse edema, indicating a diffuse axonal injury. Twelve hours after his admission, his vital signs are now:

BP 136/84
HR 100/min
RR 26
SpO_2 93%

CRITICAL THINKING QUESTIONS

1. What types of pain is V.R. suffering?
2. Can V.R. perceive pain even if he is unconscious?
3. What are V.R.'s sources of pain?
4. How will you assess V.R.'s pain?
5. V.R. is receiving a continuous infusion of morphine (10 mg/hr). The intensivist is asking you to change his morphine to a fentanyl infusion. What dosage of fentanyl will you administer to V.R.? (See Table 4-4.)
6. Which nonpharmacological methods of pain management could you use with V.R. to enhance pain control?
7. Utilize the form to write up a plan of care for V.R.

TABLE 4-4 Dosing comparison for some common opioids

| Opioid | Equianalgesic dosages | |
	Oral	Parenteral
Morphine	30 mg	10 mg
Codeine	200 mg NR	130 mg
Fentanyl*	—	100 mcg/hr (0.1 mg) is equal to 4 mg/h morphine IV
Hydromorphone	4–6 mg	1.5–2 mg
Levorphanol	4 mg	2 mg
Meperidine	300 mg NR	75–100 mg
Methadone	20 mg	10 mg
Hydrocodone	30 mg	—
Oxycodone	15–20 mg	—

Note: For comparison, a dosage of 10 mg of parenteral morphine is established.
NR = not recommended
*Fentanyl is also available in the transdermal route (Duragesic).
Sources: JCAHO, 2001; Lehne, 2004; McCaffery & Pasero, 1999; Melzack & Wall, 2003; Warfield & Bajwa, 2004.

SYNERGY MODEL	Patient Characteristics	Subjective and Objective Data	Evidence-based Interventions	Outcomes
	Resiliency			
	Vulnerability			
	Stability			
	Complexity			
	Resource Availability			
	Participation in Care			
	Participation in Decision Making			
	Predictability			

REFERENCES

Anand, K. J. S., & Craig, K. D. (1996). New perspectives on the definition of pain. *Pain, 67,* 3–6.

Aslan, F. E., Badir, A., & Selimen, D. (2003). How do intensive care nurses assess patients' pain? *Nursing in Critical Care, 8*(2), 62–67.

Bergbom-Engberg, I., & Haljamöe, H. (1989). Assessment of patients experience of discomforts during respirator therapy. *Critical Care Medicine, 17*(10), 1068–1072.

Broscious, S. K. (1999). Music: An intervention for pain during chest tube removal after open heart surgery. *American Journal of Critical Care, 8*(6), 410–415.

Bushnell, C. (1997). It's all in your head: The biology of pain. MUHC. *The McGill University Health Centre Journal.* Retrieved from www.muhc.ca/media/ensemble/vo1n03/bushnell

Carey, S. J., Turpin, C., Smith, J., Whatley, J., & Haddox, D. (1997). Improving pain management in the acute care setting. The Crawford Long Hospital of Emory University Experience. *Orthopaedic Nursing, 16*(4), 29–36.

Carroll, K. C., Atkins, P. J., Herold, G. R., Mlcek, C. A., Shively, M., Clopton, P., et al. (1999). Pain assessment and management in critically ill postoperative and trauma patients: A multisite study. *American Journal of Critical Care, 8*(2), 105–117.

Charlton, J. E. (2005). *Core curriculum for professional education in pain* (3rd ed.). Task Force on Professional Education, Seattle, WA: IASP Press.

Dunckley, P., Wise, R. G., Aziz, Q., Painter, D., Brooks, J., Tracey, I., et al. (2005). Cortical processing of visceral and somatic stimulation: Differentiating pain intensity from unpleasantness. *Neuroscience, 133,* 533–542.

Frazier, S. K., Moser, D. K., Riegel, B., McKinley, S., Blakely, W., Kim, K. A., et al. (2002). Critical care nurses' assessment of patients' anxiety: Reliance on physiological and behavioral parameters. *American Journal of Critical Care, 11*(1), 57–64.

Garbee, D. D., & Beare, P. G. (2001). Creating a positive surgical experience for patients. *AORN Journal, 74*(3), 333–337.

Gélinas, C. (2004). *Développement et validation d'une grille d'observation de douleur auprès d'une clientèle adulte de soins critiques présentant ou non une altération du niveau de conscience* (Development and validation of the Critical-Care Pain Observation Tool [CPOT] among critically ill adult patients with or without an alteration of the level of consciousness). Doctoral thesis, Faculty of Nursing, Laval University, Quebec City, Canada.

Gélinas, C. (2006). Pain and pain management. In L. D. Urden, K. M. Stacy, & M. E. Lough (Eds.), *Thelan's critical care nursing: Diagnosis and management* (5th ed., pp. 124–151). St. Louis, MO: Mosby Elsevier.

Gélinas, C., Fillion, L., Puntillo, K. A., Viens, C., & Fortier, M. (2006). Validation of the Critical-Care Pain Observation Tool in adult patients. *American Journal of Critical Care, 15*(4), 420–427.

Gélinas, C., Fortier, M., Viens, C., Fillion, L., & Puntillo, K. (2004). Pain assessment and management in critically ill intubated patients: A retrospective study. *American Journal of Critical Care, 13*(2), 126–135.

Gélinas, C., Viens, C., Fortier, M., & Fillion, L. (2005). Les indicateurs de la douleur en soins critiques [Pain indicators in critical care]. *Perspective Infirmière, 2*(4), 12–22.

Gordon, D. B., Dahl, J. L., Miaskowski, C., McCarberg, B., Todd, K. H., Paice, J. A., et al. (2005). American Pain Society recommendations for improving the quality of acute and cancer pain management: American Pain Society Quality of Care Task Force. *Archives of Internal Medicine, 165*(14), 1574–1580.

Halloran, T., & Pohlman, A. S. (1995). Managing sedation in the critically ill patient: A case study approach. *Critical Care Nurse, 15*(4), Suppl. 1–16.

Herr, K. A., & Mobily, P. R. (1991). Complexities of pain assessment in the elderly: Clinical considerations. *Journal of Gerontological Nursing, 17*(4), 12–19.

Hicks, C. L., von Baeyer, C. L., Spafford, P. A., van Korlaar, I., & Goodenough, B. (2001). The Faces Pain Scale—Revised: Toward a common metric in pediatric pain measurement. *Pain, 93,* 173–183.

Houston, S., & Jesurum, J. (1999). The quick relaxation technique: Effect on pain associated with chest tube removal. *Applied Nursing Research, 12*(4), 196–205.

International Association for the Study of Pain, Subcommittee on Taxonomy. (1979). Pain terms: A list of definitions and notes on usage. *Pain, 6,* 249–252.

Jacobi, J., Fraser, G. L., Coursin, D. B., Riker, R. R., Fontaine, D., Wittbrodt, E. T., et al. (2002). Clinical practice guidelines for the sustained use of sedatives and analgesics in the critically ill adult. *Critical Care Medicine, 30*(1), 119–141.

Jarvis, C. (2004). *Physical examination and health assessment* (4th ed.). St. Louis, MO: W.B. Saunders.

Joint Commission on Accreditation of Healthcare Organizations. (2001). *Pain: Current understanding of assessment, management, and treatments.* Oakbrook Terrace, IL: JCAHO.

Kwekkeboom, K. L., & Herr, K. (2001). Assessment of pain in the critically ill. *Critical Care Nursing Clinics of North America, 13*(2), 181–194.

Laureys, S. (2005). The neural correlate of (un)awareness: Lessons from the vegetative state. *Trends in Cognitive Sciences, 9*(12), 556–559.

Lehne, R. (2004). *Pharmacology for nursing care* (5th ed.). St. Louis, MO: W.B. Saunders.

Loeser, J. D., & Cousins, M. J. (1990). Contemporary pain management. *Medical Journal of Australia, 153,* 208–212, 216.

Lynch, M. (2001). Pain as the fifth vital sign. *Journal of Intravenous Nursing, 24*(2), 85–94.

Mateo, O. M., & Krenzischek, D. A. (1992). A pilot study to assess the relationship between behavioral manifestations and self-report of pain in postanesthesia care unit patients. *Journal of Post Anesthesia Nursing, 7*(1), 15–21.

McCaffery, M. (1979). *Nursing management of the patient with pain* (2nd ed.). Philadelphia: Lippincott.

McCaffery, M., & Pasero, C. (1999). *Pain: Clinical manual* (2nd ed.). St. Louis, MO: Mosby.

McGuire, D. B. (1992). Comprehensive and multidimensional assessment and measurement of pain. *Journal of Pain and Symptom Management, 7*(5), 312–319.

Melzack, R., & Wall, P. D. (2003). *Handbook of pain management.* Edinburgh: Churchill Livingstone.

Melzack, R. (1999). From the gate to the neuromatrix. *Pain,* Suppl. 6, S121–S126.

Melzack, R., & Casey, K. L. (1968). Sensory, motivational, and central control determinants of pain: A new conceptual model. In D. Kenshalo (Ed.), *The skin senses* (pp. 423–443). Springfield, IL: Charles C Thomas.

Melzack, R., & Wall, P. D. (1965). Pain mechanisms: A new theory. *Science, 150,* 971–979.

Menefee, L. A., & Monti, D. A. (2005). Nonpharmacologic and complementary approaches to cancer pain management. *Journal of the American Osteopathic Society, 105*(11 Suppl. 5), S15–S20.

Milbrandt, E. B., & Ely, E. W. (2005). Management of pain, anxiety, and delirium. In M. P. Fink, E. Abraham, J-L. Vincent, & P. M. Kochanek (Eds.), *Textbook of critical care* (5th ed., pp. 2057–2063). Philadelphia: W.B. Saunders.

Miller, K., & Perry, P. A. (1990). Relaxation technique and postoperative pain in patients undergoing cardiac surgery. *Heart & Lung, 19*(2), 136–146.

National Guideline Clearinghouse. (2006). Pain management. Retrieved February 14, 2006, from http://www.guideline.gov/summary/summary.aspx?ss=15&doc_id=3514&nbr=2740

Pasero, C. (2003). Pain in the critically ill patient. *Journal of Perianesthesia Nursing, 18*(6), 422–425.

Payen, J. F., Bru, O., Bosson, J. L., Lagrasta, A., Novel, E., Deschaux, I., et al. (2001). Assessing pain in the critically ill sedated patients by using a behavioral pain scale. *Critical Care Medicine, 29*(12), 2258–2263.

Pellino, T. A., Gordon, D. B., Engelke, Z. K., Busse, K. L., Collins, M. A., Silver, C. E., et al. (2005). Use of nonpharmacologic interventions for pain and anxiety after total hip and total knee arthroplasty. *Orthopaedic Nursing, 24*(3), 182–190.

Puntillo, K. A. (2001). Pain management. In H. M. Schell & K. A. Puntillo (Eds.), *Critical care nursing secrets* (pp. 339–345). Philadelphia: Hanley & Belfus.

Puntillo, K. A. (1994). Dimensions of procedural pain and its analgesic management in critically ill surgical patients. *American Journal of Critical Care, 3*(2), 116–122.

Puntillo, K. A., Miaskowski, C., Kehrle, K., Stannard, D., Gleeson, S., & Nye, P. (1997). Relationship between behavioral and physiological indicators of pain, critical care self-reports of pain, and opioid administration. *Critical Care Medicine, 25*(7), 1159–1166.

Puntillo, K. A., & Weiss, S. J. (1994). Pain: Its mediators and associated morbidity in critically ill cardiovascular surgical patients. *Nursing Research, 43*(1), 31–36.

Puntillo, K. A., White, C., Morris, A. B., Perdue, S. T., Stanik-Hutt, J., Thompson, C. L., et al. (2001). Patients' perceptions and responses to procedural pain: Results from Thunder Project II. *American Journal of Critical Care, 10*(4), 238–251.

Puntillo, K. A., Wild, L. R., Morris, A. B., Stanik-Hutt, J., Thompson, C. L., & White, C. (2002). Practices and predictors of analgesic interventions for adults undergoing painful procedures. *American Journal of Critical Care, 11*(5), 415–429.

Stanik-Hutt, J. A. (2003). Pain management in the critically ill. *Critical Care Nurse, 23,* 99–103.

Stanik-Hutt, J. A., Soeken, K. L., Fontaine, D. K., & Gift, A. G. (2001). Pain experiences of traumatically injured patients in a critical care setting. *American Journal of Critical Care, 10*(4), 252–259.

Ste-Marie, B. (2002). *Core curriculum for pain management nursing.* American Society of Pain Management Nurses. Philadelphia: W.B. Saunders.

Stuppy, D. J. (1998). The Faces Pain Scale: Reliability and validity with mature adults. *Applied Nursing Research, 11*(2), 84–89.

van de Leur, J. P., van der Schans, C. P., Loef, B. G., Deelman, B. G., Geertzen, J. H., & Zwaveling, J. H. (2004). Discomfort and factual recollection in intensive care unit patients. *Critical Care, 8*(6), R467–R473.

Warfield, C. A., & Bajwa, Z. H. (2004). *Principles and practice of pain medicine* (2nd ed.). New York: McGraw Hill.

Webb, M. R., & Kennedy, M. G. (1994). Behavioral responses and self-reported pain in postoperative patients. *Journal of Postanesthesia Nursing, 9*(2), 91–95.

Wild, L. R. (2001). Pain management: An organizational perspective. *Critical Care Nursing Clinics of North America, 13*(2), 297–309.

CHAPTER 5

Sleep Disturbances in the ICU

Catherine Vena

LEARNING OBJECTIVES

Upon completion of this chapter, the reader will be able to:

1. Discuss the importance of sleep quality and quantity on health and well-being.
2. Describe the processes that regulate sleep and waking.
3. Recognize common factors in critical care patients that disturb sleep–wake cycles.
4. Identify evidence-based interventions to promote sleep and rest in the critical care unit.
5. List optimal patient outcomes that may be achieved through evidence-based management of sleep disturbances.

Sleep, an important component of human homeostasis, is as essential as other human needs such as food or water. While much remains to be discovered about the role of sleep in health and illness, lack of adequate sleep has been linked to poor physical and mental function (Pilcher & Huffcutt, 1996). Furthermore, because sleep is important for immune, endocrine, and metabolic functions, insufficient or poorly timed sleep affects health and well-being (Akerstedt & Nilsson, 2003). Clinicians and researchers have observed sleep disruption in the intensive care unit (ICU) for at least 20 years (Gabor, Cooper, & Hanly, 2001). For the person experiencing critical illness, disturbed sleep has important implications for clinical outcomes. Therefore, it is important that nurses be proactive in assessing and promoting sleep in critically ill patients. To enhance the nurse's clinical judgment in selecting strategies to promote sleep, this chapter reviews normal sleep and sleep regulation, discusses factors that lead to disturbed sleep in the ICU, and presents evidence-based interventions to promote sleep.

OVERVIEW OF NORMAL SLEEP

We spend at least one-third of our lives asleep, yet we have little understanding of why we need sleep or what mechanisms underlie its capacities for physical and mental restoration. As late as the early 20th century, sleep was believed to be a passive, quiescent state intermediate between wakefulness and death. However, the discovery of rapid eye movements (REMs) and the identification of the dramatic effects of sleep deprivation at midcentury prompted an escalation in scientific inquiry in the field (Akerstedt & Nilsson, 2003). We now know that sleep is an active process with an inherent architecture and rhythmicity.

There are actually three distinct, functional states of the brain: waking, nonrapid eye movement (NREM) sleep, and REM sleep. The cycling of these states occurs at two levels: the basic wake/sleep cycle and the within-sleep cycle of REM and NREM sleep. Several behavioral, neuroendocrine, and central nervous system factors regulate these cycles. In optimal conditions, waking is consolidated during the day and sleeping at night. In the presence of pathology, physical illness, and/or admission to the ICU, however, wakefulness may intrude into the sleeping period and, conversely, sleep may intrude into the wake period.

Normal sleep consists of a progression through various stages defined by electroencephalographic activity, muscle tone, and eye movements (Silber, Krahn, & Morgenthaler, 2004). From an initial stage of drowsiness, an individual enters the NREM state, which has been arbitrarily divided into stages 1 through 4, roughly corresponding to sleep depth. Stages 3 and 4 are collectively termed slow-wave sleep (SWS) and are associated with the highest arousal threshold. REM sleep is characterized by electroencephalographic activity somewhat similar to stage 1 or wakefulness, and by episodic bursts of eye movements and a loss of muscle tone. While this type of sleep is often associated with dreaming, it is now known that dreaming can also occur during NREM sleep. Normal sleep architecture across the night consists of NREM alternating with REM sleep in approximately 90- to 120-minute cycles. A young adult will typically go through four to six of these cycles, as illustrated in **Figure 5-1**. Most SWS generally occurs during the first half of the night, whereas more REM sleep occurs during the second half. Stage 1 sleep represents 2% to 5% of total sleep, stage 2 represents 45% to 55%, and stages 3 and 4 account for 13% to 23%. Typically, REM sleep accounts for 20% to 25% of total sleep (Carskadon & Dement, 2005). Brief arousals punctuate normal sleep, although only the longest of these are remembered. Arousals tend to increase in frequency as sleep quality deteriorates.

As humans age, variability in sleep architecture and sleep–wake patterns increases. In general, relative to younger people, older people have more difficulty maintaining sleep and experience early-morning awakenings, resulting in more time spent in bed relative to the amount of sleep. They also have more stage 1 sleep and less stages 2, 3, and 4 sleep. While total REM time decreases by a small percentage, the proportion of time spent in REM sleep compared to total sleep remains relatively unchanged into healthy old age (Bliwise, 2005). **Figure 5-2** depicts general differences in sleep architecture between younger and older adults. Although objective changes in sleep architecture occur earlier and are more pronounced in men, women are more likely to voice subjective sleep complaints (Blazer, Hays, & Foley, 1995; Middelkoop, Smilde-van den Doel, Neven, Kamphuisen, & Springer, 1996).

While aging plays a role in changes in sleep, evidence also suggests that psychosocial factors and medical illness may be significant contributors to disturbed sleep in the elderly. In a large survey, sleep complaints were associated with respiratory symptoms, physical disability, depressive symptoms, and poor perceived health (Foley et al., 1995). Other studies have demonstrated that in the absence of psychological, medical, and social factors that precipitate disturbed sleep, the increased prevalence of sleep disturbance in elders was much less striking or even nonexistent (Bliwise, King, Harris, & Haskell, 1992; Ford & Kamerow, 1989; Gislason & Almqvist, 1987; Vitiello, Moe, & Prinz, 2002).

The Function of Sleep

The most significant response to a period of prolonged sleep loss is overwhelming sleepiness, which suggests that sleep fulfills essential needs. However, despite the rapid increase in our understanding of sleep physiology and pathology, the exact function of sleep remains unknown. Research has shown that REM and NREM sleep may serve specific biological functions. When individuals are deprived of REM sleep, they tend to spend longer periods in REM sleep during their next sleeping period. Furthermore, REM sleep after deprivation is more intense, with more eye movements occurring per minute than in normal REM sleep. Similarly, individuals who are deprived of NREM sleep spend more time in NREM sleep during a recovery sleep period. Electroencephalograms (EEGs) measuring brain activity show that rebound NREM sleep also differs from normal NREM sleep (Finelli, 2005).

While the exact function of sleep remains unclear, a number of theories have been put forth as

FIGURE 5-1 The Stages of Sleep

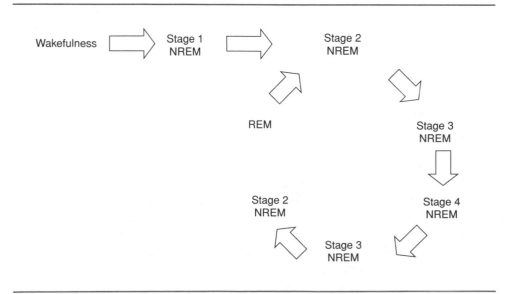

FIGURE 5-2 Sleep architecture in young versus older adults. The figures are hypnograms, which graphically represent the sleeping period, showing the timing, duration, and sequence of every sleep stage an individual has throughout each consecutive cycle. Note that REM sleep, indicated by solid areas, decreases slightly, while slow-wave sleep (Stage 4) decreases progressively with age. In addition, the elderly have increased wake time during the night.

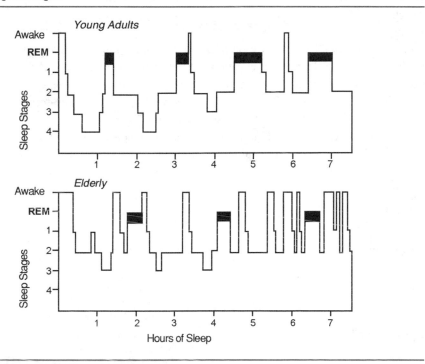

Source: Adapted with permission from Vgonstzas, A. N., & Chrousos, G. P. (2002). Sleep, the hypothalamic-pituitary-adrenal axis, and cytokines: Multiple interactions and disturbances in sleep disorders. *Endocrinology and Metabolism Clinics of North America, 31*(1), 15–36.

explanations. Some have suggested that sleep—especially NREM sleep—is necessary to reverse and/or restore biochemical and/or physiological processes through protein synthesis, cell division, and growth. Others have postulated that sleep serves to conserve energy by reducing the body's metabolic rate and temperature (Silber et al., 2004). There have also been numerous speculations on the functions of REM sleep, including brain restoration, consolidation of memory, and erasure of inappropriate memories (Siegel, 2001). Sleep appears to be important for immune and endocrine function, metabolism, and thermoregulation (McGinty & Szymusiak, 1990; Opp & Imeri, 1999). None of these theories is supported unequivocally by current evidence, however. Most likely, sleep serves many functions.

Sleep Regulation

A basic understanding of sleep regulatory mechanisms is necessary to appreciate how the sleep–wake cycle may be disrupted in patients who are admitted to the ICU. Two intrinsic processes govern physiologic sleepiness and wakefulness: process S and process C (Borbely, 1982). Process S represents

a homeostatic pressure to sleep that increases with the length of time an individual is awake and that is eliminated by sleep. Process C, the circadian rhythm, is regulated by a strong circadian pacemaker. Process C represents the propensity for wakefulness and is lowest in the early morning hours and highest at mid-day. The natural sleep–wake cycle lasts about 25 hours. However, cues from the environment entrain sleep's rhythm to a 24-hour schedule. As a result, persons depend on external cues such as exposure to light, regular meals, and social interactions to keep their diurnal cycle "on time."

Sleep propensity, sleep structure, and waking are regulated by a subtle and complex interaction of the two processes. Process C serves to maintain sleep as process S declines during the night and to maintain alertness as process S increases during the day (Borbely & Achermann, 2000, 2005). NREM sleep intensity is determined primarily by the homeostatic process (process S) and REM sleep by the circadian process (process C), while the ratio of REM to NREM sleep depends on both homeostatic and circadian factors. Factors that either interfere with or support these processes have the potential to significantly affect the timing, duration, and structure of sleep as well as daytime functioning.

SLEEP IN THE ICU

Since the late 1970s, research has confirmed that sleep is routinely disturbed in ICU patients. These findings have been identified in studies using subjective measures (patient self-report) and objective measures [polysomnography (PSG)]. Subjective measures provide information regarding a patient's perceptions of both the quantity and the quality of sleep. Often, subjective and objective measures do not show any correlation. PSG—the simultaneous recording of an EEG, electromyogram (EMG), and electrooculogram (EOG) along with respiratory patterns and pulse oximetry—is the only method of measuring sleep that yields information concerning sleep stages, arousals, abnormal movements, and disturbed breathing during sleep. Both types of studies provide data that illuminate our understanding of sleep in the ICU. Personal satisfaction with the amount of sleep and feeling refreshed after sleep are significant parts of the ICU experience. PSG analysis of sleep architecture, by contrast, provides insight into specific disruptions of the sleep–wake cycle.

Table 5-1 summarizes the research findings from studies conducted in the last decade. It appears that in a variety of ICU settings, patients commonly complain about disturbed sleep and the lack of rest. In addition, PSG studies show that sleep in the ICU is characterized by lack of consolidation (sleep is spread across the 24-hour period), increased amounts of light NREM sleep (Stage 1), marked decreases in SWS and REM sleep, and fragmentation in the form of frequent arousals and awakenings. Furthermore, in some critically ill patients, electroencephalographic features seen in normal sleep and wakefulness are absent. These patients exhibit electroencephalographic features of encephalopathy and pathological wakefulness (the behavioral appearance of wakefulness accompanied with electroencephalographic features of SWS) (Cooper et al., 2000).

Effects of Disturbed Sleep in the ICU

Sleep abnormalities described in ICU patients have important implications for patient outcomes. Frequent sleep fragmentation has been shown to produce impairment in cognitive function, including reduced attention, short-term memory, and problem-solving ability (Bonnet, 1985, 1989). Sleep fragmentation can also lead to sleepiness in the waking hours. Both sleepiness and cognitive dysfunction make it difficult for ICU

TABLE 5-1 Studies Evaluating Sleep in ICU Patients

Study	Patient Type	Method	Findings
Subjective Measures			
McKinley et al., 2002	Medical-surgical	Focus group	Three to six months after discharge, former ICU patients recalled lack of sleep and rest as contributing to anxiety and fear.
Freedman et al., 1999	Medical-surgical	Questionnaire	Perceived quality of sleep was poorer than that at home. Poor quality of sleep and daytime sleepiness were common problems in all types of ICUs.
Simini, 1999	Medical-surgical	Interview	61% reported feeling sleep deprived.
Topf & Thompson, 2001	Cardiac	Verran and Snyder-Halpern Sleep Scale	Poor-quality sleep was related to multiple stresses in the ICU.
Nelson et al., 2001	Cancer	Edmonton Symptom Assessment Scale	68% reported moderate to severe insomnia.
Polysomnographic Measures			
Gabor et al., 2001	Medical-surgical Mechanically ventilated	PSG (24 hour)	Patients had less SWS, more awakenings, and shorter sleep times. 50% of sleep was obtained during the day.
Cooper et al., 2000	Lung trauma Mechanically ventilated	PSG (24 hour)	Sleep as conventionally measured was found in only a subgroup of patients. Sleep was distributed throughout the day. REM sleep was reduced and stage 2 NREM sleep was virtually absent. Sleep was fragmented by frequent arousals and awakenings.
Gottschlich et al., 1994	Burn	PSG (24 hour)	Decreased REM and SWS. Total sleep time was adequate but was spread across the day.
Freedman et al., 2001	Medical Mechanically ventilated	PSG (24 hour)	Large variation in total sleep time among patients. Sleep was fragmented and non-consolidated. Sleep was mostly stage 1 NREM with decreased amount of stages 2, 3, 4, and REM.

patients to cooperate with complex activities and may impair the communication of important information between the patient and the ICU staff. Lack of adequate sleep may also be a precipitating factor in the development of delirium (often called "ICU psychosis"), a condition that further complicates care and is accompanied by significant morbidity (Kaneko et al., 1997). Sleep fragmentation can result in elevation of blood pressure, increases in urinary and serum catecholamines (indicators of acute stress), arrhythmias, and progression of heart failure (Leung & Bradley, 2001; Sin, Logan, Fitzgerald, Liu, & Bradley, 2000). In addition, sleep loss has been shown to produce a catabolic state leading to negative nitrogen balance, alter immune function, increase oxygen consumption and carbon dioxide production, and disrupt thermoregulation (Bonnet, 2005). Thus the lack of consolidated, restorative sleep places the ICU patient at risk for adverse outcomes.

FACTORS CONTRIBUTING TO DISTURBED SLEEP IN THE ICU

Disturbed sleeping and waking in the ICU have a multifactoral origin. In addition to personal factors, the ICU experience itself contributes to disturbed sleep. Some factors, such as sleep history and demographic factors, may predispose patients to further problems with their sleep while in the ICU. Other factors, such as psychosocial, disease-related, treatment-related, and environmental factors, may precipitate sleep–wake disturbance through interference with sleep regulatory processes (process S and process C).

Sleep History

From population-based surveys, the National Sleep Foundation (NSF) estimates that at least 34% of Americans are at risk for primary sleep disorders such as insomnia, sleep apnea, and restless legs syndrome (NSF, 2005). If true, tens of millions of Americans have undiagnosed and untreated sleep disorders. In addition, the average amount of sleep obtained by adults in the United States is 6.9 hours per weeknight. Seventy-one percent of adults say they sleep fewer than eight hours per night; 40% report sleeping fewer than seven hours (NSF). Thus a significant number of patients may come into the ICU with a preexisting sleep disorder or with chronic sleep deprivation—conditions that could feasibly worsen the effect of numerous precipitating factors present in the ICU setting.

Demographic Factors

Researchers have identified increased reports of sleep problems in elderly individuals, women, and Caucasians (Blazer et al., 1995; Bliwise, 2005; Rediehs, Reis, & Creason, 1990). Of these factors, age appears to have the most significant impact on sleep. The elderly have increased fragmentation of sleep, decreased amounts of deep sleep, and increased daytime napping that are linked to age-related changes that alter both homeostatic (process S) and circadian (process C) processes. These changes include (1) nocturia, (2) elevated autonomic activity that results in a greater susceptibility to arousal, and (3) decreased strength of circadian rhythms (Bliwise). Furthermore, primary sleep disorders such as sleep apnea (Young, Skatrud, & Peppard, 2004), periodic limb movements during sleep (Montplaisir, Allen, Walters, & Ferini-Strambi, 2005), and insomnia are more prevalent in the elderly (Benca, Ancoli-Israel, & Moldofsky, 2004). While older men have more objective changes in sleep architecture, older women are more likely to complain of sleep difficulties (Rediehs et al.). Thus elders admitted to the ICU may be at greater risk for disturbed sleep.

Psychosocial Factors

Anxiety and delirium are common in the ICU (Nelson et al., 2001; Szokol & Vender, 2001). Researchers have found that anxiety related to a general stress burden is associated with numerous changes in sleep architecture, including a reduced amount of total sleep time, difficulty getting to sleep, reduced SWS, increased microarousals and stage 1 sleep, and reduced REM density (Fuller, Waters, Binks, & Anderson, 1997; Hall et al., 2000; Kecklund & Akerstedt, 2004). These findings suggest that anxiety can interfere with process S by causing increased physiological arousal. Conversely, patients have reported that lack of sleep in the ICU contributed to their fear and anxiety (McKinley et al., 2002).

Delirium is a general impairment of cognitive processes that is characterized by a sudden onset, disorientation, impaired memory, hallucinations, and hyperactive or hypoactive behaviors (Szokol & Vender, 2001). Patients with delirium often display alterations of the sleep–wake cycle, especially agitation and inability to sleep at night and somnolence during the day (Liptzin, 1999). However, lack of sleep and loss of environmental cues have also been identified as possibly precipitating the development of delirium (Aaron et al., 1996). These findings suggest that alterations in circadian rhythms (process C) may underlie these phenomena (Meagher, O'Hanlon, O'Mahoney, Casey, & Trzepacz, 1998).

Disease-Related Factors

Chronic Illness

Many persons admitted to the ICU have exacerbations of chronic illnesses, including heart failure, lung disease, renal failure, and cancer. Because the disease process and treatments have the potential to disturb sleep regulatory processes, sleep complaints are frequent occurrences among these individuals (Parker, Bliwise, & Rye, 2000; Parker & Dunbar, 2002; Silber et al., 2004; Vena, Parker, Cunningham, Clark, & McMillan, 2004). Common complaints among patients with these conditions include difficulty getting to sleep, frequent interruptions in sleep, daytime sleepiness, and fatigue. The ICU experience brings additional stressors that can further interrupt sleep–wake cycles.

Pain

Persons in the ICU frequently experience pain (Nelson et al., 2001; Novaes, Aronovich, Ferraz, & Knobel, 1997). Disturbed sleep is a key complaint of people experiencing both acute and chronic pain (Roehrs & Roth, 2005). Researchers have discovered that areas in the brain that process pain signals also regulate NREM sleep. This phenomenon may at least partially explain the interaction between pain and poor sleep (Basbaum & Jessell, 2000). Persons with pain have reduced amounts of SWS and often experience fragmented sleep related to the arousing property of pain (Lavigne, McMillan, & Zucconi, 2005). These findings suggest alterations in process S are occurring.

Sleep-Disordered Breathing

Patients in the ICU may have any number of acute conditions that compromise their respiratory status, including trauma, sepsis, pulmonary embolus, and pulmonary edema (Silber et al., 2004). In addition, many chronic conditions such as cardiovascular disease and lung disease are accompanied by alterations in respiration (Lewis, 1999; Parker & Dunbar, 2002; Richards, Gibson, & Overton-McCoy, 2000). Sleep substantially influences respiratory control (Silber et al.). During sleep, the respiratory center becomes less responsive to both chemical and mechanical signals at the same time that voluntary control of breathing is inactivated. These effects are most pronounced during REM sleep due to increases in upper airway resistance and loss of tonic activity in the pharyngeal, laryngeal, and intercostal muscles. Altered ventilatory control during sleep may interfere with process S by eliciting marked hypoxia and hypercapnia (Douglas, 2005), conditions that have been associated with frequent arousals, poor sleep quality, and diminished SWS and REM sleep (Silber et al.). Furthermore, the effects of sleep on respiratory control have implications for maintaining stability in ICU patients.

Treatment-Related Factors

Intensive Care Technologies

Common ICU procedures—including mechanical ventilation, catheters, nasogastric tubes, indwelling monitoring devices,

and endotracheal suctioning—induce a substantial level of discomfort (Nelson et al., 2001). In addition to the presence of invasive technologies, nurses and other ICU staff must administer frequent treatments and provide around-the-clock monitoring. Both generalized discomfort and routine patient care activities can interfere with sleep homeostasis (process S) by inhibiting sleep onset and precipitating arousals.

Some treatments, such as mechanical ventilation and surgery, have also been associated with interruptions in biorhythms (process C). Research has shown that circadian rhythm markers such as melatonin, cortisol, and body temperature are altered in these patients (Frisk, Olsson, Nylen, & Hahn, 2004; Miyazaki et al., 2003; Nuttall, Kumar, & Murray, 1998; Shilo et al., 2000). In particular, rhythms of melatonin and cortisol appeared to be flat or blunted. In the case of melatonin, the normal rise in melatonin during the night—a phenomenon that promotes sleep—was either diminished or absent. Cortisol levels, which are normally low in the evening but rise rapidly in the early morning, were generally higher than normal. These findings may be related to lack of sleep, because sleep deprivation inhibits the degree to which cortisol levels fall in the evening and decreases the overall amplitude of the cirradian rhythm (Van Cauter & Spiegel, 1999). By contrast, the lowest core body temperature, which usually occurs in the early morning hours, was randomly distributed around the clock in postsurgical ICU patients (Nuttall et al.). This effect persisted for as long as three days. Given that alterations in circadian rhythms can result in shortened, irregular sleep periods and excessive daytime sleepiness (Bliwise, 1999; Cohen & Albers, 1991; Myers & Badia, 1995), these findings suggest that alterations in process C may contribute to sleep fragmentation in the ICU.

Mechanical ventilation may contribute to sleep disruption in other ways as well. Lack of synchrony between the patient and ventilator may lead to disruption of sleep (Cooper et al., 2000). The mode of ventilation may also influence sleep quality. Pressure support may lead to abnormal breathing patterns—specifically, central apneas (those arising from decreased responsiveness of the respiratory center to $PaCO_2$) (Meza, Mendez, Ostrowski, & Younes, 1998). Central apneas can cause hypoxia and hypercapnia with a consequent increase in respiratory effort—events that cause arousal from sleep. Patients with heart failure or lung disease accompanied by higher waking $PaCO_2$ levels may be particularly susceptible to this phenomenon (Parthasarathy & Tobin, 2002). Parthasarathy and Tobin found that pressure support ventilation was associated with more central apneas and arousals than assist support ventilation. They also found that the addition of dead space (extra tubing) with pressure support ventilation decreased the frequency of central apneas and sleep disruptions.

Medications

Patients in the ICU receive a number of medications that can potentially interfere with sleep or wakefulness. Impaired renal, hepatic, or neurological function in the critically ill can further sensitize patients to adverse effects from their medications. It is beyond the scope of this chapter to provide a comprehensive review of the effect of all medications on the sleep–wake cycle. **Table 5-2** summarizes the major types of drugs known to affect sleep and wakefulness that patients may receive in the ICU. While analgesics, sedatives, and hypnotics are well known for their effects on sleep and wakefulness, numerous other agents can have adverse effects on sleep regulation, but particularly those that act on the central nervous system (Schwietzer, 2005).

Environmental Factors

A comfortable environment is needed for optimal sleep. The ICU environment is not only strange and unfamiliar to patients, but also full of environmental stimuli that can adversely affect sleep. Noise, light, and ambient temperature have been shown to relate to poor sleep in the ICU.

Noise

A variety of sources, including equipment, alarms, phones, beepers, and talking, produce noise levels in critical care units that often exceed the level recommended by the Environmental Protection Agency (EPA) for acute care hospitals (EPA, 1974). Some noise related to equipment, monitors, and procedures is inevitable. However, one study identified the sources of more than 50% of peak sound levels as related to human behavior (e.g., talking, television, telephone, beepers) (Kahn et al., 1998). Nocturnal peak sound levels in a critical

care unit have been found to have a strong correlation with arousals from sleep (Aaron et al., 1996). At the same time, some researchers have noted that noise levels accounted for only 15% to 30% of arousals from sleep in ICU patients (Freedman, Kotzer, & Schwab, 1999; Gabor et al., 2003). While noise levels

TABLE 5-2 Drugs with Sleep-Impairing Properties

Category	Drug	Effects
Analgesics	Opioids	↓ REM sleep ↓ Stage II ↓ Arousal
	NSAIDs (aspirin, ibuprofen, naproxen)	↑ Stage II ↓ SWS Altered thermoregulation
Antidepressants	Tricyclic (amitryptyline, doxepin, imipramine, trimiprimine, desipramine, nortryptiline)	↓ REM, ↑ TST
	Selective serotonin reuptake inhibitors (fluoxetine, paroxetine, fluvoxamine)	↓ REM, ↓ TST
Antiemetics	Dopamine antagonists (phenothiazines, metoclopramide)	Drowsiness, sedation ↓ REM
	Anticholinergic agents (scopolomine)	Delayed REM onset ↓ REM sleep ↑ Stage II ↑ Body movement
	5-HT$_3$ antagonists (ondansetron, granisetron)	Drowsiness
Antihypertensives	Beta-adrenergic receptor antagonists (propranolol, nadolol)	Insomnia, daytime sleepiness, nightmares and vivid dreams
	Alpha-adrenergic agonist (clonidine, methyldopa)	Daytime sleepiness, insomnia, ↓ TST, ↓ SWS, REM changes
Anxiolytics	Benzodiazepines (alprazolam, diazepam, lorazepam)	↓ SWS/REM ↑ Stage II Shortened REM latency
Bronchodilators	Theophylline	↑ Arousals, ↓ TST
Corticosteroids	Prednisone, dexamethasone	Insomnia, bad dreams
Hypnotics	Benzodiazepines (flurazepam, triazolam, temazepam)	↓ SWS/REM (mild)
	Nonbenzodiazepines (zaleplon, zolpidem, zopiclone)	Minimal to no effects on SWS and REM ↓ Sleep latency

Note: REM: rapid eye movement sleep
SWS: slow-wave sleep (stage 3–4 non-REM sleep)
TST: total sleep time

Sources: Schwietzer, 2005; Silber et al., 2004.

are not the only source of sleep disruption in the ICU, they do contribute to an environment that is not conducive to rest.

Light

Regular light–dark cycles serve to "set" the biological clock and play an important role in maintaining sleep–wake cycles (Silber et al., 2004). ICUs may interrupt the normal light–dark cycle (process C) in two ways. First, patients' exposure to bright natural light may be limited by a lack of windows. Second, artificial lights may be illuminated 24 hours a day. Both exposure to bright light during the day and darkness at night are necessary to maintain a robust circadian rhythm of melatonin secretion and rest activity.

Ambient Temperature

Ambient temperature is an important determinant of sleep quality and quantity (Heller, 2005). In experimental conditions, total sleep time along with all stages of sleep were maximal when ambient temperature was thermoneutral (about 80°F). In warm environments, total sleep (including REM and NREM sleep) was reduced due to increased wakefulness. In cold environments, sleep was characterized by difficulty getting to sleep, difficulty staying asleep, increased movements, and reduction in REM sleep. Individuals vary in their sensitivity to room temperature. ICU temperatures that are lower or higher than the patient's comfort zone may interfere with process S, thereby contributing to poor sleep.

INTERVENTIONS TO IMPROVE SLEEP IN THE ICU

In light of the growing awareness of sleep disturbances and their potential adverse effects for the ICU patient, it is important that nurses implement strategies to promote sleep and rest among their patients. Because disturbed sleep is caused by multiple interacting factors, no single intervention is likely to produce the desired outcome. Given a basic understanding of the factors in the ICU that may potentially alter sleep regulatory processes, however, nurses can implement patient specific strategies to minimize disruption of sleep–wake cycles. **Table 5-3** summarizes the suggested interventions.

TABLE 5-3 Factors Related to Disturbed Sleep and Evidence-Based Interventions to Promote Sleep and Rest in the Critical Care Unit

Factors	Interventions	References
I. Sleep History A. ICU patients may have undiagnosed sleep disorders.	Include a brief sleep history on admission to the ICU. Routinely assess patients' sleep and sleeping pattern while in the ICU. Obtain patients' subjective evaluation of their sleep and level of daytime sleepiness. See **Box 5-1**.	Richards et al., 2000 Roth et al., 2002 Edwards & Schuring, 1993
II. Demographic Factors A. Elderly patients are at greater risk for sleep disturbance.	See interventions for IA.	
III. Psychosocial Factors A. Anxiety.	Assess level of anxiety. Identify contributing factors and intervene as possible. Provide back, hand, or foot massage to promote relaxation. Try other behavioral methods according to patient preferences: visual imagery, music, relaxation. Offer hypnotics/sedatives as appropriate.	Richards et al., 2000 Richardson, 2003 Treggiari-Venzi et al., 1996
IV. Disease-Related Factors A. Chronic illness: patients with chronic illnesses have a high incidence of disturbed sleep.	See assessment/monitoring interventions for IA.	
B. Pain.	Assess pain and treat aggressively.	Meuser et al., 2001
C. Sleep-disordered breathing: patients with heart or lung disease are at greater risk.	Observe for periods of apnea during sleeping periods. Consider continuous pulse oximetry monitoring (if not in place) to determine if transient episodes of hypoxia or desaturations of $\geq 5\%$ accompany apneas.	Richards et al., 2002

Factors	Interventions	References
	For patients whose oximetry alarms are triggered frequently during sleep, observe carefully to differentiate episodes of apnea from artifact.	
V. Treatment-Related Factors		
A. General discomfort related to ICU procedures.	Assess level of comfort. Comfort-promoting nursing interventions: mouth care, straightening bed, clean gown, positioning. Have family bring items the patient associates with sleep: pillows, blankets.	
B. Mechanical ventilation: may be precipitated with pressure support ventilation.	Assess for apneas. Monitor for hypoxia or frequent desaturations.	Parthasarathy & Tobin, 2002
C. Treatments may alter biorhythms.	Provide interventions to enhance normal sleep–wake rhythms. Expose patients to bright (preferably sunlight) light during the day. Keep patient rooms dark at night. Limit exposure to even dim light during the night hours. Encourage visitation from family during the day and especially at meal times. Provide time for consolidated sleep periods. Exogenous melatonin administration has been shown to enhance sleep and may serve to resynchronize the "biologic clock."	Fukuda et al., 2001 Kobayashi et al., 2001 Shilo et al., 2000
D. Medications may interrupt sleep or cause excessive drowsiness.	Monitor patient responses to drug therapy. Monitor for impaired renal and hepatic function to avoid drug toxicity from inadequate metabolism and excretion.	
VI. Environmental Factors		
A. Noise.	Put in place strategies to reduce peak sound levels. Use conference rooms for patient care planning, limit discussions near patient care areas, set beepers to vibrate, lower ring volume on telephones. Offer earplugs to patients who are sensitive to noise volumes. Institute unit quiet times, designated periods of decreased noise and patient care activity.	Kahn et al., 1998 Wallace et al., 1999 Olson et al., 2001
B. Light.	See interventions for VC.	
C. Ambient temperature.	Assess patient tolerance for ambient temperature settings. Provide extra blankets or cool room as needed.	Heller, 2005

Box 5-1
Guidelines for Sleep Assessment in the ICU

Brief Sleep History
1. Sleep Habits
   - Bedtime and arise times
   - Average length of nocturnal sleep
   - Overall quality of sleep (restorative versus nonrefreshing; light versus deep)
2. Screen for Sleep Disorders
   - Do you have difficulty falling asleep, staying asleep, or do you feel poorly rested in the morning?
   - Do you fall asleep unintentionally or have to fight to stay awake during the day?
   - Do sleep difficulties or daytime sleepiness interfere with your daily activities?

- Do work or other activities prevent you from getting enough sleep?
- Do you snore loudly?
- Do you hold your breath, have breathing pauses, or stop breathing in your sleep?
- Do you have restless or "crawling" feelings in your legs at night that go away if you move your legs?
- Do you have repeated rhythmic leg jerks or leg twitches during your sleep?
- Do you have nightmares, or do you scream, walk, punch, or kick in your sleep?
- Do the following things disturb you in your sleep: pain, other physical symptoms, worries, medications, or other (specify)?
- Do you feel sad or anxious?

3. Ongoing Sleep Assessment
   - Overall perceived quality of sleep
   - Amount of sleep during the nocturnal period and during the day
   - Perceived number of arousals from sleep
   - Evidence of breathing disorder, apneas, or unusual movements during sleep
   - Level of daytime sleepiness

Sources: Roth et al., 2002; Richards et al., 2000.

SUMMARY

Critical care units provide patients with life-saving care. However, the environment is not always optimal for healing. Patients admitted to the ICU are susceptible to severe sleep disturbances that have the potential to impair tissue repair, immune function, endocrine function, and metabolism—conditions that influence overall morbidity and mortality rates. Factors that underlie sleep disturbances may include both predisposing factors, such as sleep history and demographic factors, and precipitating factors, such as psychosocial, disease-related, treatment-related, and environmental conditions. These factors have the potential to disrupt sleep regulatory mechanisms. Nurses can promote optimal sleep for patients in the ICU by recognizing which factors may be operable in individual patients and implementing strategies to minimize disruption in sleep.

Nurses can help ensure attainment of optimal patient outcomes such as those listed in **Box 5-2** through the use of evidence-based interventions.

Box 5-2
Optimal Patient Outcomes

- Sleep patterns in expected range
- Expressed satisfaction with comfort
- Uninterrupted patterns of sleep
- Reported decrease in anxiety
- Enhanced coping strategies

CASE STUDY

A 42-year-old is admitted to the ICU status post gastric bypass procedure. The patient has a history of hypertension, diabetes, morbid obesity, and obstructive sleep apnea and did not tolerate weaning from mechanical ventilation in the postanesthesia care unit. The patient uses a CPAP mask at home for sleep apnea. Upon admission, the patient has stable vital signs and is receiving intravenous fluids at 150 mL/hr.

The patient is rested overnight on the ventilator and has acceptable weaning parameters the next morning. The patient is successfully extubated. Three hours post extubation, the ICU notes that the SpO_2 drops from 93% to 85% while the patient is asleep and on nasal cannula at 3 L/min. Breath sounds are diminished at the bases bilaterally. Other vital signs remain unchanged. The patient has no behavioral signs of pain or discomfort while asleep.

CRITICAL THINKING QUESTIONS

1. What are the possible causes of the decreased saturation in this patient?
2. What interventions are indicated for this patient?
3. How can the ICU nurse promote optimal sleep in this patient?
4. What disciplines should be consulted to work with this client?
5. What types of issues may require you to act as an advocate or moral agent for this patient?
6. How will you implement your role as a facilitator of learning for this patient?
7. Utilize the form to write up a plan of care for one client in the clinical setting who is exhibiting a sleep disturbance.
8. Write a case example from the clinical setting. Rate the patient as a level 1, 3, or 5 on each characteristic. Identify the level of nurse characteristics needed in the care of this patient.
9. Take one patient outcome for a patient experiencing sleep disturbance and list evidence-based interventions found in a literature review for this patient.

Synergy Model to Develop a Plan of Care

	Patient Characteristics	Subjective and Objective Data	Evidence-based Interventions	Outcomes
SYNERGY MODEL	Resiliency			
	Vulnerability			
	Stability			
	Complexity			
	Resource Availability			
	Participation in Care			
	Participation in Decision Making			
	Predictability			

Online Resources

American Academy of Sleep Medicine, education website: www.sleepeducation.com
National Sleep Foundation: www.sleepfoundation.com
Sleepnet: www.sleepnet.com

REFERENCES

Aaron, J. N., Carlisle, C. C., Carskadon, M. A., Meyer, T. J., Hill, N. S., & Millman, R. P. (1996). Environmental noise as a cause of sleep disruption in an intermediate respiratory care unit. *Sleep, 19*(9), 707–710.

Akerstedt, T., & Nilsson, P. M. (2003). Sleep as restitution: An introduction. *Journal of Internal Medicine, 254,* 6–12.

Basbaum, A. I., & Jessell, T. M. (2000). The perception of pain. In E. R. Kandel, J. H. Schwartz, & T. M. Jessell (Eds.), *Principles of neuroscience* (4th ed., pp. 472–491). New York: McGraw-Hill.

Benca, R. M., Ancoli-Israel, S., & Moldofsky, H. (2004). Special considerations in insomnia diagnosis and management: Depressed, elderly, and chronic pain populations. *Journal of Clinical Psychiatry, 65*(Suppl. 8), 26–35.

Blazer, D. G., Hays, J. C., & Foley, D. J. (1995). Sleep complaints in older adults: A racial comparison. *Journals of Gerontology Series A—Biological Sciences & Medical Sciences, 50*(5), M280–M284.

Bliwise, D. L. (1999). Sleep and circadian rhythm disorders in aging and dementia. In F. W. Turek & P. C. Zee (Eds.), *Regulation of sleep and circadian rhythms* (pp. 487–525). New York: Marcel Dekker.

Bliwise, D. L. (2005). Normal aging. In M. H. Krieger, T. Roth, & W. C. Dement (Eds.), *Principles and practice of sleep medicine* (4th ed., pp. 24–38). Philadelphia: Elsevier Saunders.

Bliwise, D. L., King, A. C., Harris, R. B., & Haskell, W. L. (1992). Prevalence of self-reported sleep in a health population aged 50–65. *Social Science & Medicine, 34*(1), 49–55.

Bonnet, M. H. (1985). Effect of sleep disruption on sleep, performance, and mood. *Sleep, 8*(1), 11–19.

Bonnet, M. H. (1989). Infrequent periodic sleep disruption: Effects on sleep, performance, and mood. *Physiology and Behavior, 45*(5), 1049–1055.

Bonnet, M. H. (2005). Acute sleep deprivation. In M. H. Kryger, T. Roth, & W. C. Dement (Eds.), *Principles and practice of sleep medicine* (pp. 51–66). Philadelphia: Elsevier Saunders.

Borbely, A. A. (1982). A two-process model of sleep regulation. *Human Neurobiology, 1*(3), 195–204.

Borbely, A. A., & Achermann, P. (2000). Sleep homeostasis and models of sleep regulation. In M. H. Kryger, T. Roth, & W. C. Dement (Eds.), *Principles and practice of sleep medicine* (3rd ed., pp. 377–390). Philadelphia: W.B. Saunders.

Borbely, A. A., & Achermann, P. (2005). Sleep homeostasis and models of sleep regulation. In M. H. Kryger, T. Roth, & W. C. Dement (Eds.), *Principles and practice of sleep medicine* (4th ed., pp. 405–417). Philadelphia: Elsevier Saunders.

Carskadon, M. A., & Dement, W. C. (2005). Normal human sleep: An overview. In M. H. Krieger, T. Roth, & W. C. Dement (Eds.), *Principles and practice of sleep medicine* (4th ed., pp. 13–23). Philadelphia: Elsevier Saunders.

Cohen, R. A., & Albers, H. E. (1991). Disruption of human circadian and cognitive regulation following a discrete hypothalamic lesion: A case study. *Neurology, 41*(5), 726–729.

Cooper, A. B., Thornley, K. S., Young, G. B., Slutsky, A. S., Stewart, T. E., & Hanly, P. J. (2000). Sleep in critically ill patients requiring mechanical ventilation. *Chest, 117*(3), 809–818.

Douglas, N. J. (2005). Respiratory physiology: Control of ventilation. In M. H. Kryger, T. Roth, & W. C. Dement (Eds.), *Principles and practice of sleep medicine* (4th ed., pp. 224–231). Philadelphia: Elsevier Saunders.

Edwards, G. B., & Schuring, L. M. (1993). Pilot study: Validating staff nurses' observations of sleep and wake states among critically ill patients, using polysomnography. *American Journal of Critical Care, 2*(2), 125–131.

Environmental Protection Agency. (1974). *Information on levels of environmental noise requisite to protect public health and welfare with an adequate margin of safety.* Washington, DC: Government Printing Office.

Finelli, L. A. (2005). Sleep deprivation: Cortical and EEG changes. In C. A. Kushida (Ed.), *Sleep deprivation: Basic science, physiology, and behavior* (pp. 223–264). New York: Marcel Dekker.

Foley, D. J., Monjan, A. A., Brown, S. L., Simonsick, E. M., Wallace, R. B., & Blazer, D. G. (1995). Sleep complaints among elderly persons: An epidemiologic study of three communities. *Sleep, 18*(6), 425–432.

Ford, D. E., & Kamerow, D. B. (1989). Epidemiologic study of sleep disturbance and psychiatric disorders: An opportunity for prevention? *Journal of the American Medical Association, 262,* 1479–1484.

Freedman, N. S., Gazendam, J., Levan, L., Pack, A. I., & Schwab, R. J. (2001). Abnormal sleep/wake cycles and the effect of environmental noise on sleep disruption in the intensive care unit. *American Journal of Respiratory & Critical Care Medicine, 163*(2), 451–457.

Freedman, N. S., Kotzer, N., & Schwab, R. J. (1999). Patient perception of sleep quality and etiology of sleep disruption in the intensive care unit. *American Journal of Respiratory & Critical Care Medicine, 159*(4 Pt 1), 1155–1162.

Frisk, U., Olsson, J., Nylen, P., & Hahn, R. G. (2004). Low melatonin excretion during mechanical ventilation in the intensive care unit. *Clinical Science, 107*(1), 47–53.

Fukuda, N., Kobayashi, R., Kohsaka, M., Honma, H., Sasamoto, Y., Sakakibara, S., et al. (2001). Effects of bright light at lunchtime on sleep in patients in a geriatric hospital II. *Psychiatry & Clinical Neurosciences, 55*(3), 291–293.

Fuller, K. H., Waters, W. F., Binks, P. G., & Anderson, T. (1997). Generalized anxiety and sleep architecture: A polysomnographic investigation. *Sleep, 20*(5), 370–376.

Gabor, J. Y., Cooper, A. B., Crombach, S. A., Lee, B., Kadikar, N., Bettger, H. E., et al. (2003). Contribution of the intensive care unit environment to sleep disruption in mechanically ventilated patients and healthy subjects. *American Journal of Respiratory & Critical Care Medicine, 167*(5), 708–715.

Gabor, J. Y., Cooper, A. B., & Hanly, P. J. (2001). Sleep disruption in the intensive care unit. *Current Opinion in Critical Care, 7,* 21–27.

Gislason, T., & Almqvist, M. (1987). Somatic diseases and sleep complaints. *Acta Medica Scandinavica, 221*(5), 475–481.

Gottschlich, M. M., Jenkins, M. E., Mayes, T., Khoury, J., Kramer, M., Warden, G. D., et al. (1994). The 1994 clinical research award. A prospective clinical study of the polysomnographic stages of sleep after burn injury. *Journal of Burn Care & Rehabilitation, 15*(6), 486–492.

Hall, M., Buysse, D. J., Nowell, P. D., Nofzinger, E. A., Houck, P. R., Reynolds, C. F. I., et al. (2000). Symptoms of stress and depression as correlates of sleep in primary insomnia. *Psychosomatic Medicine, 62*(2), 227–230.

Heller, H. C. (2005). Temperature, thermoregulation, and sleep. In M. H. Kryger, T. Roth, & W. C. Dement (Eds.), *Principles and practice of sleep medicine* (4th ed., pp. 292–304). Philadelphia: Elsevier Saunders.

Kahn, D. M., Cook, T. E., Carlisle, C. C., Nelson, D. L., Kramer, N. R., & Millman, R. P. (1998). Identification and modification of environmental noise in an ICU setting. *Chest, 114*(2), 535–540.

Kaneko, T., Takahashi, S., Naka, T., Hirooka, Y., Inoue, Y., & Kaibara, N. (1997). Postoperative delirium following gastrointestinal surgery in elderly patients. *Surgery Today, 27*(2), 107–111.

Kecklund, G., & Akerstedt, T. (2004). Apprehension of the subsequent working day is associated with a low amount of slow wave sleep. *Biological Psychiatry, 66,* 169–176.

Kobayashi, R., Fukuda, N., Kohsaka, M., Sasamoto, Y., Sakakibara, S., Koyama, E., et al. (2001). Effects of bright light at lunchtime on sleep of patients in a geriatric hospital. *Psychiatry & Clinical Neurosciences, 55*(3), 287–289.

Lavigne, G. J., McMillan, D., & Zucconi, M. (2005). Pain and sleep. In M. H. Kryger, T. Roth, & W. C. Dement (Eds.), *Principles and practice of sleep medicine* (4th ed., pp. 1246–1265). Philadelphia: Elsevier Saunders.

Leung, R. S., & Bradley, T. D. (2001). Sleep apnea and cardiovascular disease. *American Journal of Respiratory & Critical Care Medicine, 164,* 2147–2165.

Lewis, D. A. (1999). Sleep in patients with respiratory disease. *Respiratory Care Clinics of North America, 5*(3), 447–460.

Liptzin, B. (1999). What criteria should be used for the diagnosis of delirium? *Dementia and Geriatric Cognitive Disorders, 10,* 364–367.

McGinty, D., & Szymusiak, R. (1990). Keeping cool: A hypothesis about the mechanisms and functions of slow-wave sleep. *Trends in Neurosciences, 13*(12), 480–487.

McKinley, S., Nagy, S., Stein-Parbury, J., Bramwell, M., & Hudson, J. (2002). Vulnerability and security in seriously ill patients in intensive care. *Intensive & Critical Care Nursing, 18*(1), 27–36.

Meagher, D. J., O'Hanlon, D., O'Mahoney, E., Casey, P. R., & Trzepacz, P. T. (1998). Relationship between etiology and phenomenologic profile in delirium. *Journal of Geriatric Psychiatry and Neurology, 11,* 146–149.

Meuser, T., Pietruck, C., Radbruch, L., Stute, P., Lehmann, K. A., & Grond, S. (2001). Symptoms during cancer pain treatment following WHO-guidelines: A longitudinal follow-up study of symptom prevalence, severity and etiology. *Pain, 93,* 247–257.

Meza, S., Mendez, M., Ostrowski, M., & Younes, M. (1998). Susceptibility to periodic breathing with assisted ventilation during sleep in normal subjects. *Journal of Applied Physiology, 85,* 1929–1940.

Middelkoop, H. A., Smilde-van den Doel, D. A., Neven, A. K., Kamphuisen, H. A., & Springer, C. P. (1996). Subjective sleep characteristics of 1,485 males and females aged 50–93: Effects of sex and age, and factors related to self-evaluated quality of sleep. *Journals of Gerontology Series A—Biological Sciences & Medical Sciences, 51*(3), M108–M115.

Miyazaki, T., Kuwano, H., Kato, H., Ando, H., Kimura, H., Inose, T., et al. (2003). Correlation between serum melatonin circadian rhythm and intensive care unit psychosis after thoracic esophagectomy. *Surgery, 133*(6), 662–668.

Montplaisir, J., Allen, R. P., Walters, A. S., & Ferini-Strambi, L. (2005). Restless legs syndrome and periodic limb movement disorder. In M. H. Kryger, T. Roth, & W. C. Dement (Eds.), *Principles and practice of sleep medicine* (4th ed., pp. 839–852). Philadelphia: Elsevier Saunders.

Myers, B. L., & Badia, P. (1995). Changes in circadian rhythms and sleep quality with aging: Mechanisms and interventions. *Neuroscience and Biobehavioral Reviews, 19*(4), 553–571.

National Sleep Foundation. (2005). Sleep in America. Retrieved July 16, 2005, from http://www.sleepfoundation.org/hottopics/index.php?secid=16&id=245

Nelson, J. E., Meier, D. E., Oei, E. J., Nierman, D. M., Senzel, R. S., Manfredi, P. L., et al. (2001). Self-reported symptom experience of critically ill cancer patients receiving intensive care. *Critical Care Medicine, 29*(2), 277–282.

Novaes, M., Aronovich, A., Ferraz, M., & Knobel, E. (1997). Stressors in the ICU: Patients' evaluation. *Intensive Care Medicine, 23,* 1282–1285.

Nuttall, G. A., Kumar, M., & Murray, M. J. (1998). No difference exists in the alteration of circadian rhythm between patients with and without intensive care unit psychosis. *Critical Care Medicine, 26*(8), 1351–1355.

Olson, D. M., Borel, C. O., Laskowitz, D. T., Moore, D. T., & McConnell, E. S. (2001). Quiet time: A nursing intervention to promote sleep in neurocritical care units. *American Journal of Critical Care, 10*(2), 74–78.

Opp, M. R., & Imeri, L. (1999). Sleep as a behavioral model of neuroimmune interactions. *Acta Neurobiologiae Experimentalis, 59,* 45–53.

Parker, K. P., Bliwise, D. L., & Rye, D. B. (2000). Hemodialysis disrupts basic sleep regulatory mechanisms: Building hypotheses. *Nursing Research, 49*(6), 327–332.

Parker, K. P., & Dunbar, S. B. (2002). Sleep and heart failure. *Journal of Cardiovascular Nursing, 17*(1), 30–41.

Parthasarathy, S., & Tobin, M. J. (2002). Effect of ventilator mode on sleep quality in critically ill patients. *American Journal of Respiratory & Critical Care Medicine, 166*(11), 1423–1429.

Pilcher, J. J., & Huffcutt, A. I. (1996). Effects of sleep deprivation on performance: A meta-analysis. *Sleep, 19*(4), 318–326.

Rediehs, M. H., Reis, J. S., & Creason, N. S. (1990). Sleep in old age: Focus on gender differences. *Sleep, 13*(5), 10–24.

Richards, K. C., Anderson, W. M., Chesson, A. L., Jr., & Nagel, C. L. (2002). Sleep-related breathing disorders in patients who are critically ill. *Journal of Cardiovascular Nursing, 17*(1), 42–55.

Richards, K. C., Gibson, R., & Overton-McCoy, A. L. (2000). Effects of massage in acute and critical care. *AACN Clinical Issues, 11*(1), 77–96.

Richardson, S. (2003). Effects of relaxation and imagery on the sleep of critically ill adults. *Dimensions of Critical Care Nursing, 22*(4), 182–190.

Roehrs, T., & Roth, T. (2005). Sleep and pain: Interaction of two vital functions. *Seminars in Neurology, 25*(1), 106–116.

Roth, T., Zammit, G., Kushida, C. A., Doghramji, K., Mathias, S. D., & Wong, J. M. (2002). A new questionnaire to detect sleep disorders. *Sleep Medicine, 3*(2), 99–108.

Schwietzer, P. K. (2005). Drugs that disturb sleep and wakefulness. In M. H. Kryger, T. Roth, & W. C. Dement (Eds.), *Principles and practice of sleep medicine* (4th ed., pp. 499–518). Philadelphia: Elsevier Saunders.

Shilo, L., Dagan, Y., Smorjik, Y., Weinberg, U., Dolev, S., Komptel, B., et al. (2000). Effect of melatonin on sleep quality of COPD intensive care patients: A pilot study. *Chronobiology International, 17*(1), 71–76.

Siegel, J. M. (2001). The REM sleep-memory consolidation hypothesis. *Science, 294,* 1058–1063.

Silber, M. H., Krahn, L. E., & Morgenthaler, T. I. (2004). *Sleep medicine in clinical practice.* London: Taylor & Francis.

Simini, B. (1999). Patients' perceptions of intensive care. *Lancet, 354*(9178), 571–572.

Sin, D. D., Logan, A. G., Fitzgerald, F. S., Liu, P. P., & Bradley, T. D. (2000). Effects of continuous positive airway pressure on cardiovascular outcomes in heart failure patients with and without Cheyne-Stokes respiration. *Circulation, 102,* 61–66.

Szokol, J. W., & Vender, J. S. (2001). Anxiety, delirium, and pain in the intensive care unit. *Critical Care Clinics, 17*(4), 821–842.

Topf, M., & Thompson, S. (2001). Interactive relationships between hospital patients' noise-induced stress and other stress with sleep. *Heart & Lung, 30*(4), 237–243.

Treggiari-Venzi, M., Borgeat, A., Fuchs-Buder, T., Gachoud, J. P., & Suter, P. M. (1996). Overnight sedation with midazolam or propofol in the ICU: Effects on sleep quality, anxiety and depression. *Intensive Care Medicine, 22*(11), 1186–1190.

Van Cauter, E., & Spiegel, K. (1999). Circadian and sleep control of endocrine secretion. In F. W. Turek & P. C. Zee (Eds.), *Neurobiology of sleep and circadian rhythms.* New York: Marcel Dekker.

Vena, C., Parker, K. P., Cunningham, M., Clark, J., & McMillan, S. C. (2004). Sleep-wake disturbances in people with cancer. Part I: An overview of sleep, sleep regulation, and effects of disease and treatment. *Oncology Nursing Forum, 31*(4), 735–746.

Vgontzas, A. N., & Chrousos, G. P. (2002). Sleep, the hypothalamic-pituitary-adrenal axis, and cytokines: Multiple interactions and disturbances in sleep disorders. *Endocrinology and Metabolism, 31*(1), 15–36.

Vitiello, M. V., Moe, K. E., & Prinz, P. N. (2002). Sleep complaints cosegregate with illness in older adults: Clinical research informed by and informing epidemiological studies of sleep. *Journal of Psychosomatic Research, 53,* 555–559.

Wallace, C. J., Robins, J., Alvord, L. S., & Walker, J. M. (1999). The effect of earplugs on sleep measures during exposure to simulated intensive care unit noise. *American Journal of Critical Care, 8*(4), 210–219.

Young, T., Skatrud, J., & Peppard, P. E. (2004). Risk factors for obstructive sleep apnea in adults. *Journal of the American Medical Association, 291*(16), 2013–2016.

CHAPTER 6

Infections in the ICU

Janet Eagan

LEARNING OBJECTIVES

Upon completion of this chapter, the reader will be able to:

1. Identify the risk factors for infection in the ICU.
2. Describe transmission of infection.
3. Review common healthcare-associated infections.
4. Outline infection control and prevention strategies.
5. List optimal patient outcomes that may be achieved through evidence-based prevention and management of infection.

Healthcare-associated infections (HAIs), previously known as nosocomial infections, are the fourth leading cause of death among hospitalized patients (Kohn, Corrigan, & Donaldson, 2000). Data from the Centers for Disease Control and Prevention (CDC, 2004) report a nosocomial infection rate of 5%, of which 10% are bloodstream infections (BSIs), and an attributable mortality rate of 15% (Wenzel & Edmond, 2001).

Many reasons exist for increased infection risk in patients in the intensive care unit (ICU). Patients are there for prolonged periods of time and are exposed to hospital flora or organisms, which may lead to serious infection. Prolonged exposure frequently leads to colonization with bacteria and other pathogens and can happen rapidly. Patients become exposed and colonized by a variety of methods. The most common mechanisms of spread of organisms are linked to carriage on the hands of healthcare workers, contamination of the environment, and use and duration of certain antibiotics.

PATIENT RISK FACTORS FOR INFECTION

Table 6-1 lists some of the risk factors leading to HAI. Impaired host defense includes extremes of age. Elderly persons often have an ineffective cough, predisposing them to aspiration pneumonia. Loss of natural barriers also predisposes elderly patients to infections such as cellulitis and pressure ulcers. Many elderly experience age-related decline in immune function, which decreases their antibody response and cell-mediated immunity. An abnormal immune response may be either genetic or acquired. These conditions diminish the body's ability to fight infection.

One of the problems most commonly related to HAI is malnutrition. Protein calorie malnutrition has been associated with poor immune function, which in

TABLE 6-1 Common Risk Factors Leading to HAI

Impaired host defense
Severity of illness
Length of stay
Invasive devices
Colonization and cross-infection

Source: Rubinson, Diette, Song, Brower, & Krishnan, 2004.

turn increases the individual's risk of systemic infection (Dulger et al., 2002). In a study of 138 adult patients who did not take food by mouth for 96 hours or longer after admission to a medical ICU, daily caloric intake was recorded for each patient. Conclusions of the study were that caloric intake of less than 25% of the American College of Chest Physicians' recommendations was associated with as increased risk of nosocomial BSI among medical ICU patients (Rubinson, Diette, Song, Brower, & Krishnan, 2004). Clearly, nutritional support must be part of the patient assessment and plan for critically ill patients.

Severity of illness as a risk factor for HAI includes underlying diseases or comorbid illnesses, such as diabetes, cancer, renal failure, neutropenia, cirrhosis, altered consciousness, and pressure ulcers. Length of stay in the hospital increases the risk of HAI due to the duration of ICU exposure. Exposure risks in the ICU include invasive devices, environmental contamination, and cross-contamination by healthcare workers' (HCWs) poor hand hygiene techniques. The contaminated hands of HCWs become the vehicles for transfer of resistant pathogens from patient to patient.

Invasive devices breach the integrity of skin and mucous membranes. They include vascular devices such as central venous catheters, hemodialysis catheters, urinary catheters, surgical drains, oral/nasal endotracheal tubes, gastric tubes, and ventriculostomy and intracranial pressure monitoring devices. The longer the invasive device remains in place, the greater the risk for infection. The device days (the number of days a device is in place) of an ICU is one measure of the unit's invasive practices that constitutes an extrinsic risk factor for HAI. Device days consist of the total number of ventilator days, central line days, and urinary catheter days.

Colonization occurs when organisms adhere to epithelial or mucosal cells and then persist at the site of attachment. The presence of underlying disease and invasive medical devices allows the colonizing organism to bypass normal defense mechanisms and proliferate until an active infection occurs. Patients who are highly colonized with pathogenic hospital organisms become the major reservoir of pathogens, thereby increasing the risk of cross-transmission to others.

MODES OF TRANSMISSION

There are three modes of HAI transmission (see **Table 6-2**). Airborne transmission occurs by dissemination of airborne droplet nuclei containing infectious microorganisms, which remain suspended in the air for long periods of time. These droplets may be inhaled by susceptible hosts when the air supply is shared. A few microorganisms are known to be transmitted by the airborne route: *Mycobacterium tuberculosis,* measles, and varicella-zoster virus (chickenpox). Airborne transmis-

TABLE 6-2 Modes of HAI Transmission

Airborne
Droplet
Contact
  • Direct
  • Indirect

sion requires special air handling and ventilation in airborne infectious isolation (AII) rooms. AII rooms are under negative pressure to the hallway to prevent dispersal of infectious microorganisms. Staff must wear respiratory protection with N-95 or higher respirators during care of these patients.

Droplet transmission occurs when droplets are propelled short distances (less than 3 feet through the air) and deposited on the conjunctivae, nasal mucosa, or mouth. Respiratory droplets are generated when an infected person coughs, sneezes, or talks; they may also be generated during procedures such as suctioning, bronchoscopy, and cough induction. Droplet precautions require a private room and surgical masks for close patient contact.

Contact transmission is the most common mode of HAI transmission and may be broken out into two forms: direct contact and indirect contact. Direct contact transmission occurs when microorganisms are transferred directly from one person to another. Examples include scabies from skin-to-skin contact and blood from a sharps injury. Herpetic whitlow is seen in the ICU when staff members do not wear gloves while providing oral care to a patient who has herpes simplex virus (HSV) and the HSV is transmitted from the patient to the finger of the HCW.

HAI transmission most frequently occurs via indirect contact—that is, transmission of the infectious agent through a contaminated object or person. The environment and hands of HCWs are the most common vehicles. The patient's environment is often contaminated with microorganisms. A recent study demonstrated that after a patient leaves the ICU, numerous environmental areas may be cultured and test positive for vancomycin-resistant enterococcus (VRE). Bed rails, monitors, table tops, sink handles, intravenous (IV) poles, and the medical record all had VRE present (Hayden, 2000). VRE can live up to seven days if not cleaned properly.

Contact precautions always include the use of gloves and gowns for direct patient contact. Hand hygiene is an important aspect of all isolation categories in addition to standard precautions. Standard precautions include infection control practices and use of personal protective equipment (PPE) for all healthcare personnel when having contact with all patients regardless of patient diagnosis or infection status. These precautions apply to blood; all body fluids, secretions, and excretions except sweat; nonintact skin; and mucous membrane. The use of standard precautions during patient care is determined by the HCW–patient interaction and extent of blood, body fluid, or pathogen contact. PPE includes gloves, gowns, and face shields.

ANTIBIOTIC-RESISTANT INFECTIONS IN CRITICALLY ILL ADULTS

Antibiotic-resistant bacteria thrive among critically ill patients. Broad-spectrum antibiotic use can frequently lead to selection of multidrug-resistant organisms (MDRO). In the ICU, patient-to-patient transmission of antibiotic-resistant organisms is common. Several factors contribute to the spread of these pathogens. First, the quick pace and urgent nature of critical care often do not allow for hand hygiene. Second, pathogenic organisms are carried from patient to patient on unwashed hands of HCWs. Finally, additional sources of transmitted infections in ICUs may include patients' files, faucets, and placement in a contaminated room (one that has not been adequately cleaned) (Blanc et al., 2004; Graham, Quinlan, & Rank, 1997; Martinez, Ruthazer, Hansjosten, Barefoot, & Snydman, 2004; Panhotra, Saxena, & Al-Mulhim, 2005).

Gram-positive organisms such as *Staphylococcus aureus* and enterococci are commonly associated with central line bloodstream or surgical site infections. Resistant strains include methicillin-resistant *S. aureus* (MRSA) and VRE. Gram-negative bacilli are frequently associated with ventilator-associated pneumonia (VAP) and catheter-associated urinary tract infections. Among the gram-negative organisms that can develop resistance are *Pseudomonas aeruginosa*, *Enterobacter* spp., and *Klebsiella pneumoniae*. Resistant *Acinetobacter baumanii* has recently become a significant respiratory pathogen seen in ICU patients. Patients with MDRO are placed on contact precautions, which require the use of private rooms, gloves, and gowns for direct patient care.

COMMON INFECTIONS IN THE ICU

Four categories of infections are common in the ICU: BSIs, urinary tract infections, lower respiratory tract infections, and pneumonia.

Catheter-Related Bloodstream Infections

Intravascular devices have historically been the primary source of BSIs. Approximately 80,000 catheter-related BSIs occur in ICUs each year in the United States (Mermel, 2000). However, recent data suggest that the use of intravascular catheters that are impregnated with chlorhexidine and silver sulfadiazine may decrease the incidence of catheter-related colonization (Jaeger et al., 2005). Catheter-related BSIs are associated with significant morbidity, prolonged hospitalization, and increased costs.

Intravascular devices essential for administration of medications and IV fluids are frequently employed in the ICU. There are two types of intravascular devices: short term and long term. Short-term devices include peripheral venous, arterial, and central single- and multiple-lumen catheters. Long-term devices include tunneled central venous catheters (CVCs) and implantable intravascular devices. Peripheral catheters have rarely been associated with BSIs, whereas CVCs account for the majority of catheter-related BSIs. Risk factors include the number of lumens and the site of insertion. Neutropenia is an independent risk factor for catheter-related infections in adult cancer patients (Penzak, Gubbins, Stratton, & Anaissie, 2000). In the ICU, central venous access might be needed for extended periods of time, patients might be colonized with hospital-acquired organisms, and the catheter might be manipulated multiple times per day for administration of IV fluids, drugs, and blood products. In one study, administration of blood products through CVCs was a risk factor for catheter-related BSIs (Hanna & Raad, 2001). Migration of skin organisms at the insertion site into the cutaneous catheter tract with colonization of the catheter tip is the most common route of infection for peripherally inserted, short-term catheters. Contamination of the catheter hub contributes substantially to intraluminal colonization of long-term catheters.

Table 6-3 lists several measures to reduce the risk for infection.

TABLE 6-3 Prevention of Catheter-Related Bloodstream Infections

Site of catheter insertion: The amount of skin flora at the catheter insertion site is a major risk factor for catheter-related BSI. Recommendations are that CVCs be placed in a subclavian site instead of a jugular or femoral site to reduce the risk for infection.

Hand hygiene: Good hand hygiene can be achieved through the use of an antibacterial soap or an alcohol-based product.

Aseptic technique: Insertion of catheters requires use of maximal sterile barrier precautions (cap, mask, sterile gown, sterile gloves, and large sterile drape).

Skin antisepsis: Prior to insertion of catheter, skin should be prepped with 2% chlorhexidine (CHG)-based preparation.

Dressing changes: Use 2% CHG to disinfect the skin and either sterile gauze or a sterile transparent semi-permeable dressing to cover the catheter site. Change the dressing when visibly bloody or soiled at least once a week.

Source: O'Grady et al., 2002.

Healthcare-Associated Pneumonia

Pneumonia is an important cause of mortality in ICUs. The incidence of pneumonia in ICU patients ranges from 7% to 40%; this HAI adds an estimated $40,000 to the cost of a typical hospital admission (Tablan, Anderson, Besser, Bridges, & Hajjeh, 2004). Mortality from VAP is 46% (Ibrahim, Tracy, Hill, Fraser, & Kollef, 2001). By definition, VAP is an airway infection that developed more than 48 hours after the patient was intubated; it is the most common HAI developing in mechanically ventilated patients. The mean interval between intubation and VAP is 3.3 days (Leroy & Soubrier, 2004).

Etiology of VAP

The leading pathogenic hypothesis in VAP is oropharyngeal or gastric colonization by enteric gram-negative bacilli. This invasion is followed by aspiration of contaminated secretions (Leroy & Soubrier, 2004).

Risk Factors

Risk factors for VAP include both nonmodifiable and modifiable issues. Nonmodifiable risk factors include chronic obstructive lung disease, severity of illness, patient age and gender, history of head trauma, coma, acute respiratory distress syndrome, and type of surgery. Modifiable risk factors include type of stress ulcer prophylaxis used, the frequency of ventilator circuit changes, enteral nutrition, sinusitis, supine body position, use of antibiotics, subglottic secretion aspiration, and low endotracheal tube cuff pressures.

Prevention of VAP

VAP prevention includes the use of semirecumbent positioning, subglottic secretions, oscillating beds, enteral feeding methods, frequent ventilatory circuit changes, and use of metoclopramide. The best practices include (1) elevation of the head of the bed to between 30 and 45 degrees; (2) daily "sedation vacation" and assessment of readiness to extubate; (3) peptic ulcer disease (PUD) prophylaxis; and (4) deep venous thrombosis (DVT) prophylaxis. **Table 6-4** lists specific nursing care measures to prevent VAP.

Urinary Tract Infections

Most patients who are hospitalized in the ICU receive an indwelling urinary catheter to monitor urine output. Catheter-associated urinary tract infection (CAUTI) is the leading cause of HAI and is linked to significant morbidity, mortality, and additional hospital costs. Use of a silver alloy hydrogel-coated urinary catheter prevents urinary tract infections (Rupp et al., 2004). In the ICU, CAUTI account for 17.6% of HAI. The most significant risk factor for infection is the duration of catheter-

TABLE 6-4 Nursing Measures to Prevent VAP

1. Use standard precautions
2. Hand hygiene: Decontaminate hands before and after contact with a patient who has an endotracheal or tracheostomy tube in place, and before and after contact with any respiratory device that is used on the patient, whether or not gloves are worn.
3. Wear gloves for handling respiratory secretions.
4. Wear a gown if soiling with respiratory secretions from a patient is anticipated.
5. Perform tracheostomy care using aseptic techniques.
6. Use a sterile, single-use catheter when using the single suction system for suctioning.
7. There is no recommendation about wearing sterile rather than clean gloves when suctioning.
8. Use sterile water for rinsing respiratory equipment.
9. Do not routinely change breathing circuits or ventilator tubing.
10. Do not use large-volume room air humidifiers.

Source: Tablan, Anderson, Besser, Bridges, & Hajjeh, 2004.

ization. Other strategies to prevent CAUTI include (1) use of aseptic technique for insertion of the catheter; (2) removing the catheter as soon as possible; (3) use of a closed sterile drainage system; (4) securing the catheter to prevent movement and urethral traction; (5) avoidance of catheter irrigation; (6) using the sample port for specimen collection (never open the system); and (7) maintaining a free flow of urine into the drainage bag (Hampton, 2004). Data also suggest that, although possibly more costly, intermittent catheterization may be associated with a decreased incidence of urinary tract infections, as compared with use of indwelling catheters (Niël-Weise & van der Broek, 2005). Nurses can utilize a bladder scanner to identify those patients who are truly in need of catheterization. Unnecessary catheterizations can be prevented and risk of infection minimized by catheterizing only patients who have postvoid residual greater than 250 mL.

Surgical Site Infections

Patients are often at risk for surgical site infection. Recent statistics show medical/surgical ICUs from major teaching hospitals have significantly higher infection rates than ICUs from all other hospitals (CDC, 2004). Strategies to prevent surgical site infections may include incision care with sterile dressing, aseptic technique, and sterile packing. Sterile gloves and equipment should be used when changing dressings on any type of surgical incisions.

Fungal Infections

Increases in severity of illness, the use of invasive devices or procedures, and the administration of antimicrobial agents have resulted in an increase in the incidence of fungal infections. *Candida albicans* accounts for approximately 50% of candidal BSIs. Approximately 50% of all candidal infections occur in surgical ICUs. The ICU patients at highest risk for candidal infections in one study included those with diabetes mellitus, new-onset hemodialysis, use of total parenteral nutrition, use of broad-spectrum antibiotics, or any combination of these factors (Paphitou, Ostrosky-Zeichner, & Rex, 2005).

INFECTION CONTROL AND PREVENTION STRATEGIES

Good hand hygiene is the most effective infection control measure. Compliance with hand hygiene protocols is very low, however—especially in ICUs. Observational studies conducted in hospitals demonstrated that hand washing adherence in the ICU for HCWs was 23.1%. Following an educational intervention in one study, the adherence rate increased to 64.5% (Rosenthal, Guzman, & Safdar, 2005). The average number of times HCWs wash their hands varies markedly between hospital wards. Reasons cited for the low compliance rate include heavy workload, lack of familiarity with procedures, failure to realize the need for hand hygiene, and the emergent aspect of the work flow. Transmission of healthcare-associated pathogens from one patient to another via the hands of HCWs requires organisms present on the patient's skin or shed onto inanimate objects to be transferred to the hands of HCWs. When hand washing is not done, the contaminated hands of the caregiver may come in direct contact with another patient or inanimate object that will, in turn, come into direct contact with another patient. The importance of hand hygiene has been known since the 1800s, when Semmelweiss proved reduction in maternal mortality by physician compliance with hand washing.

Guidelines for hand hygiene in healthcare settings have been recently published (Boyce & Pittet, 2002). Recommendations include that hands be washed with soap and water when visibly soiled, contaminated with proteinaceous material, or before eating or after using a restroom. Hand washing includes the use of either a non-antimicrobial soap and water or an antimicrobial soap and water. When hands are not visibly soiled, an alcohol-based hand rub may be used for hand hygiene in all of the following clinical situations:

- Before direct contact with patients
- Before donning sterile gloves when inserting a central intravascular catheter
- Before inserting an indwelling urinary catheter, peripheral vascular catheter, or other invasive device
- After contact with a patient's intact skin
- After contact with body fluids or excretions, mucous membranes, nonintact skin, and wound dressings
- After contact with inanimate objects in the immediate vicinity of the patient
- After removing gloves
- During patient care if moving from a contaminated body site to a clean body site

Two major foci for prevention of HAI transmission in the ICU are hand hygiene and glove/gown use. Despite evidence that transmission of microorganisms by the hands of HCWs is a major cause of HAIs, especially with resistant organisms, previous studies have found that HCWs in ICUs perform hand washing only one-third of the time (Boyce & Pittet, 2002).

Understaffing and overcrowding in the ICUs can adversely impact HAI-related outcomes. One study of patients in a surgical ICU found that primary BSIs were more likely to have received care during times when there was a lower nurse–patient ratio and a higher proportion of "floating" rather than dedicated nursing staff (Robert et al., 2000).

PATIENT OUTCOMES

Nurses can help ensure attainment of optimal patient outcomes such as those listed in **Box 6-1** through the use of evidence-based interventions.

SUMMARY

Patients are at high risk for HAI, particularly when they are in the ICU. ICU infections with resistant pathogens increase both morbidity and mortality rates. Prevention strategies focus on the use of protective measures and early identification of HAIs. To protect their patients, critical care nurses must be aware of all policies and procedures that reinforce aseptic patient care techniques. Familiarity with high-risk procedures and infection control prevention strategies will help prevent transmission of potentially deadly microorganisms in the ICU.

Box 6-1
Optimal Patient Outcomes

- White blood cell count in expected range
- Absence of signs and symptoms of infection
- Vital signs in expected range
- Increased knowledge of infection control practices
- Fever not present

Strategies to decrease the risk of catheter-related infections that are backed by the strongest evidence include training of healthcare providers who insert and maintain catheters, use of a sterile barrier during insertion, use of 2% chlorhexi-dine for skin asepsis, not routinely replacing central venous catheters, and use of antiseptic/antibiotic-impregnated short-term central venous catheters if the infection rate is high despite the former measures (O'Grady et al., 2002).

CASE STUDY

A 76-year-old man who had a radical cystectomy for bladder cancer is admitted to the ICU. He is orally intubated with an 8-mm endotracheal tube at the 22-cm mark. The ventilator settings are assist control at FIO_2 of .40, rate 12, TV 500, PEEP 5 cm. Respiratory secretions are scant and clear. The patient is alert and nods his head appropriately when asked questions. He nods yes when asked if he has pain. His abdomen is distended with no audible bowel sounds $\times$ 4 quadrants. Urinary drainage is managed by an ileoconduit. Urine is bloody and has drained 100 mL during the last hour. The patient has an IV of NS at 125 mL/hr. Antibiotics are scheduled every 12 hours to decrease bowel flora. A nasogastric tube is in place to keep the bowel decompressed postoperatively. Bilateral pneumatic compression stockings are ordered. When the patient's wife comes to visit, she questions the nurse about the patients in the rooms next to him because they are on respiratory isolation. The nurse reassures the wife that there is no cause for concern. However, the nurse knows that the two patients on respiratory isolation have pneumonia caused by resistant *Acinetobacter*.

CRITICAL THINKING QUESTIONS

1. Which disciplines should be consulted to work with this patient and the staff?

2. How will you implement your role as a facilitator of learning for the staff?

3. Describe this patient's risk factors for infection.

4. How should staff assignments be designed?

5. Identify patient outcomes specific to the patient's potential for an infection.

6. Design the assessment based on the Synergy Model and the case study by utilizing the table. Consider each patient characteristic in relation to the patient's risk for infection.

7. Write a case example from the clinical setting highlighting one patient characteristic of a patient at risk for infection. Explain how the characteristic was observed through subjective and objective data.

SYNERGY MODEL	Patient Characteristics	Data to Assess	Evidence-Based Interventions
	Resiliency		
	Vulnerability		
	Stability		
	Complexity		
	Resource availability		
	Participation in care		
	Participation in decision making		
	Predictability		

Online Resources

MRSA infections in the ICU: www.jama.ama-assn.org

Epidemiology, prevalence, and sites: www.medscape.com

Healthcare-associated MRSA (HA-MRSA): www.cdc.gov/ncidod/hip/aresist

Central line–associated bloodstream infections: www.qualitytools.ahrq.gov/qualityreport

AACN—VAP Practice Alert (2004): www.aacn.org

AACN—Preventing Catheter-Related Bloodstream Infections:
http://www.aacn.org/AACN/practiceAlert.nsf/vwdoc/PracticeAlertMain

REFERENCES

Blanc, D. S., Nahimana, I., Petignat, C., Wenger, A., Bille, J., & Francioli, P. (2004). Faucets as a reservoir of endemic *Pseudomonas aeruginosa* colonization/infections in intensive care units. *Intensive Care Medicine, 30*(10), 1964–1968.

Boyce, J. M., & Pittet, D. (2002). Guideline for hand hygiene in health-care settings. Recommendations of the Healthcare Infection Control Practices Advisory Committee and the HICPAC/SHEA/APIC/IDSA Hand Hygiene Task Force. Society for Healthcare Epidemiology of America/Association for Professionals in Infection Control/Infectious Diseases Society of America. *MMWR Recommendations and Reports, 51*(RR-16), 1–45, quiz CE41–44.

Centers for Disease Control and Prevention. (2004). National Nosocomial Infections Surveillance (NNIS) system report, data summary from January 1992 through June 2004, issued October 2004. *American Journal of Infection Control, 32*(8), 470–485.

Dulger, H., Arik, M., Sekeroglu, M. R., Tarakcioglu, M., Nolan, T., Cesur, Y., et al. (2002). Pro-inflammatory cytokines in Turkish children with protein-energy malnutrition. *Mediators of Inflammation, 11*(6), 363–365.

Graham, P. S., Quinlan, G. A., & Rank, J. A. (1997). Nosocomial legionellosis traced to a contaminated ice machine. *Infection Control and Hospital Epidemiology, 18*(9), 637–640.

Hampton, S. (2004). Clinical skills. Nursing management of urinary tract infections for catheterized patients. *British Journal of Nursing, 13*(20), 1180, 1182–1184.

Hanna, H. A., & Raad, I. (2001). Concise communication. Blood products: A significant risk factor for long-term catheter-related bloodstream infections in cancer patients. *Infection Control and Hospital Epidemiology, 22*(3), 165–166.

Hayden, M. K. (2000). Insights into the epidemiology and control of infection with vancomycin-resistant enterococci. *Clinical Infectious Disease, 31*(4), 1058–1065.

Ibrahim, E. H., Tracy, L., Hill, C., Fraser, V. J., & Kollef, M. H. (2001). The occurrence of ventilator-associated pneumonia in a community hospital: Risk factors and clinical outcomes. *Chest, 120*(2), 555–561.

Jaeger, K., Zenz, S., Juttner, B., Ruschulte, H., Kuse, E., Heine, J., et al. (2005). Reduction of catheter-related infections in neutropenic patients: A prospective controlled randomized trial using chlorhexidine and silver sulfadiazine-impregnated central venous catheters. *Annals of Hematology, 84*(4), 258–262.

Kohn, L. T., Corrigan, J. M., & Donaldson, M. S. (Eds.). (2000). *Safety activities in health care organizations* (pp. 266–271). Washington, DC: National Academy Press.

Leroy, O., & Soubrier, S. (2004). Hospital-acquired pneumonia: Risk factors, clinical features, management, and antibiotic resistance. *Current Opinion in Pulmonary Medicine, 10*(3), 171–175.

Martinez, J. A., Ruthazer, R., Hansjosten, K., Barefoot, L., & Snydman, D. R. (2004). Role of environmental contamination as a risk factor for acquisition of vancomycin-resistant enterococci in patients treated in a medical intensive care unit. *Archives of Internal Medicine, 163*(16), 1905–1912.

Mermel, L. A. (2000). Prevention of intravascular catheter-related infections. *Annals of Internal Medicine, 132*(5), 391–402.

Niël-Weise, B. S., & van der Broek, P. J. (2005). Urinary catheter policies for long-term bladder drainage. *Cochrane Database of Systematic Review,* 1, CD004201.

O'Grady, N. P., Alexander, M., Dellinger, E. P., Gerberding, J. L., Heard, S. O., Maki, D. G., et al. (2002). Guidelines for the prevention of intravascular catheter-related infections. *Infection Control and Hospital Epidemiology, 23*(12), 759–769.

Panhotra, B. R., Saxena, A. K., & Al-Mulhim, A. S. (2005). Contamination of patients' files in intensive care units: An indication of strict handwashing after entering case notes. *American Journal of Infection Control, 33*(7), 398–401.

Paphitou, N. I., Ostrosky-Zeichner, L., & Rex, J. H. (2005). Rules for identifying patients at increased risk for candidal infections in the surgical intensive care unit: Approach to developing practical criteria for systematic use in antifungal prophylaxis trials. *Medical Mycology, 43*(3), 235–243.

Penzak, S. R., Gubbins, P. O., Stratton, S. L., & Anaissie, E. J. (2000). Investigation of an outbreak of gram negative bacteremia among hematology-oncology outpatients. *Infection Control and Hospital Epidemiology, 21*(9), 597–599.

Robert, J., Fridkin, S. K., Blumberg, H. M., Anderson, B., White, N., Ray, S. M., et al. (2000). The influence of the composition of the nursing staff on primary bloodstream infection rates in a surgical intensive care unit. *Infection Control and Hospital Epidemiology, 21*(1), 12–17.

Rosenthal, V. D., Guzman, S., & Safdar, N. (2005). Reduction in nosocomial infection with improved hand hygiene in intensive care units of a tertiary care hospital in Argentina. *American Journal of Infection Control, 33*(7), 392–397.

Rubinson, L., Diette, G. B., Song, X., Brower, R. G., & Krishnan, J. A. (2004). Low caloric intake is associated with nosocomial bloodstream infections in patients in the medical intensive care unit. *Critical Care Medicine, 32*(2), 350–357.

Rupp, M. E., Fitzgerald, T., Marion, N., Helget, V., Puumala, S., Anderson, J. R., et al. (2004). Effect of silver-coated urinary catheters: Cost-effectiveness and anti-microbial resistance. *American Journal of Infection Control, 32*(8), 445–450.

Tablan, O. C., Anderson, L. J., Besser, R., Bridges, C., & Hajjeh, R. (2004). Guidelines for preventing health-care–associated pneumonia, 2003: Recommendations of CDC and the Healthcare Infection Control Practices Advisory Committee. *MMWR Recommendations and Reports, 53*(RR3), 1–36.

Wenzel, R. P., & Edmond, M. B. (2001). The impact of hospital-acquired bloodstream infections. *Emerging Infectious Diseases.* Retrieved February 10, 2006, from www.cdc.gov/ncidod/eid/vol7no2/wenzel.htm

Response to Diversity

PART III

CHAPTER 7

Gerontological Issues in Critical Care

Diane J. Mick

LEARNING OBJECTIVES

Upon completion of this chapter, the reader will be able to:

1. Explain the influence of increasing numbers of older adults on provision of intensive care services.
2. Analyze the risk of ageism related to ICU care for older adults.
3. Describe the special needs of older adults in intensive care settings.
4. Compare and contrast pathophysiological findings between older and younger critically ill patients.
5. Utilize clinical judgment in classifying nursing priorities for providing care for critically ill older patients.
6. Correlate older patients' clinical presentation with their baseline functional status to set appropriate goals for posthospital outcomes.

Health care for older adults has remained a prominent concern in nursing and medical practice during the past 20 years (Churchill, 2005; Eichler, Kong, Gerth, Mavros, & Jonsson, 2004; Rellos, Falagas, Vardakas, Sermaides, & Michalopoulos, 2006; Wood & Ely, 2003). The population is successfully aging due to improvements in health care, technology, and medications. At the same time, the need for health care increases with advancing age. Older adults account for 60% of all visits to cardiologists, 53% of visits to urologists, 48% of all patients in intensive care units (ICUs), and 63% of all patients with a diagnosis of cancer (Berman et al., 2005; O'Neill & Barry, 2003).

In 1900, only about 3 million people in the United States had lived to the age of 65. By 1990, more than 33 million people had celebrated their 65th birthdays, an increase of more than 1000%. During the 20th century, life expectancy at birth increased to 79 years for women and 74 years for men. In the final decade of the 20th century, the number of older adults in the United States increased by another 12%. Statistics now show that the oldest old—those aged 85 and older—are the most rapidly growing subgroup of the older population. Add aging baby boomers (born between 1946 and 1964) to the mix, and one in five Americans will be 65 years or older by the year 2030 (Administration on Aging, 2005; American Federation for Aging Research, 2002; U.S. Census Bureau, 2001).

Which factors have triggered the increase in the older population? And what does the potential for escalating numbers of critically ill older patients mean for ICU nurses? A major factor underlying the growth of the older population is the marked decline in mortality from stroke, myocardial infarction, and diabetes (Kane, Ouslander, & Abrass, 2003). Take a minute to think about the vast progress in health care that occurred during the 20th century. Insulin, antibiotics, renal dialysis, and cardiopulmonary bypass were developed and became available during this time period. All of these treatments and interventions have played a major role in the lengthening of life. The widespread availability of new-generation cardiac medications and diagnostic procedures also has contributed to previously undreamed-of health and longevity. There is even a website where you can calculate your own potential for living to a ripe old age, based on your present age, health history, and family history. It is located at www.agingresearch.org/calculator/.

Are we ready to step up to the challenge of the graying of the ICU unit, and to provide evidence-based nursing care for an influx of older patients? Increasing numbers of older persons are being admitted to ICUs with diagnoses ranging from exacerbations of chronic illnesses such as heart failure (HF), chronic obstructive pulmonary disease (COPD), and renal insufficiency, to new onset of catastrophic health problems and trauma due to both home-related incidents and injury-resultant accidents that occurred outside the home.

How can we best ensure that we can put into practice those essential steps that will provide optimal patient outcomes for these older individuals through an ICU hospitalization, and then help restore these elders to an acceptable level of health and function after discharge? One answer lies in our development of a fundamental understanding of the factors and influences that underlie a person's inherent ability to live safely and successfully in the community, even prior to development of illness and admission to the hospital.

PREDICTING OUTCOMES FOR ELDERS FOLLOWING CRITICAL ILLNESS

Research-based evidence plays an important role in helping to identify predictors that explain individual patient outcomes after hospitalization for a critical illness. The increasing health needs of older persons, combined with technological advances and improvements in our ability to support failing organ systems for prolonged periods, have resulted in rapid growth in ICU admission rates of persons aged 65 and older (O'Neill & Barry, 2003). Because half of all general ICU patients are aged 65 years and older (Berman et al., 2005), changes are taking place in how society thinks about aggressiveness of health care and how we define acceptable outcomes from critical illness, particularly for older persons.

Since the 1980s, bioethicists have debated the extent to which older adults as a group are suited to rationing of health care generally and of intensive care specifically (Abbo, 2005; Badger, 2005; Newacheck & Benjamin, 2004). These bioethicists have used as their rationale the need to conserve technological resources and, therefore, have developed many arguments to support excluding older patients from intensive care, essentially in an effort to save healthcare dollars. With this approach, chronological age sometimes is used to explain the presence of negative conditions and circumstances such as poor prognosis, cognitive impairment, decreased quality of life, and limited life expectancy (Melia, 2001; O'Neill & Barry, 2003; Perloff & Perloff, 2004). There is a risk that these attributed characteristics, whether real or not, might become the basis for clinical decisions to withhold ICU treatment from seriously ill older individuals. Such decisions may result in illness, unnecessary suffering, and untimely death.

More recent research into long-term functional outcomes for elders after ICU hospitalization has corroborated findings from earlier studies, which demonstrated that a patient's baseline functional status (i.e., level of independence prior to hospital admission) plays a major role in that person's recovery (Ai-Ping, Lee, & Lim, 2005; de Rooij, Abu-Hanna, Levi, & de Jonge, 2005; Rozzini et al., 2005; Williams et al., 2005), while illness severity at the time of admission to the ICU explains mortality (Chelluri et al., 2001; Williams et al.). A further examination of healthcare literature reveals other stories about outcomes for older critically ill patients, ranging from reports of a complete rebound in physical functioning at three months posthospitalization for aged cardiac surgery patients (Barnason, Zimmerman, Anderson, Mohr-Burt, & Nieveen, 2000) to accounts of no differences in functional recovery between younger and older ICU patients at six weeks posthospitalization (Welsh, Thompson, & Long-Krug, 1999). Interestingly, many older patients who survive intensive care are more satisfied with their quality of life, as compared to younger patients with similar functional status following intensive care (Hendry & McVittie, 2004; Mick & Ackerman, 2002, 2004). It is unclear whether, during the recovery process from critical illness, older persons actually do fully recover their previous functional status, or whether they recalibrate their expectations and are willing to accept a lower level of function than was present during their prehospitalization state. One interpretation of this finding is that some older persons who were very socially active prior to their illness now are happy to have survived their critical illness and may be satisfied to remain in their own homes, carrying out their usual activities, rather than being placed in an alternative type of living situation, such as an assisted living facility or a long-term care institution (Mick & Ackerman, 2004).

As a person ages, we can expect the number of chronic conditions and related disabilities suffered by that individual to increase. Many older individuals require more assistance with activities of daily living (ADL) than do younger individuals (Carson, 2003). However, even in view of the physical limitations imposed by frailty, a considerable proportion of the older population describes their lives as robust and independent (Carson; Mick & Ackerman, 2004). Consequently, it is important for ICU nurses to be aware of how pathophysiological presentations among critically ill elders differ from those observed in younger and middle-aged patients, and how slow and steady progress is key to recovery for older adults. Being able to correlate these differences in clinical presentation with expectations for outcomes following critical illness, and working with patients and families to achieve their goals related to survival and discharge, are additional important tasks for critical care nurses.

PATHOPHYSIOLOGY AND AGING

Age-related changes in physiology can be difficult to recognize because they are often related to the development of chronic conditions that occur as a part of aging. The wear-and-tear theory of aging is one popular theory of aging (Ebersole, Hess, Touhy, & Jett, 2005). In this theory, the body is regarded as an energy field or machine, with structures and functions that can become overused and eventually wear out. An individual's energy for coping and adapting to illness and disability partially determines the impact of wear and tear on the body (American Federation for Aging Research, 2002). Although the physiologic reserve of all organ systems diminishes with age, the rate of physiologic decline is not the same for all older people. Because older individuals are more different than alike, it often is difficult to identify a specific age when an irreversible downturn in health occurs. People who live to old age frequently demonstrate enhanced metabolic capacity and an ability to manage stress well, which involves both biology (body) and psychology (mind) (Kane, Ouslander, & Abrass, 2003). However, in the presence of physiological stress resulting from either traumatic injury or acute illness, older patients may be unable to activate full hemodynamic and metabolic responses because their reserve for meeting physiological demands has decreased (Chelluri, 2001; Luggen & Meiner, 2001; McKinley et al., 2000; Phelan, Cooper, & Sangkachand, 2002; Thomas, Slogoff, Smith, & Evers, 2003). In such a situation, knowledgeable ICU nurses have an opportunity to make a difference not only in older patients' hospital course, but also in their posthospitalization recovery trajectory. We know that mortality rates increase with age, but acute physiologic disturbances, such as the development of infection, systemic inflammatory response syndrome (SIRS), and sepsis, have a greater influence on death as an outcome than does age alone (Chelluri).

The following sections present information that will help you relate physiological signs and symptoms during an older patient's critical illness to how well the patient functioned physically at home prior to hospitalization. Having such information about older patients' baseline health, along with knowledge of their prehospitalization physical and mental functioning, provides us with a very valuable means for predicting both in-hospital and post-discharge requirements, such as the need for physical and occupational therapy. This information also helps us forecast how rapidly an older person will progress in regaining an acceptable level of health and functioning following hospitalization (Rice & Fineman, 2004). The following sections contain age-specific perspectives that relate to the body systems reviewed elsewhere in this textbook. *Clinical Pearls* follow each individual system category.

Oxygenation and Ventilation

Changes that have occurred in the pulmonary system as a result of aging may affect the ability of the older individual to combat critical illness. Anatomical and physical changes found on examination of older patients require different assessment strategies for managing both oxygenation and ventilation. Some of these age-related changes include a decrease in maximal inspiratory and expiratory capacity, work capacity, and chest wall compliance secondary to rib cage calcification (Chelluri, 2001; Forciea, Lavizzo-Mourey, Schwab, & Raziano, 2004; Luggen & Meiner, 2001). Lungs become stiff as a person ages, and compliance is diminished because of a decrease in elastic recoil. A decrease in alveolar surface area, with an accompanying decline in surfactant production, leads to higher residual lung volumes and causes air to become trapped in smaller airways (Epstein, Peerless, Martin, & Malangoni, 2002). Auscultation of breath sounds in an older individual reveals decreased air exchange in the lung bases due to this air trapping and reduced lung expansion (Phelan et al., 2002). Forced expiratory volume in one second, as an indication of flow, drops a minimum of 20 mL per year after 25 years of age. Closing volume decreases by 20% between 20 and 80 years of age (Forciea et al.).

Increases in alveolar-arterial oxygen difference, ventilation to perfusion mismatch (approximately 4 mL per decade), and progressive reduction in arterial oxygen tension (PaO_2) (normal PaO_2 of 70 mm Hg by 80 years of age) result in altered gas exchange (Kane et al., 2003). Because there is a decrease in arterial oxygen tension but minimal accompanying change in carbon dioxide tension, arterial blood gas values for older patients will appear "abnormal" when compared to standard values established for younger and middle-aged patients. Changes in pH typically are related to pulmonary pathology or metabolic alterations rather than to the aging process itself. Physiologic changes also result in a slower clinical response to the administration of oxygen (Reuben et al., 2005). An older individual's ability to maximize oxygen consumption in response to stress is diminished due to a decrease in muscle mass, respiratory muscle strength, and altered mechanics (Kane et al.; Reuben et al.). In fact, the only sign or symptom of pneumonia in an older individual may be an increased respiratory rate (Emory University Center for Health in Aging, 2005).

Older critically ill patients have greater than normal oxygen demands due to the enhanced energy requirements associated with the stress of acute illness, blood and fluid loss, surgery, wound healing, and hospitalization itself. Early recognition of alterations in the oxygen transport variables of delivery, consumption, and extraction ratio (the percentage of oxygen used by the tissues) can assist in the prevention and treatment of tissue hypoxia (Reuben et al., 2005). Higher than normal levels of oxygen delivery are required to meet these patients' increased oxygen demands, to prevent tissue hypoxia, and to correct tissue oxygen debt. When ICU nurses monitor the results of goal-directed therapy to confirm that these results coincide with progress in serial measurements of oxygen delivery, consumption, and oxygen extraction ratio, the survival rate of critically ill older individuals can be significantly improved (Reuben et al.).

Differentiating between age-related respiratory decline and true respiratory dysfunction presents a challenge for ICU nurses. Changes in respiratory function triggered by the aging process, together with limitations from illness severity and ICU activity restrictions, place older people at risk for complications. For all these reasons, our older patients require vigilant observation and monitoring.

Cardiovascular Function

Considerable differences in cardiovascular function become apparent during aging, but the exact modifications seen often depend on an individual's race, ethnicity, gender, and decade of life. Cardiovascular functioning is affected by development of atherosclerotic and vascular changes that occur with aging. These changes may result in stiffening of the arteries, with increases in wall tension, diastolic and systolic blood pressures, and peripheral vascular resistance (Chelluri, 2001). Stiffening of valves may impede aortic outflow, contributing to a change in systolic blood pressure (Kennedy-Malone, Fletcher, & Plank, 2004). Naturally occurring age-related fluid and electrolyte alterations may play a role in higher resting blood pressures. Sodium excretion is diminished due to a decline in the glomerular filtration rate (GFR) as a person ages, resulting in elevated intravascular volume.

Documentation of an older patient's baseline blood pressure measurement will provide essential information for inter-

---

TABLE 7-1 Respiratory Clinical Pearl

The classic triad of dyspnea, chest pain, and hemoptysis as an indicator for the presence of pulmonary embolus (PE) occurs in less than 20% of older patients. In an older patient, PE should be considered in the presence of any of these presenting symptoms, alone or in combination: chest pain, hemoptysis, hypotension, hypoxia, shortness of breath, syncope, or tachycardia (Forciea, Lavizzo-Mourey, Schwab, & Raziano, 2004).

TABLE 7-2 Metabolic Clinical Pearl

A change in the base deficit, as a marker of oxygen debt, is a known parameter of injury during treatment of shock states. It helps to discern whether resuscitation efforts are adequate. Values of −6 mmol/L to −9 mmol/L have been associated with a 25% mortality rate in older patients (MacLeod, Lynn, McKenney, Jeroukhimov, & Cohn, 2004). Serial monitoring of the base deficit, via arterial blood gas analysis, may be useful in assessing the adequacy of oxygen transport in older critically ill patients.

---

preting cardiac assessment findings. A blood pressure reading that appears to be normotensive, based on what would be expected for a middle-aged person, actually may be hypotensive for that particular older patient, due to the effect of medications or to otherwise unidentified pathology. Sudden development of relative hypotension in an older individual may herald an impending acute problem. Many older persons live comfortably with what would be considered to be an elevated blood pressure in a younger or middle-aged person. When an older person's blood pressure is either abruptly or gradually adjusted to a lower level via medications, the change in intravascular mechanisms may result in syncope, or even hypotensive manifestations of a transient ischemic attack (TIA) or a low-flow cerebrovascular accident (CVA), caused by suddenly diminished cerebral perfusion.

Cell loss in the sinoatrial (SA) and atrioventricular (AV) nodes, the bundle of His, and bundle branches begins in the second decade of life (Kane et al., 2003; Kennedy-Malone et al., 2004). The sinus rate also may decrease over time as both sympathetic and parasympathetic stimulation are slowed or blocked (Kennedy-Malone et al.). As a person ages, the heart often increases in size due to the increase in workload, with a resultant thickening of the left ventricle. Older persons increase their cardiac output by augmenting stroke volume, whereas younger individuals increase cardiac output by increasing heart rate (Chelluri, 2001). Volume depletion is poorly tolerated because the older heart is more dependent on preload for optimal cardiovascular function (Chelluri; Forciea et al., 2004). Development of fibrosis influences the mechanics of the cardiac conduction system, resulting in a blunted (less than expected) increase in heart rate associated with stress; as a consequence, the resting heart rate is lower in older individuals (Kane et al.). The response to adrenergic stimulation is diminished because the receptors are less able to accept stimulation, although their number and density do not change. In older patients, this diminished response may result in a reduced response to inotropic medications, manifested by a lesser-than-expected increase in heart rate, left ventricular ejection fraction (EF), and cardiac output (Forciea et al.; Reuben et al., 2005).

Cardiac reserve is substantially diminished by age 70 (Kane et al., 2003). The lack of reserve may not affect the daily functioning of a healthy older individual, but when the same older person experiences physiological stress, such as hypoperfusion states (dysrhythmias, hypovolemia, or sepsis), this age-related lack of cardiac reserve becomes apparent via cardiac dysfunction (Kane et al.; Reuben et al., 2005). Otherwise healthy older patients who suddenly become acutely ill are more likely to demonstrate a decreased EF that is lower than their own normal EF, accompanied by decreased stroke volume and cardiac output. These measurements will be further truncated in the presence of myocardial infarction (Forciea et al., 2004). Critically ill older individuals also are at higher risk for ventricular and atrial ectopy. Determination of systemic cardiovascular dysfunction in older individuals must be individualized and based on assessment of factors that include preexisting cardiac function and evidence of adequate end-organ perfusion, including level of consciousness, urine output, and hemodynamic stability (de Rooij et al., 2005).

Renal Function

Age-related changes in renal structure and function become apparent when a decrease in physiological renal reserve becomes evident (Forciea et al., 2004; Kennedy-Malone et al., 2004). Renal mass, blood flow, and creatinine clearance decrease with age. However, normal-appearing serum creatinine levels may be misleading cues to renal function in older persons because skeletal muscle mass decreases with aging. In contrast, creatinine clearance is decreased by 33% in individuals 75–84 years of age as compared to individuals 25–34 years of age (Chelluri, 2001). For this reason, dosages of drugs eliminated via the kidney should be adjusted in older patients based on calculated creatinine clearance rather than on serum creatinine values alone (Fordyce, 1999). The kidneys' ability to concentrate urine is decreased due to a reduction in medullary hypertonicity, whereas their diluting ability is decreased due to the reduction in renal mass (Chelluri).

The most significant structural change affecting function is the reduction of kidney size as a person ages (400 g at 40 years of age but only 250 g by 80 years of age) (Ritz, 2001). The cortex is most dramatically affected, resulting in lessening of glomerular structure and function. The GFR decreases by as much as 50% by age 60 due to reductions in the size, number,

TABLE 7-3 Cardiovascular Clinical Pearl

Both patients and healthcare providers frequently attribute symptoms of HF such as dyspnea, exercise intolerance, and dry, hacking cough to a syndrome of aging, resulting in inadequate recognition and management of a treatable condition (Heart Failure Society of America, 2002). The high prevalence of HF in older persons often is associated with age-related changes in ventricular function, particularly diastolic dysfunction. Risk factors for HF (e.g., hypertension, diabetes, and hyperlipidemia) are not always treated aggressively in older adults. Older adults commonly take over-the-counter medications for unrelated ailments (e.g., nonsteroidal anti-inflammatory preparations) that exacerbate HF due to sodium retention (American College of Cardiology/American Heart Association, 2005). Healthcare providers as well as patients will benefit from increased knowledge and recognition of the signs and symptoms of HF in older adults.

and function of nephrons as well as changes in blood flow (649 mL/min in the fourth decade of life but only 289 mL/min on average in the ninth decade) (Ritz).

The kidney's response to vasopressin does not change significantly as a person ages (Heart Failure Society of America, 2002). Acid load is not effectively excreted by the aging kidney, partially as a result of a decrease in ammonia generation aided by the liver (Kane et al., 2003). Sodium wasting is slightly increased due to a decreased response to beta-adrenergic stimulation and decreased aldosterone response. The level of atrial natriuretic peptide (ANP) in the circulation is increased, which also contributes to sodium wasting. Potassium excretion is decreased due to a diminished renin/aldosterone response. Medications such as beta blockers, angiotensin-converting enzyme (ACE) inhibitors, and potassium-sparing diuretics can contribute to hyperkalemia. Impairment of the actual sensation of thirst, sodium wasting, and inability to sufficiently excrete water load are all factors that contribute to abnormalities of sodium and water homeostasis in older persons (Chelluri, 2001; Kane et al.).

Criteria for determining renal failure in critically ill older individuals should be based on an assessment of renal reserve and the assumption that older individuals have either some degree of preexisting renal dysfunction or chronic renal insufficiency. Because renal blood flow is diminished, older individuals are more sensitive to physiologic alterations such as dehydration, hypotension, and sepsis. Because lifelong exposure to potentially nephrotoxic substances has already taken place, acute renal failure is more likely to occur in the early phase of critical illness for older patients (Chelluri, 2001; Ritz, 2001).

Contrary to known and accepted physiological findings regarding renal insufficiency or impending renal failure in a younger or middle-aged adult, some consensus has been reached that blood urea nitrogen (BUN) levels in older patients may be more useful in reflecting actual changes in renal function than serum creatinine values alone (Chelluri, 2001; Ritz, 2001). Although BUN levels must be examined in the context of hydration status, protein intake, and renal blood flow, dietary protein intake by itself is unlikely to be the chief cause for an elevated BUN in an otherwise healthy and well-hydrated older person. Therefore, an elevated BUN value in an older person may be helpful for identifying renal failure (Ritz). When it has been determined that an older critically ill individual requires dialysis for survival, the need for this intervention may be considered an early warning sign for multiple organ dysfunction syndrome (MODS) (Mick & Ackerman, 2004).

Neurological System

Although brain size decreases as a person ages, intelligence does not decline with age. However, cognitive responses to stimuli slow as a person becomes older, beginning at around age 25 years. Researchers have demonstrated that performance on timed tasks peaks in the third decade and then decreases throughout the rest of one's life (Kane et al., 2003). Likewise, hearing, vision, memory, motor efficiency, and strength diminish with advancing age. Normal cerebral perfusion decreases from 80 mL/min/100 g at age 30 years to 40 mL/ min/100 g at age 70 years (Kane et al.).

In a critically ill older individual, pathology of any organ system can precipitate neurological dysfunction. Decreased

---

TABLE 7-4 Renal Clinical Pearl

The proportion of intracellular water (ICW) in body cell mass is lower and the volume of extracellular water (ECW) is expanded in older critically ill patients, signifying that cellular dehydration is in progress, via the loss of protein and potassium (Ritz, 2001; Ritz et al., 2003). With aggressive fluid resuscitation, critically ill older patients take longer to mobilize ECW than younger patients do. This difference in response suggests that prolonged ECW expansion may contribute to poorer outcomes in older critically ill patients. Understanding the effects of aging on the renal system may help guide development of new therapies for limiting the loss of body protein during critical illness.

---

cardiac output, impaired gas exchange, and electrolyte imbalances can all cause changes in level of consciousness, sometimes resulting in confusion or coma. Lethargy and confusion are hallmarks of infection and illness among older persons. Confusion and delirium can result from problems with sensory input, a common occurrence in a brightly lit and noise-infused ICU. Because hearing and vision may already be compromised, these changes may affect the older person's ability to process and understand the physical milieu of the ICU. Delirium occurs in as many as 60% of older hospitalized patients and is a frequent hospital complication for these patients (Kennedy-Malone et al., 2004). Sleep deprivation and factors such as metabolic disorders or fluid-electrolyte imbalances may also contribute to the development of delirium during critical illness (Reuben et al., 2005). Additionally, the incidence of nonconvulsive status epilepticus has been reported to be high among older critically ill individuals, so it may be regarded as an additional marker of illness severity (Clark & Halm, 2003).

Older individuals who have a preexisting cognitive or functional impairment are more vulnerable to acute confusion. To standardize clinical assessment and to track patients' cognitive status, critical care nurses should use an instrument to assess confusional states and then plan care accordingly. The Confusion Assessment Method (CAM) is a tool for clinical evaluation that enables providers to compares scores over a period of time, to determine improvement or deterioration, and to alter the plan of care accordingly (Ely et al., 2001). The CAM diagnostic algorithm includes four facets of confusion: (1) acute onset and fluctuating course, (2) inattention, (3) disorganized thinking, and (4) altered level of consciousness (Ely et al.; Nakasato, Servat, Amador, & Teasdale, 2005). To classify a patient as confused or delirious, both the first and second facets must be demonstrated, as well as either the third or fourth facet. The CAM-ICU (Confusion Assessment Method for the Intensive Care Unit), a modified version of the CAM recommended for use by the Society of Critical Care Medicine (Ely et al.), is utilized for assessing delirium in mechanically ventilated patients and those otherwise unable to communicate. Consistent and appropriate monitoring for the development of acute confusional states ultimately will help to improve patient care and outcomes.

Gastrointestinal Tract and Nutrition

Knowledge of normal gastrointestinal (GI) function for an older adult underpins understanding of how the gut functions during critical illness. Motility, secretory function, and absorption capabilities decrease with age, but there is no significant impairment of function within the GI tract in a healthy older adult (Chelluri, 2001). Liver size also decreases with age. Under stressful conditions, the liver may not be able to increase its synthetic and metabolic functions. Lean body mass and energy expenditure—even with ongoing activity—decrease with age, primarily due to changes in body composition, including the previously mentioned decrease in ICW due to proteolysis (Ritz et al., 2003). Glucose tolerance decreases, and the incidence of diabetes increases by 0.5% to 1% in individuals 65 years of age or older (Chelluri). An increase in insulin resistance contributes to glucose intolerance, though this condition may be modifiable through diet and exercise. Malnutrition is common in older individuals due to decreased intake that may occur secondary to decreased appetite, presence of clinical depression, and (sometimes) unavailability of food (Alverdy, Laughlin, & Licheng, 2003). Critical illness increases metabolic needs, placing malnourished older patients at higher risk of complications.

The GI tract plays a critical role in the operation of the body's immune system; half of all systemic immune cells are contained within this area (Schmidt & Martindale, 2001). Gut-associated lymphoid tissue is responsible for identifying foreign antigenic material within the intestines and for mounting cell-mediated and humoral responses as needed (Schmidt & Martindale). Unfortunately, in a critically ill older individual, reduction in peristalsis, gastric acid secretion, and mucus production throughout the gut contributes to bacterial overgrowth and injury, and it may provide a portal for bacteria to enter the systemic circulation (Fink, 2003). As splanchnic blood flow to the gut decreases, an older person's GI tract becomes impaired, further limiting nutrient absorption and resulting in destruction of gastric mucosa (Cook et al., 2001; Fink). As a result of these changes in mucosal integrity, critically ill older individuals are likely to develop acute GI bleeding. Given that these patients already have a diminished physiologic reserve, GI bleeding can be a root cause of higher morbidity and mortality among critically ill elders (Hazzard, Blass, Ettinger, Halter, & Ouslander, 1999; Kane et al., 2003). During acute illness, constipation also may contribute to intolerance to tube feedings, abdominal distention, pain, bacterial colonization, and bowel obstruction (Kennedy-Malone et al., 2004).

The combined influence of the stress of critical illness and associated gut starvation may exacerbate intestinal atrophy and decreased gastric motility. Reduced transit time through the small bowel can result in malabsorption, ileus formation, and further damage to gastric mucosa (Cook et al., 2001; Fink, 2003). Hypoperfusion to the gut may, in turn, lead to early stress

TABLE 7-5 Gastrointestinal Clinical Pearl

"Failure to thrive" in older persons can be caused by malnutrition, chronic disease, thyroid disease, pernicious anemia, liver dysfunction, electrolyte imbalances, terminal disease, and extreme old age (Kennedy-Malone et al., 2004). Measurement of indicators of nutritional status, such as serum albumin and total protein, as well as simple observation of an older individual's physical appearance help to guide therapy.

ulcer formation. Accordingly, blood product transfusion may be warranted in the case of severe GI bleeding (Kane et al., 2003).

Another potential problem for critically ill elders may be the acute onset or exacerbation of diverticulitis, an inflammatory condition that involves perforation of one or more colonic diverticula, or herniations of the mucosa through the muscularis of the colon (Alverdy et al., 2003). An estimated 70% of older adults will develop diverticulosis by age 85, with the prevalence rising to 80% for adults in their nineties. Approximately 30% of elders with diverticulosis go on to develop diverticulitis, which takes the most severe course in older compromised adults. Surgical intervention (i.e., colectomy) is necessary in about 25% of patients with diverticulitis (Alverdy et al.).

Hormonal Function

Hormonal changes related to age can prove difficult to interpret. Although the adrenocorticotropic hormone (ACTH) response remains intact in older persons, the incidence of thyroid abnormalities increases with age (Chelluri, 2001). Cortisol secretion and excretion decrease with age, as do aldosterone and renin levels. Thermoregulation is impaired with advancing age (Kane et al., 2003). External factors such as overall fitness, alcohol consumption, medications, and smoking may potentially contribute to problems with thermoregulation. Due to their decreased perception of and response to cold and hot weather conditions, older individuals are at high risk for developing heat stroke, hyperthermia, and hypothermia. The febrile response to injury and infection is decreased in older persons, and mortality has been found to be higher in older patients without a febrile response (Forciea et al., 2004).

The pancreas loses secretory cells as a person ages, with a concurrent increase in fatty tissue. Although amylase and bicarbonate levels remain relatively consistent over time, lipase and trypsin levels may decline substantially over time. Bile secretion remains stable when nutritional intake is adequate, while bilirubin values increase with age (Chelluri, 2001). The significant decrease in growth hormone levels with advancing age is responsible for the loss of muscle mass and sluggish protein synthesis observed during critical illness (Forciea et al., 2004). Age-related hormonal and metabolic dysfunction may limit the capacity of an older individual to generate the physiological response necessary to combat challenges to homeostasis during critical illness.

Immunity and Infection

Immune competence declines with advancing age. Over time, changes in the immune system result from extrinsic factors such as environmental exposures, medications, comorbid conditions, and malnutrition (Hazzard et al., 1999). Intrinsic factors such as normal age-related suppression of the thymus gland's function, alterations in lymphocyte proliferation and differentiation, alterations in macrophage activity, and increased formation of auto-antibodies may also explain the decrease in immunocompetence observed in older individuals (Angus et al., 2001; Martin, Mannino, & Moss, 2006). The state of immune senescence, or slowing down, is manifested by changes in T cells and cell-mediated immunity. Recent evidence suggests a decrease in T-cell proliferation with advancing age (Chelluri, 2001). In summary, these overall changes in immune function lead to a decline in the formation of high-affinity antibodies that otherwise generate long-lasting memory immune responses after vaccinations, and the expression of delayed hypersensitivity reactions to antigens encountered earlier in life (Angus et al.; Chelluri). As a consequence, vaccinations that were given to an individual 50 or more years earlier may no longer provide protection against disease, both because the earlier chemical composition of a vaccine may have not been sufficiently potent to protect an individual until old age, and because causative agents for diseases may have mutated over time, thereby rendering earlier vaccines ineffective. An older individual who may have mounted a rapid hypersensitivity reaction to bee venom or exposure to poison ivy in the past, for example, may not exhibit symptoms of anaphylaxis until 12 to 24 hours after exposure. This delay in response may confound identification of the offending agent and lead to a delay in appropriate and aggressive treatment.

An imbalance in cytokine production is thought to be responsible for the immunologic changes observed in old age. Positive changes in the immunologic profile—for example, high T-cell proliferation after stimulation, high B-cell numbers, and a low CD8:CD4 cell ratio—are a predictor of better survival rates in very old individuals (Chelluri, 2001; Paz & Martin, 2006). By contrast, a decline in peripheral lympho-

TABLE 7-6 Immunity Clinical Pearl

The diagnosis of sepsis may be delayed in more than 20% of older patients because their clinical presentation may be subtle and atypical (Reuben et al., 2005). Signs and symptoms of systemic infection in an older person may include changes in mental or functional status, weakness, malaise, confusion, anorexia, falls, normothermia or hypothermia, failure to thrive, drowsiness, unexplained hypoglycemia or hyperglycemia, acidosis, and alterations in hemostasis (Fordyce, 1999; Reuben et al.).

cyte count has been shown to be a poor prognostic indicator in otherwise healthy older individuals (Forciea et al., 2004).

Areas of the body usually occupied by innocuous organisms may become colonized with potential pathogens during old age. Benign prostatic hyperplasia (BPH) predisposes older men to urinary infection by promoting urinary stasis (Kennedy-Malone et al., 2004). The presence of urinary catheters, as well as decreased urine acidification from declining renal function, may cause urinary tract infections in older individuals (Reuben et al., 2005). Skin and mucous membranes may become thin and more readily colonized by bacterial organisms. Oral flora may be similarly altered. Colonization of the oropharynx with gram-negative organisms such as *Klebsiella, E. coli,* and *Enterobacter* has been shown to occur in older patients (Martin et al., 2006). Patients who are bedridden and who have concomitant respiratory, cardiac, or neoplastic disease are at the greatest risk for developing oropharyngeal colonization (Forciea et al., 2004). Mucociliary transport mechanisms and cough and clearance functions are depressed in older patients; these depressed functions, combined with gram-negative oropharyngeal colonization, lead to higher rates of hospital-acquired pneumonia (Kane et al., 2003). Older age and widespread use of H_2-receptor blockers have been shown to lessen the gastric acidity that can lead to gastric bacterial overgrowth and aspiration pneumonia (Chelluri, 2001; Reuben et al.).

Pain Management for Critically Ill Elders

Pain is a common occurrence in older individuals, although pain never can be regarded as a "normal" finding (American Geriatrics Society, 2002). In the ICU, an older individual's chronic pain may underlie additional acute procedural pain. Pain is regarded as a multidimensional subjective experience with sensory, cognitive, and emotional dimensions (Horgas, 2003). Pain among older adults is a common experience made complex by the presence of different types, multiple locations, and varying causes of pain (Davis & Srivastava, 2003). A comprehensive pain history is essential, concurrent with a review of cognitive function and baseline physical function (Wells, Kaas, & Feldt, 1997).

Although invasive ICU procedures such as insertion of central venous catheters or chest tubes may produce episodic pain and discomfort for older patients, it is likely that a state of chronic pain underlies these acute pain exacerbations in elderly patients. Older adults may have pain that results not only from degenerative processes, but also from diagnostic and therapeutic procedures (Davis & Srivastava, 2003). In nursing practice, identification and treatment of pain related to musculoskeletal disorders may seem obvious; attention also needs to be paid to pain caused by neurodegenerative disorders as well as circulatory-related pain from the vascular problems often experienced by older adults. Instituting effective pain management requires a thorough assessment, appropriate intervention, and systematic reassessment (Davis & Srivastava). Healthcare providers and patients alike often have insufficient knowledge about pain management, and clinicians sometimes have the mistaken belief that pain is a normal part of aging (Panda & Desbiens, 2001).

The most fundamental categorization of pain is according to its duration (Davis & Srivastava, 2003). Acute pain results from an injury, surgery, or disease-related tissue damage (Flahaerty, 2003). Autonomic activity is associated with acute pain, with symptoms that may include tachycardia and diaphoresis. In contrast, chronic pain endures past the normal duration of healing from tissue damage, and autonomic activity is not always present. Chronic pain also may be related to musculoskeletal changes associated with aging or sequelae of a previous injury (e.g., undiagnosed vertebral fracture). When it goes unrecognized or untreated, chronic pain can lead to functional loss, reduced quality of life, and mood and behavior changes (Davis & Srivastava; Flahaerty).

Because no objective measure or biological marker of pain exists, simply worded questions and easily understandable tools are most effective for assessment of pain in older adults. In the ICU, older patients may have transitory or permanent sensory deficits and cognitive impairments that result in difficulty recalling and reporting the presence of pain (Davis & Srivastava, 2003; Herr, 2002). Nevertheless, the difficulty that some older patients have in quantifying their pain does not mean that it is not real and present. ICU nurses can contribute to pain management by exploring the use of different words that an older individual may use to describe or quantify pain, such as "discomfort" or "aching" (Davis & Srivastava). Subjective instruments such as the Visual Ana-

TABLE 7-7 Pain Management Clinical Pearl

Whenever possible, clinicians should strive to adopt a preventive approach to pain management. Around-the-clock dosing, premedication prior to a painful treatment or event as well as with turns or bathing, and administering the next dose before the previous dose wears off are essential techniques for preventing pain (Kennedy-Malone et al., 2004; Panda & Desbiens, 2001).

logue Scale (VAS) and the Faces Scale (see Chapter 4) have been found to be effective in assessing pain in older adults, although it is important to utilize visually enlarged versions of these scales to ensure that the older patient is responding appropriately when differentiating levels of pain (Stolee et al., 2005). The VAS requires the ability to discriminate subtle differences in pain intensity; it may be difficult for some older individuals to complete (Davis & Srivastava). The Faces Scale places facial expressions on a scale of 0 to 6, where 0 = smile and 6 = crying grimace. It has been found to be effective in representing pain intensity among cognitively impaired elders (Davis & Srivastava; Herr).

Other observed behaviors, including facial grimacing and physical movements, such as rubbing, bracing, and guarding, have been found to be suggestive of pain in older patients (Davis & Srivastava, 2003). In the ICU, tracking of these behaviors, in combination with surveillance of hemodynamic changes, such as increased heart and respiratory rate, and restlessness are reliable indicators of pain in a sedated or mechanically ventilated patient. A consistent approach that includes regular assessment, use of a standardized tool by all care providers when feasible, and consistent documentation of findings will allow clinicians to document pain intensity and location, to quantify change, to evaluate success of treatment, and to communicate findings to other providers (Davis & Srivastava).

Physical Restraints in the ICU

Preserving patient well-being by maintaining the integrity of technological devices in the ICU is almost exclusively the responsibility of nurses. ICU nurses are most protective of those devices for which unintentional or intentional removal is perceived as life-threatening: endotracheal tubes, arterial catheters, intra-aortic balloon pumps, dialysis catheters, and central venous catheters (Happ, 2001; Vance, 2003). Restraints in the ICU setting have long provided the illusion that precautions were being taken, and the rationale for their use has been cited as prevention of injury to patients, either self-inflicted or inadvertent. Under the guise of "treatment interference protocols," restraint use in ICUs has continued, despite Joint Commission on Accreditation of Healthcare Organizations (JCAHO) standards that seek to limit use of physical restraints (JCAHO, 2001). Decisions to restrain ICU patients are classified according to the potential outcomes of treatment or device interference: (1) life-threatening outcomes resulting from interference with endotracheal tubes or pulmonary artery catheters; (2) minor consequences causing discomfort or local tissue trauma, such as those resulting from interference with a urinary drainage system; and (3) nuisance consequences attributed to such things as interference with monitor leads and blood pressure cuffs (Happ; Vance).

The Importance of Functional Status Assessment

Frail older adults who are "living on the edge" with marginal functional capacity are at risk for falling off that edge into a cascade of illness and functional decline when admitted to the ICU (Rice & Fineman, 2004). The decrease in physiologic reserve associated with normal aging leaves older adults vulnerable to rapid decompensation when faced with catastrophic illness.

Baseline recording of older patients' activity level, mental status, and cognition *over the previous four weeks* is critical for fully understanding an individual's risk for functional decline and poor outcome. Assessment via standardized instruments of other areas such as pain, energy, sleep, presence of anxiety or depression, and emotional health can provide keys to understanding individuals' perceptions of health as well as their goals for health (Chelluri, 2001; Mick & Ackerman, 2004). Questions should be asked to gather information that provides a complete picture of the older patient's home life, related to independence or dependence in ADLs such as bathing, dressing, transferring, toileting, continence, and eating (Sato, Demura, Minami, & Kasuga, 2002), as well as information on instrumental activities of daily living (IADLs), such as balancing a checkbook, shopping for groceries, preparing meals, doing housework, and taking public transportation (Owsley, Sloane, McGwin, & Ball, 2002). Collectively, this body of information provides insight into older patients' expectations for their own recovery and return to daily life.

Changes in physical and mental functioning during hospitalization, however slight, should be examined for clinical significance. How will these changes in functioning affect an older person's recovery trajectory?

Arguments against provision of intensive care for older adults often are based on presumptions of frailty and dependence after discharge (Bo et al., 2003; Joly et al., 2003; Kapp, 2002; Reiter-Theil, 2003). However, these presumptions can be proven false by continuing research into interventions that will maximize outcomes for hospitalized older adults. Approaches to care that focus on assessment of known risk factors related to frailty and preexisting comorbidities will help clarify the appropriate use of inpatient preventive strategies. Collaboration with other healthcare disciplines, such as physical and occupational therapy, will ensure successful outcomes from ICU hospitalization as well as a return to a satisfactory level of health and physical functioning for older adults (McCloskey, 2004; Mick & Ackerman, 2002, 2004).

SUMMARY

Nurses who care for older critically ill patients must have a rehabilitative and restorative philosophy that values such basic care interventions as ensuring a safe environment and providing good nutrition, meticulous skin and oral care, and bladder retraining, as much as the implementation of more high-tech tasks, as they strive to prevent functional decline for these patients (Rice & Fineman, 2004; Teel & Leenerts, 2005). The existing cohort of elderly persons was brought up in an era when displaying emotions or asking for help was considered unacceptable (Forti, Johnson, & Graber, 2000). When ICU nurses are able to anticipate concerns of older patients and continue to seek responses from them beyond silence or acquiescence, essential insights for providing individualized care will emerge.

ICU hospitalizations for catastrophic or critical illness are not necessarily terminal events. Ongoing functional assessment will help to illuminate the impact of chronicity on an older person's capacity for self-care and may help to guide healthcare decision making regarding use of critical care resources. Accordingly, ensuring equitable access to essential intensive care services, without fears of age-based limitation of health care, will help to ensure the autonomy that is central to older adults' achievement of a fulfilling and productive old age.

CASE STUDY

S.C., an 86-year-old community-dwelling married male, is brought to the emergency department (ED) at 1700 by his daughter, an RN, on the recommendation of his family physician. S.C.'s chief complaint is an oral temperature of 39.5°C and, according to his daughter, "change in mental status." S.C. had a right-sided herniorraphy four weeks ago that was performed in the same-day surgery. S.C. is a retired Internal Revenue Service counselor and a World War II veteran. He lives in a two-story home with his spouse of 62 years. S.C. is functionally independent and has a documented desire for full resuscitation.

In the ED, S.C.'s vital signs were as follows:

- Temp 39.5°C
- HR 62
- RR 16
- BP 112/68
- O_2 sat 96% on room air
- Glasgow Coma Score 14, somnolent

S.C.'s past medical history includes recent-onset of neurogenic bladder of unknown etiology, which required that he straight-catheterize his bladder every six hours, benign prostatic hyperplasia, degenerative disc disease, osteoarthritis, and hypercholesterolemia. His past surgical history reveals only a transurethral resection of the prostate and his recent right-sided herniorraphy.

S.C. is allergic to penicillin, with a past reaction of urticaria and upper airway swelling. He has no known food, latex, or environmental allergies. His medications at home include the following drugs:

- ASA 81 mg po daily
- Oxaprozin (Daypro®) 600 mg po daily
- Doxazosin mesylate (Cardura XL®) 2 mg po daily
- Atorvastatin calcium (Lipitor®) 20 mg po daily
- Propoxyphene napsylate (Darvon®) one tablet po q 6–8 h prn
- Docusate sodium (Colace®) 100 mg po at hs

S.C.'s status on admission to the ED includes slowed mentation, increased temperature, and no other presenting symptoms. His history of present illness (HPI) reveals that he has been to a follow-up surgeon's office visit that day, and that his daughter drove him 15 miles each way. S.C. has been away from home for approximately four hours and ate lunch at a family-style restaurant. No problems were apparent during the day. Around 5 P.M., his daughter noticed that S.C. was flushed, diaphoretic, and sleepy, with slowed mentation. She measured his oral temperature and found that it was 39.5°C. When S.C.'s daughter called his family physician, the doctor recommended that she transport her father to the ED.

Results of S.C.'s physical examination by the ED nurse practitioner are as follows:

Neuro and HEENT

- Awakens to verbal stimuli
- Oriented × 3 when fully awake
- Negative Babinski
- PERRLA; naso/oropharynx clear
- Cranial nerves II–XII grossly intact

Neck and Chest

- No lymphadenopathy
- Thyroid not enlarged
- No carotid bruits
- Jugular vein nondistended
- Chest clear
- No anatomical deformity

continues

Cardiovascular and Abdomen

- $S_1 S_2$; no murmur, gallop, or rub
- Face and trunk flushed, skin warm and moist
- Abdomen soft, tenses abdomen on exam
- No pulsatile masses, no organomegaly
- Positive rebound tenderness in suprapubic area
- Healing surgical scar right inguinal area

Genitourinary

- Uncircumcised penis; no redness or drainage
- Testes descended bilaterally, firm, no tenderness on palpation, no swelling
- Anal sphincter normal tone
- Brown stool present in vault; guaiac negative

Extremities

- No gross deformities
- All peripheral pulses present and strong
- No edema
- Back: no gross deformities

Social History

- Retired from IRS, college educated, married
- One daughter, two stepchildren in Florida
- Daughter lives 260 miles away
- Daughter is healthcare provider
- Does not drink alcohol
- Quit smoking in 1953
- Walks approximately 1.5 miles daily on high school track
- Literacy tutor, reading and GED prep

Family History

- Parents emigrated from Poland in 1905
- Father died in 1959 at age 77 of prostate cancer
- Mother died in 1969 at age 81 of complications of recurrent CVAs
- Family history is positive for breast cancer, esophageal cancer, and paranoid schizophrenia (three female siblings)
- One male sibling died in World War II

Initial Serum Laboratory Findings

- WBC 13.1
- Hgb 10.4
- Hct 31
- Plt 300
- INR 1.0
- Troponin T #1 > 1.0
- Na 139
- K 4.4
- Cl 104
- CO_2 27
- BUN 22
- Creat 0.9
- Glucose 84

Urinalysis

- Dark yellow, cloudy
- Specific gravity 1.035
- Protein, glucose, ketones negative
- Hemoglobin +3
- Casts 5–10

- WBCs too numerous to count
- Bacteria 20–30
- Mucus, moderate amount

Impression
- UTI /urosepsis
- Rule out cardiac event

Orders at 1800
- To Clinical Decision Unit (CDU) for urosepsis/rule out myocardial infarction
- Acetaminophen (Tylenol®) 650 mg po now
- Blood cultures × 2
- Urine C & S
- Second troponin in 3 hours
- ECG now
- IV 0.9% NS @ 40 mL/hr
- Ciprofloxacin (Cipro®) 200 mg IV q 12 hr

These orders were initiated in the CDU, a 23-hour unit in the ED. By 2010, three hours after arriving to the ED, SC has developed severe, diffuse stabbing pain in his posterior chest, radiating to his neck and left arm. SC rates this pain as a 10/10. His heart rate has increased to 96 beats per minute, and his blood pressure is 166/88 in his left arm and 160/80 in his right arm. His respiratory rate is 22, and oxygenation saturation, measured by digital pulse oximeter, is 94% on room air.

Second Complete Physical Exam
- Glasgow Coma Score 15, awake, alert, restless, MAE
- No JVD; no carotid bruits
- Chest clear
- $S_1 S_2$, no murmur, gallop, rub
- Abdominal exam unchanged; no pulsatile masses
- Has not voided
- Rectal exam unchanged
- Electrocardiogram: ST segment elevation in leads II, III, and aVF

Differential Diagnoses
- Evolving inferior MI
- Systemic inflammatory response syndrome (SIRS)
- Urosepsis
- Dissecting abdominal aortic aneurysm

A more in-depth discussion of SIRS appears in Chapter 51. Because S.C.'s objective clinical findings include four of the criteria for SIRS (urinary tract infection, ischemic myocardium, temperature of 40°C, and leukocytes of 13,100 cells/mm³, S.C. meets the criteria not only for an initial diagnosis of SIRS, but also for a diagnosis of sepsis/urosepsis.

New Orders
- Stat chest x-ray
- O_2 @ 2L via nasal cannula
- Insert large-bore IV or CVC
- NTG SL 0.4 mg SL q 5 min × 3 until BP 140/80 or pain relieved
- Cardiac telemetry
- Noninvasive BP q 3 min
- To cardiac catheterization lab for emergent cardiac catheterization

S.C.'s Decision

At this point, S.C. declines cardiac catheterization. When presented with the alternatives of an emergent transesophageal electrocardiogram to rule out aortic dissection, and to determine ventricular wall motion and EF, S.C. also declines. He is offered the option of a CT scan to rule out a dissecting aortic or thoracic aneurysm, to be followed by an echocardiogram to examine ventricular wall motion and ejection fraction, but he declines those options as well. Even though S.C. has documented

continues

his desire for full resuscitation, he makes an independent and informed decision not to pursue any diagnostic tests because he is unwilling to undergo angioplasty or coronary revascularization, even if these measures are warranted.

After further discussion with his daughter, S.C. eventually agrees to undergo a CT scan of his chest and abdomen, as well as an echocardiogram. The CT of his chest and abdomen is negative for acute pathology, and the echocardiogram shows left ventricular hypokinesis with an estimated EF of 58% and no evidence of coronary thrombosis.

Determining the Underlying Cause for S.C.'s Infection–Sepsis–Myocardial Infarction

For the past four weeks, S.C. had been straight-catheterizing his bladder at home, following an inability to void spontaneously since his herniorraphy. The visiting nurses observed his technique and had found no problems. However, unknown to the visiting nurses, S.C. was using and reusing disposable enemas on a daily basis to move his bowels. S.C. had been lubricating the previously used enema tips in the jar of sterile lubricant that had been provided to him for use when straight-catheterizing his bladder. Ultimately, it was determined, via results from his inpatient urine culture and sensitivity, that his urine contained *Enterobacter* and *E. coli*, presumably from his own bowel, and that he had inadvertently infected himself via transmission of GI bacteria from his bowel to his own bladder.

S.C.'s Trajectory

During S.C.'s 20-hour stay on the CDU, with subsequent transfer to the ICU for two days, his diagnosis is documented as an uncomplicated inferior myocardial infarction with urinary tract infection urosepsis.

S.C.'s spouse noted that he had been experiencing "chest pressure" for several months, but he had dismissed it as a "normal part of aging" and attributed his symptoms to "wear and tear," as explained to him by his primary care provider (PCP). S.C. had not reported this symptom during any subsequent office visit, to any consultants, or to the anesthesiologist prior to his hernia surgery four weeks earlier.

Why had S.C. dismissed his cardiac symptoms? In the past, when he had discussed various musculoskeletal aches or pains with his PCP, S.C.'s physician would say, "What do you expect for an old guy?" Even as a seemingly good-natured joke, this age-related generalization caused S.C. to believe that any symptom, whether severe or minor, would not be taken seriously and that his PCP would regard it as either an unimportant or untreatable sign of old age.

Another issue of nursing concern in this case is the likelihood that information overload may have taken place during his discharge instructions after S.C.'s hernia surgery. The fact that S.C., an educated and active individual, did not realize that the jar of sterile lubricant provided for his straight-catheterizations was to be used for that purpose and none other may reflect the fact that we take for granted that patients understand and retain all critical information for their successful self-care at home when we send them on their way.

Happy Trails

At the time of his discharge to home from the ICU, S.C. is switched to oral antibiotics, and arrangements are made for follow-up care by the visiting nurse service and for in-home cardiac rehabilitation for four weeks. The Area Agency on Aging is contacted to open a case on S.C. and his spouse, to determine whether all of their day-to-day needs can be met independently or with temporary in-home assistance. At his 10-week visit to the cardiologist's office, S.C. states that he has returned to doing everything that he likes to do, including walking on the high school track and resuming literacy tutoring. This apparent return to his baseline level of function likely was prompted by factors that include his levels of physical and mental activity prior to these recent hospitalizations, his marriage of 62 years, and his desire to regain his ability to be a contributing member of society at the age of 86.

CRITICAL THINKING QUESTIONS

1. Think of some case examples from your clinical experience in which the severity of an older patient's illness was a better predictor of outcome than his or her age. Does a person's age always have a direct impact on his or her hospital course?

2. Name some measurable physiological parameters that differ between middle-aged patients and older patients. How would knowledge of these differences affect your planning for an older patient's care in the ICU?

3. Carrying out a baseline functional assessment will provide insight into how well an older person might progress during an ICU hospitalization. What are some components of a baseline functional assessment?

4. Identify physical exam findings and laboratory and diagnostic test results from S.C.'s case study that you did not expect to observe in an 86-year-old individual.

5. Which disciplines should be consulted to collaborate with this client?

6. What kinds of issues might require you to act as an advocate or moral agent for this patient?

7. How will you implement your role as a facilitator of learning for this patient?

8. Utilize the form to write up pertinent data and a plan of care for a patient with HF in the clinical setting. Rate the patient as a level 1, 3, or 5 on each characteristic. Identify the level of nurse characteristics needed in the care of this patient.

9. Take one patient outcome for an aging patient and list evidence-based interventions found in a literature review for this patient.

Synergy Model to Develop a Plan of Care

	Patient Characteristics	Subjective and Objective Data	Evidence-based Interventions	Outcomes
SYNERGY MODEL	Resiliency			
	Vulnerability			
	Stability			
	Complexity			
	Resource Availability			
	Participation in Care			
	Participation in Decision Making			
	Predictability			

Online Resources

AGS Foundation for Health and Aging:
http://www.healthinaging.org/public_education/what_is_geriatrics.php

American Geriatrics Society:
http://www.americangeriatrics.org/links/index.shtml

Hartford Institute for Geriatric Nursing:
www.hartfordign.org/

REFERENCES

Abbo, E. D. (2005). Controlling health care costs. *New England Journal of Medicine, 352*(4), 415–416.

Administration on Aging. (2005). Statistics. Retrieved September 30, 2005, from http://www.aoa.dhhs.gov/prof/Statistics/statistics.asp

Ai-Ping, C., Lee, K. H., & Lim, T. K. (2005). In-hospital and 5-year mortality of patients treated in the ICU for acute exacerbation of COPD: A retrospective study. *Chest, 128*(2), 518–524.

Alverdy, J. C., Laughlin, R. S., & Licheng, M. D. (2003). Influence of the critically ill state on host–pathogen interactions within the intestine: Gut-derived sepsis redefined. *Critical Care Medicine, 31,* 598–607.

American College of Cardiology/American Heart Association. (2005). Guideline update for the diagnosis and management of chronic heart failure in the adult. Retrieved September 30, 2005, from http://www.acc.org/clinical/guidelines/failure/hf_index.htm

American Federation for Aging Research, Theories of Aging Information Center. (2002). Retrieved September 30, 2005, from http://www.infoaging.org/b-the-4-random.html#wear

American Geriatrics Society Panel on Persistent Pain in Older Persons (AGS). (2002). Clinical practice guidelines: The management of persistent pain in older persons. *Journal of the American Geriatrics Society, 46,* 635–651.

Angus, D. C., Linde-Zwirble, W. T., Lidicker, J., Clermont, G., Carcillo, J., & Pinsky, M. R. (2001). Epidemiology of severe sepsis in the United States: Analysis of incidence, outcome, and associated costs of care. *Critical Care Medicine, 29,* 1303–1310.

Badger, J. M. (2005). Factors that enable or complicate end-of-life transitions in critical care. *American Journal of Critical Care, 14*(6), 513–521.

Barnason, S., Zimmerman, L., Anderson, A., Mohr-Burt, S., & Nieveen, J. (2000). Functional status outcomes of patients with a coronary artery bypass graft over time. *Heart & Lung, 29,* 33–46.

Berman, A., Mezey, M., Kobayashi, M., Fulmer, T., Stanley, J., & Thornlow, D. (2005). Gerontological nursing content in baccalaureate nursing programs: Comparison of findings from 1997 and 2003. *Journal of Professional Nursing, 21,* 268–275.

Bo, M., Raspo, S., Massaia, M., Cena, P., Bosco, F., Fabris, F., et al. (2003). A predictive model of in-hospital mortality in elderly patients admitted to a medical intensive care unit. *Journal of the American Geriatrics Society, 51,* 529–533.

Carson, S. S. (2003). The epidemiology of critical illness in the elderly. *Critical Care Clinics, 19*(4), 605–617.

Chelluri, L. (2001). Critical illness in the elderly: Review of pathophysiology of aging and outcome of intensive care. *Journal of Intensive Care Medicine, 16,* 114–127.

Churchill, L. R. (2005). Age-rationing in health care: Flawed policy, personal virtue. *Health Care Analysis, 13*(2), 137–146.

Clark, B., & Halm, M. A. (2003). Postprocedural acute confusion in the elderly: Assessment tools can minimize this common condition. *American Journal of Nursing, 103,* 64UU–64AA3.

Cook, D. J., Griffith, L. E., Walter, S. D., Guyatt, G. H., Meade, M. O., Heyland, D. K., et al. (2001). Canadian Critical Care Trials Group. The attributable mortality and length of intensive care unit stay of clinically important gastrointestinal bleeding in critically ill patients. *Critical Care, 56,* 368–375.

Davis, M. P., & Srivastava, M. (2003). Demographics, assessment, and management of pain in the elderly. *Drugs & Aging, 20,* 23–57.

de Rooij, S. E., Abu-Hanna, A., Levi, M., & de Jonge, E. (2005). Factors that predict outcome of intensive care treatment in very elderly patients: A review. *Critical Care, 9*(4), R307–R314.

Ebersole, P., Hess, P., Touhy, T., & Jett, K. (2005). *Gerontological nursing and healthy aging* (2nd ed.). St. Louis, MO: Elsevier Mosby.

Eichler, H. G., Kong, S. X., Gerth, W. C., Mavros, P., & Jonsson, B. (2004). Use of cost-effectiveness analysis in health-care resource allocation decision-making: How are cost-effectiveness thresholds expected to emerge? *Value Health, 7*(5), 518–528.

Ely, E. W., Margolin, R., Francis, J., May, L., Truman, B., Dittus, R., et al. (2001). Evaluation of delirium in critically ill patients: Validation of the Confusion Assessment Method for the Intensive Care Unit (CAM-ICU). *Critical Care Medicine, 29,* 1370–1379.

Emory University Center for Health in Aging. (2005). Geriatric pearls. Retrieved September 30, 2005, from http://www.cha.emory.edu/reynolds program/big/pearls

Epstein, C. D., Peerless, J., Martin, J., & Malangoni, M. (2002). Oxygen transport and organ dysfunction in the older trauma patient. *Heart & Lung, 31,* 315–326.

Fink, M. P. (2003). Intestinal epithelial hyperpermeability: Update on the pathogenesis of gut mucosal barrier dysfunction in critical illness. *Current Opinion in Critical Care, 9,* 143–151.

Flahaerty, E. (2003). Try this: Best practices in nursing for older adults from the Hartford Institute for Geriatric Nursing. Assessing pain in older adults. *MedSurg Nursing, 12,* 332–333.

Forciea, M. A., Lavizzo-Mourey, R., Schwab, E. P., & Raziano, D. B. (2004). *Geriatric secrets* (3rd ed.). St. Louis, MO: Elsevier.

Fordyce, M. (1999). *Geriatric pearls.* Philadelphia: FA Davis.

Forti, E. M., Johnson, J. A., & Graber, D. R. (2000). Aging in America: Challenges and strategies for health care delivery. *Journal of the Health and Human Services Administration, 23*(2), 203–213.

Happ, M. B. (2001). Preventing treatment interference: The nurse's role in maintaining technologic devices. *Heart & Lung, 29,* 60–69.

Hazzard, W. R., Blass, J. P., Ettinger, W. H., Halter, J. B., & Ouslander, J. G. (1999). *Principles of geriatric medicine and gerontology* (4th ed.). New York: McGraw-Hill.

Heart Failure Society of America. (2002). Retrieved September 30, 2005, from http://www.abouthf.org/questions_symptoms.htm

Hendry, F., & McVittie, C. (2004). Is quality of life a healthy concept? Measuring and understanding life experiences of older people. *Qualitative Health Research, 14*(7), 961–975.

Herr, K. (2002). Chronic pain in the older patient: Management strategies. *Journal of Gerontological Nursing, 28,* 28–34.

Horgas, A. L. (2003). Pain management in elderly adults. *Journal of Infusion Nursing, 26,* 161–165.

Joint Commission on Accreditation of Healthcare Organizations (JCAHO). (2001). *Comprehensive accreditation manual for hospitals: The official handbook.* Oakbrook Terrace, IL: Joint Commission Resources.

Joly, D., Anglicheau, D., Alberti, C., Nguyen, A. T., Touam, M., Grunfeld, J. P., et al. (2003). Octogenarians reaching end-stage renal disease: Cohort study of decision-making and clinical outcomes. *Journal of the American Society of Nephrology, 14,* 1012–1021.

Kane, R. L., Ouslander, J. G., & Abrass, I. B. (2003). *Essentials of clinical geriatrics* (5th ed.). New York: McGraw Hill.

Kapp, M. B. (2002). Health care rationing affecting older persons: Rejected in principle but implemented in fact. *Journal of Aging, Society, & Policy, 14,* 27–42.

Kennedy-Malone, L., Fletcher, K. R., & Plank, L. M. (2004). *Management guidelines for nurse practitioners: Working with older adults.* Philadelphia: FA Davis.

Luggen, A. S., & Meiner, S. E. (2001). *NGNA core curriculum for gerontological nursing* (2nd ed.). St. Louis, MO: Mosby.

MacLeod, J., Lynn, M., McKenney, M. G., Jeroukhimov, I., & Cohn, S. M. (2004). Predictors of mortality in trauma patients. *American Surgeon, 70*(9), 805–810.

Martin, G. S., Mannino, D. M., & Moss, M. (2006). The effect of age on the development and outcome of adult sepsis. *Critical Care Medicine, 34*(1), 15–21.

McCloskey, R. (2004). Functional and self-efficacy changes of patients admitted to a geriatric rehabilitation unit. *Journal of Advanced Nursing, 46*(2), 186–193.

McKinley, B. A., Marvin, R. G., Cocanour, C. S., Marquez, A., Ware, D. N., & Moore, F. A. (2000). Blunt trauma resuscitation: The old can respond. *Archives of Surgery, 135,* 688–695.

Melia, K. M. (2001). Ethical issues and the importance of consensus for the intensive care team. *Social Science Medicine, 53*(6), 707–719.

Mick, D. J., & Ackerman, M. H. (2002). New perspectives on advanced practice nursing case management for aging patients. *Critical Care Nursing Clinics of North America, 14,* 281–291.

Mick, D. J., & Ackerman, M. H. (2004). Critical care nursing for older adults: Pathophysiological and functional considerations. *Nursing Clinics of North America, 3,* 473–493.

Nakasato, Y., Servat, J., Amador, F., & Teasdale, T. A. (2005). Delirium in the older hospitalized patient. *Journal of the Oklahoma State Medical Association, 98*(3), 113–116.

Newacheck, P. W., & Benjamin, A. E. (2004). Intergenerational equity and public spending. *Health Affairs (Millwood), 23*(5), 142–146.

O'Neill, G., & Barry, P. (2003). Training physicians in geriatric care: Responding to critical need. *Public Policy and Aging Report, 13,* 17–21.

Owsley, C., Sloane, M., McGwin, G., & Ball, K. (2002). Timed instrumental activities of daily living tasks: Relationship to cognitive function and everyday performance assessments in older adults. *Gerontology, 48*(4), 254–265.

Panda, M., & Desbiens, N. A. (2001). Pain in elderly patients: How to achieve control. *Consultant, 41,* 1597–1604.

Paz, H. L., & Martin, A. A. (2006). Sepsis in an aging population. *Critical Care Medicine, 34*(1), 234–235.

Perloff, J. K., & Perloff, M. (2004). Coronary artery bypass: A user's manual. *American Journal of Cardiology, 94*(2), 172–177.

Phelan, B. A., Cooper, D. A., & Sangkachand, P. (2002). Prolonged mechanical ventilation and tracheostomy in the elderly. *AACN Clinical Issues, 13,* 84–93.

Reiter-Theil, S. (2003). The ethics of end-of-life decisions in the elderly: Deliberations from the ECOPE study. *Clinical Anaesthesiology, 17,* 273–287.

Rellos, K., Falagas, M. E., Vardakas, K. Z., Sermaides, G., & Michalopoulos, A. (2006). Outcome of critically ill oldest-old patients (aged 90 and older) admitted to the intensive care unit. *Journal of American Geriatrics Society, 54*(1), 110–114.

Reuben, D. B., Heer, K. A., Pacala, J. T., Pollock, B. G., Potter, J. F., & Semla, T. P. (2005). *Geriatrics at your fingertips* (7th ed.). New York: American Geriatrics Society.

Rice, D. P., & Fineman, N. (2004). Economic implications of increased longevity in the United States. *Annual Review of Public Health, 25,* 457–473.

Ritz, P., and Investigators of the Source Study and of the Human Nutrition Research Centre–Auvergne. (2001). Chronic cellular dehydration in the aged patient. *Journal of Gerontology Series A—Biological Science and Medical Science, 56*(6), M349–M352.

Ritz, P., Salle, A., Simard, G., Dumas, J. F., Foussard, F., & Malthiery, Y. (2003). Effects of changes in water compartments on physiology and metabolism. *European Journal of Clinical Nutrition, 57* (Suppl. 2), S2–S5.

Rozzini, R., Sabatini, T., Cassinadri, A., Boffelli, S., Ferri, M., Barbisoni, P., et al. (2005). Relationship between functional loss before hospital admission and mortality in elderly persons with medical illness. *Journal of Gerontology Series A—Biological Science and Medical Science, 60*(9), 1180–1183.

Sato, S., Demura, S., Minami, M., & Kasuga, K. (2002). Longitudinal assessment of ADL ability of partially dependent elderly people: Examining the utility of the index and characteristics of longitudinal change in ADL ability. *Journal of Physiology, Anthropology, and Applied Human Science, 21*(4), 179–187.

Schmidt, H., & Martindale, R. (2001). The gastrointestinal tract in critical illness. *Current Opinion in Clinical Nutrition and Metabolic Care, 4,* 547–551.

Stolee, P., Hillier, L. M., Esbaugh, J., Bol, N., McKellar, L., & Gauthier, N. (2005). Instruments for the assessment of pain in older persons with cognitive impairment. *Journal of the American Geriatrics Society, 53*(2), 319–326.

Teel, C. S., & Leenerts, M. H. (2005). Developing and testing a self-care intervention for older adults in caregiving roles. *Nursing Research, 54*(3), 193–201.

Thomas, R. P., Slogoff, M., Smith, F. W., & Evers, B. M. (2003). Effect of aging on the adaptive and proliferative capacity of the small bowel. *Journal of Gastrointestinal Surgery, 7,* 88–95.

U.S. Census Bureau. (2001). Sixty-five plus in the United States, 1999. Retrieved September 30, 2005, from http://www.census.gov/prod/1/pop/p23-190/p23-190.html

Vance, D. L. (2003). Effect of a treatment interference protocol on clinical decision-making for restraint use in the intensive care unit: A pilot study. *AACN Clinical Issues, 14,* 82–91.

Wells, N., Kaas, M., & Feldt, K. (1997). Managing pain in the institutionalized elderly: The nursing role. In D. I. Mostofsky & J. Lomranz (Eds.), *Handbook of pain and aging* (pp. 129–151). New York: Plenum Press.

Welsh, C. H., Thompson, K., & Long-Krug, S. (1999). Evaluation of patient-perceived health status using the Medical Outcomes Survey Short-Form 36 in an intensive care unit population. *Critical Care Medicine, 27,* 1466–1471.

Williams, T. A., Dobb, G. J., Finn, J. C., & Webb, S. A. (2005). Long-term survival from intensive care: A review. *Intensive Care Medicine, 31*(10), 1306–1315.

Wood, K. A., & Ely, E. W. (2003). What does it mean to be critically ill and elderly? *Current Opinion in Critical Care, 9,* 316–320.

CHAPTER 8

Cultural Issues in Critical Illness

Renee Twibell   Debra Siela   Terri Townsend

LEARNING OBJECTIVES

Upon completion of this chapter, the reader will be able to:

1. Relate the key terminology to culturally diverse critically ill patients.

2. Explain the importance of nurses' cultural self-assessment.

3. Outline a cultural assessment plan for critically ill patients.

4. Describe strategies for communicating effectively across cultures.

5. Discuss concepts for safe medication administration in transcultural care.

6. Design care that integrates cultural differences in space, time orientation, social organization, environmental control, and biological variations.

7. Identify principles for utilizing the Synergy Model for culturally competent care during critical illness.

Suppose for a moment that you are a nurse of Asian-Pacific origin who works in an intensive care unit (ICU) on the West Coast of the United States. Your patient today is an alert, middle-aged female in respiratory failure. She is visiting your city from rural Tennessee.

In the patient's room, you find eight family members sitting on the floor. Soft prayer and singing grow gradually louder, as monitor alarms sound and the patient becomes restless. The family interrupts a scheduled bedside bronchoscopy, requesting that no procedures be conducted until the pastor arrives. The patient nods vigorously in agreement. Your frustration peaks when you find the family offering sips of herbal tea to the patient, who is intubated and restricted from taking anything by mouth (NPO). Because you are a polite, nondirect person by nature, you simply ask the family to wait a little longer to offer fluids. Escaping from the room, you sigh, doubting that you are the best nurse for this assignment. How can you plan effective care when the patient and family are so unlike you?

Nurses strive to provide high-quality care to every patient, regardless of his or her cultural background. However, with increasing frequency, nurses are caring for patients from cultural backgrounds that are markedly different from their own. Clinical agencies now require nurses to be competent in transcultural care. The Joint Commission on Accreditation of Healthcare Organizations (2005), the American Nurses Association (2005), *Healthy People 2010* (2005), and Office of Minority Health (2005) set U.S. expectations and recommendations for cultural and linguistic competence. Cultural and linguistic competence implies that healthcare providers and organizations can understand and respond effectively to the cultural and linguistic needs brought by patients to the healthcare setting (Office of Minority Health). For example, culturally diverse patients may need interpreter staff, translated written materials, clinical and support staff who know how to ask about and negotiate cultural issues, appropriate food choices, and other measures. Addressing cultural diversity has the potential to improve patient outcomes as well as the efficiency and cost-effectiveness of healthcare delivery (Office of Minority Health).

The increasing demand for culturally competent care is fueled by shifts in demographics worldwide. A recent census (U.S. Census, 2002) confirmed that minority groups are growing rapidly and account for the following percentages of the U.S. population:

- Hispanics/Latinos: 12.5%
- African Americans/Blacks: 12.3%
- Asian/Pacific Islanders: 3.6%
- American Indians/Eskimo Natives: 1%

Minority groups are predicted to account for more than 40% of the U.S. population by 2050. In contrast, members of minorities currently account for less than 12% of all U.S. nurses. Both now and in the future, nurses must be competent to care for patients from cultures that differ from their own (**Figure 8-1**).

A nurse's failure to address cultural preferences can result in poor outcomes for patients and healthcare systems alike. Wasted resources, legal risk, and human suffering increase when cultural aspects of care are mismanaged (Purnell & Paulanka, 2003). For example, when nurses do not recognize symptoms of culturally bound, genetic disorders, illness may be prolonged and intensified. To develop competence in transcultural nursing, nurses should take the following steps:

- Pursue an understanding of cultural concepts and terms
- Develop an effective approach to cultural assessment
- Plan, implement, and evaluate culturally competent care for critically ill patients

CULTURAL CONCEPTS

All people have one or more cultures. A culture is a dynamic composite of customs, beliefs, social norms, values, and physical traits that are characteristic of a racial, religious, or social group

FIGURE 8-1 Nurses Care for Patients from Varying Cultural Backgrounds

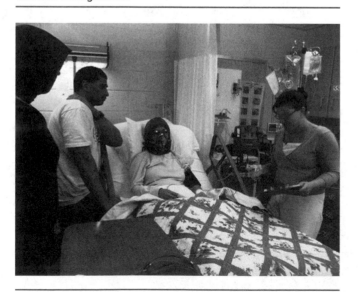

(Merriam-Webster, 2005). Culture is learned and passed on to future generations. When members of ethnic groups and cultures relocate geographically, they may adopt the ways of their new environment yet also maintain some native cultural practices.

As nurses assess their own ethnocentric beliefs and stereotypes, they begin to grasp the effects of culture on human lives. When nurses develop cultural awareness, they can assess and appreciate patients' cultural backgrounds. Eventually, nurses learn to meet patient needs in a culturally competent manner. Through cultural brokerage, nurses provide effective transcultural nursing care and contribute to optimal patient outcomes (see **Table 8-1**).

The term *culture* typically implies that people share a geographic origin or genetic traits. However, other types of cultures exist, such as cultures of hearing-impaired persons, obese

TABLE 8-1 Key Cultural Terms

Cultural awareness: the process through which nurses learn to recognize and respect the cultural beliefs and values of others, while acknowledging their own personal biases and values.

Cultural brokerage: the deliberate use of culturally competent strategies to bridge or mediate between the patient's culture and the healthcare system (Dochterman & Bulechek, 2004).

Cultural competence: the ability of healthcare providers to meet the cultural needs of patients.

Cultural values: Aspects of a particular culture that are accepted as important, such as health.

Culture: a pattern of behaviors and beliefs that develop over time and are shared by all members of a particular group.

Ethnic/ethnicity: membership in a group that shares a social and cultural heritage. Members of ethnic groups may have similar languages, histories, customs, religions, and a sense of identity.

Ethnocentricism: the belief or perception that one's own cultural beliefs are best and others' customs are inferior or wrong.

Race: groups of people who share a common ancestry and physical characteristics such as skin color, blood group, bone structure, and other biological variations.

Stereotype: the perception or assumption that all members of a cultural group are alike and share the same beliefs and values, without determining whether an individual fits the assumption.

Subcultures: groups within a culture that do not share all the aspects of that culture. Examples of subcultures include Japanese, Korean, and Vietnamese members of the Asian culture.

Transcultural nursing: a specialty of nursing focused on the delivery of culturally competent care, incorporating the patient's culture into the plan of care to achieve the best outcomes.

persons, lesbians, professional athletes, and critical care nurses. Patients may belong to more than one culture. While this chapter focuses on critically ill patients with distinct ethnic cultures, the principles described here can be utilized by nurses caring for patients from all types of cultures.

CULTURAL ASSESSMENT

Nurses' Self-Assessment

The first step toward cultural competence is for nurses to examine their own cultural backgrounds and biases. As nurses reflect on their personal life patterns, they may begin to realize that other cultures have equally acceptable worldviews and ways of being. A variety of cultural assessment tools can be used for both self-reflection and patient assessment (Dennis & Small, 2003; Giger & Davidhizar, 2004; Purnell & Paulanka, 2003; Spector, 2004).

Cultural Assessment of Patients

When conducting cultural assessments, it is important for nurses to show genuine interest in patients, to see "their world—not mine," and to be open to learning (Ryan, Twibell, Brigham, & Bennett, 2001). The Giger and Davidhizar Transcultural Assessment Model (see **Figure 8-2**) has guided nurses in a variety of settings (psychiatry, surgery, obstetrics, and ambulatory care) and countries (France and Canada) (Giger & Davidhizar, 2004). The questionnaire may take 45 minutes to complete with a stable patient. During critical illness, patients may require multiple time-sensitive interventions, leaving little time for thorough cultural assessments. Nurses need a guide for the quick assessment of key cultural factors. The Critical Care Version of the Transcultural Assessment Model can be completed in a staggered time frame, depending on the patient's stability. The questions are arranged to provide essential cultural information quickly (see **Table 8-2**).

CULTURAL FACTORS IN PLANNING CARE

The Synergy Model in Transcultural Care

Patient satisfaction is highest when nurses and patients have the same cultural background (Laveist & Nuru-Jeter, 2002).

However, cultural concordance is rarely possible due to the small number of minority nurses in the United States. When the nurse's and patient's cultures differ, the following factors should be considered:

- How fluent is the nurse in speaking and understanding the patient's language?
- What resources are available for communication support?
- How much does the nurse know about the patient's culture?
- Are value conflicts apparent between the patient and the nurse?
- How compatible are the patient's and nurse's cultures of origin?
- Are same-gender nurse–patient assignments culturally preferred?
- To what extent does the nurse possess a capacity for flexibility and creativity?

It is equally important for the nurse caring for patients from different cultures to recognize that not all people who come from the same country or who practice the same religion will be the same in terms of their belief systems and practices. It is essential to ask individual patients about their care preferences.

FIGURE 8-2 The six cultural dimensions of the Giger and Davidhizar Transcultural Assessment Model include communication, space, social organization, time, environmental control, and biological variations

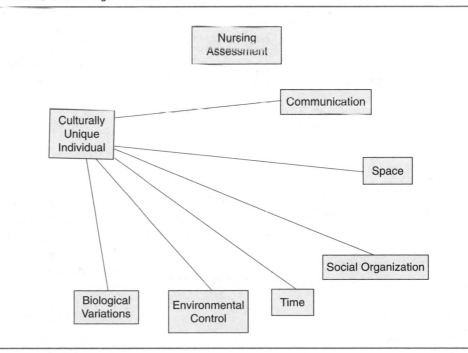

Source: Reprinted from *Transcultural nursing: Assessment and intervention* by J. Giger and R. Davidhizar, 2004, p. 7, with permission from Elsevier.

TABLE 8-2 Transcultural Assessment Model: Critical Care Version

* Complete within first hour of admission
** Complete within first day after admission
*** Complete when patient is stable

1. What is your race/cultural group?**
   - Place of birth***
   - Time in this country (if born elsewhere)***
2. Communication
   - Response to touch (receptive, startles)?*
   - Primary language spoken?*
   - Secondary language spoken?*
   - Usual voice quality (loud, soft)?***
     - Usual pronunciation (clear, slurred, dialect)?***
   - Use of nonverbal communication (gestures, body movement, expressions)?***
   - How do you discuss something important with your family?***
3. Social organization
   - Would you like for me to contact a chaplain or spiritual resource person?*
   - What is the patient's normal state of health (good, fair, poor)?*
   - How often do you have visitors in your home?***
   - What is the family's typical behavior when a family member is ill?***
   - Do you believe in a Supreme Being?***
   - How do you worship?***
4. Environmental control
   - What do you typically do, if anything, to assist in your healing process?**
   - Do you believe in bad luck or fate as a cause of illness?***
   - How do you use folk medicine, cultural practices, or home remedies?***
   - Do you feel that you have treatment choices?***
5. Space
   - Preferred personal distance in conversation*
6. Time
   - How many hours of sleep do you usually get per night?***
   - Does the patient grasp the importance of taking medications/treatments on time?***
7. Biological variations
   - What diseases or illnesses are common in your family?**
   - Do you have a genetic susceptibility to disease?***
   - What are your food preferences/dietary practices?***
   - What are your coping mechanisms when ill?***

Source: Adapted from Giger, J., & Davidhizar, R. (2004). *Transcultural nursing: Assessment and intervention.* St. Louis, MO: Mosby, pp. 10–12.

Communication

Effective communication among nurses, patients, and families is vital, especially during critical illness. Language barriers pose a major obstacle to culturally competent care (**Figure 8-3**).

FIGURE 8-3 Language Barriers Can Be a Major Obstacle in Culturally Competent Care

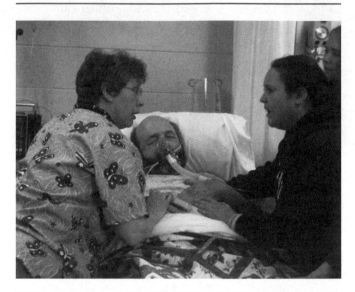

Currently, more than 300 languages are spoken in the United States, and more than 44 million adults do not speak English as a primary language (U.S. Census, 2002). When a patient speaks a few key English words, the nurse may assume erroneously that the patient fully understands what is being said. The nurse must also recall that, even within groups that speak the same language, meanings and pronunciations may vary. For example, patterns of speech differ markedly between persons from the southern and northeastern United States. Similarly, there are up to 111 languages and 8 distinct dialects spoken in the Philippines (Pacquiao, 2005). A patient born on one island may not understand a Filipino nurse from another island.

Use of Interpreters

Nurses can utilize interpreters to enhance the exchange of information and reduce patients' feelings of anxiety. Hospital employees and students from universities may be more effective interpreters than patients' family members. Family members may be reluctant to communicate some vital information to patients. For example, Mexican families do not discuss the genito-urinary tract or sexual issues across genders or age groups (Chang & Harden, 2002). Japanese and Arab Muslim families may not inform patients about their prognosis.

Nonverbal Communication

Voice intonation, gestures, eye contact, and use of touch vary among cultural groups. Because Asians and American Indians tend to speak in a soft voice, the nurse may be viewed as rude or boisterous if the volume is loud (Giger & Davidhizar, 2004). Gesturing with a wave may mean "goodbye" or "come here." In white cultures, the average length of eye contact is 3 to 10 seconds (Giger & Davidhizar); longer eye contact tends to produce anxiety. Likewise, members of some cultures (e.g., Asians and Native Americans) redirect their eyes down when thinking or paying attention and believe that long eye contact is a sign of rudeness. Appalachians avoid eye contact, because it is felt to indicate hostility. Muslim women may avoid eye contact as a sign of modesty (Luckmann, 2000). For Native Americans, even minimal eye contact is disrespectful (Galanti, 2004). Southern Europeans and Hispanics find frequent touching to be reassuring and comforting. Conversely, Northern Europeans and Asians prefer little or no touching (Giger & Davidhizar). A restless patient who seems to be resisting treatments may actually be trying to withdraw from unwanted touching.

Education

Education is most effective when it is clearly conveyed in a caring manner. In addition, patients are most likely to adhere to plans of care when those plans include cultural practices, such as home remedies, food preferences, and spiritual beliefs (Stewart, Meredith, Brown, & Galajda, 2000). The nurse should determine culturally appropriate methods of communication and preferred learning styles. For example, a Hmong patient who is starting hemodialysis may disregard written dietary instructions but follow verbal instructions.

Space

Cultural preferences for space surrounding a person's body vary across three zones:

- Intimate zone, 0–18 inches, for comfortable communication and protective messages
- Personal zone, 18–36 inches, used by friends and in some counseling interactions
- Social or public zone, 3–6 feet, used in impersonal business

White patients of European descent prefer the largest amount of personal space and may become uncomfortable if a nurse talks to them within the intimate zone. Native Americans, Appalachians, Japanese, and Mexicans prefer space between the personal zone and the social zone for most interactions. In contrast, Hispanics and Arabics prefer the least amount of personal space. A Brazilian patient who is isolated for infection control may lack the accustomed interpersonal stimulation. In such a case, the nurse should plan to enter the room and touch the patient frequently (Giger & Davidhizar, 2004).

Environmental Control

Environmental control refers to a person's ability to control nature and influence the environment, including his or her own health. Many white cultures believe that individuals influence health by preventive behaviors, such as diet and exercise. Some Hispanics, Appalachians, and Puerto Ricans, who believe that health is externally controlled, are less likely to take preventive actions and therefore may be more critically ill by the time they seek health care (Giger & Davidhizar, 2004).

Cultural Health Practices

When a patient enters the healthcare system with a critical illness, nurses should assess what traditional, cultural remedies have been tried and support them, if possible. Cultural health practices are classified into four categories: (1) practices that are beneficial, such as the Hispanic tradition of balancing "hot" and "cold" diseases, foods, and medications; (2) neutral practices that do not affect health, such as pregnant women avoiding scissors that might be associated with deformities in the unborn child; (3) uncertain practices that have ambiguous or unknown effects on health—for example, the swaddling of infants; and (4) dysfunctional health practices that are harmful and that the nurse should target for change, such as the ingestion of clay, cornstarch, and other non-edible substances (Galanti, 2004; Giger & Davidhizar, 2004).

Folk Medicine

Folk medicine may be motivated by traditional or religious beliefs. The Asian practices of coin rubbing and cupping are directed toward drawing an illness out of the body. When the skin is rubbed vigorously with a coin or suctioned into a warm cup, discolorations appear, suggesting that the illness has been brought to the surface. If a nurse is unaware of such rituals, delays in diagnosis can result. For example, an unconscious Korean man was brought to an acute care unit. No interpreter was available to aid in communication with his family. The clinical staff assumed that the red welts on his chest were related to his unconscious state, when they were actually due to cupping. The patient died before he could be accurately diagnosed as having a head injury (Galanti, 2004).

Some cultures rely on folk healers, shamans, or priests to treat illnesses. The nurse can show respect for the patient's cultural beliefs by arranging for a visit from a traditional healer.

Treatment of fevers varies among cultures. Whites believe that the body must be cooled to reduce a fever. Other cultures, such as Japanese, African Americans, and Hispanics, prefer to "sweat out" the fever by using extra blankets and drinking hot liquids.

Patients may wear a rosary, cord, special jewelry, and garments that have a spiritual significance. Medicine pouches worn around the neck may contain herbs or amulets that protect the wearer from evil spirits. Mormons wear undergarments that signify God's protection. Cambodians protect their children from death by placing cords around the wrist (Galanti, 2004). The nurse should remove these items only when no alternative exists and then keep the items near the bedside.

Time Orientation

Cultures may be past, present, or future oriented (Giger & Davidhizar, 2004). A culturally competent nurse will assess time orientation, communicate clearly about time-sensitive matters, and wisely shape the expectations of patients and families (see **Table 8-3**).

Social Organization

Family

The family is the most important social group in many cultures. Research indicates that nurses rank family issues as a primary concern in acute care settings (**Figure 8-4**). Nurses specifically report feeling anxious when large numbers of family members visit (Coffman, 2004). Asians, African Americans, and Hispanics particularly value family presence during critical illness (Urden, Stacy, & Lough, 2002). Gypsy, Asian, and Middle Eastern families believe they bring healing by their presence. Traditionally, Chinese men view it as a duty to provide care for family members during their hospitalization.

FIGURE 8-4 Nurses Report Increased Anxiety When Multiple Family Members Visit Critically Ill Patients of Varying Cultural Backgrounds

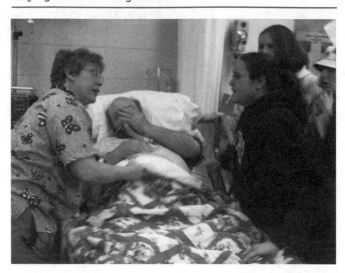

Nurses can include family members in selected aspects of care, even during critical illness. For example, family members can feed stable patients and provide massages. The nurse must carefully instruct families about what they can do safely. When families choose to give care, patients are expected to graciously accept it. Unfortunately, American nurses who do not understand an Asian patient's desire to be passive in the sick role may become frustrated when trying to teach self-

TABLE 8-3 Cultural Differences in Time Orientation

Orientation	Culture	Intervention Example
Past	Native American	A nurse integrates tribal traditions and ancestral rituals when caring for an intubated Navajo patient who needs early mobilization.
Present	Mexican, Chinese, African American, low socio-economic groups	When an Appalachian patient resists repositioning to prevent pressure ulcers, the nurse collaborates with the "granny woman" to engage the patient in a turning schedule.
		A Puerto Rican patient is scheduled for a cardiac catheterization at 8:00 A.M. The nurse instructs him to arrive at the hospital "as soon as daylight begins, before you do any work."
Future	White	A nurse reframes the expectations of a white attorney who becomes flushed and hypertensive when his discharge is delayed.

care. In such cases, education should be directed to family members.

Decision Making in Critical Illness

The nurse must determine how patients and families make decisions. Whites, and more recently African Americans, value patient participation; alternatively, the patient may choose a decision maker. Some Hispanic, Asian, and Arabic families do not tell patients about their illnesses or involve patients in decision making. In Middle Eastern, Italian, and Hispanic cultures, the father or oldest brother may publicly make decisions, but he may be greatly influenced by older females in the family (**Figure 8-5**).

Biological Variations

Disease Risk

Incidence of disease varies among ethnic groups. For example, some ethnic groups have a higher genetic risk for coronary artery disease (CAD) than others. Black and Hispanic women are at greater risk for CAD than are white women. A large percentage of Native Americans, both men and women, have at least one CAD risk factor (American Heart Association, 2004). Native Americans also have 7 to 15 times the rate of tuberculosis compared to whites. Influenza is more common in Native Americans and African Americans than in whites (Ignatavicious & Workman, 2006). The incidence of diabetes mellitus is 1.5 to 2 times greater for African Americans, Native Americans, and Mexicans than for whites.

African Americans have a higher incidence of cancer and a higher death rate from cancer than do whites. Since 1960, cancer incidence has increased 27% for African Americans but only 12 percent for whites. Lung cancer, which ranks first in frequency for African Americans and whites, is the fourth most frequent cancer seen in Asians and Hispanics (American Cancer Society, 2005).

Drug Therapy

Effects of drugs vary among ethnic groups due to differences in drug metabolism. For example, compared to whites, Chinese are twice as sensitive to the effects of the beta blocker propranolol (Inderal®) on blood pressure and heart rate. African Americans may require higher doses of angiotensin converting enzyme (ACE) inhibitors to treat hypertension compared to whites. African Americans achieve better blood pressure control when a diuretic is added to a first-line ACE inhibitor, angiotensin receptor blockers, or beta blocker. ACE inhibitors for heart failure may not be as effective in African Americans as they are in whites. Nurses must anticipate differing effects from antihypertensive drug classes across cultural groups.

Similarly, nurses must be aware that, compared to whites, all ethnic groups are more sensitive to the effects of central nervous system (CNS) drugs and require lower doses. Asians metabolize CNS drugs more slowly than do other groups and therefore require lower doses of antidepressants. African Americans achieve higher blood levels of antidepressants more quickly and experience more side effects than do whites. Asians have a lower dose/optimal response threshold for haloperidol (Haldol®) than do whites, while Chinese in particular require lower doses of haloperidol (Burroughs, Maxey, Crawley, & Levy, 2002).

Codeine is often prescribed to treat pain. Ten percent of a dose of codeine is metabolized to morphine, prompting analgesia. Five to ten percent of whites and 1% of Asians lack the enzyme that converts codeine to morphine, making codeine a poor choice for some patients. If patients are not achieving pain control from codeine, the nurse should consider other analgesics (Burroughs et al., 2002).

Ten percent of African Americans and many Near Eastern and Mediterranean males have a glucose-6-phosphate dehydrogenase enzyme (G6PD) deficiency. This genetic variation increases the risk for hemolysis if the patient receives aspirin, sulfanilamide, or primaquine.

FIGURE 8-5 Male Family Members Make Healthcare Decisions in Some Cultures

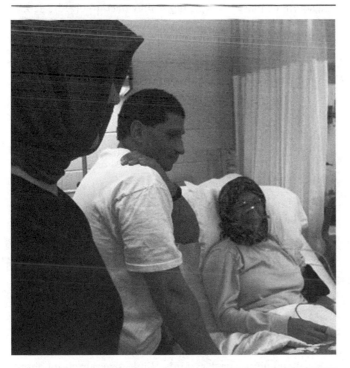

Discomfort

The expression of symptoms, such as dyspnea, nausea, fatigue, and pain, are rooted in cultural norms. Some cultures will mask symptoms, whereas others will visibly demonstrate discomfort. Asians may reject pain medication all together. Nurses must anticipate their patients' comfort needs and determine each patient's desired approach to manage discomforting symptoms.

End-of-Life Issues

Organ Donation

Critical care nurses must communicate carefully about organ donation. Gypsy cultures believe that the soul remains active in a physical shape for one year after death, so the body must remain intact. Similarly, some Asians, Arabs, Orthodox Jews, and Native Americans resist organ donation because they want the body to be buried intact. Some people of Vietnamese heritage, however, believe in cremation and will agree to organ donation in some circumstances. African Americans typically donate organs only for immediate family. Jehovah Witnesses do not favor organ donation. Filipino families rarely agree to organ donation unless a close family member is involved (Glanville, 2005; Kulwicki, 2005; Nowak, 2005; Pacquiao, 2005; Purnell & Kim, 2005; Selekman, 2003; Sharts-Hopko, 2005; Still & Hodgins, 2005).

Autopsies

When communicating about autopsies, the culturally competent nurse blends medical and legal imperatives with families' cultural preferences. Jewish families may allow autopsies but will want all body parts to be returned for burial. Religious Jewish families will usually not consent to autopsy, believing the body should be buried whole (Selekman, 2003). Mexicans believe that an autopsy may hurt the soul of the deceased, because the soul lingers near the body after death. Muslim families may not consent to autopsy (Misra-Hebert, 2003).

Advance Directives

The nurse must advocate for end-of-life (EOL) decisions that are congruent with the patient's values. Minority groups may not prepare advance directives. Some groups prefer no lifesaving interventions and simply want God's will or karma to occur. In one study, most Mexican Americans believed "the health system controls treatment," trusted the system "to serve patients well," believed advance directives "help staff know or implement a patient's wishes," and wanted "to die when treatment is futile." In that same study, most African Americans believed "the health system controls treatment," few trusted the system "to serve patients well," and most believed they should "wait until very sick to express treatment wishes" (Perkins, Geppert, Gonzales, Cortez, & Hazuda, 2002). Ideally, family conferences about EOL issues will include a support person from the patient's cultural group(s). Similarly, ethics committees should include representatives from a variety of cultures.

Grief Responses

Nurses should become familiar with the common grief responses of the predominant cultural groups in their service area. A culturally competent response at the time of death communicates caring and fosters consumer loyalty. Nurses should provide a place and adequate time for grief rituals. Some people emit loud verbal responses when death occurs and thus will benefit from dedicated "mourning places." Whites often want to be present at the time of death. Whites, Mexicans, Orthodox Jews, and Vietnamese families want to be with the body after death and may wash the body. Native Americans will not touch the body and believe that a window must be open at the time of death.

Gender Differences in Transcultural Care

Nurses must assess transcultural gender roles and beliefs and integrate patients' and families' preferences into care plans. Gender differences occur in caregiving, decision making, social contact, modesty, and healthy behaviors. In some cultural groups, touch is permitted only between members of the same sex, so nurse–patient assignments may need to be adjusted.

Evidence for Transcultural Care

Research studies and expert opinions suggest that culturally competent care improves patient outcomes and positively influences health decisions (see **Table 8-4**). Nurses can use with confidence several evidence-based nursing strategies (see **Table 8-5**). However, more research is needed to rigorously test transcultural interventions (Brach & Fraseririnco, 2000).

Guidelines for Transcultural Care

Nurses should incorporate cultural assessment information into interdisciplinary plans of care. The following primary principles guide the delivery of culturally competent care:

- As a priority, the nurse should arrange for communication support through interpreters, signage translation, and culturally appropriate teaching materials. The nurse should document in patient records the language assessment and support provided.
- The nurse must not stereotype patients according to their cultural backgrounds. While generalizations about

TABLE 8-4 Summary of Key Research on Transcultural Care

Research Study	Findings
Cooper-Patrick et al., 1999; Ferguson et al., 1998; Morales, Cunningham, Brown, & Liu, 1999; Laveist & Nuru-Jeter, 2002	Racial concordance between healthcare providers and patients results in higher patient satisfaction.
Carrasquillo, Orav, Brennan, & Burstin, 1999; Hampers, Cha, Gutglass, Binns, & Krug, 1999; Sarver & Baker, 2000	Lack of interpreters and lack of culturally appropriate education result in low patient satisfaction, poor adherence to health plans, and low-quality outcomes.
Bernstein, Mutschler, & Bernstein, 2000; Betancourt, Green, & Carrillo, 2002; Chen & Rankin, 2002; Fernandez, DeBor, Candreia, Wagner, & Stewart, 1999; Weber & Reilly, 1997	Culturally sensitive interventions are effective in changing health behaviors.
Baker, Hayes, & Fortier, 1998; David & Rhee, 1997; Derose & Baker, 2000; Stewart,1995; Stewart, Meredith, Brown, & Galajda, 2000; Tocher & Larson, 1998	Poor communication between patient and healthcare providers reduces trust, lowers patient satisfaction, increases morbidity, and reduces compliance with plans of care. Health outcomes were equivalent for English-speaking patients and non-English-speaking patients who had interpreters.
Smith, 2003	Nurses' knowledge and self-efficacy increased after cultural education. Improvements were sustained.
Maioco, 1999	Nurses' personal experiences were the primary factors in "juggling" complex cultural decisions.
Mohrmann et al., 2000	Educational materials must be culturally appropriate for optimal compliance.
Shelfer, Escarce, & Schulman, 2000	Nurses and physicians may have cultural biases that affect management of patients and symptoms.

TABLE 8-5 Evidence-Based Transcultural Care

Strategy	Strength of Evidence
Develop culturally synergistic nurse–patient relationships, including racial concordance	B
Devote adequate time to open discussion with patient and family about cultural preferences	B
Arrange for professional interpreter; document in patient records	B
Incorporate the family in the roles that they desire and choose	D
Integrate cultural routines and values with the nursing plan of care	B
Utilize culturally appropriate teaching approaches with patients	A
Nurses' performance of culturally competent care improves with education	C

Note: Strength of Evidence Rating Scale
A = Randomized control trials.
B = Non-experimental research, replicated.
C = Descriptive research or non-experimental research, unreplicated.
D = Expert opinion.
Source: Data from U.S. Department of Health and Human Services. *Healthy People 2010: Understanding and improving health.* 2nd ed. Washington, DC.

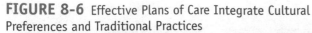

FIGURE 8-6 Effective Plans of Care Integrate Cultural Preferences and Traditional Practices

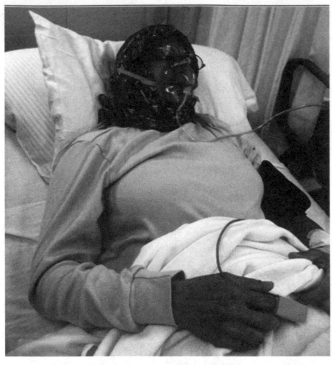

cultures can be suggested, patients may differ in important ways from their broad cultural group.

- The nurse must resist labeling patient behavior as "non-compliant." Poor communication or culturally insensitive care may contribute to nonadherence, rather than simply being a patient's blatant refusal to participate in aspects of care.
- The nurse should integrate patients' preferred cultural routines into the plan of care when it is safe to do so

(**Figure 8-6**). For example, if a patient requests prayer and "laying on of hands" for healing, ensure that those participating can touch the patient appropriately and that privacy is provided. If a patient desires modesty at all times, be sure the patient stays discreetly covered during dressing changes and physical assessments. Maintenance of meaningful rituals during critical illness communicates caring, enhances satisfaction, and may boost the immune system.

- The nurse should incorporate the family in care by clarifying the roles that they desire. Determine who will participate in decision making, who will attend teaching sessions, who will provide care after discharge, and who wishes to be present should life-threatening events occur.

EVALUATING CULTURAL CARE

Outcomes for culturally competent care flow from the design of interventions. For example, outcomes for strategies to enhance verbal communication include the ability to express and receive accurate messages (Dochterman & Bulechek, 2004). Nurses also should evaluate culturally competent care by monitoring system-level outcomes (Brach & Fraseririnco, 2000) (see **Table 8-6**).

SUMMARY

Thorough self- and patient assessments are essential for culturally competent care. The Critical Care version of the Transcultural Nursing Assessment Model (Giger & Davidhizar, 2004) guides assessment during critical illness. Evidence-based care includes using professional interpreters, integrating cultural practices into the plan of care, and designing culturally appropriate educational methods. The outcomes of transcultural care are reduced human suffering, healthy communities, and improved economies of healthcare systems.

TABLE 8-6 Target Outcomes and Sample Indicators of Culturally Competent Care

Target Outcome	Sample Indicators
Effective Patient Education Health education is tailored to patient's culture.	**Patient:** Verbalizes accurate information **System:** Reduced readmission rates, increased patient satisfaction with education
Fewer Diagnostic Delays and Errors When professionals understand patients, treatment is timely.	**Patient:** Exchanges messages appropriately **System:** Reduced mortality, fewer unnecessary procedures, reduced length of stay
Reduction in Medication Errors Healthcare providers reconcile medications and integrate folk remedies appropriately.	**Patient:** Verbalizes accurate drug regimen, expresses satisfaction with integrated plan **System:** Reduced length of stay, reduced medication errors and adverse reactions, reduced readmissions
Improved Adherence with Care Plan An acceptable plan of care is negotiated with patients.	**Patient:** Articulates willingness to adhere; condition is stable or progressing on follow-up visits **System:** Reduced length of stay, reduced readmissions, reduced pressure ulcers and falls rates, increased smoking cessation rate, reduced morbidity and mortality
Improved Patient/Nurse Satisfaction Patients and nurses respond positively to culturally competent care.	**System:** Improved patient and nurse satisfaction scores, increased customer loyalty rate, increased nurse retention, increased recruitment and retention of nurses from minority groups

CASE STUDY

R.O., age 23, is mechanically ventilated after emergency surgery for a ruptured appendix. Her two-day history of abdominal pain was erroneously treated as *empacho*, a Hispanic folk disease. The *curandero* vigorously massaged her abdomen, which increased her pain and nausea. When lemon juice on her skin did not reduce the fever, R.O.'s father sent her to the clinic. Postoperatively, she is septic. Her assigned physician, who is from Pakistan, just arrived to order medications. R.O.'s large family is at the bedside continuously, praying and patting her body. Despite patient-controlled analgesia, R.O. moans continuously and refuses to answer questions.

CRITICAL THINKING QUESTIONS

1. As R.O.'s nurse, what clinical inquiry will be needed to obtain a cultural assessment?

2. Utilizing clinical judgment, list three interventions for R.O.'s care.

3. What aspects of care will you discuss in collaborating with the physician?

4. What disciplines should be consulted to work with R.O.?

5. How will you implement your role as a facilitator of learning for this patient and the staff?

6. Utilize the form to develop a plan of care for R.O. Rate the patient as a level 1, 3, or 5 on each characteristic. Identify the level of nurse characteristics needed in the care of this patient.

7. Develop 10 cards with frequently used questions in Spanish by going to www.babelfish.altavista.com.

Using the Synergy Model to Develop a Plan of Care

SYNERGY MODEL	Patient Characteristics	Level 1, 3, or 5	Subjective and Objective Data	Evidence-based Interventions	Outcomes
	Resiliency				
	Vulnerability				
	Stability				
	Complexity				
	Resource availability				
	Participation in care				
	Participation in decision making				
	Predictability				

Online Resources

Center for Cross-Cultural Healthcare:
www.crosshealth.com

Consumer health brochures in multiple languages:
http://medstat.med.utash/edu/24languages

National Center for Cultural Competence: http://gucchd.georgetown.edu/nccc (assessment tools)

Provider's guide to quality and culture: http://erc.msh.org (video clips, audio clips)

Resources for cross-cultural healthcare:
www.diversityRx.org

Transcultural Nursing Society:
www.tcns.org

University of South Dakota School of Nursing:
www.usd.edu/med/nursing/care/care.cfm
(CD-ROM available with pre-test and post-test on nursing care of Lakota Indians)

Multimedia Spanish language translator:
http://www.hhcc.arealahec.dst.nc.us

Translation of large pieces of text:
www.babelfish.altavista.com

Virtual medical conversation in Spanish:
http://idrama.com/medspanish_LP.htm

Office of Minority Health:
www.omhrc.gov

REFERENCES

American Cancer Society. (2005). Retrieved from www.cancer.org

American Heart Association. (2004). *Heart disease and stroke statistics—2003 update.* Dallas, TX: American Heart Association.

American Nurses Association. (2005). Retrieved from http://nursingworld.org/readroom/position/ethics/etcldv.htm

Baker, D., Hayes, R., & Fortier, J. (1998). Interpreter use and satisfaction with interpersonal aspects of care for Spanish-speaking patients. *Medical Care, 36*(10), 1461–1470.

Bernstein, J., Mutschler, P., & Bernstein, E. (2000). Keeping mammogram appointments: Motivation, health beliefs, and access barriers experienced by older minority women. *Journal of Midwifery and Women's Health, 45*(4), 308–313.

Betancourt, J., Green, A., & Carrillo, J. (2002). Cultural competence in health care: Emerging frameworks and practical approaches. The Commonwealth Fund. Retrieved from http://www.cmwf.org

Brach, C., & Fraseririnco, I. (2000). Can cultural competency reduce racial and ethnic health disparities? A review and conceptual model. *Medical Care Research and Review, 57,* 181–217.

Burroughs, V., Maxey, R., Crawley, L., & Levy, R. (2002). Cultural and genetic diversity in America: The need for individualized pharmaceutical treatment. Retrieved July 10, 2005, from www.npcnow.org

Carrasquillo, O., Orav, E. J., Brennan, T. A., & Burstin, H. (1999). Impact of language barriers on patient satisfaction in an emergency department. *Journal of General Internal Medicine, 14,* 82–87.

Chang, M., & Harden, J. (2002). Meeting the challenge of the new millennium: Caring for culturally diverse patients. *Urologic Nursing, 22*(6), 372–377.

Chen, J. L., & Rankin, S. H. (2002). Using the resiliency model to deliver culturally sensitive care to Chinese families. *Journal of Pediatric Nursing, 17*(3), 157–166.

Coffman, M. J. (2004). Cultural caring in nursing practice: A meta-synthesis of qualitative research. *Journal of Cultural Diversity, 11*(3), 100–109.

Cooper-Patrick, L., Gallo, J. J., Gonzales, J. J., Vu, H. T., Powe, N. R., Nelson, C., et al. (1999). Race, gender and partnership in the patient–physician relationship. *Journal of the American Medical Association, 282*(6), 583–589.

David, R., & Rhee, M. (1997). The impact of language as a barrier to effective healthy care in an underserved urban Hispanic community. *Journal of General Internal Medicine, 12,* 123.

Dennis, B. P., & Small, E. B. (2003). Incorporating cultural diversity in nursing care: An action plan. *The American Black Nursing Foundation Journal, 14*(1), 17–26.

Derose, K., & Baker, D. (2000). Limited English proficiency and Latinos' use of physician services. *Medical Care Research, 57*(1), 76–91.

Dochterman, J., & Bulechek, G. (2004). *Nursing interventions classification (NIC).* St. Louis, MO: Mosby.

Ferguson, J., Weinberger, M., Westmoreland, G., Mamlin, L., Segar, D., Greene, J., et al. (1998). Racial disparity in cardiac decision making. *Archives of Internal Medicine, 158*(13), 1450–1453.

Fernandez, M., DeBor, M., Candreia, M., Wagner, A., & Stewart, K. (1999). Evaluation of ENCORE: A community-based breast and cervical cancer screening program. *American Journal of Preventative Medicine, 16,* 35–49.

Galanti, G. (2004). *Caring for patients from different cultures* (3rd ed.). Philadelphia: University of Pennsylvania Press.

Giger, J., & Davidhizar, R. (2004). *Transcultural nursing: Assessment and intervention* (4th ed.). St. Louis, MO: Mosby.

Glanville, C. L. (2005). People of African American heritage. In L. D. Purnell & B. J. Baulanka (Eds.), *Transcultural health care: A culturally competent approach* (2nd ed., pp. 40–53). Philadelphia: F.A. Davis.

Hampers, L. C., Cha, S., Gutglass, D. J., Binns, H. J., & Krug, S. E. (1999). Language barriers and resource utilization in a pediatric emergency department. *Pediatrics, 103,* 1253–1256.

Healthy People 2010. (2005). U.S. Department of Health and Human Services, Office of Disease Prevention and Health Promotion. Retrieved from www.healthypeople.gov

Ignatavicious, D., & Workman, M. (2006). *Medical-surgical nursing: Critical thinking for collaborative care.* St. Louis, MO: Mosby.

Joint Commission on Accreditation of Healthcare Organizations. (2005). Retrieved from www.jcaho.org/about+us/hlc/about_hlc.htm

Kulwicki, A. D. (2005). People of Arab heritage. In L. D. Purnell & B. J. Baulanka (Eds.), *Transcultural health care: A culturally competent approach* (2nd ed., pp. 90–105). Philadelphia: F.A. Davis.

Laveist, T. A., & Nuru-Jeter, A. (2002). Is doctor–patient race concordance associated with greater satisfaction with care? *Journal of Health and Social Behavior, 43*(3), 296–306.

Luckmann, J. (2000). Transcultural communication building blocks: Beliefs, behavior, and communication. *Transcultural communication in health care* (pp. 42–58). Canada: Delmar.

Maioco, G. (1999). *Decision-making process nurses use to provide culturally sensitive care.* Unpublished dissertation. Salt Lake City, UT: University of Utah.

Merriam-Webster Online Dictionary. (2005). www.m-w.com

Misra-Hebert, A. D. (2003). Physician cultural competence: Cross-cultural communication improves care. *Cleveland Clinic Journal of Medicine, 70*(4), 289–303.

Mohrmann, C., Coleman, E., Coon, S., Lord, J., Heard, J., Cantrell, M., et al. (2000). An analysis of printed breast cancer information for African American women. *Journal of Cancer Education, 15*(1), 23–27.

Morales, L., Cunningham, W., Brown, J., & Liu, H. (1999). Are Latinos less satisfied with communication by health care providers? *Journal of General Internal Medicine, 14,* 409–417.

Nowak, T. T. (2005). People of Vietnamese heritage. In L. D. Purnell & B. J. Baulanka (Eds.), *Transcultural health care: A culturally competent approach* (2nd ed., pp. 327–343). Philadelphia: F.A. Davis.

Office of Minority Health. (2005). Assuring cultural competence in health care: Recommendations for national standards and an outcomes-focused research agenda. Retrieved October 5, 2006, from http://www.omhrc.gov/clas/

Pacquiao, D. F. (2005). People of Filipino heritage. In L. D. Purnell & B. J. Baulanka (Eds.), *Transcultural health care: A culturally competent approach* (2nd ed., pp. 138–159). Philadelphia: F.A. Davis.

Perkins, H. S., Geppert, C. M., Gonzales, A., Cortez, J. D., & Hazuda, H. P. (2002). Cross-cultural similarities and differences in attitudes about advance care planning. *Journal of General Internal Medicine, 17*(1), 48–57.

Purnell, L. D., & Kim, S. (2005). People of Korean heritage. In L.D. Purnell & B.J. Baulanka (Eds.), *Transcultural health care: A culturally competent approach* (2nd ed., pp. 249–263). Philadelphia: F.A. Davis.

Purnell, L. D., & Paulanka, B. J. (2003). *Transcultural health care: A culturally competent approach* (2nd ed.). Philadelphia: F.A. Davis.

Ryan, M., Twibell, R., Brigham, C., & Bennett, P. (2001). Learning to care for clients in their world, not mine. *Journal of Nursing Education, 39*(9), 401–408.

Sarver, J., & Baker, D. (2000). Effect of language barriers on follow-up appointments after an emergency department visit. *Journal of General Internal Medicine, 15*(4), 256–264.

Selekman, J. (2003). People of Jewish heritage. In L. D. Purnell & B. J. Baulanka (Eds.), *Transcultural health care: A culturally competent approach.* (2nd ed., pp. 234–248). Philadelphia: F.A. Davis.

Sharts-Hopko, N. C. (2005). People of Japanese heritage. In L. D. Purnell & B. J. Baulanka (Eds.), *Transcultural health care: A culturally competent approach* (2nd ed., pp. 218–233). Philadelphia: F.A. Davis.

Shelfer, S., Escarce, J., & Schulman, K. (2000). Race and sex differences in the management of coronary artery disease. *American Heart Journal, 139*(5), 848–857.

Smith, L. (2003). Evaluation of an educational intervention to increase cultural competence among registered nurses. *Journal of Cultural Diversity, 8*(2), 50–63.

Spector, R. (2004). *Cultural diversity in health and illness* (6th ed.). Upper Saddle River, NJ: Prentice Hall.

Stewart, M. A. (1995). Effective physician–patient communication and health outcomes: A review. *Journal of the Canadian Medical Association, 152*(9), 1423–1432.

Stewart, M., Meredith, L., Brown, J., & Galajda, J. (2000). The influence of older patient–physician communication on health and health-related outcomes. *Clinical Geriatric Medicine, 16*(1), 25–36.

Still, O., & Hodgins, D. (2005). Navajo Indians. In L. D. Purnell & B. J. Baulanka (Eds.), *Transcultural health care: A culturally competent approach* (2nd ed., pp. 279–293). Philadelphia: F.A. Davis.

Tocher, T., & Larson, E. (1998). Quality of diabetes care for non-English speaking patients: A comparative study. *Western Journal of Medicine, 168,* 504–511.

Urden, L., Stacy, K., & Lough, M. (2002). *Thelan's critical care nursing diagnosis and management* (4th ed.). St. Louis, MO: Mosby.

U.S. Census. (2002). United States Census Bureau. Retrieved from www.census.gov

Weber, B., & Reilly, B. (1997). Enhancing mammography use in the inner city: A randomized trial of intensive case management. *Archives of Internal Medicine, 157*(20), 2345–2349.

CHAPTER 9

Complementary Therapies in the ICU

Michael Neville

LEARNING OBJECTIVES

Upon completion of this chapter, the reader will be able to:

1. List rationales for patients' use of complementary therapies.

2. Describe the use of selected complementary therapies in the ICU.

3. Discuss nursing implications for patients taking herbal remedies prior to an ICU admission.

4. List optimal patient outcomes that may be achieved through the use of complementary therapies.

Complementary and alternative therapy (CAT) is employed by patients for the prevention and treatment of illness despite the fact that there are "no plausible biomedical explanations" for its usefulness (Krucoff et al., 2005, p. 211). The National Center for Complementary and Alternative Medicine (NCCAM) has divided CAT into several categories: *alternative medical systems* (e.g., Native American medicine, aromatherapy, tai chi), *mind–body interventions* (e.g., relaxation, guided imagery, exercise), *biologically based therapies* (e.g., megavitamins, herbs, diet), *manipulative and body-based methods* (e.g., acupressure, massage, chiropractic), and *energy therapies* (e.g., electromagnetic/magnet, therapeutic touch) (Gaskill, 2004; Lindquist, Tracy, Savik, & Watanuki, 2005).

The use of CAT in adults has become increasingly popular in the United States. Wahner-Roedler and colleagues (2005) noted in 1991 that as many as 34% of subjects surveyed in the United States were using CAT. The percentage increased to approximately 42% by 1997. During the 1990s, Americans made more visits to complementary therapy providers than to their primary care physicians (O'Brien King, 1999). Adults who were more likely to use CAT included those with more education, a poor health status, a history of a worldview-altering transformational experience, higher incomes, feministic ideals, dedication to environmentalism, and interests in growth, psychology, and spirituality (Hayes & Alexander, 2000; Moenkhoff, Baenziger, Fischer, & Fanconi, 1999). Psychological factors such as personality traits, perceived social support and strain, and coping strategies have also been shown to influence the use of CAT in adults (Honda & Jacobson, 2005).

CAT use in infants and pediatric patients has neither been widely used nor studied (Mark & Barton, 2001; Moenkhoff et al., 1999). More published literature is available about the use of CAT in critically ill neonates, particularly the use of touch. Parents often want to do everything possible for their sick children and may ask for "natural therapies" in hopes of avoiding adverse reactions (Mark & Barton). Factors most associated with the use of CAT in pediatric patients include severity of illness in the child and parental use of CAT (Highfield, McLellan, Kemper, Risko, & Woolf, 2005).

Some use CAT because it is viewed as "natural," but CAT is not necessarily innocuous. Adverse effects "may be experienced as the result of unsafe use, overuse, unanticipated harm, or interactions between CAT and other traditional prescribed or CAT therapies" (Lindquist et al., 2005, p. 63). In some instances, the use or misuse of CAT may be the very reason the patient seeks medical care (Meghani, Lingquist, & Tracy, 2003).

Controversy exists regarding the use of CAT in critically ill patients. Greater numbers of patients and their families are requesting that clinicians consider adding these therapies to traditional treatments during hospitalization or requesting that providers continue home-initiated CAT during hospitalization (Gaskill, 2004; Lindquist et al., 2005). While critical care nurses may be resistant to consider CAT in an "already stressful, high-tech, and chaotic setting," they may also feel pressure to satisfy patients' requests and be in tune with societal demands (Meghani et al., 2003, p. 138). Few data exist regarding the specific use of CAT in critically ill patients, and "even less information is available about the safety and efficacy of the nurse's use of nontraditional therapies for problematic conditions in critically ill patients" (Lindquist et al., pp. 64, 66).

A survey of 2,740 Ohio nurses in 1997 was developed by the Ohio Board of Nursing to assess nurses' self-rated knowledge level about CAT, use of CAT for self and for patients, perceptions of CAT efficacy, and referral patterns for CAT. This survey revealed that the most frequently used CATs nurses used on themselves were prayer (81%), diet (74%), and herbs (41%). Respondents indicated that they most frequently used diet (38%) and prayer (30%) for their patients. They also indicated that dietary advice (43%) and prayer (30%) offered by clergy members were the CATs most frequently provided to their patients by referral (O'Brien King, 1999).

CAT encompasses many modalities of treatment, and all cannot be discussed here. Consequently, this chapter will be limited to the deeper exploration of therapeutic touch, music therapy, prayer/spirituality, and herbal therapies.

THERAPEUTIC TOUCH

"A person may be born blind, deaf, and mute, but in order to live, the skin—constituting 20% of the body weight—must respond to touch" (Das, 2005, p. 240). Das stated that as language breaks down in the midst of physical pain, touch, which is most closely allied to affect and emotion, fills in the gap. Depending on the culture, touching may be a sign of caring, friendliness, affection, or disrespect (see Chapter 8 on cultural issues).

One trial examined the occurrence of touch by healthcare professionals. The frequency of *nonproprietary* and *proprietary* *touches* was compared in 900 hospital personnel, including medical doctors, residents, interns, senior medical students, junior medical students, registered nurses, senior nursing students, junior nursing students, sophomore nursing students, licensed vocational nurses, aides, and orderlies. The investigators noted that 72% of touches were performed by personnel between 18 and 33 years; females touched 85% more than males; 73% of touches were performed by Caucasians; the patient's hand was the part of the body most frequently touched; and patients in "good or fair" condition garnered 70% of the given touches whereas those with conditions labeled "serious or poor" were given far fewer touches. Finally, it was noted that registered nurses touched patients more frequently (154 touches) than others in the study. Junior nursing students placed second on the list, touching 73 times (Barnett, 1972).

The practice of *healing touch* or *therapeutic touch (TT)* builds on previous statements about the importance of touch, but is based on "clearing, aligning, and balancing the human energy system" (Jones & Kassity, 2001, p. 761). Some healthcare providers treat mental or physical disease from an energy-based perspective (Jones & Kassity), which takes the view that the illness is the result of the patient's entire energy field. Caregivers work to restore the appropriate balance between the patient and his or her environment's energy systems. Placement of hands above or directly on the patient's body in specific and intentional ways is the process used to promote healing (Wardell & Weymouth, 2004).

Less formalized or structured nursing continuing education programs on TT were begun in the early 1980s. More formalized programs were offered by the American Holistic Nurses Association (AHNA) in 1989, and then endorsed by Healing Touch International, Inc., in 1996 (Wardell & Weymouth, 2004). Many thousands have completed training courses in countries around the world and are now using these techniques in private practices, operating rooms, and pain centers (Wardell & Weymouth).

A 2004 literature review by Wardell and Weymouth indicated that the use of TT on immune disorders (e.g., human immunodeficiency virus (HIV), cancer, mental health disease, cardiovascular conditions, and pain has been examined through research. The use of TT in the elderly and pediatric patients has also been studied (Gregory & Verdouw, 2005; Ireland, 1998; Ireland & Olson, 2000; Woods, Craven, & Whitney, 2005). Researchers reported that subjects with immune disorders receiving TT had reductions in pain, anxiety, and stress. Improvements in HIV patients were weaker, being seen only during the follow-up phase many weeks after the treatment. Findings in cancer patients were variable. Some cancer patients reported clinically significant subjective improvements in well-being, mood, fatigue, interpersonal relationships, blood pressure control, and pain reduction. Mental health studies of TT use were exploratory and were too limited to provide strong conclusions. TT use in post-traumatic stress disorder (PTSD) patients deserves further exploration, because preliminary data appear promising (Wardell & Weymouth, 2004). Cardiovascular patients treated with TT had positive trends toward improvements, but no significant changes in outcomes were noted (Krucoff et al., 2001). Results from use of TT in pain sufferers were positive—seven of the nine studies included in the literature review demonstrated pain reduction.

Data have questioned the effectiveness of TT (Cox & Hayes, 1999a). Several studies, however, have suggested that TT promotes relaxation and comfort in patients in the intensive care unit (ICU), leading to improved sleep (Richards, Nagel, Markie, Elwell, & Barone, 2003). It was therefore concluded that TT is safe for critically ill patients and should be performed by ICU nurses who have received specialized training. It is further noted that TT could contribute to the psychological well-being of patients in the ICU, because it promotes relaxation, comfort, and a sense of peace (Cox & Hayes, 1999b).

MUSIC THERAPY

The rhythmic sounds that promote "relaxation, communication, healing, and feelings of well-being" are found in music and date back to Aristotle and Pythagoras, who taught that musical instruments could "erase negative emotions such as worry, fear, sorrow, and anger" (Kowalak & Mills, 2002, p. 348). Music has also been reported to affect blood pressure, lower stress levels, enhance memory in Alzheimer's disease patients, and decrease acute postoperative and chronic pain (Fugh-Berman, 1997; Pelletier, 2000). Although music therapy has grown in popularity and may be viewed as a cost-effective intervention, the appropriate length of time, "optimal dosages," and best choices of music are less clear and deserve more research (Pelletier).

A study of critically ill ventilated patients in the ICU examined the ability of adjunctive music therapy to reduce anxiety and increase relaxation. Twenty-four mechanically ventilated subjects matched for APACHE II scores were randomized into one of three groups (New Age, classical, or no music) and wore padded headphones for 30 minutes twice daily for two sessions. Investigators found that the subjects in the New Age group had the largest reductions in clinical parameters, except heart rate during session 1. Subjects in the no-music group had the largest reductions in mean heart rate during the first session, but also had the largest increases in heart rate during the second session. Blood pressure reduc-

tions were greatest in the classical and New Age groups during the second session (Sabatini, 2005).

Aragon and colleagues (2002) evaluated the use of live harp music in vascular and thoracic surgical patients. Patient satisfaction (measured by a 4-item questionnaire) and physiological measures (heart rate, diastolic and systolic blood pressures, oxygen saturation, and respiratory rate) were recorded at baseline, 0, 5, 10, 15, and 20 minutes after the initiation of harp playing. Measurements at 5 and 10 minutes after conclusion of harp playing were also taken. Investigators concluded that the harp music had positive effects on perception of pain, anxiety, and satisfaction. Statistically significant changes in oxygen saturation and systolic blood pressure were noted; other physiologic parameters showed a downward trend, albeit without statistical significance.

Another study comparing the effects of silence and "white noise" on coronary care unit patients found that although both were effective in lowering stress responses, 30 minutes of uninterrupted rest was most beneficial. While music may be useful in a critically ill patient, silence and 6 to 8 hours of uninterrupted sleep are also important (Fugh-Berman, 1997). Therefore, nurses should organize care to provide long periods of quiet time to promote rest and sleep. A more in-depth discussion of sleep disturbances in the ICU patient appears in Chapter 5.

PRAYER AND SPIRITUALITY

A recent study suggests that those who believe in God and pray during times of illness have better health outcomes than those who do not (Harris et al., 1999). Whether faith somehow bolsters or improves hormonal, immunologic, or autonomic responses to stress remains a mystery. Although modifications in health curricula are being made to prepare clinicians for the growing interest of their patients in the connections between medicine and spirituality, spiritual variables remain largely uninvestigated in the scientific literature (Aviles et al., 2001). Many debates exist regarding the differences between prayer and spirituality. It has been suggested that religion is "a belief system that embodies a philosophy, or religion is a part of spirituality, or religion is an organized system of beliefs and practices that are designed to bring the believer closer to God" (Holt-Ashley, 2000, pp. 61–62).

Spirituality, by contrast, has been defined as "the search for meaning and purpose, a part of a person that involves the intangible nonphysical world, or the quest for answers about life and meaning that may lead to practices and religious doctrine" (Holt-Ashley, 2000, p. 62). Prayer is commonly associated with religion or spirituality. Scientists have attempted to derive its origins or its power, but "science raises more questions than it answers about prayer, because science cannot measure the [immeasurable]" (Holt-Ashley). Many have attempted anyway. In fact, 212 published trials have evaluated the effects of spiritual factors on outcomes in health care. Of these, 75% report a positive effect, 17% no effect, and 7% a negative effect (Aviles et al., 2001).

Nurses often "talk about God, talk about religious beliefs, provide active listening, read scripture, discuss meaning and purpose of life, and pray with patients" (Cavendish, Konecny, Luise, & Lanza, 2004, p. 27). Although much literature exists regarding prayer use by nurses, most refer to specific prayers written by nurses or to the personal use of prayer by nurses to positively influence their own work rather than the use of prayer as a patient "intervention." One group of nurses prays daily for their patients and for themselves in a medical ICU setting. They meet 15 minutes before work each day for this activity because they believe that patients want and need prayer. The author studying this nurses group concluded that by involving patients in the spiritual realm, nurses can offer richer support to patients and their families. "Nurses in MICUs who pray for themselves and for their patients can expect positive outcomes" (Holt-Ashley, 2000, p. 67).

Two recently published, randomized, controlled trials examined the benefits of intercessory prayer in patients with coronary disease. The primary objective in one trial, which randomized 990 patients to a "prayer group" versus a "usual care" group, was to determine whether intercessory prayer reduced overall lengths of stay (LOS) and the adverse event rate (Harris et al., 1999). The other trial randomized 799 subjects to control versus intercessory prayer groups to determine the effects of prayer on cardiovascular disease progression after hospital discharge. Intercessors in both trials were community volunteers who either agreed with a particular statement of faith or belonged to a local religious or community group (Aviles et al., 2001). Intercessor groups were formally organized in the Harris trial groups into 15 teams of 5 members, whereas intercessor group sizes in the Aviles trial were less formally organized and ranged in number from 1 to 65 members. Intercessors in the Harris trial were requested to pray daily for "a speedy recovery with no complications" for 28 days (LOS was 28 days or less for 95% of their participants); a weighted and summed coronary care unit course score (MAHI-CCU) was used to evaluate patient outcomes. Investigators in the Aviles trial asked intercessors to pray at least once weekly for 26 weeks and compared groups with respect to the following end points: rehospitalization for cardiac disease, coronary revascularization, and emergency department visit for cardiovascular disease, cardiac arrest, or death. Participants in the Harris trial in the prayer group had lower mean weighted and

unweighted MAHI scores than those in the usual-care group; differences in hospital LOS between the groups were not significant. Results from the Aviles trial revealed that a primary end point at 26 weeks had occurred in 25.6% of the intercessory prayer subjects and 29.3% of the control group; investigators found no significant differences between the groups. Therefore, the Aviles trial did not show intercessory prayer to improve medical outcomes after hospitalization in a coronary care unit.

In a recent study, 748 subjects were enrolled in a trial that compared four interventions: (1) music/imagery/touch (MIT) with intercessory prayer (IP), (2) IP only, (3) MIT only, and (4) neither therapy. Subjects in all groups received percutaneous coronary intervention (75%) or elective catheterization (99%) in nine U.S. centers. Investigators compared MIT and IP with regard to primary (combined in-hospital major cardiac events and 6-month cardiac readmissions or death) and secondary (6-month major cardiovascular events, 6-month death or readmission, and 6-month mortality). Researchers found no significant differences between the four groups with respect to primary and secondary end points; a slight decrease in 6-month mortality was noted in those receiving both MIT and IP (Krucoff et al., 2005).

HERBS

Herbal therapy dates back as far as 466–377 B.C. and was used by Hippocrates in his teaching and practice (Jones & Kassity, 2001). Herbal therapies are widely used today by many in addition to or in place of traditional or prescription medications. According to a report by the World Health Organization, as many as "75% of the global population—most of the developing world—depends on botanical medicines for their basic health care needs" (Jones & Kassity, p. 763). A 2004 NCCAM survey determined that as many as 20% of the U.S. population had used "natural therapies" (Barnes, Powell-Griner, McFann, & Nahin, 2004).

The NCCAM survey (Barnes et al., 2004) found that the herbs most likely to be used by Americans included echinacea (40.3%), ginseng (24.1%), ginkgo biloba (21.1%), garlic supplements (19.9%), glucosamine (14.9%), St. John's wort (12.0%), peppermint (11.8%), fish oils (11.7%), ginger (10.5%), and soy supplements (9.4%). Survey participants cited many reasons for trying herbal remedies, including back pain (16.8%), head cold (9.5%), neck pain (6.6%), joint pain (4.9%), and arthritis (4.9%).

Although specific data about the use of herbs in critically ill patients are lacking, it is feasible that preadmission use of herbal preparations in these patients resembles that of the general population. An OVID search from 1977 to the present revealed no randomized, controlled trials on the intentional use of herbs to treat illness in ICU patients. Another literature search resulted in 14 citations, 5 of which were related to medicinal use of these agents. One clinical trial (Lau et al., 2005) highlighted the use of an herbal agent for management of severe acute respiratory syndrome (SARS) in a Hong Kong hospital. The researchers of this pilot study concluded that there is a good potential of using traditional Chinese medicine supplements to prevent the spread of SARS. Another study (Bostelmann et al., 2002) explored the use of an herb, *Esberitox N*, for its immunomodulatory effects in hepatitis B seroconversion. No clinical trials documenting the use of the aforementioned commonly used herbal preparations were found.

While clinicians in some hospitals are encouraged or permitted to prescribe herbal therapies, herbal therapy use in other hospitals is strongly discouraged or is even banned. In any case, it is important for healthcare providers to realize that some herbal therapies, when combined with traditionally prescribed drugs, increase the risk for potentially life-threatening interactions. Consequently, it is vitally important that they query the patient or family specifically about these therapies during patient assessments. For example, ginkgo, ginseng, and garlic all have coagulation-modifying properties and may act synergistically when combined with anticoagulant drugs such as warfarin (Coumadin®), heparin, clopidogrel (Plavix®), and enoxaparin (Lovenox®), resulting in hemorrhage (Anonymous, 2002). Clearly, a large number of patients use herbal remedies. These agents have a potential to interact with medications prescribed during an ICU admission. Such interactions can be hazardous. Nurses have a responsibility to ask whether use of herbal remedies is occurring when obtaining a patient history and physical (Smith, Ernst, Ewings, Myers, & Smith, 2004).

PATIENT OUTCOMES

Nurses can help ensure attainment of optimal patient outcomes such as those listed in **Box 9-1** through the use of evidence-based interventions.

Box 9-1
Optimal Patient Outcomes

- Reported satisfaction with symptom control
- Physical comfort in expected range
- Reported physical and psychological well-being
- Perceived control of health beliefs

SUMMARY

Despite the lack of scientific support, patients will likely continue to pursue TT, music therapy, prayer/spirituality, herbal remedies, and other forms of CAT. The motivation to use CAT will increase over the coming years. The 2004 NCCAM survey revealed that 54.9% of respondents sought CAT because they thought it would help their condition if it was combined with conventional medicine; 50.1% thought it would be interesting to try; 27.7% thought that conventional medicine would not help their condition; 25.8% used CAT because a conventional medical professional recommended it; and 13.2% found conventional medicine too expensive (Barnes et al., 2004).

It is imperative that nurses continue to increase their knowledge base regarding CAT. "If we think of (healing) as a larger or smaller room, it appears evident that most people learn to only know a corner of the room, a place by the window, a strip of floor on which they walk up and down." CAT is undoubtedly one way to "know a larger room" (Jones & Kassity, 2001, p. 750).

CASE STUDY

T.M., a 67-year-old female, was admitted to the ICU from a nursing home with a diagnosis of suspected pneumonia. She is on 4 liters by nasal cannula with an oxygen saturation of 92%. Her past medical history includes a previous myocardial infarction, migraine headaches, depression, and isolated systolic hypertension. The nurse asks T.M.'s family what medications T.M. is taking and discovers the following pre-admission agents: ECASA 325 mg daily, nifedipine (Procardia XL®, Adalat-CC®) 90 mg twice daily, and paroxetine (Paxil®) 20 mg daily.

CRITICAL THINKING QUESTIONS

1. When using your clinical judgment during the completion of an admission history, what additional questions to the family should the nurse consider? Using the table below, identify questions to elicit further understanding of the patient characteristics during an admission history.

2. What types of CAT discussed in this chapter might be considered in addition to traditional therapies (e.g., antibiotics) to treat T.M.?

3. What types of CAT (give specific examples if possible) are especially dangerous if combined with T.M.'s current medication regimen?

4. How will you implement your role as a facilitator of learning for this patient?

5. Identify one outcome for this patient and list evidence-based interventions to ensure optimal patient outcomes.

Patient Characteristics	Questions to Ask the Patient during an Admission History
Resiliency	
Vulnerability	
Stability	
Complexity	
Resource availability	
Participation in care	
Participation in decision making	
Predictability	

SYNERGY MODEL

Online Resources

National Center for Complementary and Alternative Medicine:
www.nccam.org

American Holistic Nurses Association:
www.ahna.org

Bandolier:
www.jr2.ox.ac.uk/bandolier/booth/booths/altmed.html

Official Organization for Therapeutic Touch:
www.therapeutictouch.org

American Music Therapy Organization:
www.musictherapy.org

Focus on Alternative and Complementary Therapies:
http://journals.medicinescomplete.com/journals/fact/current

REFERENCES

Anonymous. (2002). Herbs and the heart. *Harvard Heart Letter, 12*(11), 2–3.

Aragon, D., Farris, C., & Byers, J. F. (2002). The effects of harp music in vascular and thoracic surgical patients. *Alternative Therapies in Health and Medicine, 8*(5), 52–60.

Aviles, J. M., Whelan, E., Hernke, D. A., Williams, B. A., Kenny, K. E., O'Fallon, W. M., et al. (2001). Intercessory prayer and cardiovascular disease progression in a coronary care unit population: A randomized controlled trial. *Mayo Clinic Proceedings, 76*(12), 1192–1198.

Barnes, P., Powell-Griner, E., McFann, K., & Nahin, R. (2004). Complementary and alternative medicine use among adults. *Advance Data, 343,* 1–19.

Barnett, K. (1972). A survey of the current utilization of touch by health team personnel with hospitalized patients. *International Journal of Nursing Studies, 9*(4), 195–209.

Bostelmann, H. C., Bodeker, R. H., Dames, W., Henneicke-von Zepelin, H. H., Siegers, C. P., & Stammwitz, U. (2002). Immunomodulation by herbal agents. A double-blind study in a medical university hospital involving a hepatitis B vaccine adjuvant model. *Fortschritte der Medizin, 120*(4), 119–123.

Cavendish, R., Konecny, L., Luise, B. K., & Lanza, M. (2004). Nurses enhance performance through prayer. *Holistic Nursing Practice, 18*(1), 26–31.

Cox, C., & Hayes, J. (1999a). Physiologic and psychodynamic responses to the administration of therapeutic touch in critical care. *Intensive and Critical Care Nursing, 15*(6), 363–368.

Cox, C., & Hayes, J. (1999b). Experiences of administering and receiving of therapeutic touch in intensive care. *Intensive and Critical Care Nursing, 15*(5), 283–287.

Das, S. (2005). The impotence of sympathy: Touch and trauma in the memoirs of the First World War nurses. *Textual Practice, 19*(2), 239–262.

Fugh-Berman, A. (1997). *Alternative medicine: What works.* Baltimore: Williams & Wilkins.

Gaskill, M. (2004). Forces of nature. Retrieved May 23, 2005, from http://www.nurseweek.com/news/features/04-08/alternative_print.html

Gregory, S., & Verdouw, J. (2005). Therapeutic touch: Its application for residents in aged care. *Australian Nursing Journal, 12*(7), 23–25.

Harris, W. S., Gowda, M., Kolb, J. W., Strychacz, C. P., Vacek, J. L., Jones, P. G., et al. (1999). A randomized, controlled trial of the effects of remote, intercessory prayer on outcomes in patients admitted to the coronary care unit. *Archives of Internal Medicine, 159*(19), 2273–2278.

Hayes, K. M., & Alexander, I. M. (2000). Alternative therapies and nurse practitioners: Knowledge, professional experience, and personal use. *Holistic Nursing Practice, 14*(3), 49–58.

Highfield, E. S., McLellan, M. C., Kemper, K. J., Risko, W., & Woolf, A. D. (2005). Integration of complementary and alternative medicine in a major pediatric teaching hospital: An initial overview. *Journal of Alternative and Complementary Medicine, 11*(2), 373–380.

Holt-Ashley, M. (2000). Nurses pray: Use of prayer and spirituality as a complementary therapy in the intensive care setting. *AACN Clinical Issues, 11*(1), 60–67.

Honda, K., & Jacobson, J. S. (2005). Use of complementary and alternative medicine among United States adults: The influences of personality, coping strategies, and social support. *Preventive Medicine, 40*(1), 46–53.

Ireland, M. (1998). Therapeutic touch with HIV-infected children: A pilot study. *Journal of the Association of Nurses in AIDS Care, 9*(4), 68–77.

Ireland, M., & Olson, M. (2000). Massage therapy and therapeutic touch in children: State of the science. *Alternative Therapies in Health and Medicine, 6*(5), 54–60, 62–63.

Jones, J. E., & Kassity, N. (2001). Varieties of alternative experience: Complementary care in the neonatal intensive care unit. *Clinical Obstetrics and Gynecology, 44*(4), 750–768.

Kowalak, J. P., & Mills, J. (2002). *Professional guide to complementary and alternative therapies.* Springhouse, PA: Springhouse.

Krucoff, M., Crater, S. W., Gallup, D., Blankenship, J. C., Cuffe, M, Guarneri, M., et al. (2005). Music, imagery, touch, and prayer as adjuncts to individual cardiac care: The monitoring and actualization of Noetic trainings (MANTRA) II randomized study. *Lancet, 336,* 211–218.

Krucoff, M. W., Crater, S. W., Green, C. L., Maas, A. C., Seskevich, J. E., Lane, J. D., et al. (2001). Integrative Noetic therapies as adjuncts to percutaneous intervention during unstable coronary syndromes: A monitoring and actualization of Noetic training (MANTRA) feasibility pilot. *American Heart Journal, 142*(5), 760–769.

Lau, J. T., Leung, P. C., Wong, E. L., Fong, C., Cheng, K. F., Zhang, S. C., et al. (2005). The use of an herbal formula by hospital care workers during the severe acute respiratory syndrome epidemic in Hong Kong to prevent severe acute respiratory syndrome transmission, relieve influenza-related symptoms, and improve quality of life: A prospective cohort study. *Journal of Alternative and Complementary Medicine, 11*(1), 49–55.

Lindquist, R., Tracy, M. F., Savik, K., & Watanuki, S. (2005). Regional use of complementary and alternative therapies by critical care nurses. *Critical Care Nurse, 25*(2), 63–75.

Mark, J. D., & Barton, L. L. (2001). Integrating complementary and alternative medicine with allopathic care in the neonatal intensive care unit. *Alternative Therapies in Health and Medicine, 7*(4), 134–135.

Meghani, N., Lindquist, R., & Tracy, M. F. (2003). Critical care nurses' desire to use complementary alternative modalities (CAM) in critical care and barriers to CAM use. *Dimensions of Critical Care Nursing, 22*(3), 138–144.

Moenkhoff, M., Baenziger, O., Fischer, J., & Fanconi, S. (1999). Parental attitude towards alternative medicine in the paediatric intensive care unit. *European Journal of Pediatrics, 158,* 12–17.

O'Brien King, M. (1999). Complementary, alternative, integrative: Have nurses kept pace with their clients? *MEDSURG Nursing, 8*(4), 249–256.

Pelletier, K. R. (2000). *The best alternative medicine.* New York: Simon & Schuster.

Richards, K., Nagel, C., Markie, M., Elwell, J., & Barone, C. (2003). Use of complementary and alternative therapies to promote sleep in critically ill patients. *Critical Care Nursing Clinics of North America, 15*(3), 329–340.

Sabatini, R. (2005). The effects of music twice daily on various outcomes in mechanically ventilated ICU patients: An AACN-funded study. *American Journal of Critical Care, 14*(3), 255.

Smith, L., Ernst, E., Ewings, P., Myers, P., & Smith, C. (2004). Co-ingestion of herbal medicines and warfarin. *British Journal of General Practice, 54*(503), 439–441.

Wahner-Roedler, D. L., Elkin, P. L., Vincent, A., Thompson, J. M., Oh, T. H., Loehrer, L. L., et al. (2005). Use of complementary and alternative medical therapies by patients referred to a fibromyalgia treatment program at a tertiary care center. *Mayo Clinic Proceedings, 80*(1), 55–50.

Wardell, D. W., & Weymouth, K. F. (2004). Review of studies of healing touch. *Journal of Nursing Scholarship, 36*(2), 147–154.

Woods, D. L., Craven R. F., & Whitney, J. (2005). The effect of therapeutic touch on behavioral symptoms in persons with dementia. *Alternative Therapies in Health and Medicine, 11*(1), 66–74.

Clinical
Judgment

PART IV

Cardiovascular

CHAPTER 10

Cardiac Anatomy and Physiology and Assessment

Deborah Becker

THE CARDIOVASCULAR SYSTEM

The roles of the cardiovascular system are to pump blood throughout the body to deliver oxygen to the cells, organs, muscles, and tissues; and to eliminate carbon dioxide. A basic understanding of the anatomy and physiology of the heart will assist the intensive care unit (ICU) nurse in correlating the physical findings with functioning of the heart.

The Heart

The adult heart is about the size of a closed fist and sits on the left side of the thorax in front of the lungs. The heart is a pump with four chambers: the right atrium (RA), the right ventricle (RV), the left atrium (LA), and the left ventricle (LV) (see **Figure 10-1**). The two atria are the upper chambers of the heart and are smaller in size than the ventricles. The two ventricles are the larger, lower chambers of the heart and are responsible for the pumping that the heart does. The left ventricular wall is about twice as thick as the right ventricular wall because it needs to generate enough force to pump the blood through the entire body, while the right ventricle needs to generate only enough force to pump the blood through the pulmonary vasculature (Guyton & Hall, 2006).

The heart also has four valves. The valve between the right atrium and the right ventricle is the tricuspid valve. The pulmonic valve is located between the right ventricle and the pulmonary artery. The valve between the left atrium and the left ventricle is known as the bicuspid or mitral valve, and the aortic valve is located between the left ventricle and aorta (see Figure 10-1). The triscuspid and mitral valves are collectively referred to as atrioventricular (AV) valves, based on their location in the heart. The AV valves have fibrous strands called chordae tendineae on their leaflets that attach to papillary muscles located on the respective ventricular walls (see Figure 10-1). When the ventricles contract, the papillary muscles also contract and generate enough pressure to prevent the valves from bulging back into the atria and becoming incompetent. The pulmonic and aortic valves, also known as the semilunar valves because of the shape of the valve leaflets, do not have chordae tendineae. All of the valves, under normal conditions, serve as gates controlling the flow of blood from one part of the heart to the next and ensuring that blood moves only in the forward direction (Guyton & Hall, 2006).

FIGURE 10-1 Anatomy of the Heart

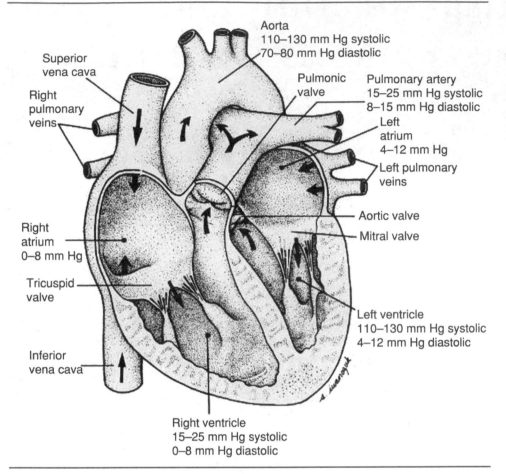

Aorta
110–130 mm Hg systolic
70–80 mm Hg diastolic

Superior
vena cava

Right
pulmonary
veins

Pulmonic
valve

Pulmonary artery
15–25 mm Hg systolic
8–15 mm Hg diastolic

Left
atrium
4–12 mm Hg

Left pulmonary
veins

Aortic valve

Mitral valve

Right
atrium
0–8 mm Hg

Tricuspid
valve

Left ventricle
110–130 mm Hg systolic
4–12 mm Hg diastolic

Inferior
vena cava

Right ventricle
15–25 mm Hg systolic
0–8 mm Hg diastolic

Source: Reprinted from Darovic: *Hemodynamic Monitoring,* 3/e, 2002, with permission from Elsevier.

The Cardiovascular System

The heart is connected to the vascular system, a network of arteries, arterioles, capillaries, venules, and veins that transport the blood from the heart to the rest of the body. The cardiovascular system is designed to transport oxygen and nutrients to the cells of the body and to remove carbon dioxide and metabolic waste products from the body. The cardiovascular system is made up of two major circulatory systems that act in concert. The right side of the heart pumps blood to the lungs through the pulmonary artery and pulmonary capillaries, and then returns the oxygenated blood to the left atrium through the pulmonary veins. The left side of the heart pumps blood from the heart to the rest of the body through the aorta, arteries, arterioles, and systemic capillaries, and then returns blood to the right atrium through the venules and the two great veins, the inferior and superior vena cavae (Guyton & Hall, 2006).

Basic Cardiac Physiology

A basic understanding of cardiac physiology is essential to interpreting the physical findings during a cardiac exam. Each beat of the heart consists of two phases: diastole and systole. During diastole, the ventricles are filling with blood from the atria. The atria are contracting so as much blood as possible can be moved to the ventricles. It is also during diastole that the coronary arteries become perfused with blood. During systole, the ventricles contract, moving blood forward to either the lungs or the rest of the body. During systole, the atria are relaxed and filling with blood. Diastole lasts longer so that ventricular and coronary artery filling may take place. This process repeats itself with each heartbeat (Guyton & Hall, 2006).

The nurse must also understand the physiology associated with the heart sounds of S_1, S_2, S_3, and S_4. S_1 occurs near the beginning of (ventricular) systole when the tricuspid and mitral valves close. The closing of these two valves and the increased pressure in the ventricular walls as they contract should occur simultaneously. Any splitting of the S_1 sound as the valves close should be considered pathological. S_2 occurs near the end of systole when the pulmonic and aortic valves close. The closing of these two valves occurs with beginning of backward flow in the pulmonary artery and aorta, respectively, as the ventricles relax. These two valves can close simultaneously or with a slight gap between them under normal physiologic circumstances. S_3 occurs at the end of the rapid filling period of the ventricle, during the beginning of diastole. S_3, if heard, should occur 120 to 170 milliseconds after S_2. S_4, if heard, corresponds to atrial contraction occurring at the end of ventricular diastole.

The entire cardiac cycle is often broken down into seven phases. These seven phases contain information on the aortic, left ventricular, and left atrial pressures, along with ventricular volume, heart sounds, and the electrocardiogram

(ECG) (Guyton & Hall, 2006). **Figure 10-2** is a visual depiction of the seven phases:

- Atrial contraction
- Isovolumetric contraction
- Rapid ejection
- Reduced ejection
- Isovolumetric relaxation
- Rapid filling
- Reduced filling

Circulation

It is important to understand blood flow through the heart so as to understand the overall function of the heart and to recognize how changes in electrical activity affect peripheral blood flow.

Deoxygenated blood from the body returns to the heart via the superior and inferior vena cavae and is emptied into the right atrium. The right atrium is extremely distensible (i.e., able to stretch to accommodate the volume of blood). Blood then moves through the triscupid valve into the right ventricle, which is also a highly distensible chamber. From the right ventricle, blood passes through the pulmonic valve, and into the pulmonary artery. It becomes oxygenated as it travels through the pulmonary circulation, contacting alveoli and exchanging gases. Blood then moves through the pulmonic vein into the left atrium, a chamber that is less distensible to the amount of blood returning to it but is nevertheless able to accommodate this volume. From the left atrium, blood travels through the mitral valve into the left ventricle. During systole, blood is pumped through the aortic valve, through the aorta and into the arteries, arterioles, and capillaries throughout the whole body.

Blood supply to the heart muscle itself occurs during diastole. Blood enters the coronary sulcus arising from the aorta where it enters both the right and left coronary arteries. The right and left coronary arteries branch into other arteries, arterioles, and capillaries that bring oxygen and nutrients to the muscle walls of the heart so it can function properly (Guyton & Hall, 2006).

Cardiac Output

Cardiac output is defined as the amount of blood ejected from the left ventricle per minute. Cardiac output is a product of stroke volume and heart rate. Stroke volume is the amount of blood ejected from the left ventricle with each heartbeat. Normal stroke volume is approximately 70 mL. Normal cardiac output ranges between 4 and 8 L/min.

FIGURE 10-2 The Cardiac Cycle

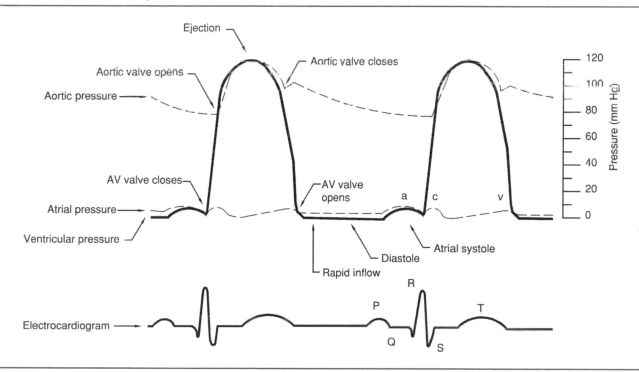

Source: Illustrated by James R. Perron.

Changes in the normal heartbeat can affect cardiac output. For example, when a patient becomes tachycardic (defined as a heart rate exceeding 100 beats per minute), the amount of time the left ventricle has to fill during diastole is lessened, which in turn diminishes the amount of stroke volume and leads to a reduction in cardiac output. An increase in heart rate also increases the workload of the heart and increases oxygen consumption. In contrast, bradycardia (defined as a heart rate of less than 60 beats per minute) allows for more filling of the ventricle to occur. However, the left ventricle fills only during the first two-thirds of diastole. Therefore, more time does not make a difference and can result in a reduction in cardiac output (Guyton & Hall, 2006). (Dysrhythmias will be discussed later in this chapter.)

Nervous System Innervation of the Heart

Two branches of the autonomic nervous system supply the heart— the sympathetic system and the parasympathetic system. Nervous system innervation provides adrenergic and cholinergic responses by the heart as the body's needs change.

The sympathetic nervous system responds to the body's needs for more movement and action. By increasing the heart rate, contractility of the heart muscle, automaticity of the pacemaker cells of the heart, and AV nodal conduction, the body appropriately responds to situations that require the fight-or-flight response.

The parasympathetic nervous system responds to situations where the body needs to reduce its rate of movement and action. Parasympathetic nervous system innervation causes the heart rate to slow down and reduces the rate of conduction of the AV node.

Electrophysiology

Two types of cardiac cells exist: electrical and myocardial. Electrical cells are distributed throughout the heart in an orderly fashion and make up the conduction system of the heart. The electrical cells possess specific properties that assist in generating and conducting the electrical impulse throughout the heart—namely, automaticity, excitability, and conductivity. Automaticity is the ability of the cell to spontaneously generate and discharge an electric impulse. Excitability is the ability of the cell to respond to an electrical impulse. Conductivity is the ability of the cell to transmit an electrical impulse to another cell (Guyton & Hall, 2006).

Depolarization and Repolarization

Cardiac cells, when at rest, are considered to be polarized, meaning that no electrical activity is occurring. The cell membrane of the cardiac cell separates different concentrations of ions, such as sodium, potassium, and calcium; this state is called the resting potential. Once an electrical cell generates an electrical impulse (through the property of automaticity of the specialized cardiac cells), the impulse causes the ions to cross the cell membrane and produces an action potential. This change in cell electronegativity is known as depolarization. The movement of the ions across the cell membrane through the sodium, potassium, and calcium channels is the impetus for the cardiac cells and muscle. Depolarization with corresponding contraction of the myocardial muscle moves as a wave through the heart. Once the cell has been depolarized, the ions then return to their previous resting state, a process known as repolarization. This phase correlates to the relaxation of the myocardial muscle.

The movement of ions across the cell membrane generates a new action potential curve with each electrical impulse received. **Figure 10-3** shows the action potential with its five phases of 0 to 4. Phase 4 is the resting phase, when the cell is ready to receive an electrical stimulus. Phase 0 is characterized by a tall upstroke. During this phase, the cell receives an impulse, depolarizes, and begins to contract. In phase 1, contraction occurs and the cell begins an early, rapid, partial repolarization. Phase 2 is the plateau phase; contraction is completed and the cell begins to relax and repolarizes during

FIGURE 10-3 The Action Potential, Phases 0–4

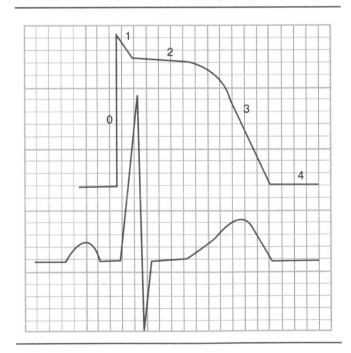

this phase. Phase 3 is the downslope, the final phase of rapid repolarization. Phase 4 is the resting phase, the period between action potentials when the cell is ready to receive an electrical stimulus and start the cycle all over again (Guyton & Hall, 2006).

Refractory and Supernormal Periods

The absolute refractory period is the period in which no stimulus, no matter how strong, can cause another depolarization. The onset of phase 0 begins the absolute refractory period, and it extends midway through phase 3. This period corresponds to the onset of the Q wave and ends at the peak of the T wave of the ECG tracing. The relative refractory period, also known as the vulnerable period of repolarization, is when the cell is partially repolarized. During this period, a very strong stimulus could cause the cell to become depolarized again, even though the cell has not completely repolarized. This period correlates with the second half of phase 3 and corresponds to the downslope of the T wave of the ECG.

A supernormal period can occur briefly from the very end of phase 3 into the early part of phase 4. During the supernormal period, a weaker than normal stimulus can cause a depolarization. On the ECG, this corresponds to the end of the T wave, just before the cell returns to its resting potential. The supernormal period is not a normal period in a healthy heart. Figure 10-3 shows the action potential and its relationship to the ECG tracing.

DYSRHYTHMIA INTERPRETATION

The ECG is the highly useful recording of electrical impulses produced and conducted by cardiac cells. The cardiac impulse produces a weak electrical current that spreads through the entire body and can be recorded on the body surface. An ECG tracing can reveal the anatomical location of the heart; chamber size; rhythm and conduction disturbances; extent, location, and progression of a myocardial infarction; electrolyte dis-

turbances; and drug effects. It cannot tell us about the mechanical performance of the heart, however. The 12-lead ECG should always be interpreted in conjunction with the clinical findings. The ECG strip generated by a monitor can provide a snapshot of what is happening in the heart. If a change is noted on a strip, a 12-lead ECG should be obtained and should be correlated to physical findings.

Electrode Placement and Skin Care

To ensure accurate and high-quality rhythm strips for interpretation, proper lead placement is essential; see **Figure 10-4**. It is important not to place the electrodes on ribs, the clavicle, tendons, or major muscle mass, because a poor-quality tracing will result. Optimal placement is on the intercostal spaces. Electrodes must adhere completely to the skin. It may be necessary to shave hair at the site for electrode placement. If artifact still appears on the tracing and electrodes are adhering well to the skin, the electrodes should be removed, the skin cleansed by rubbing briskly with alcohol, and the electrodes replaced.

FIGURE 10-4 Placement of ECG Leads

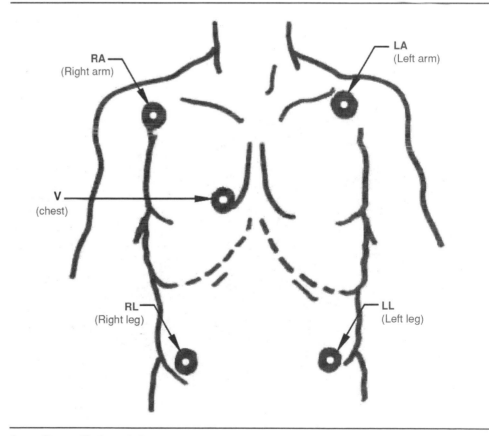

Source: Illustrated by James R. Perron.

Conduction System

The conduction system consists of five components:

- Sinoatrial (SA) node
- AV node
- Bundle of His
- Right and left bundle branches
- Purkinje fibers

As shown in **Figure 10-5**, the SA node is located in the upper wall of the right atrium near the inlet of the superior vena cava. It consists of cells specialized for automaticity or self-excitation. The SA node, which is also referred to as the dominant or primary pacemaker of the heart, discharges at an inherent rate of 60 to 100 times per minute (Guyton & Hall, 2006).

Intra-atrial tracts of nervous tissue extend from the SA node throughout the atria. The tract extending from the SA node to the left atrium is called Bachmann's bundle. Once an impulse is initiated, it is conducted through the atria. The muscle cells then depolarize and produce a P wave on the ECG.

Under normal circumstances, electrical activity is followed by muscle contraction—in this case, contraction of the right and left atria. The impulse moves down the intra-atrial pathways to the AV node.

The AV node and bundle of His make up the AV junction. The AV node is located in the bottom of the right atrium near the interatrial septum. Its major function is to triage atrial signals for transmission to ventricles, allowing only the strongest stimuli to pass and delaying ventricular excitation to allow for adequate ventricular filling. In the ECG, this delay in electrical activity is represented by the isoelectric line following the P wave and before the QRS complex. Although the nodal tissue itself has no pacemaker cells, the tissue surrounding it, known as junctional tissue, contains latent pacemaker cells that can fire at an inherent rate of 40 to 60 beats per minute. If the SA node fails to generate an electrical impulse, the junctional tissue could stimulate the heart to beat.

The bundle of His is located below the AV node, is part of the AV junction, and extends into the ventricles next to the interventricular septum. The main function of the bundle of His is to rapidly conduct the impulse through the ventricles. The bundle of His ultimately divides into right and left bundle branches.

The bundle branches are located in the intraventricular system. The right bundle branch extends into the right ventricle and sends the impulse to the Purkinje fibers located deep in the wall of the right ventricle. The left bundle branch splits off from the right bundle branch and goes through the intraventricular system on the left side. The left bundle branch has two distinct fascicles: the anterior and the posterior. Because of the size of the left ventricle and the need for the ventricles to depolarize simultaneously, the two fascicles are able to send the electrical impulses faster and more efficiently to the Purkinje fibers of the left ventricle.

Purkinje fibers extend from the bundle branches deep into the ventricular muscle. Once the

FIGURE 10-5 The Conduction System

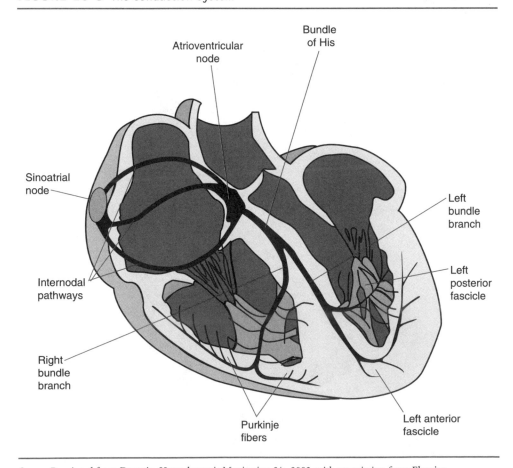

Source: Reprinted from Darovic: *Hemodynamic Monitoring*, 3/e, 2002, with permission from Elsevier.

impulse reaches the Purkinje fibers, ventricular depolarization occurs with subsequent ventricular contraction. The impulse transmission down the ventricular conduction system is recorded as the QRS complex on the ECG. As discussed earlier, the repolarization of the cells follows this phase, resulting in ventricular relaxation and producing a T wave on the ECG. The ventricular system also contains cells that are capable of automaticity. The inherent discharge rate in the ventricles is less than 40 beats per minute. If both the SA and AV nodes failed to fire, the ventricles should generate a heartbeat (Guyton & Hall, 2006).

Configuration of the Normal ECG

The electrical impulse generated in the SA node is conducted throughout the heart, causing the cells to depolarize and subsequently repolarize. These changes in electronegativity produce corresponding changes throughout the body. The cardiac monitor, through the use of leads placed on the skin, can detect these changes. As the impulse travels through the heart, electrical signals are transmitted through the skin (Thaler, 2003).

As the impulse travels from the SA node through the intra-atrial pathways and Bachmann's bundle to the AV node, the cells are depolarized. This depolarization of the atria is represented by the P wave on the ECG. If a P wave is not present or is abnormally shaped, it implies either that the impulse was not generated by the SA node or that something has altered the intra-atrial pathways (Thaler, 2003). Once the impulse reaches the AV node, it is held there until the ventricles are ready to receive the impulse. The period from the beginning of the P wave to the beginning of the QRS complex is designated the PR interval; it represents the time it takes for the impulse to reach the ventricles. Normally the PR interval is 0.12 to 0.20 second.

As the impulse reaches the bundle of His and is transmitted down the bundle branches and Purkinje fibers, a QRS complex is generated. From where the Q wave leaves the baseline to the point where the complex returns to baseline is referred to as the ventricular or QRS complex. The time it takes to transmit the impulse through the ventricle resulting in depolarization is normally 0.04 to 0.12 second. A longer time period would indicate a change from the normal transmission of the signal through the ventricles (Thaler, 2003).

The QRS complex is made up of two or three waves: the Q wave, the R wave, and the S wave. The Q wave may or may not be present in a normal ECG tracing; it is defined as the first negatively deflected wave after the PR interval. The R wave is defined as the first positively deflected wave after the PR interval. The S wave is defined as the negatively deflected wave that follows the first positive deflection. The R^1 wave is the second positive deflection, and the S^1 wave is the second negative deflection. When a complex consists exclusively of a Q wave, it is called QS even though there is no downward S wave. The term "QRS complex" is also used as a collective noun to describe the ventricular complex despite the waves that actually compose it (Thaler, 2003).

The ST segment is the interval occurring at the end of the QRS complex and the beginning of the T wave. This segment represents complete depolarization of the ventricles and the beginning of repolarization. Generally this segment is fairly isoelectric or flat. If a deviation greater than 0.5 mm from baseline is noted, an abnormality exists and may indicate cardiac ischemia.

The T wave represents the repolarization phase of the ventricles. Typically the T wave is deflected in the same direction as the majority of the QRS complex, meaning that if the QRS is mainly positively deflected, the T wave should likewise be positively deflected. The QT interval represents the total duration of ventricular depolarization and repolarization. It is measured from the end of the PR interval to where the T wave returns to baseline. A normal QT interval ranges from 0.42 to 0.48 second. The QT interval varies with age, gender, and heart rate. It shortens with tachycardia, lengthens with bradycardia, and may also vary due to drug effects. An additional wave, the U wave, may be found after the T wave; it is deflected in the same direction as the T wave. The U wave is seen with potassium deficiency and may be noted when the heart rate is slow enough for it to be picked up by the monitor (Thaler, 2003).

Ectopic Beats and Dysrhythmias

Any cardiac impulse originating from other than the SA node is considered abnormal and is referred to as an ectopic beat. Ectopic beats can originate in the atria, the AV junction, or the ventricles. They are named based on their point of origin. For example, a beat generated from the ventricle is called a premature ventricular complex (PVC). Sometimes after an ectopic beat occurs, there may a compensatory delay as the heart recovers.

Ectopic beats occur for two reasons. The first reason is the premature activation of another cardiac cell. Impulses may occur prematurely before the sinus node recovers enough to initiate another beat; these beats are called premature beats and are named for the area of the heart from which the beat originated. Increased automaticity, reentry, or retrograde conduction can produce premature beats. A dysrhythmia can occur if a cell's automaticity is increased or decreased. Reentry and retrograde conduction are discussed in depth later.

The second reason why ectopic beats may occur is an abnormality of the conduction system. Cells capable of automaticity may start discharging impulses that are perceived by the rest of the heart as coming from the pacemaker. This site then takes over control.

In cases where the SA node firing is excessively slow or fails altogether, cells from areas of ectopic beats serving a protective function initiate a cardiac impulse before prolonged cardiac standstill can occur. These beats, which are referred to as escape beats, fill in for the failed SA node. If they did not beat, there would be no rhythm at all. When analyzing a rhythm strip, a delay before the escape beat occurs would be present. This delay shows that the ectopic site was expecting the SA node to fire, but when the SA node did not fire, this site took over. If the SA node fails to resume function, the ectopic site will assume the role of the pacemaker and sustain a cardiac rhythm, referred to as an escape rhythm.

As mentioned earlier, reentry and retrograde conduction may cause ectopic beats to occur. In reentry, re-excitation of a previously depolarized region of cardiac tissue occurs when a single impulse continues for one or more cycles, sometimes resulting in ectopic beats or tachyarrhythmias (Thaler, 2003). In retrograde conduction, an impulse generated from below the AV node is transmitted backward toward the AV node. This conduction usually takes longer than normal and can cause the atria and ventricles to be out of synchronization with the other (Thaler).

Sinus Disturbances

Sinus rhythm is the normal rhythm generated by the SA node and conducted normally through the conduction system, at a rate between 60 and 100 beats per minute. A rate faster than 100 beats per minute is referred to as tachycardia; a rate below 60 beats per minute is said to be bradycardic. Sometimes, slight variations in the rate of sinus rhythm can occur relative to respiratory cycle. The rate increases with inspiration and decreases with expiration, for example. This kind of sinus arrhythmia typically occurs without any significance. **Figure 10-6** shows sinus rhythm, sinus bradycardia, and sinus tachycardia.

Sinus pause or sinus arrest can occur when the SA node fails to initiate an impulse for a period of time. Sinus pause is said to occur when the SA node fails to fire for a short period of time, usually less than 3 seconds in duration. If the duration is greater than 3 seconds, then the lack of SA node firing is referred to as sinus arrest. In either case, it is important to remember that no ventricular contraction is occurring and, therefore, no blood pressure is being generated. The patient may complain of lightheadedness and dizziness from this loss of circulation. If it lasts too long, the patient may develop cardiac arrest. If the patient is symptomatic, a pacemaker may be needed (Thaler, 2003).

FIGURE 10-6 (a) Normal Sinus Rhythm; (b) Sinus Bradycardia; (c) Sinus Tachycardia

(a)

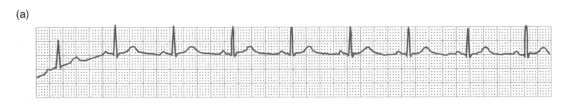

(b)

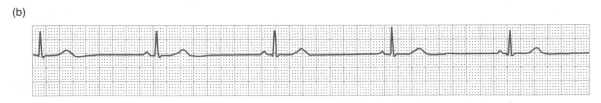

(c)

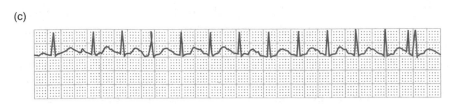

Atrial Dysrhythmias

An irritable focus in the atria may release a stimulus that is conducted through the AV node and into the ventricles prematurely. This is known as a premature atrial contraction (PAC). When analyzing the rhythm strip, a PAC appears as a beat that occurs earlier than expected and has a P wave that is either normal or different in contour. Occasionally a PAC can continue to fire at a rapid rate greater than 150 beats per minute; this situation is referred to as atrial tachycardia. In this case, the P wave can still be distinguished, but again its contour appears different than that of normal sinus rhythm (Thaler, 2003).

When the SA node is replaced by an extremely irritable focus in the atrium that stimulates the atria to contract between 200 to 360 times per minute, the situation is referred to as atrial flutter. In atrial flutter, the atrial wave generated by this rapid firing is no longer referred to as a P wave, but now appears to be saw-tooth in nature and is called a flutter wave. The ventricle usually does not respond to such a rapid rate due in part to the AV node doing its job and due in part to the ventricular response being blocked so that it is one-half or one-fourth of the atrial rate (Thaler, 2003).

On occasion, the atria may become so irritable that multiple foci in the atrium begin to fire impulses at rates between 300 and 600 times per minute. The atrial activity is chaotic in

this case, and no distinguishable P waves can be found. The ventricular rate in response to the rapid atrial activity becomes variable. This rhythm is referred to as atrial fibrillation. If the ventricular rate is greater than 100 beats per minute, it is referred to as uncontrolled atrial fibrillation; however, if the rate is between 60 and 100 beats per minute, it is considered controlled. **Figure 10-7** shows supraventricular tachycardia, atrial fibrillation, and atrial flutter rhythm strips.

Junctional Dysrhythmias

In the event that the SA node does not fire, the AV junctional tissue may replace the pacemaker activity of the SA node. The inherent rate of the AV junctional tissue is between 40 and 60 beats per minute. The location in the AV junctional tissue where the impulse is generated will determine whether a P wave is noted on the ECG strip. The P wave may be (1) upright; (2) inverted, indicating that the impulse came from low in the AV junctional tissue and thereby depolarized the atria in a retrograde fashion; or (3) indistinguishable, indicating that it occurred at the same time the QRS wave was generated. Because the ventricle is a larger chamber, the QRS wave is dominant and the P wave is buried in the QRS complex. Junctional rhythms can be either bradycardic or tachycardic. If the rhythm is below the inherent rate of 40 beats per minute, then it is referred to as junctional

FIGURE 10-7 (a) Supraventricular Tachycardia; (b) Atrial Fibrillation; (c) Atrial Flutter

(a)

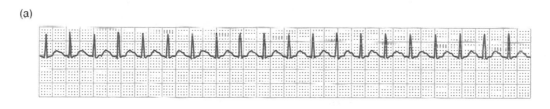

(b)

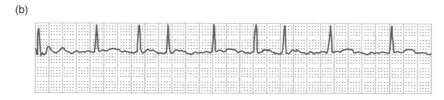

(c)

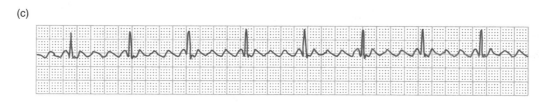

bradycardia. If the rate is greater than 60 beats per minute, it is referred to as junctional tachycardia (Thaler, 2003).

Premature junctional contractions (PJC) may also occur. In this case, the ectopic site is located in the AV junctional tissue. The site fires earlier than the next sinus beat is expected, and depolarization of the atria and ventricle occurs. If, however, the SA node does not fire when expected and the AV node notices that an impulse was not generated, the AV node may initiate a stimulus. In such a case, the junctional beat occurs later than normal and is referred to as an escape beat. This beat attempts to maintain the patient's hemodynamic status. If this beat were not generated, sinus pause or sinus arrest could occur (Thaler, 2003).

Occasionally, sites in both the atria and the junctional tissue become irritable and stimulate impulses. In this case, the rhythm strip will show complexes that are generated from the variety of ectopic sites. This rhythm is referred to as wandering atrial pacemaker (Thaler, 2003). **Figure 10-8** shows premature junctional contraction, a junctional rhythm, and an accelerated junctional rhythm.

Ventricular Dysrhythmias

An irritable site in the ventricle may generate an impulse that stimulates the myocardium prematurely. Because this impulse is generated below the AV node, the atria are not stimulated and, therefore, no P wave is noted nor does atrial contraction occur. Because the ectopic site is not part of the conduction system, the impulse is generated from cell to cell, taking longer to depolarize the ventricular tissue. Hence, the shape of the QRS widens and duration of the QRS complex increases. Sometimes PVCs occur in patterns. Bigeminy, trigeminy, and quadrageminy are PVCs that occur every second, third, and fourth beat, respectively. PVCs that occur in groups of two are referred to as pairs or couplets; those occurring in groups of three are referred to as triplets.

Similar to the junctional tissue, ventricular cells may fire when they notice that an impulse from above was supposed to fire, but did not. In this case, the site is again trying to maintain hemodynamic stability. The ventricular beat generated is referred to as a ventricular escape beat. The inherent rate for an idioventricular rhythm is 20 to 40 beats per minute. An accelerated idioventricular rhythm has a rate of 40 to 100 beats per minute.

In some cases, ventricular ectopic sites may become extremely irritable and begin to fire at rates greater than 100 beats per minute, assuming the work of the SA node. In this case, the ventricular focus usually takes over at a rate greater than 140 beats per minute. This rhythm is referred to as ventricular tachycardia. Ventricular tachycardia may cause the patient to become lightheaded and dizzy and, in some cases, to enter cardiac arrest. These effects mostly occur because the atria are not providing the blood volume to the ventricles as they do in sinus

FIGURE 10-8 (a) Premature Junctional Contraction; (b) Junctional Rhythm; (c) Accelerated Junctional Rhythm

(a)

(b)

(c)

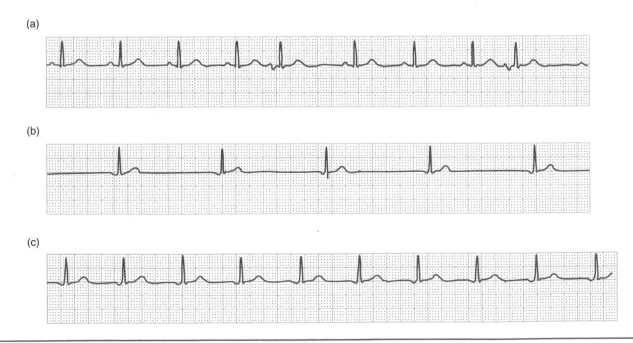

rhythm. This loss of coordinated atrial contraction is often referred to as loss of atrial kick. The result may be a 20% to 30% loss of cardiac output, which in many cases may cause patients to become symptomatic (Darovic, 2004).

An extremely rapid, regular ventricular rhythm that does not allow for adequate perfusion is ventricular flutter. Ventricular flutter is often seen as a transitional rhythm from ventricular tachycardia to ventricular fibrillation. In ventricular flutter, the ventricular rate ranges between 150 and 300 beats per minute. At this rate, a significant loss of cardiac output is experienced.

If left to continue, or in some cases occurring without progression from a less significant ventricular dysrhythmia, ventricular fibrillation is rapid, chaotic ventricular activity that does not allow for adequate perfusion. It is often seen as irregular undulations of varying configuration and amplitude on the ECG. This rhythm is accompanied by loss of consciousness, apnea, and pulselessness. If treatment is not provided immediately, death may ensue within 3 to 5 minutes.

In some instances, there may be an absence of any rhythm or beats. This situation is referred to as cardiac arrest, cardiac standstill, or asystole. The rhythm is noted to have no QRS complexes and appears to be a finely undulating line going across the paper on the ECG. This rhythm is accompanied by loss of consciousness, apnea, and pulselessness, and it may lead to death if left untreated. **Figure 10-9** shows premature ventricular contractions, ventricular escape rhythm, ventricular tachycardia, and ventricular fibrillation rhythm strips.

Atrioventricular Heart Blocks

Sometimes the AV node abnormally delays the sinus impulse, a delay referred to as AV block. The most benign case is first-degree AV block, in which the sinus impulse is delayed at a constant duration. The PR interval is greater than 0.20 second in duration throughout the rhythm. Conduction through the ventricles is normal (Thaler, 2003).

There are two types of second-degree heart blocks: Mobitz Type I, also known as Wenckebach, and Mobitz Type II. In Mobitz Type I, the sinus impulses are increasingly delayed each time they pass through the AV node, until finally an impulse is completely blocked and not conducted to the ventricles. This type of block is characterized by a progressive prolongation of the PR interval until a ventricular complex is dropped. Then the cycle repeats itself. Although it is typically considered a minor dysrhythmia, Mobitz Type I can be a precursor to Mobitz Type II or to complete heart block.

FIGURE 10-9 (a) Premature Ventricular Contraction; (b) Ventricular Tachycardia; (c) Ventricular Fibrillation

(a)

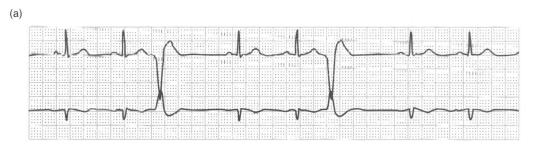

(b)

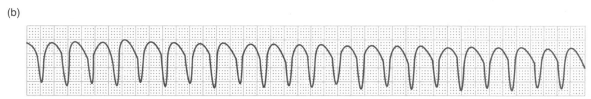

(c)

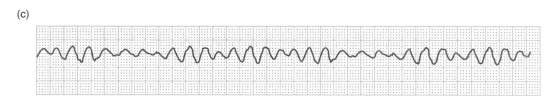

Second-degree heart block, type II (Mobitz Type II), occurs when the sinus impulse is consistently blocked as it passes through the AV node. Cyclically, a sinus impulse is completely blocked at the AV junction, preventing its conduction into the ventricles. This type of block is characterized by a constant PR interval with P waves that are periodically not conducted to the ventricles. This unstable rhythm may lead to third-degree or complete heart block when the loss of ventricular contraction leads to hemodynamic instability.

Third-degree or complete heart block occurs when every sinus impulse is blocked at the level of the AV node, causing the atria and ventricles to beat independently of each other. This type of block is characterized by a regular atrial rhythm occurring independently of either a junctional or a ventricular rhythm. The ECG strip appears to have both P waves and QRS complexes marching across the paper at regular rates. Because there is no synchronization of the atria with the ventricles, however, the result is a significant reduction in cardiac output and slow pulse (Thaler, 2003). This situation is considered an emergency and often requires placement of a pacemaker. **Figure 10-10** shows rhythm strips of the heart block rhythms.

Understanding the functioning of the conduction system and the complications that can potentially occur when dysrhythmias arise is instrumental to understanding the significance of physical assessment findings related to heart rhythm and cardiac output.

CARDIAC ASSESSMENT

Cardiac assessment not only includes checking vital signs and pulses, but also includes obtaining a health history, identifying risk factors, and performing a thorough cardiovascular physical examination. ICU nurses who accurately perform a cardiac assessment are able to connect the anatomy and physiology to the findings obtained on the physical assessment and in the health history. This skill takes time and practice to achieve.

FIGURE 10-10 (a) First-Degree AV Block; (b) Second-Degree AV Block, Type I; (c) Type I Wenckebach; (d) Third-Degree AV Block

(a)

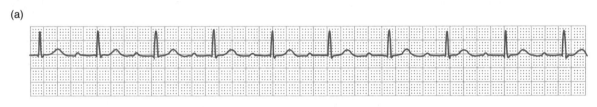

(b)

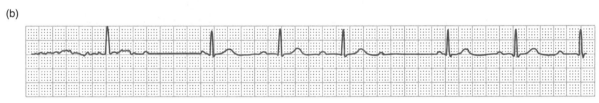

(c)

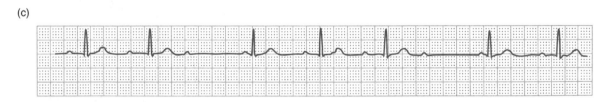

(d)

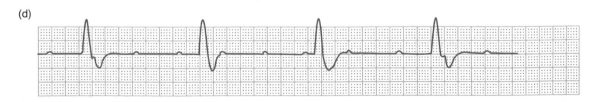

Source: Illustrated by James R. Perron.

Health History

Obtaining a health history is the first step in performing the cardiac assessment. Information regarding the patient's chief complaint, symptoms, and history of present illness are important to obtain to help the ICU nurse understand why the patient sought medical care. Included in the health history are the patient's past medical history, family history, social history, list of medications, and presence of any allergies. Several barriers may potentially impede the ability to obtain a complete and accurate health history. If the patient is unable to respond to questions, family members, significant others, friends, other care providers, the patient's primary physician, and old medical records may be able to provide essential information.

Identification of Risk Factors

An essential part of the cardiac assessment is identification of risk factors for coronary artery disease. Risk factors are classified as modifiable or nonmodifiable and are described in detail in Chapter 12. These risk factors should be considered during the cardiac assessment.

Signs and Symptoms of Cardiovascular Disease

It is extremely important that the ICU nurse be able to recognize the signs and symptoms of cardiovascular disease. Although cardiac disease is not always the cause of the symptom, cardiovascular reasons must always be considered because of the vital role the cardiovascular system plays in maintaining the well-being of an individual. **Table 10-1** lists common signs and symptoms associated with cardiac disease. When obtaining information regarding the symptoms exhib-

TABLE 10–1 Signs and Symptoms of Cardiac Disease

Chest discomfort: pain, squeezing, pressure, weight on chest, tightness (not always present in women)

Shortness of breath

Diaphoresis

Pain radiating to left arm or jaw, or back

Lightheadedness or dizziness

Nausea, vomiting, or both

Palpitations

Fatigue (more common in women)

Inability to perform activities of daily living (more common in women)

ited by the patient, it is important to gather details regarding the onset, duration, characteristics, associated symptoms, precipitating factors, and factors alleviating the symptoms to assist in determining the cause of the patient's complaint (Bicking & Szilagyi, 2004).

Physical Examination

The physical examination of a patient with a cardiovascular-related complaint must be performed in a systematic manner so as not to skip any important elements. Following are the components of this systematic review, including explanations of each element's importance and how to perform it.

General Appearance

Observation of the patient's general appearance begins upon meeting the patient and continues throughout the physical examination. Note the patient's overall skin color, posture, level of consciousness, grooming, and amount of distress. Obtaining the patient's height and weight is the next step; this information allows drug calculations and fluid requirements to be performed if necessary.

Vital Signs

Measurement of vital signs includes obtaining a temperature, blood pressure, pulse rate, and respiratory rate. Temperature in the cardiac patient may provide a picture of how much work the patient must do to maintain the current hemodynamic status.

Assess the patient's pulse rate and quality. If the patient's heart rate is irregular, auscultate an apical rate for a full minute while palpating a peripheral pulse. Determine whether all impulses auscultated are being perfused to the periphery. Patients with atrial fibrillation or premature beats, such as premature ventricular contractions, may not perfuse every beat, thereby resulting in a pulse rate less than the apical rate auscultated. This difference is referred to as the pulse deficit.

Measuring blood pressure should be done in both arms. A difference of 5 to 10 mm Hg is acceptable. Usually, the higher blood pressure is the one recorded. A difference of greater than 10 mm Hg between arms may indicate arterial obstruction or occlusion to the side with the lower reading. A significant difference in blood pressure measurement between each arm is often seen in patients with an aortic aneurysm or dissection (Seidel, Ball, Dains, & Benedict, 2003).

Occasionally blood pressure or Korotkoff sounds are not easily heard. In this case, a Doppler device may be used to listen to the sounds and obtain the measurement. Only the systolic measurement can be obtained via this method.

Orthostatic blood pressure measurements are taken with the patient lying down, sitting up, and standing. They are indicated when patients complain of lightheadedness, dizziness, vertigo, or syncope upon standing or position change. Orthostatic hypotension is said to be present if a 20 mm Hg drop in systolic pressure and an increase in heart rate are associated with a postural change. Orthostatic blood pressure measurements are taken first with the patient in the supine position. Wait 2 to 3 minutes after each position change before taking the next blood pressure measurement. With each blood pressure measurement, record a pulse rate as well. If the patient does not tolerate a change in position, return the patient to the previous position and record the symptoms observed by you and reported by the patient (Rushing, 2005).

Skin

Color.   Color of the skin and mucous membranes is assessed to determine the presence of cyanosis, pallor, jaundice, or redness. Cyanosis is a bluish color that indicates less than optimal oxygenation. It can be classified as peripheral or central. When assessing for peripheral cyanosis, examine the extremities, nail beds, and nose. Causes of peripheral cyanosis include heart failure, shock, exposure to cold, and anxiety. To assess for central cyanosis, examine the mucous membranes, lips, and conjunctivae (areas that are typically warm and well perfused). Causes of central cyanosis include congenital right-to-left shunts. Patients with darker skin may be more difficult to assess for color changes. Therefore, it is suggested that conjunctivae, sclerae, buccal mucosa, tongue, lips, nail beds, palms, and soles of the feet be assessed (Seidel et al., 2003).

Temperature and Moisture.   When assessing the patient's perfusion state, it is important to touch the patient's skin and assess for both temperature and moisture level. Assess the bilateral upper and lower extremities simultaneously, comparing perfusion of the right and left sides of the body. Skin temperature is usually evaluated as cold, cool, normal, warm, or hot.

Capillary Refill.   Another way of evaluating arterial circulation is by compressing the nail bed, causing it to blanch, releasing it, and then timing how long it takes for the nail bed to pink up again. Normal capillary refill usually occurs within 2 seconds.

Carotid Arteries

Inspection.   The patient is first placed in the supine position with the head of the bed at a 30° angle. The neck is inspected for signs of visible pulsations. A pulsating mass or bulge may be an indication of a kinked carotid artery.

Palpation.   Next the carotid artery is palpated. This is done by standing on the same side of the patient for which the artery will be palpated. The arterial pulsation is found by locating the thyroid cartilage and sliding the fingers down the side of the neck about halfway between the thyroid cartilage and the sternocleidomastoid muscle. Because applying too much pressure on the carotid artery may cause vagal nerve stimulation, resulting in a decrease in heart rate, the carotid artery is palpated on the lower portion of the neck. Additionally, both carotid arteries are never palpated at the same time, because this may cause a reduction in blood flow to the brain. Upon palpation, attention should be paid to the quality of the pulsation, noting whether the pulse is full, bounding, or weak. If a thrill (a vibrating feeling much like that of a purring cat) is noted, it may indicate the presence of arterial narrowing.

Auscultation.   Auscultation of the carotid artery should be performed when patients are suspected of having cardiac or cerebrovascular disease. A carotid bruit is said to be present if a sound much like that of a murmur, but produced by turbulent blood flow in the vessel, is heard. A bruit is an indication of arterial narrowing.

Jugular Veins

The neck veins are normally flat when the patient is sitting erect, but may become visible when the patient is supine. Jugular venous distention is an abnormal finding indicating that the central venous pressure is elevated. Because of the presence of valves, which prevent backflow of blood, venous distention may be present when central venous pressure is normal.

To assess the patient for jugular venous distention, stand to the right of the patient. Place the patient supine with the head of the bed at a 30° angle. Keep the patient's neck in a relaxed position but slightly turned to the left. Expose the patient's neck area and chest so that the sternal notch or Angle of Louis is visible. Identify the external and internal jugular veins. The external jugular vein lies superficially and is typically easier to visualize than the internal jugular vein. The internal jugular vein lies anterior to the external jugular vein and parallel to the carotid artery and trachea. Upon finding the internal jugular vein, note the highest point where pulsations are found (Bicking & Szilagyi, 2004).

Heart

The examination of the heart is performed with the patient lying supine, with the head of the bed at a 30° angle and with the examiner to the right of the patient. The patient's chest should be exposed. It is important to respect the patient's privacy and to attempt to keep the patient as covered as possible without interfering with the examination.

Inspection.   Inspect the patient's precordium for pulsations, and attempt to visualize the point of maximal impulse (PMI) or area of apical impulse. These pulsations may be seen more easily with the use of tangential light. The PMI should be located in the fifth intercostal space (ICS) at the mid-clavicular line. Locating the PMI allows for an approximation of the size of the heart. If the heart is enlarged, then a displacement of the PMI is expected. The PMI, if visualized, is the only normal pulsation to be found on the precordium. Any additional pulsations should be identified and described by using anatomical reference lines and intercostal spaces. Identifying their location provides insight into the possible cause of the abnormality. For instance, a lift or heave of the left sternal border indicates right ventricular hypertrophy.

Palpation.   Palpate the patient's precordium for pulsations and thrills, using the palm of your hand and fingertips. Systematically palpate key areas of the chest that correspond to key areas of the underlying heart. **Figure 10-11** indicates the five key areas of palpation. Palpation should begin at the second ICS, right sternal border; progress to the second ICS, left sternal border (LSB); then to Erb's point at the third intercostal space, LSB; then to the fifth ICS, LSB; and then to the fifth ICS, mid-clavicular line, where the PMI is located. The last area palpated should be the epigastric area. While palpating, note any pulsations or vibrations. If any is felt, describe the sensation and the location where it was found. As mentioned earlier, a thrill is a vibratory sensation usually caused by the turbulent flow of blood through diseased valves, whereas pulsations are felt as tapping sensations (Seidel et al., 2003).

The PMI is a normal pulsation usually felt as a tapping sensation, approximately 2 cm in diameter. If the left ventricle is hypertrophied or the entire heart is enlarged, the PMI may be displaced, indicating the change in the heart's size. A medial shift of the PMI may be present with a downward shift in the diaphragm, as seen with chronic obstructive pulmonary disease or left-to-right mediastinal shifts.

Auscultation.   After inspecting and palpating, the next step is auscultation of the heart. Although it is often tempting to auscultate the heart from the beginning of the examination, valuable information would be lost without the inspection and palpation of the precordial area. Both the bell and the diaphragm of the stethoscope are used to auscultate the heart.

The bell of the stethoscope is used to hear low-pitched sounds (S_3, S_4, and diastolic murmurs due to ventricular filling) and should be pressed lightly against the chest wall. The diaphragm of the stethoscope is used to hear high-pitched sounds (S_1, S_2, and murmurs due to stenosis) and should be pressed firmly against the chest wall. It is important not to press the bell of the stethoscope too firmly against the skin; otherwise, it will act as a diaphragm and block out the low-pitched sounds (Bicking & Szilagyi, 2004).

Auscultation of the heart is performed in the same five areas of the heart as mentioned earlier. Beginning in the aortic area and progressing through the pulmonic area, Erb's point, the tricuspid area, and mitral area, auscultation should concentrate first on listening for normal heart sounds and then on detecting heart murmurs. At each of the five areas, time

FIGURE 10-11 Key Areas for Heart Auscultation

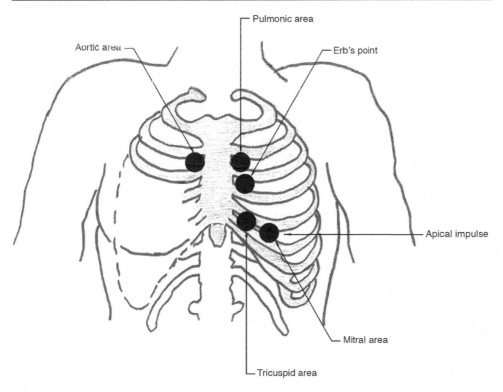

Source: Reprinted from Urden: *Priorities in Critical Care Nursing,* 4/3, 2003 Mosby, with permission from Elsevier.

should be taken to listen for each heart sound (S_1 and S_2) and to assess the time between sounds. Variations in the heart sounds include louder or softer sounds, presence of extra sounds, or splitting of sounds.

First Heart Sound.   The first heart sound, S_1, is produced by the closure of the mitral and tricuspid valves. Normally the mitral valve closes slightly earlier than the tricuspid valve due to the higher pressure gradient present in the left ventricle. The two components of S_1 are referred to as M_1 and T_1, signifying the closure of the mitral valve followed by the tricuspid valve, respectively. However, S_1 is typically heard as one sound.

S_1 marks the end of diastole and the beginning of ventricular systole. Upon auscultation of the heart sounds, S_1 is considered the "lub" and is a high-pitched sound. It will be heard loudest at the apex of the heart, at the fifth intercostal space, mid-clavicular line, due to the close proximity of the mitral and tricuspid valves (Seidel et al., 2003).

Second Heart Sound.   The second heart sound, S_2, is produced by the closure of the pulmonic and aortic valves. S_2 signifies the end of systole and beginning of diastole. S_2 is heard loudest at the base of the heart, at the second intercostal space, left or right sternal border. S_2 is referred to as the "dub" and is higher in pitch and shorter in duration than S_1.

A split S_2 occurs when the aortic and pulmonic valves do not close at the same time. Normal, physiologic splitting of S_2 may happen on inspiration because of increased venous return to the heart, delaying the closure of the pulmonic valve. In contrast, pathologic splitting of S_2 is suspected when the split sound persists throughout respiration, appears on expiration, and disappears on inspiration (Seidel et al., 2003).

Third Heart Sound.   The third heart sound, S_3, is produced after S_2 by the rapid filling of the ventricle during early diastole. The sounds produced are often compared to saying the word "Ken-tuck-ee"—illustrating the normal S_1, followed by the S_2, and followed by a quick extra sound, the S_3. An S_3 may be a normal finding in children and young adults. Decreased ventricular compliance or increased volume, as is seen in heart failure, may result in the vibration of the ventricle during diastole, causing a pathologic S_3 sound. A pathologic S_3 may be referred to as a ventricular gallop (Seidel et al., 2003).

Fourth Heart Sound.   The fourth heart sound, S_4, is produced during atrial contraction and represents the atria's forceful contraction to send blood to the ventricles at the end of diastole, often referred to as the "atrial kick." The S_4 sound occurs just before S_1, as a result of reduced left or right ventricular compliance. The S_4 sound is often compared to saying the word "Ten-nes-see," representing S_4, S_1, S_2. These sounds are often referred to as an atrial gallop. On the rare occasion that both an S_3 and an S_4 are present, the sounds generated are known as a summation gallop (Seidel et al., 2003).

Murmurs.   Murmurs are sounds generated by the turbulent flow of blood. Oftentimes, valvular disorders will produce murmuring of the normal S_1 and S_2 sounds. The murmur is produced when blood flows back through a valve that is incompetent, causing regurgitation of blood back into the chamber from which it came. A murmur may also be produced if blood flow is forced through a stenotic valvular area. Blood flow through an abnormal opening, such as a ventricular septal defect, or blood flow through normal structures at faster than normal speed may cause murmurs as well.

Recognizing the presence of a murmur is the first step. Further classifying murmurs and describing their unique characteristics are considered advanced skills for ICU nurses. Murmurs are classified by where in the cardiac cycle they are heard, also referred to as timing, such as systolic or diastolic, or continuous. More specific classifications describe when in that part of the cardiac cycle the murmur begins. For example, holosystolic murmurs start with S_1 and end at S_2.

The intensity of murmurs is rated on a scale from I to VI, where the numbers represent the loudness of the sounds heard upon auscultation. Grade I corresponds to a faint, hardly discernible sound, as opposed to Grade IV, where the murmur is loud, and Grade VI, where the murmur can be heard without using a stethoscope (Bicking & Szilagyi, 2004).

Pattern, pitch, quality, and radiation are also considered when assessing murmurs. Terms such as crescendo (moving from quiet to loud), decrescendo (moving from loud to soft), crescendo-decrescendo (moving from soft to loud and back to soft again), or plateau (staying at the same intensity throughout) describe the pattern of the murmur. Pitch is described as low, medium, or high, depending on the velocity of the blood flow. Higher-velocity flows create high-pitched murmurs. Quality and radiation are also considered when describing murmurs. Quality is described as blowing, rumbling, harsh or musical. Whether the murmur radiates to other areas of the chest, neck, or abdomen is noted as well (Bicking & Szilagyi, 2004).

Extra Heart Sounds.   Murmurs arise when valves are supposed to be closing. Alternatively, sounds can also occur when valves open. An "opening snap" may be produced by the mitral valve and heard in early diastole. An "ejection click" of the semilunar valves (pulmonic and aortic) may be heard in early systole upon opening. Mechanical prosthetic valves produce loud clicks as they open and close. This clicking is expected—when it is not heard, in fact, it is a sign that the valve may have clots or vegetation on it. Such a finding should be reported to the physician.

Pericardial Friction Rubs. A pericardial friction rub can be heard when the parietal and visceral pericardia rub together, typically a sign of inflammation of the linings. The sound produced is a harsh, grating sound classically described as a scratching sound or the sound of sandpaper. If a pericardial friction rub is suspected, it can be best heard at the third intercostal space, left sternal border. Having the patient sit up, lean forward, and exhale can intensify the sound to make it easier to hear. It is important to distinguish between a pericardial friction rub and a pleural rub. If the patient is able to cooperate, you can ask the patient to hold his or her breath. If the sound continues to be produced, it is most likely a pericardial friction rub and not a pleural rub (Bicking & Szilagyi, 2004).

Extremities

When assessing the extremities, the ICU nurse should inspect, palpate, and, if necessary, auscultate. First, inspect the extremities for color, hair distribution, and presence of any edema. Next, palpate the extremities, noting temperature of the skin. It is important to assess both left and right extremities at the same time, comparing one to the other.

Pulses. The common sites for palpating pulses include the carotid, brachial, radial, femoral, popliteal, dorsalis pedis, and posterior tibial arteries. Pulses are assessed for rate, rhythm, contour, amplitude (strength), and equality, bilaterally. Contour is assessed using either the carotid artery or the brachial artery. A smooth, sudden upstroke after S_1 is expected. Amplitude of the pulse is noted next. On a scale of 0 to 4, 0 refers to absent; 1 refers to diminished or barely palpable; 2 refers to normal; 3 refers to full or increased; and 4 refers to bounding (Seidel et al., 2003). Sometimes pulse amplitude is performed based on a 0 to 3 or 0 to 2 scale. Therefore, it is im-

portant to note the scale being used when documenting your findings (Bicking & Szilagyi, 2004).

Bruits. Peripheral arteries can become occluded with atherosclerotic material. Depending on the extent of atherosclerosis, blood flow through the lumen may meet resistance, resulting in a turbulent blood flow at the area of partial occlusion. If auscultated, this turbulence is referred to as a bruit. Presence of a bruit may indicate reduced blood flow to the area distally and may require attention, especially if the patient complains about intermittent claudication. Presence of a bruit should be documented when one is found.

Edema. Edema is the presence of fluid in the interstitial space. It is assessed by pressing the skin against an underlying bone on the dorsum of the foot, behind the medial malleolus and at the pretibial area. Firm pressure is applied for 5 seconds and then released. Edema should be assessed in the sacral area and other dependent areas in bedridden patients. This condition is measured on a 4-point scale, where slight edema is documented as 1+ and the most severe edema is documented as 4+. An indentation in the skin after pressure is released is referred to as pitting edema. Slight pitting edema is present when the indentation quickly disappears after pressure is released, as opposed to severe pitting edema, which may take 2 to 5 minutes before the indentation disappears (Bicking & Szilagyi, 2004).

SUMMARY

The primary function of the cardiopulmonary system is oxygen delivery. It is essential for the ICU nurse to understand electrical activity and pumping action of the heart, identify aberrancies, and anticipate the clinical significance of changes in structure and function.

CRITICAL THINKING QUESTIONS

1. Why is it essential to begin cardiopulmonary resuscitation in a patient who is experiencing ventricular fibrillation?
2. If a patient has atrial fibrillation with an atrial rate greater than 200 beats per minute and a ventricular rate less than 60 beats per minute, why might the patient need a pacemaker inserted?
3. Why do some patients with bradycardia have signs of impaired cardiac output whereas others do not? How does the body compensate for a decrease in heart rate?
4. Which symptoms might you anticipate finding in a patient with supraventricular tachycardia? Why?
5. Describe the flow of blood from the systemic circulation through the heart, and back to the systemic circulation.
6. Define stroke volume and cardiac output.
7. Correlate what occurs electrically and mechanically in the heart (i.e., what is occurring when each of the waves appears on the ECG rhythm strip paper or on the monitor).

Online Resources

Adult Cardiac Anatomy:
http://user.gru.net/clawrence/vccl/chpt2/adult.htm

American Heart Association:
www.americanheart.org

Cardiac Assessment:
www.coconino.edu/mbaker/divisionpage/Nursing%20Presentations/CardiacAssessment-BCC-CCTP.htm

Cardiovascular Physiology Concepts:
http://www.cvphysiology.com/Heart%20Disease/HD001.htm

REFERENCES

Bicking, L. S., & Szilagyi, P. G. (2004). *Bates' guide to physical examination and history taking* (8th ed.). Philadelphia: Lippincott Williams & Wilkins.

Darovic, G. O. (2004). *Handbook of hemodynamic monitoring* (2nd ed.). St. Louis, MO: Elsevier.

Guyton, A. C., & Hall, J. E. (2006). *Textbook of medical physiology* (11th ed.). Philadelphia: Elsevier.

Rushing, J. (2005). Assessing for orthostatic hypotension. *Nursing, 35*(1), 30.

Seidel, H. M., Ball, J. W., Dains, J. E., & Benedict, G. W. (2003*). Mosby's guide to physical examination* (5th ed.). St. Louis, MO: Mosby.

Thaler, M. S. (2003). *The only ECG book you will ever need* (4th ed.). Philadelphia: Lippincott Williams & Wilkins.

CHAPTER 11

Hemodynamic Monitoring

Kim Blount

LEARNING OBJECTIVES

Upon completion of this chapter, the reader will be able to:

1. Describe the physiologic basis for hemodynamic monitoring.
2. List clinical conditions that alter hemodynamic parameters.
3. List indications for hemodynamic monitoring.
4. Describe technical factors that affect the accuracy of hemodynamic value measurement.
5. Discuss nursing interventions used in the care of patients with hemodynamic monitoring catheters.

Hemodynamic monitoring is a fascinating technology that has been utilized in the care of critically ill patients for more than 30 years. The word *hemodynamic* can be divided into two parts: *hemo*, meaning "blood," and *dynamic*, meaning "ever changing." Therefore, hemodynamic monitoring is the bedside measurement of the ever-changing pressure of blood flow through the cardiac, pulmonary, and systemic vasculature via invasive catheters. Placement of pulmonary artery catheters (PACs) for the purposes of hemodynamic monitoring has become a common, but controversial, practice in contemporary intensive care units (ICUs).

Invasive hemodynamic monitoring is utilized when more than standard vital signs assessment is required to monitor perfusion status (Adams, 2004). When used accurately and with sound clinical judgment, proper hemodynamic management may result in improved patient outcomes, lower mortality rates, and better quality of life after critical illness (Connors et al., 1996).

All patients who enter ICUs are at risk for developing impaired tissue perfusion related to loss of blood volume and alterations in vascular tone, vascular integrity, and cardiac function. Conditions such as traumatic injury, acute myocardial infarction, heart failure, massive blood volume loss, systemic infection, and surgical interventions are contributing factors that affect the delicate balance of both tissue perfusion and oxygenation.

The bedside clinician should remain keenly aware that each patient's response to critical illness is unique. Each measurement obtained during hemodynamic monitoring is also unique to that particular patient, at that particular time, and to that particular situation.

The overall goal of collaborative care during critical illness is to provide adequate oxygen delivery to the tissues and to sustain life until homeostasis and healing can occur. Nursing care of patients with hemodynamic monitoring requires a combination of knowledge, skills, experience, and attitudes to accurately interpret hemodynamic measurements for positive outcomes. This chapter focuses on basic-level hemodynamic education such as the physiologic basis of hemodynamic monitoring, tools used to measure hemodynamics, waveform components, technical factors that affect the accuracy of invasive hemodynamic measurements, and interpretation of values.

PHYSIOLOGIC BASIS OF HEMODYNAMIC MONITORING

In a perfect world, with each millisecond of life, many red blood cells travel throughout the pulmonary vasculature, heart, and systemic vascular tree for the purpose of feeding each and every cell of the body with life-sustaining oxygen. Blood flows in a continuous, predictable circuit: to the lungs, which maintain oxygen supply; to the heart, which pumps oxygen-rich blood to organ systems; and to the systemic vasculature, which provides an uninterrupted conduit through which blood travels. Because blood flow is predictable, invasive catheters can be utilized to gather internal relevant information on whether one of these intricate systems has been altered by disease processes.

Physical assessment findings and values obtained through hemodynamic monitoring are compared to established normal parameters for each system in that particular patient. Once parameters are analyzed, the bedside clinician is able to determine which alterations are occurring and offer possibilities for treatment to maintain cellular oxygen delivery and oxygen utilization by the tissues. If cells are unable to obtain and utilize oxygen for aerobic metabolic processes, they will become hypoxemic and anaerobic. Unless oxygen delivery and utilization resume, organ dysfunction, organ failure, and death can occur. Cellular oxygenation is dependent on three main physiologic processes: pulmonary gas exchange, oxygen delivery, and oxygen consumption (Johnson, 2004). These processes are the physiologic basis of hemodynamic monitoring.

Pulmonary Gas Exchange

Before blood is delivered to the tissues, it must be loaded with oxygen. The pulmonary system's main function is to provide oxygen to the blood plasma. Room (ambient) air is inhaled and humidified via the nose and the trachea. The percentage of oxygen in room air is 21%, and the pressure of oxygen in the ambient air is generally about 150 mm Hg. This pressure is represented by the abbreviation PO_2 (partial pressure of oxygen). At 21% FiO_2 or about PO_2 of 150 mm Hg, oxygen enters the nose, is conducted down the airways into the terminal bronchioles, and lastly enters the alveoli, where gas exchange occurs. The PO_2 when it reaches the alveolus is lower than when it first entered the nose due to the humidification process that occurs as the air is being conducted to the alveolus.

The PO_2 in the alveolus is about 100 mm Hg (i.e., PaO_2 of 100 mm Hg). Oxygen moves from an area of high concentration to one of low concentration. A pulmonary capillary, which has both a venous end and an arteriole end, surrounds each alveolus. The blood returning to the alveolus is the venous portion and has a partial pressure of about 45 mm Hg (PvO_2). Because the PO_2 in the venous portion of the capillary is less than the pressure in the alveolus, oxygen diffuses across the alveolar capillary membrane and into the blood plasma. The oxygen measurement in the arterial end of the capillary will reach about 80 to 100 mm Hg (PaO_2). This concept of oxygen diffusion is paramount in maintaining the availability of oxygen to the blood plasma. Any disease process or injury that impairs respiratory function or alveolar integrity will, by necessity, alter the PaO_2. The role of bedside clinicians in the pulmonary gas exchange process is to assess respiratory function (discussed in Chapter 20).

Cardiac Output

Cardiac output (CO) is the amount of blood pumped by the heart every minute (Urban, 2004). It is the driving force behind oxygen delivery. Once oxygen diffusion has taken place and hemoglobin is loaded with oxygen for transport, the blood must be propelled forward into the aorta and dispersed via the complex vascular tree to all vital organ systems and cells within the body. CO is represented by the mathematical formula CO = HR (heart rate) $\times$ SV (stroke volume). The normal value is expressed in liters per minute. The normal value range for CO is 4 to 8 L/min (Darovic, 2002). Any factor that affects heart rate will alter the CO equation, and thus perfusion and oxygen delivery to the cells. **Figure 11-1** depicts the two major components of oxygen delivery (DO_2); arterial oxygen content (CaO_2) and CO.

A measurement called cardiac index is a more precise value in determining tissue perfusion. This value takes into consideration the perfusion across a person's body surface area (height and weight). The formula for cardiac index is Cardiac index (CI) = Cardiac output (CO)/Body surface area (BSA). The normal cardiac index is in the 2.5–4.2 L/min/m^2 range (Darovic, 2002). Indexed values should be used when applicable for further individualization of hemodynamic assessment and treatment of the clinical condition.

Stroke volume is the amount of blood ejected by the ventricle with each beat. Normal value ranges for stroke volume are 60 to 130 mL/beat. There are three components of stroke volume: preload, afterload, and contractility.

Preload

Preload is the amount of stretch or volume in the ventricle at the end of diastole. To eject blood during ventricular systole, the ventricle must be "preloaded" with blood before ejection. Preload occurs during the diastolic phase of the cardiac cycle and refers to the ability of the ventricle to stretch and fill with blood and the ability of the pulmonary vasculature and sys-

FIGURE 11-1 Oxygen Delivery

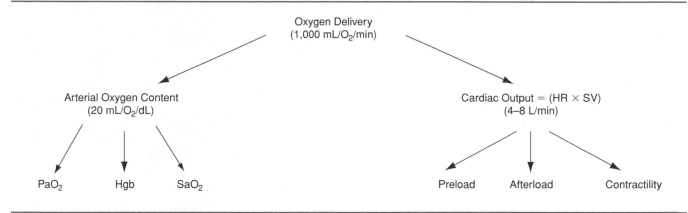

temic vasculature to return blood to the heart. This hemodynamic parameter is determined by the amount of volume in the vascular space, the amount of venous return, and the amount of blood in the ventricle at the end of diastole.

End diastole is the phase of the cardiac cycle in which the ventricle is the most full of blood. As blood fills the heart, it exerts pressure on the atrial and ventricular musculature. The size of the ventricle and the degree of ventricular stretch or compliance limit the amount of blood it can accept. Certain disease states, such as heart failure and cardiomyopathy, restrict the ability of the heart to stretch. In these conditions, addition of small amounts of fluid to the vascular system can produce larger changes in preload value measurements (Brandsetter et al., 1998). **Table 11-1** describes some disease processes and factors that affect the amount of both right and left ventricular preload.

Right atrial preload measurement is obtained by monitoring pressures in the right atrium or central veins. Thus bedside clinical measurement of right atrial preload is the mean right atrial pressure (RAP) or central venous pressure (CVP). CVP monitoring is typically ordered as a marker of the patient's volume status. Unfortunately, it correlates poorly with this status and does not predict a patient's response to fluid bolus (Rhodes, Grounds, & Bennett, 2005).

Left ventricular preload or left ventricular end diastolic pressure (LVEDP) reflects the amount of volume in the left ventricle at the end of filling (diastole). LVEDP can be obtained indirectly by placing a catheter in the left atrium. Another indirect measurement of left ventricular preload can be obtained by inflating the balloon of a PAC and "wedging" the catheter in a small branch of the pulmonary artery (PA), thereby occluding blood flow in that segment of the PA (Urban, 2004). This pressure reading is termed pulmonary artery occlusive pressure (PAOP); it is also called pulmonary capillary wedge pressure (PCWP) and pulmonary artery wedge pressure (PAWP) (Forrester, Diamond, Chatterjee, & Swan, 1976a, 1976b).

Afterload

Afterload is the amount of resistance the ventricle must overcome to eject the volume of blood into the pulmonary or systemic vasculature (Urban, 2004). Right ventricular afterload is present in pulmonary vascular beds, and left ventricular afterload is present in the aorta and systemic vasculature. For example, if asked to push 60 mL of fluid through a garden hose or a drinking straw, which device would have the least resistance and more easily accept the 60 mL of fluid? The garden hose, because its diameter is larger than the diameter of the straw. This is the principle of afterload. The larger the diameter of the vessel, the less the resistance (afterload) to blood flow. Afterload affects the amount of contractile tension the myocardium must generate to open the pulmonic/aortic valve and eject blood volume into the vasculature. Vascular resistance exists in the vessels that accept blood from the ejecting ventricle—that is, "after" the load of blood is ejected.

The right heart vascular resistance originates from the pulmonary vascular beds and is known as pulmonary vascular resistance (PVR). PVR is a calculated hemodynamic value. This number is obtained by placing hemodynamic measurements such as CO, mean pulmonary artery pressure, and PAOP in a formula and calculating the value. Right heart afterload is influenced by the amount of vasodilation or vasoconstriction in the pulmonary beds, the amount of volume placing pressure on the pulmonary beds, disease processes that alter alveolar distention and pulmonary vascular function, and the effects of positive pressure mechanical ventilation (Johnson, 2004). The left heart vascular resistance

TABLE 11-1 Clinical Conditions That Alter Preload

Right Atrial Preload: CVP	
Increase	**Decrease**
Intravascular volume gain	Intravascular volume loss
• Volume overload (fluid boluses)	• Hemorrhage
• Renal failure	• Diuresis
• Fluid shifts	• Third spacing
Heart failure: loss of contractility	• Dehydration: diarrhea, vomiting, excessive NG drainage
• RV failure secondary to LV failure/mitral valve disease	↓ Venous return
• RV failure r/t RV infarct	• Peripheral pooling
• Cardiomyopathy	• Reverse Trendelenburg
• RV failure r/t ↑ pulmonary vascular resistance: COPD, hypoxia, massive PE, ARDS, shock states	Systemic venous dilation: neurogenic and early septic shock, vasodilators
↓ RV compliance r/t cardiac tamponade/pericardial effusion	↑ Heart rate, loss of atrial kick, irregular rhythm
↑ Systemic venous return	↑ Myocardial contractility
• Vasoconstriction: hypothermia, shock states, vasopressors	• Hyperdynamic disease states
Valve disease: pulmonic valve stenosis	• Drugs: positive inotropes

Left Ventricular Preload: PAOP	
Increase	**Decrease**
Intravascular volume gain	Intravascular volume loss
• Volume overload (fluid boluses)	• Hemorrhage
• Renal failure	• Diuresis
• Fluid shifts	• Third spacing
Heart failure	• Severe dehydration
• LV Failure r/t LV infarct	↓ Pulmonary venous return
• Cardiomyopathy	Pulmonary venous dilation
• LV r/t ↑ systemic vascular resistance, shock states	↓ Heart rate, loss of atrial kick, irregular rhythm
↓ LV compliance r/t cardiac tamponade, pericardial effusion	↑ Myocardial contractility
↑ Pulmonary venous return	• Hyperdynamic disease states
Valve disease: aortic valve stenosis	• Drugs: positive inotropes

Note: ↑ = increase, ↓ = decrease, RV = right ventricular, LV = left ventricular, COPD = chronic obstructive pulmonary disease, PE = pulmonary embolus, ARDS = acute respiratory distress syndrome.
Sources: Darovic, 2002; Adams, 2004.

originates from the aorta and systemic vasculature; it is estimated by calculating a hemodynamic measurement known as systemic vascular resistance (SVR). Left ventricular afterload is influenced by atherosclerosis, disease processes that alter vascular tone, and pharmacologic medications that alter vascular tone (Urban, 2004). **Table 11-2** lists right and left heart resistances and clinical conditions that can alter them.

Contractility

Contractility is the inherent ability of the cardiac muscle fibers to contract and eject blood into pulmonary or systemic vasculature. Any disease process or injury that alters blood return to the heart (preload), vascular resistance (afterload), or the ability of the heart to contract (contractility) will alter stroke volume, CO, and tissue perfusion.

The heart muscle consists of multiple cardiac units called myofibrils. Each myofibril, in turn, consists of functional units called sarcomeres. The sarcomeres are the contractile units of the heart. When activated by electrical stimulus and electrolytes such as calcium, each sarcomere shortens. When multiple sarcomeres shorten, the myofibril contracts. As multiple myofibrils contract simultaneously, the ventricular muscle tissue contracts and exerts pressures on the blood in the ventricles (Darovic, 2002). This buildup of myocardial tension (squeeze) signals the onset of ventricular systole. The pressure in the ventricles builds until the pressure in the ventricle exceeds the pressure in the PAs or aorta.

At this time, the aortic and pulmonic valves open, and the ventricle ejects a percentage of the preload blood volume into the pulmonary or systemic vasculature. The per-

TABLE 11-2 Clinical Conditions That Alter Afterload

Clinical Conditions That Alter Right-Sided Afterload (PVR)	
Increase PVR	**Decrease PVR**
Hypoxia: Number 1 Cause	Drug therapies: vasodilators
Obstruction: acute pulmonary embolism—cor pulmonale, mitral stenosis	Correction of hypoxemia or acidosis
↓ Pulmonary compliance	Exercise (slight SNS stimulation, producing vasodilation)
• Cardiogenic: pulmonary edema	
• Non-cardiogenic: ARDS	
• Fluid volume overload	
Vasoconstriction: acidemia, hypoxia	
Pulmonary HTN	

Clinical Conditions That Alter Left-Sided Afterload (SVR)	
Increase SVR	**Decrease SVR**
Volume loss/hypoperfusion (compensatory—causes vasoconstriction)	Arterial vasodilatation
Arterial vasoconstriction	• Drugs: vasodilators and some inotropes; alpha and calcium channel blockers
• Hypothermia	• Shock states: septic, anaphylactic, neurogenic
• Drugs: alpha vasopressors and some inotropes	• Anesthesia
• LV heart failure	• Hyperthermia
• Shock states: hypovolemic and cardiogenic	
• Stress, anxiety	
Atherosclerosis: narrows blood vessels ↑ resistance to flow	

Note: ↑ = increase, ↓ = decrease, ARDS = acute respiratory distress syndrome, HTN = hypertension, SNS = sympathetic nervous system, LV = left ventricular.
Sources: Adams, 2004; Darovic, 2002.

centage of blood ejected by the ventricle is known as the ejection fraction (EF). Left ventricular EF is commonly reported as part of several diagnostic tests, such as an echocardiogram. Clinical conditions that affect contractility are listed in **Table 11-3**.

Contractility of the myofibrils is affected by the amount of preload. This phenomenon is commonly known as the Frank-Starling law. Starling proposed that contractility could be improved with the addition of volume to the ventricle. As volume is added to the ventricle, the sarcomeres stretch, causing the actin and myosin filaments to spread farther apart and resulting in greater recoil and strength in the subsequent contraction. For example, the farther one stretches a rubber band, the greater the recoil and the farther the rubber band will travel when released. However, the rubber band has a breaking point at which the fibers will be stretched too far, break, and fail to travel any distance.

The same principle applies to the actin and myosin filaments in the sarcomere. At a certain point, adding volume to the ventricle will no longer create a stronger contraction. At that moment, the heart will simply fail to develop enough tension to open cardiac valves and eject blood volume. In these circumstances, stroke volume, contractility, and tissue oxygen perfusion will decrease. Patients who experience hypovolemia and low preload values will benefit from volume resuscitation (Leeper, 2003). Those who experience hypervolemia from congestive heart failure are less likely to benefit from volume resuscitation.

Afterload also affects contractility: The higher the afterload, the more myocardial tension the ventricle must generate. Increased afterload increases myocardial work, contractility, and myocardial oxygen demand. As long as a ventricle remains healthy and is able to compensate for the increased afterload, stroke volume will be maintained. However, disease processes can alter the compensatory ability of the ventricle, leading to a decreased stroke volume and CO. Lower afterload parameters are preferred in patients with heart failure to decrease myocardial workload, decrease myocardial oxygen consumption, and improve contractility.

TABLE 11-3 Clinical Conditions That Alter Contractility

Increase Contractility	Decrease Contractility
Hyperdynamic states	• Hypodynamic states
• Shock states	• Late sepsis r/t release of myocardial depressant factors
• Hyperthyroidism	• Cardiogenic shock
↑ Preload, ↑ afterload	• Myocardial infarction
Positive inotropes: exogenous catecholamines	• Hypercarbia
• Beta stimulants	↓ Preload, ↓ afterload
• Phosphodiesterase inhibitors	Negative inotropes
Endogenous catecholamine release	• Beta blockers
• SNS	• Calcium channel blockers
• Metabolic rate	Electrolyte imbalance
• Exercise	• Hyponatremia
• Stress, pain, anxiety	• Hyperkalemia
Electrolyte levels	• Hypocalcemia
• ↑ Calcium levels	• Hypomagnesemia
Functional myocardium	↓ O$_2$ supply: anaerobic metabolism
	Loss of functional myocardium > 40%
	Right heart: ↑ PVR; pulmonary edema
	Severe metabolic acidosis

Note: ↑ = increase, ↓ = decrease, ARDS = acute respiratory distress syndrome, SNS = sympathetic nervous system.
Sources: Adams, 2004; Darovic, 2002.

Heart Rate

Heart rate is the number of times the heart beats per minute. The normal heart rate is 60 to 100 beats per minute. Factors affecting heart rate include baroreceptors, chemoreceptors, metabolic needs, myocardial oxygen supply, and the autonomic nervous system. Any condition that disrupts the normal heart rate and regular rhythm will alter CO (see **Figure 11-2** for factors that alter heart rate). Rhythms such as atrial fibrillation, bradycardia, and ventricular fibrillation either decrease or increase heart rate and, in turn, alter the normal CO values.

Cardiac Reserve

When cells require more oxygen for metabolic processes, such as during exercise and under stress conditions caused by disease, the body will autoregulate blood flow and CO and increase oxygen delivery to meet the greater oxygen demand. This ability to compensate for insults points out the resiliency of the body to restore basic level of function. For example, the kidneys optimize circulating blood volume by increasing or decreasing the excretion of sodium and water as well as altering vascular tone (Adams, 2004). This compensatory ability

FIGURE 11-2 Factors That Alter Heart Rate

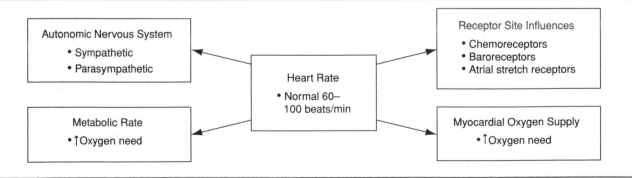

to increase CO and oxygen delivery is called cardiac reserve. During these types of situations, CO may increase 5 to 10 times the normal value (Darovic, 2002). Unfortunately, in the critically ill patient, the ability to increase oxygen delivery may be altered and the patient may not be able to meet the oxygen demand of the cells, putting the cells and organs into oxygen debt.

Oxygen Delivery

Hemoglobin and SaO$_2$

Once oxygen is present in blood plasma, it must become attached to a hemoglobin molecule for its transport to systemic cells. Hemoglobin's affinity for oxygen is illustrated in a graph known as the oxygen hemoglobin dissociation curve. It exemplifies conditions when oxygen is more likely to be released or dissociated from the hemoglobin molecule (i.e., release of oxygen to the tissues). Thus the saturation of the hemoglobin molecule with oxygen is predictable in certain conditions. The body needs oxygen released from hemoglobin at the tissue level. If hemoglobin holds on to oxygen and does not release it, the oxygen will not be available to the cells. Certain conditions—for example, acidosis, alkalosis, hypo-hyperthermia, and decreased amounts of a protein called 2,3-diphosphoglycerate (DPG)—either increase or decrease the hemoglobin molecule's ability to bind, carry, and release oxygen to the tissues. For example, receiving multiple units of blood decreases levels of DPG, thereby decreasing hemoglobin's ability to release oxygen to the tissues. Therefore, even though cells may demand oxygen, hemoglobin may not release it. This places the cells into oxygen debt. Alterations in pH balance such as acidosis can cause hemoglobin to easily release oxygen to the tissues. It is the role of the bedside clinician to determine whether any of these conditions that alter oxygen delivery to cells exist in the particular patient. Figure 11-1 depicts the two major components of oxygen delivery (DO$_2$): arterial oxygen content (CaO$_2$) and cardiac output (CO). (See **Box 11-1**.)

Mixed Venous Oxygen Saturation

Mixed venous oxygen saturation (SvO$_2$/ScvO$_2$) measurements reflect the percentage of oxygen that was taken (or extracted) by the body (Headley, 1998; Johnson, 2004). These measurements cannot determine individual supply or consumption of oxygen by individual organs. Fiber optic catheters use a technique called reflection spectrometry to measure this hemodynamic parameter. Optical filaments in the catheter transmit light and receive reflected light from the blood vessel—either the pulmonary artery (SvO$_2$) or the superior vena cava–central

---

Box 11-1

Glossary of Hemodynamic Terms

PaO$_2$: Partial pressure of oxygen in the alveolus

Hgb: Hemoglobin

SaO$_2$: Arterial oxygen saturation

Preload: The amount of stretch or volume in the ventricle at the end of diastole

Afterload: The amount of resistance the ventricle must overcome to eject the volume of blood into the pulmonary or systemic vasculature

Contractility: The inherent ability of the cardiac muscle fibers to contract and eject blood into pulmonary or systemic vasculature

Stroke volume: The amount of blood ejected by the ventricle with each beat

---

vein (ScvO$_2$). These data are processed in a computer, and a number value is displayed. Normal SvO$_2$ values range from 60% to 80%. Normal ScvO$_2$ values are similar to the SvO$_2$ values, albeit slightly higher (Johnson).

ScvO$_2$ is an emerging technology that is listed in the Society of Critical Care Medicine's treatment protocols for the Surviving Sepsis Campaign. SvO$_2$/ScvO$_2$ values provide one of the most rapid bedside methods of assessing tissue perfusion and oxygenation currently being used in ICUs (Ott, Johnson, & Ahrens 2001; Rivers et al., 2001). Oxygen-rich blood reflects a greater amount of light than desaturated blood. Normal values indicate that the oxygen supply meets the oxygen consumption by the tissues. SvO$_2$/ScvO$_2$ values less than 50% indicate anaerobic metabolism and cellular hypoxia. Changes in SvO$_2$/ScvO$_2$ values of more than 5% that last for a few minutes indicate an alteration in oxygen delivery or oxygen consumption (Jersurum, 2004).

There are essentially four determinants of SvO$_2$/ScvO$_2$: CO, hemoglobin, SaO$_2$, and oxygen consumption. A decline in CO, hemoglobin, and/or SaO$_2$ will reduce oxygen delivery to the tissues (see **Table 11-4**). If oxygen demands are not met and cells do not have enough oxygen to carry out their metabolic processes, the cells will become hypoxic and begin to dysfunction. This cellular hypoxemia can lead to organ dysfunction and a condition known as multiple organ dysfunction syndrome (MODS). Patients who suffer from systemic hypoxemia have high morbidity and mortality rates (Rivers et al., 2001).

TABLE 11-4 Clinical Conditions That Alter SvO_2/$ScvO_2$ Values

Upward Number Value Trends	
Conditions	**Example**
O_2 supply exceeds O_2 demand ($\downarrow$ tissue utilization of O_2)	Septic shock Hypothermia Cyanide poisoning Pharmacologic paralysis
Technical problems with SvO_2 reading	Wedged PAC Clots on the catheter tip Noncalibrated
Alteration in O_2 delivery ($\uparrow$ CO or $\uparrow$ oxygen tension)	Hyperoxia, $\uparrow FiO_2$ Excessive inotropic therapy

Downward Number Value Trends	
Conditions	**Example**
O_2 demand exceeds O_2 supply ($\uparrow VO_2$/tissue utilization) $\downarrow$ CO $\downarrow$ Hgb $\downarrow SaO_2$	Movement, shivering, fever, pain Shock, hypotension, hypovolemia, dysrhythmias, $\uparrow$ PEEP Anemia, hemorrhage, carbon monoxide poisoning Hypoventilation, intrapulmonary shunts, ARDS, atelectasis, pneumonia, ventilator disconnect, disconnect from O_2 source, respiratory failure

Note: $\uparrow$ = increase, $\downarrow$ = decrease, O_2 = oxygen, SvO_2 = mixed venous oxygen saturation, $ScvO_2$ = central mixed venous oxygen saturation, CO = cardiac output, Hgb = hemoglobin, SaO_2 = arterial oxygen saturation, ARDS = acute respiratory distress syndrome, PEEP = positive end expiratory pressure, FiO_2 = fraction of inspired oxygen, VO_2 = oxygen consumption, PAC = pulmonary artery catheter.
Sources: Adams, 2004; Darovic, 2002.

Oxygen Consumption

For metabolic processes to function normally, each cell within the organ system must consume oxygen. The amount of oxygen extracted from the blood and consumed at the tissue level is 20% to 25% of the overall amount delivered (Johnson, 2004). Oxygen consumption is increased by factors such as endotracheal suctioning, linen changes, general nursing care, and dressing changes (Johnson). Increased oxygen consumption causes the body to mount a compensatory response in an attempt to increase oxygen delivery and maintain the new balance. The sympathetic nervous system releases endorphins to increase heart rate, blood pressure, and CO. Respiratory rate and depth rise to increase air conduction to the alveoli. If the body does not maintain its resiliency, oxygen debt will occur and cells will begin to dysfunction. Without adequate availability of oxygen, cells will begin to use glucose for energy, a condition called anaerobic metabolism.

Byproducts of anaerobic metabolism include lactic acid and hydrogen peroxide. If oxygenation is not restored, the cells will die. If enough cells are altered, normal organ function will be inhibited. Acute renal failure, changes in mental status, liver dysfunction, and gut dysfunction are all indications that the organ system is experiencing an oxygen imbalance. Performing serial lactic acid levels is one recommended way to monitor cellular oxygenation (Rivers et al., 2001). Elevated lactic acid levels indicate anaerobic metabolism and oxygen debt. In critically ill patients, sedation therapy may be undertaken to decrease oxygen consumption by decreasing skeletal muscle movement. As part of this treatment, oxygen consumption values are monitored with a PAC in conjunction with other hemodynamic parameters.

PHYSICAL ASSESSMENT

Constant vigilance is required to assess subtle changes in tissue perfusion and oxygenation. Clinical assessment of heart rate and stroke volume can assist the ICU nurse in determining the problem parameter and selecting the appropriate treatment to optimize oxygen delivery. The bedside clinician's role in monitoring CO is to monitor the patient for potential and actual alterations in the three stroke volume components and the heart rate.

Tools for Measuring Parameters

Intra-arterial Catheters

Use of an intra-arterial catheter in critically ill patients offers several benefits. First, the accuracy of mean arterial pressure (MAP) calculations can result in improved management of hemodynamically unstable patients. Indications for placement of an arterial line include accurate and frequent blood pressure monitoring as well as drawing of blood for arterial blood gases (ABGs) (Rhodes et al., 2005). This step is especially important in patients who are receiving vasoactive agents that require titration. The arterial line is the preferred method for monitoring blood pressure in patients who are experiencing hypoperfusion and hypotension states. Cuff blood pressure measurements are unreliable in these clinical conditions because compensatory vasoconstriction can cause Korotkoff sounds to vary during manual blood pressure measurement (Darovic, 2002). By contrast, arterial lines are designed to continuously monitor arterial waveforms as well as systolic, diastolic, and MAPs.

The most common insertion site is the radial artery, which allows free movement of arms and legs. If the radial artery is not available, insertion sites such as the femoral, dorsalis pedis, brachial, and axillary arteries may be utilized to monitor arterial pressures. The patient's clinical status, the integrity of the selected artery, the presence of circulation beyond the proposed cannulation site, and clinical staff preference are taken into consideration prior to insertion of the line (Lough, 2006). Possible complications associated with hemodynamic monitoring include vascular insufficiency distal to the insertion site, hemorrhage, infection, and thromboembolism. Nursing interventions for care of patients with intra-arterial lines focus on the prevention of complications such as thrombosis, vessel spasm, infection, line disconnection, and bleeding.

Central Venous Access

Generally, central venous access devices are used when peripheral sites are not accessible due to such factors as trauma, vascular inflammation, and loss of vascular integrity. Central venous lines aid in the delivery of large fluid volumes for fluid resuscitation, provide access for a PAC or transvenous pacing, and enable monitoring of the amount of blood returning to the right heart from the systemic circulation. Both single-lumen and multilumen central catheters are available. Central venous catheters are also used in hemodynamic monitoring as an alternative to the PAC. These catheters directly measure pressures in the central veins (CVP) as deoxygenated blood from the body returns to the heart. Possible complications from central venous line insertion and monitoring include

hemorrhage, pneumothorax, vascular erosions, catheter-related sepsis, and thromboembolic events.

Pulmonary Artery Catheter

The PAC is inserted into a central vein and threaded into the heart. It is 110 cm long, with markings at 10-cm increments along the length of the catheter. Use of the PAC in the treatment of critically ill patients has been controversial ever since this device's development (Prentice & Ahrens, 2001). Discussions concerning the cost versus the benefit of the catheter have been ongoing as the result of trends toward managed care, cost containment, and further research studies. Research studies have reported contradictory results, with findings ranging from a rise in mortality and cost of care, to reports of positive patient outcomes (Connors et al., 1996; Yu et al., 2003).

Because the controversy associated with the PAC has not yet been resolved, the decision of whether to insert a PAC is the responsibility of ICU professionals, who must analyze clinical assessment data and diagnostic information to determine the most beneficial approach to treatment. Clinical conditions indicated for the placement of a PAC to aid in treatment decisions include, but are not limited to, (1) monitoring of pump function (e.g., with cardiogenic shock, heart failure, cardiomyopathy, myocardial infarction, or valvular dysfunction); (2) assess fluid volume status (e.g., following trauma or surgery or with patients in renal failure); (3) determine pulmonary function (e.g., with acute lung injury, acute respiratory distress syndrome, or chronic obstructive pulmonary disease); or (4) assess oxygenation status (e.g., in patients with sepsis or MODS).

PACs are inserted via central veins such as the femoral vein, the subclavian vein, the brachial vein, and—the most common site—the jugular vein. The anatomy of the PAC is depicted in **Figure 11-3**.

Since the introduction of the PAC in 1970, advances in technology have created sophisticated catheters that can monitor the right ventricular EF, pace the heart, provide continuous monitoring of CO, and provide quantitative values for the body's delivery and consumption of oxygen (Ott et al., 2001). No matter the sophistication of the PAC, every catheter always has four ports in common. Depending on the manufacturer, some PACs have other ports (see **Table 11-5**).

When the catheter balloon is inflated, it acts as a buoy to carry or "float" the catheter to a narrower branch of the PA. The catheter will eventually not be able to migrate any farther due to the diameter of the balloon being larger than that of the pulmonary artery branch. At that point, the catheter is "wedged" in place. Wedging refers to occluding all forward

FIGURE 11-3 Pulmonary Artery Catheter

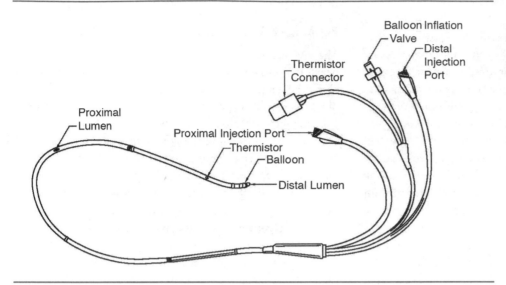

Source: Illustrated by James R. Perron.

flow of blood through a small PA. When wedged in place, the catheter values reflect the amount of blood in the left ventricle at the end of filling (LVEDP). Balloon inflation is limited to 10 or 15 seconds to minimize the PA complications that can develop from a wedged catheter.

After obtaining a wedge pressure, the syringe should be allowed to passively release the air in the balloon. Once the balloon has been deflated, the ICU nurse should note the return of the PA waveform. The syringe should be removed from the port, the air removed, and the syringe placed back on the port with the gate clamp or gate stopcock in the "off" position. This procedure is recommended to maintain patient safety and inadvertent wedging of the balloon. **Table 11-6** lists potential complications associated with PA catheter monitoring, etiology, nursing management, and outcomes of optimal care.

Maintaining Accuracy

Transducer Systems

The accuracy of the hemodynamic measurement is only as good as the integrity of the technology and the clinician interpreting the data (Adams, 2004). Pressure values are obtained by translating waves of pressure into measurable numbers. Transducers, monitoring cables, and bedside hemodynamic monitors are the three pieces of equipment that accomplish this task.

A transducer is a fluid-filled interface between the catheter tip and monitor. Transducer systems are disposable, are made of stiff noncompliant tubing, and contain a com-

puter chip that converts pressure signals to energy signals. The transducer is connected to the monitor via a cable. Once the energy signal is received by the monitor, it is translated into understandable waveforms and pressure values by the bedside computer and the measurements are then displayed on the monitor screen. The integrity of the transducer system must be maintained for accurate waveforms and values.

Transducers are flushed with normal saline, heparinized saline, or dextrose depending on the preference of the center. Heparin-induced thrombocytopenia (HIT) may be a complication of utilizing heparinized saline as a flush solution (AACN, 2004; Warkentin & Greinacher, 2004). As a consequence, some centers prefer not to use heparin in their flush solutions. Dextrose solutions may also affect lab values; the purpose of the invasive line must therefore be taken into consideration prior to flushing the line and hanging the flush solution bag. The fluid is placed in a pressure infusion cuff and is pressurized to 300 mm Hg. With the bag at this pressure, fluid infuses at a rate of 3 mL/hr.

Leveling and Zeroing the Transducer System

The transducer is leveled and zeroed prior to obtaining hemodynamic measurements. It is leveled with an anatomical location called the phlebostatic axis. With the patient in the supine position, the phlebostatic axis is located at the intersection of the fourth intercostal space and the midpoint of the anterior–posterior diameter. This axis corresponds to the level of the right atrium for PA, central venous, and left atrial pressure readings and to aortic root pressure for arterial lines (Gawlinski, 1997). **Figure 11-4** depicts the position of the phlebostatic axis. A carpenter's level or laser light level may be used to attain accurate parallel level with the phlebostatic axis. Transducers are leveled whenever the head of the bed elevation changes, when the patient shifts from supine to side lying, and after transport.

Zeroing the transducer refers to opening the reference stopcock to air and calibrating the monitor to atmospheric pressure. By using the "zero" reference calibration, the force of atmospheric pressure on the transducer is negated. This process enables the device to accurately obtain pressures within

TABLE 11-5 Pulmonary Artery Catheter Ports

Port	Where Port Opens	What It Measures	What Can Be Infused Through It/ What It Can Be Used for
Distal	PA	PAP, PAOP, and, indirectly, LAP	Only NS, heparinized NS, or D_5W on a pressure bag to maintain patency of the catheter. Can be used to obtain mixed venous blood samples.
Proximal	RA	RAP, CVP	Crystalloids. Because the proximal port can be used to measure CO, administration of vasoactive agents through this port is not ideal. To measure CO, the infusion would have to be stopped, interrupting the medication, and the patient would be receiving a bolus of the vasoactive agent that is left in the catheter during the first CO measurement. Administration of blood or blood products is not ideal because there is a potential for the catheter to become clogged. Parenteral nutrition is not ideal for the same reason.
Balloon	Tip of catheter, in the PA	PAOP when temporarily inflated	Nothing infused. Used only to obtain wedge pressures.
Thermistor	Tip of catheter, in the PA	Core temperature	Nothing infused. Used only to obtain core temperature and in determination of bolus cardiac output.
RV (not available in all catheters)	RV	Not used for measurement; port available for insertion of a transvenous temporary pacemaker is required	Can be used to administer small amounts (up to 50 mL/hr) of fluid. Vasoactive agents and parenteral nutrition may also be administered, if rate does not exceed 50 mL/hr.
Proximal infusion (not available in all catheters)	RA	Not used for measurement; used as an extra infusion port	Crystalloids, colloids, parenteral nutrition, vasoactive agents, blood, and blood products may all be infused. Continuous infusion is not required.

Note. PA = pulmonary artery, PAP = pulmonary artery pressure, PAOP = pulmonary artery occlusive pressure, LAP = left atrial pressure, RAP = right atrial pressure, CVP = central venous pressure, CO = cardiac output, RV = right ventricle, RA = right atrium.

the blood vessels. Transducers and monitoring equipment may drift away from zero, just as home weight scales often drift away from zero. Follow the institution's policy or manufacturer's recommendation for leveling and zeroing lines.

Head of Bed/Backrest Elevation Effects on Waveform Readings

Research indicates patients may be positioned with backrest elevation up to 60° as long as the air–fluid interface of the stopcock is level with the phlebostatic axis with no significant difference in readings (AACN, 2004) of CVP/RAP, PA pressures, or PAOP readings.

Hydrostatic Pressure

The pressure exerted by the weight of the fluid within the catheter and connecting tubing is known as hydrostatic pressure. This pressure is proportional to the height of the fluid in the column. If the transducer is higher than the phlebostatic axis, the pressure will be lower. Transducers lower than the phlebostatic axis will make the pressure value appear (incorrectly) higher. Every inch of discrepancy between transducer and the phlebostatic axis results in an approximate 2 mm Hg error in the reading (AACN, 2004; Darovic, 2002).

Square Wave Testing: Assessing Dynamic Response

Transducer systems vibrate (oscillate) as a result of pulsatile waves being transmitted from the catheter lumen through the tubing to the monitor. Every system has its own natural frequency. Compare this phenomenon to the natural sound frequency of guitar strings. Tight and thin guitar strings resonate at a higher frequency and give very high-pitched, high-frequency sounds. Loose and thick guitar strings resonate at a

TABLE 11-6 Possible Complications of PAC Monitoring

Complication	Etiology	Nursing Intervention	Outcomes
Bleeding	—initial line insertion —line disconnect —incorrectly turned stopcocks —pressure tubing not secured	—Ensure tubing and stopcocks are applied securely —Ensure that stopcocks are in the correct positions —Secure the catheter to prevent accidental dislodgement.	Patient will not sustain blood loss to PA catheter placement.
Air Embolism	—obtaining central access —loose connections —air bubbles in pressure tubing	—Position patient in Trendelenburg during PA catheter insertion —Prime pressure tubing prior to connecting —Check connections —Monitor lines for air bubbles —Management of air embolism is in Chapter 22	Patient will not sustain an air embolism as a result of PA catheter placement.
Pulmonary Artery Rupture	—pulmonary hypertension —anticoagulation —improper balloon inflation —improper catheter position —flushing catheter while balloon is inflated —continuous wedge measurement —balloon inflation with fluid —catheter migration into the pulmonary artery	—No more than 1.5 cc of air to inflate balloon —Inflate slowly & stop inflation once PAOP waveform appears —Limit inflation to 10 to 15 seconds —Allow balloon to deflate before drawing catheter back —Do not flush the catheter when the balloon is inflated —Prevent inadvertent wedging —Monitor PAP waveform	Patient will not sustain pulmonary artery rupture.
Catheter Knotting	—frequent reposition of catheter —insertion with deflated balloon —right ventricular hypertrophy	—Avoid catheter manipulation —Inflate balloon during insertion	Patient will not sustain catheter knotting while PA catheter is in place.
Clot Formation	—low flow state —inadequate anticoagulation —coagulopathies —blood clot formation on catheter —inadequate flushing of the catheter	—Maintain flush bag pressured to 300 mm Hg —Use heparin-coated catheters if available —Utilize no more than 1.5 cc of air to inflate balloon —Observe for blood return in balloon port —Report to MD if blood from port noted	Patient will not sustain a balloon rupture while PA catheter is in place. Patient will not sustain a clot from PA catheter.
Ventricular Dysrhythmias	—catheter in contact with right ventricle	—Monitor cardiac rhythm during insertion —Encourage rapid insertion while catheter is floated through right ventricle —Perform ongoing assessment of PA catheter waveforms —Monitor for ectopy	Patient will not sustain ventricular arrhythmias associated with PA catheters.
Infection	—lack of sterile technique during insertion —lack of sterile technique during dressing changes —loss of occlusiveness of dressing —nonadherence to dressing change and tubing change protocols —manipulation of caps	—Ensure adherence to sterile technique during insertion —Adhere to evidence-based standards to dressing and tubing changes —Monitor integrity of dressing for occlusiveness —Avoid touching male end of caps when zeroing the system	Patient will not develop an infection related to PA catheter.

FIGURE 11-4 The Phlebostatic Axis

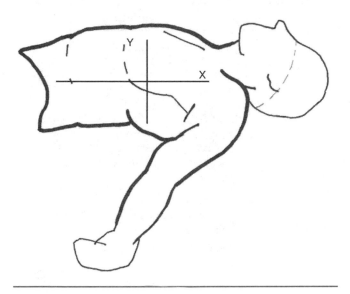

Source: Illustrated by James R. Perron.

lower frequency and give a low-pitched, low-frequency sound. Transducer systems are affected by their own set of factors, just as the sounds from guitar strings are affected by the thickness and tightness of the strings.

ICU nurses can test the frequency response of the system by completing a procedure known as square wave test or dynamic response test. Poor dynamic response will affect readings, making them appear either lower or higher than actual. Performing a dynamic response test is an important troubleshooting step when waveforms and numbers do not appear appropriate.

To perform a square wave test or dynamic response test, quickly squeeze and release the fast-flush device of the pressure waveform you are testing (if using a "pig-tail" fast flush device, quickly pull and release it). This results in a "square wave" in place of the waveform. If the dynamic response is appropriate, one or two oscillations will appear below the baseline.

TROUBLESHOOTING SYSTEMS

Troubleshooting hemodynamic monitoring lines takes experience and practice. **Table 11-7** represents common monitoring problems, causes of these problems, and nursing interventions.

Cardiac Output Measurement

The thermodilution method for obtaining CO is the gold standard in bedside hemodynamic monitoring. The bolus CO method uses an injectate solution (D_5W or NS) that is cooler

than body temperature. The injectate can be either iced or room temperature. Room-temperature injectate is preferred over iced injectate in contemporary CO measurement.

The injectate is given as a bolus into the right atrium via the proximal port of the PAC. The temperature change in the blood is measured downstream by the thermistor located on the distal tip of the catheter. The resultant change in blood temperature over time is recorded and displayed as a thermodilution curve. Bedside monitors with computer systems analyze the temperature/time curve and display a numeric value.

Intermittent thermodilution CO is used to measure ventricular blood flow at a given point in time. At least three measurements are taken, and then three COs within 0.5 L/min of each other are averaged to reflect the average flow rate. Several system-related factors can cause inaccurate CO measurements during this procedure and must be taken into account (Headley, 1998):

- Use the correct computation constant (type of catheter, amount of injectate, temperature of injectate).
- Avoid wrapping your hand around the syringe prior to instillation of fluid, so as not to warm it. This can affect accuracy of the measurement.
- Steadily push the syringe plunger.
- Inject fluid at the end of expiration.
- Inject fluid in less than 4 seconds.
- Wait 1 minute between each injection.
- The head of the bed's elevation should be less than 45°, with the patient in a supine position (Lough, 2006).
- Use a consistent injectate volume (10 mL, 5 mL, or 3 mL) per institution policy or patient fluid volume status. A menu is available on the cardiac monitor to help ensure accurate CO measurement.

Historically, it has been recommended that all CO measurements be taken with the patient in the supine position and a zero-degree head of bed elevation (Giuliano, Scott, Brown, & Olson, 2003). Often, a patient's condition necessitates that the head of the bed be elevated. Research has reported that performing a CO at a 20° elevation is accurate. Accuracy of CO measurements up to at least 20° and even greater elevations in some cardiac patient populations has been reported (Driscoll, Shannanhan, Crommy, Foong, & Gleeson, 1995; Giuliano et al.). The thermodilution CO method is not accurate, however, in the presence of a "wedged" catheter, tricuspid valve regurgitation, dysrhythmias, intracardiac shunts, severe mitral valve regurgitation, and right ventricular assist devices.

Continuous cardiac output (CCO) devices use thermal energy pulses to determine ventricular blood flow. Instead of averaging one to three measurements intermittently, these de-

TABLE 11-7 Critical Thinking: Troubleshooting Hemodynamic Monitoring Lines

Problem	Possible Cause	Prevention/Intervention
No waveform	• No power supply • Transducer not connected to pressure monitoring cable • Stopcock turned off to patient • Tubing kinked or compressed • Loose connections • Wrong pressure scale • Monitor module not connected • Catheter occlusion (clots, kink in catheter itself, catheter up against vessel wall)	• Check power supply, cable connections, and module • Check for loose connections • Check stopcock position • Check tubing for kinks • Use appropriate pressure scale • Check catheter position • If a clot is suspected, try to aspirate; if line will not flush, do not force it, but notify physician
Blood backup into the system	• Loose connections or leak in flush-bag pressure system • Stopcock in wrong position, no dead-ender caps • Low flush-bag pressure	• Dead-ender caps • Check connections • Stopcock in right position • Pressure bag: 300 mm Hg
Catheter artifact	• Electrical interference • Patient movement/respiration	• Ensure all lines are grounded
Catheter whip	• PAC: from force of contraction of RV in hyperdynamic conditions such as sepsis, anemia, excessive catecholamines, or catheter close to pulmonary valve • Arterial: hyperdynamic state, small vessel	• Perform dynamic response testing to check for appropriate dampening of system • Have physician reposition the catheter if needed; obtain CXR
Waveform drifting	• Temperature change in IV solution/catheter • Drifting from zero	• Zero monitor • Be aware of temperature
Unable to flush	• Stopcock in wrong position • Kinks in the tubing • Inadequate pressure for bag inflation • Clot in catheter	• Check stopcock position • Remove kinks • Ensure appropriate bag inflation • Aspirate: same rules as for waveform
Overdamped waveform Causes underestimation of pressures	• Air bubbles in system • Kinks in tubing/catheter • Blood backup in tubing/catheter • Catheter tip occlusion (clot, catheter up against vessel wall)	• Remove air bubbles and inspect tubing routinely • Remove kinks in tubing • Check catheter position • Observe for blood backup • Maintain pressure bag and continual flush system • Test dynamic response
Underdamped waveform Causes overestimation of pressures	• Tubing too long, greater than 4 feet • Excessive number of stopcocks or connectors	• Test dynamic response • Tubing length no longer than 4 feet, minimize stopcocks (have approximately three per line) • Noncompliant tubing
Inappropriate pressures with proper waveform	• ↓ Pressures: transducer higher than reference point • ↑ Pressures: transducer lower than reference point • Drift from zero	• Level and zero system

↑ = Increase, ↓ = Decrease.

vices heat passing blood with a thermal filament every few seconds. The temperature of the heated blood is measured in determining the CO. All CO measurements obtained during a 3- to 6-minute time frame are averaged and then displayed on the bedside monitor. Advantages to CCO include the elimination of user technique inconsistencies and the continuously updated measurement of CO. CCO catheters do not use injectate solutions and therefore conserve fluid intake for patients on fluid restriction (Headley, 1998).

Waveform Interpretation

Pulmonary Artery Catheter Waveforms

The PAC is a flow-directed catheter. When inflated, the balloon at its distal tip acts as a buoy to carry the catheter forward in the direction of blood flow. During its insertion, the distal port is monitored and waveforms appear in order as the catheter is advanced into the PA. Waveforms reflect mechanical events and pressure changes within the cardiac chambers and the pulmonary vasculature. Each chamber of the heart varies in terms of its pressure values and waveform components. These waveforms and pressure readings identify the placement of the catheter for the clinician. When properly in place, the distal port of the PAC "sits" in the PA and the proximal port of the PAC "sits" in the right atrium (see **Figure 11-5**). Once positioned correctly in the PA, the balloon is deflated and continual monitoring ensues. The bedside clinician monitors these waveforms and values for changes.

Right atrial waveforms are low-pressure waveforms that indicate atrial contraction (a wave), tricuspid valve closure (c wave), and bulging of the tricuspid valve into the atrium during right ventricular contraction (v wave). When normal anatomy and pressure values exist, these waves are essentially the same height. To negate the effects of intrathoracic pressure changes during respiration, the pressure measurement is taken on the waveform in the middle of the wave at the end of expiration (Rhodes et al., 2005). This will produce a mean value of 0 to 8 mm Hg (see Figure 11-5). This

waveform is monitored intermittently or continuously via the proximal port.

The right ventricular (RV) waveform has a systolic peak and a diastolic low (see Figure 11-5). The most readily identified difference between the PA waveform and the RV waveform is the dicrotic notch. The dicrotic notch on the PA waveform represents closure of the pulmonic valve and its associated pressure changes within the PA. Because that physiologic process does not occur in the RV, the dicrotic notch is absent in the RV waveform. RV systolic pressures range from 15 to 30 mm Hg, and RV diastolic pressures from 0 to 10 mm Hg. The RV waveform is seen both during insertion and during migration of the distal tip back into the right ventricle. It is therefore an important waveform to recognize. Irritation of the ventricle can occur when the stiff catheter tip brushes against the ventricular wall; this problem causes arrhythmias such as premature ventricular contractions and ventricular tachycardia.

PA pressure waveforms are monitored via the distal port of the PAC. Components of the PA waveform resemble those of an arterial line waveform: a systolic peak, dicrotic notch (pulmonic valve closure), and diastolic low. The main difference between PA pressures and systemic pressures is the numerical value. Normal PA systolic pressures are 15 to 30 mm Hg, and PA diastolic pressures are 8 to 15 mm Hg.

PAOP is monitored from the distal port of the PAC with the balloon at the tip of the catheter inflated. Once the balloon is inflated, the waveform changes from a PA pressure waveform to a flattened or "damped" PAOP waveform. The balloon is intermittently inflated to decrease the risk of PA rupture from prolonged PA occlusion (AACN, 2004). Components of this waveform are similar to the right atrial a, c, and v waves, except that the mechanical events causing the waves occur on the left side of the heart instead of the right. The PAOP waveform is measured at the end of expiration in the middle of the waveform. Monitors are not able to take into account the respiratory variation that occurs with inspiration and expiration. Because of this limitation, bedside monitor

FIGURE 11-5 Pulmonary Artery Catheter Waveforms

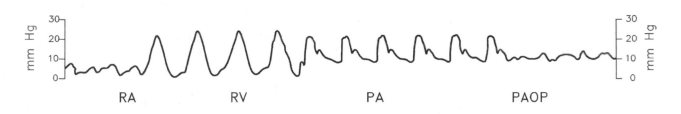

Source: Illustrated by James R. Perron.

digital readings may vary more than 4 mm Hg at a time with respiratory variation, which may sometimes lead to inaccurate pressure measurement and inappropriate patient treatment (Ahrens & Schallon, 2001). It is good practice to print the waveform, take note of the respiratory variation, and read the pressure value from the graph paper.

As an adjunct to mechanical ventilation, positive end expiratory pressure (PEEP) will keep alveoli open and place pressure on the pulmonary capillary beds. Elevated alveolar pressure elevates both PA pressures and PAOP. Because PAOP measurements rely on a steady column of uninterrupted blood flow, a PEEP greater than 10 mm Hg can artificially elevate PAOP.

Intra-arterial Waveform

Components of the intra-arterial pressure waveform reflect the mechanical movements of blood from the ventricles into the vasculature as well as blood pressure changes during systole and diastole (see **Figure 11-6**). The highest point on the systemic waveform—called the systolic peak—reflects the ventricular ejection and stroke volume. A notch on the downstroke of the waveform—called the dicrotic notch—represents the closing of the aortic valve. The dicrotic notch signifies the end of ventricular systole and the beginning of diastole. The remainder of the waveform represents diastolic run-off, which occurs as blood is perfused down the arterial tree. Figure 11-6 depicts a normal arterial waveform. Arterial waveforms and resultant blood pressures vary with insertion site. Systolic pressures become higher and diastolic pressures become lower as the blood vessels become smaller and more distal to the heart,

FIGURE 11-6 Intra-arterial Waveforms

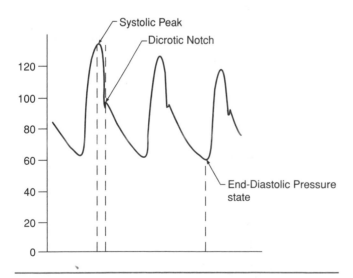

Source: Illustrated by James R. Perron.

such as in the dorsalis pedis artery. The appearance of the dicrotic notch changes the farther down the arterial tree.

MAP is utilized to assess the average pressure in the arterial beds across the vasculature. It reflects the perfusion pressure throughout the cardiac cycle. MAP in the range of 70–90 mm Hg is considered ideal (Lough, 2006). CO and vascular resistance determine MAP. As CO and stroke volume decline, systemic afterload increases to compensate for the deficit. Because the body's main goal is organ perfusion, compensatory mechanisms are activated to maintain a "normal" MAP. If tissue perfusion is not maintained, organ systems will begin to malfunction. Decreasing urine output, decreasing level of consciousness, and capillary refill time of more than 3 seconds are all signs of decreased end-organ perfusion.

CLINICAL INQUIRY AND DECISION MAKING

ICU nurses acquire knowledge of hemodynamic monitoring throughout their careers. Nurses new to the ICU must understand that interpretation of hemodynamic waveforms and their associated values takes time and practice. As the number of patient interactions accumulates with experience, clinical judgment skills will grow. It can be said that hemodynamic number values are only as good as the person who interprets the data. Care should be taken to avoid pitfalls that cause technical inaccuracies in value measurement.

Bedside practitioners must use noninvasive assessment techniques such as patient observation, palpation, and auscultation to gather information about a patient's vulnerability to a situation, and the complexity of the illness, and choose treatment while working collaboratively so as to bring about stabilization of vitals signs and body processes. The physical assessment data are combined with the hemodynamic measurements and then compared to a known set of standards, and a conclusion is drawn regarding how a disease process or traumatic event is affecting the patient's dynamic processes. It is always good critical thinking practice to ask why, how, and what. Here are some recommendations to assist with value interpretation:

Basic Information
- What is the patient's current diagnosis?
- Perform a baseline systems assessment.
- Obtain past medical history (e.g., heart failure, chronic obstructive pulmonary disease (COPD), peripheral vascular disease).
- How does the past medical history affect the plan of care for this patient?
- How would you focus your assessment?

Interpreting Values
- Trend the data. Do you have multiple readings over time?

- Are hemodynamic measurements within normal limits for the patient and his or her condition?
- Are hemodynamic measurements higher than normal, within normal limits, or lower than normal?
- In which direction are measurements trending: up or down?
- Ensure that appropriate techniques are used in gathering data.
- Check the transducer system for inaccuracies.

Interpreting Changes
- Do the patient's clinical signs and symptoms match the number values?
- Has the patient's system assessment changed?
- Is end-organ perfusion adequate?
- Has the patient's condition changed with a nursing intervention?
- Has the patient's condition changed with a medical intervention (e.g., fluid administration, diuretic administration, pharmacologic intervention)?
- Why might the changes be occurring? What is the pathophysiology of the disease process?

SUMMARY

Hemodynamic parameters are used in conjunction with clinical factors to help guide the treatment of disease process to a positive outcome. It is good and thorough practice to collect multiple data sets so that you can detect trends in values instead of rendering a treatment decision based on only one set of hemodynamic measurements. Accurate gathering of hemodynamic values and comparison of those values to the physiologic condition are paramount to cost-effective, outcome-driven therapies. Various types of invasive monitoring devices and methods of hemodynamic measurement provide the bedside clinician with insight into the blood flow and oxygen dynamics of critically ill individuals. Each piece of technology is selected to meet the monitoring needs for the individual patient's situation. Accurate monitoring techniques are employed to prevent errors in hemodynamic measurement. As our knowledge of the human body and technology grow, the ability to measure and interpret hemodynamic parameters will be enhanced.

CASE STUDY

Mr. L. is a 46-year-old patient who was admitted to the ICU yesterday with complaints of crushing substernal chest pain while attending the big Sunday football game at the local stadium. He reported diaphoresis and nausea during the chest pain event. Stadium staff called 911, and Mr. L. came to the attention of the local EMS advanced life support units. Paramedics administered oxygen, nitroglycerin, and aspirin at the scene with minimal relief of Mr. L.'s chest pain. In collaboration with the base hospital physicians, it was decided that Mr. L. needed immediate attention by cardiology to return adequate blood flow to his heart. He was transported to the Heart Center for further treatment and evaluation.

Mr. L. has a past medical history of diabetes, hypertension, and COPD. He is overweight by 40 pounds and smokes at least one pack of cigarettes per day. Mr. L. is divorced and currently resides with his girlfriend of 2 years. He has two daughters, both in their mid- to late twenties and not married. He states that he drinks socially, about two to three beers at a time, mostly on the weekends. He denies any substance abuse.

Once in the emergency department, a 12-lead ECG was performed and revealed a 4-mm ST-segment elevation in the anterior leads that corresponded to the left anterior descending coronary artery. Lab work revealed positive cardiac markers, indicating Mr. L. had suffered a myocardial infarction. He was rushed to the cardiac catheterization lab, where he received a diagnostic cardiac catheterization and coronary intervention with a drug-eluting stent. The physician placed a right jugular continuous cardiac output catheter with oximetric (SvO$_2$) capability. Mr. L. has a right femoral arterial line. He is on 6 L/min nasal oxygen. Once he was stabilized from the intervention, he was transported via stretcher to the ICU for continued monitoring and treatment.

On admission to the ICU, Mr. L. is groggy from the conscious sedation he received in the cardiac catheterization lab. However, he wakes when his name is called and he follows all commands. At this time he has no complaints of chest pain. He does state that he is hungry, he needs to urinate, and his right groin is sore from the catheter. The ICU nurse connects him to a cardiac monitor for rhythm analysis. His hemodynamic PAC line and arterial line are also connected to the monitor via the transducer for continual monitoring of hemodynamic waveforms (arterial, PAP, CVP) and blood pressure monitoring. A pulse oximeter is placed on his finger to monitor oxygen saturation.

Hemodynamic measurements were taken on arrival at 1600, again during the night at 0100, and then again at 0330 when Mr. L. began to complain of shortness of breath and a feeling of impending doom. His physical assessment at 0330 revealed diminished bilateral breath sounds with crackles in the bases, diaphoresis, tachypnea, dyspnea, and capillary refill of more than 3 seconds, with pale nail beds. Mr. L.'s urine output had diminished from 100 mL/h to 15 mL/h. He was anxious and scared, and stated he didn't want to die. The hemodynamic data are listed below for your interpretation.

Parameter	Admission/Cath Lab (1600 hours)	During the Night (0100 hours)	0330
Temperature	99.2°F		100.0°F
Heart rate	89	92	115
Blood pressure (mean)	120/78 (92)	110/80 (90)	80/60 (67)
PAP	35/20 (25)	42/24 (29)	48/30 (36)
CVP	6	10	12
PAOP	10	22	28
BSA	1.8		
SvO_2	70%	66%	58%
CO	5.0	4.2	2.5
CI	2.7	2.3	1.38
SV	56	46	22
SVI	31	26	12
PVR	240	133	256
SVR	1,376	1,523	1,760
RVSWI	8	6.7	1.3
LVSWI	35	24	9

CRITICAL THINKING QUESTIONS

1. Interpret the physical assessment data at 0330. What is Mr. L.'s priority problem?

2. In the hemodynamic measurement table, determine whether the hemodynamic parameters are higher than normal, within normal limits, or lower than normal for each of the three time frames. (*Hint:* place a ↑ or ↓ arrow beside values that are higher or lower than normal or an "=" mark beside values that are within normal limits.)

3. Trend the values. Did any hemodynamic values change? If so, which ones? In which direction did they change: up, down?

4. Are there any pathophysiologic processes occurring with Mr. L. that would cause these changes in his assessment and hemodynamic parameters? If so, what are they?

5. Using the Synergy Model, in what level (1, 3, or 5) would you place each patient characteristic for Mr. L. at 0330?

Note: Much information is presented in this case study. You as the bedside clinician must sort through the information one piece at a time to put the entire puzzle together. The nursing knowledge base for the care of this patient would include the following elements:

- Cardiac risk factors and their impact on the patient's disease process
- The American Heart Association's Standards for Treatment of Patients with Acute Coronary Syndrome/Acute MI
- Possible complications from an anterior wall myocardial infarction
- Hemodynamic waveform and value interpretation
- Expected hemodynamic value changes due to pathophysiology of acute myocardial infarction

6. What disciplines should you consult to work with this client?

7. What types of issues may require you to act as an advocate or moral agent for this patient?

8. How will you implement your role as a facilitator of learning for this patient?

Using the Synergy Model to Develop a Plan of Care

	Patient Characteristics	Level (1, 3, 5)	Subjective and Objective Data	Evidence-based Interventions	Outcomes
SYNERGY MODEL	Resiliency				
	Vulnerability				
	Stability				
	Complexity				
	Resource availability				
	Participation in care				
	Participation in decision making				
	Predictability				

CRITICAL THINKING QUESTIONS

1. Write up a plan of care for one client in the clinical setting for a patient requiring hemodynamic monitoring. Rate the patient as a level 1, 3, or 5 on each characteristic. Identify the level of nurse characteristics needed in the care of this patient.
2. Take one patient outcome for this patient and list evidence-based interventions for this patient.

Online Resources

Cleveland Clinic Center for Continuing Education, Hemodynamic Monitoring:
www.clevelandclinicmeded.com/micu/hemodynamic.htm

Hemodynamic Monitoring, Medi-Smart:
medi-smart.com/cc-hemo.htm

Posey, A., Hemodynamic Monitoring, An Introduction:
www.rnceus.com/course_frame.asp?exam_id=46&directory=hemo

Pulmonary Artery Catheter Education Project:
www.pacep.org

REFERENCES

Adams, K. (2004). Hemodynamic assessment: The physiologic basis for turning data into clinical information. *AACN Clinical Issues, 15*(4), 534–546.

Ahrens, R., & Schallon, L. (2001). Comparison of pulmonary artery and central venous pressure waveform measurements via digital and graphic measurement methods. *Heart & Lung, 30,* 26–38.

American Association of Critical Care Nursing. (2004). Pulmonary artery pressure monitoring. *AACN Practice Alert.*

Brandsetter, R. D., Grant, G. R., Estilo, M., Rahim, M., Singh, K., & Gitler, B. (1998). Swan-Ganz catheter: Misconceptions, pitfalls, and incomplete user knowledge—an identified trilogy in need of correction. *Heart & Lung, 27*(4), 218–222.

Connors, A. F., Spreoff, T., Dawson, N. V., Thomas, F., Harrell, F. E., Wagner, N., et al. (1996). The effectiveness of right heart catheterization in the initial care of critically ill patients. *Journal of the American Medical Association, 276,* 889–897.

Darovic, G. O. (2002). *Hemodynamic monitoring: Invasive and noninvasive clinical application* (3rd ed.). Philadelphia: Saunders.

Driscoll, A., Shannanhan, A., Crommy, L., Foong, S., & Gleeson, A. (1995). The effect of patient position on the reproducibility of cardiac output measurements. *Heart & Lung, 24,* 38–44.

Forrester, J. S., Diamond, G., Chatterjee, K., & Swan, H. J. (1976a). Medical therapy of acute myocardial infarction by application of hemodynamic subsets: First of two parts. *New England Journal of Medicine, 295,* 1356–1362.

Forrester, J. S., Diamond, G., Chatterjee, K., & Swan, H. J. (1976b). Medical therapy of acute myocardial infarction by application of hemodynamic subsets: Second of two parts. *New England Journal of Medicine, 295,* 1404–1413.

Gawlinski, A. (1997). Facts and fallacies of patient positioning and hemodynamic measurement. *Journal of Cardiovascular Nursing, 12*(1), 1–15.

Giuliano, K. K., Scott, S. S., Brown, V., & Olson, M. (2003). Backrest elevation and cardiac output measurement. *Nursing Research, 52*(4), 242–248.

Headley, J. (1998). Invasive hemodynamic monitoring: Applying advanced technologies. *Critical Care Nursing Quarterly, 21*(3), 73–84.

Jersurum, J. (2004). Protocols for practice—SvO$_2$ monitoring. *Critical Care Nurse, 24*(4), 73–76.

Johnson, K. (2004). Diagnostic measures to evaluate oxygenation in critically ill adults. *AACN Clinical Issues, 15*(4), 506–524.

Leeper, B. (2003). Monitoring right ventricular volumes: A paradigm shift. *AACN Clinical Issues, 14,* 208–219.

Lough, M. E. (2006). Cardiovascular diagnostic procedures. In L. D. Urden, K. M. Stacy, & M. E. Lough (Eds.), *Thelan's critical care nursing: Diagnosis and management* (5th ed., pp. 319–426). St. Louis, MO: Elsevier.

Ott, K., Johnson, K., & Ahrens, K. (2001). New technologies in the assessment of hemodynamic parameters. *AACN Clinical Issues, 15*(2), 41–55.

Prentice, D., & Ahrens, T. (2001). Controversies in the use of pulmonary artery catheter. *Journal of Cardiovascular Nursing, 15*(2), 1–5.

Rhodes, A., Grounds, R. M., & Bennett, E. D. (2005). Hemodynamic monitoring. In M. P. Fink, E. Abraham, J-L. Vincent, & P. M. Kochanek (Eds.), *Textbook of critical care* (5th ed., pp. 735–739). Philadelphia: Saunders.

Rivers, E., Nguyen, S., Havstad, J., Ressler, A., Muzzin, R., Knoblich, E., et al. (2001). Early goal-directed therapy in the treatment of severe sepsis and septic shock. *New England Journal of Medicine, 345*(19), 1368–1377.

Urban, N. (2004). Integrating the hemodynamic profile with clinical assessment. *AACN Clinical Issues, 4*(1), 161–179.

Warkentin, T. E., & Greinacher, A. (2004). Heparin–induced thrombocytopenia: Recognition, treatment, and prevention: The seventh ACCP conference on Antithrombotic and Thrombolytic Therapy. *Chest, 126*(Suppl. 3), 311S–337S.

Yu, D. T., Platt, R., Lanken, P. N., Black, E., Sands, K. E., Schwartz, J. S., et al. (2003). Relationship of pulmonary artery catheter use to mortality and resource utilization in patients with severe sepsis. *Critical Care Medicine, 31*(12), 2734–2741.

CHAPTER 12

Coronary Artery Disease

Barbara Hutton Borghardt

Upon completion of this chapter, the reader will be able to:

1. Describe the pathophysiology of coronary artery disease.

2. Discuss the assessment for patients with ischemic heart disease.

3. Describe pharmacological management for the patient with coronary artery disease.

4. List optimal patient outcomes that may be achieved through evidence-based management of coronary artery disease.

Coronary artery disease (CAD) is a significant health problem and cause of death in the United States today. More than 500,000 Americans die each year from CAD, and approximately 6.8 million people suffer from angina pectoris. In 2004, 600,000 patients experienced a myocardial infarction (MI), and 450,000 patients had a recurrent MI (AHA Journal Report, 2004). Many of these deaths may have been preventable. Despite the advances in diagnosis, technology, and treatment, many patients with CAD remain undiagnosed or delay treatment, resulting in increased morbidity and mortality.

CAD exists along a continuum that progresses from stable angina pectoris, to unstable angina, to myocardial injury, and MI. Many of the therapeutic modalities used in the treatment of CAD are designed to prevent MI or to limit the infarct size. These modalities help to preserve functioning myocardial muscle and preserve the quality of life (Berra & Klieman, 2003).

THE CORONARY ARTERIES

The coronary arteries, which arise from the ascending aorta, supply the heart muscle with oxygen and nutrients. They travel over the epicardial (outermost) layer of the heart and branch many times as they invade the endocardial (innermost) layer (see **Figure 12-1**). Because the heart is beating continuously, it requires a continuous supply of oxygen and nutrients to maintain its muscular activity, which is supplied by the coronary arteries. **Box 12-1** describes the coronary arteries and the areas of the heart each supplies.

PATHOPHYSIOLOGY OF CORONARY ARTERY DISEASE

Development of Atherosclerotic Lesions

Although CAD can occur for many reasons, the most common cause is atherosclerosis. Approximately 80% of MIs are the result of atherosclerotic plaques (Morton, 2005). Over time, a series of pathological changes known as atherosclerosis occur within the coronary artery. Atherosclerosis results in a progressive narrowing of the lumen of the vessel, which in turn limits the ability of the coronary artery to deliver oxygen and nutrients to the area of the heart that it supplies.

FIGURE 12-1 The Coronary Arteries: (a) Anterior View and (b) Posterior View

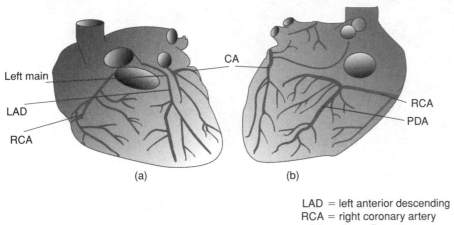

(a)   (b)

LAD = left anterior descending
RCA = right coronary artery
CA = circumflex artery
PDA = posterior descending artery

monocytes (white blood cells) migrate to the area of the injury, move into the intima (under the endothelial layer), and differentiate into macrophages. The macrophages ingest the lipid particles that find their way into the intima and become foam cells.

As the lesion becomes larger, many of the foam cells die and produce a necrotic core within the plaque covered by a collagenous fibrous cap (Kaul, McAleer, & Steingart, 2005; Libby, 2004–2005a). Cytokines and growth factors encourage smooth muscle cells to move into the developing lesion and divide, resulting in the formation of the atherosclerotic plaque (Libby).

These changes are believed to begin with an injury to the endothelial (innermost) layer of the vessel wall. Factors such as hypertension, vasoconstriction, hyperlipidemia, hyperglycemia, and smoking have all been implicated in the development and progression of the disease (Baird, 2001; Morton, 2005).

Lipoprotein particles, which are molecules that bind with fats (cholesterol and triglycerides), allowing those fats to be transported throughout the body, adhere to the endothelial wall of the vessel and undergo oxidative and chemical changes. A local inflammatory response ensues in which

See **Figure 12-2**.

As blood flow to the heart muscle becomes increasingly restricted, chest pain may develop. Atherosclerotic lesions, however, often remain asymptomatic until the lesion restricts 60% to 70% of blood flow (Morton, 2005). Whether symptoms of pain occur may depend on the development of collateral circulation. This response to a slow-growing lesion occurs when smaller arteries, which connect to larger vessels, dilate and grow. New capillaries may develop in the area in response to pressure changes and ischemia (Gardner & Altman, 2005; Morton).

Box 12-1
The Coronary Arteries

The left main coronary artery arises from the aorta and quickly branches to form the left anterior descending (LAD) and the left circumflex artery (LCA). The LAD supplies the anterior surface of the left ventricle (LV), medial anterior surface of the right ventricle (RV), lower one-third of the posterior surface of the RV, and most of the intraventricular septum. The LCA supplies the lateral wall, apical portion of the posterior wall of LV, sinus node (in 45% of people), and atrioventricular node (in 10% of people).

The right coronary artery (RCA) supplies most of the RV, part of the posterior wall of the LV, the sinus node (in 50% of people), the atrioventricular node (in 90% of people), and part of the intraventricular septum.

In 80% to 90% of the population, the RCA gives rise to the posterior descending artery (PDA). This percentage of the population is said to be *right dominant*. In about 7% of the population, the LCA gives rise to the PDA; this group is the *left dominant* population. In another 7%, both the LCA and the RCA give rise to the PDA. This is the *co-dominant* population. The PDA supplies the posterior wall of the right and left ventricles.

Source: Carter & Ellis, 2005.

FIGURE 12-2 Process of Atherosclerosis: Normal Coronary Artery; Fatty Streak; Growing Atheroma Lesion; Plaque Disruption

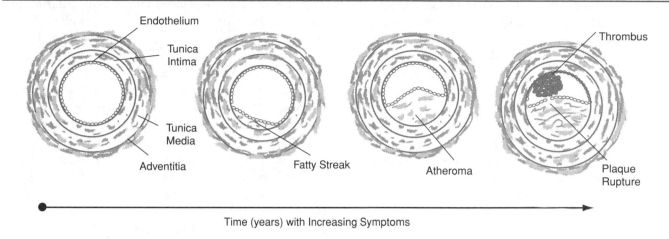

Time (years) with Increasing Symptoms

Inflammation plays a significant role in all stages of plaque development. This inflammation is meant to be protective and to heal the injury. Unfortunately, many of the chemical mediators of inflammation result in further progression of the disease. The inflammatory process leaves behind biomarkers, such as C-reactive protein (CRP) that can be measured as predictors of CAD (see "Markers of Inflammation") later in this chapter (Kaul et al., 2005).

Atherosclerosis is a slowly progressing disease. It does not undergo a steady or linear progression over time, however (Virmani et al., 2005). In the presence of significant risk factors, atherosclerosis will produce more severe lesions earlier in life. For this reason, there is a growing focus on improving the diet and health practices of children with hyperlipidemia and hyperglycemia (Kavey et al., 2003).

Plaque Rupture and Thrombus Formation

Inflammatory processes and sheer stress appear to weaken the fibrous cap and, at any time during its development, the atherosclerotic plaque may become unstable and rupture (Hawley, 2004; Kaul et al., 2005). Rupture appears to occur more often with moderate-size lesions, rather than the previously suspected larger lesions (Gardner & Altman, 2005; Hawley).

Plaque disruption exposes the lipid-rich foam cells to blood flow within the vessel's lumen. These cells are highly prone to platelet adhesion to the site of the rupture. The clotting cascade is initiated, leading to the formation of fibrin. Platelets adhere to the fibrin mesh, creating a thrombus (Gardner & Altman, 2005). Thrombus development will produce a significant change in the patency of the artery, because it may fully or partially occlude the lumen. Persons with

stable angina may experience a progression in their symptoms to unstable angina or MI.

RISK FACTORS

Risk factors are behaviors or conditions that increase the likelihood of CAD. Some risk factors, such as smoking or hypertension, are modifiable; others, such as age and genetic predisposition, are not. The effect of risk factors is cumulative. The more risk factors a person has, the greater the possibility of developing CAD (AHA Scientific Position, 2005).

Nonmodifiable Risk Factors

Family History and Ethnicity

Family history is a significant nonmodifiable risk factor for CAD and is most likely related to genetic alterations in lipid metabolism and environmental factors (Newton & Froelicher, 2005). The risk is greater if a parent or sibling had CAD, especially if that person developed the disease before the age of 50. Until the age of 70, CAD death rates are highest among black males. After the age of 70, white men have the highest death rate. Black women have higher death rates than white women, but after the age of 80, white women move into second place behind white men in terms of death rates from this cause (Newton & Froelicher).

Gender and Estrogen

Men are much more likely to have CAD than are premenopausal women. After menopause, however, the percentage of women with CAD begins to rise rapidly, and in the seventh decade of life becomes nearly equal to the percentage of men with CAD (Becker, 1999). Loss of the protective mechanism of estrogen, which produces higher levels of high-density lipoproteins (HDL), is believed to be the cause (Morton, 2005). Recent data suggest that women who are 10 to 12 years postmenopausal and are taking combined (estrogen and progesterone) hormone replacement therapy have an increased risk of heart disease (Rossouw et al., 2002). Postmenopausal women who are taking estrogen-only hormone replacement therapy do not have an increased risk for heart disease but do have an increased risk of stroke (U.S. Department of Health and Human Services, 2004). Premenopausal women who smoke or use birth control pills, however, have a significantly higher risk for CAD than those who do not (Assman et al., 1999).

Advancing Age

Persons of advancing age are more prone to show signs of CAD. CAD develops sporadically over decades. As age increases, so does the likelihood of further development of the atherosclerotic plaque. More than 80% of persons who die from CAD are 65 years of age or older (AHA Scientific Position, 2005).

Modifiable Risk Factors

Cholesterol/Lipoproteins/Triglycerides

The most firmly established modifiable risk factor is the relationship between CAD and alterations in cholesterol, triglycerides, and lipoprotein levels. Cholesterol, a molecule produced by the liver, is an important part of the composition of cell membranes. It adds structure and stability to the cell membrane and regulates its permeability to water. Cholesterol is an important base from which hormones, steroids, and bile salts are built (Davidson, 2002).

Triglycerides, a major source of fat energy used by the body, are composed of a glycerol molecule connected to three fatty acid chains. Monounsaturated and polyunsaturated fats tend to lower total cholesterol levels. Saturated fats elevate total cholesterol levels and have been implicated in the atherogenic process (Becker, 1999).

Lipoproteins bind with fats, allowing them to be transported throughout the body. They are named according to their density. Low-density lipoproteins (LDL) consist of two types: small, dense particles and larger, less dense particles. The smaller particles appear to be able to penetrate the endothelial space of the vessel wall more easily than the larger particles, and are more likely to undergo oxidation than the larger particles—both properties that promote atherogenesis (Fair & Berra, 2005).

HDLs are known to be protective and prevent atherosclerotic changes. Two mechanisms may be responsible for this protective effect. First, HDLs undergo less oxidation than LDLs. Second, HDLs increase the transport of cholesterol to the liver to be cleared in bile. Low levels of HDL are found to contribute to CAD risk (Libby, 2004–2005b).

A serum profile that measures total cholesterol, triglycerides, and HDL and LDL cholesterol should be assessed after a 9- to 14-hour fast (Assman et al., 1999; Davidson, 2002). Total cholesterol levels should be maintained at less than 200 mg/dL and triglycerides at less than 150 mg/dL. Ideally, LDL levels should be less than 130 mg/dL, or less than 100 mg/dL for people who are at high risk for CAD. HDL levels of less than 30 to 40 mg/dL are associated with a higher risk of CAD (Berra & Klieman, 2003; Fair & Berra, 2005).

Diabetes/Hyperglycemia

Even when modified by diet, oral hypoglycemics, and/or insulin, diabetes carries a significantly increased risk of CAD. Approximately two-thirds of persons with diabetes will die from complications of heart or blood vessel disease (Morton, 2005). Chronic hyperglycemia is thought to increase the production of free radicals in the bloodstream, which can be counteracted by antioxidants. If, however, the antioxidant supply in the body is used up, glycated proteins form, leading to vascular damage. Diabetics are also prone to develop diabetic dyslipidemia, a condition associated with insulin resistance and resulting in abnormal lipoprotein molecules that are very atherogenic (Libby, 2004–2005b).

Hypertension

Hypertension, defined as a systolic blood pressure greater than 140 mm Hg and a diastolic pressure greater than 90 mm Hg, is associated with a three- to four-fold increase in the risk of CAD. Hypertension may be influenced by age, hereditary factors, renal function, sodium intake, obesity, and medications such as steroids (Becker, 1999). It is felt to promote atherosclerotic changes to the vessel wall by sheer stress and endothelial dysfunction (Braunwald, 2001).

Smoking

Cigarette smokers are two to three times more likely to die from CAD than are nonsmokers. Fortunately, this is a modifiable risk. Indeed, 5 to 15 years after quitting, previous smokers will have the same risk of developing CAD as nonsmokers. Smokers have a much greater chance of dying from sudden death than do nonsmokers (World Health Organization, 1998).

Inactivity

Leading a sedentary lifestyle can have deleterious effects on health. Physical inactivity is comparable to hypertension, smoking, or high cholesterol as a CAD risk (World Health Organization, 1998). Regular physical exercise can prevent the development of CAD. In addition, regular exercise reduces other atherosclerotic risk factors such as hypertension, hyperglycemia, high cholesterol and triglyceride levels, and overweight (Thompson et al., 2003).

Overweight/Obesity

Obesity is often associated with other CAD risk factors such as hypertension, hyperglycemia, and lipoprotein disorders. Thus considerable debate has arisen regarding whether it is a risk factor for CAD on its own (Gola, Bonadonna, Doga, Mazziotti, & Giustina, 2005). More recent evidence has shown that when the other risk factors are controlled, obesity still carries a higher risk for CAD (Braunwald, 2001; Stevens, Cai, Everson, & Thomas, 2003).

Metabolic Syndrome

Persons with at least three of the following diagnostic criteria for metabolic syndrome are at 1.5 to 3 times greater risk for developing cardiovascular disease and diabetes (Isomaa et al., 2001; Stevens et al., 2003). They have a greater mortality rate than the general population (AHA Statistical Fact Sheet, 2005; Isomaa et al.). The criteria (AHA Statistical Fact Sheet) are:

> Waist circumference > 40 inches for men or > 35 inches for women
>
> Serum triglyceride level > 150 mg/dL
>
> HDL cholesterol < 40 mg/dL for men or < 50 mg/dL for women
>
> Blood pressure > 130/85
>
> Fasting blood sugar > 110 mg/dL

MARKERS OF INFLAMMATION

Given that all stages of the atherosclerotic process and plaque rupture are associated with inflammation, certain markers of inflammation may be able to predict CAD or the probability of an impending cardiac event. Predicting when people are at risk may be of great value for individuals whose conventional risk factors are inconclusive or who have no signs or symptoms of their ischemic heart disease (ICD). People with elevated markers may benefit from early therapy with aspirin and statins to reduce their risk (Casey, 2004; Rosenson & Koenig, 2003).

C-Reactive Protein

CRP is a peptide produced by the liver in response to inflammation. During the inflammatory response, the serum level of CRP may rise by 25% or more from baseline (Duffy & Salerno, 2004). CRP levels are also known to be elevated in certain immune disorders, such as rheumatoid arthritis and systemic lupus, and in infections (Casey, 2004). Highly sensitive CRP, a blood assay designed to detect smaller fluctuations in CRP levels, has been used to detect inflammation and minute tissue damage (Rosenson & Koenig, 2003). In persons who have experienced unstable angina or an MI, elevated levels appear to predict the possibility of a recurrent event (Flutterman & Lemberg, 2002). For maximum effectiveness as a predictor, it is suggested that two CRP levels be obtained two weeks apart, and their results averaged. See **Table 12-1** for interpretation of CRP results.

Other Markers of Inflammation

In addition to CRP, other inflammatory markers are under current investigation and may prove useful in predicting CAD:

- Fibrinogen levels
- Homocysteine levels
- Interleukin-6 (IL-6)
- CD 40 ligand
- Lipoprotein (a)

BLOOD SUPPLY AND DEMAND

In addition to the atherosclerotic process, other factors can contribute to the development of myocardial ischemia, injury, and infarction. Because the heart requires a constant blood supply, it must maintain a delicate balance between the blood supply it receives and the blood supply it demands. With atherosclerosis, blood supply to an area of the heart muscle will diminish as the lesion grows larger. No symptoms may be present until other factors upset the balance of supply and demand; these factors are listed in **Figure 12-3**.

TABLE 12-1 C-Reactive Protein Levels

Level	Degree of Risk
< 1.0 mg/L	Low
1.0–3.0 mg/L	Average
> 3.0 mg/L	High

Source: Casey, 2004.

FIGURE 12-3 Factors Affecting Blood Supply and Demand

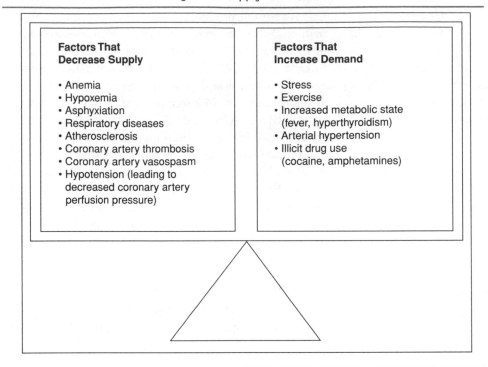

Factors That Decrease Supply

- Anemia
- Hypoxemia
- Asphyxiation
- Respiratory diseases
- Atherosclerosis
- Coronary artery thrombosis
- Coronary artery vasospasm
- Hypotension (leading to decreased coronary artery perfusion pressure)

Factors That Increase Demand

- Stress
- Exercise
- Increased metabolic state (fever, hyperthyroidism)
- Arterial hypertension
- Illicit drug use (cocaine, amphetamines)

Source: Gardner & Altman, 2005.

Many of the medications used in the treatment of IHD will increase blood supply to the heart muscle or decrease its demand for oxygen. Nitrates and calcium channel blockers (CCBs), for example, cause vasodilation of the coronary arteries, which in turn improves blood supply. Beta-adrenergic blockers, by contrast, decrease the workload of the heart by reducing both heart rate and contractility of the heart muscle.

With IHD, patients can have chronic/stable angina or acute coronary syndromes (ACS). ACS are discussed in Chapter 14.

Angina Pectoris

Angina pectoris is the term used to describe the chest pain or discomfort caused by lack of oxygen (ischemia) to the heart muscle (Baird, 2001). Unfortunately, not all persons with ischemia will experience chest pain—although pain is undesirable, it is an important warning sign of myocardial ischemia (Ryan, Devon, & Johnson Zerwic, 2005). Typically, the pain of angina will occur when myocardial oxygen demand rises, such as during times of stress or exercise. With the presence of atherosclerotic plaques, the artery is unable to supply enough blood to meet the increased demand, resulting in ischemia.

Stable/chronic angina is characterized by pain or discomfort that is predictable and does not change in intensity, dura-

tion, or frequency. Usually it is precipitated by stress, exertion, or exercise and has not changed over a period of several months.

The chest pain accompanied by IHD may be described in several ways. It is helpful to use the acronym O-P-Q-R-S-T to obtain an accurate description of the pain (Becker, 1999). See **Box 12-2**.

In addition, assessment should include what the patient usually does to relieve pain. Patients with angina are typically instructed to rest and take sublingual or buccal spray nitroglycerin. If they have taken three doses without relief, they are instructed to seek medical help.

Differential Diagnosis of Ischemic Heart Disease

Other disorders in which chest pain is a symptom may mimic IHD and confound the diagnosis. **Table 12-2** lists some of the more common disorders.

Electrocardiographic Changes in Ischemic Heart Disease

In IHD, the electrocardiogram (ECG) has been the most frequently used assessment tool, and it remains a standard in the diagnosis of myocardial ischemia, injury, and infarction. The use of the ECG has several limitations, however. First, preexisting cardiac diseases, such as bundle branch blocks and left ventricular hypertrophy, may obscure new ECG changes, making the diagnosis of a new event difficult. Second, ECG changes with ischemia revert to normal when the anginal episode is over and may be missed during the initial assessment of the patient. Third, it may be difficult to determine the age of a cardiac event based on ECG findings. Fourth, neurological disorders, pericarditis, and electrolyte abnormalities may be misinterpreted as IHD (Pyne, 2004).

Ischemia refers to an area of the heart muscle to which blood supply is compromised. Patients with angina will experience ischemic changes on their ECG, including ST-segment depression and T-wave inversion that return to normal when the episode is over. Changes to the myocardial muscle are reversible at this point.

Box 12-2

The O-P-Q-R-S-T Assessment for Pain

O *Other symptoms.* What other symptoms accompanied the pain? Patients may report numbness and tingling in the hands or fingers, faintness, excessive sweating, shortness of breath, extreme fatigue, anxiety, nausea, vomiting, and palpitations. Patients who experience these signs and symptoms, along with atypical chest pain, are more likely to delay seeking treatment. Women, diabetics, and the elderly are more likely to experience atypical symptoms.

P *Precipitating factors.* What activity was the patient involved in during or just prior to the onset of the pain? Did the patient awaken from sleep? Was there emotional or physical stress involved? Did the pain occur after a large meal? Being out in cold weather, for example, often triggers anginal attacks.

Q *Quality of the pain.* The pain may be described in a variety of ways. Most commonly, the pain is crushing, suffocating, heavy, or squeezing. It may also be burning, stabbing, or just a dull ache. Many patients with MI report the pain as the worst they have ever experienced.

R *Region (location) of pain.* Where is the pain located? Most commonly, the pain is substernal or retrosternal, or on the left side of the chest. Atypical pain may be located posteriorly between the scapula, epigastric area, shoulders, and, rarely, ears. In addition, the pain may radiate to the neck, down the arms, into the jaw, or to the left shoulder.

S *Severity.* The patient should be asked to rate the pain on a scale of 0 to 10, where 0 means no pain and 10 is the worst pain ever experienced. Also, is this pain similar or worse than any other previous episodes of pain?

T *Time.* What time did the pain begin? How long did it last? How does this episode compare to the length of time of previous episodes? Has the pain been occurring with increasing frequency and/or for longer periods of time?

Sources: Becker, 1999; Braunwald, 2003; Ryan, Devon, & Johnson Zerwic, 2005.

TABLE 12-2 Differential Diagnosis of Ischemic Heart Disease

Esophageal/gastric disorders: Esophageal spasm or reflux; peptic ulcer disease. Usually relieved by antacids, food, or milk products.

Costochondritis: Pain on palpation of the anterior chest over the costochondral joints.

Acute pericarditis: Inflammation of the pericardial sac surrounding the heart. Sharp pain, aggravated by breathing, relieved by sitting forward.

Pulmonary embolus: A blood clot to the lung may produce chest pain, usually on inspiration; associated with dyspnea and impaired oxygen saturation.

Dissecting aortic aneurysm: A medical emergency; a tear in the intimal layer of the aorta causes blood to separate the underlying areas. Pain is severe and retrosternal. Blood pressure may be different in each arm.

Pneumothorax: Partial or complete collapse of a lung or lobe of a lung. Usually characterized by a sharp pain and diminished breath sounds over the affected area with diminished chest movement.

Source: Braunwald, 2001.

Injury refers to prolonged, intense ischemia of the myocardial muscle. Striking ECG changes of ST-segment elevation are present, and the patient may experience unstable angina or infarction. Changes to the myocardial muscle may or may not be reversible at this point, depending on the length of time and degree of the injury.

Infarction refers to death of myocardial muscle and is not reversible (Brady, Aufderheide, Chan, & Perron, 2001). Developement of Q waves is noted on the ECG.

TREATMENT OF CHRONIC STABLE ANGINA AND SUSPECTED OR KNOWN CAD

The goals of treatment in patients with chronic stable angina or in patients with known or suspected CAD are twofold: (1) to prevent progression of the disease that will lead to MI and death, and (2) to improve the quality of life through control of symptoms (Snow et al., 2004). These treatments involve both lifestyle modifications and pharmacological intervention.

Lifestyle Alterations

Modifying lifestyle is, perhaps, the most difficult intervention. After a work-up to determine which risk factors need to be addressed, an individualized plan is put into place with the help of healthcare professionals. The plan typically includes the following elements:

- Stress management and relaxation techniques.
- Dietary modifications—to institute a low-cholesterol, low-saturated-fat diet with an increase in fiber, with follow-up on serum cholesterol and triglyceride levels continuing until the levels are stable. For diabetics, improved management of hyperglycemia with close follow-up of recorded fingerstick blood sugars is necessary.
- Smoking cessation programs.
- Activity alterations—to become less sedentary and utilize physician-guided exercise programs that will be increased gradually as tolerated.
- Blood pressure modification—to incorporate behaviors that will lower blood pressure, including a lower-sodium diet, exercise, stress reduction, and medications, if necessary.
- Weight reduction—to undergo supervised weight reduction through diet and exercise.
- Patient education—to recognize the symptoms related to ischemia or progressing angina, such as increasing chest pain, decreased exercise tolerance, orthopnea, shortness of breath, fatigue, sweating, dizziness, and palpitations (Baird, 2001; DeeBene & Vaughan, 2005).

Pharmacological Management

Lipid-Lowering Medications

- Statins limit the rate of cholesterol production and the inflammatory response in atherosclerosis (Ehrenstein, Jury, & Mauri, 2005; Fair & Berra, 2005). Statins have been the most effective of the lipid-lowering agents. Side effects include gastrointestinal intolerance, headache, and elevations in liver enzymes.
- Bile acid–binding resins increase intestinal excretion of bile acids, which results in increased production of bile acids by the liver. Because liver stores of cholesterol are reduced, an increased number of LDL receptors are produced, resulting in lower blood cholesterol levels.
- Cholesterol absorption inhibitors prevent the absorption of cholesterol from the intestine, resulting in lower serum cholesterol and LDL levels, and higher HDL levels.
- Niacin (vitamin B_3), in large doses, blocks the release of free fatty acids from fat tissues, resulting in lower triglyceride and LDL levels; it also raises HDL levels.
- Fibric acid derivatives have been effective in treating high triglyceride levels, which may increase HDL levels as well.

Antiplatelet Medications

Aspirin is given for its antithrombogenic effect through platelet inhibition, and to reduce the inflammatory response in atherosclerosis (Awtry & Loscalzo, 2000), in doses of 81 to 360 mg daily. If the patient cannot tolerate aspirin therapy, thienopyridines, such as clopidogrel (Plavix®) or ticopidine hydrochloride (Ticlid®), may be used instead (DeeBene & Vaughan, 2005).

Angiotensin-Converting Enzyme Inhibitors

Angiotensin-converting enzyme (ACE) inhibitors, which block the conversion of angiotensin I to angiotensin II, result in arterial vasodilation and lower blood pressure. The ultimate effect is to decrease myocardial oxygen demand by decreasing the workload of the heart. Long-term use may stabilize atherosclerotic endothelium in the coronary arteries, preventing plaque rupture and decreasing the risk of left ventricular failure (DeeBene & Vaughan, 2005; Snow et al., 2004).

Nitrates

Nitrates relieve the symptoms of chest pain or discomfort by promoting vasodilation in the coronary arteries and in collateral vessels. These peripheral venous and arterial vasodilators lower blood pressure and decrease the amount of blood returning to the heart, thereby relieving the symptoms of heart failure (Cannon & Braunwald, 2004–2005).

Beta-Adrenergic Blocking Agents

Beta blockers inhibit the effect of sympathetic stimulation by the catecholamines epinephrine and norepinephrine on beta receptors. This effect results in lower heart rate, contractility, and blood pressure, which in turn decreases myocardial oxygen demand. A slower heart rate allows for improved coronary artery perfusion, which increases blood supply to the heart muscle. Beta blockers are antidysrhythmics as well, so they may prevent dysrhythmias in an ischemic heart.

Calcium Antagonists (Calcium Channel Blockers)

If patients are unable to tolerate beta blockers, CCBs may be utilized. These agents, which block the action of calcium, have several effects: (1) coronary artery (CA) and systemic arteriole vasodilatation; (2) decreased contractility of the heart (negative inotropy); and (3) decreased heart rate and conduction through the atrioventricular (AV) node. These drugs increase myocardial oxygen supply by promoting CA vasodilation and by slowing heart rate, thereby allowing for longer diastolic perfusion time. In addition, they decrease myocardial oxygen demand by slowing the heart rate, decreasing contractility, and lowering blood pressure.

Patient teaching is an essential component for patients receiving any type of pharmacotherapy for angina and CAD. The importance of follow-up must be stressed. For patients taking lipid-lowering medications, liver enzymes and cholesterol profiles will be followed. Patients should report feelings of extreme tiredness, fatigue, or muscle aches because myopathies may result. Patients taking antiplatelet medications should be instructed to report any signs of bleeding. While taking CCBs, beta blockers, and ACE inhibitors, routine checks of blood pressure are performed. Patients may be taught to take their pulse daily, and as a guide to exercise.

PATIENT OUTCOMES

Nurses can help ensure attainment of optimal patient outcomes such as those listed in **Box 12-3** through the use of evidence-based interventions.

SUMMARY

Care of the cardiac patient can be complex and challenging and takes place in a wide range of settings. Nurses working in intensive care units will care for patients with cardiovascular disease. Support, encouragement, and education are all necessary tools to help patients through the difficult time of adjusting to a new diagnosis and possibly an altered lifestyle.

Box 12-3
Patient Outcomes

- Adherence to treatment plan
- Activity tolerance
- Physical comfort within expected range
- Seeks health-related information from a variety of sources to develop health strategies
- Describes strategies to maximize health
- Modifiable risk factors for CAD will be minimized or eliminated
- Angina not present

CASE STUDY

Mr. K. is a 59-year-old obese male with a history of familial hyperlipidemia and smoking. For the past month, he has been experiencing episodes of chest pressure or "twinges" with exertion that typically last 3 to 5 minutes. Six months ago, he was told that his serum glucose was elevated, but he has not had time to follow up. He now presents to the emergency department with complaints of increasing chest pain occurring and lasting for 5 to 10 minutes. He has no pain at this time. His vital signs are BP 106/70, HR 92, and RR 22; his ECG and troponin are within normal limits.

CRITICAL THINKING QUESTIONS

1. What known risk factors have contributed to Mr. K.'s condition?
2. Based on Mr. K.'s symptoms, what is the most likely diagnosis?
3. Which medications and interventions do you think are appropriate at this time?
4. Discuss possible treatment modalities for Mr. K.'s condition.
5. Discuss areas of patient teaching Mr. K. will need for discharge and lifestyle modifications in which he will require support.
6. How will you implement your role as a facilitator of learning for this patient?

Using the Synergy Model to Develop a Plan of Care

	Patient Characteristics	Subjective and Objective Data	Evidence-based Interventions	Outcomes
SYNERGY MODEL	Resiliency			
	Vulnerability			
	Stability			
	Complexity			
	Resource availability			
	Participation in care			
	Participation in decision making			
	Predictability			

CRITICAL THINKING QUESTIONS

1. Write a case example from the clinical setting highlighting one patient characteristic. Explain how the characteristic was observed through subjective and objective data.

2. Utilize the form to write up a plan of care for one client with CAD in the clinical setting. Rate the patient as a level 1, 3, or 5 on each characteristic.

3. Take one patient outcome for this patient and list evidence-based interventions for this patient.

Online Resources

American Heart Association:
www.americanheart.org

Braunwald's Heart Disease: A Textbook of Cardiovascular Medicine, 7th ed. (2005):
http://home.mdconsult.com

REFERENCES

AHA Journal Report. (January 1, 2004). American Heart Association Heart Disease and Stroke Statistics. Retrieved April 26, 2005, from www.americanheart.org

AHA Scientific Position: Risk Factors and Coronary Heart Disease. (2005). American Heart Association. Retrieved May 18, 2005, from www.myamericanheart.org

AHA Statistical Fact Sheet 2005 Update. (2005). American Heart Association. Retrieved May 18, 2005, from www.americanheart.org

Assman, G., Carmena, R., Cullen, P., Fruchart, J. C., Jossa, F., Lewis, B., et al. (1999). Coronary heart disease: Reducing the risk. *Circulation, 100,* 1930–1938.

Awtry, E. H., & Loscalzo, J. (2000). Aspirin. *Circulation, 101*(10), 1206–1218.

Baird, M. S. (2001). Acute coronary syndromes. In P. L. Swearington & J. Hicks Keen (Eds.), *Manual of critical care nursing* (4th ed., pp. 247–264). St. Louis, MO: Mosby.

Becker, D. (1999). Coronary artery disease. In L. Bucher & S. Melander (Eds.), *Critical care nursing* (pp. 201–227). Philadelphia: W. B. Saunders.

Berra, K., & Klieman, L. (2003). National Cholesterol Education Program: Adult Treatment Panel III—new recommendations for lifestyle and medical management of dyslipidemia. *Journal of Cardiovascular Nursing, 18*(2), 85–92.

Brady, W. J. Jr., Aufderheide, T. P., Chan, T., & Perron, A. D. (2001). Diagnosis and treatment of acute myocardial infarction: Electrocardiographic diagnosis of acute myocardial infarction. *Emergency Medicine Clinics of North America, 19*(2). Retrieved June 17, 2001, from http://home.mdconsult.com

Braunwald, E. (2001). *A textbook of cardiovascular medicine* (6th ed.). W. B. Saunders. Available at http://home.mdconsult.com

Braunwald, E. (2003). Application of current guidelines to the management of unstable angina and non ST-elevation MI. *Circulation, 108*(Suppl. III), III-28–III-37.

Cannon, C. P., & Braunwald, E. (2004–2005). Unstable angina and non-ST elevation MI. In D. L. Kasper, E. Braunwald, A. S. Fauci, S. L. Hauser, D. L. Longo, J. L. Jameson, et al. (Eds.), *Harrison's principles of internal medicine* (16th ed.). McGraw-Hill (Harrison's Online). Retrieved May 18, 2005, from www.accessmedicine.com

Carter, T., & Ellis, K. (2005). Right ventricular infarction. *Critical Care Nurse, 25*(2), 52–62.

Casey, P. (2004). Markers of myocardial injury and dysfunction. *AACN Clinical Issues, 15*(4), 547–557.

Davidson, D. (2002). Understanding cholesterol. *Nursing Spectrum.* Retrieved May 20, 2005, from http://community.nursingspectrum.com

DeeBene, S., & Vaughan, A. (2005). Acute coronary syndromes. In S. L. Woods, E. S. Sivarajan Froelicher, S. Underhill Motzer, & E. J. Bridges (Eds.), *Cardiac nursing* (5th ed., pp. 550–584). Philadelphia: Lippincott Williams & Wilkins.

Duffy, J. R., & Salerno, M. (2004). New blood test to measure heart attack risk: C-reactive protein. *Journal of Cardiovascular Nursing, 19*(6), 425–429.

Ehrenstein, M. R., Jury, E. C., & Mauri, C. (2005). Statins for atherosclerosis—as good as it gets? *New England Journal of Medicine, 352*(1), 73–75.

Fair, J. M., & Berra, K. A. (2005). Lipid management in coronary heart disease. In S. L. Woods, E. S. Sivarajan Froelicher, S. Underhill Motzer, & E. J. Bridges (Eds.), *Cardiac nursing* (5th ed., pp. 897–915). Philadelphia: Lippincott Williams & Wilkins.

Flutterman, L. G., & Lemberg, L. (2002). Novel markers in the acute coronary syndrome: BNP, IL-6, PAPP-A. *American Journal of Critical Care, 11*(2), 168–172.

Gardner, P., & Altman, G. (2005). Pathophysiology of acute coronary syndrome. In S. L. Woods, E. S. Sivarajan Froelicher, S. Underhill Motzer, & E. J. Bridges (Eds.), *Cardiac nursing* (5th ed., pp. 541–549). Philadelphia: Lippincott Williams & Wilkins.

Gola, M., Bonadonna, S., Doga, M., Mazziotti, G., & Giustina, A. (2005). Cardiovascular risk in aging and obesity: Is there a role for GH. *Journal of Endocrinology Investigation, 28*(8), 759–767.

Hawley, D. A. (2004). What's new in acute coronary syndromes? *Nursing Clinics of North America, 39,* 815–828.

Isomaa, B., Almgren, P., Tuomi, T., Forsen, B., Lahti, K., Nissen, M., et al. (2001). Cardiovascular morbidity and mortality association with metabolic syndrome. *Diabetes Care, 24,* 683–689.

Kaul, P., McAleer, E. P., & Steingart, R. M. (2005). New biomarkers for myocardial infarction and unstable angina. *Clinical Advisor, 8*(1), 35–38.

Kavey, R. W., Daniels, S. R., Lauer, R. M., Atkins, D. L., Hayman, L. L., & Taubert, K. (2003). American Heart Association guidelines for primary prevention of atherosclerotic cardiovascular disease beginning in childhood. *Circulation, 107,* 1562–1570.

Libby, P. (2004–2005a). Pathogenesis of atherosclerosis. In D. L. Kasper, E. Braunwald, A. S. Fauci, S. L. Hauser, D. L. Longo, J. L. Jameson, et al. (Eds.), *Harrison's principles of internal medicine* (16th ed.). McGraw-Hill (Harrison's Online). Retrieved May 18, 2005, from www.accessmedicine.com

Libby, P. (2004–2005b). Prevention and treatment of atherosclerosis. In D. L. Kasper, E. Braunwald, A. S. Fauci, S. L. Hauser, D. L. Longo, J. L. Jameson, et al (Eds.), *Harrison's principles of internal medicine* (16th ed.). McGraw-Hill (Harrison's Online). Retrieved May 18, 2005, from www.accessmedicine.com

Morton, P. G. (2005). Acute myocardial infarction. In P. G. Morton, D. K. Fontaine, C. M. Hudak, & B. M. Gallo (Eds.), *Critical care nursing: A holistic approach* (8th ed., pp. 422–447). Philadelphia: Lippincott Williams & Wilkins.

Newton, K. M., & Froelicher, E. S. (2005). Coronary heart disease risk factors. In S. L. Woods, E. S. Sivarajan Froelicher, S. Underhill Motzer, & E. J. Bridges (Eds.), *Cardiac nursing* (5th ed., pp. 809–824). Philadelphia: Lippincott Williams & Wilkins.

Pyne, C. (2004). Classification of acute coronary syndromes using the 12-lead electrocardiogram as a guide. *AACN Clinical Issues, 15*(14), 558–567.

Rosenson, R. S., & Koenig, W. (2003). Utility of markers in the management of coronary artery disease. *American Journal of Cardiology, 92*(Suppl.), 10i–18i.

Rossouw, J. E., Anderson, G. L., Prentice, R. L., LaCroix, A. Z., Kooperberg, C., Stefanick, M. L., et al. (2002). Risks and benefits of the estrogen plus progestin in healthy post menopausal women. Principal results of the Women's Health Initiative randomized controlled trial. *Journal of the American Medical Association, 288*(3), 321–333.

Ryan, C. J., Devon, H. A., & Johnson Zerwic, J. (2005). Typical and atypical symptoms: Diagnosing acute coronary syndromes accurately. *American Journal of Nursing, 105*(2), 34–36.

Snow, V., Barry, P., Fihn, S. D., Gibbons, R. J., Owens, D. K., Williams, S. V., et al. (2004). Primary care management of chronic stable angina and asymptomatic suspected or known coronary artery disease: A clinical practice guideline from the American College of Physicians. *Annals of Internal Medicine, 141,* 562–567.

Stevens, J., Cai, J., Everson, K. R., & Thomas, R. (2003). Fitness and fatness as predictors of mortality from all causes and from cardiovascular disease in men and women in the U.S. *Circulation, 107,* 2096–2101.

Thompson, P. D., Buchner, D., Pina, I. L., Balady, G. I., Williams, M. A., Marcus, B. H., et al. (2003). Exercise and physical activity in the prevention and treatment of atherosclerotic cardiovascular disease. *Circulation, 107,* 3109–3123.

U.S. Department of Health and Human Services. (2004). NIH asks participants in Women's Health Initiative estrogen-alone study to stop study pills, begin follow-up phase. Retrieved October 4, 2005, from www.nhlbi.nih.gov/neu/press

Virmani, R., Kolodgie, F. D., Burke, A. P., Finn, A. V., Gold, H. K., Tulenko, T. N., et al. (2005). Atherosclerotic plaque progression and vulnerability to rupture: Angiogenesis as a source of intraplaque hemorrhage. *Arteriosclerosis Thrombosis Vascular Biology, 25*(10), 2054–2061.

World Health Organization. (1998). The tobacco epidemic: A crisis of startling dimensions. World Health Organization Statement for World No-Tobacco Day. May 31, 1998. Retrieved June 17, 2006, from www.ritobaccocontrolnet.com/whoepide.htm

CHAPTER 13

Hypertension

James R. Steele   Sonya R. Hardin

LEARNING OBJECTIVES

Upon completion of this chapter, the reader will be able to:

1. Discuss the epidemiology of hypertension.
2. Explain the underlying physiology of hypertension.
3. Differentiate between hypertensive urgency and hypertensive emergency.
4. Discuss the treatment modalities for hypertension.
5. Recognize assessment data indicative of hypertension.
6. Identify pharmacologic strategies in managing hypertensive crisis.
7. Design an educational plan for the hypertensive patient.
8. List optimal patient outcomes that may be achieved through evidence-based management of hypertension.

The National Center for Health Statistics (2005) estimates that 42.3 million people have hypertension in the United States. An additional 7.7 million people have been told by their physician on two or more occasions that they had hypertension (but had pressures below 140/90 when checked during the survey). This gives a total of 50 million hypertensive people in the United States alone and does not include patients who currently are being treated but who do not achieve the desired level of control.

According to the American Heart Association (2005), people with uncontrolled or under-controlled hypertension are three times more likely to develop coronary artery disease, six times more likely to develop congestive heart failure (CHF), and seven times more likely to suffer a stroke compared with their nonhypertensive counterparts. According to Fields et al. (2004), the incidence of hypertension has increased for both males and females in general, as well as with age. Given these trends, a nurse can expect to provide care to more patients with a history of hypertension as a comorbidity factor or in an emergent stage.

PATHOPHYSIOLOGY

According to Beevers, Lip, and O'Brien (2001), blood pressure is a balance between peripheral resistance and cardiac output. Individuals maintain a specific level of circulating blood and cardiac output to sustain normal life functions. Most elevations are due to increased peripheral resistance—while the body is attempting to maintain a constant cardiac output, the heart must work harder. Elevation in peripheral resistance is primarily due to contraction of the smooth muscle layer surrounding the smaller arterioles as a result of increased intracellular calcium. Over time, this contraction leads to muscular hypertrophy, similar to the muscle mass increase associated with weight lifting. Eventually this increased muscle mass in the arteriole walls becomes permanent and irreversible. It is possible that such arteriole hypertrophy is a defense mechanism designed to protect the capillary beds from damage secondary to the higher pressures on the arterial side of the cardiovascular system.

To better understand hypertension and hemodynamic principles, understanding of the concepts of preload and afterload is needed. Preload is the tension applied to the walls of the heart as it stretches during diastole (ventricular filling). The volume of blood is translated to the actual ventricular tension experienced. Preload is the stretch applied to the heart before it starts to contract so it is associated with filling. You can indirectly measure preload by measuring filling pressures and end diastolic volume (EDV). An increase in preload is usually accomplished by an increase in EDV, which is usually caused by an increase in fluid or in filling pressures. The increased pressure will increase the volume, which will in turn increase the wall tension and thus increase contractile force. Heart failure is often associated with fluid retention and therefore increased vascular pressures; these effects increase filling pressures so that you have a larger than normal EDV (increased preload). A stiff heart due to hypertension will require higher than normal EDV to fill the heart, so the filling pressures are consequently higher. The filling volume of the left ventricle, or the preload, is affected by factors that influence blood return to the heart and mechanical properties of the heart.

Afterload refers to the wall tension on the heart needed to eject the blood. If arterial pressure increases, ventricular pressure must increase as well. The wall tension in the heart must increase to overcome the greater arterial pressure. If the patient has a stenotic aortic valve, there is high resistance and the ventricular pressure must increase to eject blood. Consequently, the wall tension must increase to generate enough pressure to perform this task. Afterload is increased by resistance to ejection of blood by the left ventricle due to peripheral vascular resistance or aortic impedance. In aortic stenosis, there is usually low arterial pressure as a compensatory mechanism to reduce the afterload and preserve the heart function.

Physiological Mechanism of Hypertension

The primary physiological mechanism of hypertension is induced by an abnormal sodium transport mechanism across the cell wall due to a defect in or inhibition of the sodium–potassium pump (Na^+, K^+-ATPase) or due to increased permeability to sodium. The net result is increased intracellular sodium, which makes the cell more sensitive to sympathetic stimulation. Na^+, K^+-ATPase may also be responsible for pumping norepinephrine back into the sympathetic neurons to inactivate the sodium–potassium pump. Thus inhibition of this mechanism could conceivably enhance the effect of norepinephrine.

Stimulation of the sympathetic nervous system raises blood pressure, usually to a greater extent in hypertensive or pre-hypertensive patients than in normotensive patients. Whether this hyperresponsiveness resides in the sympathetic nervous system itself or in the myocardium and vascular smooth muscle that this system innervates is unknown, but this stimulation can often be detected before sustained hypertension develops. A high resting pulse rate, which can be a manifestation of increased sympathetic nervous activity, is a well-known predictor of subsequent hypertension.

One theory of the mechanism of hypertension revolves around the renin-angiotensin-aldosterone system. The juxtaglomerular apparatus in the kidneys helps regulate volume and pressure. Renin forms in the granules of the juxtaglomerular apparatus cells and then catalyzes conversion of the protein angiotensinogen to angiotensin I. This inactive product is cleaved by a converting enzyme—mainly in the lungs but also in the kidneys and brain—to angiotensin II. Angiotensin II is a potent vasoconstrictor that also stimulates release of aldosterone. Aldosterone causes retention of sodium and water by the kidneys, thereby increasing blood pressure by enhancing circulating volume.

Plasma renin activity (PRA) is usually normal in patients with primary hypertension but is suppressed in about 25% of cases and elevated in about 15% of cases. Hypertension is more likely to be accompanied by low renin levels in blacks and elderly individuals. Although angiotensin is generally acknowledged to be responsible for renovascular hypertension, at least in the early phase, there is no consensus regarding the role of the renin-angiotensin-aldosterone system in patients with primary hypertension, even in those with high PRA.

Most likely, the cause of hypertension is a function of more than one of these physiological mechanisms—an idea that gives rise to the mosaic theory. The mosaic theory states that multiple factors sustain elevated blood pressure, even though an aberration of only one was initially responsible for the hypertension. The interaction between the sympathetic nervous system and the renin-angiotensin-aldosterone system could potentially be the culprit. The sympathetic innervation of the juxtaglomerular apparatus in the kidney releases renin; angiotensin stimulates autonomic centers in the brain to increase sympathetic discharge. Angiotensin also stimulates production of aldosterone, which leads to sodium retention; this excessive intracellular sodium enhances the reactivity of vascular smooth muscle to sympathetic stimulation, and the cycle continues fulfilling itself, with no control mechanism to stop it.

Primary and Secondary Hypertension

In the majority of people with high blood pressure (more than 90%), a single specific cause is not known. This type of disease is termed essential or primary high blood pressure, and it is a heterogeneous disorder related to dietary, genetic, and neurohormonal factors. Secondary hypertension accounts for approximately 5% to 10% of all cases. An identifiable cause underlies secondary hypertension. **Table 13-1** shows some of the identifiable mechanisms of secondary hypertension.

TABLE 13-1 Mechanisms of Secondary Hypertension

Diagnosis	Mechanism
Renal artery stenosis	↑ SVR, ↑ cardiac output
Chronic renal failure	↑ Renal perfusion and restoration of glomerular filtration
Primary hyperaldosteronism	↑ Aldosterone, ↑Na^+, ↑ H_2O
Stress	↑ Angiotension II, ↑ catecholamines
Sleep apnea	Sympathetic activation and hormonal changes, obesity
Hyperthyroidism/ hypothyroidism	↓ Vasodilator metabolites
Pheochromocytoma	↑ Catecholamines
Aortic coarctation	↑ Renin, activation of renin-angiotension-aldosterone system
Medications	Oral contraceptives, over-the-counter decongestants, non-steroidal anti-inflammatory drugs, and cocaine

Source: Klabunde, 2004.

In a recent study, researchers did not find a linear association between caffeine consumption and hypertension in women but did find the incidence of hypertension to be increased among women who consumed sugared and diet colas. Further study is needed to clarify the role of colas in the incidence of hypertension (Winkelmayer, Stampfer, Willett, & Curhan, 2005).

URGENT AND EMERGENT HYPERTENSION

In the intensive care unit (ICU), a patient may develop or initially present with urgent or emergent hypertension. The distinction between urgent and emergent hypertension helps to classify treatment and can relate to the presence of primary or secondary hypertension.

Urgent hypertension is a severe blood pressure elevation without any evidence of progressive organ dysfunction. In such a case, the blood pressure can be slowly lowered over a 24-hour period of time. Urgent hypertension is usually treated with oral agents such as beta blockers, angiotensin-converting enzyme (ACE) inhibitors, and calcium channel blockers, and requires the nurse in the ICU to monitor the blood pressure every hour. In the past, nifedipine (Procardia®) was given sublingually to quickly bring down the blood pressure. Significant adverse effects of sudden and severe decrease in blood pressure

have been reported with this regimen, however, so it is now recommended that nifedipine be avoided.

In emergent hypertension, an immediate admission to the ICU will be required to monitor the blood pressure and to administer intravenous antihypertensive therapy. Typically, the patient will present with a blood pressure greater than 220/120 mm Hg. Emergent hypertensive pathology can include hypertensive encephalopathy, intracranial hemorrhage, acute coronary syndrome, acute pulmonary edema, drug overdose, acute renal failure, or a dissecting aneurysm.

A hypertensive emergency is clinically defined as including end-organ damage or dysfunction including CHF, renal failure, hypertensive encephalopathy, hematuria, and retinal hemorrhage. The diagnosis is not based on the absolute level of blood pressure (Graber, 2004). The goal of treatment is to decrease the mean arterial pressure and minimize organ hypoperfusion. Blood pressure should be lowered by 30% in 30 minutes and by 25% within 2 hours. Ultimately, within 6 hours, a diastolic pressure of 100–105 mm Hg should be obtained.

Individuals with chronic hypertension may not tolerate a "normal" blood pressure, so it is important to act judiciously when lowering blood pressure. Three drugs are typically recommended to control an emergent hypertensive patient: nitroprusside (Nipride®), nitroglycerin, and labetalol (Normdyne®). These drugs require frequent assessment of the blood pressure between titration and following administration.

Nitroprusside (Nipride) should be started at an infusion rate of 0.5 mcg/kg/min and titrated until the desired blood pressure reduction is achieved. The average dose is 0.3 to 10 mcg/kg/min. This highly potent arterial and venous dilator can be used in all hypertensive emergencies, although it is not the drug of choice for preeclampsia. Infusion of nitroprusside can cause cyanide toxicity. Therefore, long-term use of nitroprusside or high infusion rates requires assessment for metabolic acidosis. The late sign of elevated serum thiocyanate levels or red blood cell (RBC) cyanide concentrations greater than 4 mcg/kg/min for as little as 2 to 3 hours may result in detectable metabolic changes.

Nitroglycerin is typically started at 10 mcg/min. The dose is increased by 10 to 20 mcg/min until the desired effect is obtained. Nitroglycerin is a potent venous and arterial dilator, depending on the infusion rate, and has its maximum effect on capacitance vessels.

Labetalol (Normodyne®, Trandate®) is given as an initial bolus of 20 mg intravenously. The usual effective dose is 20 to 80 mg every 10 minutes for a total of 300 mg. It can also be administered as a continuous infusion of 2 mg/min. The infusion should be stopped when blood pressure control is achieved. Labetalol is a combined alpha blocker and beta blocker (primarily a beta blocker). It does not change cerebral blood flow and is probably the drug of choice in hypertension secondary to increased intracranial pressure. It is especially useful in catecholamine-mediated hypertension (e.g., pheochromocytoma) and avoids the reflex tachycardia seen with nitroglycerin and nitroprusside. The time of onset is 5 minutes, with maximum response occurring in 10 minutes. The drug has an 8-hour duration.

Table 13-2 provides information on the parenteral antihypertensive agents that may be utilized during emergent hypertension.

NURSING MANAGEMENT

When a hypertensive patient is admitted to the ICU, the nurse will obtain a history of events leading up to the admission, including signs and symptoms (headache, seizure, chest pain, dyspnea, and edema) associated with the hypertensive emergency, and all current medications including both prescription and nonprescription drugs. The patient should be questioned on his or her level of compliance with prescribed antihypertensive medications as well as any use of recreational drugs. A history of comorbid conditions—specifically those related to prior or current neurologic, cardiac, and renal conditions—should be obtained.

Laboratory studies required for the hypertensive patient include a urinalysis and chemistry panel, and electrocardiogram (ECG). The urinalysis may reveal evidence of renal disease through such findings as proteinuria, RBCs, or cellular casts. The chemistry panel could indicate electrolyte abnormalities (e.g., hypokalemia or hypomagnesemia). A 12-lead ECG provides evidence of cardiac ischemia and/or left ventricular hypertrophy. Abnormal findings should be reported to the physician or nurse practitioner.

The major nursing intervention is vigilance in monitoring blood pressure. Consistent elevation should be reported to prevent end-organ damage and to ensure timely intervention with antihypertensives. During the emergent hypertension, parenteral infusions to control blood pressure will require blood pressures to be taken every 15 minutes during periods of titration. A change in dose of a parenteral agent requires a repeat blood pressure in 15 minutes. Once a parenteral infusion has been titrated to the level needed to manage the blood pressure, hourly readings are appropriate for most patients. When weaning patients from antihypertensive agents, frequent blood pressures of every 15 minutes are warranted. Typically parenteral infusions are replaced with oral agents to control blood pressure in primary hypertension. Continuous assessment for signs and symptoms of stroke, cardiac events, and end-organ damage is needed during an ICU stay.

Prior to patient transfer out of the ICU, the nurse should assess for orthostatic hypotension. During the first time the patient is out of the bed, a standing or sitting blood pressure should be documented to facilitate pharmacological manage-

TABLE 13-2 Parenteral Antihypertensive Infusions for Emergent Hypertension

Drug	Class	Initial Dose	Infusion	Maximum Dose
Enalapril (Vasotec®)	ACE inhibitor	1.25 mg IV push over 5 minutes every 6 hours		20 mg/day
Esmolol (Brevibloc®)	Beta blocker	500 mcg/kg over 1 minute	50–200 mcg/kg/min	200 mcg/kg/min
Labetalol (Trandate®, Normodyne®)	Beta blocker	20 mg over 1 minute	0.5–2.0 mg/min	2400 mg/day
Nitroprusside (Nipride®)	Vasodilator	0.3 mcg/kg/min	Titrate	10 mcg/kg/min
Nitroglycerin (Tridil®, Nitrobid®)	Nitrate	10–20 mcg/min	Titrate	200 mcg/min
Nicardipine (Cardene®)	Calcium channel blocker	5 mg/hr	Titrate	15 mg/hr
Fenoldpam (Corlopam®)	Dopamine (D$_1$) agonist	0.1 mcg/kg/min	Titrate	0.5 mcg/kg/min

ment by the physician or nurse practitioner. Monitoring for patient falls is important with the ICU patient who is on antihypertensive agents, given the potential for orthostatic hypotension. Patients should be instructed to call prior to transfer back to the bed and should be cautioned regarding the side effects of fatigue, lethargy, and sleep deprivation associated with some antihypertensives.

NURSING MANAGEMENT BASED ON MEDICAL DIAGNOSIS

Postoperative Hypertension

Postoperative hypertension is an acute, transient increase in blood pressure that develops within 30 to 90 minutes following a surgical procedure and typically lasts for 4 to 8 hours after surgery. It is defined as a systolic blood pressure greater than 160 mm Hg or a diastolic blood pressure greater than 90 mm Hg (Lewis, 2002).

High blood pressure is a frequent complication after surgery. However, formal guidelines for the treatment of postoperative hypertension have not been developed. It has also been recognized that postoperative hypertension is much more common in patients who have existing hypertension prior to the surgery.

The cool temperatures in the operating room and the exposure of internal organs to cold ambient temperatures are the primary reasons for patients developing generalized hypothermia. Hypothermia leads to generalized peripheral vasoconstriction as a compensatory mechanism to retain body heat. After leaving the operating room, these cold, volume-depleted patients often are hypertensive until they warm to temperatures above 36.5°C. When body temperature increases, the patient experiences generalized vasodilation, and hypovolemia becomes apparent. The use of intermittent doses of vasodilating drugs to control the intraoperative and immediate postoperative hypertension produces unpredictable responses in terms of both effect and duration.

Temperature is not the only factor complicating blood pressure control after surgery. The treatment of hypertension must also include interventions that address pain, hypoxemia, and any other underlying physiological disturbances that affect the blood pressure (Ramsey, Neil, Sullivan, & Perfelto, 1999).

Acute Aortic Dissection

As soon as a diagnosis of acute aortic dissection is suspected, intravenous antihypertensive therapy should be initiated. Systolic blood pressure should be decreased to approximately 110 mm Hg until the patient can be taken to the operating room. Patients with aortic dissection require close observation of vascular pressures, urine output, mental status, and neurologic

signs. If the patient becomes suddenly hypotensive, it suggests aortic rupture and requires emergent surgical repair. Upon return from the operating room, the patient will require close observation to maintain a normotensive state. This will be accomplished with the use of pharmacological interventions.

Hypertension after a Cerebrovascular Accident

After a stroke, cerebral autoregulation is impaired. There is no evidence that hypertension has a deleterious effect on the outcome of ischemic strokes during the acute phase. Lowering the blood pressure in patients with cerebral ischemia, however, may result in further ischemic injury. Thus the common practice of lowering blood pressure is potentially dangerous. The current recommendation is that hypertension in the setting of acute ischemic stroke should be treated rarely and cautiously. It is generally recommended that antihypertensive therapy be reserved for patients with a diastolic pressure greater than 120 to 130 mm Hg, aiming to reduce the pressure by no more than an arbitrary figure of 20% in the first 24 hours following the stroke (Varon & Marik, 2000).

In patients with intracerebral hemorrhage, the value of early antihypertensive therapy in preventing rebleeding or reducing vasogenic edema has not been demonstrated. A rapid decline in blood pressure within the first 24 hours after an intracerebral hemorrhage has been linked to increased mortality (Varon & Marik, 2000).

Hypertensive Crisis in End-Stage Renal Disease

Hypertension is also a complication of chronic renal failure. The cause of hypertension is an increase in extracellular volume secondary to sodium retention by the diseased kidney, plus vasoconstriction due to increased activity of the renin-angiotensin system. These patients may require emergent ultrafiltration to control their blood pressure (Varon & Marik, 2000).

Prior to Discharge

Management of hypertension in the community begins prior to discharge from the hospital with understanding of the blood pressure goals identified in the Seventh Report of the Joint National Committee on Prevention, Detection, Evaluation, and Treatment of High Blood Pressure (JNC-7). The JNC-7 guidelines provide an evidence-based approach to the prevention and management of hypertension. The key messages of this report are as follows:

- In individuals older than age 50, systolic blood pressure of greater than 140 mm Hg is a more important cardiovascular disease risk factor than elevated diastolic blood pressure.

- Beginning at a blood pressure of 115/75, cardiovascular risk doubles with each increase in blood pressure of 20 mm Hg in systolic pressure and/or 10 mm Hg in diastolic pressure.
- Individuals who are normotensive at age 55 have a 90% risk of developing hypertension that requires intervention.
- Most hypertensive patients will require two or more antihypertensive medications.

Uncomplicated hypertension consists of elevated blood pressure without the presence of other cardiovascular risk factors—namely, smoking, elevated cholesterol, sedentary lifestyle, obesity, and known diabetes. In these cases, the initial therapy begins with a thiazide diuretic, either alone or combined with drugs from other classes. The JNC-7 report also delineates specific high-risk conditions that are compelling indications for the use of other antihypertensive drug classes such as ACE inhibitors, angiotensin-receptor blockers, beta blockers, and calcium channel blockers.

The JNC-7 recommendations also stipulate when two or more antihypertensive medications should be used to achieve target blood pressure goals. For patients whose blood pressure is more than 20 mm Hg above the systolic blood pressure goal or more than 10 mm Hg above the diastolic blood pressure goal, initiation of therapy using two agents—one of which usually will be a thiazide diuretic—is recommended. The stated goals are a sustained blood pressure of 140/90 mm Hg. The goals are more stringent for diabetics and renal patients; their goal is pressure less than 130/80 mm Hg. **Table 13-3** lists some of the drugs prescribed to manage hypertension.

TABLE 13-3 Medications for Hypertension

Drug Category	Mechanism	Precautions
Thiazide diuretics	Effective alone and useful in offsetting the fluid retention caused by other agents.	Monitor hypokalemia, arrhythmias, and gout
Loop diuretics	More effective in patients with impaired renal function.	Monitor hypokalemia and arrhythmias
Anxiety medications	Stress is often linked to high blood pressure. Calming patients and quieting their emotions help lower blood pressure.	Monitor respirations
Alpha blockers	Control nerve impulses to the smooth muscles surrounding blood vessels, allowing them to relax. This reduces the resistance that blood must flow against.	Monitor for congestive cardiac failure
Beta blockers	Target beta receptors in the heart and blood vessels: beta$_1$ receptors in the heart and beta$_2$ receptors in the lungs (remember—you have one heart and two lungs). Act predominantly on the beta$_1$ receptors in the heart, making the heart pump at a slower rate and with less force.	Use with caution in individuals with asthma, bronchospastic disease, heart failure, and peripheral vascular disease
Angiotensin-converting enzyme inhibitor	Prevent the formation of angiotensin II, the hormone that causes blood vessels to constrict. Cause the blood vessels to relax, thereby lowering blood pressure.	Monitor for dry cough
Angiotensin II type 1 receptor blockers	Antagonize the action of angiotensin II by displacing it from its receptor. Inhibit angiotensin II–induced vascular smooth muscle contraction, aldosterone release, and adrenal and presynaptic catecholamine release, among other effects.	Use with caution in renovascular disease
Calcium channel blockers	Control the flow of calcium into cells. Help the heart and blood vessels relax.	Monitor for second- or third-degree heart block, heart failure
Vasodilators	Relax the muscles around the blood vessels, reducing resistance to blood flow.	Monitor blood pressure, orthostatic pressure, and peripheral edema

Source: National Heart, Lung, and Blood Institute, 2005.

Abrupt discontinuation of treatment with a short-acting sympathetic blocker (e.g., clonidine or propranolol) can lead to severe hypertension. In addition to drug therapy withdrawal, increased adrenergic activity can lead to severe hypertension in a variety of other clinical settings: the use of sympathomimetic drugs such as cocaine, amphetamines, or phencyclidine; the combination of a monoamine oxidase inhibitor and the ingestion of tyramine-containing foods (e.g., aged cheeses, some aged or cured meat, draft beer, soy sauce); pheochromocytoma; and autonomic dysfunction (e.g., Guillian-Barré syndrome) (Varon & Marik, 2000).

The JNC-7 made the recommendations shown in **Figure 13-1** regarding treatment of hypertension. **Table 13-4** presents the JNC-7 definitions of blood pressure levels in adults (ages 18 years and older).

The JNC-7 stresses that the keys to managing hypertension are lifestyle changes and use of antihypertensive agents. Prior to discharge, patients will need education and oral antihypertensive agents with follow-up appointments with their primary care provider.

PATIENT EDUCATION

Blood pressure–related risk reduction efforts have almost uniformly revolved around hypertension detection and treatment. Unfortunately, noncompliance with antihypertensive agents results in numerous hospital admissions annually. Such noncompliance is associated with high drug costs, lack of physical symptoms that might prompt patients to seek treatment, and misunderstandings about hypertension. Education targeted at high-risk populations, such as African Americans, persons with high blood pressure, persons with a family history of hypertension, and individuals with one or more lifestyle factors that contribute to age-related increases in blood pressure, should form the focus for intervention strategies.

Intervention programs conducted in community-based and practice-based settings indicate that the desired lifestyle changes are potentially feasible. These lifestyle factors to be addressed include a high sodium intake, excessive consumption of calories, stress, physical inactivity, excessive alcohol consumption, and deficient intake of potassium. Achievement of intervention goals has, however, been constrained by a number of societal barriers, including a lack of satisfactory food choices and the absence of a national campaign to foster adoption of the population-based and targeted intervention strategies necessary to prevent high blood pressure.

The National High Blood Pressure Education Program is positioned to provide leadership for such a campaign. Goals of this campaign should include increased efforts to promote consumption of foods that are lower in sodium and calorie content and higher in potassium content; physical activity; and moderation in alcohol consumption. Finally, additional attention needs to be focused on research questions related to the

FIGURE 13-1 Decision Tree for Drug Treatment

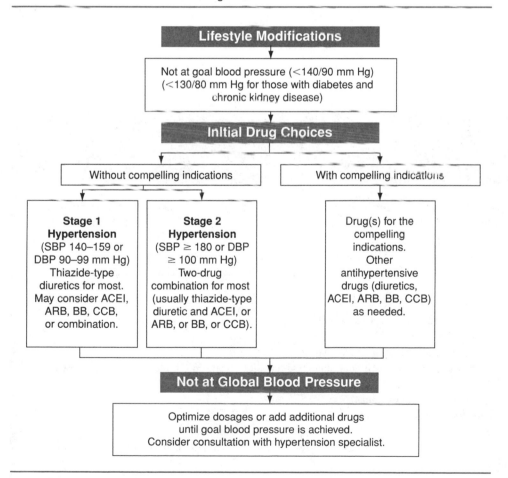

Source: Chobanian et al., 2003.
ACEI = angiotension-converting enzyme inhibitor; ARB = angiotension receptor blocker; BB = beta blocker; CCB = calcium channel blocker.

TABLE 13-4 Categories of Blood Pressure Levels in Adults

| | Blood Pressure Level (mm Hg) | | |
	Systolic		Diastolic
Normal	< 120	and	< 80
Prehypertension	120–139	or	80–89
High Blood Pressure			
Stage 1 hypertension	140–159	or	90–99
Stage 2 hypertension	≥ 160	or	≥ 100

Source: Chobanian et al., 2003.

prevention of high blood pressure. Increased understanding of the management of hypertension in the ICU setting is needed to establish protocols specific to each underlying cause.

PATIENT OUTCOMES

Nurses can help ensure attainment of optimal patient outcomes such as those listed in **Box 13-1** through the use of evidence-based interventions.

SUMMARY

Over 40 million people in the United States have hypertension. While the exact causes of hypertension are unknown, several etiologic factors have been identified. The primary treatment of hypertension is lifestyle modification. However, several classifications of medication are on the market for treatment. Control of hypertension is essential to avoid complications that can impact quality of life and survival.

Box 13-1
Patient Outcomes

- Describes strategies to maximize health
- Performs prescribed health behaviors
- Blood pressure in expected range
- Absence of sequela released to disease process

CASE STUDY

B.D. is a 61-year-old African American male who was admitted to the ICU through the emergency department after presenting with a 3-day history of blurred vision, nausea, and vomiting. His blood pressure was 210/136 in both arms. B.D. later admitted that he had experienced some difficulty in expressing what he was feeling to his wife. He also stated that he had noticed some difficulty standing up, with diminished strength to his left side, when he decided to seek treatment today.

On physical exam, B.D.'s point of maximal intensity was displaced to the left, he had bilateral crackles at the bases, and he had 2+ pitting edema to his lower extremities.

1. What lab tests should be ordered and why?
2. What would be considered critical lab values for this patient?
3. What would the initial treatment involve?
4. What critical issues would you need to assess for and/or avoid?

The labs come back with an increased creatinine, high potassium, and low bicarbonate in the blood sample and RBCs and protein in the urine.

5. What actions should be taken based on these values?
6. What additional life-threatening condition do you think B.D. is developing?
7. What therapies would you expect to be initiated after the blood pressure is stabilized?

B.D. is stabilized and will be discharged to home in the next few days. His care team has decided to keep him in the ICU for monitoring and discharge planning.

8. What issues would you address in your discharge planning?
9. How would you validate B.D.'s knowledge levels?
10. When do you think he would need follow-up appointments?

CRITICAL THINKING QUESTIONS

1. What are the possible etiologies for development of hypertension?
2. What is the proper sequencing of therapies, both modalities and medicines, based on the latest national standard for treatment of hypertension?
3. Which medications are used in particular patient subpopulations and why?
4. What are the possible long-term negative outcomes of uncontrolled hypertension?
5. Where would you refer your patient and family to get the most current information on living with and controlling high blood pressure?
6. Write a case example from the clinical setting highlighting one patient characteristic. Explain how the characteristic was observed through subjective and objective data of a patient experiencing a hypertensive crisis.
7. Write a case example from the clinical setting. Rate the patient as a level 1, 3, or 5 on each characteristic. Identify the level of nurse characteristics needed in the care of this patient.
8. Identify an ongoing clinical trial for patients experiencing hypertension (see the website www.clinicaltrials.gov). Identify the criteria to be a subject in the research study and the risks involved.

Using the Synergy Model to Develop a Plan of Care

Patient Characteristics	Levels 1, 3, or 5	Subjective and Objective Data	Evidence-based Interventions	Outcomes
Resiliency				
Vulnerability				
Stability				
Complexity				
Resource availability				
Participation in care				
Participation in decision making				
Predictability				

Online Resources

Virtual Hospital University of Iowa: http://www.vh.org/index.html

An Introduction to Hypertension: http://www.about-hypertension.com/

Hypertension Tutorial: http://www.nlm.nih.gov/medlineplus/tutorials/hypertension/htm/index.htm

A Guide to Lowering High Blood Pressure: http://www.nhlbi.nih.gov/hbp/treat/bpd_type.htm

REFERENCES

AHA Statistical Fact Sheet 2005 Update. (2005). Retrieved June 17, 2006, from www.americanheart.org

Bales, A. (1999). Hypertensive crisis. *Postgraduate Medicine, 105*(5), 119–135.

Beevers, G., Lip, G., & O'Brien, E. (2001). The ABC of hypertension: The pathophysiology of hypertension. *British Medical Journal, 322,* 912–916.

Chobanian, A. V., Bakris, G. L., Black, H. R., Cushman, W. C., Green, L. A., Izzo, J. L., et al. (2003). The seventh report of the Joint National Committee on Prevention, Detection, Evaluation, and Treatment of High Blood Pressure (JNC7). *Journal of the American Medical Association, 289*(19), 2560–2571.

Fields, L. E., Burt, V. L., Cutler, J. A., Hughes, J., Rocella, E. J., & Sorlie, P. (2004). The burden of adult hypertension in the United States 1999 to 2000: A rising tide. *Hypertension, 44*(4), 398–404.

Graber, M. A. (2004). Emergency medicine. In M. Graber & M. L. Lanternier (Eds.), *Family practice handbook* (4th ed., pp. 23–72). St. Louis, MO: Mosby.

Klabunde, R. E. (2004). *Cardiovascular physiology concepts.* Philadelphia: Lippincott Williams & Wilkins.

Lewis, K. (2002). Pharmacological review of postoperative hypertension. *Journal of Pharmacy Practice, 15*(2), 135–146.

National Center for Health Statistics. (2005). Retrieved October 29, 2005, from http://www.cdc.gov/nchs/index.htm

National Heart, Lung, and Blood Institute of the National Institutes of Health. (2005). Retrieved October 29, 2005, from http://www.nhlbi.nih.gov/

Ramsey, S. D., Neil, N., Sullivan, S. D., & Perfelto, E. (1999). An economic evaluation of the JNC hypertensive guidelines using data from a randomized controlled trial. Joint National Committee. *Journal of the American Board of Family Practice, 12*(2), 105–114.

Varon, J., & Marik, P. E. (2000). The diagnosis and management of hypertensive crises. *Chest, 118*(1), 214–227.

Winkelmayer, W. C., Stampfer, M. J., Willett, W. C., & Curhan, G. C. (2005). Habitual caffeine intake and the risk of hypertension in women. *Journal of the American Medical Association, 294,* 2330–2335.

CHAPTER 14

Acute Coronary Syndrome

Barbara Hutton Borghardt

Acute coronary syndrome (ACS) is a term used to describe ischemic coronary events in which the patient is at risk for developing myocardial damage. Under the heading of ACS are three conditions: unstable angina, non-ST-elevation myocardial infarction (NSTEMI), and ST-elevation myocardial infarction (STEMI). Because there is a propensity for chronic angina to become unstable, it will be discussed here as well. It should be noted, however, that relatively few patients with acute myocardial infarction (AMI) will experience chronic/stable angina as a precursor. In fact, the first symptom in approximately 50% of these patients is sudden death (Fass, 2003).

UNSTABLE ANGINA

Unstable angina is characterized by chest pain that has increased in intensity, and that may have increased in duration and frequency. The pain generally lasts longer than 10 minutes. If the pain is of new onset, it is usually described as severe. This type of angina requires immediate intervention, because it may be pre-infarction angina and the myocardial muscle is at risk for damage (Becker, 1999).

Printzmetal's (variant, vasospastic) angina is characterized by chest pain or discomfort that is unrelated to exercise or exertion. The pathogenesis of this pain differs from that of the atherosclerotic lesions of stable angina: It results from a vasospasm of a large epicardial coronary artery. The pain may occur at rest and at the same time of day, often in the morning. Patients who experience vasospasm may have atherosclerotic changes or normal coronary arteries (Becker, 1999). The pain is usually described as severe, and electrocardiographic (ECG) changes mimic an impending myocardial infarction (ST-segment elevation). These changes usually revert to normal when the pain subsides.

MYOCARDIAL INFARCTION

Myocardial infarction (MI) refers to necrosis (death) of a portion of myocardial muscle due to decreased blood supply. It may result from coronary artery stenosis, thrombosis, and/or vasospasm. A diseased heart that suddenly increases its demand for oxygen because of stress or exercise may also suffer MI damage. MIs are characterized according to their ECG changes: non-ST-elevation MI (NSTEMI), which is the most common type, or ST-elevation MI (STEMI).

In NSTEMI, blood supply is disrupted to the heart muscle due to plaque rupture with a non-occlusive thrombus, vasospasm, or an imbalance between oxygen supply and demand (Antman & Braunwald, 2004–2005). The infarcted area does not completely transverse the total thickness of the ventricular wall, but rather remains confined to the subendocardial (innermost) portion of the wall (see **Figure 14-1**). In a STEMI, the plaque rupture with thrombus formation may be totally occlusive. The infarcted area completely transverses the thickness of the ventricular wall (see **Figure 14-2**). The ECG changes noted will be ST-segment elevation with subsequent Q-wave formation in the majority of cases.

While it is possible to have no pain or atypical symptoms with MI, the pain is usually severe and lasts longer than 20 to 30 minutes. The pain may begin at rest or with exercise, but, unlike angina, it does not subside when the patient rests (Antman & Braunwald, 2004–2005).

ASSESSMENT OF THE PATIENT

When ischemic heart disease (IHD) is suspected, several assessment tools are used to obtain the diagnosis. Traditionally, the 12-lead ECG has been the gold standard. Although it is still heavily relied on, it has limitations in its ability to detect transient changes. For this reason, history, physical assessment, and diagnostic tests are performed as well.

History

Careful history should be obtained from the patient and/or family. Information to be gathered includes age, present illness, family history of illness, and assessment risk factors, including lifestyle risk factors. Family history of heart disease should arouse suspicion. History of the present symptoms should be explored. Although chest pain is the most common symptom, other symptoms, such as exertional dyspnea or fatigue, may have been present prior to the pain. Probing the past and present medical history for unexplained symptoms, diabetes, thyroid dysfunction, recreational drug and alcohol use, and medications the patient is taking should be part of the initial inquiry. In addition, if not already available, baseline vital signs and mental status should be assessed. Chest pain accompanied by IHD may be described in several ways, as discussed in Chapter 12.

Physical Assessment

An essential part of the patient assessment is the physical evaluation. Often the exam will appear normal, but evidence of atherosclerotic changes in peripheral blood vessels may sometimes include carotid bruits, diminished pulses in the lower extremities, and aortic aneurysm. A systolic murmur may be present with valvular or papillary muscle dysfunction. The additional heart sounds of S_3 and S_4 may indicate left ventricular (LV) dysfunction. A pericardial friction rub may be heard post MI.

The appearance of a patient having an acute MI is variable. The individual may be pale, diaphoretic, and very frightened. The skin may be cool and clammy with diminished pulses. The symptoms of ischemia do not always correlate with the severity of the disease, however (Braunwald, 2001). If neurological changes are present, they can range from minor confusion and memory impairment to more obvious confusion. Subtle changes are more likely to be noticed by family members who know the patient well, rather than by staff personnel.

Vital signs should be assessed and compared to baseline. Cardiac monitoring should be instituted and a 12-lead ECG performed as soon as possible. Abnormalities in heart rate and rhythm are noted as well as any deviation in blood pressure from baseline. With acute MI, patients may have bradycardia or tachycardia, or they may have atrial or ventricular dysrhythmias. Blood pressure can be elevated, or low from poor heart function, or from medications.

FIGURE 14-1 Localization of Infarction: (a) Anterior Wall, (b) Septal Wall, (c) Lateral Wall, and (d) Inferior Wall

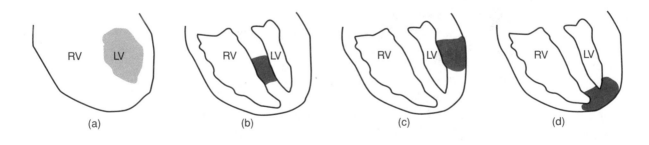

(a)   (b)   (c)   (d)

FIGURE 14-2 NSTEMI versus STEMI

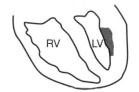
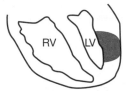

Non-ST-segment
elevation myocardial
infarction

ST-segment
elevation myocardial
infarction

Assessment of respiratory rate and breath sounds will help to determine whether LV performance is poor. Crackles may be heard, especially in the lower lung fields, or throughout the lungs as heart failure increases. Occasionally, wheezes may be heard with increased pulmonary congestion.

Signs and symptoms of right ventricular failure may be noted with a right ventricular ischemia or infarct. They include neck vein distention, hepatojugular reflux, and increasing peripheral edema along with hypotension (Carter & Ellis, 2005).

DIAGNOSTIC TESTS

Electrocardiographic Changes in Ischemic Heart Disease

In cases of IHD, the ECG has been the most frequently used assessment tool, and it remains a standard in the diagnosis of myocardial ischemia, injury, and infarction. The utility of the ECG may be limited due to a number of reasons. First, pre-existing cardiac diseases, such as bundle branch blocks and left ventricular hypertrophy, may obscure the new ECG changes, making the diagnosis of a new event difficult. Second, ECG changes with ischemia tend to revert to normal when the anginal episode is over and may be missed during the initial assessment of the patient. Third, it may be difficult to determine the age of a cardiac event based on ECG findings. Finally, neurological disorders, pericarditis, and electrolyte abnormalities may be misinterpreted as IHD (Pyne, 2004).

Ischemic heart disease and its corresponding ECG changes are described in **Box 14-1**. **Box 14-2** describes ECG changes that are considered significant for ACS.

The 12-lead ECG allows us to view the heart from 12 different angles and can assist us in determining which areas of the left ventricle are affected by ischemia and/or infarction. Ischemia will cause abnormalities in the electrical current through the muscle, and areas of infarction will be electrically silent. **Table 14-2** reveals the ECG leads in which changes will occur with infarction of different areas of the heart.

Specific Biomarkers for Myocardial Infarction

Serum biomarkers indicative of myocardial muscle damage will be elevated in the presence of MI. Elevations are noted within a predictable time frame after the damage has occurred. Patients, however, may present for medical attention later than their symptoms arise, thereby missing the opportunity to demonstrate ECG changes and biomarker elevations. Along with a 12-lead ECG,

---

Box 14-1

Common Cardiac Conditions and Their Associated ECG Changes

Ischemia refers to compromise to the blood supply of an area of the heart muscle. Patients with angina experience ischemic changes on their ECG, including ST-segment depression and T-wave inversion, which return to normal when the episode is over. Changes to the myocardial muscle are reversible at this point.

Injury refers to prolonged, intense ischemia of the myocardial muscle. Striking ECG changes of ST-segment elevation are present, and the patient may experience unstable angina or an infarction at this time. Changes to the myocardial muscle may or may not be reversible at this point, depending on the length of time and degree of the injury.

Infarction refers to death of myocardial muscle and is not reversible. For NSTEMI, ECG changes are similar to ischemia but last longer, at least 24 hours. For STEMI, ST elevation with the development of Q waves will be noted. In the precordial (chest) leads, a loss of normal R-wave progression may be noted. **Table 14-1** shows the ECG changes associated with unstable angina/NSTEMI and STEMI.

TABLE 14-1 ECG Changes with Acute Coronary Syndrome

Condition	Pathophysiology	ECG Changes
Normal heart	None	Normal ECG
Angina	• Atherosclerotic plaque > 60% to 70% stenosis • Imbalance of supply and demand • Ventricular hypertrophy • Valvular disease • Cardiomyopathy	Inverted T wave ST-segment depression Tall, peaked T waves
Unstable angina/NSTEMI	• Plaque rupture with thrombus, subtotal occlusion • Vasospasm • Imbalance of supply and demand • Total occlusive thrombus with collateral circulation • Obstructive lesion	T-wave inversion ST-segment depression
STEMI	• Plaque rupture with occlusive thrombus	ST-segment elevation

TABLE 14-1 ECG Changes with Acute Coronary Syndrome—continued

Condition	Pathophysiology	ECG changes
STEMI	• Plaque rupture with occlusive thrombus	Significant Q wave

Loss of R-wave progression in anterior leads

V1   V2   V3

V4   V5   V6

Box 14-2

Significant ECG Changes in Acute Coronary Syndrome

T wave changes: Flat or inverted T waves, may be biphasic. Peaked T waves.

ST-segment depression: To be considered significant, the ST depression should be at least 1 mm below the isoelectric line, and last for 0.08 second after the end of the QRS.

ST-segment elevation: ST segments that are 1 mm above the isoelectric line and appear in two contiguous leads.

Q waves: Significant Q waves are more than 0.04 second wide and at least ¼ the size of the R wave in that lead.

serum markers should be drawn as soon as possible, preferably within one hour of presentation. Because these blood tests are readily available, and their results can be obtained quickly, they are essential for providing a diagnosis for ACS.

Troponin is a structural protein found involved in muscular contraction. The troponins that are specific to cardiac muscle are troponins I and T. Troponin C is found in both cardiac and skeletal muscle. When the cells of the heart muscle become damaged, troponin levels will begin to rise in the bloodstream at 4 to 10 hours, peaking at 14 to 24 hours after the event. Troponin levels will remain elevated for 10 to 14 days, making a diagnosis possible for patients who may have delayed seeking treatment. These proteins appear to be more sensitive and specific than *creatine kinase* (CK) in terms of their ability to detect myocardial necrosis. Troponins are not normally found in the blood, and their concentrations can reach more than 20 times their baseline range, allowing for the detection of even small infarct areas. The amount of troponin elevation does correlate with the size of the infarction. Troponins are the preferred biomarker in the diagnosis of ACS (Antman & Braunwald, 2004–2005; Casey, 2004).

TABLE 14-2 ECG Changes with Infarcted Heart Wall

Area of Infarction	ECG Changes
Anterior wall	Leads V2, V3, and V4.
Anteroseptal wall	Leads V1, V2, and V3.
Anterolateral wall	Leads V4, V5, and V6.
High lateral wall	Leads I and AVL.
Inferior wall	Leads II, III, and AVF.
Posterior wall	ST-segment depression in V1 and V2, with tall R waves in the same leads. In addition, ST-segment elevation in the posterior chest leads V7 through V9 is indicative of posterior wall infarction.
Right ventricular (RV) wall	Infarction occurs in about half of patients with inferior/ posterior infarction. ST-segment elevation in the inferior leads and V1 may be noted. Right-sided chest leads may be applied V1R to V6R, with V4R being the most sensitive lead. ST-segment elevation in the right-sided leads is indicative of RV infarction.

Sources: Carter & Ellis, 2005; Pyne, 2004; Ozdemir, Altunkeser, Addullah, Odzil, & Gok, 2003.

CK is a cellular enzyme found in the tissues of the heart, brain, skeletal muscle, and, to a lesser extent, smooth muscle (Casey, 2004; Reen, 2005). CK is released into the bloodstream after damage to these tissues has occurred. Of the three CK isoenzymes (CK-MM, CK-MB, and CK-BB), only CK-MB is predominately found in the heart. CK-MB levels will begin to rise 3 to 4 hours after myocardial damage, will peak in 12 to 24 hours, and will return to normal in 3 to 4 days. Generally, CK-MB levels are drawn on admission, then every 8 hours for 3 times or until the levels noticeably decrease. CK-MB has been further fractionated into CK-MB1 and CK-MB2. If the ratio of CK-MB2 to CK-MB1 is greater than 1.5, it is suggestive of an MI (Casey).

Other laboratory tests may be performed as well:

- Myoglobin.
- Serum lipid measurements: total cholesterol, low-density lipoprotein (LDL) and high-density lipoprotein (HDL), and triglycerides.
- Complete blood count (CBC). The white blood cell (WBC) count may be elevated in cases of ACS. Anemia may precipitate cardiac ischemia. Platelet count should be checked prior to invasive procedures to alert the healthcare provider to the potential for bleeding.
- Serum electrolytes. Abnormal potassium and magnesium levels can result in dysrhythmias. Blood urea nitrogen (BUN)/creatinine is checked prior to initiating procedures and medications and to determine renal function. Low serum glucose can imitate a cardiac syncopal event, or the blood sugar may be elevated in diabetics due to stress.
- Arterial blood gas (ABG)—may be measured to evaluate oxygenation and ventilation.

- Coagulation studies such as PT/PTT, INR, fibrinogen, and fibrin split products—provide baseline coagulation status in the event that thrombolytic therapy or invasive procedures become necessary.
- Liver function tests.

Imaging Studies

A *two-dimensional echocardiogram* may reveal new myocardial wall motion abnormalities that may occur with ischemia or after an MI, and give an estimate of LV ejection fraction (the percentage of blood that is ejected in relation to the amount that is present in the left ventricle at the end of filling). It may also reveal valve dysfunction, pericarditis, pericardial effusions, septal defects, papillary muscle dysfunction, ventricular aneurysm, or thrombus formation within a heart chamber (Nishimura, Gibbons, Glockner, & Tajik, 2004–2005).

In a *transesophageal echocardiogram (TEE)*, the patient swallows an endoscopic transducer that allows for a clearer ECG picture. Because a TEE involves esophageal intubation and sedation of the patient, it requires careful monitoring during and after the procedure (Baird, 2001).

A *chest radiograph* is of limited value but may rule out other causes of chest pain such as pneumothorax. It may also reveal an enlarged heart due to pericarditis or effusion, aortic aneurysm, aortic dissection, ventricular aneurysm, and pulmonary vascular congestion due to heart failure.

Stress testing is used to diagnose IHD and records a person's 12-lead ECG before, during, and after exercise. This test is usually done for patients who have chest pain with exertion, but not with rest. A positive stress test reveals ST-segment depression

(Selwyn & Braunwald, 2004–2005). Stress testing can help to determine whether a patient is at high risk for an acute coronary event (Nishimura et al., 2004–2005).

Nuclear imaging studies (myocardial perfusion scan) involve injecting a radioactive tracer into the bloodstream. As the tracer decays, it emits gamma rays that are recorded by a specialized camera. These tracers allow for the detection of myocardial blood flow. The two most common tracers are thallium-201 (^{201}Tl) and ^{99m}Tc-sestamibi (Cardiolite®). Damaged myocardial cells will not absorb these tracers and will appear as "cold spots." These scans cannot reveal the age of an infarct (Nishimura et al., 2004–2005).

Stress perfusion imaging is done both at rest and while the heart is under stress. ^{201}Tl is given at rest to evaluate myocardial blood flow; then ^{99m}Tc-sestamibi or ^{99m}Tc-tetrofosmin (Myoview®) is given during stress. The stress state of the heart is achieved either through exercise or with use of pharmacological agents such as with dipyridamole (Persantine®) or adenosine (Adenocard®). During stress, regions of the heart supplied by normal coronary arteries will receive twice the amount of tracer received by areas supplied by diseased vessels (Soine & Hanrahan, 2005).

Stress echocardiography is an echocardiogram done as the patient exercises or is given dobutamine (Dobutrex®) to stress the heart. Wall motion abnormalities may be present with exercise (as ischemia is induced) that are not noted with the resting heart (Selwyn & Braunwald, 2004–2005).

In a *multiple gated acquisition (MUGA) scan*, a small amount of the patient's blood is labeled with technetium pertechnetate and re-injected into the bloodstream. Images of wall motion are obtained at various points during the cardiac cycle. MUGA scans evaluate left and right ventricular function and identify abnormalities of the left ventricle (Soine & Hanrahan, 2005).

In *positron emission tomography (PET)*, a positron-emitting radiotracer is injected into the bloodstream and broken down into high-energy photons, which are detectable by PET imaging. Stress PET imaging allows for the measurement of coronary blood flow and helps to determine viability of muscle, because it can distinguish areas of ischemia from areas of infarction (Morton, 2005; Soine & Hanrahan, 2005).

Magnetic resonance imaging (MRI) can assist in determining the size and location of an infarct. In addition, it can distinguish ischemic, but viable, portions of the heart muscle from areas of necrosis (Braunwald, 2001).

Cardiac Catheterization and Angiography

Cardiac catheterization is done to evaluate ventricular and valvular performance, and for purposes of angiography to determine the patency of the coronary arteries and the extent of atherosclerotic disease. Both right and left heart catheterization may be performed.

In left heart catheterization, an introducer sheath is inserted into a large artery—usually the femoral, but the radial and brachial may be used as well. Under fluoroscopy, a catheter is threaded into the sheath and advanced into the left ventricle. Pressure readings within the heart chambers and across the valves are recorded to determine ventricular and valvular function. At this point, a *ventriculogram* may be done, in which a contrast medium is injected into the ventricular cavity to evaluate wall motion.

With angiography, iodine-based contrast agents are injected into the opening of the coronary arteries and contrast flow is filmed at various angles. The results are useful for determining the presence and extent of atherosclerotic disease and the best course of treatment (Baim & Grossman, 2004–2005)

Cardiac catheterization also allows for percutaneous interventional procedures, such as stent placement or balloon angioplasty. It will be performed prior to coronary artery bypass graft (CABG) surgery to direct surgical procedures (Baim & Grossman, 2004–2005; Scanlon et al., 1999).

COMPLICATIONS OF MYOCARDIAL ISCHEMIA AND INFARCTION

Heart Failure

Both myocardial ischemia and infarction can produce alterations in LV function. Most commonly, this will occur to patients after a STEMI to the anterior wall, which is the largest portion of the left ventricle. Generally, the degree of damage correlates with the degree of LV failure and symptoms (Gardner & Altman, 2005).

After an MI, an area of necrosis renders the heart unable to pump blood normally. This area undergoes stretching and thinning, especially along the edges of the infarct. Eventually, the non-infarcted tissue will begin to lengthen, producing an overall enlargement of the LV chamber, which further impedes the heart's function (Antman & Braunwald, 2004–2005). Heart failure is discussed in more detail in Chapter 15.

Cardiogenic Shock

Cardiogenic shock is a serious complication that occurs in 7% to 8% of patients with MI and carries a mortality rate of 50% (Antman and Braunwald, 2004–2005; Hochman, 2003). It is characterized by a low perfusion state that follows from cardiac dysfunction (Doven et al., 2004). Although it may be present on admission, cardiogenic shock most often develops within hours after admission (Laurent & Shinn, 2005). Cardiogenic shock is described in more detail in Chapter 18.

Dysrhythmias

Dysrhythmias are the most common cause of death after an MI, usually occurring in the first few hours post MI (Antman & Braunwald, 2004–2005). Ischemia and injury to the heart muscle can produce metabolic disturbances and alter impulse propagation along conduction pathways. The result: atrial and ventricular dysrhythmias, heart blocks, and brady-dysrhythmias. The most common dysrhythmias seen are premature ventricular contractions (PVCs), supraventricular tachycardia, sinus tachycardia, atrial fibrillation, atrial flutter, paroxysmal atrial tachycardia, and bradycardias, including heart blocks. A detailed description of dysrhythmias appears in Chapter 10.

Left Ventricular Aneurysm

After an MI, the area of necrosis stretches, while the remaining functional cells shorten in an effort to increase stroke volume. The result is a dilating or "ballooning" out of the infarcted area, especially during systole. LV aneurysm may result in heart failure and mural thrombus formation within the pooled blood of the aneurysm. Clinical manifestations include chest pain, heart failure, ventricular dysrhythmias, persistent ST elevation on ECG, and a double or displaced apical pulse. Treatment includes management of heart failure and dysrhythmias, anticoagulation, and/or surgical aneurysmectomy (Antman & Braunwald, 2004–2005; Martinez, 2003).

Septal Defect

Acute septal rupture occurs with an MI to the anterior-septal area of the LV in approximately 2% of patients within the first week post MI. The septal rupture results in an abnormal communication between the left and right ventricles. Because pressures are much higher in the LV, blood is shunted into the lower-pressure RV. The thin-walled RV, which is now subjected to higher pressure, dilates, resulting in increased pulmonary pressures. Cardiac output drops, leading to LV failure. Signs and symptoms include chest pain, biventricular failure, low blood pressure, and a loud holosystolic murmur. Treatment includes inotropic agents, nitroprusside (Nipride®), intravenous (IV) nitroglycerin, or angiotensin-converting enzyme (ACE) inhibitors. An intra-aortic balloon pump (IABP) may be used as well while the patient waits for emergency surgical repair (Martinez, 2003).

Acute Mitral Valve Regurgitation

Mitral valve regurgitation (MVR) usually occurs within the first week after an NSTEMI or an inferior wall MI and is the result of dysfunction or rupture of the papillary muscle. Signs and symptoms may range from mild, with a new onset of a systolic murmur, to severe, with a sudden onset of shortness of breath, pulmonary edema, and hypotension. Treatment of mild MVR involves correcting the ischemia with nitroglycerin and/or revascularization. Severe MVR will require afterload-reducing agents such as nitroprusside or intravenous nitroglycerin, inotropic agents, ACE inhibitors, and dysrhythmia control. IABP may be necessary before surgical repair (DeeBene & Vaughan, 2005).

Pericarditis

Pericarditis, an inflammation of the sac that surrounds the heart, occurs in 6% to 20% of patients with a large transmural MI. It can occur either in the hospitalized patient or several weeks post MI (Dressler's syndrome). The incidence of pericarditis is lower in patients who receive thrombolytic therapy. Symptoms include chest pain, low-grade fever, pericardial friction rub, and ST-segment elevation in most ECG leads. Treatment includes high-dose aspirin. Patients should be monitored for the development of pericardial tamponade (Martinez, 2003).

TREATMENT OF ACUTE CORONARY SYNDROME

When patients present to the hospital with ACS, a rapid response is necessary to ensure quick diagnosis and treatment. Fewer delays in treatment will help to preserve functioning myocardial muscle, resulting in fewer complications and decreasing morbidity and mortality from this cause.

Patients will undergo risk stratification in the emergency department to determine the likelihood that symptoms are related to ACS. Patients with *high risk* are those with two of the following criteria: persistent, typical chest pain that is increasing in frequency and duration; chest pain that lasts longer than 20 minutes or occurs at rest; any signs and symptoms of heart failure; hemodynamic instability or dysrhythmias; age 75 years or older; an ECG with ST-segment changes or new bundle branch block; and an elevated cardiac marker such as troponin, myoglobin, or CK.

Patients with an *intermediate risk* are those who have one of the following criteria: rest angina lasting less than 20 minutes; history of MI, cardiovascular accident (CVA), or coronary bypass surgery; age 70 years or older; ECG changes of T-wave inversion or pathological Q waves; and slightly elevated cardiac markers.

Patients with a *low risk* meet all of the following criteria: new onset of angina within the past two weeks; normal ECG, or unchanged ECG with chest pain; and normal cardiac markers (Braunwald, 2003; Hawley, 2004).

Patients suspected of experiencing an acute coronary event are placed on continuous cardiac monitoring and given supplemental oxygen therapy via nasal cannula at 2–4 L/min. With ECG changes, bed rest is encouraged and, if not contraindicated, the patient is given chewable aspirin at a dose of 160 to 325 mg.

Anti-ischemic and Cardioprotective Therapy

Anti-ischemic and cardioprotective strategies are used to relieve pain and ischemia in the early phase of ACS. These therapies protect the heart by mechanisms that limit the extent of damage to the muscle by increasing the blood supply to the muscle and decreasing the heart's demand for oxygen at the critical time of infarction.

Management of Chest Pain

Persistent chest pain should be treated with nitroglycerin (NTG). Initially, NTG may be given via buccal spray or sublingually every 5 minutes for a total of three doses. If the pain is still unrelieved, an IV drip may be started at 5–10 mcg/min, and titrated up in 10 mcg increments until pain is relieved or for a maximum dose of 75–100 mcg/min. Hypotension may be a limiting factor with NTG use, and blood pressure should be monitored frequently as the dose is titrated. Before receiving NTG, patients should be queried regarding their use of sildenafil citrate (Viagra®).

Morphine sulfate 2–4 mg is usually effective in relieving pain and may need to be administered repeatedly every 5–10 minutes. Hypotension may result and can be treated with a fluid bolus (Antman & Braunwald, 2003–2004).

Pharmacological Treatment

Beta-Adrenergic Blockers.   The actions of beta blockers are the same as when they are used for angina, but the agents are initially given intravenously, followed by oral doses. Beta blockers have been shown to limit infarct size and reduce mortality (Kloner & Rezkella, 2004). Conditions that may limit their use are hypotension, bradycardia, heart blocks, conduction defects, and moderate to severe heart failure (Antman & Braunwald, 2003–2004). Patients with bronchospastic airways may be unable to tolerate beta blockers or may need beta$_1$-selective agents.

Calcium Channel Blockers.   Calcium channel blockers are used if beta blockers are not tolerated or with dysrhythmias. Unlike beta blockers, they have not been shown to decrease mortality in acute MI (Kong, Blazing, & O'Connor, 2000). Their actions are the same as for angina, and these agents are usually given intravenously followed by oral doses. Calcium channel blockers may be used for atrial dysrhythmias. Their use is limited in patients with moderate to severe LV failure, and with heart blocks.

Angiotensin-Converting Enzyme Inhibitors.   See the discussion of angina for ACE inhibitors' mechanisms of action. Early use of ACE inhibitors in hospitalized patients with MI has been shown to reduce mortality rates. ACE inhibitors should be avoided in patients who are hypotensive or in renal failure.

Antithrombotic Therapy

Antithrombotic agents, which include antiplatelet and antithrombin agents, are important in the treatment of both unstable angina and MI. These agents help to establish and maintain the patency of the coronary arteries. They help to prevent the secondary complications of reinfarction, mural thrombus, or pulmonary embolism from deep-vein thrombosis (Antman & Braunwald, 2004–2005).

Aspirin.   Aspirin (ASA) is given in doses of 81 to 160 mg/day for platelet inhibition. Clopidogrel (Plavix®) may be prescribed if patients are unable to tolerate aspirin. Recent evidence suggests that patients with UA/NSTEMI benefit from the concomitant use of ASA and clopidogrel to reduce the risk of death, MI, or CVA (Antman & Van de Werf, 2004).

Glycoprotein IIb/IIIa Inhibitors.   After plaque rupture, glycoprotein (GP) receptors, which are located on the surfaces of platelets, bind with fibrinogen and promote coronary thrombus formation. GP IIb/IIIa inhibitors bind to the GP receptor and prevent platelet aggregation and thrombus formation. These agents are often given as adjunctive therapy with heparin or ASA for patients undergoing percutaneous coronary intervention (PCI) (Diehl-Oplinger & Begliomini, 2004). Patients should be monitored for bleeding while they are receiving GP IIb/IIIa inhibitors. These agents are given as an IV bolus, followed by an IV infusion for 12 to 72 hours.

Unfractionated Heparin.   The anticoagulant unfractionated heparin (UFH) exerts its effects by preventing the conversion of prothrombin to thrombin, which in turn prevents the conversion of fibrinogen to fibrin. While UFH cannot dissolve existing clots, it may prevent their extension, and it has some antiplatelet activity as well. UFH is given as an 80 units/kg bolus, then an IV infusion starting at 10 units/kg and finally titrated to a PTT 1.5–2 times normal (Matura & Mengo, 2003).

Low-Molecular-Weight Heparin.   Low-molecular-weight heparin (LMWH) is administered twice daily via the subcutaneous route. It has a longer half-life and a longer anticoagulatory effect than UFH. Unlike with IV heparin, however, its effects cannot be reversed quickly for procedures or for bleeding.

Direct Thrombin Inhibitors.   These agents bind directly to thrombin to exert their anticoagulation effects. They are used for patients who are unable to tolerate heparin.

Warfarin Sodium (Coumadin®).   Coumadin is an oral anticoagulant that competes with vitamin K and diminishes the production of clotting factors essential for clot formation.

Statins.   Statins were discussed in Chapter 12. Results of a recent study suggest that administration of statins within 24
hours of an MI may decrease the short-term death rate by
more than 50%. It is further suggested that statins may decrease myocardial inflammation, which occurs immediately
after an MI (see www.sciencedirect.com/science?).

Revascularization Procedures

Revascularization procedures involve the restoration of blood
flow through the coronary artery to limit damage to the heart
muscle (Wong & White, 2000).

Thrombolytic therapy involves the use of agents that will
dissolve the fibrin clot in an occluded or nearly occluded coronary artery so as to restore blood flow. The success rates for this
therapy have depended largely on the time from the onset of
symptoms to the initiation of treatment. The goal is to institute thrombolysis as early as possible, preferably within 30
minutes of arrival to the hospital, and 2 to 4 hours from the
onset of symptoms (DeeBene & Vaughan, 2005). Some patients may still benefit, however, even up to 12 hours after the
onset of symptoms (Antman & Braunwald, 2004–2005).
Thrombolytics are given intravenously.

Patients selected are those with chest pain associated with
ST-segment elevations in two contiguous leads (two leads that
represent the same area of the heart), a new left bundle branch
block, or evidence of a posterior wall MI (DeeBene & Vaughan,
2005). Patients receive IV heparin for 48 hours as well as ASA.
Following this procedure, patients are monitored for evidence
of bleeding, intracranial bleeding, and reperfusion dysrhythmias such as PVCs, ventricular tachycardia, or heart blocks.
Reocclusion of the coronary artery occurs in approximately
10% of patients, resulting in the reappearance of chest pain
and ECG abnormalities (Wong & White, 2000). Contraindications to receiving thrombolytics include a history of hemorrhagic CVA at any time, ischemic CVA within the past year,
marked hypertension, and aortic dissection (Antman &
Braunwald, 2004–2005).

Percutaneous Coronary Interventions (PCIs) are procedures designed to open stenosed coronary arteries. As with
cardiac catheterization, a catheter is inserted through an introducer sheath that has been placed into a large peripheral artery,
usually the femoral artery. The catheter is then advanced into
the heart, specifically into the coronary artery, while a
guidewire allows for the introduction of balloons or stents.
These procedures may be performed in patients who have sta-

ble angina, who cannot achieve relief of symptoms through
medical therapy, or who are in the acute phases of unstable
angina and MI. Mostly, PCI is done for patients with single- or
double-vessel disease, because patients with multiple-vessel disease will require surgical intervention (Selwyn and Braunwald,
2004–2005). A local anesthetic is given at the insertion site,
and patients receive light sedation during the procedure.

Careful monitoring of heart rate and rhythm, blood pressure, respiratory rate, and oxygen saturation are required during
the procedure. Following the PCI, patients may have the sheath
remain in place for 4 to 6 hours, or less time if a vascular closure
device is utilized. After the sheath's removal, manual pressure is
followed by a pressure dressing and the patient is assessed every
15 minutes for 1 to 2 hours for bleeding or hematoma at the
site. In addition, distal limb circulation is evaluated by checking
pulses, capillary refill, and skin color. Patients may be required
to remain on bed rest up to 6 hours after sheath removal with
minimal head elevation (Reynolds, Waterhouse, & Miller, 2001).

Patients will continue on antiplatelet and antithrombin
therapy post PCI. In addition to bleeding at the access site,
bleeding may occur into the retroperitoneal space. In such a
case, the patient usually complains of back and groin pain. If
this condition is left untreated and undiagnosed, the patient's
hemoglobin level will decrease and hypotension may result.
Other potential complications include coronary artery perforation, allergic reactions to the contrast dye, dysrhythmias,
coronary artery vasospasm, and restenosis (Deelstra, 2005).

Several techniques are utilized as PCIs:

Percutaneous transluminal coronary angioplasty (PTCA).
After guidewire insertion into the coronary artery (CA),
a catheter with a deflated balloon is placed across the
atherosclerotic lesion. The balloon is then inflated, resulting in the disruption of the plaque and stretching of
the vessel wall, which in turn enlarges the diameter of the
vessel. This procedure is not used as frequently due to
complications of vessel dissection, abrupt vessel closure, and restenosis (Baim & Grossman, 2004–2005).

Cutting balloon angioplasty. The balloon utilized for this
procedure has microscopic blades that make incisions
in the plaque for easier compression when the balloon
is inflated and rotated (Deelstra, 2005).

Directional atherectomy/rotational atherectomy. Directional
atherectomy involves the use of a rotating cutter that
debulks the plaque and collects plaque fragments in the
nosecone area of the device. Rotational atherectomy
("Rotoblator") uses a very-high-speed rotating ellipti-
cal burr with an abrasive surface that selectively cuts
plaque rather than normal elastic endothelium. It is

done in stages using increasingly larger rotating burrs (Deelstra, 2005).

Laser angioplasty. A laser uses photochemical processes to ablate tissue that it comes in contact with. This type of angioplasty is often used for the more difficult to reach distal coronary arteries (Baird, 2001).

Intercoronary stenting. Stenting is done in approximately 85% of all PCIs. Stents are metallic mesh walls inserted into the CA (see **Figures 14-3** and **14-4**) (Baim & Grossman, 2004–2005). Drug-eluting stents have recently been introduced, in which the stent is coated with an agent that prevents stent thrombosis and proliferation of tissue into the stent. With drug-eluting stents, the rate of restenosis has diminished to less than 10% (Baim & Grossman).

Coronary artery bypass grafting (CABG). CABG is discussed in Chapter 17.

INTERVENTIONS OF THE CRITICAL CARE CARDIAC PATIENT

The cardiac patient typically has problems related to pain, cardiac output, oxygenation, and anxiety. Specific nursing interventions for these four major patient problems are discussed here. Patients in the acute phase of unstable angina/MI are admitted to the intensive care unit (ICU), which offers expert nursing and medical care. The ICU utilizes special equipment for monitoring and for treatments as well as specialized medications. Expert observation allows personnel to promptly detect and treat complications.

Interventions for Pain

- Provide a calm environment along with reassurance.
- Administer oxygen at 2–4 L/min via nasal cannula.
- Encourage verbalization of pain by patient.
- Note the characteristics of pain (see Box 12-2, on the use of the O-P-Q-R-S-T assessment).
- Administer NTG sublingually or buccal spray ×3.
- Administer NTG drip in recommended doses.
- Administer morphine sulfate as needed in recommended doses.
- Note the response to treatment and monitor for side effects (e.g., hypotension).
- Notify the physician if pain is not improved or becomes worse.
- Perform an ECG daily and as needed with episodes with pain.
- Assess activity limitations related to pain, fatigue, or dyspnea, and modify activities accordingly.
- Maintain activity limitations until the patient is hemo dynamically stable and free from pain.
- Obtain cardiac marker levels as indicated (e.g., troponin, CK).
- Administer medications to increase myocardial oxygen supply, such as nitroglycerin, and calcium channel blockers.
- Administer medications to decrease myocardial oxygen demand, such as beta blockers and ACE inhibitors.

Interventions for Impaired Cardiac Output

- Provide for continuous cardiac monitoring with individualized alarms. Note any changes in the ST segment or T wave indicative of ischemia, injury, or infarction.
- Monitor heart rate and rhythm, blood pressure, mean arterial pressure, respiratory rate, and urine output, and record these data every hour and with changes.
- Monitor the patient following administration of medications, especially for changes in blood pressure and heart rate and rhythm.

FIGURE 14-3 Balloon Deflated for Stent Placement

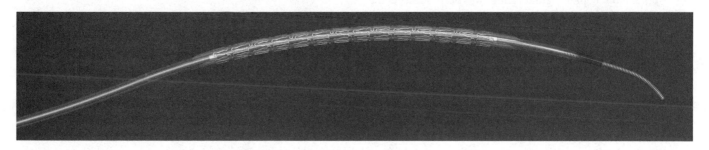

Source: With permission from Guidant Corporation, Indianapolis, IN.

FIGURE 14-4 Balloon Inflated for Stent Placement

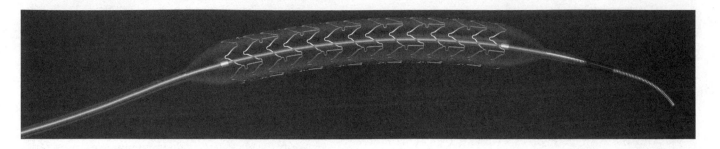

Source: With permission from Guidant Corporation, Indianapolis, IN.

- With a pulmonary artery catheter, monitor pulmonary artery tracing continually for detection of permanent pulmonary artery wedge or catheter displacement into the RV. Monitor for decreased pulmonary artery pressures and decreased cardiac output (CO), which may indicate hypovolemia. Monitor for increased pulmonary artery pressures and decreased CO, which may indicate heart failure.
- Maintain accurate intake and output measures and daily weights.
- Notify the physician of any dysrhythmias and administered antidysrhythmics as per protocol.
- Administer inotropic agents, vasopressors, and vasodilator agents as per protocol with careful monitoring of vital signs and hemodynamic monitoring, especially on initiation of therapy and with changes. Titrate doses until the desired hemodynamic effect is achieved.
- Monitor for clinical manifestations of left-sided heart failure/pulmonary edema: S_3, S_4 heart sound, dyspnea, cough, crackles, or wheezes auscultated over lung fields, decreasing oxygen saturation, decreasing CO and rising pulmonary artery catheter pressures, and increased systemic vascular resistance (SVR).
- Monitor for clinical manifestations of right-sided heart failure: equalization of PAOP and RA pressures, hypotension, hepatojugular reflux, and peripheral edema.
- Monitor for complications of acute MI, and notify the physician if any are suspected.
- Administer antithrombotic therapy—that is, ASA, antiplatelet, or heparin therapy to prevent or limit thrombus formation. Monitor coagulation studies, and observe for obvious or occult bleeding.
- Monitor serum electrolytes, BUN, and creatinine daily and as needed.
- Prepare the patient and family for diagnostic tests, PCI, or surgical intervention by explaining the procedures and encouraging questions. Provide drawings, demonstrations, and videos to assist in the learning process.
- Monitor pulses, color, capillary refill, and temperature in the affected limb after cardiac catheterization or PCI as per protocol.
- Provide a low-fat, low-sodium diet along with measures to increase appetite.

Interventions for Oxygenation

- Administer oxygen therapy with nasal cannula (4–6 L/min) as indicated to maintain oxygen saturation (SpO_2) > 92%.
- Monitor for increasing respiratory distress: increased respiratory rate and work of breathing, shortness of breath, decreased SpO_2, pallor, cyanosis of nail beds and lips, cough, or wheezing.
- Provide ventilatory support if needed, along with sedation to maintain comfort with intubation.
- Perform a chest radiograph daily and as needed for acute changes.
- Assess breath sounds every 4 hours and as needed. Notify the physician of any changes.
- Monitor ABGs as needed with changes in the patient's condition and/or ventilator settings.

Interventions for Anxiety

- Explain all procedures and invite questions. Use diagrams, drawings, and handouts to assist in learning.
- Encourage family involvement in the patient's care.
- Assess for signs and symptoms of anxiety: increased heart rate, respiratory rate and blood pressure; restlessness; pressured speech; and inability to focus.
- Encourage verbalization of fears regarding the diagnosis and any potential or actual loss of function.
- Begin coordination of discharge planning with emphasis on support for the patient and family.

PATIENT OUTCOMES

Nurses can help ensure attainment of optimal patient outcomes such as those listed in **Box 14-3**.

SUMMARY

Care of the cardiac patient can be complex and challenging. Acute management, prevention of complications, support and encouragement, and education are necessary tools to help patients through the difficult time of adjusting to a new diagnosis and possibly an altered lifestyle.

Box 14-3

Outcomes for Patients with Acute Coronary Syndrome

- Pain not present
- Absence of sequela of disease process
- Knowledge of disease process and health care regimen
- Adherence to treatment plan
- Hemodynamic status—no deviation from expected range
- Adjustment to required changes in lifestyle

CASE STUDY

S.H. is a 56-year-old man who came to the emergency department (ED) with a report of substernal chest pain. The pain was non-radiating and was accompanied by diaphoresis and nausea. The pain started 60 minutes prior to the patient's arrival in the ED. His past medical history was significant for diabetes, hypertension, and hypercholesterolemia. Vital signs upon arrival in the ED were BP 162/74, HR 98, RR 22, and temperature 98.6°F. Oxygen saturation was 94% on room air. A 12-lead ECG was obtained and revealed ST-segment elevation in leads II, III, and aVF. S.H. received oxygen at 4 L/min via nasal cannula, sublingual nitroglycerin, aspirin, and a heparin bolus and subsequent continuous infusion. Cardiac enzymes and troponin levels were drawn and sent to the lab.

S.H. was taken for emergent cardiac catheterization and possible intervention. The heart catheterization revealed a near-occlusive lesion in the right coronary artery. S.H. underwent PTCA and stent placement. He was started on heparin to prevent clot formation at the stent and was transferred to the ICU for monitoring. Serial ECGs and cardiac enzymes were obtained. Significant lab values were as follows: CK-MB = 146 ng/mL (normal ≤ 5.0 ng/mL) and troponin I level = 16.0 ng/mL (> 1.5 is indicative of MI). S.H.'s ST segments were less elevated later that evening.

S.H. was discharged from the ICU five days after PTCA and was discharged home two days later.

CRITICAL THINKING QUESTIONS

1. Based on his symptoms, ECG, and biomarker findings, what is the most likely diagnosis for S.H.?
2. Would S.H. be considered at high, intermediate, or low risk for experiencing ACS? What symptoms or findings is this based on?
3. Based on S.H.'s vital signs, which medications do you think are appropriate at this time?
4. Explain which tests S.H. may undergo to confirm the diagnosis.
5. Which disciplines should be consulted to work with this client?
6. How will you implement your role as a facilitator of learning for this patient?

7. List all of the subjective and objective data for each patient characteristic and identify the degree to which that characteristic is manifested (i.e., level 1, 3, or 5). Then choose appropriate interventions that will result in optimal patient outcomes. Complete the chart below.

8. Utilize the form to write up a plan of care for one cardiac client in the clinical setting. Rate the patient as a level 1, 3, or 5 on each characteristic. Identify the level of nurse characteristics needed in the care of this patient.

9. Take one patient outcome for a cardiac patient and list evidence-based interventions found in a literature review for this patient.

Using the Synergy Model to Develop a Plan of Care

	Patient Characteristics	Level 1, 3, or 5	Subjective and Objective Data	Evidence-based Interventions	Outcomes
SYNERGY MODEL	Resiliency				
	Vulnerability				
	Stability				
	Complexity				
	Resource availability				
	Participation in care				
	Participation in decision making				
	Predictability				

Online Resources

ACC/AHA 2002 Guidelines Update for the Management of Patients with Unstable Angina:
www.americanheart.org/presenter.jhtml

Interactive Case—ACS: www.mdchoice.com/cme/coronary3/frame.asp

Diagnosis of ACS: www.aafp.org/afp/20050701/119.html

Advances in the Approach to ACS: www.hosppract.com/issues/2000

REFERENCES

Antman, E. M., & Braunwald, E. (2004–2005). ST-segment elevation MI. In D. L. Kasper, E. Braunwald, A. S. Fauci, S. L. Hauser, D. L. Longo, J. L. Jameson, et al. (Eds.), *Harrison's principles of internal medicine* (16th ed.). McGraw-Hill (Harrison's Online). Retrieved May 18, 2005, from www.accessmedicine.com

Antman, E. M., & Van de Werf, F. (2004). Pharmacoinvasive therapy for ST-elevation myocardial infarction. *Circulation, 109*(21), 2480–2486.

Baim, D. S. (2004–2005). Percutaneous coronary revascularization. In D. L. Kasper, E. Braunwald, A. S. Fauci, S. L. Hauser, D. L. Longo, J. L. Jameson, et al. (Eds.), *Harrison's principles of internal medicine* (16th ed.). McGraw-Hill (Harrison's Online). Retrieved May 18, 2005, from www.accessmedicine.com

Baim, D. S., & Grossman, W. (2004–2005). Diagnostic cardiac catheterization and angiography. In D. L. Kasper, E. Braunwald, A. S. Fauci, S. L. Hauser, D. L. Longo, J. L. Jameson, et al. (Eds.), *Harrison's principles of internal medicine* (16th ed.). McGraw-Hill (Harrison's Online). Retrieved May 18, 2005, from www.accessmedicine.com

Baird, M. S. (2001). Acute coronary syndromes. In P. L. Swearington & J. Hicks Keen (Eds.), *Manual of critical care nursing* (4th ed., pp. 247–264). St. Louis, MO: Mosby.

Becker, D. (1999). Coronary artery disease. In L. Bucher & S. Melander (Eds.), *Critical care nursing* (pp. 201–227). Philadelphia: W.B. Saunders.

Braunwald, E. (2001). *A textbook of cardiovascular medicine* (6th ed.). Philadelphia: W.B. Saunders. Available at http://home.mdconsult.com

Braunwald, E. (2003). Application of current guidlines to the management of unstable angina and non ST-elevation MI. *Circulation, 108*(Suppl. III), III-28–III-37.

Carter, T., & Ellis, K. (2005). Right ventricular infarction. *Critical Care Nurse, 25*(2), 52–62.

Casey, P. (2004). Markers of myocardial injury and dysfunction. *AACN Clinical Issues, 15*(4), 547–557.

DeeBene, S., & Vaughan, A. (2005). Acute coronary syndromes. In S. L. Woods, E. S. Sivarajan Froelicher, S. Underhill Motzer, & E. J. Bridges (Eds.), *Cardiac nursing* (5th ed., pp. 550–584). Philadelphia: Lippincott Williams & Wilkins.

Deelstra, M. H. (2005). Interventional cardiology techniques. In S. L. Woods, E. S. Sivarajan Froelicher, S. Underhill Motzer, & E. J. Bridges (Eds.), *Cardiac nursing* (5th ed., pp. 585–600). Philadelphia: Lippincott Williams & Wilkins.

Dichl Oplinger, L., & Begliomini, R. (2004). Using glycoprotein inhibitors for acute coronary syndrome. *Nursing, 34*(9), 32cc1–32cc4.

Doven, O., Akkus, M. N., Camsari, A., Pekdemir, H., Cicek, D., Kanik, A., et al. (2004). Impact of intensive strategy for the management of patients with cardiogenic shock after acute myocardial infarction. *Coronary Artery Disease, 15*(6), 361–366.

Fass, A. E. (2003). Perspectives in the management of chronic coronary artery disease. *Heart Disease: A Journal of Cardiovascular Medicine, 5*(6), 365–367.

Gardner, P., & Altman, G. (2005). Pathophysiology of acute coronary syndrome. In S. L. Woods, E. S. Sivarajan Froelicher, S. Underhill Motzer, & E. J. Bridges (Eds.), *Cardiac nursing* (5th ed., pp. 541–549). Philadelphia: Lippincott Williams & Wilkins.

Hawley, D. A. (2004). What's new in acute coronary syndromes? *Nursing Clinics of North America, 39*, 815–828.

Hochman, J. S. (2003). Cardiogenic complicating acute myocardial infarction: Expanding the paradigm. *Circulation, 107*(24), 2998–3002.

Kloner, R. A., & Rezkella, S. H. (2004). Cardiac protection during acute myocardial infarction: Where do we stand in 2004? *American Journal of Cardiology, 44*(2), 276–286.

Kong, D. F., Blazing, M. A., & O'Connor, C. M. (2000). Advances in the approach to acute coronary syndromes. *Hospital Practice*. Retrieved July 29, 2005, from www.hosppract.com

Laurent, D., & Shinn, J. A. (2005). Acute heart failure and shock. In S. L. Woods, E. S. Sivarajan Froelicher, S. Underhill Motzer, & E. J. Bridges (Eds.), *Cardiac nursing* (5th ed., pp. 659–688). Philadelphia: Lippincott Williams & Wilkins.

Martinez, J. A. (2003). Complications of acute myocardial infarction. *Emergency Medicine, 35*(7), 20–32.

Matura, L. A., & Mengo, D. F. (2003). Guidelines for the diagnosis and management of unstable angina and non ST-segment elevation MI. *Internet Journal of Advanced Nursing Practice, 6*(1). Retrieved May 3, 2005, from www.ispub.com

Morton, P. G. (2005). Acute myocardial infarction. In P. G. Morton, D. K. Fontaine, C. M. Hudak, & B. M. Gallo (Eds.), *Critical care nursing: A holistic approach* (8th ed., pp. 422–447). Philadelphia: Lippincott Williams & Wilkins.

Nishimura, R. A., Gibbons, R. J., Glockner, J. F., & Tajik, A. J. (2004–2005). Non-invasive cardiac imaging: Echocardiography, nuclear cardiology, and MRI/CT imaging. In S. L. Woods, E. S. Sivarajan Froelicher, S. Underhill Motzer, & E. J. Bridges (Eds.), *Cardiac nursing* (5th ed., pp. 628–688). Philadelphia: Lippincott Williams & Wilkins.

Ozdemir, K., Altunkeser, B. B., Addullah, I., Odzil, S., & Gok, H. (2003). New parameters in identification of RV myocardial infarction and proximal RCA occlusion. *Chest, 124*(1), 219–226.

Pyne, C. (2004). Classification of acute coronary syndromes using the 12-lead electrocardiogram as a guide. *AACN Clinical Issues, 15*(14), 558–567.

Reen, S. (2005). Laboratory tests using blood. In S. L. Woods, E. S. Sivarajan Froelicher, S. Underhill Motzer, & E. J. Bridges (Eds.), *Cardiac nursing* (5th ed., pp. 265–295). Philadelphia: Lippincott Williams & Wilkins.

Reynolds, S., Waterhouse, K., & Miller, K. H. (2001). Patient care with percutaneous transluminal coronary angioplasty. *Nursing Management, 32*(9), 51–54, 56.

Scanlon, P. J., Faxon, D. P., Audet, A. M., Carabello, B., Dehmer, G. J., Eagle, K. A., et al. (1999). ACC/AHA guidelines for coronary angiography: Executive summary and recommendations: A report of the American Task Force on Practice Guidelines (Committee on Coronary Angiography) *Circulation, 99*(17), 2345–2357.

Selwyn, A. P., & Braunwald, E. (2004–2005). Ischemic heart disease. In D. L. Kasper, E. Braunwald, A. S. Fauci, S. L. Hauser, D. L. Longo, J. L. Jameson, et al. (Eds.), *Harrison's principles of internal medicine* (16th ed.). McGraw-Hill (Harrison's Online). Retrieved May 18, 2005, from www.accessmedicine.com

Soine, L., & Hanrahan, M. (2005). Nuclear and other imaging studies. In S. L. Woods, E. S. Sivarajan Froelicher, S. Underhill Motzer, & E. J. Bridges (Eds.), *Cardiac nursing* (5th ed., pp. 319–325). Philadelphia: Lippincott Williams & Wilkins.

Wong, C. K., & White, H. D. (2000). Medical treatment for acute coronary syndromes. *Current Opinion in Cardiology, 15*, 441–462.

CHAPTER 15

Heart Failure

Sara Paul   Kismet D. Rasmusson

LEARNING OBJECTIVES

Upon completion of this chapter, the reader will be able to:

1. Describe the pathophysiology of heart failure.

2. Identify assessment data utilized in clinical judgment for patients with heart failure.

3. Discuss the medical and nursing management of heart failure.

4. Delineate appropriate patient and family teaching strategies for the acutely ill heart failure patient.

5. Recognize resources available to the nursing and healthcare community to further assist in care and education of the heart failure patients and their families.

6. List optimal patient outcomes that may be achieved through evidence-based management of heart failure.

Heart failure (HF) is a major cause of morbidity and mortality in the United States, with more than 5 million people being diagnosed with this disease (American Heart Association, 2005). It is defined as a failure of the heart's pump, resulting in a decrease in cardiac output (the amount of blood ejected by the heart each minute) (Heart Failure Online, 2005). Each year, there are approximately 550,000 newly diagnosed cases of HF and nearly 1 million related hospital discharges for this cause (American Heart Association). As the U.S. population ages, the prevalence of HF will increase. Survival rates for HF have improved over recent years due to medical and technological advances; as a consequence, the incidence of people living with chronic HF has continued to climb. Patients with chronic advanced HF often have comorbidities such as ischemic heart disease, diabetes, and hypertension (Krum & Gilbert, 2003). As many as 40% of patients with HF are readmitted within six months of hospital discharge. Common reasons for frequent readmissions include noncompliance with diet or medications, ischemia, myocardial infarction, angina, arrhythmias, worsening azotemia, poorly controlled blood pressure, alcohol abuse, and comorbidities (e.g., pneumonia, pulmonary embolism, sepsis) (Hoyt & Bowling, 2001).

Patients with decompensated HF are admitted to the intensive care unit (ICU) for hemodynamic stabilization. Some patients in HF are also admitted to exclude acute coronary syndrome (ACS) as the etiology of the HF (Lettman, Sites, Shofer, & Hollander, 2002); HF is a complication of ACS. A more in-depth discussion of ACS appears in Chapter 14.

PATHOPHYSIOLOGY

The most common cause of HF is ischemic coronary artery disease, although chronic hypertension is also a common etiology. **Table 15-1** lists causes of HF. Risk factors for developing HF are similar to those for developing ischemic heart disease: advanced age, coronary artery disease, hypertension, male gender, hypercholesterolemia, diabetes, cigarette smoking, myocardial infarction, and family history. A more in-depth discussion of risk factors for heart disease appears in Chapter 12.

At one time, HF was simply thought to be a problem of a weak heart pump. However, scientific discoveries over the past 25 years have shown that HF results from a much more complex process. As listed in Table 15-1, an initial insult causes stress to

---

TABLE 15-1 Causes of Heart Failure

1. Ischemic heart disease/myocardial infarction
2. Chronic hypertension
3. Aortic valve regurgitation or stenosis
4. Mitral valve regurgitation or stenosis
5. Dilated "idiopathic" cardiomyopathy (unknown cause)
6. Hypertrophic cardiomyopathy
7. Viral myocarditis
8. Bacterial myocarditis
9. Collagen disease: rheumatoid arthritis, lupus, progressive systemic sclerosis
10. Sarcoidosis
11. Metabolic factors: diabetes, malnutrition, thiamine deficiency, obesity, thyroid disease, hyperthyroidism, hypothyroidism, carcinoid
12. Toxins: alcohol, cocaine, radiation, drugs, chemotherapy agents, heavy metals
13. Neuromuscular disease: muscular dystrophy
14. Others: amyloidosis, peripartum cardiomyopathy
15. Congenital heart disease
16. Chronic arrhythmias
17. Chronic anemia

Sources: Baran & Gomberg-Maitland, 2002; Stevenson, 2004.

---

the heart. In response to that stress, neurohormones and other intrinsic molecules that are usually inactive in the body become active and take effect on the heart muscle, changing the shape of the heart over time. The term for this change in shape is ventricular remodeling (Paul, 2003). A healthy heart is shaped like the bottom half of a football standing on end—a sort of cone shape. After ventricular remodeling, the heart is more spherically shaped, like a basketball. At some point, patients become symptomatic with shortness of breath, fatigue, and swelling in the feet and ankles. The transition to symptomatic HF occurs independently of the patient's hemodynamic status. Continued activation of these harmful neurohormones in the body may explain why HF continues to progress over time, regardless of which problem initiated the HF.

There are two types of HF: systolic and diastolic. Systolic HF occurs when the contractility of the ventricles is weakened. Diastolic HF occurs when the heart pump strength is not diminished, but rather the ventricle's ability to fill during diastole is reduced because it is fibrotic and not distensible. Nearly 50% of all HF is diastolic; however, most research in HF has been done in patients with systolic HF. Although patients with diastolic HF have lower mortality rates than their counterparts with systolic HF, their symptoms are similar (Senni & Redfield, 2001).

PATIENT HISTORY AND PHYSICAL EXAM

Pertinent Questions for HF Patients

The patient's cardiac history is an important aspect of the assessment and is vital to the plan of care. It is important to learn about the patient's history of heart disease and any surgery or cardiac interventions the patient has undergone in the past, such as pacemaker or defibrillator implant, catheterization procedures, or congenital heart defect repair. The nurse should ask the patient about other cardiovascular illnesses such as dysrhythmias, myocardial infarction, hypertension, stroke, and peripheral vascular disease. It is also important to determine any pertinent family history of premature coronary heart disease, sudden death, or cardiomyopathy. Pertinent noncardiac illnesses to ask about include diabetes, hypercholesterolemia, and lung disease.

Many of the symptoms that are associated with HF are nonspecific and could easily apply to other conditions. For that reason, it is important to ask specific questions that focus on differentiating the cause of the patient's symptoms. **Table 15-2** lists pertinent questions to ask HF patients during a nursing assessment. Patients diagnosed with HF present with typical symptoms easily remembered by using the Heart Failure Society of America's acronym FACES: Fatigue, Activities limited, Chest congestion, Edema, and Shortness of breath (www.hfsa.org).

Expected Exam Findings in Heart Failure

Physical assessment techniques include visual inspection, palpation, and auscultation of the patient. The physical examination should be performed beginning at the patient's head, working down toward the feet (Paul & Glotzer, 2004). Visually, the patient must be assessed for signs of HF including altered level of consciousness, respiratory distress, jugular venous distention, cyanosis, and peripheral edema. Tachypnea with minimal exertion, such as climbing onto the exam table, may indicate decompensated or end-stage HF. Palpation of the precordium in patients with HF may typically reveal an enlarged and laterally displaced point of maximum apical impulse. A lift or thrill may be felt along the left sternal border in some patients with HF. Often, a third heart sound (S_3) is heard, as well the murmur of mitral regurgitation (holosystolic murmur heard at the apex, often radiating to the axilla) (Carabello, 2004).

Irregularities in the cardiac rhythm are common in patients with HF. More than 80% of patients with HF and cardiomyopathy have atrial fibrillation or ventricular dysrhythmias (e.g., premature ventricular contraction, ventricular tachycardia, accelerated idioventricular rhythm, and ventricu-

TABLE 15-2 Pertinent Questions for Heart Failure Patients

1. Have you been hospitalized or seen in the emergency department recently?
2. What types of activities or exercises do you perform?
3. How many days per week do you perform this exercise?
4. How many minutes are you able to do this exercise without stopping?
5. When you feel that you must stop exercising, is it because you are short of breath or is it because your legs are tired?
6. How much fluid do you drink each day?
7. What are some examples of foods that you eat?
8. Do you become short of breath at rest? With exertion?
9. Do you have a cough? Is it dry or productive? Is it worse when lying down?
10. Do you become short of breath when you lie down flat? Does it help to prop your head up on pillows? If so, how many pillows?
11. Do you wake up from your sleep feeling like you're smothering?
12. Do you get swelling in your ankles or abdomen?
13. Do you ever feel your heart fluttering, racing, or skipping beats? If so, how long does that last? Do you have any other symptoms when that happens?
14. Do you ever get dizzy? If so, does it get to the point where you feel like you're going to pass out? Do you have any other symptoms with the dizziness?
15. Do you ever get chest pain? If so, is it at rest or with activity? How long does it last? Does it radiate to another part of your body? What do you do to relieve it?
16. What prescription medications and dosages do you take?
17. What over-the-counter medications do you take?

Source: Paul & Glotzer, 2004.

lar fibrillation) (Podrid & Ganz, 2005). Rales, wheezes, or decreased breath sounds may be auscultated in the lungs, although the absence of these abnormalities does not rule out pulmonary edema. Some patients with HF may cough or become dyspneic when moved to the reclined position if pulmonary edema is present.

Palpation of the abdomen is performed to assess for ascites or hepatomegaly. The legs and feet are examined to assess for the presence of edema, cyanosis, and peripheral pulses. The strength of peripheral pulses should be noted in the assessment.

Diagnostic Tests

The goals of diagnostic testing for HF are to establish the diagnosis, identify the underlying pathology, and identify abnormalities that may be treated, such as coronary artery

disease. Diagnostic tests may help to establish other conditions that mimic, contribute to the development of, or worsen HF, such as severe anemia, renal dysfunction, thyroid disorders, liver disease, and hemochromatosis. **Table 15-3** lists diagnostic tests for HF and the possible findings.

PHARMACOLOGIC TREATMENT

Acute Decompensated Heart Failure

Treatment goals for acute decompensated HF focus on symptom relief and support of hemodynamic function. For patients with pulmonary edema or other significant edema, treatment options such as intravenous diuretics and vasodilating drugs may be necessary (Stevenson, 2004). Vasodilator action is achieved with nitroglycerin (Nitrostat®), nitroprusside (Nipride®), or nesiritide (Natrecor®). Recombinant human B-type natriuretic peptide (nesiritide) is a cardiac hormone. It may be useful in the management of acute decompensated HF because it acts as an arterial and venous dilator, inhibits the renin-angiotensin-aldosterone system (RAAS), and has antisympathetic action. This latter action is important because patients with HF cannot tolerate increases in heart rate (Baran & Gomberg-Maitland, 2002). Nesiritide also acts as a diuretic and promotes excretion of sodium by the kidneys (Norton & Kesten, 2005). Data suggest that nesiritide promotes and maintains hemodynamic stability as well. Side effects that ICU nurses need to observe for are asymptomatic and symptomatic hypotension. Both of these side effects are treated by decreasing the rate of the infusion (Strain, 2004). A recent meta-analysis claims that nesiritide increases mortality (Sackner-Bernstein, Kowalski, Fox, & Aaronson, 2005). More data are needed on this issue before any definitive conclusion is reached.

Cool extremities, poor mentation, and reduced blood pressure are all signs of reduced cardiac output and hypoperfusion related to severely decompensated HF. If the patient is hemodynamically unstable, cardiac function may be supported with intravenous inotropic agents such as dobutamine (Dobutrex®), dopamine (Intropin®), or milrinone (Primacor®) (**Table 15-4**). Long-term or intermittent use of these medicines remains controversial, but may be used chronically in patients awaiting cardiac transplantation or receiving palliative care. Palliative care is discussed in Chapter 60.

Pharmacologic management and technology are used to manage HF in the ICU. Use of intravenous diuretics is a primary intervention. Calcium channel blockers, beta blockers, nesiritide, and angiotensin-converting enzyme (ACE) inhibitors have a place as well. Likewise, intra-aortic balloon pumps (IABPs) and ventricular assist devices may be considered; these technologies are discussed in more depth in

TABLE 15-3 Diagnostic Tests for Heart Failure

Test	Finding	Suspected Diagnosis
Electrocardiogram	Acute ST-T wave changes	Myocardial ischemia
	Tachyarrhythmias	Thyroid disease or HF due to rapid ventricular rate
	Bradyarrhythmias	HF due to low heart rate
	Previous MI (i.e., Q waves)	HF due to reduced LV performance
	Low voltage	Pericardial effusion
	Left ventricular hypertrophy	Cardiomyopathy
Chest x-ray	Cardiomegaly	Dilated cardiomyopathy; rule out pericardial effusion
	Increased pulmonary venous congestion (interstitial, alveolar edema)	Right ventricular failure; pulmonary edema
CBC	Anemia	HF due to or aggravated by decreased oxygen carrying capacity
Urinalysis	Proteinuria	Nephrotic syndrome
	Red blood cells or cellular casts	Glomerular nephritis
Serum creatinine	Elevated	Volume overload due to renal failure
Electrolytes	Low sodium (<135 mEq/L)	Activated renin-angiotensin system
	Low potassium	Increased risk of arrhythmia
Serum albumin	Decreased	Increased extravascular volume (edema) due to hypoalbuminemia
T4 and TSH	Abnormal T4 or TSH	HF due to or aggravated by hypo/hyperthyroidism
B-type natriuretic peptide (BNP)	Elevated level >100 pg/mL	May indicate fluid volume overload in HF exacerbation
N-terminal pro-brain natriuretic peptide (NT-pro-BNP)	Elevated >125 pg/mL. Values differ between men & women. Values increase with aging	Precursor to BNP. Indicates the presence of early cardiac dysfunction
Echocardiogram	Normal ejection fraction	Possibly diastolic HF
	Decreased ejection fraction	Systolic HF
	Abnormal ventricular wall motion	Possible ischemia/infarct
	Abnormal valve function	Mechanical cause of HF
Pulmonary artery occlusive pressure	>20 mm Hg	Elevated LV filling pressures, indicating HF exacerbation
Cardiac catheterization or thallium scan	Coronary occlusion or myocardial ischemia	Coronary artery disease

Note: MI = myocardial infarction; HF = heart failure; LV = left ventricular; TSH = thyroid stimulating hormone.
Source: Hunt et al., 2005.

Chapters 16 and 17. Placement of a pulmonary artery catheter may also be considered (Baran & Gomberg-Maitland, 2002).

Chronic Heart Failure

Standardized guidelines for the management of chronic HF have been published by the American Heart Association and the American College of Cardiology (Hunt et al., 2005). These evidence-based guidelines were developed by HF experts, and are based on the results of clinical trials involving patients with systolic HF (**Table 15-5**). Recently, a National Institute of Aging–funded study conducted by Kitzman (2005) sought to examine the role of decreased aortic distensibility in the pathophysiology of exercise intolerance in elderly patients with diastolic HF and determine whether aortic distensibility, exercise intolerance, and quality of life can be improved with enalapril, an ACE inhibitor (http://crisp.cit.nih.gov).

ACE inhibitors are the cornerstone of HF therapy, even in asymptomatic HF patients (Captopril Multicenter Research Group, 1983; CONSENSUS Trial Study Group, 1987; Investigators for SOLVD, 1991). These drugs both block the

TABLE 15-4 Drugs Used in the Management of Acute Decompensated Heart Failure

Drug	Dose/Bolus	Starting Effective Range
Diuretic		
Furosemide	Bolus 40–80 mg	5–10 mg/hr
Vasodilators		
Nesiritide	Bolus 2 mcg/kg	0.005–0.03 mcg/kg/min
Nitroglycerin	20 mcg/min	40–400 mcg/min
Nitroprusside	10 mcg/min	30–350 mcg/min; <4 mcg/kg/min
Inotropic Agents		
Dobutamine	2.5 mcg/kg/min	2–10 mcg/kg/min for vasodilation and increased contractility
Dopamine	1–2 mcg/kg/min	2–5 mcg/kg/min for vasodilation and increased contractility
	4–5 mcg/kg/min	6–15 mcg/kg/min for vasoconstriction and increased contractility
Milrinone	Optional bolus 50–75 mcg/kg over 10 min	0.10–0.75 mcg/kg/min; usual dose 0.5 mcg/kg/min

activation of the RAAS and reduce blood pressure. Research has shown that symptoms improve, hospitalizations decrease, and HF mortality is reduced with use of ACE inhibitors. Survival is improved by delaying the progression of the disease and reversing ventricular remodeling. Adverse reactions commonly associated with ACE inhibitors include dizziness, fatigue, nausea, diarrhea, cough, hyperkalemia, angioedema, and renal impairment.

Angiotensin-receptor blockers (ARBs) have significant benefits similar to ACE inhibitors and are an alternative therapy to ACE inhibitors (Pfeffer et al., 2003; Pitt et al., 2000; Wong et al., 2002). ARBs do not block the activation of the RAAS, but rather block angiotensin from entering cardiac cells, thereby preventing the detrimental effects of the RAAS. Adverse effects associated with ARBs are similar to those for ACE inhibitors. Patients who are unable to take an ACE inhibitor or an ARB due to side effects may instead take a nitrate, such as isosorbide dinitrate (Isordil®), in combination with hydralazine hydrochloride (Apresoline®). This drug combination has been shown to reduce mortality in HF, although ACE inhibitors and ARBs remain the preferred drugs.

Beta blockers are a class of medications that have been proven to reduce HF morbidity and mortality by blocking norepinephrine, which is released by the sympathetic nervous system (Hjalmarson et al., 2000; Packer et al., 2001). Improvements of ventricular function have been seen in patients with severe systolic HF. Beta blockers should be started at the lowest possible dose when patients are not retaining fluid, then increased as tolerated every two weeks. These drugs are contraindicated in patients with asthma or bronchospastic airway disease, bradycardia, cardiogenic shock, or decompensated HF. Common adverse reactions include fatigue, dizziness, depression, dyspnea, bradycardia, palpitations, edema, syncope, hypotension, heart block, and bronchospasm.

Diuretics are used for HF patients who have edema or "congestive" symptoms. When necessary, diuretics control symptoms of cough, shortness of breath, edema, and ascites. While they have not been shown to reduce morbidity or mortality in HF, these drugs clearly reduce fluid retention. Patients must be monitored for changes in renal function, potassium levels, and magnesium levels. Electrolyte supplements should often accompany diuretic therapy. Patients taking diuretics may become dehydrated, so they should be assessed for fluid volume status frequently. For patients with significant symptoms of pulmonary edema, intravenous loop diuretics enhance diuresis and improve symptoms. Adverse reactions of diuretics include dehydration, fluid and electrolyte imbalance, gastrointestinal (GI) upset, dizziness, orthostatic hypotension, jaundice, rash, hyperuricemia, tinnitus, and photosensitivity. Patients on diuretics should be educated about self-management techniques that will improve diuretic therapy, such as fluid and sodium restriction.

Digoxin (Lanoxin®) has been shown to improve symptoms, quality of life, and exercise tolerance in HF (Digitalis Investigation Group, 1997) and is typically added to augment other HF therapies. It improves cardiac contractility and has mild neurohormone-blocking properties. Lower doses of digoxin should be used in elderly patients, in patients with renal dysfunction, and in patients with a lower body mass index. Adverse reactions that may occur with digoxin include heart block, dysrhythmias, GI effects (nausea, anorexia, vomiting, diarrhea), and central nervous system (CNS) effects (confusion, visual or mental disturbances, headache, weakness, dizziness).

Aldosterone antagonists are potassium-sparing diuretics that contribute to blocking of the RAAS. When they are used in conjunction with standard medical therapy for patients with continued significant HF symptoms (NYHA classes III–IV), reductions in mortality, reductions in hospital admissions, and improved functional class have been seen (Pitt et al., 2003). Lab monitoring of renal function and potassium levels is essential within one week of initiating an aldosterone

TABLE 15-5 Major Clinical Trials of Medications Used to Treat Chronic Heart Failure

Clinical Trial	Drug Tested	Target or Mean Dose
Angiotensin-Converting Enzyme Inhibitors		
Studies of Left Ventricular Dysfunction (SOLVD)	Enalapril versus placebo	10 mg twice a day
Survival and Ventricular Enlargement (SAVE)	Captopril versus placebo	50 mg three times a day
Acute Infarction Ramipril Efficacy (AIRE)	Ramipril versus placebo	5 mg twice a day
Trandolapril Cardiac Evaluation Study (TRACE)	Trandolapril versus placebo	4 mg a day
Assessment of Treatment with Lisinopril and Survival (ATLAS)	Low- versus high-dose lisinopril	2.5–5 mg versus 32.5–35 mg
Angiotensin-Receptor Blockers		
Evaluation of Losartan in the Elderly (ELITE II)	Losartan versus captopril	50 mg a day (losartan) versus 50 mg three times a day (captopril)
Valsartan Heart Failure Trial (Val-HeFT)	Valsartan versus placebo	160 mg twice a day
Candesartan in Heart Failure Assessment of Reduction in Morbidity and Mortality (CHARM-Added)	Candesartan versus placebo	32 mg a day
CHARM-Alternative	Candesartan	32 mg a day
Beta Blockers		
Metoprolol CR/XL Randomized Intervention Trial in Congestive Heart Failure (MERIT-HF)	Metoprolol CR/XL	159 mg a day
Cardiac Insufficiency Bisoprolol Study (CIBIS-II)	Bisoprolol	7.5 mg a day
Carvedilol Prospective Randomized Cumulative Survival (COPERNICUS)	Carvedilol	37 mg a day
Aldosterone Antagonists		
Randomized Aldactone Evaluation Study (RALES)	Spironolactone versus placebo	25 mg a day
Eplerenone Post-Acute Myocardial Infarction Heart Failure Efficacy and Survival Study (EPHESUS)	Eplerenone versus placebo	Up to 50 mg a day
Isosorbide Dinitrate/Hydralazine		
African American Heart Failure Trial (A-HeFT)	Isosorbide dinitrate/hydralazine added to standard HF therapy	120 mg isosorbide dinitrate/ 225 mg hydralazine in 3 divided daily doses
Digoxin		
Digitalis Investigation Group (DIG)	Digoxin versus placebo	0.125–0.25 mg a day

Sources: Eichhorn & Bristow, 2004; Pitt et al., 1999; Pitt et al., 2003; Konstam & Patten, 2004; Taylor et al., 2004.

antagonist because these drugs may increase the patient's serum potassium level. Patients on these drugs should generally not receive potassium supplementation, even if they are also taking diuretics. Adverse reactions include breast pain, hyperkalemia, hyponatremia, GI disturbance, headache, rash, confusion, ataxia, impotence, hirsutism, menstrual changes, and gastric ulcers.

In a study of African Americans with advanced HF, BiDil®—a combination drug containing isosorbide dinitrate and hydralazine—was found to decrease mortality and hospitalizations and improve quality of life (Taylor et al., 2004). The

combination also boosted the amounts of nitric oxide in the blood, a substance that is found in lower levels in African Americans. BiDil is the first drug to target a specific racial group—in this case, African Americans. Side effects of this medication include hypotension, tachycardia, headache, dizziness, and systemic lupus erythematosus–like symptoms (Nitromed, 2005).

Drugs that should be avoided in patients with HF include nonsteroidal anti-inflammatory agents (NSAIDs), antihistamines, certain calcium channel blockers, and antiarrhythmic drugs other than amiodarone hydrochloride (Cordarone®)

and dofetilide (Tikosyn®). These medications can aggravate symptoms of HF.

Diastolic Heart Failure

Pharmacologic treatment for patients who have diastolic HF is empirical, based on the results of case studies and small clinical trials. As yet, there have been no large drug trials addressing the management of diastolic HF. The goals for treating patients with diastolic HF are the same as for patients with systolic HF—to help them feel better, have more energy, and live longer. The same drugs that are used in systolic HF may be used in diastolic HF, such as ACE inhibitors, ARBs, beta blockers, and diuretics. Digoxin should probably be avoided unless the patient has atrial fibrillation, but patients with diastolic HF may take calcium channel blockers to slow the heart rate and lower blood pressure. Standardized guidelines for the management of diastolic HF are not yet available.

NONPHARMACOLOGIC TREATMENT

Acute Decompensated Heart Failure

In hospitalized patients with acute decompensated HF, an IABP may be used to increase blood flow to the heart muscle and decrease the heart's workload. A balloon in the aorta inflates when the heart relaxes, propelling blood forward toward the periphery, while at the same time pushing blood backward into the coronary arteries. The balloon deflates quickly when the aortic valve opens and left ventricular contraction begins, creating a suction that "pulls" the blood out of the ventricle, thereby assisting forward blood flow and increasing cardiac output. This greatly reduces the workload on the heart by reducing myocardial oxygen consumption and allowing the heart an opportunity to recover. IABP therapy is often used in patients with cardiogenic shock and acute decompensated HF due to acute myocardial infarction (Laham & Aroesty, 2005). A more in-depth discussion about IABP appears in Chapter 17.

A left ventricular assist device (LVAD) may be used in an individual with acute myocardial infarction to support the patient's circulation until the heart improves enough to allow the patient to undergo cardiac surgery (American Heart Association, 2006). Traditionally, LVADs have been reserved for use in very sick HF patients awaiting cardiac transplantation. More recently, they have been used as long-term therapy in patients with cardiogenic shock or severe left ventricular failure. The Randomized Evaluation of Mechanical Assistance for the Treatment of Congestive Heart Failure trial evaluated whether mechanical LVADs could be an effective alternative for patients who are ineligible for heart transplantation (Stevenson et al., 2004). This trial compared patients with severe HF who received therapy with LVADs to patients who received optimal medical therapy. The trial results supported the concept that LVADs could be used as permanent therapy in HF patients who did not qualify for heart transplantation. Survival time and quality of life were improved in patients on LVAD therapy versus those receiving medical therapy. More information can be found on LVADs in Chapter 16.

Chronic Heart Failure

Device therapy for chronic HF has advanced considerably in recent years. In some HF patients, depolarization between the right and left ventricles is delayed, causing the two ventricles to contract in a dyssynchronous fashion. This abnormal contraction of the ventricles impairs the ability of the heart to eject blood efficiently and may increase mitral valve regurgitation (Littmann & Symanski, 2000). By implanting pacemaker leads in both the right and left ventricles and pacing the ventricles to contract simultaneously, blood flow is improved and mitral regurgitation is decreased. This type of pacemaker is known as a biventricular pacemaker, or cardiac resynchronization therapy, because both right and left ventricular contraction are physiologically synchronized by the pacemaker. Recent studies have suggested that cardiac resynchronization therapy improves outcomes in patients with chronic HF after optimal medical therapy has been achieved (Bristow et al., 2004; Cleland et al., 2005; Kadish et al., 2004).

Patients with HF are at higher risk for sudden arrhythmic cardiac death as compared to the general population. Clinical trials have shown that implantable cardioverter-defibrillators (ICDs) reduce mortality in patients who have systolic HF. The Multicenter Automatic Defibrillator Implantation Trial showed that patients who had coronary artery disease, nonsustained ventricular tachycardia, and systolic HF had reduced mortality compared with similar patients receiving conventional antiarrhythmic therapy (Moss et al., 1996). Recently, the Defibrillators in Non-Ischemic Cardiomyopathy Treatment Evaluation trial showed that patients with HF who do not have coronary artery disease may also benefit from prophylactic implantation of an ICD (Kadish et al., 2004). In this study, the risk of sudden death from arrhythmia was significantly reduced in HF patients who received an ICD.

Procedures may also be performed if the patient's HF has a correctable cause, such as ischemic coronary disease or heart valve dysfunction. In some cases, surgical therapy may be done to delay or avoid the need for cardiac transplantation, particularly given that the supply of donor hearts for transplant does not meet the demand. **Table 15-6** lists corrective procedures that might be performed in appropriate patients with HF (Albert, 2003).

Heart transplantation has evolved during the last three decades to become a well-accepted treatment for some patients with end-stage HF (Smith, Farroni, Baillie, & Haynes, 2003). Indications for heart transplantation include the following conditions (Koerner, Durand, Lafuente, Noon, & Torre-Amione, 2000):

- Severe end-stage HF despite optimal medical management
- Refractory angina pectoris not amenable to revascularization
- Life-threatening ventricular arrhythmias uncontrolled with medical and surgical interventions
- Cardiac tumor confined to the myocardium and absence of metastasis

There are many restrictions and contraindications to heart transplantation, and not all end-stage HF patients are appropriate candidates. Additionally, organ donation is not agreeable to all citizens. Consequently, the number of patients in need of transplant far exceeds the pool of donors.

PATIENT AND FAMILY EDUCATION

Medical treatment of HF is only one portion of the overall plan of care for patients with HF. Patients must make important lifestyle changes that will improve their symptoms and may also improve their disease state. It is the nurse's role to make sure that patients and their family members are educated about HF and understand the actions that will promote self-care. Topics that should be included in patient and family education are listed in **Table 15-7**.

PATIENT OUTCOMES

Nurses can help ensure obtainment of optimal patient outcomes, such as those listed in **Box 15-1**, through the use of evidence-based interventions.

TABLE 15-6 Possible Surgical/Interventional Procedures for Heart Failure

1. Coronary artery revascularization with bypass surgery or percutaneous coronary angioplasty or stent placement
2. Mitral or aortic valve repair or replacement
3. Dor procedure (reconstruction surgery to reshape the ventricle from a spherical shape to cone shape) (http://jtcs.ctsnetjournals.org/cgi/content/full/124/5/886)
4. Arrhythmia ablation for incessant tachyarrhythmias
5. Cellular transplantation—implantation of skeletal muscle cells into the myocardium to regenerate and reinforce structure and function (investigational) (www.med.umich.edu/opm/newspage/2002/musclecell.htm)

TABLE 15-7 Patient and Family Education for Living with Heart Failure

1. Dietary sodium restriction: 2,000–3,000 mg daily sodium intake
2. Fluid intake restricted to 64 ounces per day
3. Daily weight monitoring
4. Smoking cessation
5. Elimination/limitation of alcohol intake
6. Weight loss if appropriate
7. Reduced fat and cholesterol intake if at risk for coronary artery disease
8. Take medications as prescribed
9. Do not take nonsteroidal anti-inflammatory drugs (e.g., ibuprofen, naproxen)
10. Immunization with influenza and pneumococcal vaccines
11. Report signs and symptoms of worsening condition to healthcare provider, such as:
    a. Weight gain > 3 pounds over 3 days or 5 pounds in a week
    b. Pressure or pain in the chest
    c. Increased shortness of breath or fatigue
    d. Dizziness or syncope
    e. Increased swelling in feet, ankles, legs, or abdomen
    f. Palpitations or heart "racing" sensation
    g. Rapid heart rate > 120 beats per minute
    h. Poor appetite, nausea, vomiting, abdominal pain

SUMMARY

HF is a major cause of morbidity and mortality in the United States. Innovations in technology and clinical trials are attempting to improve quality of life and patient outcomes.

Box 15-1
Optimal Patient Outcomes

- Ejection fraction within expected range
- Adventitious breath sounds not present
- Performs activities of daily living consistent with energy and tolerance
- Vital signs in expected range in response to activity
- Neck vein distention not present
- Reduced hospital readmission
- Body weight stable
- Modifies lifestyle to decrease risk factors

CASE STUDY

Mr. P. was a 28-year-old male, who presented to a clinic for presence of cardiomegaly (enlarged heart) on his chest x-ray. He had no known medical problems and had been healthy as a child into adulthood. He did not smoke, drink alcohol, or use illicit drugs. He took no medications other than occasional acetaminophen. He began feeling fatigued about a month prior to his referral. When he developed a cough, he sought treatment by his primary care provider. Pneumonia was diagnosed, and he received a course of antibiotics. Mr. P.'s symptoms did not improve over the next two to three weeks, however. In fact, in addition to his cough, he began feeling significant shortness of breath with exertion and woke up nightly feeling air-hunger and anxious.

Mr. P. returned to his primary care physician, who ordered a chest x-ray on hearing rales. Cardiomegaly and pleural effusions were diagnosed. He was then referred for cardiology evaluation.

Physical Exam

Vital signs: BP 102/54, heart rate 118, weight 82 kg, SpO$_2$ 92% on room air

General: No acute distress at rest, but dyspneic with mild activity

HEENT: Unremarkable

Lungs: Bilateral crackles R > L, slight inspiratory wheeze

CV: Heart rate regular, tachycardic, II/VI holosystolic murmur at the left lower sternal border radiating to the axilla, visible and bounding apical pulse, visible jugular venous distention, no lower-extremity edema

Abdomen: Soft, tender to palpation in the right upper quadrant, active bowel sounds

Musculoskeletal, Neuro, Psych: Unremarkable

Diagnostic Tests Performed

Echocardiogram: Showed an ejection fraction of 18% (indicating severely depressed cardiac contractility), moderate to severe mitral valve regurgitation, significant four-chamber cardiac dilatation

ECG: Sinus tachycardia; large-amplitude QRS complexes across the precordial leads, enlarged and biphasic P waves, QRS and PR intervals normal

Labs: Sodium 142, potassium 3.9, creatinine 1.6, BUN 42, calcium 8.7, chloride 110, glucose 72, BNP 1280, TSH 1.7; urinalysis, CBC, fasting lipids all WNL

Diagnosis: Severely reduced left ventricular function, accounting for Mr. P.'s clinical symptoms

Stress thallium was ordered to rule out coronary artery disease as the cause. The likely etiology is idiopathic dilated cardiomyopathy, New York Heart Association class III–IV. Cardiac transplantation was discussed if symptoms worsened or if Mr. P. failed medical therapy.

Mr. P. was started on a diuretic [furosemide (Lasix®) 40 mg daily], an ACE inhibitor [enalapril (Vasotec®) 2.5 mg twice daily], an aldosterone blocker [spironolactone (Aldactone®) 25 mg daily], and digoxin 0.25 mg daily.

He was given HF self-management instruction with a prescription to attend a more in-depth patient education class. Mr. P. was instructed to take appropriate medications and monitor his BP daily. He was to notify his doctor or nurse if his systolic BP was less than 90 mm Hg and to monitor his weight daily (target is a 2-pound loss per day or a target of a 4-pound loss over the next two days). He was also told to limit sodium to 2 grams daily and limit fluids to 2 liters daily. He was notified about when to call for worsening symptoms and follow up in two days. Mr. P. was recommended to take time off from work.

Follow-up

At his next visit, Mr. P.'s symptoms were improved, yet he still coughed when he reclined. The furosemide dose was doubled. Labs were stable. The enalapril dose was not changed. Mr. P. was to return in one week.

Over time, his cough, jugular vein distention, and shortness of breath improved. Carvedilol (Coreg®) was introduced at a starting dose of 3.125 mg twice a day. Mr. P. was instructed when to call for worsening symptoms. He was seen every two weeks to increase his carvedilol dose until he reached the maximum dose of 25 mg twice a day.

Two months later, a repeat echocardiogram showed Mr. P.'s left ventricular ejection fraction had improved to 40%. Six months after the repeat echocardiogram, the ejection fraction had improved to 60%, which is within the normal range. Mr. P. was able to stop taking furosemide, digoxin, and spironolactone, but remained on his ACE inhibitor (enalapril) and beta blocker (carvedilol) for life. He required no cardiac device therapy and was no longer in need of a heart transplant. He returned to work and regained his quality of life.

CRITICAL THINKING QUESTIONS

1. What is the benefit of using diuretics in heart failure patients?
2. What is the benefit of using ACE inhibitors and beta blockers in heart failure patients?
3. What is the role of an aldosterone blocker in the treatment of heart failure?
4. What should we teach patients with heart failure about taking care of themselves?
5. Utilize the form to write up the data and a plan of care for a patient with heart failure in the clinical setting. Rate the patient as a level 1, 3, or 5 on each characteristic. Identify the level of nurse characteristics needed in the care of this patient.
6. Take one patient outcome for a patient and list evidence-based interventions found in a literature review for this patient.

Using the Synergy Model to Develop a Plan of Care

	Patient Characteristics	Level 1, 3, or 5	Subjective and Objective Data	Evidence-based Interventions	Outcomes
SYNERGY MODEL	Resiliency				
	Vulnerability				
	Stability				
	Complexity				
	Resource availability				
	Participation in care				
	Participation in decision making				
	Predictability				

Online Resources

American Heart Association: www.americanheart.org

Update of the ACC/AHA Guidelines for the Evaluation and Management of Chronic Heart Failure in the Adult, originally published in 2001: http://www.americanheart.org/presenter.jhtml?identifier=3032845

Heart Failure Society of America: www.hfsa.org

ADHERE Registry: www.adhereregistry.com

UCSD Practical Guide to Clinical Medicine: http://medicine.ucsd.edu/clinicalmed/heart.htm

CHF Patients.Com: www.chfpatients.com

Cardiovascular Exam Web Sites:

- www.blaufuss.org/tutorial/
- http://uisvideo2.med.unc.edu/mpar/cardiovascex.ram
- www.familypractice.com/heartlab/heartlab.htm
- www.med-ed.virginia.edu/courses/pom1/videos/cardiac.cfm
- www.meddean.luc.edu/lumen/MedEd/medicine/pulmonar/pd/contents.htm
- www.wilkes.med.ucla.edu/inex.htm
- www.cvtoolbox.com/cvtoolbox2/physexam/physexam.html

Journal of Cardiac Failure (online): http://journals.elsevierhealth.com/periodicals/yjcaf

The Heart.Org: www.theheart.org

Cardiology OnLine: www.cardiologyonline.com

Heart Failure Online: www.heartfailure.org

National Heart Lung and Blood Institute, Heart Failure: www.nhlbi.nih.gov/health/public/heart/other/hrtfail.htm

REFERENCES

Albert, N. (2003). Surgical management of heart failure. *Critical Care Nursing Clinics of North America, 15,* 477–487.

American Heart Association. (2005). *Heart disease and stroke statistics—2005 update.* Dallas, TX: American Heart Association.

American Heart Association. (2006). Left ventricular assist device. Retrieved on February 16, 2006, from http://www.americanheart.org/presenter.jhtml?identifier=4599

Baran, D. A., & Gomberg-Maitland, M. (2002). Confronting heart failure in the ICU: The treatment challenge: Signs and symptoms guide the treatment. *Journal of Critical Illness, 17*(10), 381–386.

Bristow, M., Saxon, L., Boehmer, J., Krueger, S., Kass, D., DeMarco, T., et al. (2004). Cardiac resynchronization therapy with or without an implantable defibrillator in advanced chronic heart failure. *New England Journal of Medicine, 350,* 2140–2150.

Captopril Multicenter Research Group. (1983). A placebo-controlled trial of captopril in refractory chronic congestive heart failure. *Journal of the American College of Cardiology, 2,* 755–763.

Carabello, B. (2004). Valvular heart disease. In L. Goldman & D. Ausiello (Eds.), *Cecil textbook of medicine* (22nd ed., pp. 431–441). Philadelphia: Saunders.

Cleland, J., Daubert, J., Erdmann, E., Freemantle, N., Gras, D., Kappenberger, L., et al. (2005). The effect of cardiac resynchronization on morbidity and mortality in heart failure. *New England Journal of Medicine, 352,* 1539–1549.

CONSENSUS Trial Study Group. (1987). Effects of enalapril on mortality in severe congestive heart failure. Results of the Cooperative North Scandinavian Enalapril Survival Study (CONSENSUS). *New England Journal of Medicine, 316,* 1429–1435.

Digitalis Investigation Group. (1997). The effect of digoxin on mortality and morbidity in patients with heart failure. *New England Journal of Medicine, 336,* 525–533.

Eichhorn, E., & Bristow, M. (2004). Antagonism of beta adrenergic receptors in heart failure. In D. L. Mann (Ed.), *Heart failure* (pp. 619–635). Philadelphia: Saunders.

Heart Failure Online. Retrieved September 16, 2005, from www.heartfailure.org

Hjalmarson, A., Goldstein, S., Fagerberg, B., Wedel, W., Waagstein, F., Kjekshus, J., et al., for the MERIT-HF Study Group. (2000). Effects of controlled-release metoprolol on total mortality, hospitalizations, and well-being in patients with heart failure: The Metoprolol CR/XL Randomized Intervention Trial in congestive heart failure. *Journal of the American Medical Association, 283,* 1295–1302.

Hoyt, R. E., & Bowling, L. S. (2001). Reducing readmissions for congestive heart failure. *American Family Physician, 63*(3), 1593–1598, 1600.

Hunt, S., Abraham, W., Chin, M., Feldman, A., Francis, G., Ganiats, T., et al. (2005). ACC/AHA 2005 guideline update for the diagnosis and management of chronic heart failure in the adult: A report from the American College of

Cardiology and the American Heart Association Task Force on Practice Guidelines. Retrieved August 23, 2005, from http://www.acc.org/clinical/guidelines/failure/index.pdf

Investigators for SOLVD. (1991). Effect of angiotensin converting enzyme inhibition with enalapril on survival in patients with reduced left ventricular ejection fraction and congestive heart failure: Results of the treatment trial of the Studies of Left Ventricular Dysfunction (SOLVD): A randomized double blind trial. *New England Journal of Medicine, 325,* 293–302.

Kadish, A., Dyer, A., Daubert, J., Quigg, R., Estes, M., Anderson, K., et al. (2004). Prophylactic defibrillator implantation in patients with nonischemic dilated cardiomyopathy. *New England Journal of Medicine, 350,* 2151–2158.

Kitzman, D. (2005). Exercise intolerance in elderly diastolic heart failure. Retrieved September 15, 2005, from http://crisp.cit.nih.gov/crisp/

Koerner, M., Durand, J., Lafuente, J., Noon, G., & Torre-Amione, G. (2000). Cardiac transplantation: The final therapeutic option for the treatment of heart failure. *Current Opinion in Cardiology, 15,* 178–182.

Krum, H., & Gilbert, R. (2003). Demographics and concomitant disorders in heart failure. *Lancet, 362,* 147–158.

Laham, R. J., & Aroesty, J. M. (2005). Intraaortic balloon pump counterpulsation. Retrieved February 16, 2006, from http://patients.uptodate.com/topic.asp?file=chd/24375

Lettman, N. A., Sites, F. D., Shofer, F. S., & Hollander, J. E. (2002). Congestive heart failure patients with chest pain. Incidence and predictors of acute coronary syndrome. *Academic Emergency Medicine, 9*(9), 903–909.

Littmann, L., & Symanski, J. (2000). Hemodynamic implications of left bundle branch block. *Journal of Electrocardiology, 33*(Suppl.), 115–121.

Moss, A., Hall, W., Cannom, D., Daubert, J., Higgins, S., Klein, H., et al. (1996). Improved survival with an implantable defibrillator in patients with coronary disease at high risk for ventricular arrhythmia. *New England Journal of Medicine, 335,* 1933–1940.

Nitromed, Inc. (2005). BiDil dosage and administration package insert. Lexington, MA.

Norton, C. K., & Kesten, K. (2005). An update on the treatment of heart failure using biventricular pacing and intravenous nesiritide. *Journal of Emergency Nursing, 31*(1), 76–79, 117–123.

Packer, M., Coats, A., Fowler, M., Katus, H., Krum, A., Mohacsi, P., et al. (2001). Effect of carvedilol on survival in severe chronic heart failure. *New England Journal of Medicine, 344,* 1651–1658.

Paul, S. (2003). Ventricular remodeling. *Critical Care Nursing Clinics of North America, 15,* 407–411.

Paul, S., & Glotzer, J. (2004). Clinical evaluation of the heart failure patient. Retrieved August 24, 2004, from http://www.aahfn.org/ce/ce_20/ce_3_study_guide.pdf

Pfeffer, M., Swedberg, K., Granger, C., Held, P., McMurray, J., Michelson, E., et al. (2003). Effects of candesartan on mortality and morbidity in patients with chronic heart failure: The CHARM-Overall programme. *Lancet, 362,* 759–766.

Pitt, B., Poole-Wilson, P., Segal, R., Martinez, F., Dickstein, K., Camm, A., et al. (2000). Effect of losartan compared with captopril on mortality in patients with symptomatic heart failure: Randomized trial—the Losartan Heart Failure Survival Study (ELITE II). *Lancet, 355,* 1582–1587.

Pitt, B., Remme, W., Zannad, F., Neaton, J., Martinez, F., Roniker, B., et al., for the Eplerenone Post-Acute Myocardial Infarction Heart Failure Efficacy and Survival Study Investigators. (2003). Eplerenone, a selective aldosterone blocker, in patients with left ventricular dysfunction after myocardial infarction. *New England Journal of Medicine, 348,* 1309–1321.

Podrid, P. J., & Ganz, L. I. (2005). Ventricular arrhythmias in heart failure and cardiomyopathy. Retrieved February 16, 2006, from http://patients.uptodate.com/topic.asp?file=hrt_fail/14585

Sackner-Bernstein, J. D., Kowalski, M., Fox, M., & Aaronson, K. (2005). Short-term risk of death after treatment with nesiritide for decompensated heart failure: A pooled analysis of randomized controlled trials. *Journal of the American Medical Association, 293*(15), 1900–1905.

Senni, M., & Redfield, M. (2001). Heart failure with preserved systolic function. A different natural history? *Journal of the American College of Cardiology, 38,* 1277–1282.

Smith, L., Farroni, J., Baillie, B., & Haynes, H. (2003). Heart transplantation: An answer for end-stage heart failure. *Critical Care Nursing Clinics of North America, 15,* 489–494.

Stevenson, L. (2004). Management of acute decompensation. In D. Mann (Ed.), *Heart failure: A companion to Braunwald's heart disease* (pp. 579–594). Philadelphia: Saunders.

Stevenson, L., Miller, L., Desvigne-Nickens, P., Ascheim, D., Parides, M., Renlund, D., et al. (2004). Left ventricular assist device as destination for patients undergoing intravenous inotropic therapy: A subset analysis from REMATCH (Randomized Evaluation of Mechanical Assistance in Treatment of Chronic Heart Failure). *Circulation, 110,* 975–981.

Strain, W. D. (2004). Use of the recombinant human B-type natriuretic peptide (BNP) (nesiritide) in the management of acute decompensated heart failure. *International Journal of Clinical Practice, 58*(11), 1081–1087.

Taylor, A., Ziesche, S., Yancy, C., Carson, P., D'Agostino, R., Ferdinand, K., et al. (2004). Combination of isosorbide dinatrate and hydralazine in blacks with heart failure. *New England Journal of Medicine, 351,* 2049–2057.

Wong, M., Staszewsky, L., Latini, R., Barlera, S., Volpi, A., Chiang, Y. T., et al. (2002). Valsartan benefits left ventricular structure and function in heart failure: Val-HeFT echocardiographic study. *Journal of the American College of Cardiology, 40,* 970–975.

Cardiac Assist Devices

Shannon L. Deluca   Dana F. Kay   Cathy Clark

LEARNING OBJECTIVES

Upon completion of this chapter, the reader will be able to:

1. Define the current applications for ventricular assist devices (VADs).

2. Describe the types of assist devices.

3. Discuss the medical and nursing management of patients with VADs.

4. Identify key elements to be included in patient and family teaching.

5. Discuss common postoperative complications.

6. List indications for cardiac pacing.

7. Analyze the nursing management of patients with pacemakers.

8. List indications for implantable cardioverter defibrillators (ICDs).

9. Describe the nursing management of patients with ICDs.

10. List optimal outcomes that may be achieved through evidence-based management of patients with cardiac assist devices.

Despite a growing number of medical advances in heart failure treatment strategies, the number of deaths continues to rise each year. An estimated 40% of patients die within one year after diagnosis (Hipken, Rogers, & Jones, 2004). Patients with New York Heart Association (NYHA) class III to IV heart failure symptoms, including shortness of breath with minimal activity or at rest, have extremely poor quality of life and an estimated 50% one-year mortality. An in-depth discussion of heart failure appears in Chapter 15.

When all medical options fail, patients can be referred for surgical alternatives such as circulatory support and cardiac transplantation. Transplant is indicated in patients with NYHA class IV heart failure who have less than a 50% chance of survival for one year on optimal medical management, have no other life-threatening systemic disease, and can comply with a complex medication regimen (Bosen, 2003). However, the limited number of donor hearts significantly constrains the availability of this option, with only 3,500 procedures being performed each year among the 30,000 patients listed for cardiac transplant (Christensen, 2000). Further discussion of cardiac transplantation appears in Chapter 17.

With the demand for donor hearts exceeding the supply and many patients with late-stage heart failure being considered unsuitable candidates for transplant, alternatives such as ventricular assist devices (VADs), implantable cardioverter-defibrillators (ICDs), and pacemakers are used as a way to restore normal blood flow, rate, and rhythm and to improve quality of life.

VAD BASICS

VADs are artificial mechanical pumps that take over the function of the failing ventricle and pump blood to the body. These devices decrease the workload of the heart, restore normal blood flow to the body, and decrease or eliminate heart failure symptoms. These goals are accomplished by aiding the pumping action of either or both ventricles (the pumping chambers of the heart) if they are not strong enough to adequately pump blood (U.S. Food and Drug Administration [FDA], 2005; Health-cares.net, 2005). VADs can be used to support the right ventricle (right ventricular assist device, RVAD), the left ventricle (LVAD), or both ventricles (BiVAD). Because the left ventricle (LV) is the major pumping chamber, LVADs are the most common type of assist device (Christensen, 2000).

In all except one of the available models (discussed later), a VAD does not replace the heart. Rather, it works with the patient's heart to pump blood through the systemic circulation (FDA, 2005).

All current VADs are preload dependent, meaning that the amount of blood returning to the heart is the amount of fluid pumped. When functioning in auto mode, VADs will pump as fast as the preload of the pump allows. Although artificial pumps, the devices function much like the native heart. For optimal VAD function, there must be adequate preload or volume in the pump. VADs, like the heart, are sensitive to impedance to flow. As a consequence, hypertension and mechanical obstruction must be avoided. Most of the devices discussed in this chapter provide pulsatile flow similar to the native heart and operate asynchronously to the native heart rate. Therefore, it is important to remember the patient's pulse will be synchronous with the VAD rate—not the heart rate on the electrocardiogram (ECG). To comprehend VAD therapy, an understanding of VAD terminology is necessary (see **Table 16-1**).

TABLE 16-1 VAD Terminology

Auto mode: The device pumps at a variable rate depending on the preload of the pump. Sensors inside the pump detect when the pump is full and activate the driver to cause systole. This mode is preferred while the patient is being supported because it simulates physiologic conditions, allowing the pump flow to change with the patient's level of activity and demands of the body.

Axial/rotary: Consists of high-speed, axial flow, rotary blood pump with no pulsatile action. Significantly smaller. May be suitable for a wide range of patients, including children.

Blood pumping chamber: Collects the blood until a force is created to move the blood to the rest of the body.

Bridge to recovery: VAD is placed to allow the heart to rest so myocardial recovery can take place. Eventually the VAD can be removed. Used primarily in situations such as acute heart failure due to myocarditis.

Bridge to transplant: VAD is placed to support the patient until a suitable donor heart is obtained for cardiac transplantation.

Cannula: The conduit that connects the blood-pumping chamber to the circulatory system. The inflow cannula connects the blood pump to the ventricle it is supporting. Outflow cannulas connect the blood pump to the aorta (LVAD) or the blood pump to the pulmonary artery (RVAD).

Destination therapy: VAD is placed with the intent to support the patient indefinitely.

Driveline: The cannula that connects the blood-pumping chamber to the power source of the driver.

Driver: The power source for the blood-pumping chamber. Drivers are pneumatic or electric, depending on the type of pump used.

Electrical driver: An electric motor moves the diaphragm or pusher plate inside the pump that causes the blood to move out of the pump.

Extracorporeal: The blood pump is outside the body. Because the blood pump is not implanted inside the body habitus, it can be used in smaller adults and even some children.

Fixed rate mode: The device pumps at a rate that is preset by the operator. The rate is independent of the preload or the patient's physiological demand. This mode is used during device implantation when the patient is being weaned from cardiopulmonary bypass or while weaning the patient from VAD support. It may also be used as a backup rate if the blood pump's internal sensor fails.

Intracorporeal/paracorporeal: The blood pump is inside the body. These devices require a larger body surface area, usually greater than 1.5 m^2, and therefore may be limited to adults.

Intraperitoneal: The blood pump is placed within the abdominal cavity.

Pneumatic driver: A pump powered by air pressure. Air from the drive console is pumped into the air chamber inside the blood pump, causing the diaphragm to move and expel the blood inside the blood pump.

Postcardiotomy failure: Cardiogenic shock that occurs in patients undergoing myocardial revascularization or a valve operation. It inhibits the ability to wean the patient from cardiopulmonary bypass.

Preperitoneal: The blood pump is placed in a pocket made in the patient's left upper quadrant in the rectus sheath.

Rate: Number of times the VAD empties its contents. VAD rate = patient's pulse rate.

Stroke volume: Amount of blood ejected from the pump during each pumping cycle.

VAD Output (flow): Amount of blood ejected from the pump per minute, measured in liters per minute. Considered synonymous with cardiac output.

Source: Christensen, 2000.

Basic VAD Physiology

A VAD has three major components: a pump (located either inside or outside the body), a control system, and an energy source. The energy source may be a battery or compressed air (pneumatic). The control system and energy source are found outside the body. When a patient has a VAD, blood flows from the ventricle(s) to a pump (FDA, 2005).

Left Ventricular Assist Devices

An LVAD receives blood from the LV and delivers it to the aorta (FDA, 2005). The inflow cannula is placed in the LV and connects to the blood pump; the outflow cannula connects the blood pump to the ascending aorta. Oxygenated blood travels from the lungs via the pulmonary veins to the left atrium and LV. Blood is then pulled from the LV to an "inflow cannula" to a blood pump. The pump sends blood through the "outflow cannula" to the aorta, thereby circumventing the weakened ventricle (see **Figure 16-1**) (Health-cares.net, 2005). Although some blood may continue to flow through the native LV and out the aorta, the LVAD will assume the function of the LV.

LVADs are the most common assist devices utilized in device therapy. This is not surprising, because the LV is the major pumping chamber of the heart; therefore major damage to the LV leads to systemic organ damage and significantly impairs quality of life. Because of its workload, the LV is far more likely to suffer ischemic damage from myocardial infarction. Even in cardiomyopathy, where both ventricles are weakened, the majority of patients can be supported successfully with isolated LVADs. Some degree of right ventricular failure does occur after LVAD placement but can be managed with in-

otropic therapy (medications that increase contractility) and nitric oxide (which relaxes blood vessels). Infrequently, a temporary RVAD may be needed.

Right Ventricular Assist Devices

An RVAD receives blood from the right ventricle (RV) and delivers it to the pulmonary artery (FDA, 2005). The inflow cannula is placed in the right atrium or RV and connects to the blood pump; the outflow cannula then connects the blood pump to the pulmonary artery. Venous blood flow then travels from the inferior vena cava to the right atrium. The RVAD takes over function of the failing RV (see **Figure 16-2**).

The need for isolated RV support is not as common as the need for LV support. However, RVADs may be needed to support patients with acute RV failure, such as in patients with acute RV myocardial infarction, pulmonary embolism, or RV failure in donor hearts after cardiac transplantation and post LVAD implant.

FIGURE 16-1 Left Ventricular Assist Device

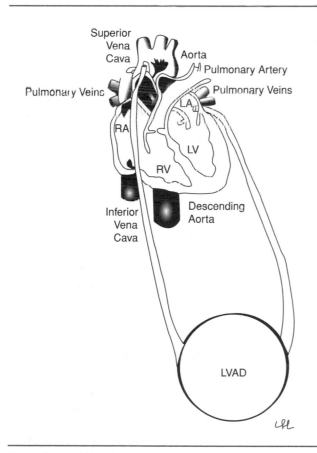

Source: Illustrated by Lydia Lemmond.

FIGURE 16-2 Right Ventricular Assist Device

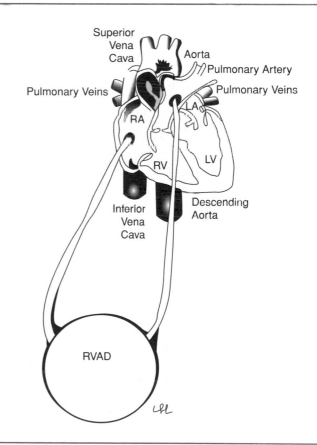

Source: Illustrated by Lydia Lemmond.

BiVentricular Assist Device

A combination RVAD/LVAD is used when both ventricles (biventricular) support is indicated (see **Figure 16-3**). Patients with biventricular infarction, intractable ventricular arrhythmias, and multiple organ dysfunction syndrome (e.g., kidney and liver dysfunction) are potential candidates for BiVADs (Goldstein & Oz, 2000). Criteria for predicting which patients will require biventricular support are not well established. Some hemodynamic indicators may be a low RV stroke work index, a lower preoperative RV ejection fraction, or low pulmonary artery pressures. Other investigators have suggested criteria other than hemodynamics as predictors of BiVAD support, such as small body surface area (BSA), female gender, non-ischemic diagnosis, preoperative ventilator support, or circulatory support (Ochiai et al., 2002).

Current Applications

VADs were initially intended to support the heart on a short-term basis until a donor heart became available for cardiac transplantation (FDA, 2005). Today, however, there are three

FIGURE 16-3 Combination RVAD/LVAD (BiVAD)

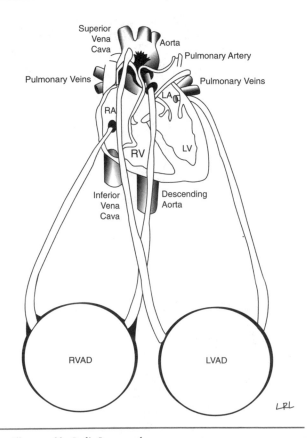

Source: Illustrated by Lydia Lemmond.

main applications for VADs: bridge to transplant, bridge to recovery, and destination therapy.

Bridge to Transplant

Each year, a number of patients die while awaiting cardiac transplantation. Critically ill patients who once would have died while waiting are allowed time to recover with a VAD bridge to transplant. In this circumstance, the VAD will take over all or most of the work of the heart until a transplant can be performed. This allows the patient to live long enough to receive a donor heart. Studies have shown that survival after transplant is equal to or greater than that for transplant patients who have not received VAD therapy (Bond, Nelson, Germany, & Smart, 2003). LVADs are now portable and can be used for weeks to months. Patients can be discharged from the hospital and have a satisfactory quality of life while awaiting cardiac transplant (American Heart Association, 2005).

Bridge to Recovery

Investigators have shown that a limited number of patients with severe heart failure can experience myocardial recovery with a device implant, thus avoiding transplantation (Cianci, Lonergan-Thomas, Slaughter, & Silver, 2003). VADs assist the heart by decreasing preload (the amount of ventricular stretch at the end of filling), reducing myocardial workload, and providing increased systemic circulation and tissue perfusion. Post-cardiotomy syndrome (fever following incision to the heart wall) and myocarditis (inflammation of heart muscle) are the most common candidates for use of a VAD as a bridge to recovery (Health-cares.net, 2005).

Destination Therapy

Until recently, VADs were used primarily by patients who required support until they were able to undergo cardiac transplantation or who were recovering from cardiac surgery (Health-cares.net, 2005). Patients with end-stage heart failure who are not transplant candidates either because of age or other relative contraindications may be evaluated for VAD implant. Some VADs are used for either destination therapy or permanent heart support (Mason & Konicki, 2003).

Patient Selection and Timing

Typical hemodynamic criteria for initiation of VAD support appear in **Table 16-2**. These criteria are important to selection of patients for VAD implant but ultimately are not the most crucial consideration. Clinical history and compliance with previous medical therapy are key components of this decision. Of note, patients with advanced heart failure can have relatively stable hemodynamics but other negative indicators such as poor

TABLE 16-2 Hemodynamic Criteria for Initiation of VAD Support

Cardiac index < 2 L/min/m²

Mean arterial pressure < 60 mm Hg

Systolic blood pressure < 90 mm Hg

Pulmonary artery occlusive pressure > 20 mm Hg

Systemic vascular resistance > 2,100 dyne/sec/cm^{-5}

Urine output < 20 mL/hr

Source: Christensen, 2005.

oxygen uptake, exercise intolerance, and persistently elevated levels of brain natriuretic peptide (Christensen, 2000). Brain natriuretic peptide is discussed in more detail in Chapter 15.

The timing of the insertion of a VAD must not be underestimated as a factor for success. Avoiding irreversible end-organ damage is the ultimate goal. Patient outcomes have been studied by classifying patients who underwent mechanical support with a VAD as a bridge to transplant into elective, urgent, and emergent categories. Outcomes were better in the elective group than in the other two groups (Miller, 2003). This finding implies that early VAD implantation improves patient survival.

To be considered for implantation of a VAD, the patient must meet specific criteria regarding blood flow, blood pressure, and general health. Poor candidates for a VAD include those with irreversible renal failure, severe disease of the vascular system of the brain, metastatic cancer, severe liver disease, clotting disorders, severe lung disease, infections that do not respond to antibiotics, or extreme youth or age (Health A to Z, 2005). Contraindications for VAD placement include recent major cerebrovascular accident, sepsis, irreversible multiple organ dysfunction syndrome, medical noncompliance, life-limiting comorbidities, and contraindications to cardiac transplantation (in the bridge-to-transplant group only) (Thoratec Corporation, 2003).

Choosing a Device

Device selection is based on the needs of the patient (Cianci et al., 2003). The choice of device is generally made by the cardiac surgeon and depends on the following factors:

- Size of the patient (BSA < 1.5 m² is typically contraindicated for intracorporeal devices)
- Previous abdominal or cardiac surgery (adhesions may prohibit successful implant)
- Univentricular or biventricular device (the majority of patients can be supported with an LVAD, a smaller group will do better with BiVAD support, and an even smaller percentage will need isolated RVAD support)
- Patient's medical history and ability to tolerate anticoagulation—many VADs require anticoagulation to decrease the risk of thromboembolism (Christensen, 2005).

Current FDA-Approved Systems

Abiomed BVS 5000

The Abiomed BVS 5000 is an extracorporeal assist device (in which blood circulation occurs outside the body) that is pneumatically driven (by compressed air) and is best used for short-term left, right, or biventricular support (see **Figure 16-4**). In 1992, it became the first heart assist device approved by the FDA

FIGURE 16-4 Abiomed BVS 5000

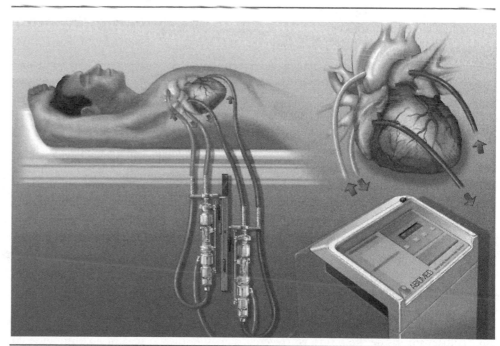

Source: Reprinted with permission from Abiomed Corporation.

for the support of post-cardiotomy failure patients. Since then, the indications for its use have been expanded to include all forms of recoverable heart failure. Patients can be supported for several weeks, but their mobility remains limited to dangling at the bedside or transferring to sitting position (Goldstein & Oz, 2000).

The pump placed at the patient's bedside consists of two chambers. The upper (atrial) chamber is gravity filled; the lower (pumping) chamber is pneumatically driven. The chambers are separated by polyurethane valves to ensure unidirectional flow. The blood pump is attached to the patient's heart with cannulas that exit the skin, allowing blood to flow to and from the pumping chambers. The patient must be anticoagulated while on this device (Christensen, 2005).

The maximum flow of the Abiomed BVS 5000 is 5.5 L/min and stroke volume is 80 mL. The height of the external pump will affect the ability of the atria to fill; the typical height is approximately 25 cm below the patient's atria. Inadequate filling may occur if the pump is placed too high; if the pump position is too low, prolonged filling may occur (Goldstein & Oz, 2000).

Abiomed AB 5000

The Abiomed AB 5000 is a short-term mechanical circulatory support system that can provide left, right, or biventricular support for patients as a bridge to recovery and bridge to transplant. It was developed for patients on the BVS 5000 who need longer support and use the same console and cannula. The AB 5000 allows for longer support time and improved patient mobility. Patients can ambulate inside hospital rooms and within the hospital (Abiomed, 2005).

Thoratec VAD

The Thoratec VAD system is an extracorporeal, pneumatically driven pump with the versatility to support patients of almost any body size. It can be used as an LVAD, RVAD, or BiVAD. It was first used in 1982 for post-cardiotomy failure and in 1984 as a bridge to cardiac transplantation. Currently, the Thoratec VAD is the only FDA-approved VAD for use as both a bridge to cardiac transplantation and a bridge to cardiac recovery (Goldstein & Oz, 2000).

The Thoratec VAD system includes a blood pump, inflow and outflow cannulas, and a pneumatic driver. It consists of a single blood-pumping sac (Christensen, 2000). Two mechanical valves on the inlet and outlet cannulas allow one-way blood flow through the pump requiring anticoagulation. Blood enters the pump with the assistance of negative pressure (vacuum) from the external console. When the blood pump is full, a fill sensor inside the pump is triggered, signaling the pneumatic console to pump in air and compress the blood from the sac.

The Thoratec VAD can be used in three separate modes: asynchronous (fixed rate), volume according to left ventricular filling volume (automated), and synchronous (timed to the patient's heart rate). The device has a maximum stroke volume of 65 mL and a maximum flow rate of 7 L/min. The volume mode is the recommended operating mode during patient support. The asynchronous mode is typically used to wean patients from the device (Christensen, 2005).

Thoratec Implantable VAD

Thoratec has also developed an implantable version of the Thoratec VAD system called the IVAD. The IVAD uses the same technology and principles of operation as the original Thoratec VAD, which is now called the PVAD. The difference is that the IVAD is made of titanium and can be implanted intracorporeally, having only a small percutaneous tube exiting the skin and connecting to the console.

Although Thoratec IVAD/PVAD patients were able to mobilize freely with these devices, they were limited by being tethered to a large device console. Recently, the Thoratec TLC-II Portable VAD Driver was released, which can be carried or pushed on a mobility cart and allows for significant improvement in patient mobility. The Thoratec TLC-II is FDA approved for discharge to home. As a consequence, Thoratec VAD patients supported either univentricularly or biventricularly can be discharged home to await cardiac transplantation or myocardial recovery (Farrar, Reichenbach, Rossi, & Weidman, 2000).

Thoratec HeartMate Implanted Pneumatic Left Ventricular Assist System (HeartMate IP)

The HeartMate IP is an intracorporeal, pneumatically driven device that is used only as an LVAD. The pump is placed intraabdominally or preperitoneally, depending on the surgeon's preference. It has FDA approval as a bridge to transplant. The blood pump is a titanium cylinder that consists of a blood chamber and air chamber separated by a flexible polyurethane diaphragm, a driveline, and inflow/outflow conduits that contain porcine valves. The HeartMate IP has been shown to have a significant nonthromboembolic event rate. This has been attributed to the unique blood-contacting surface on the titanium shell and textured polyurethane on the diaphragm (Christensen, 2000). Therefore, anticoagulation is not indicated for patients with this device. The blood pump driveline exits the patient's skin through the right lower quadrant, and the drive console shuffles air to and from the pump to move the internal diaphragm. With a stroke volume of 83 mL and a maximum pumping rate of 140 beats/min, the IP LVAD can provide flow rates of up to 12 L/min (Texas Heart Institute, 2005). The HeartMate IP is implanted in the left upper quadrant of the abdomen (Health-cares.net, 2005). An implanted Thoratec HeartMate XVE is illustrated in **Figure 16-5**.

Thoratec HeartMate XVE Left Ventricular Assist Device

This intracorporeal, electrically driven pump can be used only as an LVAD. It is the only FDA-approved device as both a bridge to transplant and destination therapy. It can be placed in the intra-abdominal or pre-peritoneal position. The HeartMate XVE has an electric motor, which is housed within the blood pump and creates the pumping action of the diaphragm. The blood pump has a stroke volume of 83 mL/beats up to 120 beats/min with a maximal blood flow rate of 10 L/min. The percutaneous tube exits the skin through the right upper quadrant.

The System Controller is a microprocessor that initiates motor function and monitors and reports system function and malfunction. It allows the pump to operate in two modes: Fixed Rate Mode or Auto Rate Mode.

World Heart Corporation's Novacor Left Ventricular Assist System

The Novacor LVAD is an intracorporeal, electrically driven pump indicated as a bridge to transplant. The blood pump is made of a fiberglass reinforced shell with two chambers (pre-chamber and pumping chamber) separated by a pusher plate. The pusher plate moves to the right and left, causing the pump to fill and empty (World Heart Corporation, 2005). The

FIGURE 16-5 Thoratec HeartMate XVE

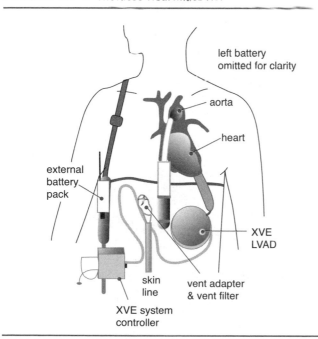

Source: Reprinted with permission from Thoratec Corporation.

pump's driveline exits the skin and is attached to an electrical controller; it can be powered through AC connection or battery powered for untethered mode. The controller regulates the pumping action of the LVAD and monitors system function. To decrease the risk of thromboembolism, patients on Novacor LVADs usually receive anticoagulants.

Future Device Therapy

Thoratec HeartMate II Left Ventricular Assist System (LVAS)

Thoratec's HeartMate II is a rotary blood pump designed to address the need for smaller, long-lasting devices for patients requiring long-term, permanent cardiac support. This LVAS consists of a high-speed axial flow rotary pump; axial flow devices have no pulsatile action from the device itself. The HeartMate II is significantly smaller than current FDA-approved devices, so it may be suitable for a wider range of patients, including both adults and children. The pump speed can provide blood flow of up to 10 L/min.

Abiomed's AbioCor Replacement Heart

This fully implantable device does not assist the native heart, but rather replaces it (see **Figure 16-6**). The AbioCor System includes two blood-pumping sacs that fill and empty alternately, supplying the pulsatile flow to the aorta and pulmonary artery. Separating the two sacs is an artificial septum that contains a hydraulic pump, which shuffles fluid back and forth, thereby moving the septum from the left to right side. This allows the blood to eject from the blood sacs to the other side. The AbioCor can provide a cardiac output of 4 to 8 L/min. This device also has a unique wireless power transfer system, allowing an external battery to be worn on the patient's waist. The battery connects to an external coil placed on the chest. Another coil is implanted inside the chest and receives the current. Therefore, no wires puncture the skin, which decreases the risk of infection (Holmes, 2003).

Potential Postoperative Concerns

Insertion of a VAD is associated with some serious complications: bleeding, development of blood clots, partial paralysis of the diaphragm, respiratory failure, renal failure, failure of the device, damage to the coronary blood vessels, stroke, and infection. Occasionally, with an LVAD, the RV begins to need assistance. If VADs are inserted in both ventricles, the heart may become so dependent on the support that they cannot be removed (FDA, 2005; Health A to Z, 2005).

- Hypovolemia (low circulating volume) can cause the pump to have inadequate preload and thus low VAD

FIGURE 16-6 The AbioCor System

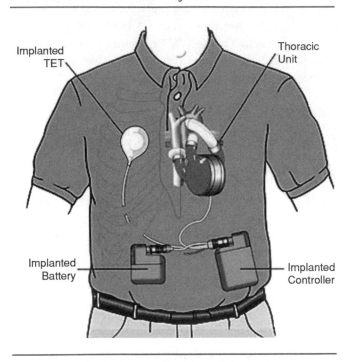

Source: Reprinted with permission from Abiomed Corporation.

flow. Fluid resuscitation is required to ensure optimal preload for VAD pumps (Central Venous Pressure [CVP] = 15–20 is usually optimal for both RVADs and LVADs), and intravenous vasoconstrictors will assist in maintaining adequate venous return.

- Bleeding is a common problem due to anticoagulation therapy and liver congestion. Bleeding occurs in as many as 30% to 50% of patients (Health A to Z, 2005). Coagulopathies may be corrected with appropriate blood products. The patient may have to return to the OR for operative-site bleeding. For bridge-to-transplant patients, leukocyte-reduced blood products (white blood cells removed) should be utilized to minimize antigen exposure.
- Tamponade is evidenced by poor VAD filling, low VAD output, and increased filling pressures. Urgent transport to the OR while the patient is supported with fluid resuscitation and inotropic therapy may be required.
- Arrhythmia treatment should be the same as for any other patient, utilizing cardioversion and antiarrhythmic agents. Although some arrhythmias may not cause immediate hemodynamic compromise, they may compromise VAD filling, reduce flow, and increase the risk of clot formation.

- Right heart failure is a common occurrence after LVAD implantation secondary to RV dysfunction and increased pulmonary vascular resistance. Treatment includes inotropic therapy, nitric oxide (pulmonary vasodilator), or insertion of an RVAD.
- Infection is a common complication that has been identified as a major cause of death in all device patients. Over the last several years, several basic principles have been shown to reduce the incidence of infection and should be strictly adhered to. See **Table 16-3** for infection control guidelines.

CARE OF THE PATIENT WITH A VAD

Pre-implantation

Evaluation of the patient prior to implantation includes careful assessment of comorbidities and risk factors. It will include lab data (e.g., coagulation factors, renal and liver function tests), evaluation of RV failure, hemodynamic status, pulmonary function, and renal function.

Nutrition has recently been identified as one of the most important factors in overall outcomes for these patients. A full screening for malnutrition includes serum albumin and pre-albumin. Malnutrition seen in severe heart failure (cardiac cachexia) predisposes the individual to skeletal muscle atrophy and impaired wound healing with increased risk for infection. Nutritional support should be initiated immediately in at-risk patients and continued into the postoperative phase until the patient has adequate caloric intake.

TABLE 16-3 General Infection Control Guidelines

- Dressings over driveline exit sites must be kept clean and dry at all times.
- Sterile dressing to driveline exit site must be changed at least daily using strict aseptic technique. *Note:* Dressings should be changed more frequently when increased drainage is observed.
- Immobilize driveline or exit cannulas with abdominal binders continuously. This prevents trauma to the exit site and helps to develop tissue ingrowth around the driveline, which promotes formation of a skin barrier. Trauma to exit sites significantly increases the risk of infection.
- Remove monitoring lines as soon as possible to decrease the risk of infection.
- Notify the physician of a temperature change (< 36°C [96.9°F] or > 38.5°C [101.4°F]) or other signs and symptoms of driveline infection (redness, increase in drainage, foul odor, or skin separation from driveline).
- Ensure adequate nutrition (maintain albumin > 2.5). This is essential for the healing process to occur.

Psychiatric/Neurocognitive Evaluation

Key factors in the assessment of substance abuse include alcohol, tobacco, and nonprescription drugs. The assessment of a patient's medical compliance with medications and appointments is also essential. Evaluation of an available support network is equally as important in patients undergoing VAD therapy as it is in patients who are being considered for cardiac transplantation. A caregiver who is committed to the patient and will provide adequate emotional support is necessary for successful VAD implant candidates.

Education

The patient and family must be educated by the cardiologist, implant surgeon, and VAD coordinator prior to the implant procedure on the risks and benefits of the assist device. These risks include postoperative bleeding, thromboembolism, infection, and renal failure. Optimally, the patient and family should view videos, see the actual device, and meet a patient who has undergone a VAD implant. Fears related to the loss of independence, financial stressors, change in body image, and loss of control need to be addressed prior to the implant. The VAD coordinator takes an active role in supporting the patient and family with education to ensure that they make an informed decision.

Post-implantation

Hemodynamic parameters and lab values must be monitored closely. Extubation and removal of vascular access lines should be performed as early as possible. Weaning of inotropic support should be done with caution, paying careful attention to VAD flow rates. Some LVAD patients may require long-term inotropic support.

The physical assessment of patients with assist devices should cover the elements listed in **Table 16-4**.

Extracorporeal pumps (e.g., Abiomed BVS 5000 and Thoratec VAD system) must be assessed at regular intervals to ensure that the pumps are filling and emptying completely. Blood pumps are assessed by determining that the sac found within the blood pump completely inflates and deflates with blood. It is also important to examine the blood sacs with a flashlight to confirm complete emptying of the blood sacs and to establish that there are no clots.

Intracorporeal pumps (e.g., the HeartMate XVE, Thoratec IVAD, and Novacor) require less bedside assessment of function and have alarms that alert the nurse to system malfunction. Nurses must be trained on pump operation, device alarms, and responding to emergencies.

Rehabilitation of the VAD patient begins the day of implantation. Because early ambulation may decrease hospital length of stay and decrease morbidity and mortality, physical and occupational therapists are essential members of the VAD team, providing fitness and self-care activities.

For patients with devices approved for discharge to home, teaching is initiated prior to implantation. This ensures safe home discharge for these patients. **Table 16-5** lists topics that should be included in discharge teaching.

Prior to discharge, patients and their caregivers must be able to demonstrate their ability to carry out the procedures without hesitation. Escorted and unescorted visits away from the hospital are incorporated to help patients and caregivers increase confidence and proficiency in device management (Hipkin et al., 2004).

Conclusion

Table 16-6 compares the various VADs. Newer generations of VADs are smaller and mechanically more basic. Many of these devices are totally implantable. Destination therapy is a reality and becoming more common. VADs are becoming accepted as valid alternatives to living with end stage heart failure. In the future, they may be utilized as replacements for the heart to alleviate the supply/demand imbalance for donor organs (Hunt, 2005).

TABLE 16-4 VAD Physical Assessment

- Pump function
- Vital signs
- Pump rate, stroke volume, mode of operation (fixed or auto)
- Mental status, level of consciousness
- Driveline exit site appearance
- Proper connection of driveline to pump controller

TABLE 16-5 Discharge Teaching

The discharge process includes education of local physicians and nurses, emergency responders, and emergency department staff. Their training includes device operation, emergency management protocols, and contact numbers for the VAD team.
- Device operation and management
- Daily maintenance
- Alarm recognition
- Troubleshooting strategies
- Emergency procedures
- Changing batteries

TABLE 16-6 Comparison of Ventricular Assist Devices

Device	FDA Approval	Length of Support	Type of Support	Anticoagulation	Discharge to Home
Abiomed BVS 5000	Yes	Weeks (up to 90 days)	LVAD, RVAD, BiVAD	Yes	No
Abiomed AB 5000	Yes	Months	LVAD, RVAD, BiVAD	Yes	No
Thoratec VAD	Yes	Long term (500 days)	LVAD, RVAD, BiVAD	Yes	Yes; on TLC II driver
Thoratec HeartMate XVE	Yes	Long term (years)	LVAD	No	Yes
Novacor	Yes	Long term (years)	LVAD	Yes	Yes
Thoratec HeartMate II	No, currently in clinical trials	Long term (years)	LVAD	Yes	Yes
Abiocor	No, currently in clinical trials	Long term	Total heart replacement	No	Yes

Note: LVAD = left ventricular device, RVAD = right ventricular assist device, BiVAD = biventricular assist device

IMPLANTABLE HEMODYNAMIC MONITORING SYSTEMS

As care becomes more sophisticated for managing individuals with heart failure, practitioners need current information regarding the pressures of the heart for optimally managing therapy. Recently, technological advances have provided an implantable device for this purpose produced by Medtronic, Inc. This device, which is known as the Chronicle,™ is similar to a conventional pacemaker. It is implanted in a pectoral pocket on the upper left side of the chest under local anesthesia. A right ventricular lead is placed to facilitate the collection of data. A program is used to retrieve the data, or a telephone-size device in the home can be utilized to transmit data to a central computer through the Internet. These data are the same as those provided by a pulmonary artery catheter. Each patient carries a small device called an external pressure reference to utilize when calibrating the Chronicle to the changes of barometric pressures.

Potential complications during the insertion of this device include dysrhythmias, thrombosis, tamponade, hematoma, lead fracture, pneumothorax, and infection. Once the patient is recovered and returned to the intensive care unit (ICU), the nurse should do gentle, passive range-of-motion exercises to prevent a frozen shoulder while being careful not to displace the lead. The head of the bed should be elevated 30 degrees to minimize swelling. Patients will complain of soreness and eventually pain on movement when the anesthesia dissipates. A major limitation of this device is that the battery is good for only three years. Many heart failure patients can live many years with close monitoring and management. Future models could potentially have a longer life expectancy. Data suggest that this device can reduce hospitalizations by enabling therapy to be customized based on the data the Chronicle yields (Wadas, 2005).

PACEMAKERS

In 2003, more than 197,000 pacemakers were implanted in patients in the United States (Gregoratos, 2005). Pacemakers deliver electrical current to the heart to stimulate depolarization. These devices may be permanent or temporary, depending on the clinical situation. Permanent pacemakers are used when the heart's own pacemaker cells can no longer function properly. Temporary pacing is indicated when the clinical situation may be reversible. For example, patients with electrolyte imbalances, in the acute phase of Lyme disease, following drug overdose, or postanesthesia hypothermia may require only temporary pacing (Gregoratos). **Box 16-1** lists possible indications for cardiac pacing.

Temporary Pacemakers

Temporary pacemakers may be transthoracic, transvenous, or epicardial. The type of pacemaker gives a clue as to where and how it is placed.

Transthoracic (or Transcutaneous) Temporary Pacemakers

Transthoracic pacemakers are used externally. They generate electrical stimuli that pace the heart through external elec-

Box 16-1
Possible Indications for Cardiac Pacing

- Symptomatic bradydysrhythmias
- Symptomatic tachycardias (e.g., supraventricular tachycardia, atrial flutter, atrial fibrillation)
- Chronic heart failure
- Second degree heart block, type II
- Second-degree heart block, type I (occasionally)
- Third-degree (Complete) heart block
- Asystole (if early onset)
- Sick sinus syndrome
- Sinus arrest
- Bundle branch block (right, left, left anterior hemiblock, left posterior hemiblock)
- Prophylactically during surgery in patients with a history of acute coronary syndrome or cardiac dysrhythmias

Sources: Gregoratos et al., 2002; Overbay & Criddle, 2004; Rajappan & Fox, 2003.

trodes that adhere to the chest wall. Correct placement of the pads is essential. The packaging of the pads usually contains a diagram meant to facilitate correct positioning. The anterior (front) pad is placed just to the left of the sternum. The posterior (back) pad is placed on the patient's back to the left of the spine. This placement is often referred to as a "heart sandwich" in the clinical setting. The electrodes must adhere firmly

to the skin. Shaving or otherwise removing chest hair may be required on males. Breasts may need to be lifted to help ensure firm placement of the pads on the chest.

Once the pads are attached to the chest, they are attached to an instrument cable and the cable is attached to the pacing machine. It is essential to ascertain that all connections are secure.

Once connected, the pacing rate is set. The usual rate is 60 beats per minute, but this is determined based on the patient's baseline heart rate and a rate that is needed to maintain adequate cardiac output. Next, the milliamps (mA) or output is set. This represents how much electricity will be delivered through the pads to the heart to stimulate depolarization. Setting the output starts at 0 mA and slowly titrates it upward until capture is obtained. Capture is both an electrical and a mechanical event; it is the ability of the electrical impulse to initiate a cardiac response. Capture is detected on the ECG and is manifested by a pacemaker spike followed by a P wave (if an atrial pacing wire is in place), QRS complex (if the ventricle is being paced), or both a P wave and QRS complex (if a dual-chamber pacemaker is in place) (Overbay & Criddle, 2004).

You have achieved 100% capture when an appropriate cardiac response follows each pacemaker spike. **Figure 16-7** shows 100% capture of a ventricular pacer, and **Figure 16-8** shows 100% capture of a dual pacer.

Transthoracic pacing is a potential source of great discomfort for the patient. The critical care nurse should ensure the patient is receiving adequate analgesia and sedation when this treatment modality is in use. Nursing care of patients with transthoracic pacemakers also entails assessment to evaluate pulses, mental status, heart rhythm, pacemaker activity, percentage of time the pacemaker is in use (versus the patient's inherent heart rhythm), and hemodynamic response (Overbay & Criddle, 2004).

FIGURE 16-7 100% Capture of a Ventricular Pacer

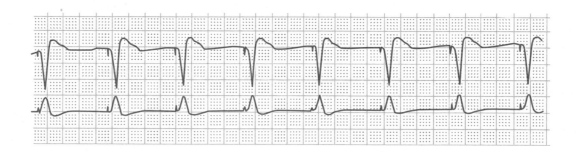

FIGURE 16-8 100% Capture of Dual Chamber Pacemaker

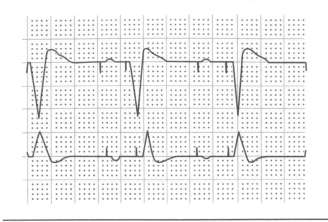

Transvenous Temporary Pacemakers

A transvenous pacemaker includes a wire whose tip delivers an electrical impulse to the endocardium in the right atrium or RV. This wire is connected to a battery-powered pulse generator (Bacoka, 2001). It is usually threaded through a central venous catheter introducer in the subclavian or jugular vein.

There are several components of transvenous pacing. Three types of pulse generators are used: single-chamber atrial pacers, single-chamber ventricular pacers, and dual-chamber pacers [formerly known as atrioventricular (AV) sequential pacemakers], which pace both the atrium and the ventricle (Overbay & Criddle, 2004). Single-chamber atrial pacers can be used in patients to enhance heart rate if the cardiac conduction system is still intact. Ventricular pacers are designed for patients with normal contractility that requires an increase in heart rate. Dual-chamber pacemakers are used to obtain optimal cardiac output (Overbay & Criddle).

When transvenous pacemaker wires are in place, they remain in direct contact with the endocardium. There are two types of pacemaker wires—unipolar and bipolar. With a unipolar wire, only the negative electrode is in direct contact with the heart. With a bipolar wire, both negative and positive electrodes lie within the heart (Overbay & Criddle, 2004).

The ICU nurse will assist the physician with insertion of a transvenous pacemaker. In this procedure, the patient is connected to a 12-lead ECG monitor. The distal pin of the pacemaker wire is connected to the V1 lead with an alligator clamp. The physician then inserts the pacemaker wire into the desired heart chamber, usually the RV. When the pacemaker is in place, the pacing generator is connected to pacing wires. The proximal and distal electrodes are connected at the positive (+) and negative (−) areas, respectively, on the pulse generator.

As with transthoracic pacemakers, the rate is set to maintain adequate cardiac output. In patients who have experienced cardiac arrest, the initial rate may be set for 80 beats/min. For patients requiring overdrive pacing to slow a rapid heart rate, pacing rates are initially set slightly higher than the patient's rapid rate and gradually titrated down to break the rapid rhythm (Overbay & Criddle, 2004).

The mA is set to obtain 100% capture (Overbay & Criddle, 2004). The amount of output (mA) needed to reach this state will be significantly less for a transvenous wire than for a transthoracic pacemaker, and may be as low as 1.5 to 3 mA (as compared with 40 to over 100 mA for the transthoracic pacemaker). The output level may require modification because an endothelial sheath forms around the tips of the electrodes. As a failsafe measure intended to prevent loss of capture, the output is set 1.5 to 3 times higher than is initially required for capture (Overbay & Criddle).

Possible complications of transvenous pacemaker insertion include pneumothorax, local trauma to the insertion site, failure to obtain central access, myocardial perforation, cardiac perforation, cardiac tamponade, and dysrhythmias. The most feared complication when the catheter is actually in place is infection (Overbay & Criddle, 2004; Rajappan & Fox, 2003).

Nursing care of patients with a temporary invasive pacemaker requires monitoring cardiac and hemodynamic status, providing site care, monitoring for correct functioning of the pacemaker, determining the percentage of time the patient is using the pacemaker (e.g., by counting the number of times the pacemaker fires in one minute), and observing for changes that would necessitate modifications in pacemaker settings. Common causes of pacemaker malfunctions include battery failure, displacement of the pacer catheters, new drugs, electrolyte imbalances, loose connections, or electromagnetic interference.

Two problems are commonly associated with pacemakers—failure to capture (**Figure 16-9**) and failure to sense (**Figure 16-10**). When failure to capture occurs, there is a pacemaker spike but no subsequent depolarization of the ventricle (no wide QRS immediately following the pacemaker spike). The main cause of failure to capture is inadequate mA. It may also be related to a low battery or a lead problem such as loss of contact with the heart chamber, a break, or displacement. Failure to capture may also be caused by conditions such as hyperkalemia, ischemia, or medications [e.g., amiodarone (Cordarone®)] (Roppolo, Keelen, & Simonson, 2006). When this situation occurs, the patient is assessed and then connections and settings are checked to detect disconnections, broken wires, or other mechanical issues. If the patient is hemodynamically unstable as a result of the loss of capture, the mA is increased until capture is restored. Positioning the patient on the left side may also

FIGURE 16-9 Failure to Capture

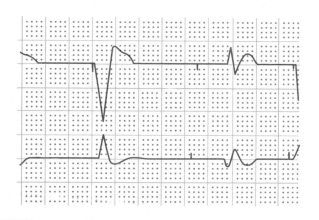

promote capture if it improves contact between the electrode and myocardial tissue (Overbay & Criddle, 2004). Symptomatic patients may exhibit any number of cardiac symptoms, including bradycardia, tachycardia, heart blocks, diaphoresis, dyspnea, weakness, dizziness, fainting, chest heaviness or pain, edema, and even cardiac arrest (Yeo & Berg, 2004).

When failure to sense occurs, it means that the pacemaker did not sense that the patient's inherent rhythm kicked in, so it generated a pacer spike. This condition will be manifested as a pacemaker spike within the patient's inherent rhythm. A ventricular capture following the pacer spike may or may not occur. Depending on where the pacemaker fires, a lethal arrhythmia (e.g., ventricular fibrillation) may arise. Failure to sense can occur when the sensitivity setting is too low (Roppolo et al., 2006). Sensitivity is the ability of the pulse generator to detect and recognize impulses that the patient's myocardial tissue is generating on its own. The sensitivity setting is measured in millivolts (mV) and is initially set at about 2 to 5 mV. Failure to sense can also be caused by displacement of the electrode. When this situation occurs, the patient may be repositioned on the left side in an effort to improve contact between the electrode and the myocardium. If this does not remedy the problem, the sensitivity needs to be increased by decreasing the mV; the generator will then detect beats that occur at lower levels. Conversely, if the pacemaker is detecting beats that are not actually occurring (inappropriate sensing), the sensitivity threshold must be increased to block out artifact. This increase is accomplished by increasing the mV (Overbay & Criddle, 2004).

Another potential problem is pacemaker failure. This problem may arise due to a malfunction or disruption of mechanical components, poor myocardial function from electrolyte disturbances, myocardial scarring, or any factors that affect electrical impulse conduction or cardiac contractility (Overbay & Criddle, 2004).

Epicardial Pacing

The third method of temporary invasive pacing involves directly stimulating the epicardium. This type of pacing is initiated after cardiac surgery. Postoperatively, electrodes are lightly sutured to the epicardium before the thorax is closed. These pacing wires are pulled through the skin and secured to the external chest wall, where they remain ready for attachment to a temporary pacing generator as needed. A patient may have a single set or double set of electrodes, but each set of electrodes includes two wires that protrude from an incision in the chest wall. When dual-wire sets are used, one pair paces the ventricles and the other pair is attached to the atrium. In each pair of wires, one lead is positive and the other (typically the shorter of the two wires) is negative; however, practice varies among institutions. Ventricular pacing wires exit through the left side of the sternum; atrial pairs are placed on the right side (Bethea et al., 2005). Having identifying labels on the wires is helpful. If no labels are present, ascertaining which wire is which (and marking the wires accordingly) can save precious time later if an emergency situation arises.

Epicardial wires usually remain under a dressing for the first 48 hours following cardiac surgery. Once the dressings are removed, care of the site should be performed daily. The site is cleaned with saline and assessed for redness or drainage. The wires must be taped securely to the skin to prevent their accidental removal (Overbay & Criddle, 2004).

Capture and sensitivity threshold testing should be performed every 12 to 24 hours to help prevent failure to capture and to promote optimal pacemaker function. The atrium and the ventricle are tested separately. Threshold testing should

FIGURE 16-10 Failure to Sense

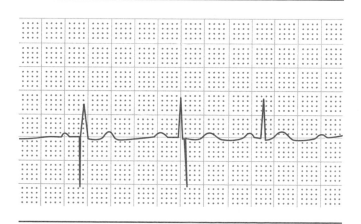

not be performed on patients who require use of the pacemaker more than 90% of the time (Overbay & Criddle, 2004). As with transvenous pacemakers, epicardial wires may develop an endothelial sheath around their tips, so that more mA may be required for capture and fewer millivolts to sense (Overbay & Criddle).

Permanent Pacemakers

Permanent pacemakers are placed either transvenously or epicardially (the former type is more common). They are implanted under the skin on the chest wall and may be seen in different places on the trunk. In the early 1970s, pacemakers were larger and easily palpated. Current models may be as small as a half-dollar and difficult to feel. Before a decision is made to insert a permanent pacemaker, it should be determined that the underlying condition cannot be reversed.

Permanent pacemakers may stimulate the atrium, ventricle, or both chambers of the heart. Programming information can be found on the cards that patients carry with them. In 1974, a nomenclature code was developed to help understand how pacemakers function (see **Table 16-7**). This code has since been replaced by a more advanced one. The most common method of programming is that specified by the North American Society of Pacing and Electrophysiology (NASPE), now better known as the NASPE/BPEG Generic Pacemaker Code.

The pacemaker will be adjusted to the patient's particular needs in terms of rate (maximum and minimum), mode (demand or asynchronous), electrical output sense-pace indicator, and AV interval (see **Box 16-2**).

Biventricular Pacemakers

A biventricular pacemaker is used in remedying symptoms associated with chronic heart failure. This device is employed in addition to pharmaceutical treatments that the patient may already be utilizing and is usually not activated until later in the illness. The purpose of biventricular pacing is to help the heart beat in synchrony once again. Two pacemaker wires are inserted into the heart: one in the RV and the other located via the tortuous coronary sinus to the posterior ventricular wall.

TABLE 16-7 (a) ICHD Pacemaker Codes

Chamber Paced	Chamber Sensed	Response
V: Ventricle	V: Ventricle	I: Inhibited
A: Atrium	A: Atrium	T: Triggered
D: Dual (both A and V)	D: Dual (both A and V)	D: Dual (both I and T)
0: None	0: None	0: None

Source: Pacemaker Study Group, 1974.

(b) The Revised Five-Position ICHD Code

Position	I	II	III	IV	V
Category	Chamber(s) paced	Chamber(s) sensed	Mode of response(s)	Programmable functions	Special antitachyarrhythmia functions
Letters used	V: Ventricle A: Atrium D: Double*	V: Ventricle A: Atrium D: Double* 0: None	T: Triggered I: Inhibited D: Double* 0: None R: Reverse	P: Programmable M: Multiprogrammable C: Communicating 0: None	B: Bursts N: Normal rate S: Scanning E: External
Manufacturer's designation only	S: Single chamber	S: Single chamber	Comma optional here	Comma optional here	Comma optional here

*Double = inhibited and triggered.
Source: Pacemaker Study Group, 1983.

Box 16-2
Permanent Pacemaker Settings and Terminology

Rate: The number of impulses needed to stimulate the heart to beat effectively, to prevent symptom occurrence, and to maintain cardiac output.

Mode (demand or asynchronous): Tells the pacemaker when to pace the heart and is based on the patient's current heart rate and rhythm. A demand pacemaker works when the heart rate falls below or exceeds a certain rate; this is the usual mode that is utilized in most pacemakers. Some individuals' devices may be programmed to work in asynchronous mode, which means that the device paces at the same rate regardless of what the rate or rhythm is.

Output: The amount of energy required to engage depolarization; it is measured in milliamps. The farther away that the electrical energy is from the heart muscle, the more energy it takes to make the pacemaker work.

Sensitivity: The ability of the pacemaker to sense when a heartbeat should be initiated. This value is measured in millivolts.

AV indicator: Seen only with dual-chamber pacemakers. It measures the stimulation distance between the atrium and the ventricle.

Inhibited: A pacemaker stimulus is not fired if the pacemaker senses an intrinsic beat from the patient.

Triggered: A pacing stimulus is activated in response to sensed intrinsic activity or a lack of an inherent response. (For example, ventricular pacing can be triggered in response to a paced P wave. In this case, the P wave stimulates a ventricular response. Atrial pacing can also be triggered by lack of an inherent P wave.)

Source: Jacobson & Gerity, 2005.

The benefits of this type of pacing are that the patient will obtain greater comfort, be at decreased risk for dysrhythmias, and have a heart that pumps more effectively (Lane, Mayet, & Peters, 2003).

IMPLANTABLE CARDIOVERTER-DEFIBRILLATORS

In 2003, more than 64,000 ICDs were implanted in patients in the United States (Gregoratos, 2005). **Box 16-3** lists indications for ICD insertion. These devices are used in patients with recurrent, sustained ventricular tachycardia or fibrillation (American Heart Association, 2006). The ICD leads are placed inside the heart or on the heart surface to help resynchronize the heart rhythm through the delivery of electrical shocks. When the leads detect ventricular tachycardia or ventricular fibrillation, the ICD provides a shock to the heart to restore normal cardiac rhythm (American Heart Association). The amount of voltage that is supplied is determined by the severity and type of patient's cardiac condition. Low voltage may be used in patients who have atrial fibrillation, whereas higher voltages may be used in patients who have a history of ventricular fibrillation. As with pacemakers, each individual receives a card with the voltage information on it along with the manufacturer, model number of the device, and heart rate at which the shocks occur. Two benefits of having an ICD are that it reduces the chance of sudden cardiac death, resulting in decreased mortality, and that it decreases the usage of antiarrhythmic medications in some patients (Gollob & Seger, 2001).

The leads of newer ICD models sense the cardiac rhythm and sometimes pace the heart, as needed. These devices can

Box 16-3
ICD Indications

- History of sudden cardiac arrest
- History of sustained ventricular fibrillation or ventricular tachycardia from structural heart disease or, in those patients who don't have heart disease, failure to respond to other treatments
- History of symptomatic ventricular fibrillation or ventricular tachycardia during a cardiac study
- Myocardial infarction with poor ejection fractions ($\leq 30\%$) one month after the event and three months after coronary artery bypass graft

Source: Gregoratos et al., 2002.

overdrive-pace a rapid rhythm or provide backup pacing, as described earlier in this chapter for slow cardiac rhythms (American Heart Association, 2006).

Two of the major causes of improper shocks from an ICD are lead fractures and loose connections to the device (Gollob & Seger, 2001). If repeated shocks occur due to malfunctioning, placement of a magnet over the ICD will disrupt the device. That is, holding the magnet over the generator for 20 to 30 seconds will disrupt the ICD (Stone & McPherson, 2004).

In addition, data suggest that patients with implantable cardio defibrillators may have a poor quality of life due to anxiety and depression. This is related to discharges of the device (Thomas et al., 2006).

The ICU nurse should teach patients to watch for signs and symptoms of infection after new pacemaker or ICD implantation, including redness, tenderness, swelling and/or warmth (on the ipsilateral side of leads), drainage from the suture line, or fever. Patients should also be taught to carry ICD and pacemaker identification cards at all times, to obtain a MedicAlert® bracelet or necklace, and to avoid electromagnetic interference, which can cause malfunctioning of the device (see **Box 16-4**). It is also recommended that if patients have questions about equipment or appliances, they should check with the manufacturer prior to operation or contact the American Heart Association (Yeo & Berg, 2004). With the

widespread use of personal digital assistant (PDA) devices, some questions have arisen about whether they can affect ICDs and pacemakers. Tri, Trusty, and Hayes (2004) conducted a test on ICDs in conjunction with PDAs and found no electromagnetic interference.

The ICU nurse must provide information to patients who have newly implanted ICDs or pacemakers about checking the device's functioning, battery life, initial follow-up with the physician, and driving (automobile) concerns. The latter is primarily a concern with patients with ICDs. Patients with noncommercial driver's licenses can resume driving in six months. The longer restrictions are associated with those patients who had an ICD implanted for symptomatic tachyarrhythmias that could lead to sudden death. The highest risk of possible shock from the ICD is observed in the first month after implantation. Aircraft and commercial drivers should not drive after implantation of an ICD, but may do so after pacemaker implantation (Moss, Daubert, & Zareba, 2002). Gollob and Seger (2001) also recommend that operators of heavy machinery no longer do so after implantation of an ICD.

PATIENT OUTCOMES

Nurses can help ensure attainment of optimal patient outcomes such as those listed in **Box 16-5** through the use of evidence-based interventions.

SUMMARY

Advanced technology has allowed individuals with cardiac problems to live more comfortable lives with the use of VADs, pacemakers, and ICDs. Nurses need to be knowledgeable about the purposes, benefits, and side effects of these devices and provide thorough patient education to ensure optimal patient outcomes.

Box 16-4
Possible Sources of Electromagnetic Interference for ICDs and Pacemakers

- Large stereo speakers
- Chain saws
- Car engines
- Arc welding
- Security antitheft gates (e.g., in airports, banks, or stores)
- Digital cell phones
- Magnetic resonance imaging
- Radiation treatments
- Transcutaneous electrical nerve stimulation
- Short-wave or microwave electrocautery

Source: Yeo & Berg, 2004.

Box 16-5
Optimal Patient Outcomes

- Uses effective coping strategies
- Knowledge of post care
- Vital signs in expected range
- Demonstration of positive self-regard
- Performance of self-care tasks
- Adjustment to changes in health status

CASE STUDY

A 33-year-old male with a two-year history of heart failure secondary to idiopathic cardiomyopathy is in the process of an out-patient heart transplant evaluation. He presents for a routine follow-up appointment. A 20-pound weight gain over four weeks was noted. The patient reports sleeping in the recliner for the last two nights secondary to paroxysmal nocturnal dyspnea (patient awakens gasping and must sit or stand to get his breath). The patient's mother also reports his poor appetite, nausea, and abdominal fullness. The patient denies missing any medications. He has been following a strict low-sodium diet at home.

Vital signs: HR 132, BP 86/68, RR 24, weight 110 kg, SpO$_2$ 90% on room air

General: Dyspneic with conversation

HEENT: Unremarkable

Lungs: Clear to auscultation (*Note:* This is not an unusual sign in patients with chronic heart failure.)

CV: Prominent S$_3$ gallop, visual jugular venous distention, 2+ pitting edema to knees bilaterally

Abdomen: Large, soft, tender to palpation in the right upper quadrant; hypoactive bowel sounds; positive for ascites

Neuro, psych: Patient is anxious and fidgety

Home medication list:

- Furosemide (Lasix®) 120 mg twice daily
- Potassium chloride (K-lor®) 40 mEq twice daily
- Lanoxin (Digoxin®) 0.125 mg daily
- Carvedilol (Coreg®) 12.5 mg twice daily
- Ramipril (Altace®) 5 mg daily
- Spironolactone (Aldactone®) 25 mg daily

Diagnostic tests:

- Echocardiogram: LV severely dilated and depressed systolic function with ejection fraction estimated at 10%; RV chamber is enlarged and hypokinetic
- ECG: Sinus tachycardia
- Labs: Sodium 130 mEq/L, potassium 3.7 mEq/L, BUN 32 mg/dL, creatinine 1.2 mg/dL, calcium 9.2 mEq/dL, chloride 105 mEq/L, glucose 85 mg/dL, BNP 1680 pg/mL

Impression/Plan

This patient has NYHA class IV heart failure and should be placed on the maximal oral medication regimen. The patient was admitted to the ICU for worsening congestive heart failure. Intravenous milrinone (Primacor®) was started at 0.375 mcg/kg/minute. The furosemide dose was changed to 160 mg IV twice daily.

Two days later on hospital rounds, the patient was noted to be increasingly short of breath at rest and anxious. His weight was stable but not down despite the increased dose of intravenous diuretics. His poor appetite persisted. The physical exam was unchanged from pre-admission, except the patient's lungs now had basilar crackles. His cardiac transplant evaluation was completed, and he was listed for cardiac transplant as status IB.

Inpatient Procedures Performed

A pulmonary artery catheter was inserted. Initial hemodynamic parameters were as follows (refer to Chapter 11 for more information on each of these parameters and normal values): Cardiac Output 3.8 L/min; Cardiac Index 1.6 L/min/m^2; CVP 15 mm Hg; Pulmonary Artery Pressures (PAP) 45/30 mm Hg; Mean PAP 35 mm Hg; Pulmonary Artery Occlusive Pressure 30 mm Hg; BP 82/58; Mean Arterial Pressure 66 mm Hg; Systemic Vascular Resistance 1120 dynes/sec/cm^{-5}; RVSWI 6.5 g/m^2/beat.

After conferencing, the medical team decided an LVAD should be placed as a bridge to cardiac transplantation. The patient and family were educated on the pros and cons of device therapy. They were given a booklet explaining the function of the device and a video of the implant and discharge process.

A VAD was implanted the next day. The patient experienced a moderate degree of right heart failure postoperatively, which was managed with a combination of intravenous milrinone, dobutamine (Dobutrex®), and nitric oxide. The patient was weaned from these medications over the next three days. Nutritional support was initiated immediately postoperatively, and physical therapy was consulted on postoperative day 1.

After a four-day ICU stay, the patient was transferred to the VAD unit where discharge teaching was initiated. He was first hesitant about discharging to home with the LVAD to wait for transplant; by day 10, however, he and his family became more enthusiastic. Prior to discharge, his energy level was back to normal. With the guidance of physical therapy, the patient was walking almost one mile daily. His appetite improved and, although he did have some complaints of fullness after eating large meals, his nutritional status returned to normal.

After completing a long list of competencies and several short excursions out of the hospital, the patient was discharged to home with his VAD. After 63 days of support, the patient received a successful heart transplant.

CRITICAL THINKING QUESTIONS

1. What is the benefit of an LVAD in this patient?
2. What were the indicators for device therapy in this case study?
3. List key elements to be included in the nursing assessment of LVAD patients.
4. List four common psychosocial concerns of the potential VAD patient.
5. Name common postoperative complications following VAD implantation and the nursing interventions utilized to decrease them.
6. Which disciplines should be consulted to work with this client?
7. What types of issues may require you to act as an advocate or moral agent for this patient?
8. How will you implement your role as a facilitator of learning for this patient?

Using the Synergy Model to Develop a Plan of Care

	Patient Characteristics	Level 1, 3, or 5	Subjective and Objective Data	Evidence-based Interventions	Outcomes
SYNERGY MODEL	Resiliency				
	Vulnerability				
	Stability				
	Complexity				
	Resource availability				
	Participation in care				
	Participation in decision making				
	Predictability				

CRITICAL THINKING QUESTIONS

1. Utilize the form to write up a plan of care for one client with a ventricular assist device, implantable cardioverter-defibrillator, or pacemaker in the clinical setting. Rate the patient as a level 1, 3, or 5 on each characteristic. Identify the level of nurse characteristics needed in the care of this patient.

2. Take one patient outcome for a patient with a VAD, implantable cardioverter-defibrillator, or pacemaker and list evidence-based interventions for this patient.

Online Resources

Expert Panel Review of the NHLBI Total Artificial Heart Program, The National Heart, Lung, and Blood Institute, Willman VL. June 1998–November 1999: www.nhlbi.nih.gov/resources/docs/tah-rpt.htm

FDA Approves Heart Assist Pump for Permanent Use, Press release # P02-48, U.S. Food and Drug Administration, November 6, 2002: www.fda.gov/bbs/topics/NEWS/2002/NEW00851.html

National Institutes of Health: www.nhlbi.nih.gov/meetings/workshops/nextgen-vads.htm

Up to Date: http://patients.uptodate.com/topic.asp?file=chd/28782

REFERENCES

Abiomed. (2005). Retrieved October 26, 2005, from www.abiomed.com

American Heart Association. (2005). Retrieved October 25, 2005, from www.americanheart.org/presenter.jhtml?identifier=4599

American Heart Association. (2006). Implantable cardioverter defibrillator. Retrieved February 24, 2006, from www.americanheart.org/presenter.jhtml?identifier=11227

Bacoka, J. (2001). Emergency transvenous pacemaker insertion. Nursing, 31(9), 96.

Bethea, B. T., Salazar, J. D., Grega, M. A., Doty, J. R., Fitton, T. P., Alejo, D. E., et al. (2005). Determining the utility of temporary pacing wires after coronary artery bypass surgery. Annals of Thoracic Surgery, 79(1), 104–107.

Bond, A. E., Nelson, K., Germany, C. L., & Smart, A. N. (2003). The left ventricular assist device. American Journal of Nursing, 103(1), 32–40.

Bosen, D. M. (2003). New strategies for treating patients with heart failure. Nursing, 33(12), 44–47.

Christensen, D. M. (2000). The ventricular assist device. Nursing Clinics of North America, 35(4), 945–959.

Christensen, D. M. (2005). Ventricular assist devices. Retrieved October 25, 2005, from http://nursing.advanceweb.com

Cianci, P., Lonergan-Thomas, H., Slaughter, M., & Silver, M. (2003). Current and potential applications of left ventricular assist devices. Journal of Cardiovascular Nursing, 18(1), 17–22.

Farrar, D., Reichenbach, S., Rossi, S., & Weidman, J. R. (2000). Development of an intracorporeal Thoratec Ventricular Assist Device for Univentricular or Ventricular Support. American Society for Artificial Organs Journal, 46(3), 351–353.

Goldstein, D. J., & Oz, M. C. (2000). Cardiac assist devices. Armonk, NY: Futura Publishing.

Gollob, M. H., & Seger, J. J. (2001). Current status of the implantable cardioverter-defibrillator. Chest, 119(4), 1210–1221.

Gregoratos, G. (2005). Indications and recommendations for pacemaker therapy. American Family Physician, 71(8), 1563–1570.

Gregoratos, G., Abrams, J., Epstein, A. E., Freedman, R. A., Hayes, D. L., Hlatky, M. A., et al. (2002). ACC/AHA/NASPE 2002 guideline update for implantation of cardiac pacemakers and antiarrhythmia devices: Summary article. Circulation, 106, 2145–2161.

Health A to Z. (2005). Retrieved October 25, 2005, from www.healthatoz.com

Health-cares.net. (2005). Retrieved October 25, 2005, from www.healthcares.net

Hipkin, M., Rogers, P., & Jones, I. (2004). Care of patients with heart failure and the use of ventricular assist devices. Professional Nurse, 19(12), 34–36.

Holmes, E. C. (2003). The AbioCor totally implantable replacement heart. Journal of Cardiovascular Nursing, 18(1), 23–29.

Hunt, S. A. (2005). Cardiac transplantation and prolonged assisted circulation. In D. Kasper, E. Braunwald, A. Fauci, S. Hauser, D. Longo, & J. Jameson (Eds.), Harrison's principles of internal medicine (16th ed., pp. 1378–1380). New York: McGraw-Hill.

Jacobson, C., & Gerity, D. (2005). Pacemakers and implantable defibrillators. In S. L. Woods, E. S. Sivarajan Froelicher, S. U. Motzer, & E. J. Bridges (Eds.), Cardiac nursing (5th ed., pp. 709–755). Philadelphia: Lippincott Williams & Wilkins.

Lane, R. E., Mayet, J., & Peters, N. S. (2003). Biventricular pacing for heart failure. British Medical Journal, 326, 944–945.

Mason, V. F., & Konicki, A. J. (2003). Left ventricular assist devices as destination therapy. AACN Clinical Issues, 14(4), 488–497.

Miller, L. W. (2003). Patient selection for the use of ventricular assist devices as a bridge to transplantation. Annals of Thoracic Surgery, 75, S66–S71.

Moss, A. J., Daubert, J., & Zareba, W. (2002). MADIT-II: Clinical implications. Cardiac Electrophysiology Review, 6(4), 463–465.

Ochiai, Y., McCarthy, P. M., Smedira, N. G., Banbury, M. K., Navia, J. L., Feng, J., et al. (2002). Predictors of severe right ventricular failure after implantable left ventricular assist device insertion: Analysis of 245 patients. *Circulation, 106*(12 Suppl. 1), I-198–202.

Overbay, D., & Criddle, L. (2004). Mastering temporary invasive cardiac pacing. *Critical Care Nurse, 24*(3), 25–32.

Pacemaker Study Group, Inter-Society Commission for Heart Disease Resources (ICHD). (1983). Optimal resources for implantable cardiac pacemakers. *Circulation, 68,* 226A–244A.

Pacemaker Study Group, Inter-Society Commission for Heart Disease Resources (ICHD). (1974). Implantable cardiac pacemakers: Status report and resource guidelines. *Circulation, 50,* A21–A35.

Rajappan, K., & Fox, K. F. (2003). Temporary cardiac pacing in district general hospitals—sustainable resource or training liability? *Quality Journal of Medicine, 96*(11), 783–785.

Roppolo, L. P., Keelen, G., & Simonson, R. B. (2006). Emergency pacing. *Emergency Medicine Reports.* Retrieved February 24, 2006, from www.emronline.com/emrarchives.html

Stone, K. R., & McPherson, C. A. (2004). Assessment and management of patients with pacemakers and implantable cardioverter defibrillators. *Critical Care Medicine, 32*(4 Suppl.), S155–S165.

Texas Heart Institute. (2005). Thoratec HeartMate II LVAS. Retrieved October 26, 2005, from www.texasheartinstitute.org

Thomas, S. A., Friedmann, E., Kao, C. W., Inguito, P., Metcalf, M., Kelley, F. J., et al. (2006). Quality of life and psychological status of patients with implantable cardio-defibrillators. *American Journal of Critical Care, 15*(4), 389–398.

Thoratec Corporation. (2003). *Patient and Device Selection Criteria Unique to the Thoratec VAD System and HeartMate LVAS* [brochure]. Pleasanton, CA: Author.

Tri, J. L., Trusty, J. M., & Hayes, D. L. (2004). Potential for personal digital assistant interference with implantable cardiac devices. *Mayo Clinic Proceedings, 79*(12), 1527–1530.

U.S. Food and Drug Administration. (2005). Retrieved October 26, 2005, from www.fda.gov/hearthealth/treatments/medicaldevices/vad.htm

Wadas, T. (2005). The implantable hemodynamic monitoring system. *Critical Care Nurse, 25*(5), 14–24.

World Heart Corporation. (2005). Retrieved October 26, 2005, from www.worldheart.com

Yeo, T. P., & Berg, N. C. (2004). Counseling patients with implanted cardiac devices. *Nurse Practitioner, 29*(12), 58, 61–65.

CHAPTER 17

Cardiac Surgery and Heart Transplant

Mary Zellinger

LEARNING OBJECTIVES

Upon completion of this chapter, the reader will be able to:

1. Discuss the various types of cardiac surgery: conventional bypass, beating heart cardiac surgery, and minimally invasive cardiac surgery.

2. Describe the preoperative teaching for the cardiac surgery patient.

3. Relate the nursing care for postoperative cardiac surgery patients to the Synergy Model.

4. Discuss the complications of post–cardiac surgery and evidence-based interventions.

5. Explain the criteria utilized for identifying candidates for heart transplantation.

6. Discuss the nursing assessment and interventions for the postoperative transplant patient.

7. List optimal outcomes that may be achieved through evidence-based management of the patient undergoing cardiac surgery or heart transplant.

Cardiovascular disease remains a leading cause of death in the United States. Despite significant advances in preventive measures and early medical intervention, the extent of disease often requires invasive procedures such as angioplasty, stenting, and cardiac surgery. The field of cardiac surgery has undergone dramatic changes since its inception in the 1950s and will likely continue to evolve to offer patients the best options for many types of cardiac dysfunction in the future.

The interest in surgically addressing cardiac dysfunction dates back to the late 1800s, when surgeons attempted to repair traumatic cardiac damage. Other attempts—with varied degrees of success—continued throughout World War II (Stephenson, 2003). The challenge of performing this procedure on a beating heart proved too great, and attempts were generally abandoned until the introduction of the cardiopulmonary bypass machine in the 1950s. This system enabled cardiac surgeons to divert blood flow away from the heart so that its motion could be suspended, thus offering the opportunity to operate on a motionless organ while ensuring adequate protection to other organs and tissues.

Cardiac surgery off pump, although attempted by Vineberg in 1951 with questionable results, gained renewed interest in the early 1990s as surgeons searched for ways to avoid the complications of cardiopulmonary bypass, and technologic advances made it possible. More recently, minimally invasive cardiac surgery has been performed on patients with specific types of lesions, such as in the left anterior descending artery, which can be exposed and bypassed with a left internal mammary artery via a left thoracotomy without the support of bypass and without a sternotomy (opening the chest wall). As advances continue to be made using this technique, outpatient cardiac surgery comes closer to a reality.

PREOPERATIVE WORKUP

Once the decision for cardiac surgery has been made, the patient is referred to a cardiac surgeon for evaluation and scheduling. If possible, lab specimens are obtained in an outpatient area prior to the hospital admission date. A chest radiograph and electrocardiogram (ECG) are also performed if these have not been obtained within the previous 30 days. Preoperatively, the patient will meet with an anesthesiologist so that personal data can be obtained, especially information about the patient's medical history, medications, and allergies that may affect the operative process.

PREOPERATIVE EDUCATION

Information about how to prepare for the procedure itself and education about the immediate postoperative recovery period is provided during the preoperative consult. The day prior to surgery, the patient will shower twice with a special antimicrobial soap, and once again the morning of surgery. The shower incorporates a 10-minute "scrub" with the soap brush in the area between neck and groin or neck and knees, depending on which type of surgery is planned. Proper use of the incentive spirometer is reviewed, because this will help maintain adequate respiratory function in the postoperative period. The patient will not be permitted anything by mouth (NPO) starting at midnight the night before surgery, except for small sips of water with medications, as directed by the physician. Certain types of medications, such as anticoagulants, must be held for five to seven days prior to surgery, unless specifically ordered by the physician, to prevent excess bleeding in the perioperative period. The patient should be as well rested as possible in the days before surgery.

The patient will be given a book or video to review that contains information about what to expect in the immediate postoperative period, during the entire hospitalization, and during the post-hospital discharge recovery period. Knowing what to expect—for instance, in the intensive care unit (ICU) regarding monitors and tubes and activity progression—helps both the patient and family prepare. Finally, anticipating that the recovery process may entail emotional ups and downs will enable the patient to cope with these fluctuations more easily as they occur. If assistance is anticipated for recovery, the nurse will contact the social worker to meet with the patient and family to begin planning (see **Box 17-1**).

Many times, patients will remain in the hospital after the cardiac event that requires intervention. If a patient has certain coronary blockages (e.g., significant left main coronary occlusion) or requires heparin, nitroglycerin, or other supportive medications, then continuous monitoring is needed until the procedure can be performed.

THE DAY OF SURGERY

On the morning of surgery, the patient will take one additional shower with the antimicrobial soap. Clipping of hair from body surfaces will reduce the potential for nosocomial infection and is done either before the patient leaves for the preoperative holding area (POHA) or once in the operating room (OR). The chest is clipped from nipple to nipple and neck to

---

Box 17-1

Reasons for Social Service Consult

The patient:
- Has financial issues
- Needs equipment at home
- Needs labs drawn at home
- Needs IV antibiotics at home
- Lives out of state
- Lives alone
- Has home care needs
- Requests assessment of discharge needs
- Needs assessment of financial issues related to home care
- Has significant other as a dependent

---

umbilicus. Both sides of the groin should be clipped unless a dressing is in place. If the patient is to have bypass grafts, both legs from ankles to groin and from midline on top of the leg to midline underneath the leg will be clipped.

The patient may receive a sedative before arriving in the POHA. Once in the POHA, various intravenous (IV) lines and catheters are inserted as specified by the anesthesiologist. An arterial line will be inserted so that the blood pressure can be continuously monitored as intraoperative and postoperative fluctuations due to autonomic nervous system stimulation, volume changes, and cardiac manipulation may occur. A large-bore IV line is used so that fluid may be delivered rapidly if necessary. Either a central line or a pulmonary artery catheter will be placed so that cardiac filling pressures can be followed and treatment adjusted accordingly.

OPERATING ROOM

After the patient is moved to the OR, the anesthesiologist will sedate and intubate the patient. Once the patient is intubated and fully anesthetized, an antibacterial agent is again used and applied from midline to midline and neck to knees. After sterile drapes are applied, the surgical procedure is initiated.

On-Pump Coronary Artery Bypass Graft

Because most cardiac surgical procedures are performed via a mediasternotomy incision, a special saw is used to cut the sternal bone, chest retractors are inserted, and the chest is opened. Once the chest and pericardium are opened, the two cardiopulmonary bypass (CPB) cannulae are inserted into the heart. One cannula is passed into the right atrium to divert blood returning there to the pump; the second is placed in the aorta for blood return from the pump. The membrane oxygenator in the pump removes carbon dioxide, the heat exchanger controls blood temperature, and the blood is oxygenated prior to return to the aorta. Catheters are also inserted into the coronary arteries to deliver cardioplegic solution to the myocardium. The cardioplegic solution contains electrolytes and blood in a hypothermic environment; as this solution circulates throughout the heart, it will stop, or arrest, the heart. The solution is injected frequently throughout the procedure to maintain this arrested state so that the surgeon can work on a nonmoving organ. An icy slush is continuously applied to the heart to keep it cold and decrease myocardial oxygen demand throughout the procedure. Cardiac surgery performed via CPB has proven to be safe and effective. By arresting the heart, the surgeon has the benefit of working on a nonmoving organ, and adequate cerebral perfusion is maintained. The cardiac arrest also allows for optimal visualization of the target site for a precise anastomosis.

Although still the gold standard for cardiac surgery, on-pump cardiac surgery is associated with many complications. Because the blood flows along bypass tubing (an artificial environment), a diffuse inflammatory process may be initiated that may cause multiple problems postoperatively. Adverse neurologic events with a 3% to 4% rate of stroke and permanent pulmonary dysfunction are a few of the other complications that may result (Cleveland, Shroyer, Chen, Peterson, & Grover, 2001). Because of these potential problems, off-pump cardiac surgery has attracted renewed interest and has been performed by many surgeons since the 1990s.

Off-Pump Cardiac Surgery

"Beating heart" or off-pump coronary artery bypass (OPCAB) graft surgery has gained popularity in the last several years due to advances made in technology and mechanical stabilization systems. These stabilization devices allow an immobilized target site for the performance of the vascular anastomosis. Potentially, OPCAB surgery can be done on lesions in any coronary artery. Although it is estimated that 80% of all coronary artery bypass grafts (CABGs) in the United States can be done off-pump safely and effectively, most patients referred for OPCAB are either young and healthy, or older and sicker patients who would not tolerate CPB (Lorenz & Coyte, 2002). Early graft patency equivalent to that in on-pump cases has been demonstrated in early clinical outcomes and follow-up catheterization. Additionally, data show a decreased need for blood transfusions postoperatively, decreased length of stay, and decreased costs associated with OPCAB (Lorenz & Coyte).

Once the pericardium is opened, stabilization devices are applied to the heart so that the area with the lesion can be kept as still as possible. Because the heart continues beating, blood flow to the other organs and tissues is maintained. However, occurrence of anginal pain within one year of surgery has been documented, perhaps because of the different degrees of revascularization (Moshkovitz, Lusky, & Mohr, 1995).

Minimally invasive direct coronary artery bypass (MIDCAB) surgery via a small left anterior thoracotomy without CPB was popularized in 1995. Since then, this procedure has been performed in many centers worldwide. Mid-term results of studies indicate excellent patency rates of the left internal mammary artery (LIMA) to the left anterior descending artery (Finkelmeier, 2000). The procedure has been modified since 1995 to make it less invasive by using two or three 5-mm incisions to harvest the LIMA via standard thoracscopic techniques (hand-held), with a voice-activated robotic camera system (AESOP), or using full robotic technology (Zeus or DaVinci) (Finkelmeier).

The endoscopic atraumatic CABG procedure is a modification of the MIDCAB that avoids rib spreading, instead using a smaller intercostal muscle incision to perform the LIMA to the left anterior descending (LAD) anastomosis on the beating heart. The widespread acceptance of these procedures has been limited by the relatively small number of patients with single-vessel coronary artery disease limited to the left anterior descending artery.

Choices for Conduits

Multiple choices are available as conduits for bypass grafting. The greater saphenous vein graft is commonly used. One benefit of using this vein is that its removal from the leg does not compromise circulation to the leg; the lesser saphenous vein and tributaries will assume the venous drainage from the leg. The vein can be removed from the leg in two ways. In the first technique, the surgeon makes an incision over the course of the vein, harvesting it from ankle to thigh. The saphenous grafts are attached to the aorta and coronary arteries in a reverse fashion so that blood from the aorta to the coronary arteries flows with the venous valves, not against them (Finkelmeier, 2000).

A newer approach is to remove the vein endoscopically. In this technique, two small incisions are made in the leg and a tunnel is created inside the leg down the length of the saphenous vein. Carbon dioxide gas is used to inflate the tunnel as the branches leading to the vein are sealed off. The vessel is then divided at two ends and removed through the small incision (Finkelmeier, 2000). These small incisions are less painful for the patient during the postoperative period.

Because venous valves may interfere with adequate blood flow, using arteries is the preferred option for grafts when possible. The internal mammary artery remains an optimal graft. The LIMA comes off the left subclavian and can be left attached here, decreasing the need for multiple anastomoses. Used in this manner, it is called a pedicle graft. The distal end of the artery is dissected away from the thoracic wall and attached distal to the occlusion of the targeted coronary artery. Another option is to remove the LIMA from the subclavian and use it as a free graft if additional length is needed. The right internal mammary artery can also be used, although it is employed less frequently and is most often used as a free graft (Finkelmeier, 2000).

The radial artery is another vessel that may be used as a conduit. Because there is collateral blood flow to the hand via the ulnar artery, the radial artery can be removed without fear of compromising blood flow to the hand. Benefits of the radial graft are the availability and visibility of the artery. The gastroepiploic and inferior epigastric artery may also be used, but these arteries are used much less frequently because of the risk of contamination during harvesting. Under extreme conditions, a fetal umbilical artery may be used (Finkelmeier, 2000). Finally, the search continues for an artificial conduit that will have the same vasoresponsive properties as autologous grafts.

Valve Surgery

Surgery to address valve disease—particularly that involving the mitral valve—has evolved from absolute replacement to attempted repair as often as possible. No prosthetic valve is as good as the native valve, so all attempts are made to repair the valve instead of replacing it.

Repair techniques can be performed on stenotic or incompetent valves. An annuloplasty is a procedure performed on the valve annulus, the ring of tissue that supports the valve leaflets. A valvuloplasty refers to the reconstruction of one or more components of the valve—namely, the leaflets, annulus, chordae tendineae, and/or papillary muscles that anchor the leaflets to the heart wall. Stenotic valves may require cutting or separating the valve leaflets to increase the valve orifice. Incompetent valves, causing regurgitation, may be repaired by shortening the supporting structures to allow the valve to close tightly, or by inserting one of a variety of prosthetic rings to reshape a deformed valve. Balloon valvuloplasty is a procedure done in the cardiac catheterization lab that involves threading a balloon-tipped catheter through a large artery into the narrowed valve opening. The balloon is inflated, thereby enlarging the valve opening (Finkelmeier, 2000). Less invasive techniques to repair the cardiac valves continue to be investigated.

Minimally Invasive Cardiac Surgery

Minimally invasive cardiac operations are now performed for a number of procedures, which traditionally required an 11- to 12-inch sternotomy. Oftentimes, the operation can be done through 8- to 10-centimeter mini-thoracotomy incisions. The main benefit is cosmetic; however, some evidence suggests that postoperative recovery is quicker with the minimally invasive procedures, primarily because there is less surgical trauma with a smaller incision. This type of approach is being used for a number of procedures, including aortic valve replacement, mitral valve repair or replacement, tricuspid valve procedures, repair of atrial septal defects, and surgical ablation of atrial fibrillation (Finkelmeier, 2000).

Mitral valve repair techniques are also being addressed in the catheterization lab. The EVEREST clinical trial (Endovascular Valve Edge-to-Edge REpair STudy) is investigating the safety and efficacy of the Evalve devices in treating patients diagnosed with moderate to severe mitral regurgitation (MR), as compared to surgical repair of MR. A tiny clip, delivered by a catheter and deployed in the heart to repair a malfunctioning and leaking mitral valve, is designed to secure the valve's leaflets near the center of the valve so that blood leakage is minimized and the heart pumps more efficiently (Finkelmeier, 2000). This procedure may decrease complications, decrease length of stay in the hospital, and significantly reduce healthcare costs.

When necessary, valve replacement can be done with any one of a variety of prostheses, each of which has its own advantages and disadvantages. Mechanical valves are extremely durable, lasting a patient's lifetime, and are constructed from materials such as Dacron, titanium, and pyrolytic carbon. The disadvantage to using a mechanical valve is the long-term need for anticoagulation to prevent formation of blood clots on the prosthesis. Biological valves do not require lifelong anticoagulation, but their durability is not as great as that of mechanical valves. Bioprosthetic valves are made of tissue taken from pigs, cows, or human donors. Allografts, which are taken from human cadavers, have excellent hemodynamics. These valves are procured, treated with antibiotic solution, and frozen until needed for surgery, at which time they are thawed and implanted. Finally autografts, which consist of tissue from the patient's own body, can be used, as in the Ross procedure. During this surgical procedure, the patient's pulmonary valve is removed and used to replace the aortic valve, and then an allograft is used to replace the pulmonic valve. The pulmonary autograft in the aortic position is superior to bioprostheses, which tend to degenerate after only a few years in patients younger than age 35, because of the autograft's greater longevity (Finkelmeier, 2000).

IMMEDIATE POSTOPERATIVE ASSESSMENT

Upon completion of the cardiac surgery, chest tubes are placed into the pleural and/or mediastinal spaces to collect pooled blood. The patient is then transported to a postanesthesia care unit or ICU that specializes in recovery of cardiac surgery patients. Staff caring for the patient are educated and competent in stabilizing, weaning, extubating, and progressing the patient along the path toward recovery, while monitoring the patient closely for any potential complications.

Prior to leaving the OR, the anesthesiologist may call to give a brief report to the nurse who will be caring for the patient. This report includes information about the procedure itself, any complications encountered, medications received, most recent lab values, medical history, allergies, and specific orders. Upon arrival to the unit, the patient is connected to the ventilator via an endotracheal tube by the respiratory therapist, who then checks for bilateral breath sounds. The nurse attaches the patient to the cardiac monitor and obtains initial vital signs: heart rate, blood pressure, temperature, SpO_2, $ETCO_2$, and central venous pressure (CVP). If the patient has a pulmonary artery catheter, the pulmonary artery systolic, diastolic, mean, and occlusive or wedge pressures, as well as the cardiac output/index, are obtained. The nurse verifies which fluids and vasoactive medications are being delivered, checking for dosage, rate, and accurate delivery. Any required adjustments based on vital signs will be made. A quick head-to-toe assessment is performed, including sedation level and neurologic status, breath sounds, heart sounds, and adequacy of pulses. Vital signs are obtained on a frequent basis for the first several hours, as the hemodynamic status changes and requires fluid and medication titration. The head of bed should be elevated due to the potential for aspiration (Grap et al., 2005). A warm blanket is placed over the patient if the temperature is low to enhance the warming process.

Labs obtained in the immediate postoperative period include electrolytes, arterial blood gas, complete blood count, coagulation profile, and bleeding times. A chest radiograph is performed to verify endotracheal tube placement and check pulmonary status, and an ECG is obtained to check for ischemia.

IMMEDIATE POSTOPERATIVE MONITORING

In the immediate postoperative period, maintaining hemodynamic stability is the priority. A cardiac index of $2.5-4 L/min/m^2$ will be sustained by normalizing heart rate and stroke volume. Many variables may increase heart rate in the postoperative period. Most often, hypovolemia and pain are issues that need to be assessed. Once hypovolemia is ruled out or resolved, the patient should be closely assessed for the presence of pain. Despite sedation, the nurse may need to use a valid and reliable instrument to assess for pain in cognitively impaired patients. Dysrhythmias that may be seen in the postoperative period include premature ventricular contractions or ventricular tachycardia from electrolyte imbalance, or cardiac irritability from intraoperative manipulation (Finkelmeier, 2000). Ventricular fibrillation, although rare, may also occur and is treated aggressively according to standards developed by the American Heart Association.

Atrial fibrillation is a common occurrence in the postoperative patient. Its etiology may include atrial stretch from volume overload, pericarditis, metabolic/electrolyte disturbances, and surgical manipulation. Early treatment with amiodarone (Cordorone®) or another atrial antiarrhythmic may be helpful. Amiodarone is a Class III antiarrhythmic agent that prolongs the duration of the myocardial cell action potential and refractory period and possesses mild alpha-, beta-, and calcium channel blocking effects. It has been shown to be effective in decreasing the incidence of atrial fibrillation (Stamou et al., 2001).

Bradycardia and heart block may sometimes occur postoperatively. Patients who have had valve surgery are more at risk for this complication due to the manipulation performed around the conduction system during surgery. Medications and hypothermia may also cause some degree of bradycardia postoperatively (Finkelmeier, 2000). If epicardial pacing wires were placed during surgery, they can be connected to an external pacemaker for temporary pacing. A higher heart rate stimulated by a pacemaker will enhance cardiac output when stroke volume is decreased. Epicardial pacing wires can be used to help determine types of dysrhythmias by analyzing the atrial ECG and to treat atrial tachyarrhythmias by rapid atrial pacing. If epicardial wires were not placed, a ventricular pacing wire may be inserted via a specially designed pulmonary artery catheter. Finally, transvenous pacing wires may be inserted or transcutaneous pads may be applied. If possible, atrial pacing is preferred because of the atrial kick, which contributes 25% to 30% of cardiac output (Finkelmeier).

Adequate stroke volume should be ensured. Variables that affect stroke volume—preload, afterload, and contractility—often are affected in the intraoperative and postoperative period. Preload may be altered as the patient undergoes the rewarming process, which may cause vasodilation and a drop in preload. Bleeding from chest tubes or third spacing that results from the inflammatory process may also decrease preload and, therefore, decrease cardiac output. Blood pressure, cardiac filling pressures, urinary output, and signs of dehydration must be evaluated. Adjustments to volume administration are frequently necessary. Volume repletion is accomplished with crystalloids (e.g., lactated Ringer's solution, normal saline), or colloids (e.g., albumin, blood, blood products) as determined by the patient's lab results. If preload is too high, diuretics and vasodilators such as nitroglycerin may be used.

An increased afterload may result from hypovolemia, hypothermia, pain, anxiety, or increased catecholamine stimulation from the surgical procedure. Along with volume repletion and a hyperthermia unit to warm the patient, vasodilators such as nicardipine (Cardene®) that work directly on the arterial system will be beneficial. Pain medication may have some vasodilator effects. A decreased afterload may be the result of significant arterial vasodilation and may be treated with vasoconstrictor agents [e.g., norepinephrine (Levophed®)].

Decreased contractility in the postoperative period may be the result of an increase or a decrease in preload, an increase in afterload, or factors that affect the myocardial contractility directly (e.g., ischemia, right or left ventricular failure, and aneurysms). The ECG must be closely analyzed for any changes. Electrolyte imbalances and tamponade (which will be addressed later) may also affect contractility. Electrolyte disturbances may result from diuresis, preoperative vomiting, acidosis, alkalosis, renal dysfunction, or decreased preoperative oral intake.

Once preload and afterload are adjusted to enhance contractility, other interventions such as electrolyte replacement and treatment of tamponade are completed. If contractility requires augmentation, positive inotropic medications are initiated. Pharmacologic support can be provided by drugs such as epinephrine, dobutamine (Dobutrex®), and milrinone (Primacor®). If additional support is needed, an intra-aortic balloon pump (IABP) is added (Reid & Cottrell, 2005).

The IABP can increase cardiac output by as much as one liter and may be necessary to support the patient through an acute event. The IABP is a catheter that is typically inserted into the femoral artery and advanced into the descending thoracic aorta. The tip of the catheter sits distal to the take-off of the subclavian artery so as not to interfere with cerebral perfusion, and above the renal artery, so as not to interfere with renal perfusion. The catheter is triggered by the patient's ECG to inflate immediately after the closure of the aortic valve and to deflate immediately prior to the opening of the aortic valve. When the catheter balloon (typically 30 or 40 mL) inflates, it displaces the same amount of blood, forcing the blood up to the head, down the coronaries, and distal to other organs and tissues; this principle is known as counterpulsation. The frequency of balloon assistance is set to assist each cardiac cycle or less often (e.g., 1:2, 1:3, 1:4, or 1:8), depending on how much

cardiac support is needed. In many ways, displacing blood has an action similar to that of a vasodilator: It decreases afterload for the left ventricle, making it easier for the heart to pump (Reid & Cottrell, 2005).

Accurate timing of the catheter is imperative. If timed to inflate or deflate incorrectly, the pumping action of the catheter may cause more cardiac dysfunction. If the catheter is inflated too early during ventricular systole, it will produce a significantly higher pressure for the heart to pump against, increasing afterload and myocardial workload. If it inflates too late, the full benefit of the pump will not be obtained. If the catheter is timed to deflate too late, it will still be inflated during the beginning of ventricular systole, again increasing workload to the left ventricle. If the catheter deflates too early, the pressure in the aorta has time to rise back up so that no beneficial effect is obtained. Accurate timing via the arterial waveform is essential and will determine whether the benefit of decreasing afterload and increasing coronary artery perfusion is obtained, which is the purpose of using the IABP (see **Figure 17-1**).

After explaining the purpose of the IABP, the ICU nurse will prepare the patient for IABP insertion. A thorough assessment prior to insertion provides a hemodynamic and physical baseline and documents the need for therapy. The assessment should include skin color, temperature, capillary refill time, quality of pulses in both legs, and baseline sensation and movement. A neurologic check and all hemodynamic variables should also be obtained.

There are several contraindications to IABP use. If the patient has aortic valve insufficiency, blood will be pushed back into the heart when the balloon inflates during diastole, increasing left ventricular workload. A dissecting aortic aneurysm is another contraindication because the catheter may perforate the side of the aorta during its insertion. Relative contraindications include end-stage cardiomyopathy unless the IABP is being used as a bridge to transplant, severe atherosclerosis, end-stage disease, and abdominal aortic aneurysms. If inotropic and counterpulsation therapy are not adequate to maintain cardiac index, a ventricular assist device (VAD) may be used. (VADs are discussed later in this chapter and Chapter 16.)

Following blood glucose levels closely is imperative for many reasons in the postoperative period. Hyperglycemia has been associated with a significantly higher rate of infection and can result in white blood cell function impairment, electrolyte swings, dehydration, and an increased urine output due to hyperosmolar diuresis (Levetan, 2000). An increase in blood glucose may be seen in both diabetic and nondiabetic patients. It results from the release of catecholamines, cortisol, and glucagon during surgery; a de-

FIGURE 17-1 Intra-aortic Balloon Pump. A: Balloon Deflated. B. Balloon Inflated

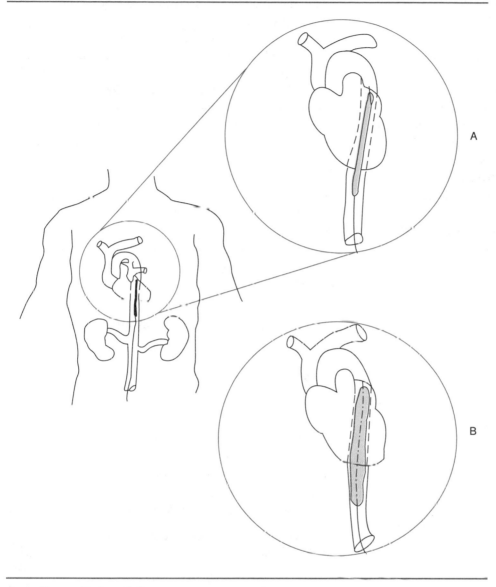

Source: Illustrated by James R. Perron.

carbon dioxide production, increases oxygen consumption by two to five times the resting state, and increases myocardial workload. There are many causes of shivering. Anesthesia may promote heat loss by depressing the regulatory system; drugs may produce vasodilation and suppress neuromuscular activity, thereby antagonizing warming mechanisms. In addition, during surgery, temperature decreases may result from the administration of the cold cardioplegic solution into the aortic root (Seifert, 2002). Early detection of shivering is important to avoid further metabolic cost to the patient. "Shivering checks" should be added to the postoperative assessment, because the muscles that shiver are typically between the neck and knees and may be covered by a blanket. Restoration of heat loss is a priority and can be accomplished with warm blankets, a hyperthermia unit, or warming IV fluids and blood products. Agents such as meperidine (Demerol®) may be administered. It is important to have IV fluids available, because as patients become warm and dilate, these fluids can be infused to maintain preload.

Postoperative bleeding is always a concern for the cardiac surgical patient. The loss of blood decreases oxygen carrying capacity to vital organs and tissues. Decreased volume will decrease preload and, therefore, stroke volume and cardiac output.

The causes of postoperative bleeding are many. The CPB circuit may cause platelet destruction as the blood circulates through it, in addition to decreasing levels of clotting factors. Inadequate hemostasis from incomplete heparin reversal or excessive protamine sulfate administration may be the cause, or a surgical bleed from a suture site may occur (Poston et al., 2005). If chest tube drainage exceeds 100mL/hr for more than 3 hours, 200 mL/hr for 2 hours, or 300 mL during the first hour,

creased utilization of glucose due to hypothermia; and failure of insulin secretion in response to hyperglycemia. The use of exogenous insulin to maintain blood glucose no higher than 110 mg/dL reduces morbidity and mortality among critically ill patients in the ICU (Finney, Zekveld, Elia, & Evans, 2003).

Shivering is another potential problem seen in the postoperative period. Shivering is a normal compensatory response to body cooling, triggered by the return of the central nervous system thermoregulatory function. It is a physiologic hazard because it increases metabolic rate, increases

the physician should be notified. Blood or blood products may be ordered if the hematocrit is low or the coagulation profile is outside the normal range, respectively. If the patient is hypertensive, the blood pressure needs to be decreased to prevent stress on suture sites, which may cause further bleeding, requiring the patient to be surgically reexplored.

Pooling of excess blood not drained from the thoracic cavity, hemorrhage, malposition or occlusion of chest tubes, and collection of blood in the mediastinum may all cause cardiac tamponade. This will result in compression of the heart, limitation of diastolic filling time, and a decrease in cardiac output. Signs and symptoms of which the ICU nurse should be cognizant include a narrowing pulse pressure, unexplained hypotension, muffled heart sounds, distended neck veins, and tachycardia. A dramatic rise in CVP and equalization of the cardiac filling pressures are cardinal signs. Other signs include evidence of decreased perfusion such as cool, clammy skin, restlessness, apprehension, and dyspnea. On a chest radiograph, a widened mediastinum or presence of a "water bottle" heart may be evident (Kaplow, 2005). A more in-depth discussion of cardiac tamponade appears in Chapter 47.

When buildup of blood in the chest occurs rapidly, causing immediate hemodynamic decompensation, the patient should be returned to the OR immediately for reexploration. If the event occurs so quickly that there is no time to move the patient to the OR, the chest will be opened at the bedside to relieve pressure and remove any clots or blood impeding cardiac function.

OPEN CHEST RESUSCITATION

If the patient is bleeding from the chest tubes, volume must be replaced with crystalloids, blood, or colloids. If the blood pressure continues to decline, the patient should be placed in modified Trendelenburg position (flat with foot of bed elevated) to increase venous return. Vasopressors (e.g., norepinephrine) may be needed to maintain blood pressure when filling pressures are adequate (Finkelmeier, 2000).

The necessary equipment for opening the chest should be brought to the bedside. This equipment includes the cardiac resuscitation tray, emergency cart, and defibrillator with internal paddles. The blood bank should be requested to send any available blood for the patient. The chest dressing is removed and the incision covered with antimicrobial wash. The surgeon and assistant, wearing sterile gowns, gloves, and masks, will open the chest wall, cut the sternal wires, insert the chest retractor, and spread the chest sternum. Setup for sterile suction must be readily available so that all excess blood can be removed from the chest for evaluation of the patient's status. If a bleeding site is identified, it will be repaired, and preparation for patient transport to the OR will occur once the hemodynamics

are stabilized. If the patient requires intra-cardiac drug administration or internal defibrillation, these can be done at the bedside (see **Box 17-2**).

Upon transport back to the OR, with the site being covered by sterile drapes during transport, the chest is cleaned out under sterile conditions, the repair reevaluated, and the chest closed. If the chest cannot be closed because of the development of cardiac or pulmonary edema, a rubber sheet, or dam, may be attached to the skin and kept in place for 24 to 48 hours or longer as necessary. The patient is then returned to the cardiac surgical ICU.

A coronary artery graft spasm is another potential, but rare complication. A transient reduction in the lumen diameter may occur to a degree sufficient to produce myocardial ischemia. ST segment elevation, transient atrioventricular (AV) block, hypotension, and intractable ventricular dysrhythmias may all be indications of a spasm (Finkelmeier, 2000). IV nitroglycerin may be helpful. It may be necessary to return the patient to the OR to replace the graft.

WEANING FROM MECHANICAL VENTILATION

Once the patient is warm and stable without significant bleeding in the chest tubes, the weaning process may begin. Sedation is weaned and, once the patient is awake and breathing spontaneously, ventilatory support is gradually decreased, weaning parameters are obtained, and the patient is extubated. Potential benefits of early extubation include reduced risk of pulmonary barotrauma, decreased incidence of ventilator-associated pneumonia, improved ventricular performance and renal function, increased patient comfort, and earlier mobilization. Early extubation also reduces both ICU and hospital length of stay (Reis,

> **Box 17-2**
> # Open Chest Cardiac Resuscitation: Sequence of Events
>
> 1. Antimicrobial wash is poured over chest
> 2. Sutures are cut (knife blade and handle)
> 3. Sternal wires are cut (wire cutters)
> 4. Rib retractors spread the chest wall
> 5. Suction—tonsil suction (on tray) to sterile tubing
> 6. Open massage or internal defibrillation (by physician)
> 7. Intra-cardiac drugs
> 8. Back to OR or close chest

Mota, Ponce, Costa-Pereira, & Guerriero, 2002). Ideally, this process is completed within four hours after arrival to the ICU.

After extubation, the patient must be encouraged to cough and deep breathe on at least an hourly basis to prevent pulmonary complications such as atelectasis and pneumonia. Within one hour post-extubation, the patient can sit on the side of the bed or in a bedside chair. The blood pressure should be checked immediately prior to sitting and then as soon as the patient is in the sitting position to check for orthostasis. Orthostasis is often an indicator of hypovolemia. While the patient is in the dangling position, the patient will support the sternum and cough several times. Also, posterior breath sounds can be auscultated while the patient is in this position.

Pain control is an important component during the weaning, extubation, and post-extubation period. Acute postoperative pain from surgical wounds is primarily inflammatory in nature and is associated with the release of chemical mediators. Inadequate analgesia, an uninhibited stress response, or both can lead to many adverse effects during the postoperative period. Physiological consequences such as autonomic nervous stimulation, the endocrine stress response, and reflex motor activity can lead to pulmonary complications because the discomfort may prevent the patient from coughing, deep breathing, and increasing activity level. Hemodynamic changes such as tachycardia, hypertension, and vasoconstriction may occur, along with an increase in metabolism and platelet activation. Inadequate pain control is associated with increased atelectasis and significantly lowers tissue oxygen levels, which can predispose the patient to infection (Milgrom & Brooks, 2004).

BEYOND THE IMMEDIATE POSTOPERATIVE PERIOD

The patient may be transferred to an intermediate care unit several hours after extubation if he or she no longer requires vasoactive support for hemodynamic stability. Most patients remain in the ICU overnight and transfer out in the morning of the next day. Once on the intermediate care unit, the patient will remain on telemetry for several days due to the potential for dysrhythmias. During the first two days, activity level is gradually increased so patients are out of bed for meals and walking at least four times a day.

Many patients after cardiac surgery experience long-term neurocognitive deficits such as impaired attention, concentration, and memory. Microembolization and hyperthermia are considered to be the primary causes of these effects. Hyperthermia increases metabolism and oxygen consumption, which can potentially increase the degree of tissue injury. Multiple methods are used to reduce microembolization, including use of filtering devices, membrane oxygenators, ultrasound, and transesophageal echocardiography to identify areas of heavy plaque. Practices that avoid hyperthermia during the rewarming phase are also utilized, such as slower rewarming (Finkelmeier, 2000).

Chest tubes remain in place for 24 to 48 hours postoperatively. Pleural effusions and pneumonia may develop because of colonization of the upper respiratory tract in intubated patients, phrenic nerve damage, and excessive crystalloid infusion. Effusions will likely resolve with time; if they persist, thoracentesis or chest tube reinsertion may be required. Lingering effusions not drained may cause lung entrapment (Finkelmeier, 2000).

Postoperative infection can be a devastating complication after cardiac surgery. A postoperative infection may develop from many sources, including sinusitis, catheter-related sepsis, pneumonia, endocarditis/pericarditis, perforated ulcer, bowel infarction from emboli, urosepsis, or a wound infection. In particular, a wound infection may result from intraoperative contamination, hematogenous spread of pathogens, or postoperative wound contamination. Strict wound care protocols should be followed. Sternal dressings should remain on for the first 48 hours. If they are heavily stained with blood, they are to be changed using sterile technique. Antimicrobial wash and sterile water or normal saline (NS) are used to cleanse the area around the incision. After 48 hours, the dressings are removed. If the patient is able to shower after that time, antimicrobial wash and water will be used; if the patient is unable to shower, the incisions are cleaned by following the same procedure.

Prophylactic antibiotics are administered for 24 hours postoperatively, with the initial dose being given in the OR within an hour of the first incision being made. Manifestations of a postoperative infection may include fever, tachycardia, tachypnea, leukocytosis, chest discomfort, and elevated C-reactive protein levels (Cleveland et al., 2001). Operative sites must be evaluated closely for erythema, pain, hardening of the skin, or drainage that is excessive, purulent, or odorous.

The diagnosis of mediastinitis is often challenging, because a general inflammatory reaction to operative trauma can also occur. The mortality rate for sternal wound infections is as high as 30% (Luckraz, Murphy, Bryant, Charman, & Ritchie, 2003). Risks for the development of these infections include redo procedures, closed chest massage, an open chest, prolonged CPB, decreased tissue perfusion, and tracheostomy. Sternal wound infections may require reexploration for debridement and reconstruction with muscle flaps.

Post-pericardiotomy syndrome is a potential complication after cardiac surgery that typically appears in the first one to two weeks postoperatively; it occurs in 18% of patients. An inflammatory process can complicate operations in which the pericardial sac is opened. The clinical presentation is variable, so the diagnosis is based on the following clinical findings: malaise, pericardial friction rub, low-grade fever persisting over several days without evidence of local infection, and chest pain. Treatment may include aspirin, indomethicin (Indocin®), non-steroidal anti-inflammatory drugs (NSAIDs) to resolve symptoms, and antacids for gastric irritation (Finkelmeier, 2000).

Peripheral nerve damage is another possible complaint of patients in the postoperative period. Brachial plexus injury during retraction of the sternum may occur, and is manifested by paresthesia involving the fourth and fifth fingers on the affected side. The numbness may persist for several months but almost always resolves on its own.

Bacterial endocarditis, if it occurs, usually develops in people with underlying cardiac defects who develop bacteremia with organisms that cause endocarditis. Bacteremia may occur spontaneously or complicate a focal infection (e.g., urinary tract infection, pneumonia, cellulitis). Blood-borne bacteremia may lodge on damaged or abnormal heart valves or on endocardium near anatomical defects (Luckraz et al., 2003). As yet, no clinical trials have been conducted in patients with underlying structural heart disease to definitely establish that antibiotic prophylaxis provides protection against development of endocarditis during invasive procedures or that endocarditis is attributable to these procedures.

PREPARATION FOR DISCHARGE

For the stable uncomplicated cardiac surgical case, length of stay will average three to four days. Hospital discharge criteria mandate that the patient be hemodynamically stable, able to provide self-care, and knowledgeable about what that self-care incorporates (see **Box 17-3**). The patient also must be knowledgeable about all prescribed medications, including their purpose, side effects, doses, and scheduling. Mandated shorter hospitalizations have compressed the amount of time available for patient education.

Postoperative issues such as fatigue, inability to focus, depression, discomfort, and narcotic use for pain management can present challenges to effective patient learning. Discharge teaching also includes content on activity progression, lifting restrictions, bathing and incision care, incisional healing sensations, potential loss of appetite, bowel changes, sleep disturbances, diet, smoking cessation, and emotions of the patient and spouse after discharge.

The patient should have a contact number to call if questions or problems arise after discharge. The primary physician or referring cardiologist will be seen within two weeks of discharge so that vital signs can be checked and the incision evaluated. The patient will return to see the cardiac surgeon four to six weeks after discharge; if the healing process has pro-

---

Box 17-3
Discharge Criteria

Vital signs are stable.
Desired discharge outcomes:
- Walks independently or with minimal assistance
- Adequate oral intake
- Pain control with oral medications
- No wound drainage
- Communicates verbally or returns to preoperative status
- Verbalizes knowledge of post-discharge self-care
- Absence of complications

---

gressed normally, the patient will be discharged from the care of the cardiac surgeon at that time. If the patient has a mediastinal incision from opening the sternum and it has healed well, the patient will be given approval to begin driving and lifting objects heavier than 5 to 10 pounds.

A comprehensive cardiac rehabilitation program with both exercise and nonexercise components is recommended to begin at this point. This program will focus on improving functional work capacity, reducing anxiety and depression, increasing a sense of well-being, promoting an understanding of coronary artery disease, and helping the patient return to normal routines. Goals of these programs include physical training and a broad spectrum of education, including cardiac disease risk factor reduction and behavior modification, to enable patients to achieve their optimal level of health and maximize their quality of life (Ivan der Peijl et al., 2004).

Options for patients requiring cardiac surgery are expanding daily, and it is imperative that nurses caring for these patients at the bedside be familiar with all of these options. Knowledge about procedures, potential complications, immediate postoperative care, educational needs, and discharge protocols are essential components for ensuring quality patient care.

CARDIAC TRANSPLANTATION

Cardiac transplantation has improved dramatically since the first procedure was performed in the late 1960s. Transplantation offers patients with no other alternatives an option for survival. Better patient selection, donor management, postoperative care, immunosuppressive agents, and evaluative techniques for infection and rejection have improved long-term outcomes of this procedure. Potential recipients for adult cardiac transplantation include individuals with isolated severe heart disease that is unresponsive to other medical therapies. Most patients have idiopathic or dilated cardiomyopathy, although hypertrophic and restrictive cardiomyopathy are also possible etiologies. Ideal candidates have no other significant medical problems and no social or behavioral problems and would be expected to lead a healthy and productive life post-transplant. Recipient contraindications include advanced age (most often older than 65 years), severe liver or kidney dysfunction, active infection, recent pulmonary infarction, severe pulmonary hypertension, and history of drug or alcohol abuse (Mancini & Gangahar, 2005).

The diagnostic evaluation for cardiac transplantation is performed by a multidisciplinary team including a physician, nurse, social worker, and psychologist and includes a physical and psychosocial evaluation, lab work, pulmonary function tests, and a right heart catheterization. Initiation of preoperative teaching is started so that the patient and significant others are knowledgeable about the process and expectations for care after transplantation.

During the preoperative waiting period, the team focuses on maintaining hemodynamic stability. The patient is placed on a national waiting list based on degree of cardiac dysfunction. Once a cardiac donor has been identified and matched with the recipient, the path to transplantation is begun.

Criteria for cardiac donors remain strict. The donor must have no severe chest trauma, no prolonged cardiac arrest, and no heart disease or infection. There must be ABO blood group compatibility, a sufficient heart size, a negative cytotoxic antibody screen, and a negative lymphocyte cross match (Mancini & Gangahar, 2005). The current shortage of available donors has forced the extension of an acceptable age for donation to approximately 55 years or younger as long as all other criteria are met.

After the donor evaluation process has been completed by the United Network for Organ Sharing (a nonprofit, scientific, and educational organization that administers the United States' only organ procurement and transplantation network), the team from the recipient hospital travels to the hospital where the donor is located to perform the cardiectomy. The donor heart will be physically evaluated, then removed, packed in ice, and transported for the transplant procedure to begin.

Most transplant procedures are orthotopic, meaning that the majority of the recipient's heart is removed and the donor heart is sewn onto the remaining part of the atrium. A heterotopic heart transplant leaves the diseased recipient heart in place to act as an accessory pump. This is rarely done, but may be an option when the recipient is hemodynamically deteriorating and the only available donor heart is smaller or has questionable function. Problems with this method include the risk of systemic emboli from clots in the poorly contracting recipient left ventricle, continuing angina related to recipient ischemic heart muscle, and the risk of infection and thrombus formation (Lenner, Padilla, Teirstein, Gaso, & Schilerog, 2001).

Care of the transplanted patient in the immediate postoperative period is similar to care of other cardiac surgical patients. In addition, assessment for the signs and symptoms of infection and rejection must be ongoing. Early complications for heart transplantation include donor organ dysfunction, acute rejection, renal failure, arrhythmia, bleeding, and infection. Late complications include accelerated coronary atherosclerosis, chronic rejection, hypertension, and malignancy. Medication-related problems are also a possibility.

Rejection is diagnosed by myocardial biopsy. At frequent intervals during the first two years, a tissue sample of myocardium is removed during a right heart catheterization. If rejection is detected, immunosuppressive drug doses are increased for a period of time to combat the rejection.

VENTRICULAR ASSIST DEVICES

A VAD is a mechanical pump that aids the left ventricle, the right ventricle, or both ventricles by providing temporary circulatory support. It decreases the workload of the heart while maintaining adequate flow and blood pressure. In the past, the VAD was most often used for patients awaiting cardiac transplant, to serve as a "bridge to transplant." In some patients with reversible forms of cardiac failure, a VAD can be implanted with the hope that it will support the heart so the heart has time to recover, with the assist device later being removed. More recently, in selected patients who are not good candidates for cardiac transplantation because of other medical complications, VADs have been inserted as permanent devices, known as "destination therapy."

Postoperative care is similar to that of other patients after cardiac surgery, with a few additions. The pump rate, flow, stroke volume, and mode of operation should be monitored. Because these patients are at risk for thromboembolism and therefore are anticoagulated, bleeding in the postoperative period is not uncommon. The pump cannula exit sites require meticulous care with sterile dressing procedures. The ICU nurse must be able to handle emergencies that arise and troubleshoot problems with the pump. Because these patients may remain in the ICU longer than other cardiac surgical cases, it is important for the nursing staff to encourage active family involvement by developing individualized patient schedules with patient input and allowing adequate uninterrupted sleep.

Once the patient is extubated, activity is increased from bedside dangling to standing and walking in the area. As soon as possible, a level of independence in VAD self-care should be obtained. VADs are discussed in more detail in Chapter 16.

PATIENT OUTCOMES

Nurses can help ensure the obtainment of optimal patient outcomes such as those listed in **Box 17-4** through the use of evidence-based interventions for patients undergoing cardiac surgery or cardiac transplantation.

SUMMARY

Caring for the cardiac surgery patient requires the involvement of a multidisciplinary team of professionals. The ideal team will consist of the nursing staff, a cardiovascular clinical nurse specialist, a nurse manager, a nurse clinician, a surgeon, a respiratory therapist, a social worker, home care, utilization management, pastoral care, nutrition, education, cardiac rehabilitation, anesthesia, and a pharmacist. This team ensures an optimal outcome for the patient through the use of critical

---

Box 17-4
Patient Outcomes

- White blood cell count within expected range
- Demonstrates understanding of the disease process
- Absence of signs and symptoms of infection
- Renal function within normal limits
- Absence of bleeding postoperatively
- Modifies lifestyle to reduce risk factors
- Angina not present
- Free of transplant rejection

---

pathways, standing orders, discharge protocols, and team meetings. Ultimately, the nurse at the bedside during the first 24 hours postoperatively requires a high level of vigilance and the ability to foresee potential complications.

CASE STUDY

A 59-year-old female with a history of hypertension, smoking two packs of cigarettes per day, and living alone collapsed in the emergency department (ED) after entering a complaint of chest pain. She was intubated and resuscitated in the ED. Once stabilized, she had a blood pressure of 220/96, obvious JVD, crackles halfway up posteriorly, and audible S_3 on auscultation. Her ECG revealed a bundle branch block and Q waves in leads II, III, and aVF. The patient's heart rate was 58. She was transferred to the ICU for treatment with heparin, nitroglycerin, and mechanical ventilation.

During the night, the patient's heart rate dropped to 40, blood pressure was 88/54, the nitroglycerin was discontinued, and the physician was notified that the patient was in complete heart block. The nurse placed the external (transcutaneous) pacemaker on the patient until the physician arrived and placed a temporary pacer and intra-aortic balloon pump. The patient was stabilized and taken to the catheterization lab for a heart catheterization. Results from the catheterization indicated an occlusion of the right coronary artery of 80% and mild disease of the left coronary artery with an occlusion of 60%. The patient was scheduled for a coronary artery bypass graft the next day.

The patient underwent cardiac surgery and returned to the cardiovascular recovery room on the ventilator, with epicardial wires taped to the chest, a midline incision, a pulmonary artery catheter and arterial catheter in place, and a chest tube to 20 cm H_2O. The patient is hypotensive with norepinephrine (Levophed®) and milrinone (Primacore®) infusions.

CRITICAL THINKING QUESTIONS

1. During the first four hours postoperatively, which complications should the nurse be alert for? What is the best management technique if a complication occurs?
2. Describe the preoperative education that should be given for a cardiac surgery patient.
3. What purpose do epicardial pacing wires serve for the postoperative cardiac surgery patient?
4. Why would you expect the patient to have a chest tube in place?
5. How would you manage pain control in a cardiac surgery patient?

6. How should you address the potential risk for a postoperative infection?

7. Would a consult to the social worker be required for this case and, if so, why?

8. Utilize the form to write a plan of care for a cardiac surgery patient in the clinical setting. Rate the patient as a level 1, 3, or 5 on each characteristic.

9. Take one patient outcome for a patient and list evidence-based interventions found in a literature review for this patient.

Using the Synergy Model to Develop a Plan of Care

	Patient Characteristics	Level 1, 3, or 5	Subjective and Objective Data	Evidence-based Interventions	Outcomes
SYNERGY MODEL	Resiliency				
	Vulnerability				
	Stability				
	Complexity				
	Resource availability				
	Participation in care				
	Participation in decision making				
	Predictability				

10. Develop a problem list of potential postoperative complications that are associated with four of the Synergy Model patient characteristics in the table below.

	Patient Characteristics	Potential Postoperative Complications
SYNERGY MODEL	Vulnerability	
	Resource availability	
	Participation in care	
	Participation in decision making	

11. Identify one nurse characteristic that would be crucial in providing care to the cardiac surgery patient and provide a rationale for choosing that characteristic as it relates to this patient population.

Online Resources

American Heart Association: www.americanheart.org

ACC/AHA Guideline Update on Perioperative Cardiovascular Surgery: www.acc.org/clinical/guidelines/perio/update/pdf/perio_update.pdf

Society of Thoracic Surgeons—Medical Specialty Society, Antibiotic prophylaxis in cardiac surgery, 2005: www.sts.org/sections/aboutthesociety/practiceguidelines/antibioticguideline/

Task force on infective endocarditis of the European Society of Cardiology by the European Society of Cardiology—Medical Specialty Society, Guidelines on prevention, diagnosis and treatment of infective endocarditis, January 2004: www.escardio.org/NR/rdonlyres/64662308-7C90-4C73-A21E

American Heart Association—Professional Association, Practice standards for electrocardiographic monitoring in hospital settings: an American Heart Association scientific statement from the Councils on Cardiovascular Nursing, Clinical Cardiology, and Cardiovascular Disease in the Young, October 26, 2004: http://circ.ahajournals.org/cgi/content/full/110/17/2721

Society of Thoracic Surgeons—Medical Specialty Society, Gender-specific practice guidelines for coronary artery bypass surgery, 2004: www.ctsnet.org/file/GenderGuidelineOct04-EASYPRINT.pdf

REFERENCES

Cleveland, J. C., Shroyer, A. L., Chen, A. Y., Peterson, E., & Grover, F. L. (2001). Off-pump coronary artery bypass grafting decreases risk-adjusted mortality and morbidity. *Annals of Thoracic Surgery, 72*(4), 1282–1288.

Finkelmeier, B. (2000). *Cardiothoracic surgical nursing* (2nd ed.). Philadelphia: Lippincott.

Finney, S. J., Zekveld, C., Elia, A., & Evans, T. W. (2003). Glucose control and mortality in critically ill patients. *Journal of the American Medical Association, 290,* 2041–2047.

Grap, M., Munro, C., Hummel, R. S., Elswick, R. K., McKinney, J. L., & Sessler, C. N. (2005). Effect of backrest elevation on the development of ventilator-associated pneumonia. *American Journal of Critical Care, 14*(4), 325–332.

Ivan der Peijl, I., Vliet Vlieland, T. P., Versteegh, M. I., Lok, J. J., Munneke, M., & Dion, R. A. (2004). Exercise therapy after coronary artery bypass graft surgery: A randomized comparison of a high and low frequency exercise therapy program. *Annals of Thoracic Surgery, 77,* 1535–1541.

Kaplow, R. (2005). Cardiac tamponade. In C. H. Yarbro, M. H. Frogge, & M. Goodman (Eds.), *Cancer nursing: Principles and practice* (6th ed., pp. 873–886). Sudbury, MA: Jones and Bartlett.

Lenner, R., Padilla, M. L., Teirstein, A. S., Gaso, A., & Schilerog, J. (2001). Pulmonary complications in cardiac transplant recipients. *Chest, 120,* 508–513.

Levetan, C. (2000). Controlling hyperglycemia in the hospital: A matter of life and death. *Clinical Diabetes, 18*(1), 17–24. Retrieved February 16, 2006, from http://journal.diabetes.org/clinicaldiabetes/v18n12000/Pg17.htm

Lorenz, B., & Coyte, K. (2002). Coronary artery bypass graft surgery without cardiopulmonary bypass: A review and nursing implications. *Critical Care Nurse, 22*(1), 51–60.

Luckraz, H., Murphy, F., Bryant, S., Charman, S. C., & Ritchie, A. J. (2003). Vacuum-assisted closure as a treatment modality for infections after cardiac surgery. *Journal of Thoracic and Cardiovascular Surgery, 125*(2), 301–305.

Mancini, M. C., & Gangahar, D. M. (2005). Heart transplantation. Retrieved November 13, 2005, from www.emedicine.com/med/topic3187.htm

Milgrom, L., & Brooks, J. (2004). Pain levels experienced with activities after cardiac surgery. *American Journal of Critical Care, 13*(2), 116–125, 183–185.

Moshkovitz, Y., Lusky, A., & Mohr, R. (1995). Coronary artery bypass without cardiopulmonary bypass: An analysis of short term and midterm outcome in 220 patients. *Journal of Thoracic Cardiovascular Surgery, 110,* 979–987.

Poston, R., Gu, J., Manchio, J., Lee, A., Brown, J., Gammie, J., et al. (2005). Platelet function tests predict bleeding and thrombotic events after off-pump coronary bypass grafting. *European Journal of Cardiovascular Surgery, 27*(4), 584–591.

Reid, M. B., & Cottrell, D. (2005). Nursing care of patients receiving intra aortic balloon counterpulsation. *Critical Care Nurse, 25*(5), 40–49.

Reis, J., Mota, J. C., Ponce, P., Costa-Pereira, A., & Guerriero, M. (2002). Early extubation does not increase complication rates after coronary artery bypass graft surgery with cardiopulmonary bypass. *European Journal of Cardiothoracic Surgery, 21*(6), 1026–1030.

Seifert, P. (2002). *Cardiac surgery: Preoperative patient care.* St. Louis, MO: Mosby.

Stamou, S. C., Hill, P. C., Sample, G. A., Snider, E., Pfister, A. J., Lowery, R. C., et al. (2001). Prevention of atrial fibrillation after cardiac surgery: The significance of postoperative oral amiodarone. *Chest, 120,* 1936–1941.

Stephenson, L. W. (2003). History of cardiac surgery. In L. H. Cohn & L. H. Edmunds (Eds.), *Cardiac surgery in the adult* (pp. 3–30). New York: McGraw-Hill.

Shock

Eric Wolak   Ernest J. Grant   Sonya R. Hardin

LEARNING OBJECTIVES

Upon completion of this chapter, the reader will be able to:

1. Define the four types of shock.

2. Describe the pathophysiologic changes as a basis for the signs and symptoms of shock.

3. Discuss the nursing assessment of the patient in shock.

4. Explain the effects of shock on the major body systems.

5. Describe the role of the nurse with appropriate interventions for patients in shock.

6. Evaluate the effectiveness of these interventions for patients in shock.

7. Compare the therapeutic and pharmacologic management of the patient with the different types of shock.

8. List optimal patient outcomes that may be achieved through evidence-based management of shock.

Shock is perhaps one of the most complicated and deadly syndromes in healthcare and is a common occurrence in intensive care unit (ICU) settings. Thus it is imperative that critical care nurses have a strong understanding of the various types of shock, their associated signs and symptoms, and the knowledge base needed to manage these challenging patients. Although shock may be classified in numerous ways, with each classification having a multitude of etiologies, the core concept is universal: Shock is an imbalance between oxygen supply and demand. This syndrome of inadequate end-organ perfusion (e.g., liver, intestines, kidneys, heart, lungs, and brain) results in a decrease in the supply of oxygen and nutrients required to maintain the metabolic needs of cell life (Doven, 2004). When the supply of oxygen and nutrients cannot meet the demand at the level needed to sustain normal cellular metabolism, the body responds initially by activating intrinsic compensatory mechanisms to improve perfusion, especially in areas of high demand such as the brain, heart, and lungs. When compensatory mechanisms fail to restore adequate perfusion, a cascade of cellular abnormalities can result in total organ dysfunction and, eventually, death.

Classification systems have been developed to define shock either by its cause or by its underlying pathophysiologic effects (Doven, 2004). One such system classifies shock syndromes according to the underlying pathology (see **Table 18-1**).

CREATING A FOUNDATION

Before we can begin our discussion of shock, it is vital to briefly review hemodynamics. Hemodynamics concerns the physical factors regulating blood flow within the circulatory system. The core concept of hemodynamics involves cardiac output (CO)/cardiac index (CI).

$$\text{Cardiac Output (CO)} = \text{Heart Rate (HR)} \times \text{Stroke Volume (SV)}$$

$$\text{Cardiac Index (CI)} = \frac{\text{Heart Rate (HR)} \times \text{Stroke Volume (SV)}}{\text{Body Surface Area (BSA)}}$$

These equations demonstrate that the CO is the amount of blood pumped by the heart each minute and that the CI is the amount of blood pumped by the heart each

TABLE 18-1 Classification of Shock Etiology and Underlying Effects

Classification	Etiology	Underlying Pathology
Hypovolemic	Hemorrhage Burns Excessive diuretic use Fluid losses (e.g., vomiting, diarrhea, nasogastric tube drainage)	Whole blood loss Plasma loss
Cardiogenic	Myocardial infarction Dysrhythmias Blunt cardiac injury End-stage cardiomyopathies • Congestive • Hypertrophic • Restrictive Valvular heart disease • Severe valvular stenosis • Acute valvular regurgitation	Loss of cardiac contractility Reduced cardiac output
Obstructive	Cardiac tamponade Tension pneumothorax Tension hemothorax	Compression of heart with obstruction to atrial filling Mediastinal shift with obstruction to atrial filling Combination of above Venous pooling—maldistribution of blood volume
Distributive	Neurogenic • Injury and disease of the spinal cord • Spinal anesthesia or epidural block • Vasomotor center depression (e.g., severe pain, drugs, hypoglycemia, emotional stress) Anaphylactic • Drugs • Insect bites/stings • Contrast media • Blood transfusions • Foods • Vaccines Septic • Infection (bacteria, virus, fungal) • Patients receiving immunosuppressive therapy • Patients with chronic disease (e.g., AIDS, cancer, diabetes) • Malnourished patients	Decrease in venous resistance Poor distribution of blood flow

Sources: Hochman, 2003; Jones, 2002; Kelly, 2005; Kumar, Abbas, & Nelson, 2005.

minute per BSA. Measurements in relation to the CI are a more accurate measure of values because this calculation takes into account the size of the body. Normal CO is 4 to 8 L/min and normal CI is 2.5 to 4 L/min/m^2. As shown in the preced-

ing equations, HR and SV are essential variables in relation to CO/CI. *Heart rate* (HR) is the number of times the heart beats each minute, which for a normal adult heart is 60 to 100 beats per minute. *Stroke volume* (SV) is the amount of blood pumped out of the heart with each beat. In an adult patient, the SV is normally 65 to 135 mL (Kumar, Abbas, & Nelson, 2005; Marino, 1998). A complete discussion of hemodynamics appears in Chapter 11.

Shock is a syndrome of poor perfusion, which is a component of CO. Thus critically ill patients in shock could have a very low CO/CI, depending on the type of shock. Suppose you are caring for a patient with a CO of 3.0 L/min and an HR of 100 beats/min. In this scenario, the patient's SV (amount of blood pumped out each beat) would only be 30 mL (3000 mL ÷ 100 beats/min = 30 mL). This is much lower than the normal SV of 65 to 135 mL. As a consequence, the tissues will not receive adequate oxygen for survival and will not function properly when they are underperfused. This is why it is very important to have a good understanding of CO in relation to shock.

Both HR and SV can be manipulated to change CO. For example, if HR increases and SV remains unchanged, CO will increase. You can see this simply by changing the numbers in the formula. Here are some examples to challenge your critical thinking regarding how HR affects CO:

1. If a patient's blood pressure is falling, what does his or her HR usually do? It usually increases to maintain the patient's CO. Do you think this is a beneficial response?

2. Suppose a patient's HR went from 100 beats/min to 80 beats/min and his SV remained at 30 mL. What would his CO be? It would be 2,400 mL/min (2.4 L/min). Do you think the patient would benefit from this decrease in HR?

3. Cardiac contraction and the subsequent opening of the aortic valve require a large amount of oxygen. Therefore, the faster the HR, the more oxygen the heart uses. Do you see how it might benefit a patient if his or her HR decreases?

4. The faster the HR, the less time there is for ventricular filling, and the less time there is for coronary arteries to perfuse (remember most of coronary artery blood flow is during diastole). Do you see how a decrease in HR might be beneficial?

5. Suppose you have a patient in complete heart block and has an HR of 40 beats/min with a blood pressure of 80/40 mm Hg. Do you think it might benefit his or her CO to increase the HR?

As demonstrated by these examples, an increase or decrease of a patient's HR can greatly affect the clinical presentation and response to therapies.

Now let's look at SV. SV determinants are preload, afterload, and contractility. Preload is the amount of stretching the cardiac muscle does prior to contraction; it is typically measured in the ICU with a pulmonary artery (PA) catheter. Right heart preload is measured by using the central venous pressure (CVP) and is normally 0 to 8 mm Hg. Left heart preload is measured by using the pulmonary artery occlusive pressure (PAOP) with normal values ranging from 8 to12 mm Hg. According to the Frank-Starling law of stretch, the more blood that enters the ventricles during diastole, the greater the stretch that muscle fibers will have; the greater the preload. This phenomenon is very effective, but works only up to a point. If the ventricles are overstretched, the strength of the contractions will decrease. Thus optimal preload gives the patient the best CO (Kumar et al., 2005; Marino, 1998).

Because the left ventricle provides the effective force of blood flow throughout the body, the term *preload* typically refers to the left side of the heart; it is also known as the PAOP or "wedge" pressure (Marino, 1998).

Afterload is the amount of work the heart has to do to eject blood. Most of the resistance the ventricle encounters is from the blood vessels, although valves, blood viscosity, and flow patterns can also have an influence. However, the principal factor determining blood flow is the diameter of the vessel, and the heart's and lungs' afterloads are usually changed through vasodilation or vasoconstriction. Many people think of afterload as blood pressure or, more correctly, as systemic

vascular resistance (SVR) on the left side of the heart and pulmonary vascular resistance (PVR) on the right side of the heart (Marino, 1998).

To really understand the meaning of SVR and PVR, you need to understand the components of their formulas. First you need to know how to figure out mean arterial pressure (MAP) and mean pulmonary artery pressure (MPAP) and what they mean. The MAP is superior to the systolic pressure for arterial pressure monitoring because it is the true driving pressure for peripheral blood flow. To calculate this value, you take the systolic value and add it to twice the diastolic value (the heart is at rest twice as long as it is ejecting), add them up, and divide by 3. To find the MPAP, we do it just like MAP, only now we take one times the PA systolic pressure and two times the PA diastolic pressure and divide by 3 (Marino, 1998). Refer to **Table 18-2** for hemodynamic reference values. The formulas for SVR and PVR are as follows:

$$SVR = \frac{MAP - CVP}{CO} \times 80 \text{ dynes/sec/cm}^{-5}$$

$$PVR = \frac{MPAP - PAOP}{CO} \times 80 \text{ dynes/sec/cm}^{-5}$$

In these formulas, the measurement of dynes/seconds /cm^{-5} is a function of work. This highlights the roles of SVR and PVR as resistance the heart must work against. Also, these formulas demonstrate the close relationship of SVR and PVR to CO. Because CO is a denominator in these formulas, when it goes up, SVR and PVR must go down. This relationship makes sense once you think about it. If the left side of the heart has more resistance to work against (increased SVR), then it will be able to force out less blood (decreased CO). Just as with CI, it is important to think of these values and factors in reference to the individual's BSA. These relationships give the systemic vascular resistance index (SVRI) and pulmonary vascular resistance index (PVRI). To calculate these indexes, you would simply replace CI in the earlier equation with CO. Refer to Table 18-2 for these reference ranges.

Having an understanding of these hemodynamic concepts is imperative to comprehend the various shock syndromes and their manifestations. By knowing how cardiac blood flow, resistance, vessel diameter, blood return, and overall fluid dynamics work synergistically, the critical care nurse is better able to understand the pathology of his or her patient and will have the tools needed to provide the most effective care.

CLASSIFICATIONS OF SHOCK SYNDROMES

There are four classifications of shock syndromes: hypovolemic, cardiogenic, obstructive, and distributive. Each of these syndromes has a unique, specific mechanism that causes alter-

TABLE 18-2 Hemodynamic Parameters

Parameter	Abbreviation	Normal Range
Central venous pressure	CVP	0–8 mm Hg
Pulmonary artery occlusive pressure	PAOP	8–12 mm Hg
Cardiac output	CO	4–8 L/min
Cardiac index	CI	2.4–4.0 L/min/m^2
Systemic vascular resistance	SVR	770–1,500 dynes/sec/cm^{-5}
Systemic vascular resistance index	SVRI	1,600–2,400 dynes/sec/cm^5/m^2
Pulmonary vascular resistance	PVR	20–120 dynes/sec/cm^{-5}
Pulmonary vascular resistance index	PVRI	200–400 dynes/sec/cm^5/m^2
Mean arterial pressure	MAP	60–105 mm Hg
Mean pulmonary artery pressure	MPAP	15–19 mm Hg
Stroke volume	SV	65–135 mL

Sources: Alderson, Schierhout, Roberts, & Bunn, 2004; Marino, 1998.

ation in tissue perfusion. Hypovolemic shock is primarily a preload problem, in which there is inadequate circulating volume. In cardiogenic shock, the heart fails to function efficiently as a pump (Krost, 2004). In obstructive shock, a blockage of the circulation tissue prevents venous return. In distributive shock, there is a maldistribution of circulating blood.

HYPOVOLEMIC SHOCK

Hypovolemic shock is the most common shock syndrome. It develops when there is a loss of plasma volume. This condition can progress to a shock state when the blood volume is insufficient to fill the intravascular space. Loss of intravascular volume can be due to either actual external fluid loss (actual hypovolemia) or internal fluid shift from the intravascular space to the interstitial or intracellular spaces (relative hypovolemia).

Actual hypovolemia occurs because of external hemorrhage, gastrointestinal volume losses, renal volume losses, or loss of plasma. Actual losses are generally easily identifiable and to some extent measurable. In contrast, in relative hypovolemia (e.g., burn injury), the fluid has not left the body, but has shifted from the intravascular space and is unavailable for circulation. Whatever the cause of hypovolemic shock, it is characterized by insufficient total vascular volume, resulting in

a decrease in preload, stroke volume, and CO. There is also circulatory insufficiency and, ultimately, inadequate tissue perfusion. Relative hypovolemia is less quantifiable than actual hypovolemia but is characterized by internal hemorrhage, third spacing of fluid, and massive vasodilation. For example, patients with cirrhosis sequester fluid in the peritoneal cavity and will have relative hypovolemic shock. Internal hemorrhages such as a hemothorax, hemorrhagic pancreatitis, a ruptured spleen, or long bone fractures may also lead to hypovolemic shock, as can severe sodium depletion, Addisonian crisis, and hypopituitarism. Lastly, massive vasodilation states such as those caused by anaphylaxis and spinal shock can create a relative hypovolemic state (Bridges, 2005; Kelly, 2005).

Burn injuries and resulting burn shock are well-known examples of relative hypovolemic shock. Interstitial tissue spaces can serve as reservoirs for fluid, particularly when there is an alteration in capillary permeability or a decrease in colloidal osmotic pressure. With larger burn injuries (i.e., greater than 20% total BSA burns), there is generalized increased capillary permeability, vasoconstriction leading to increased vascular hydrostatic pressure, decreased vascular oncotic pressure, increased interstitial oncotic pressure, and decreased interstitial hydrostatic pressure. All of these alterations cause vascular fluid to shift from the vascular space to the interstital space, resulting in massive relative hypovolemia and subsequent shock (Demling, 2005).

There are three stages of hypovolemic shock: mild, moderate, and severe. Depending on the severity and rate of the volume loss, the patient may progress through these stages slowly or rapidly. In the mild stage, the patient generally experiences a blood volume deficit ranging from 0% to 10%, or approximately 500 mL. This volume deficit creates a decrease in venous return and CO. The autonomic nervous system is activated to compensate for the volume loss; the subsequent increases in vasoconstriction and myocardial contractility are able to maintain arterial pressure and CO (Kelly, 2005).

In moderate hypovolemic shock, CO and arterial pressure fall significantly, and blood volume is reduced by 15% to 20%. There is intense arteriolar vasoconstriction and diminished blood flow to the liver, pancreas, kidneys, and gastrointestinal tract. In this stage, a general venoconstriction assists in increasing venous return to the general circulation. The sympathetic compensatory response causes tachycardia, tachypnea, peripheral vasoconstriction, pallor, diaphoresis, and restlessness (Kelly, 2005).

In severe hypovolemic shock, the blood volume deficit exceeds 25%, and small additional losses create major decreases in CO, blood pressure, and tissue perfusion. At this point, all of the compensatory mechanisms are functioning at maximum capacity, and even the brain and myocardium become subject to a fall in perfusion. The patient becomes confused, anxious, agitated, obtunded, and eventually comatose (Kelly, 2005).

The hemodynamic consequences of hypovolemic shock, whether it be actual or relative, result from the overall decrease in vascular volume. Consequently, there is less venous return to the heart, followed by decreased PA pressures, decreased PAOP, and ultimately, decreased CO (see Table 18-3). As discussed earlier, when CO is decreased, SVR increases automatically. This increase in SVR is due to stimulation of the vasomotor center in the medulla, which causes activation of the sympathetic nervous system and release of the α-adrenergic hormones epinephrine and norepinephrine and selective peripheral vasoconstriction; this cascade of events further decreases CO (Schulman, 2002). It is the decreased CO that results in poor end-organ perfusion.

Consequently, the goal of therapy in hypovolemic shock is to restore adequate circulating volume as quickly as possible. This can be accomplished most readily by infusion of replacement solutions and treatment of the cause of the hypovolemic state. Replacement fluid solutions will improve tissue perfusion and meet cellular demands (Lighthall & Pearl, 2003).

Management of patients in hypovolemic shock is dependent upon the cause. Immediate management would include placing the patient in a modified Trendelenburg position (supine with leg elevation) (Kelly, 2005). If hypovolemia is due to the loss of blood, control of the hemorrhage is a priority, followed by infusion of blood products (see Boxes 18-1, 18-2, 18-3, and 18-4). If blood products are not required, then fluid replacement will consist of either a crystalloid or colloid solution. Much debate has focused on which of these options is preferable (Johnson, 2004; Rizoli, 2003). A systematic review failed to support the use of colloids over crystalloids in the critically ill patient (Alderson, Schierhout, Roberts, & Bunn, 2004). However, fluid choice remains a clinical decision based on individual patient requirements and response.

CARDIOGENIC SHOCK

Cardiogenic shock is a syndrome that results from ineffective perfusion caused by inadequate contractility of the cardiac muscle. Unlike in hypovolemic shock, there is no decreased intravascular volume or vasodilation of the vascular space (Worthley, 2000). Both physiological and anatomical cardiac and noncardiac problems may cause pump dysfunction of the heart (see Table 18-1). The most common cardiac etiology is anatomical damage resulting from myocardial infarction and impairment of the cardiac muscle's pumping ability. Because the left ventricle is the heart's primary pump, cardiogenic shock is usually the result of left ventricular dysfunction (Krost, 2004). Left ventricular dysfunction leads to decreased CO and causes blood to back up into the pulmonary system, producing pulmonary congestion. However, the right ventricle can also be involved. In right ventricular dysfunction, the blood backs up into the venous circulation, reducing the available SV for each heartbeat (Pfisterer, 2003).

Regardless of the etiology, the end result is that SV and CO are insufficient to meet tissue and cellular needs. If an adequate increase in vascular resistance does not compensate for this decrease in CO, a drop in the MAP will occur. This will further compromise the ventricle, because adequate coronary artery blood flow requires normal blood pressure. When compensatory mechanisms are working, catecholamine release (e.g., epinephrine and norepinephrine) creates an increased systemic vascular resistance in an attempt to maintain MAP. However, this requires a fine balance, because these catecholamines may have a detrimental effect in the form of increased afterload, although increasing coronary artery perfusion also creates more resistance that the impaired ventricle must work against. Furthermore, the catecholamine-stimulated sympathetic drive increases ventricular contractility, which might also potentiate myocardial ischemia and failure (Hochman, 2003).

TABLE 18-3 Hemodynamics of Shock Syndromes

Type of Shock	CO	CVP	SVR	Pulmonary Artery Pressure	PAOP
Hypovolemic	↓	↓	↑	↓	↓
Cardiogenic	↓	↑	↑	↑	↑
Obstructive	↓	↑	↑	↓	↓
Distributive					
Neurogenic	↓	↓	NL or ↑	↓	↓
Anaphylactic	↓	↓	NL or ↑	↓	↓
Septic	NL or ↑	NL or ↓	↓	NL or ↓	NL or ↓

NL = normal
↓ = decrease
↑ = increase
Sources: Bench, 2004; Muhlberg & Ruth-Sahd, 2004.

Box 18-1

Blood Transfusion Steps

1. Check the physician's orders to determine:
   - The product to be administered
   - The number of units or volume to be administered
   - The date to be administered
   - Any special processing required
   - The duration of infusion
   - Any pre-medication orders, if indicated
2. Draw blood and send it to the lab for type and crossmatch.
3. When the patient is ready to be transfused, take the blood bank slip to the blood bank to obtain blood. Blood products must be hung within 30 minutes of leaving the blood bank refrigerator. The blood bank will usually release only one blood product at a time. *NEVER* place blood products in the refrigerator on the patient care unit.
4. For whole blood, red blood cells, or granulocytes, verify the following data in the computer and with the blood bank:
   - Blood grouping
   - Rh type
   - Number of units crossmatched
   - Number of units to be administered
   - Also check the appearance of the unit for the presence of clots, clumps, or abnormal cloudiness, and the integrity of the seals.
5. Verify informed consent has been obtained, except for emergency transfusions.
6. Establish or verify the patency of the peripheral or central venous access device. Use a 20-gauge or larger catheter to prevent lysis of red blood cells.
7. Obtain and record the patient's baseline vital signs. If febrile, notify the physician to decide whether the transfusion can wait or if the patient should receive acetaminophen as a pre-medication.
8. Two qualified health professionals trained in blood administration procedures should compare:
   - The blood product, type and Rh, blood product number, and expiration date with the blood container bag's label.
   - The blood container tag with the patient blood bracelet.
9. Give only two units per filter set. Administer within four hours after removal from blood bank. If more than six to eight units of PRBC are given, then FFP should be given with every other unit. Give one platelet transfusion for every unit of PRBC after eight units (varies among institutions).
10. Prime the filtered administration set with the blood product or 0.9% sodium chloride.
11. If a leukocyte-depletion filter is indicated, follow the manufacturer's and the blood bank's instructions for its setup. A leukocyte-depletion filter may be used to prevent repeat febrile reactions.
12. Adjust the rate of flow to 2–5 mL/min during the first five minutes of platelets or plasma infusions or 2 mL/min for the first 15 minutes for whole blood, RBC, or granulocytes. Patients should be observed closely for the first 15 minutes.
13. At the end of the first 15 minutes, obtain and record the TPR and BP. If vital signs are within normal range and the patient has no signs or symptoms of an adverse reaction, change the rate to infuse the unit within the time period specified in the physician's order.
14. At the conclusion of a blood product transfusion in which no adverse reaction occurred:
    - Obtain a post-transfusion H & H for post-count as physician ordered. Flush the blood administration set with 0.9% sodium chloride until the tubing is clear.
    - Obtain and record vital signs post infusion.
15. Disconnect and discard the empty blood product bag into a red container.

Continue to monitor the patient for signs and symptoms of an adverse reaction during the transfusion and 1 hour post transfusion. If the patient experiences a reaction while the transfusion is in progress, immediately stop the transfusion. Maintain the patency of the line with normal saline and notify the physician.

TPR = temperature, pulse, respirations
BP = blood pressure
H & H = hemoglobin & hematocrit

PRBC = packed red blood cells
FFP = fresh frozen plasma
RBC = red blood cells

Box 18-2
Transfusion Reactions

Hemolytic Transfusion Reactions

Fever, chills, flushing, nausea, burning at the intravenous (IV) line site, chest tightness, restlessness, apprehension, joint pain, back pain, tachycardia, tachypnea, hypotension, oozing from the IV site, diffuse bleeding, hemoglobinuria, shock, oliguria (in renal failure)

Nonhemolytic Febrile Reactions

Fever, chills, malaise

Anaphylactic Reaction

Symptoms usually occur with less than 10 mL of blood transfused; chills, abdominal cramps, dyspnea, vomiting, diarrhea, tachycardia, flushing, urticaria, wheezing, laryngeal edema, hypotension

Box 18-3
Blood Products

- Whole blood
- Packed red blood cells
- Granulocyte concentrates
- Platelet concentrates
- Human plasma: fresh frozen plasma/freeze-dried plasma
- Plasma protein fraction
- Human albumin 25%
- Cryoprecipitate
- Clotting factors: Factor VIII/IX
- Immunoglobulins

As demonstrated in Table 18-1, causes of cardiogenic shock include cardiomyopathy, cardiac dysrhythmias that impair the efficiency of myocardial contractions, congestive heart failure, and ventricular septal defect or rupture of the ventricular wall (Doven, 2004). In all of these situations, the heart is unable to provide adequate SV and CO/CI. For example, with cardiac dysrhythmias (e.g., premature ventricular contractions, sinus tachycardia), the amount of blood pumped out of the heart in a minute is reduced, leading to inadequate organ perfusion. Regardless of the cause, the extent of pump failure depends on the degree of heart muscle impairment and the adequacy of compensatory mechanisms.

Hemodynamically, cardiogenic shock presents with decreased CO, a result of the decreased SV. The decrease in CO is accompanied by an increase in SVR, or afterload. This increase is the result of compensatory mechanisms (e.g., catecholamine release). As the ventricle fails to eject adequate volume, the volume in the left ventricle at the end of filling (PAOP) begins to rise. This increase leads to distention of the ventricle, and elevated filling pressures are ultimately transmitted to the pulmonary bed (reflected as increased PA pressures and increased PAOP). These increased pressures can often be visualized as jugular venous distention (Hochman, 2003) (see Table 18-3). As the shock state continues and oxygen supply fails to meet demand, end-organ dysfunction ensues.

The primary dysfunction in cardiogenic shock relates to myocardial pumping ability. The major goal in treatment of this type of shock is to assist the contractility of the heart while alleviating, if possible, the cause of the pumping problem. Unlike with hypovolemic shock, a modified Trendelenburg position is not recommended in this shock state. Patients with decreased cardiac pump ability already have pulmonary congestion. If a patient is placed supine with legs elevated, there will be increased resistance for the heart to beat against, worsening tissue perfusion and pulmonary edema. To reduce afterload, patients should have head-of-bed elevation. The specific treatment modality depends on the exact cause of the impairment (e.g., acute myocardial infarction); however, an inotropic agent is often used. The purpose of using an inotropic drug, such as milrinone (Primacor®) or dobutamine (Dobutrex®), in a patient with cardiogenic shock is to improve the ability of the myocardium to contract effectively and to reduce afterload. Also, a diuretic, such as furosemide (Lasix®), is often given to reduce the pulmonary congestion (Barkman & McCay, 2002).

OBSTRUCTIVE SHOCK

Obstructive shock develops when a physical obstruction somewhere in the circulatory system impedes either the outflow or filling of the heart. As in cardiogenic shock, there is no decreased intravascular volume or vasodilation of the vascular space. The distinction from cardiogenic shock reflects the fact that the CO in obstructive shock is decreased from a drop in preload rather than from myocardial dysfunction. This can result from pulmonary embolism, dissecting aortic aneurysm, atrial tumors, pericardial tamponade, tension pneumothorax, and a ruptured diaphragm with evisceration of abdominal contents into the thoracic cavity. These events impair venous return because of the high pressures surrounding the right atrium (Podbregar, Krivec, & Voga, 2002). With a tension pneu-

Box 18-4
Blood Types

Types	Blood Can Be Given to	Blood Can Be Received from
A+	A+, AB+	A+, A−, O+, O−
O+ (almost 40% of the population has O+ blood)	O+, A+, B+, AB+	O+, O−
B+	B+, AB+	B+, B−, O+, O−
AB+ (universal recipient)	AB+	Everyone
A−	A+, A−, AB+, AB−	A−, O−
O− (universal donor; only about 7% of all people have type O negative blood)	Everyone	O−
B−	B+, B−, AB+, AB−	B−, O−
AB−	AB+, AB−	AB−, A−, B−, O−

mothorax and a ruptured diaphragm, venous return is impaired because the great veins are compressed as they enter the chest (Bench, 2004). Clinically, these patients resemble those in hypovolemic shock (see Table 18-3).

To return CO to normal and improve tissue perfusion, the obstruction must be alleviated or repaired. The ultimate treatments for obstructive shock patients are largely surgical—for example, removing the pulmonary embolus or relieving the pericardial tamponade (Yamamoto, Schroeder, Morley, & Beliveau, 2005).

DISTRIBUTIVE SHOCK

Distributive shock is characterized by an abnormal distribution of the intravascular volume. This type of shock is often complicated by loss of intravascular fluid from increased capillary permeability. Although blood volume does not change, vascular tone decreases. Three types of distributive abnormalities are observed: neurogenic, anaphylactic, and septic (Doven, 2004; O'Brien, 2005). Septic shock is described in more detail in Chapter 51.

The three types of distributive shock are all characterized by a relative hypovolemia from the massive vasodilation. This relative hypovolemia causes a decrease in preload and low CVP and PAOP (see Table 18-3). However, the effect on CO depends on the compensatory mechanisms deployed, such as increased HR (Muhlberg & Ruth-Sahd, 2004). The major therapeutic goal in treating distributive shock is to stop the cause of vasodilation and to return the circulating volume to the intravascular space to improve tissue perfusion. Intra-

vascular fluid resuscitation should occur before the administration of vasoconstrictive agents.

Neurogenic Shock

Neurogenic shock is caused by massive vasodilation as a result of loss of sympathetic vasoconstrictor tone in the vascular smooth muscles and impairment of autonomic function, resulting in vasodilation. The massive vasodilation causes pooling of blood into the venous system, decreased venous return to the heart, decreased CO, and eventually inadequate end-organ perfusion. Patients in neurogenic shock typically present with hypotension, resulting from the abnormal distribution of volume. Normally, the body attempts to compensate for this hypotension and to maintain CO by increasing HR (Schulman, 2002). However, in neurogenic shock, the body is unable to use these compensatory mechanisms because of sympathetic blockade and dominance of the parasympathetic nervous system. Therefore, the HR is slower than needed. The bradycardia and poor venous return, due to vasodilation, result in decreased SV and CO. Over time, the poor CO leads to inadequate end-organ perfusion. Thus the shock state and decreased tissue and cellular perfusion result from massive vasodilation and bradycardia.

The hemodynamic presentation of patients with neurogenic shock is very dynamic and does not follow absolutes. It is generally associated with a decrease in CVP, PA pressures, PAOP, SV, and CO/CI. As CO decreases, SVR increases (Tator, 2004) (see Table 18-3).

Several precipitating factors may lead to neurogenic shock (see Table 18-1). For example, disease or injury to the spinal cord can interrupt transmission of sympathetic nerve impulses to peripheral blood vessels. After a spinal cord injury, neurogenic shock usually lasts from hours to weeks. Spinal anesthesia can also block the transmission of impulses from the sympathetic nervous system. Depression of the vasomotor center of the medulla as a result of drugs, severe pain, or hypoglycemia can likewise decrease vasoconstrictor tone of peripheral blood vessels (Doven, 2004).

Because neurogenic shock has a multitude of causes, the treatment options vary. Fluid replacement to maintain MAP is the first line of therapy. However, due to the vasodilation, fluid requirements are extensive; thus careful monitoring of the patient during fluid administration is important to prevent the development of pulmonary edema from fluid overload. Drugs that stimulate the sympathetic nervous system may be required to increase blood pressure through vasoconstriction and increased HR. These α- and β-agonist medications include epinephrine and norepinephrine. An α-agonist causes peripheral vasoconstriction, whereas β-agonists increase HR, blood pressure cardiac contractility, and CO. As a critical care nurse, one must be diligent in monitoring these patients, because the increase in SVR and HR increases the workload of the heart and can be detrimental, sometimes leading to myocardial damage (McLlvoy, Meyer, & Vitaz, 2000).

Anaphylactic Shock

Anaphylaxis is an acute and potentially life-threatening massive allergic reaction. It occurs when a sensitized person is exposed to an antigen—that is, a substance to which the person has an allergy. The antigen enters the body and combines with immunoglobulin E antibodies on the surface of the mast cells and basophils. The reaction then causes direct damage to the adjacent vascular walls and causes cells throughout the body to release vasoactive mediators, such as histamine and prostaglandins, which trigger a systemic response. This cascade of events causes vasodilation, increased capillary permeability (causing movement of circulating fluids into the interstitial space and potentiating relative hypovolemia), reduced CO, and poor organ perfusion. Severe bronchospasms also may occur from release of these chemical mediators (Crusher, 2004).

The onset of symptoms is related to the degree of exposure to the antigen and/or the severity of the allergy. Typical symptoms include bronchospasm and laryngeal edema, rash, flushed skin, and generalized edema from increased capillary permeability. Hemodynamically, there is a decrease in blood pressure, CO/CI from the vasodilation that occurs, and a compensatory increase in HR to improve or maintain CO (see Table 18-3). Much as in neurogenic shock, the SVR may be decreased due to the decreased CO; however, although afterload may appear elevated, vasodilation is ensuing in these patients.

A patient can develop a severe allergic reaction, possibly leading to anaphylactic shock, after ingesting or being injected with an antigen to which that person has previously been sensitized. Parenteral administration of an antigen is the route most likely to cause anaphylaxis (O'Brien, 2005). However, oral, topical, and inhalation routes of administration of an antigen have been known to cause anaphylactic reactions (see Table 18-1).

The primary treatment for patients in anaphylactic shock is the administration of epinephrine. Epinephrine reverses symptoms of anaphylaxis by its effect on α- and β-receptors. Administration will reverse vasodilation and raise blood pressure. It also reduces edema, dilates the bronchioles, has a positive inotropic effect (increased contractility) on the myocardium, and inhibits further mediator response (Jones, 2002).

STAGES OF SHOCK

No matter what the initial cause of the shock state is, the end result is always the same: The tissues fail to receive oxygen and nutrients and to rid themselves of waste products. It is the inadequate tissue and cell perfusion that causes widespread disruption to cellular metabolism. Shock is a very complex syndrome, because the problem concerns not only the amount of blood volume, but also its delivery in terms of blood flow to organs and cells of the body. A number of variables may influence the course of shock, such as the age and the overall state of health of the person before the shock insult.

It is the responsibility of the nurse to prevent the development of shock. This includes early interpretation of observational and measurable data to recognize its initial development. For improved understanding and recognition of shock, it can be divided into three stages: compensated, progressive, and irreversible. These stages are not absolute, but rather should be regarded as a continuum.

Compensated Shock

The first stage of shock is termed "compensated" because the body's compensatory mechanisms are able to maintain cardiovascular dynamics and stabilize the circulation in the face of whatever defect is occurring. This is achieved through several mechanisms. The primary compensatory mechanism is mediated through the sympathetic nervous system and the adrenal glands. This response is initiated by the decrease in blood pressure, which results from decreased CO and/or vasodilation. It stimulates baroreceptors located in the aortic arch and carotid sinuses. Baroreceptors (pressure-sensitive nerve endings) respond to any decrease in arterial blood flow. A decrease in circulation causes a reduction in the pressure exerted by the blood in the artery, resulting in a decrease in the firing of the carotid sinus and aortic arch baroreceptors. Subsequently, sympathetic nervous system discharge increases, which in turn increases HR, myocardial contractility, vascular resistance, and blood pressure. This sympathetic stimulation also causes dilation of the coronary arteries, resulting in an increase in oxygen supply to the myocardium, which now has an increased oxygen demand as a result of the increase in HR and contractility (Kelly, 2005). This effect is evident in most syndromes of shock, except for neurogenic shock, in which the sympathetic system's response is blocked.

In this compensatory stage, increased resistance caused by the baroreceptors is not uniform throughout the body's organ systems. In particular, perfusion decreases in the kidneys. The diminishing blood flow to the kidneys stimulates the release of renin into the blood. In the bloodstream, renin activates angiotensinogen to produce angiotensin I, which is converted to angiotensin II by angiotensin-converting enzyme (ACE) produced by the lungs. Angiotensin II is a very powerful vasoconstrictor. Furthermore, angiotensin II stimulates aldosterone release by the adrenal cortex, which causes sodium retention (Khalaf & DeBlieux, 2001). The increased sodium reabsorption raises the serum osmolarity and stimulates the release of antidiuretic hormone (ADH) by the posterior pituitary. ADH targets kidney tubules and inhibits urine formation by increasing reabsorption of water into the circulation. As a result, less urine is produced and blood volume increases, thereby improving venous return to the heart, CO, and blood pressure (Diehl-Oplinger & Kaminski, 2004).

In the compensatory stage, the most reliable sign of the start of poor perfusion is the patient's level of consciousness. It may undergo subtle changes, usually in the form of restlessness, irritability, and/or apprehension. Furthermore, the patient's HR is moderately elevated and the quality of pulses may be either weak or bounding, depending on the degree of vasodilation and the amount of SV. Respiratory rate will be increased to compensate for the decreased tissue oxygenation. Urine output may start to decline to 0.5 mL/kg/hr or slightly less, and bowel sounds will become hypoactive due to reduced blood flow to the gastrointestinal (GI) system (Lighthall & Pearl, 2003).

Progressive Shock

As shock progresses, the body's compensatory mechanisms begin to fail. The progression of shock becomes evident at the cellular, organ, and system levels, and extensive physiological dysfunction occurs. Despite the attempt of the body to increase CO by increasing the HR and myocardial contractility, there is a decrease in CO. This decreased CO plus the peripheral vasoconstriction cause tissue hypoxia. As tissue perfusion decreases, cells switch from an aerobic metabolic state to an anaerobic state. In the anaerobic state, serum lactate levels increase, resulting in metabolic acidosis. As the shock state progresses, the rise in the lactic acid level will often correlate with the severity of the shock state. Furthermore, increased lactate levels will depress cardiac function by impairing calcium metabolism within the myocardial cells (Nguyen et al., 2004).

During this stage of shock, the adrenal medulla secretes a large amount of catecholamines. These catecholamines maintain perfusion to the brain and heart. Catecholamines also stimulate the liver to undergo glycogenolysis, releasing its glycogen stores in the form of glucose. In addition, the release of insulin by the pancreas is suppressed. Thus the brain, which does not require insulin for the utilization of glucose, has energy available for metabolism (Doven, 2004).

Patients in this stage of shock often present with deteriorating levels of consciousness. They may demonstrate progressive confusion, apathy, and decreased response to painful stimuli. Mean arterial blood pressure will be less than 60 mm Hg, or less than 25% from baseline. Tachycardia becomes noticeably evident during this stage, and peripheral pulses are weak. Respiratory rates increase in an attempt to compensate for tissue hypoxia and metabolic acidosis; due to the decreased level of consciousness, however, the depth decreases and patients appear tired and weak. Urine output continues to decrease and becomes less than 0.5 mL/kg/hr, demonstrating poor renal perfusion. The patient's mucous membranes become notably dry, and the capillary refill becomes sluggish and may exceed three seconds. Furthermore, as poor perfusion progresses, patients may become hypothermic and cool to the touch (Nguyen et al., 2004).

Irreversible Shock

Irreversible shock, the final stage, is also referred to as the refractory phase because the body systems no longer respond to treatment. As each organ system decompensates and requires more support, a point is reached where therapeutic measures are no longer effective in maintaining function. The term "irreversible" is appropriate because it is at this point that the body systems cross the line from organ dysfunction to failure. The extent of tissue damage and necrosis, the number of mediators and toxins that have been released into the systemic circulation, and the degree of acidosis are so profound that even a return of normal CO and blood pressure will not reverse the downward progression (Nguyen et al., 2004).

The signs of irreversible shock can be seen in each organ system. The patient is no longer responsive to verbal or painful stimuli and appears to be in a comatose state. CO/CI does not respond to inotropic support or fluid administration. The patient may show signs of pancreatitis, gastrointestinal bleeding, and liver failure and may not absorb or metabolize nutrition. Renal failure might require daily dialysis. The skin is cold and clammy, with a significant decrease in temperature. Cyanosis may be present and is usually observed in the lips, mucous membranes, and nail beds. However, it may be more obvious in the palms, soles, and conjunctiva (Schulman, 2002).

At this point, the vasomotor centers become so depressed that no sympathetic activity occurs. The vascular bed is generally dilated due to the central nervous system (CNS) depression, toxins, and acidosis. Deterioration will continue and death will ensue. All of the organ systems need not fail for death to occur, however. When three systems fail, patients have a 90% to 100% mortality rate (Bench, 2004).

SYSTEM PROGRESSION AND MANAGEMENT

The nursing role in the acute stages of shock involves monitoring the patient's ongoing physical and emotional status to detect subtle changes, planning and implementing nursing interventions and therapy, evaluating the patient's response to therapy, and providing emotional support to the patient and significant others. Nursing responsibilities also include judging when it is necessary to alert other healthcare team members to changes in the patient's status that may require reevaluation of treatment. Therefore, reassessment, as often as the patient's condition warrants, is important. All shock syndromes affect the various organ systems. It is this effect and the resultant response of these organ systems that produce the distinct signs and symptoms critical care nurses need to recognize so that early therapeutic management can be initiated.

Neurologic Status

As perfusion decreases, whether from decreased CO or vasodilation, blood pressure decreases, which further decreases the cerebral perfusion pressure. Although blood flow is given preference to the brain to maintain nutritional supply, with the decrease in MAP, decreased cerebral perfusion will ensue. Of all organs, the brain is both the most intricate and the most susceptible to hypoxic injury. The brain is primarily affected because it depends on glucose and oxygen to function. Although it is protected by the compensatory vasoconstriction and autoregulation, if the MAP falls below 60 mm Hg, the capacity for autoregulation decreases (Schulman, 2002).

One of the first signs of developing shock is an alteration or decrease in level of consciousness. Mental status abnormalities are associated with poor outcome, as respiratory alkalosis, hypoxemia, and electrolyte disturbances start to appear. If blood flow continues to deteriorate, autoregulation can no longer maintain normal cerebral metabolism and unconsciousness rapidly occurs. With severe degrees of reduction of blood flow, the brain becomes ischemic and irreversible brain injury develops (Nguyen et al., 2004).

Cardiovascular Status

The heart muscle relies on the delivery of oxygen and nutrients to its cells via the coronary arteries and has a very high oxygen requirement. Thus a major reduction in cardiac blood flow quickly renders the heart muscle ischemic (Pfisterer, 2003).

Blood flow to the heart during the initial stage of shock is relatively preserved due to compensatory mechanisms, even as blood flow to other organs suffers. Consequently, myocardial dysfunction occurs only if there is a reduction in coronary blood flow exceeding the limits of compensatory mechanisms. In every type of shock, blood supply to the coronary arteries begins to deteriorate. As this deterioration progresses, myocardial contractility and compliance are reduced, the heart muscle becomes dysfunctional, and the heart stops to function adequately as a pump, causing a decrease in CO. Failure of the circulatory pump increases the deficient oxygen delivery throughout the remainder of the body as well as to the heart itself. Except in cardiogenic shock, major effects on myocardial function do not occur until the late stages of shock (Hochman, 2003). However, during the later stages of shock, the increased acidosis and low oxygen levels result in a decrease in myocardial contractility and a further reduction in CO. These effects may also produce dangerous cardiac arrhythmias (Pfisterer, 2003).

Respiratory Status

Individuals in states of shock are at increased risk for developing pulmonary insufficiency, either through pulmonary edema or acute respiratory distress syndrome (ARDS). The pulmonary system can be greatly affected by shock. Decreased blood flow can cause an increase in deadspace, alter gas exchange, cause alveolar collapse, and lead to decreased compliance (Khalaf & DeBlieux, 2001). Pulmonary edema can develop as well (Auer, Berent, Weber, Lamm, & Eber, 2005).

Every patient in any state of shock is at a high risk of developing ARDS. As level of consciousness decreases, the depth of respirations becomes less. This decreased tidal volume contributes to alveolar collapse, progression of atelectasis, and subsequent emergence of ARDS (Khalaf & DeBlieux, 2001). ARDS is described in more detail in Chapter 25.

Renal Status

The renal system is considered a secondary—rather than a primary—organ when patients are in shock. Therefore, regardless of the type of shock, the kidneys are immediately affected by hypoperfusion. Typically, there is a correlation between the amount of renal blood flow and the amount of urine output. Because renal blood flow depends on CO, any change in CO directly affects urinary output. Clinically, the patient may present with urinary output less than 0.5 mL/kg/hr. Furthermore, the renin-angiotension-aldosterone system is activated, which promotes sodium and water retention (Ruffell, 2004). This permits volume conservation, allowing the body to temporarily maintain CO. With this compensatory volume retention, the specific gravity of the urine will be greater than 1.015, and the urine sodium level will be less than 20 mmol/L. This state, which is typically referred to as prerenal failure, signifies that the kidneys are still functional and are compensating for the decreased perfusion (Schulman, 2002).

As perfusion to the kidneys continues to decline, acute tubular necrosis ensues and urine output falls to anuric (< 100 mL/24 hr) levels. Because the nephron can no longer carry out its functions, urine specific gravity falls to 1.010 and urine sodium levels rise to greater than 30 mmol/L. The kidney is unable to concentrate the urine, so it is considered to be in a dysfunctional state.

Gastrointestinal Status

As CO declines, blood is shunted to areas of higher priority; perfusion is limited to secondary organs, such as the intestines. Furthermore, as a result of the vasoconstrictor effects of compensatory mediators, such as vasopressin, angiotensin II, and catecholamines, the intestines suffer an early reduction in oxygen delivery in all types of shock. If alert, the patient may complain of nausea. Bowel sounds become hypoactive, and the abdomen often becomes distended, especially in the face of increased capillary permeability and subsequent third spacing. The placement of a nasogastric tube is often needed to assist in the elimination of gastric secretions that are not moving through the intestinal system due to decreased motility. If this inadequate perfusion persists, an ischemic gut can develop, which contributes to the development of lactic acidosis (Nguyen et al., 2004). Although the stomach has decreased motility, the small intestines remain peristaltic in earlier stages of shock. Thus nutrition should be limited to post-pyloric or parenteral nutrition (Schulman, 2002).

Furthermore, the gut contains bacteria and bacterial toxins. Normally, the mucosa of the intestines creates a barrier between the intestines and the bloodstream. In shock states, the intestinal mucosa barrier loses its integrity and becomes permeable to bacteria and endotoxins. When these pathogens enter the systemic circulation, infection and multiple organ dysfunction and failure ensue (Ruffell, 2004).

The liver is a highly complex organ that has multiple functions. It plays a key role in carbohydrate and lipid metabolism as well as synthesis of various proteins such as albumin and coagulation factors. In shock, both the hepatic arterial and portal venous blood flow are reduced. In compensatory shock, adrenaline-induced glycogenolysis and gluconeogenesis result in a large release of glucose (Dettenmeier et al., 2003).

In progressive shock, all liver functions, including protein synthesis, gluconeogenesis, lactate metabolism, detoxification, and glycogen storage, are diminished. However, the liver has a considerable reserve capacity, so the functions of the liver remain conducive to life with even a 90% decrease in function. In general, the liver adapts well to shock. Liver failure is typically a factor only in the irreversible stages of shock and is more often due to multiple-organ failure (Tazbir, 2004).

MANAGING THE PATIENT WITH SHOCK

Regardless of the precipitating cause of shock, if left untreated, the patient will progress to a situation of inadequate tissue perfusion and organ failure (Tortora & Grabowski, 2003). Initial interventions should be aimed at optimizing oxygen delivery to all organs. Common interventions include adequate oxygen, fluid, and drug therapy. In all cases, the nurse needs to provide a safe environment for the patient who may be at risk due to a reducing level of consciousness and deteriorating vital signs. Close monitoring of vital signs is essential.

The nurse should also ensure that all emergency equipment is available and working. The location of the patient should be considered to ensure close observation. Psychological care of the patient and family is another vital component. Anxiety management is a key part of the treatment of the patient in shock, because there is a direct link between anxiety and the initiation of the stress response (Tortora & Grabowski, 2003). Anxiety could be related to a fear of death, the degree of technical equipment around the bedside, and the discomfort of critical illness. Information regarding the patient's condition and any interventions should be provided, and an open, honest, and supportive relationship should be developed between the nurse, patient, and significant others.

Other important nursing considerations relate to the maintenance of skin integrity, which is put at risk by poor perfusion and immobility. Thus appropriate positioning and prevention of nosocomial pressure ulcers are of high priority.

Adequate nutritional monitoring and intake are important, as the gastrointestinal tract may not be functioning normally. Furthermore, complete blood count, urea, creatinine, and electrolyte levels—all of which may become disrupted due to fluid loss and/or renal impairment—must be monitored closely. For example, increases in potassium, as can occur in renal insufficiency and failure, may cause cardiac dysrhythmias. Low hemoglobin will reduce oxygen carrying capacity, further limiting the degree of oxygen delivery to tissues (Casey, 2001). Oxygen therapy should be administered and titrated according to oxygen saturation and arterial blood gas results (Pilkington, 2004). A reduced level of consciousness and deteriorating state mean that the patient cannot attend to personal hygiene needs and will, therefore, need assistance. Effective oral hygiene is essential to ensure comfort and to prevent the development of oral and systemic infection.

Optimal tissue perfusion and transport of oxygen to the cells are the goals of therapy regardless of the classification of shock. Treatment comprises a joint effort involving all members of the critical care team working to reach optimal tissue perfusion as quickly and efficiently as possible. For the critical care nurse, involvement in this process is initiated with assessment and monitoring techniques. Proper technique and interpretation of the data will ensure quality information that can enhance care and improve patient outcomes.

NURSING MANAGEMENT OF SHOCK

The primary goal in managing shock is to provide oxygenation to the vital organs and to restore circulating blood volume. The first assessment should focus on the ABCs: airway, breathing, and circulation. An airway should be patent to provide adequate ventilation. Achieving patency may require the utilization of an oral airway, bag-valve device ventilation, or intubation. Intubation may be required in case of respiratory distress, severe hypoxemia, pronounced acidosis, or coma. If intubation is required, low tidal volumes and peak inspiratory pressures should be implemented to prevent the reduction in venous return that is associated with positive-pressure ventilation (refer to Chapter 23). The goal is to keep the oxygen saturation as high as possible to ensure adequate organ oxygenation.

The utilization of fluid resuscitation requires considering the underlying cause of the shock, because fluids can be either harmful or beneficial, depending on the etiology. For example, in hypovolemic shock, the goal is to restore the vascular volume in such conditions as trauma, diabetic ketoacidosis, bowel obstruction, or severe diarrhea and vom-

iting. Patients should receive a bolus of 1 to 2 liters of lactated Ringer's solution. The nurse should have started two large-bore intravenous (IV) lines (14- or 16-gauge or greater) and administered 250 mL IV fluid rapidly as a bolus over 15 minutes. Ongoing IV therapy is based on the response to fluid resuscitation, continuing losses, and the underlying etiology of shock. Fluid resuscitation should be utilized to provide an HR less than 100 beats/min, and a systolic blood pressure greater than 90 mm Hg. If patients do not adequately respond to fluid resuscitation, then use of vasopressors or inotropes should be considered.

In other circumstances, such as cardiogenic shock, fluid therapy can be harmful. Additional fluid loading in these patients may increase an already increased left ventricular end diastolic pressure, worsen pulmonary edema, and further decrease CO. In cardiogenic shock, treatment is targeted with early inotropic support, together with aggressive management of pulmonary edema. Another example where fluids may be harmful is in shock associated with ongoing noncompressible hemorrhage such a leaking aortic aneurysm. Such a patient should be treated with the principles of hypotensive resuscitation, by keeping the systolic blood pressure around 90 mm Hg, giving just enough fluid to maintain brain perfusion, and maintaining a MAP of 60. Blood is the choice for fluid replacement. IV fluids are not given until the patient is in the operating room to prevent dilutional coagulopathy (Roberts, Revell, Youssef, Bradbury, & Adam, 2006).

After initial resuscitation, the nurse should continue with an ongoing assessment of the ABCs, vital signs (including pulse oximetry), and level of consciousness as often as possible until the patient is stable. A urinary catheter should be inserted to monitor hourly urine output. Urine output should be at a minimum of 0.5 mL/kg/hr. A nasogastric tube is inserted to decompress the bowel and should be set for low intermittent suction.

The healthcare team should focus on identifying and managing the underlying cause of shock and treating the preexisting medical problems that may be complicating and worsening the patient's condition.

PATIENT OUTCOMES

Nurses can help ensure obtainment of optimal patient outcomes such as those listed in **Box 18-5** through the use of evidence-based interventions for patients with shock.

SUMMARY

Shock is defined as a state in which the tissue metabolic demands of the body are not being met. Physiologically, it may be either hypovolemic, cardiogenic, obstructive, or distribu-

Box 18-5
Patient Outcomes

- Vital signs and hemodynamic parameters within expected range
- Renal function within expected range
- Urine specific gravity within normal limits
- Gastrointestinal status within expected range
- Alveolar exchange of CO_2 and oxygen within expected range
- Tissue perfusion not compromised

tive. The typical situation features a decrease in blood pressure and CO. Regardless of its cause or classification, the end result of a shock state is decreased tissue and cellular perfusion and end-organ dysfunction. Although discussed here separately, shock classifications do not always exist in isolation from one another. That is, the various shock states can be the precipitating cause of another form of shock. The major therapeutic goal in treating all of the shock states is to improve tissue perfusion and achieve balance between oxygen supply and demand.

CASE STUDY 1

Mr. J.L. is a 65-year-old male who was admitted for a complaint of chest pain. A 12-lead ECG revealed ST-segment elevation in leads V1 to V4, signifying a left anterior wall infarction. Several hours later, Mr. J.L. becomes confused and lethargic. You notice neck vein distention. Auscultation of heart sounds reveals a high-pitched, grade IV systolic murmur. Auscultation of lung sounds reveals diffuse coarse crackles. Peripheral pulses have become thready to palpation. Vital signs reveal a decrease in heart rate from 100 beats/min to 70 beats/min, and his blood pressure has dropped from 130/88 mm Hg (MAP of 102 mm Hg) to 80/40 mm Hg (MAP of 53 mm Hg). Urinary output for this past hour has dropped from 1 mL/kg/hr to 0.5 mL/kg/hr.

CRITICAL THINKING QUESTIONS

1. What type of shock does this patient present with?
2. What immediate interventions should be done for this patient?
3. Which medications would you anticipate will be ordered for this patient?
4. What is the physiology behind this patient's neck vein distention and diffuse crackles?
5. What is the physiology behind this patient's decreased mean arterial pressure and urinary output?

CASE STUDY 2

A 28-year-old patient has been admitted to the ICU after a motor vehicle crash. She is intubated and sedated. She has multiple broken bones, cuts, and lacerations. After a few hours, you notice that her heart rate has climbed 20 points (from 80 beats/min to 100 beats/min). Her blood pressure has steadily been declining (from 110/70 mm Hg to 80/35 mm Hg). Her peripheral pulses are thready to palpation, and her skin is cool to touch. Her bowel sounds have become absent and her abdomen, which was soft and palpable, is now tight.

CRITICAL THINKING QUESTIONS

1. What type of shock is this patient in?
2. Where do you think this patient is bleeding?
3. Calculate this patient's mean arterial pressure.
4. What do you think is this patient's SVR?
5. What do you think is this patient's preload?
6. Which interventions would you anticipate so that this patient has improved end-organ perfusion?
7. What is the pathophysiology of this patient's increasing heart rate?

CASE STUDY 3

Mr. S.L. is a 50-year-old male who was in a house fire a month ago. He sustained 57% total body surface area burns. Recently, he has presented with a fever of 39.0°C. His heart rate has increased from 100 beats/min to 130 beats/min. His blood pressure has decreased from 108/50 mm Hg (MAP of 69 mm Hg) to 78/38 mm Hg (MAP of 51 mm Hg). Urine output has declined to 0.25 mL/kg/hr, and his most recent white blood cell count is 15,000 mm^3 (up from 8,000 mm^3 the previous day).

CRITICAL THINKING QUESTIONS

1. How does this type of shock differ from Case Study 2? Why would this patient present with this type of shock?
2. Would you anticipate this patient's urine sodium to be high or low? Why?
3. Would you anticipate this patient to have a low, normal, or high lactate level? Why?
4. Hemodynamically, what would you anticipate this patient's preload and afterload to be?
5. Which medications would you anticipate giving this patient?
6. What stage of shock do you think this patient is in? Why?

Using the Synergy Model to Develop a Plan of Care

	Patient Characteristics	Level (1, 3, 5)	Subjective and Objective Data	Evidence-based Interventions	Outcomes
SYNERGY MODEL	Resiliency				
	Vulnerability				
	Stability				
	Complexity				
	Resource availability				
	Participation in care				
	Participation in decision making				
	Predictability				

CRITICAL THINKING QUESTIONS

1. Write a case example from the clinical setting highlighting one patient characteristic. Explain how the characteristic was observed through subjective and objective data.
2. Utilize the form to write up a plan of care for one client in the clinical setting.
3. Write a case example from the clinical setting. Rate the patient as a level 1, 3, or 5 on each characteristic. Identify the level of nurse characteristics needed in the care of this patient.
4. Take one patient outcome for a patient and list evidence-based interventions found in a literature review for this patient.
5. Which disciplines should be consulted to work with this client?
6. How would you modify your plan of care for patients of diverse backgrounds?
7. What types of issues may require you to act as an advocate or moral agent for this patient?
8. How will you implement your role as a facilitator of learning for this patient?

Online Resources

The following websites offer great online modules to improve your understanding of shock:

Medi-Smart Nursing Education Resources: medi-smart.com

Haemorrahage Shock: www.surgical-tutor.org.uk

Pathophysiology of Various Shock States: compartevents.com/icem2006presentations/PRESENTATIONS/ Wednesday-June-7/critical-care-track_suat_12h00/img3.html

REFERENCES

Alderson, P., Schierhout, G., Roberts, I., & Bunn, F. (2004). Colloids versus crystalloids for fluid resuscitation in critically ill patients. *Cochrane Database of Systematic Review, 4* (CD000567).

Auer, J., Berent, R., Weber, T., Lamm, G., & Eber, B. (2005). Catecholamine therapy inducing dynamic left ventricular outflow tract obstruction. *International Journal of Cardiology, 101*, 325–328.

Barkman, A., & McCay, J. (2002). Cardiogenic shock in a patient with hypertrophic obstructive cardiomyopathy after insertion of a pacemaker. *American Journal of Critical Care, 11*(6), 537–542.

Bench, S. (2004). Clinical skills: Assessing and treating shock: A nursing perspective. *British Journal of Nursing, 13*(12), 715–721.

Bridges, E. J. (2005). Cardiovascular aspects of septic shock: Pathophysiology, monitoring, and treatment. *Critical Care Nurse, 25*(2), 14–16, 18–20, 22–24 passim.

Casey, G. (2001). Oxygen transport and the use of pulse oximetry. *Nursing Standards, 15*(47), 46–53.

Crusher, R. (2004). Anaphylaxis. *Emergency Nurse, 12*(3), 24–31.

Demling, R. H. (2005). The burn edema process: Current concepts. *Journal of Burn Care and Rehabilitation, 26*(3), 207–227.

Dettermeier, P., Swindell, B., Stroud, M., Arkins, N., & Howard, A. (2003). Role of activated protein C in the pathophysiology of severe sepsis. *American Journal of Critical Care, 12*(6), 518–524.

Diehl-Oplinger, L., & Kaminski, M. F. (2004). Choosing the right fluid to counter hypovolemic shock. *Nursing 2004, 34*(3), 52–54.

Doven, O. (2004). Infarction. *Coronary Artery Disease, 15*(6), 361–366.

Hochman, J. S. (2003). Cardiogenic shock complicating acute myocardial infarction: Expanding the paradigm. *Circulation, 107*, 2998–3002.

Johnson, K. B. (2004). Influence of hemorrhagic shock followed by crystalloid resuscitation on propofol: A pharmacokinetic and pharmacodynamic analysis. *Anesthesiology, 101*(3), 647–659.

Jones, G. J. (2002). Anaphylactic shock. *Emergency Nurse, 9*(10), 29–35.

Kelly, D. M. (2005). Hypovolemic shock: An overview. *Critical Care Nurse Quarterly, 28*(1), 2–19.

Khalaf, S., & DeBlieux, P. M. (2001). Managing shock: The role of vasoactive agents. *Journal of Critical Illness, 16*(7), 334–338.

Krost, W. S. (2004). Cardiogenic shock. *Emergency Medical Services, 33*(9), 69–73, 78, 112–113.

Kumar, V., Abbas, A., & Nelson, F. (2005). *Robbins and Cotran pathologic basis of disease* (7th ed.). Philadelphia: Elsevier Saunders.

Lighthall, G. K., & Pearl, R. G. (2003). Volume resuscitation in the critically ill: Choosing the best solution. *Journal of Critical Illness, 18*(6), 252–260.

Marino, P. L. (1998). *The ICU book* (2nd ed.). Baltimore: Williams & Wilkins.

McLlvoy, L., Meyer, K., & Vitaz, T. (2000). Use of an acute spinal cord injury clinical pathway. *Critical Care Nursing Clinics of North America, 12*(4), 521–530.

Muhlberg, A. H., & Ruth-Sahd, L. (2004). Holistic care: Treatment and interventions for hypovolemic shock secondary to hemorrhage. *Dimensions of Critical Care Nursing, 23*(2), 55–61.

Nguyen, H. B., Rivers, E. P., Knoblich, B. P., Jacobsen, G., Mazzin, A., Ressler, J. A., et al. (2004). Early lactate clearance is associated with improved outcome in severe sepsis and sepsis shock. *Critical Care Medicine, 32*(8), 1637–1642.

O'Brien, J. F. (2005). The keys to quickly identifying anaphylaxis. *Journal of Respiratory Diseases, 26*(7), 308–309, 312–316.

Pfisterer, M. (2003). Right ventricular involvement in myocardial infarction and cardiogenic shock. *Lancet, 362*, 392–394.

Pilkington, P. (2004). Humidification for oxygen therapy in non-ventilated patients. *British Journal of Nurses, 13*, 111–115.

Podbregar, M., Krivec, B., & Voga, G. (2002). Impact of morphologic characteristics of central pulmonary thromboemboli in massive pulmonary embolism. *Chest, 122*(3), 973–979.

Rizoli, S. (2003). Crystalloids and colloids in trauma resuscitation: A brief overview of the current debate. *Journal of Trauma, 54*(Suppl. 5), S82–S88.

Roberts, K., Revell, M., Youssef, H., Bradbury, A. W., & Adam, D. J. (2006). Hypotensive resuscitation in patients with ruptured abdominal aortic aneurysm. *European Journal of Vascular Endovascular Surgery, 31*(4), 339–344.

Ruffell, A. J. (2004). Sepsis strategies: An ICU package? *British Association of Critical Care Nurses, 9*(6), 257–263.

Schulman, C. (2002). End points of resuscitation: Choosing the right parameters to monitor. *Dimensions of Critical Care Nursing, 21*(1), 2–14.

Tator, C. H. (2004). Current primary to tertiary prevention of spinal cord injury. *Topics in Spinal Cord Injury and Rehabilitation, 10*(1), 1–14.

Tazbir, J. (2004). Sepsis and the role of activated protein C. *Critical Care Nurse, 24*(6), 40–45.

Tortora, G., & Grabowski, S. (2003). *Principles of anatomy and physiology* (10th ed.). New York: John Wiley & Sons.

Worthley, L. I. G. (2000). Shock: A review of pathophysiology and management. Part I. *Critical Care and Resuscitation, 2*, 55–65.

Yamamoto, L., Schroeder, C., Morley, D., & Beliveau, C. (2005). Thoracic trauma: The deadly dozen. *Critical Care Nurse Quarterly, 20*(1), 22–40.

Vascular Disorders

Rebecca Long

Upon completion of this chapter, the reader will be able to:

1. Identify signs and symptoms of a ruptured abdominal aortic aneurysm.
2. Differentiate between acute arterial and venous occlusions.
3. Identify assessment data to determine the risk for compartment syndrome.
4. Delineate appropriate patient and family teaching strategies for the patient with vascular disease.
5. Recognize resources available to the nursing and healthcare community to further assist in care and education of vascular disease for the patient and family.
6. List optimal patient outcomes that may be achieved through evidence-based management of vascular disorders.

Vascular disease can affect the arterial, venous, and lymph channels throughout the body. Conditions that occur in acute and critically ill patients include abdominal aortic aneurysm (AAA), arterial and venous occlusions of the extremities, and compartment syndrome. The etiology, assessment, management, and patient education for these challenging conditions are reviewed in this chapter. Pertinent problems and complications for patients with vascular diseases are noted as well.

ABDOMINAL AORTIC ANEURYSM

Etiology

An AAA, often referred to as a "triple A," involves a dilatation of the aortic wall in the abdomen. Atherosclerosis and weakening of the vessel media can contribute to the development of these aneurysms. Additional risk factors include alterations in collagen synthesis, male gender, family history, hypertension, diabetes, tobacco use, hypercholesterolemia, trauma, and infection.

AAA rupture is the tenth leading cause of death in men older than 55 years of age (Vascular Disease Foundation, 2005). The prevalence of AAA in adults 65 to 80 years of age is 4% to 7% (Vascular Disease Foundation). These aneurysms occur in men four to five times more frequently than women (American Heart Association, 2005). Men between the ages of 65 and 75 who are or have been smokers should have a one-time ultrasound to screen for AAA, according to a new recommendation from the U.S. Preventive Services Task Force (Fleming, Whitlock, Beil, & Lederle, 2005). Because the normal abdominal aorta measures from 2 to 2.5 cm, aortas larger than 4 cm may be palpable and are typically monitored over time through radiological exams. Once aneurysms become larger than 5 cm, early intervention is warranted, because the likelihood for rupture increases with the size of the aneurysm as well as the rapidity of growth of the dilatation. These aneurysms are targeted for surgical intervention.

Dissection of an aneurysm is life-threatening. Tearing of the vessel wall to create a *false lumen* and subsequent hemorrhage into this lumen creates a blood-filled channel that continues to grow. There is a higher incidence of rupture of abdominal aneurysms (9 per 100,000) as compared to rupture of degenerative thoracic aneurysms (3 per 100,000) (Clouse et al., 2004).

Assessment

Initially, aneurysms may be asymptomatic. They may be detected on a routine physical or when the patient is receiving a diagnostic test for a different problem [e.g., computerized tomography (CT) scan, x-ray, ultrasound, intravenous pyelogram]. As the aneurysm enlarges, bruits may become audible to the left of the umbilicus. The patient may present with abdominal, flank, or low-back pain. If the pain is unrelenting despite position changes, the aneurysm may be leaking (Gonzalez, 2005). Complaints of gastrointestinal discomfort and diarrhea may be present due to the pressure on the mesenteric artery. Leaking can also affect the spinal vertebrae and renal arteries due to a decreased flow of blood, resulting in transient paralysis and anuria.

Ultrasound of the abdomen is the first diagnostic step in determining the presence and size of an aneurysm. Typically, patients will receive an ultrasound every six months to track the progression of an aneurysm, once identified. CT scans, magnetic resonance imaging (MRI), and angiograms of the abdomen may also be used in determining aneurysmal features.

If the aneurysm has ruptured, the patient will need to be monitored for hypovolemic shock. Hypotension, tachycardia, decreased urine output, and altered mental status will be present. Peripheral pulses will be absent or diminished. Mottling over the anterior abdomen may be present or flank ecchymosis can occur.

Medical Management

Intervention is generally not indicated unless the aneurysm has reached 5.5 cm or has demonstrated rapid growth. Leaking necessitates immediate repair no matter what the size of the aneurysm. Intervention may consist of surgical resection and use of a tubular Dacron graft. Ideally, this procedure will be done electively. Endoaneurysmal repair is being undertaken with increasing frequency. Patient selection for this repair is dependent upon several factors (Hall, 2003):

- Patient selection focused on anatomy
- Medical comorbid conditions
- Clinician skill
- Hospital experience and access to various devices
- Diameter and length of AAA
- Presence of thrombus
- Coexistent aneurysmal or occlusive disease

Less invasive is the use of aortic stent grafting, in which a stent is introduced into the body through the groin by a small surgical incision. The stent in the groin is threaded through the abdominal aorta with the help of real-time x-ray images. After the graft is correctly positioned, it is released from the delivery catheter. The device self-expands to match the diameter of the arteries. With this procedure, a large incision in the abdomen is not required. Recovery after stent grafting is generally much quicker, consisting of a couple of days in the hospital followed by normal activity within six weeks.

A number of clinical trials related to AAA are identified in **Table 19-1**. These clinical trials reflect the current trends in prevention, diagnosis, and management of vascular problems.

TABLE 19-1 Clinical Trials Related to Medical Management of Abdominal Aortic Aneurysm

Leg pain study	A nationwide study is underway to test the effectiveness of an approved cholesterol-modifying medication in treatment of claudication. 1-888-LEG-HURT (1-888-534-4878) or visit www.leghurt.com.
Genetic study	Mt. Sinai and Stanford Universities are conducting a trial to understand genetic factors that influence the development of atherosclerosis in coronary or peripheral arteries.
Ultrasound study	The University of Virginia is conducting a study, "Evaluation of Large-Vessel and Microvascular Disease with Contrast Enhanced Ultrasound of Leg Skeletal Muscle," to determine whether ultrasound of the calf muscle can successfully detect peripheral artery disease (PAD).
No pain study	The National Institutes of Health is sponsoring a study on the use of nitric oxide as it relates to pain in the case of peripheral arterial insufficiency. Participants must be able to travel to Stanford University in Palo Alto, California, and must have a positive PAD diagnosis. For more information, contact John Cooke at john.cooke@stanford.edu or 650-725-3778.
Relaxation study	Harvard University will use MRI rapid acquisition with relaxation enhancement and hyperspectral imaging to identify diabetic patients at risk of foot ulceration, and to predict the failure to heal such ulcers.
MRI study	The University of Virginia is planning to develop and test MRI methods to image the arterial wall and characterize atherosclerotic plaque in PAD.

Source: Vascular Disease Foundation. (2005). Clinical trials. Retrieved March 23, 2006, from www.vdf.org/Clinical/listings.php

Nursing Management

For the asymptomatic patient with an AAA, obtaining an initial hemodynamic assessment with blood pressure and peripheral pulses is important. Any patient symptoms should be clearly noted. Monitoring for signs and symptoms of a leak is a crucial part of care and should be conducted each shift.

For the patient with AAA rupture, nursing management is targeted at preservation of tissue perfusion and stabilization of the patient until definitive treatment is arranged. Large-bore intravenous lines should be inserted to allow rapid infusions. Administration of crystalloids and/or blood will be necessary to maintain adequate circulating volume. Administration of warmed blood is preferable to optimize coagulation ability. To reduce or limit the progression of the dissection, lowering the patient's blood pressure will reduce cardiac contractility. This can be accomplished, if not contraindicated (i.e., if the patient is not hypotensive), with the administration of a beta blocker and nitroprusside (Nipride®) intravenously to reduce the patient's blood pressure. Labetalol (Trandate®) may be used in place of nitroprusside and a beta blocker. Hydralazine (Apresoline®) is contraindicated, because it may worsen the dissection.

If there is time, a urinary catheter will be inserted to monitor perfusion of the kidneys and a nasogastric tube will be inserted to decompress the stomach in preparation for surgery/endovascular repair.

One study evaluated postoperative pain in patients in the intensive care unit (ICU) following AAA repair. The researcher acknowledged that postoperative pain causes a sympathetic nervous system reaction, which may increase tissue oxygen needs. Hemodynamically unstable patients may not be able to compensate for this effect and maintain adequate tissue perfusion. As a consequence, these patients are at risk for serious complications. The researcher concluded that a continuous infusion of analgesics promoted better patient outcomes when compared with intermittent administration of opioids. Patients experienced fewer episodes of pain, less pain intensity, and fewer changes in oxygen saturation and heart rate (Stanley, 1996).

A systolic pressure of 70 to 80 mm Hg may be needed to administer analgesics as long as both cerebral and renal perfusion are maintained. As the patient's blood pressure is reduced, some pain relief may be reported because of reduced pressure on the stretched adventitia of the dilated vessel. Because of its mild vasodilating effects, morphine is the drug of choice for pain related to aortic dissection, but its effects on the patient's hemodynamics and ventilatory system must be monitored. For patients with significant hemodynamic compromise, the principle of "scoop and haul" to the surgical suite to expedite life-saving intervention is indicated. In this situation, the patient requires fluids to maintain a blood pressure and needs immediate surgical intervention.

Postoperative care includes monitoring of the patient's hemodynamic and ventilatory systems. Assessment of circulating volume and renal function through observation of blood pressure and central pressures (see Chapter 11 for more details) are critical. Observation of lab values such as hemoglobin and creatinine will be important to monitor because these patients usually require blood products postoperatively and may have a high creatinine level due to a decreased perfusion to the kidneys. Assessment of lower limb perfusion and monitoring for potential complications such as renal failure, myocardial infarction, bleeding or infection, ileus or bowel infarction, and spinal cord ischemia should be done. **Table 19-2** delineates additional nursing interventions.

Patient and Family Education

For patients with known and asymptomatic AAA, education regarding the importance of obtaining regular ultrasounds to monitor the AAA's growth is important (see **Table 19-3**). In addition, signs and symptoms of rupture should be reviewed with the patient, and the patient should know to call 911 or emergency equivalent for the area if symptoms exist. Medic Alert identifiers may be appropriate.

For patients with symptomatic or urgent intervention, psychosocial support is paramount. Such an individual often has a sense of impending doom and may be quite anxious. Calmness and emotional support for the patient and family are important. Education regarding the process of getting ready for surgery and postoperative recovery should be reviewed. Spiritual support should be offered. Balancing the physical, emotional, and spiritual needs of patients with rupture of AAA can be very challenging and yet highly rewarding.

Further education should include making the patient aware that sexual dysfunction is a complication of AAA repair. In men, this typically occurs in the form of retrograde ejaculation, not impotence. Patients usually return to work within six weeks postoperatively after a seven- to ten-day hospitalization.

ARTERIAL OCCLUSION AND VENOUS OCCLUSION

Arterial or venous occlusion is most often due to thrombosis, which involves a blood clot that partially or completely occludes the vascular system. A thrombus may develop on the intima of the vascular system, or it may migrate there from another location. Sequelae of this occlusion depend on factors such as the area either downstream (arterial) or upstream (venous) from the occluded area. Ischemia results when the metabolic needs of the tissues are not adequately met. Arterial occlusion that completely obstructs the vessel requires immediate treatment. Arterial occlusion can occur as a result of a thrombus that originated in the atrium (mural thrombi). A thrombus may also occur in the femoral, iliac, and popliteal arteries. Venous occlusion can be insidious; it can begin in the femoral or iliac veins of the legs. With the advent of central catheters, venous thrombosis has been noted to occur with increasing frequency in the arms. Deep vein thrombosis (DVT) is the term commonly used to describe thrombus in the venous system—most commonly the deep veins of the femoral, iliac, or perineal arteries.

Etiology

Atherosclerosis is the most frequent cause of arterial occlusion and is the result of a process that occurs over years. Arterial disease occurs in men between the ages of 50 and 70—twice as often as in same-age women (American Heart Association, 2005). In one study, the survival rates of patients with claudication were 94.6% at one year, 79.4% at 3 years, 67.3% at 5 years, and 37.4% at 10 years (Kobayashi et al., 2000). Arterial occlusion can also result from trauma and shearing injury. Diabetic patients have higher rates of arterial thrombosis. Tobacco use increases the rate of progression, severity, and amputation rate (Cronenwett & Rutherford, 2001).

Venous thrombosis usually includes two of the following three factors, which are collectively known as Virchow's triad:

- Slowing down of the blood flow (stasis)
- Changes or damage to venous walls (intima)
- Changes in the consistency (coagulability) of the blood

The following conditions contribute to the development of these factors:

- Recent surgery
- Recent trauma to the pelvis or a lower extremity

TABLE 19-2 Clinical Judgment for Nursing Interventions

Interventions	Clinical Judgment
1. Provide pain management	Decreases the stress on the aorta wall so that suture lines can heal.
2. Continuous electrocardiogram (ECG) and hemodynamic monitoring	Keep the patient normotensive with the use of vasodilators because hypertension can cause bleeding. Hypotension can cause organ ischemia and should be treated with fluids. Monitoring for arrhythmias is needed due to the potential for postoperative complications such as myocardial infarction.
3. Complete assessment every 1–2 hours	Close assessment of the patient is warranted the first 48 hours postoperatively to ensure that any changes in patient status can be reported and medical interventions implemented.
4. Prevent postoperative shivering	Gradual warming of the patient is warranted in the first few hours to prevent stress on the aorta.
5. Ventilator management	Oxygenation should be monitored with pulse oximetry to ensure that adequate oxygenation is maintained to prevent organ ischemia.
6. Head of bed less than 45 degrees	Keeps the head low to decrease stress on the aortic graft.
7. Monitor renal function	Ischemia to the kidneys may be indicated by low urinary output and elevated blood urea nitrogen (BUN) and creatinine levels. Interventions such as fluid boluses and diuretics are often needed to maintain renal function in the first 48 hours postoperatively.
8. Wound assessment every shift	Describing the wound and/or dressing each shift provides for continuity of care and monitors for symptoms of infection and bleeding.

- Stroke
- Cancer
- Coagulation disorders
- Heart disease
- Immobilization
- Oral contraceptives
- Vessel disease (such as varicose veins) (Bick, 2000)

Assessment

In arterial occlusion, the patient should be assessed for the following criteria (5 Ps):

- Pain—severe and more sudden onset
- Pallor—paleness of affected area
- Pulse—loss of

TABLE 19-3 Preoperative Patient Education for Patients with Ruptured AAA

- Provide orientation to the environment
- Explain the preoperative interventions such as intravenous lines, fluid administration, urinary catheter, nasogastric drainage, and frequent vital signs
- Discuss pain control
- Review the immediate postoperative interventions and environment
- Discuss spiritual needs

Source: Doenges, Moorhouse, & Geissler-Murr, 2004.

- Poikolothermia—cool or coldness of area downstream
- Paresthesias—impaired motor and sensory function

In venous occlusion, the patient should be assessed for these criteria:

- Pain—aching or throbbing; slower in onset
- Swelling below or of affected extremity
- Redness or increased temperature
- Dilation of superficial veins
- Mottling of the affected area

Medical Management

Heparin is used intravenously to prevent further clot development and to control possible embolic sources. However, if surgery or the use of epidural/intraspinal anesthesia is immediate, heparin is not used due to the risk of bleeding at the surgical site or into the spinal column that may result in paralysis.

Occlusion of the periphery is categorized by the Society for Vascular Surgery/International Society for Cardiovascular Surgery into four classes: viable, marginally threatened, immediately threatened, and irreversible changes. Implications of this stratification include the dictum that patients in more severe stages must have immediate treatment, which may include surgery or interventional radiology.

The difference between endovascular (nonsurgical) versus surgery for arterial occlusion is usually determined by the severity of the ischemia and threat to the individual's limb. Permanent neuromuscular damage can occur in 4 to 6 hours. However, some reperfusion and rescue of tissue may occur with ischemia of up to 12 hours. Amputation may be necessary if the tissue is not salvageable and if byproducts may potentially enter the systemic circulation (Cronenwett & Rutherford, 2001).

For those patients who do not exhibit severe and prolonged ischemia, thrombolysis may be attempted via a catheter in the radiology suite or operating room. If this procedure is unsuccessful, or if the patient has severe ischemia, a thromboembolectomy (removal of thrombus) will be done emergently in the operating room.

Treatment for venous occlusion typically involves bed rest and immobilization of the affected extremity, with the goal of preventing migration of the thrombus. In addition, administration of either unfractionated heparin or a low-molecular-weight heparin is done with a target international normalized ratio (INR) of 2.0 to 3.0. INR is a lab test that measures the clotting mechanism. Current evidence supports administration of a vitamin K antagonist for patients for 3 to 12 months, depending on the cause and incidence of DVT (Buller et al., 2004).

Nursing Management

Nursing care of a patient with occlusion of the arterial or venous system requires careful neurovascular assessments. Management of pain can be challenging. Oral or intravenous opioids are often ordered. Maintenance of fluid balance is also important; intravenous crystalloids may be used for this purpose, because the patient may be on nothing by mouth (NPO) status in preparation for interventions. Antibiotics will be ordered if infection is suspected. Thrombolytics may be used for venous embolism. Patients are placed on bed rest to avoid migration of the clot or due to activity intolerance. If amputation is possible, it is important to monitor the patient preoperatively for systemic sequelae of decreased tissue perfusion, such as acute tubular necrosis or sepsis. In addition, potassium values should be monitored because potassium is released into the bloodstream with cellular destruction. Serious cardiac arrhythmias can occur with excess potassium levels and are often evidenced by peaked T waves in the cardiac rhythm.

COMPARTMENT SYNDROME

Etiology

In compartment syndrome, elevated pressure occurs within a confined space in the body. This condition can be caused by increased volume within a space, such as with bleeding, edema, or fractures, or by decreased compartment size, as in the presence of casts or infiltration of intravenous fluids. Development of this syndrome results when increased amounts of pressure obliterate capillary flow, and it may lead to tissue damage if not treated. Normally, compartment pressures range from 0 to 8 mm Hg. However, if pressures reach 30 to 40 mm Hg, cellular destruction can occur. Muscle dysfunction can occur within 2 to 4 hours; permanent injury such as sensory impairment and loss of function can occur after 12 hours of elevated pressure. In one study, this syndrome was most commonly seen in fractures of the tibial or the radial shaft (McQueen &

Court-Brown (1996). Soft-tissue injury without fractures was the second most common cause of compartment syndrome. This syndrome may occur in the following conditions:

- Trauma such as a fracture, sports injury, or crush injury
- Reperfusion syndrome
- Muscle overuse or damage
- Lower-extremity surgery
- Venomous snakebite or frostbite

Assessment

Identifying patients at risk for development of compartment syndrome is of paramount importance. Regular neurovascular assessments should be performed and documented on all patients identified as being at higher risk. This assessment should observe the patient for both motor and sensory impairment. In particular, the presence of unrelenting pain out of proportion to the injury is significant (Gonzalez, 2005). Patients may have pulses despite the presence of compartment syndrome, because the large arteries are located outside the compartments. Astute nursing observation and communication of findings are key in early recognition of this syndrome. In addition, the urine should be monitored for a reddish-brown color and for the presence of myoglobin. Myoglobin is released from damaged muscle cells and can cause acute tubular necrosis, resulting in renal failure.

Determination of pressures within the compartment is done via a needle attached to a pressure system. The vascular department can assist in determination of compartmental pressures; however, diagnosis of this syndrome may be made based on clinical findings.

Medical Management

Removal of any contributory causes, such as a cast or splint, will be undertaken initially. Decompression of the compartment—called a fasciotomy—may be done surgically. The site is left open for a number of days to allow drainage of the soft tissue.

Nursing Management

Frequent neurovascular assessments are important in cases of compartment syndrome. If the patient does receive a fasciotomy, prevention of infection poses a major challenge due to the presence of the open wound. Meticulous dressing changes are required with appropriate pain management. Because tissue is left exposed following fasciotomy, it may be very sensitive to temperature and movement of air. Monitoring the nutritional status to promote wound healing is important. Finally, recognition of the emotional aspects that an open wound may have on the patient and family is important.

Patient Education

Discussion of the nature and treatment of compartment syndrome with the patient and family is indicated. Measures to prevent infection and the reason for immobilization of the affected extremity should be explained. The importance of adequate nutrition should be reviewed. Pain control can be challenging, because the affected area is often very sensitive.

PATIENT OUTCOMES

Nurses can help ensure obtainment of optimal patient outcomes such as those listed in **Box 19-1** through the use of evidence-based interventions for patients with vascular disorders.

SUMMARY

As life expectancy increases, more patients with vascular disease will require care (Fahey, 2004). In caring for patients with AAA, arterial and venous thrombosis, and compartment syndrome, nurses have opportunities to improve clinical outcomes and decrease complications and readmission rates through vigilant assessments, monitoring, and patient education.

Box 19-1
Patient Outcomes

- Peripheral pulses strong
- Adjustment to changes in health status
- Knowledge of emergency care
- Adherence to treatment plan
- Expressed satisfaction of level of comfort
- Coagulation status, no deviation from expected range
- Tissue perfusion not compromised
- Neurovascular status not compromised

CASE STUDY

A 65-year-old male was admitted to the ICU status post repair of a large infrarenal AAA (6 cm in diameter). His past medical history is significant for hypertension and recent development of back pain. He is a one-pack-per-day tobacco smoker. The AAA was diagnosed from x-rays, which were being done to evaluate his back pain. The aneurysm was palpable as a pulsating mass in his mid-abdomen.

The patient underwent endovascular repair and was transferred to the ICU postoperatively for overnight monitoring. He did not develop any signs of bleeding or infection. All distal pulses to the lower extremities remained palpable. The patient was transferred to the surgical unit the following morning and was discharged home a few days later.

CRITICAL THINKING QUESTIONS

1. Which nursing assessments would be pertinent in this case? Are there additional symptoms such as redness, warmth, or swelling?
2. What are the most likely complications that may occur postoperatively in this patient?
3. Which disciplines should be consulted to work with this client?
4. How would you modify your plan of care for patients of diverse backgrounds?
5. What type of issues may require you to act as an advocate or moral agent for this patient?
6. How will you implement your role as a facilitator of learning for this patient?
7. Based on this case study, design a plan of care utilizing the Synergy Model. The table below is provided to help guide your thinking.

Using the Synergy Model to Develop a Plan of Care

	Patient Characteristics	Subjective and Objective Data	Evidence-based Interventions	Outcomes
SYNERGY MODEL	Resiliency			
	Vulnerability			
	Stability			
	Complexity			
	Resource availability			
	Participation in care			
	Participation in decision making			
	Predictability			

Online Resources

Society for Vascular Nursing: www.svnnet.org

Society of Vascular Nursing (United Kingdom): www.svn.org.uk

American Association of Critical-Care Nurses: www.aacn.org

National Institutes of Health: www.nlm.nih.gov/medlineplus/vasculardiseases.html

American College of Chest Physicians: www.chestnet.org

Society for Vascular Surgery: www.svs.vascularweb.org

American Heart Association: www.americanheart.org

Legs for Life®, the Society of Interventional Radiology (SIR) screening for early detection and monitoring of AAA: www.legsforlife.org

AAA practice guidelines: www.mamc.amedd.army.mil/Clinical/standards/aaa_alg.htm

Prevention for AAA guidelines: www.ahrq.gov/clinic/serfiles.htm

Aneurysm repair video: http://medlineplus.nlm.nih.gov/medlineplus/aneurysms.html

REFERENCES

American Heart Association. (2005). Statistics on abdominal aortic aneurysm. Retrieved October 5, 2005, from www.americanheart.org

Bick, C. (2000). Abdominal aortic aneurysm repair. *Nursing Standard, 15*(3), 47–52, 54–56.

Buller, H., Agnelli, G., Hull, R., Hyers, T., Prins, M., & Raskob, G. (2004). The seventh ACCP conference on antithrombotic and thrombolytic therapy: Evidence-based guidelines. *Chest, 126*(3), 401S–428S.

Clouse, W. D., Hallet, J. W., Schaff, H. V., Spittell, P. C., Rowland, C. M., Ilstrup, D. M., et al. (2004). Acute aortic dissection: Population-based incidence compared with degenerative aortic aneurysm rupture. *Mayo Clinic Proceedings, 79*(2), 176–180.

Cronenwett, J., & Rutherford, R. (2001). *Decision making in vascular surgery.* Philadelphia: W.B. Saunders.

Doenges, M., Moorhouse, M., & Geissler-Murr, A. (2004). *Nurse's pocket guide.* Philadelphia: F.A. Davis.

Fahey, V. (2004). *Vascular nursing.* Philadelphia: W.B. Saunders.

Fleming, C., Whitlock, E. P., Beil, T., & Lederle, F. (2005). Screening for abdominal aortic aneurysm: A best-evidence systematic review for the U.S. Preventive Services Task Force. *Annals of Internal Medicine, 142,* 203–211.

Gonzalez, D. (2005). Crush syndrome. *Critical Care Medicine, 33*(Suppl.), S34–241.

Hall, S. (2003). Endovascular repair of abdominal aortic aneurysms. *AORN Journal, 77*(3), 631–642.

Kobayashi, M., Shindo, S., Kubota, K., Kojima, A., Ishimoto, T., Iyori, K., et al. (2000). Causes of late mortality in patients with disabling intermittent claudication. *Japanese Circulation Journal, 64*(12), 925–927.

McQueen, M. M., & Court-Brown, C. M. (1996). Compartment monitoring in tibial fractures: The pressure threshold for decompression. *Journal of Bone Joint Surgery, 78,* 99–104.

Stanley, K. L. (1996). *A comparison of acute pain responses of patients post abdominal aortic aneurysm repair receiving intermittent or continuous infusion morphine sulfate.* Unpublished doctoral dissertation. Rush University, College of Nursing.

Vascular Disease Foundation. (2005). Disease information. Retrieved October 5, 2005, from http://www.vdf.org/AAA/

Respiratory

CHAPTER 20

Respiratory Anatomy, Physiology, and Assessment

Stephen Parkman

LEARNING OBJECTIVES

Upon completion of this chapter, the reader will be able to:

1. Identify and describe the main structures of the thorax.
2. Differentiate between the primary and accessory muscles used for breathing.
3. Explain the major structures of the upper respiratory tract.
4. Discuss the major structures of the lower respiratory tract.
5. Describe the microanatomy of the respiratory system.
6. Describe the pulmonary circulatory system and explain how gas exchange occurs.
7. Perform a proper respiratory assessment.

The main purpose of the respiratory system is to provide oxygen (O_2) to the cells of the body and to remove carbon dioxide (CO_2), a waste product of cellular metabolism. To perform this vital function, the respiratory system must work in unison with the cardiovascular system. Neither system can perform its primary role without the other. Therefore, the two systems are often collectively referred to as the cardiopulmonary system. This system can be viewed as two structures with two functions that work in synchronization with each other.

ANATOMY OF THE RESPIRATORY SYSTEM

The Thoracic Cavity

The thorax is formed by the rib cage, the thoracic vertebrae, and the sternum. The trachea, esophagus, lungs, heart, and great vessels are protected by the thoracic cavity. The thoracic cavity is wider at the base than at the top. The base of the cavity is bound by the diaphragm, a dome-shaped muscle-fibrous tissue separating the thoracic and abdominal cavities (**Figure 20-1**) (Sherwood, 2004).

The rib cage is composed of 12 pairs of ribs that attach posteriorly to the 12 thoracic vertebrae. Anteriorly, only 10 pairs of ribs are attached directly to the sternum via costal cartilages. The eleventh and twelfth pairs of ribs are referred to as floating ribs or vertebral ribs because they have no connection to the sternum (**Figure 20-2**) (Scanlan, Spearman, & Sheldon, 1995).

Muscles Associated with Breathing

Various muscles of the thorax and abdomen are essential to the movement of gas into and out of the lungs. These muscles may be divided into the primary and accessory muscles of ventilation. The primary muscles of ventilation consist of the diaphragm and the intercostal muscles. Both are utilized during rest and exercise. The accessory muscles assist the primary muscles during conditions of increased ventilatory demand. The accessory muscles are composed of the scalenes, sternomastoids, pectoralis major, and abdominals (**Figure 20-3**) (Scanlan et al., 1995).

The muscles of the respiratory system create negative and positive forces, enabling inspiration and expiration to occur. The lungs have natural elastic recoil secondary to

FIGURE 20-1 Gross Anatomy of the Thorax

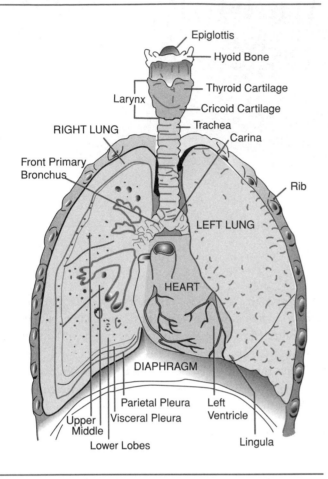

Source: Reprinted with permission from Martin, D. E., & Youtsey, J. W. (1988). *Respiratory anatomy and physiology.* St. Louis, MO: Mosby.

FIGURE 20-2 Rib Cage

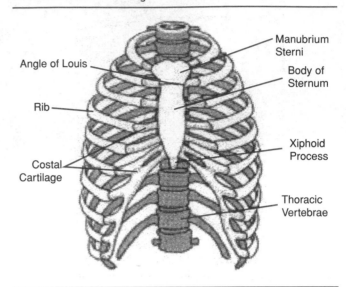

Source: Reprinted with permission from Scanlan, C. L., Spearman, C. B., & Sheldon, R. L. (1995). *Egan's fundamentals of respiratory care* (6th ed.). St. Louis, MO: Mosby.

the action of elastin, an enzyme. In addition, the many small bronchial tubes of the lungs provide airway resistance to air flow. The muscles of the respiratory system attempt to overcome the combined forces of elastic recoil and airway resistance on a breath-to-breath basis.

The primary muscles overcome recoil and resistance to create a negative pressure on inspiration and allow air flow to be drawn into the lungs. As inspiration increases in terms of air volume per unit of time, the accessory muscles will assist the primary muscles in the breathing effort. Expiration is usually passive due to the natural elastic properties of the lung under normal resting conditions. However, as the work of breathing increases, such as with exercise or increased airway resistance, primary and accessory muscles will assist with expiration. The muscles of breathing are just as important as the heart muscle. If either fails, death is soon to follow without medical intervention (Scanlan et al., 1995).

Nerve cells, which have a regulating influence on breathing, originate in the respiratory centers located in the pons and medulla of the brainstem. These nerve impulses are carried via the spinal cord to the various skeletal muscle fibers that play a role in breathing (**Figure 20-4**) (Sherwood, 2004).

Diaphragm

As mentioned earlier, the diaphragm is a dome-shaped musculo-fibrous tissue separating the thoracic and abdominal cavities. It contains several orifices that permit such structures as the esophagus, aorta, inferior vena cava, and several visceral nerves to pass through. The diaphragm facilitates breathing, vomiting, coughing, sneezing, defecation, and giving birth (Scanlan et al., 1995).

The diaphragm is innervated by the phrenic nerve, which is classified as a cervical nerve (**Figure 20-4**). This explains why patients with a cervical spinal cord injury are at risk for disruption of breathing secondary to potential damage to the phrenic nerve.

Stimulation of the muscle fibers of the diaphragm causes the diaphragm to drop downward within the thoracic cavity. This downward drop creates a negative intrathoracic pressure, pulling air into the lungs and creating inspiration. The diaphragm accounts for about 75% of the change in thoracic volume during resting inspiration. In contrast, it does not actively participate in exhalation. It returns to its resting position during the passive recoil of the lungs and thorax.

FIGURE 20-3 The Muscles of Ventilation

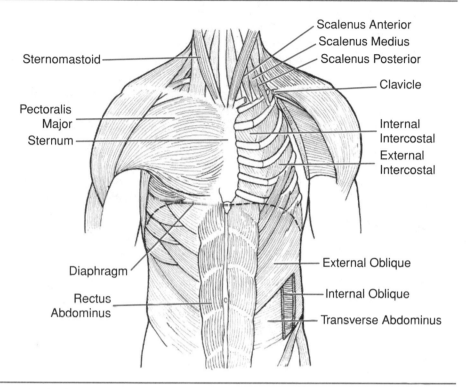

Sternomastoid

Pectoralis
Major
Sternum

Scalenus Anterior
Scalenus Medius
Scalenus Posterior

Clavicle

Internal
Intercostal
External
Intercostal

Diaphragm

Rectus
Abdominus

External Oblique

Internal Oblique

Transverse Abdominus

Source: Reprinted with permission from Scanlan, C. L., Spearman, C. B., & Sheldon, R. L. (1995). *Egan's fundamentals of respiratory care* (6th ed.). St. Louis, MO: Mosby.

Intercostal Muscles

Two sets of intercostal muscles are located between each rib, the external and internal intercostal muscles (Figure 20-3). These muscles are innervated by the intercostal nerves, which emerge from the thoracic spinal cord segment (Figure 20-4). During inspiration in relaxed breathing, the intercostal muscles generate tension, which helps to keep the ribs in constant position relative to one another. This action creates stability of the chest wall. During periods of increased work of breathing, a tremendous amount of negative pressure is created in the thorax during inspiration and, therefore, sinking of the intercostals can occur. This action is often referred to as intercostal retractions (Scanlan et al., 1995).

Scalenes, Sternomastoids, Pectoralis Major, and Abdominals

As mentioned earlier, the scalene, sternomastoids, pectoralis major, and abdominals constitute the accessory muscles of breathing (Figure 20-3). They are located within the neck, thorax, and abdominal areas. Their most important function related to breathing is to assist in ventilation when the diaphragm and intercostal muscles can no longer meet ventila-

tory demands. Patients with severe chronic obstructive pulmonary disease (COPD) rely on these muscles to assist the primary muscles on a regular basis. For individuals with healthy lungs, accessory muscles are used primarily during periods of vigorous exercise (Scanlan et al., 1995).

The Respiratory Tract

The respiratory tract is divided into an upper and lower portion. The upper tract includes the nasal and oral cavities, the pharynx, and the larynx. Its purpose is to warm, humidify, and filter inspired gas. The lower respiratory tract begins at the inferior border of the larynx at the cricoid cartilage and extends all the way to the most distal part of the lungs, the alveoli. It is devoted almost entirely to conduction and interchange of gas. However, both the upper and lower respiratory tracts serve other functions totally unrelated to ventilation, such as providing a sense of smell, phonation (producing sounds through the vocal cords), and swallowing (Sherwood, 2004).

The Upper Respiratory Tract

The upper respiratory tract serves several important respiratory functions. The nasal passages humidify inspired air and exchange heat for the respiratory system and the body. The nose, pharynx, and larynx serve as defense mechanisms for the lungs. These structures also conduct gases to and from the lungs.

The Nasal Cavity. Adults normally breathe primarily through the nose. The nasal cavity serves to defend and humidify the respiratory system. The nasal passages are lined with large hairs. The primary purpose of these hairs is to block entry of particles. In addition, the olfactory region is located within the nasal cavity. This region helps to determine whether the inspired gas is of appropriate quality for the lungs. If the gas is insufficient or polluted, a sneeze may result as the tract attempts to clean itself (Sherwood, 2004).

Bony shelves, called turbinates, are located on the lateral wall of the nasal cavity (**Figure 20-5**). The turbinates are lined

FIGURE 20-4 Nerve Impulses

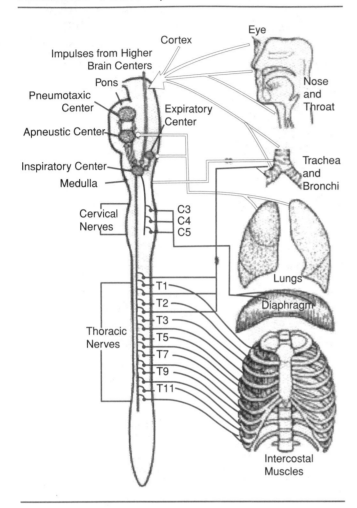

Source: Reprinted with permission from Martin, D. E., & Youtsey, J. W. (1988). *Respiratory anatomy and physiology.* St. Louis, MO: Mosby.

by highly vascular bed tissue, which consists of pseudostratified, ciliated columnar epithelial cells. The turbinates provide a large surface area for heat and moisture exchange. They heat and moisturize inspired gas close to body temperature. This process occurs until the inspired gas reaches the nasopharynx. During expiration, water vapor condenses in the nose, which retains heat and moisture for the next inspiration (Sherwood, 2004).

The Oral Cavity.   The oral cavity is involved in speech, digestion, and respiration. Adults perform mouth breathing during phonation, exercise, or when the nasal cavity is obstructed by infection or foreign material. The mucosal surfaces of the oral cavity also provide humidification and warming of inspired gases, albeit at a less efficient rate than the nasal cavity.

The mouth has protective cough and gag reflexes that help to protect the lower respiratory tract.

The Pharynx.   The pharynx is located posterior to the nasal and oral cavities. It begins behind the nasal cavity and extends down to where the airway and digestive tracts separate. The pharynx is divided into three sections: nasopharynx, oropharynx, and hypopharynx (**Figure 20-6**) (Scanlan et al., 1995).

The nasopharynx lies behind the nasal cavity. Muscles in the soft palate occlude the nasopharynx during coughing or swallowing. Also located within the nasopharynx are the Eustachian tubes and adenoid tonsils. The Eustachian tubes connect the middle ear with the nasopharynx. The adenoid tonsils contain lymphoid tissue that helps to protect entrances to the respiratory and digestive tracts.

The oropharynx is located in the back of the oral cavity. It extends from the back of the soft palate down to the base of the tongue. When the oral cavity is extended open, the oropharynx can be viewed directly. The oropharynx contains the palatine tonsil.

FIGURE 20-5 Upper Respiratory Tract

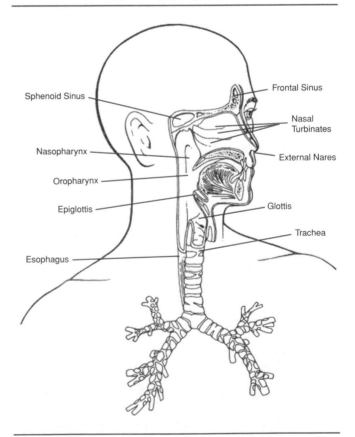

Source: Reprinted with permission from Martin, D. E., & Youtsey, J. W. (1988). *Respiratory anatomy and physiology.* St. Louis, MO: Mosby.

FIGURE 20-6 Pharynx

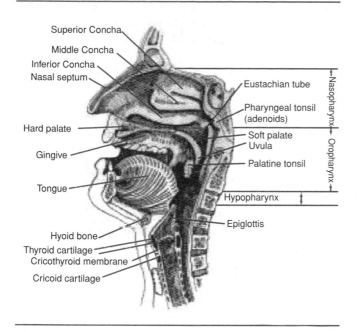

Superior Concha
Middle Concha
Inferior Concha
Nasal septum
Eustachian tube
Pharyngeal tonsil (adenoids)
Hard palate
Soft palate
Uvula
Gingive
Palatine tonsil
Tongue
Hypopharynx
Epiglottis
Hyoid bone
Thyroid cartilage
Cricothyroid membrane
Cricoid cartilage

Nasopharynx → Oropharynx →

Source: Reprinted with permission from Scanlan, C. L., Spearman, C. B., & Sheldon, R. L. (1995). *Egan's fundamentals of respiratory care* (6th ed.). St. Louis, MO: Mosby.

The portion of the pharynx between the epiglottis and the larynx is the hypopharynx. Directly below the hypopharynx is where the respiratory and digestive tracts separate. The hypopharynx changes its shape during swallowing and speech.

The Larynx. The larynx is a complex series of cartilages that are connected to bones by muscles. It is located below the pharynx and is often called the "voice box." The larynx functions as the "security gate" to the lower respiratory tract and is the point at which the respiratory and digestive tracts begin.

One structure of the larynx that is crucial to lower respiratory tract protection is the epiglottis. The epiglottis acts as the chief guardian of the laryngeal opening. This leaf-shaped cartilage extends from the base of the tongue and attaches to the hyoid bone of the larynx. During swallowing, the epiglottis is pushed down and back by the tongue and rising larynx. This motion causes the epiglottis to cover the laryngeal opening and directs food into the esophagus.

The larynx contains the thyroid and cricoid cartilages. The thyroid cartilage, which is often referred to as the "Adam's apple," serves to protect the vocal cords that lie posterior to the cartilages. The vocal cords appear as two white-colored ligaments (**Figure 20-7**). They are actually composed of muscle, ligament, and submucosal soft tissue. The open area between the vocal cords is called the glottis. Sound is produced by vi-

bration of the vocal cords as they constrict and relax as air is exhaled between them (Scanlan et al., 1995).

The Lower Respiratory Tract

The lower respiratory tract begins as the inferior aspect of the cricoid cartilage and extends to the most distal segments of the lungs, the alveoli. This part of the respiratory tract performs the most vital function of the cardiopulmonary system: It conducts respiratory gases and allows gas exchange with the blood. The lower respiratory tract starts with one large airway, the trachea, and divides hundreds of times into smaller airway branchings. These branches eventually reach millions of tiny air sacs called alveoli, where gas and blood share a common boundary.

The Trachea The trachea begins below the vocal cords at the cricoid cartilage and marks the beginning of the conducting system. This single, tubular structure measures 2.0 to 2.5 cm in diameter in the average adult. The trachea is lined with 16 to 20 C-shaped cartilaginous rings, which provide support to the airway. The trachea extends to the level of the aortic arch. At this point, the trachea bifurcates into the right and left mainstem bronchi.

The point at which the trachea bifurcates is marked by a sharp dividing cartilage. This cartilage, which is called the carina, helps to divide air flow to the right and left mainstem bronchi. The right mainstem bronchus angles off at 20 to 30 degrees from midline. The left mainstem bronchus deflects more sharply, at 45 to 55 degrees (**Figure 20-8**). As a consequence, aspirated substances have a tendency to follow the straighter course into the right mainstem bronchus (Scanlan et al., 1995).

FIGURE 20-7 Interior of the Larynx

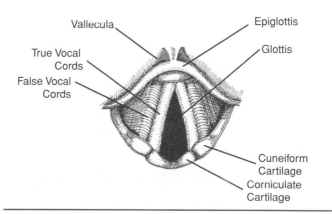

Vallecula
True Vocal Cords
False Vocal Cords
Epiglottis
Glottis
Cuneiform Cartilage
Corniculate Cartilage

Source: Reprinted with permission from Scanlan, C. L., Spearman, C. B., & Sheldon, R. L. (1995). *Egan's fundamentals of respiratory care* (6th ed.). St. Louis, MO: Mosby.

FIGURE 20-8 Angles of Mainstem Bronchi from Midline

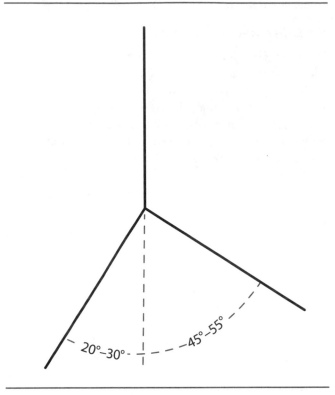

Source: Reprinted with permission from Scanlan, C. L., Spearman, C. B., & Sheldon, R. L. (1995). *Egan's fundamentals of respiratory care* (6th ed.). St. Louis, MO: Mosby.

Segmental Branches. Each mainstem bronchus divides more than 20 times. The right mainstem bronchus divides into the upper, middle, and lower lobe bronchi. The left mainstem bronchus divides into the left upper and lower lobe bronchi. The left lung does not have a middle lobe. A division of the left upper lobe, the lingual, corresponds to the right middle lobe.

The bronchi continue to divide into smaller and more numerous airways. Each branch gives rise to two lower generations. Lobar bronchi divide into segmental bronchi, segmental bronchi divide into subsegmental bronchi, and subsegmental bronchi divide into extremely small airways called bronchioles. Bronchioles measure 1 to 2 mm in diameter and are the smallest conducting airways of the lower respiratory tract. Bronchioles divide further into alveolar ducts and sacs, each containing dozens of individual alveoli. The alveoli are the site of gas exchange.

The cross-sectional area of the conducting system increases exponentially as respiratory gas travels from the trachea down to the terminal bronchioles. At the level of the terminal bronchioles, the cross-sectional area is about 20 times greater than at the trachea. Due to this increase in cross-sectional area, the velocity of respiratory gas flow decreases during inspiration. When inspired respiratory gas reaches the alveoli, its average velocity is about the same as the rate of diffusion. This provides an excellent environment for gas exchange.

Microanatomy of the Conducting Airways

The walls of the conducting airways are all very similar in structure (**Figure 20-9**). All conducting airways are lined with pseudostratified, ciliated columnar epithelial cells. In addition, basal cells in the walls differentiate into ciliated and goblet cells.

Each ciliated cell is lined with about 200 microscopic hairlike projections called cilia. The cilia whip back and forth in a rhythmic manner about 20 strokes per second. In this way, they propel foreign material and mucus up toward the pharynx so that these substances can be expelled (Martin & Youtsey, 1988).

The conducting airways also contain bronchial glands, mast cells, capillaries, smooth muscle, and elastic tissue. The bronchial glands connect to the bronchial surface via long, narrow ducts. Bronchial glands are the major source of respiratory tract secretions in normal, healthy lungs. Their number increases significantly in diseases such as chronic bronchitis. Mast cells are also located within the conducting airways. When stimulated by certain triggers, mast cells can release a potent substance called histamine. Histamine causes vasodilation and bronchoconstriction of the smooth muscle. This type of reaction is often seen in asthma (Scanlan et al., 1995).

Microanatomy of the Terminal Airways and Alveoli

The terminal bronchioles occur at about the seventeenth generation of bronchi. After the terminal bronchioles, the respiratory bronchioles appear. The respiratory bronchioles are referred to as the transitional area of the lung. They lie between zones dedicated solely to conduction and zones dedicated solely to gas exchange. The respiratory bronchioles have some alveolar sacs, so a small amount of respiratory gas exchanges with the blood.

Respiratory bronchioles terminate into alveolar ducts. These ducts are long corridors with clusters of 10 to 16 air sacs, or alveoli, attached to their sides. The alveolus is the final anatomical unit within the respiratory system and the primary site of gas exchange. The alveoli are 240 microns in diameter and number about 300 million in the two lungs. The lungs' surface area is comparable to the size of a tennis court.

The two predominant cells found in the alveolus are alveolar type I and type II cells (**Figure 20-10**). Alveolar type I cells account for about 90% of the alveolar surface area, but only 40% of the total number of alveolar cells. They are very thin, flat cells. Alveolar type II cells are more numerous than type I cells, but because of their shape, they occupy less than 5%

FIGURE 20-9 Sketch of a Microscopic View of the Conducting Airways

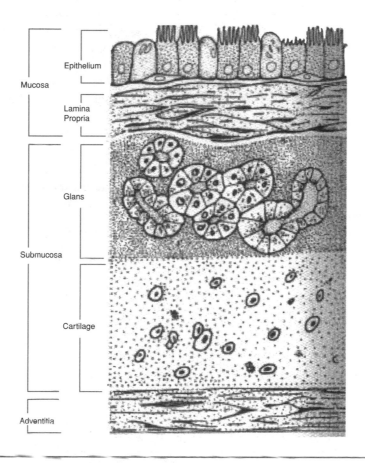

Source: Reprinted with permission from Scanlan, C. L., Spearman, C, B., & Sheldon, R. L. (1995). *Egan's fundamentals of respiratory care* (6th ed.). St. Louis, MO: Mosby.

Pulmonary Circulation and Gas Exchange

The heart and lungs function together as one unit to supply the body's cells with oxygen and to remove carbon dioxide, the waste product of cellular metabolism. The body is continually using oxygen and producing carbon dioxide. Ventilation and pulmonary perfusion must be at an optimal level for gas exchange to occur. This crucial exchange takes place at the alveolar-capillary membrane.

Pulmonary circulation is the movement of blood from the heart, to the lungs, and back to the heart again. It is just one phase of the overall circulatory system. The pulmonary circulation and the lungs work together in unison to achieve optimal gas exchange. Therefore, if either system fails, the other system must work harder to maintain adequate oxygen consumption and carbon dioxide removal.

Two systemic veins, the superior and inferior vena cava,

of the alveolar surface area. These cells produce a surface-tension–lowering substance called pulmonary surfactant. Pulmonary surfactant coats the alveolar walls, reduces surface tension, and improves alveolar compliance, which in turn leads to alveolar stability and reduces the likelihood of alveolar collapse. Pulmonary surfactant is composed of lipids and proteins, with the lipid portion being the key factor in reducing alveolar surface tension. Type II cells proliferate in cases of lung injury and give rise to new type I cells (Scanlan et al., 1995).

A third cell type, the alveolar macrophage, is also found in alveoli. Alveolar macrophages are about 15 to 30 microns in diameter. Their job is to keep the alveoli clean and sterile. Macrophages are bactericidal and can ingest foreign particles. Macrophage activity can be weakened in the presence of cigarette smoke, hypoxia, hyperoxia, ozone, and corticosteroid ingestion.

bring carbon dioxide–rich blood back to the heart, entering the right atrium. The right atrium fills with carbon dioxide–rich blood and then contracts, pushing the blood through the tricuspid valve into the right ventricle. The right ventricle fills and then contracts, pushing the blood into the two pulmonary arteries, which branch to each lung. The pulmonary arteries segment off into tiny vessels called capillaries. These millions of capillaries share extremely thin walls with alveoli called the alveolar-capillary membrane (**Figure 20-11**). It is at this membrane that the removal of carbon dioxide and the intake of oxygen into the capillaries take place. This exchange occurs because of partial pressure gradients and diffusion.

The fresh, oxygen-rich blood enters the four pulmonary veins and then returns to the heart, reentering through the left atrium. The oxygen-rich blood then passes through the mitral valve into the left ventricle. The left ventricle contracts, forcing the blood to exit through the aortic valve and into the main

FIGURE 20-10 Microscopic View of Alveolar Cellular Composition

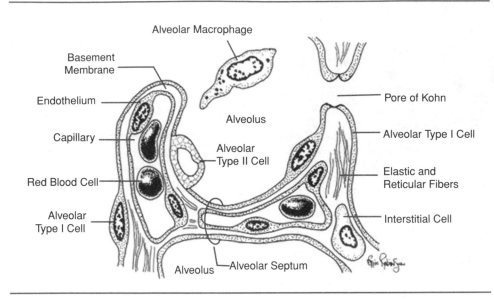

Source: Reprinted with permission from Scanlan, C. L., Spearman, C. B., & Sheldon, R. L. (1995). *Egan's fundamentals of respiratory care* (6th ed.). St. Louis, MO: Mosby.

artery called the aorta. The forceful contraction of the left ventricle forces the blood through the aorta to begin its journey throughout the body. A large majority of oxygen is carried through the blood bound to red blood cells called hemoglobin. Hemoglobin carries oxygen to the cells, where carbon dioxide diffuses from the tissues to the capillaries. Carbon dioxide–rich and deoxygenated blood is then returned to the right atrium via the superior and inferior vena cava and the cycle starts again (Des Jardins & Burton, 2001).

ASSESSMENT OF THE RESPIRATORY SYSTEM

A thorough physical examination of the chest and lungs is essential when performing an assessment of the respiratory system. The physical examination should be conducted in a consistent manner. The general examination steps are as follows: inspection, palpation, percussion, and auscultation.

Inspection

Inspection is the process of obtaining a large amount of information about the clinical status of the patient through a visual inspection. An inspection is based on observing the chest shape, the breathing rate and pattern, and the skin and mucous membranes. Inspection of these three categories can give a quick clinical picture of the patient from a respiratory standpoint (Wheeldon, 2005).

Chest Shape

Chest shape is determined by the anteroposterior (AP) diameter of the thoracic cavity. The AP diameter normally increases gradually with age but may prematurely increase in patients with certain types of COPD. This abnormal increase in AP diameter is often referred to as a barrel chest. In healthy adults, there is a 45-degree angle of articulation be-

FIGURE 20-11 A Normal Alveolar-Capillary Membrane

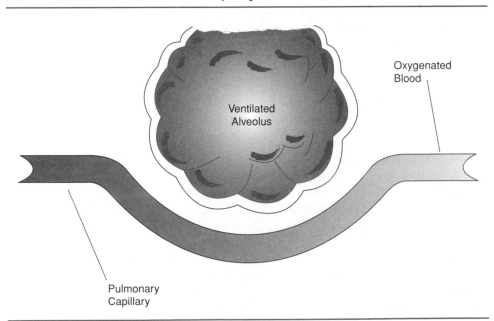

Source: Reprinted with permission from Scanlan, C. L., Spearman, C. B., & Sheldon, R. L. (1995). *Egan's fundamentals of respiratory care* (6th ed.). St. Louis, MO: Mosby.

tween the ribs and spine. However, when the AP diameter increases, the ribs appear horizontal in the thoracic cavity (Oakes, 2004).

Respiratory Rate and Pattern

At rest, the healthy adult has a consistent respiratory rate and rhythm of breathing. The normal respiratory rate of an adult is 12 to 20 breaths per minute. A normal inspiratory-to-expiratory ratio (I:E) is 1 second for inspiration and 2 seconds for expiration. A normal pulse oximetry level is 95% to 100%. Patients with COPD will require prolonged expiration of usually 3 to 4 seconds. Several types of abnormal breathing patterns may occur depending on the disease state of the patient, as seen in **Table 20-1** (Oakes, 2004).

Any respiratory abnormalities that increase the work of breathing may cause the accessory muscles of breathing to become active. With an increase in the work of breathing, the following may occur:

- A change in rate and depth of breathing
- A change in I:E ratio
- Retractions of the intercostal spaces during inspiration
- Nasal flaring
- Pursed-lip breathing
- Patient sitting upright, leaning forward
- Diaphoretic, clammy
- Unable to talk in complete sentences

Skin and Mucous Membranes

The skin and mucous membranes should be observed as part of the inspection. Cyanosis of mucous membranes is a good indicator of poor oxygenation. If the patient is being poorly oxygenated, the mucosal membranes of the nose and mouth will appear blue in color. Furthermore, patients in a chronic hypoxic state may have clubbing of the digits.

Patients with cardiopulmonary disease, such as congestive heart failure or pulmonary hypertension, may present with edema in the legs or ankles in an exacerbated state.

Palpation

Palpation is the process of touching the chest wall to evaluate underlying structures. It is performed to evaluate vocal fremitus, estimate thoracic expansion, and assess the skin and subcutaneous tissues of the chest.

Vocal fremitus refers to the vibrations created by the vocal cords during speech; these vibrations are transmitted down through the chest wall. The feeling of these vibrations on the chest wall is referred to as tactile fremitus. To assess tactile fremitus, the patient is asked to repeat the words "ninety-nine" while the examiner feels the anterior, lateral, and posterior chest wall. The vibrations of tactile fremitus may be increased, decreased, or absent depending on the disease state of the lung (**Table 20-2**) (Oakes, 2004).

Thoracic expansion is assessed by placing both of the examiner's hands on the patient's posterior chest at the level of T9 or T10 and observing movement of the hands during a deep inspiration. The normal chest wall expands symmetrically during deep inhalation. Diseases such as COPD, which affects both lungs, can cause a bilateral reduction in chest expansion. Diseases that may affect only one lung, such as atelectasis, pleural effusion, or pneumothorax, may cause unilateral expansion.

Palpation can be used to examine for subcutaneous emphysema (also known as crepitus). This condition arises when air leaks from the lung into the subcutaneous tissues. Fine

---

TABLE 20-1 Abnormal Breathing Patterns

Pattern	Characteristics	Causes
Apnea	No breathing	Respiratory or cardiac arrest
Biot's	Irregular breathing with long periods of apnea	Increased intracranial pressure
Cheyne-Stokes	Irregular type of breathing; breaths increase and decrease in depth and rate with periods of apnea	Central nervous system diseases; drug overdose
Kussmaul's	Deep and fast	Metabolic acidosis
Apneustic	Prolonged inhalation	Brain damage
Paradoxic	Sinking in of the abdominal wall with each inspiratory effort	Muscle fatigue
Asthmatic	Prolonged exhalation	Obstruction to air flow out of lungs

Sources: Oakes, 2004; Wheeldon, 2005.

TABLE 20-2 Causes of Abnormal Tactile Fremitus

Increased Fremitus Vibrations	Decreased Fremitus Vibrations
Areas of consolidation:	Bronchial obstruction with
Atelectasis	mucus plug or foreign object
Fibrosis	Pneumothorax
Infarct	Pleural effusion
Pneumonia	COPD
Tumor	Muscular or obese chest wall

Source: Oakes, 2004.

TABLE 20-3 Normal Breath Sounds

Type	Description
Vesicular	Normal sound over most of lungs
Bronchovesicular	Normal sound over upper half of sternum
Bronchial	Normal sound over the trachea

Source: Oakes, 2004.

bubbles in the subcutaneous tissues produce a crackling sensation when palpated (Des Jardins & Burton, 2001). Subcutaneous emphysema may be palpated in the following conditions: high positive end-expiratory pressure (PEEP) setting, pneumothorax, pneumomediastinum, around chest tube sites, and barotraumas.

Percussion

Percussion is the process of tapping on a surface in an effort to evaluate the size and density of the underlying structure. Percussion of the chest wall produces a sound and a palpable vibration useful in evaluating underlying lung tissue. Percussion is performed by placing the distal portion of the middle finger of the nondominant hand firmly on the chest wall while striking this finger behind the nail bed or the distal interphalangeal joint.

Percussion notes are commonly referred to as resonance, dullness, or hyperresonance. Resonance is heard over a normal lung. Dull percussion notes are heard in patients with chest disorders such as pleural effusion, atelectasis, or consolidation. When the chest is percussed over areas of trapped gas, a hyperresonant note is produced. These sounds are described as loud, low in pitch, and long in duration; they are commonly heard in patients with asthma, emphysema, or pneumothorax (Des Jardins & Burton, 2001).

Auscultation

Auscultation, using a stethoscope, over the thorax is performed to identify normal or abnormal lung sounds. Normal breath sounds are described in **Table 20-3**. Abnormal sounds or vibrations produced by the movement of air in the lungs are termed adventitious sounds. Adventitious breath sounds are described in **Table 20-4**.

SUMMARY

The respiratory system is a complex unit whose primary role is to provide gas exchange on a breath-to-breath basis. For this to occur, the respiratory system must extend beyond the anatomical boundaries of the lungs. The thoracic cavity stabilizes and protects the lungs. Various muscles of the thorax and abdomen are essential to the movement of gas into and out of the lungs. Motor neurons innervate the muscles of ventilation.

TABLE 20-4 Adventitious Breath Sounds

Type	Description	Location	Common Causes
Crackle	High-pitched crackling during inspiration	Alveoli, bronchioles	Pulmonary edema, pneumonia
Wheeze	Musical-high pitched usually during expiration but may occur during inspiration	Bronchi, bronchioles	Asthma, bronchitis, tumor, foreign body
Stridor	Loud, high-pitched crowing in upper airway	Upper airway obstruction	Croup, epiglottitis, laryngospasm, foreign body
Rub	During inspiration, loud, harsh, grating vibration	Pleural space rub	Pleurisy

Source: Oakes, 2004.

The upper respiratory tract humidifies and filters the gas that enters the lungs. The lower respiratory tract provides the arena for gas and capillary blood to interact and acts as a defense ground against foreign microbes.

The respiratory system responds quickly to changing physiologic demands. When the system becomes compromised due to disease, trauma, or infection, it is more difficult to meet physiologic demands. The clinician must assess and identify signs and symptoms of respiratory compromise and treat the patient accordingly to restore normal function.

Patient assessment is a major role for the intensive care unit (ICU) nurse. In addition to the four steps of the respiratory assessment described previously, an expanded assessment can help ensure patients receive appropriate care. Nurses in the ICU are well positioned to be able to perform a comprehensive respiratory assessment on their patients (Cox & McGrath, 1999). The questions asked by the ICU nurse should provide information that paints a complete picture of the patient's respiratory status. The focus of the assessment is described in **Table 20-5**.

TABLE 20-5 Respiratory Assessment

Presence of respiratory distress at time of assessment[*]
(description, SpO_2, vital signs, accompanying symptoms [mental status changes, anxiety], possible precipitating cause)

Past medical history

Family history (e.g., asthma)

History of respiratory symptoms (e.g., shortness of breath, productive or nonproductive cough, orthopnea, allergies)

Description of sputum (if applicable)

Use of respiratory medications (prescription or over-the-counter)

Use of oxygen at home

[*]If the patient is in respiratory distress, defer comprehensive assessment until the patient is stabilized.
Sources: Cox & McGrath, 1999; Des Jardins & Burton, 2001.

CRITICAL THINKING QUESTIONS

1. What are the primary muscles of ventilation?
2. What function does the upper respiratory tract serve?
3. What is the primary purpose of alveolar type II cells?
4. Where is the respiratory center of the brain located?
5. If a patient aspirates, which lung is likely to become infected? Why?
6. What are the four steps of a respiratory assessment?
7. What type of chest shape is a COPD patient likely to have?
8. What types of physical signs may a patient in respiratory distress exhibit?

Online Resources

The R.A.L.E. Repository—sound recordings: www.rale.ca/repository.htm

Anatomy and Physiology of the Respiratory System:
http://www.le.ac.uk/pathology/teach/va/anatomy/case2/frmst2.html

REFERENCES

Cox, C. L., & McGrath, A. (1999). Respiratory assessment in critical care units. *Intensive Care Medicine, 15*(4), 226–234.

Des Jardins, T., & Burton, G. G. (2001). The physical examination and its basis in physiology. In T. Des Jardins & G. G. Burton (Eds.), *Clinical manifestations and assessment of respiratory disease* (4th ed., pp. 17–56). St. Louis, MO: Mosby.

Martin, D. E., & Youtsey, J. W. (1988). *Respiratory anatomy and physiology.* St. Louis, MO: Mosby.

Oakes, D. (2004). Bedside patient assessment. In D. Oakes, *Clinical practitioner's pocket guide to respiratory care* (6th ed., pp. 1–15). Orono, ME: Health Educator Publications.

Scanlan, C. L., Spearman, C. B., & Sheldon, R. L. (1995). Functional anatomy of the respiratory system. In G. Ruppel & J. Tesoriero (Eds.), *Egan's fundamentals of respiratory care* (6th ed., pp. 178–212). St. Louis, MO: Mosby.

Sherwood, L. (2004). *Human physiology.* Belmont, CA: Brooks/Cole—Thomson Learning.

Wheeldon, A. (2005). Respiratory assessment. Exploring nursing roles: Using physical assessment in the respiratory unit. *British Journal of Nursing, 14*(10), 571–574.

Wilkins, R. L., Krider, S. J., & Sheldon, R. L. (2000). *Clinical assessment in respiratory care* (4th ed.). St. Louis, MO: Mosby.

Respiratory Monitoring

Dianna Levine

Respiratory monitoring (see **Table 21-1**) entails continuous and thorough physical assessment for vulnerable patients. It includes monitoring changes in mental status because confusion and restlessness can be caused by hypoxia of the central nervous system (CNS). Cardiac monitoring can reveal cardiac dysrhythmias that may indicate impending respiratory insufficiency. Monitoring ventilation includes noting the patient's respiratory rate, rhythm, chest excursion, and breath sounds. The character of pulmonary secretions should be monitored (tenaciousness, color, and smell). To ensure that air enters the alveolus unencumbered, the patient is hydrated to liquefy secretions and chest physical therapy is done to mobilize the secretions. Coughing is encouraged. If patients are unable to clear their airway, they may be suctioned. Coughing and deep breathing prevent atelectasis. Monitoring fluids is a primary goal so that euvolemia (normal volume status) is maintained and fluid overload is prevented. The effects of medications are monitored, such as dilators that are given for bronchospasm and diuretics that are used to treat or prevent pulmonary edema. The aim of all these interventions is to ensure that air reaches the alveolar capillary membrane so that gas exchange can take place.

For gas exchange to occur, blood must circulate through the pulmonary capillaries. Perfusion of blood can be impaired by low pressures or by a block in the pulmonary vasculature. Blood pressure is monitored and, when needed, vasopressors are administered in an attempt to provide perfusion to the alveolar capillary bed and provide sufficient circulation to transport blood to the cells throughout the body. As part of this effort, the patient is monitored for signs of thrombophlebitis. Prevention protocols are also instituted. One aim of these protocols is to protect lung perfusion because most pulmonary emboli originate from a clot formation that travels from the lower extremities (Church, 2001).

Monitoring hemoglobin provides information about the oxygen-carrying capacity of the blood. With airway patency and perfusion maintained, how well the gases have diffused across the alveolar-capillary membrane is monitored. This monitoring entails the use of pulse oximetry (SpO_2 monitoring), arterial blood gases (ABGs), and, to a lesser extent, capnography ($EtCO_2$ [end-tidal CO_2] monitoring). This chapter focuses on these three monitoring modalities, their indications for use, their limitations,

TABLE 21-1 Terms to Know

Respiration: The exchange of oxygen and carbon dioxide by the lung.

Ventilation: Movement of air between the atmosphere and the alveolus.

Perfusion: The flow of blood through the lungs.

Diffusion: The mechanism for transfer of gases at the alveolar-capillary membrane.

Hypoxia: Reduced oxygen in the tissues.

Hypoxemia: Reduced oxygen in the blood.

Atelectasis: Collapse of the alveoli.

and the interpretation of their values. The ultimate goal is to provide adequate cellular oxygenation. Appropriate and timely recognition of changes and management will promote positive patient outcomes.

SpO$_2$ MONITORING (SATURATION OF PERIPHERAL O$_2$)

Pulse oximetry has become a standard for monitoring the respiratory status of patients in critical care. Pulse oximetry is indicated for any patient at risk for respiratory compromise and is used to monitor the effects of oxygen therapy. In the intensive care unit (ICU), a pulse oximeter is usually a component of a monitoring system and provides continuous information about changes in oxygen saturation and pulse rate. It is commonly measured on a finger, an earlobe, or the bridge of a nose, using a probe suitable for the site that is chosen.

Pulse oximetry has the advantage of being noninvasive, easy to use, and cost-effective. It consists of a probe that is placed on a vascular area such as a finger or an earlobe. The probe or sensor contains two light-emitting diodes—one red and one infrared—and a photodetector. The photodetector is placed opposite to the light source. It can determine the amount of light that is absorbed by both frequencies. The infrared light detects both oxyhemoglobin (hemoglobin saturated by oxygen) and deoxygenated hemoglobin (hemoglobin that is without oxygen) (Grap, 2002).

The sensor monitors the arteriolar vascular bed's pulsation. It transfers this information to a screen that displays a waveform generated by this pulsatile force. An audible tone is produced with each pulse detected. The oximeter takes from 3 to 10 seconds to stabilize before revealing the patient's SpO$_2$ (oxygen saturation), which is displayed as a percentage. A normal value is considered to be 97% to 99% for a healthy person. An SpO$_2$ of 90% or less usually indicates respiratory failure, ne-

cessitating the administration of supplemental oxygen (Carroll, 2003a). A patient with a chronic respiratory disease, however, might tolerate lower oxygen saturations. For each patient, the desired parameter at which to notify the physician should be specified and alarms set appropriately. Pulse oximetry results of 70% or lower may not be accurate (Grap, 2002).

The technology for respiratory monitoring became available in critical care in the 1980s. Prior to that time, monitoring for cyanosis was the assessment parameter indicative of perfusion and oxygenation. Cyanosis, a late indicator of respiratory failure, occurs when the SpO$_2$ decreases to a level of 80% to 85% (Giuliano & Higgins, 2004). The advent of pulse oximetry was a welcome development, and today this technology is a standard monitoring modality in the ICU. Healthcare professionals, however, were not always informed about its limitations (see **Box 21-1**). Until recently, educational deficits have been recognized in staff members who commonly used this technology.

Knowing the limitations of respiratory monitoring can prevent unwarranted dependence on the use of this monitoring technique as the sole intervention. Monitoring of the patient's overall status should be a prime consideration. Alarms should be individualized according to the goal of therapy for the patient. Limits should be designated as being within 5% of the patient's acceptable baseline (Schutz, 2001); however, a low alarm of less than 90% can place the patient in jeopardy. If multiple changes in oxygen saturation occur instantaneously, it usually indicates a technical problem rather than a change in the patient's condition; in such a case, the equipment should be checked. Oxygen saturation can also decrease with patient activity. When a pulse oximeter is applied, the site should be warm, proximal pulses should be present, and capillary refill should be brisk. The probe site should be periodically evaluated to prevent skin breakdown.

Patients should be informed that the pulse oximeter is only one way that their oxygenation is being monitored and that the values displayed will vary depending on the position of the sensor, the amount of light in the room, or their activity. Alarms are often set off by these extraneous factors rather than oxygenation saturations that are below desirable limits.

ARTERIAL BLOOD GAS MONITORING

ABG (see **Table 21-2**) monitoring provides a comprehensive picture of oxygenation, ventilation, and acid–base balance. It is also used to initiate therapy and to monitor the effectiveness of therapy. An arterial blood specimen is taken using a heparinized syringe. All air bubbles are removed. The specimen is immediately taken to the lab to be analyzed, often on ice to slow oxygen metabolism. To ensure accuracy of the results and their subsequent interpretation and appropriate interventions,

Box 21-1
Limitations of Pulse Oximetry

1. Pulse oximetry does not give information about the amount of hemoglobin, so overall oxygen content is not available through this kind of monitoring (Carroll, 2003b). The patient can have an SpO$_2$ of 99% but have tissue hypoxia because the individual does not have enough hemoglobin to adequately oxygenate tissues. If hemoglobin levels are high, the patient may have enough oxygen to meet the metabolic demands of the body but not all the hemoglobin molecules may be saturated, leading to a low SpO$_2$ value.
2. Pulse oximetry does not give information about how well the patient eliminates carbon dioxide. Carbon dioxide is the major waste product of cellular metabolism and is regulated by the lungs. It contributes to the patient's acid–base status. High levels of carbon dioxide are caused by hypoventilation; low levels are caused by hyperventilation.
3. Carbon monoxide has an affinity for hemoglobin and displaces oxygen. It gives a bright red color to the blood that is detected by pulse oximetry as oxygen, leading to a falsely high SpO$_2$ reading. Patients who smoke cigarettes are affected, as are patients who are admitted for smoke inhalation.
4. Methemoglobinemia is a condition that can be caused by nitrate administration, inhaled nitric oxide, or topical anesthetics. It produces abnormal hemoglobin that cannot bind with oxygen. If methemoglobin is present, the SpO$_2$ values will be distorted (Giuliano & Higgins, 2004).
5. Motion artifact (interference) can affect the accuracy of pulse oximetry. Rhythmic movement such as seizure activity, tremors, or shivering can cause falsely high pulse/heart rate detection. This problem can be identified by noting a difference between the patient's radial pulse and the pulse detected by the oximeter. If this problem is encountered, the probe can be placed on the ear using an appropriate sensor. New-generation pulse oximeters minimize motion interference.
6. Patients who are hypotensive may develop vasoconstriction of their extremities as the body attempts to shunt blood to the vital organs. When perfusion is compromised in the extremity, the pulse is weak and will not be detected by the pulse oximeter. Readings either are absent or falsely low.
7. Cool extremities cause vasoconstriction and poor pulse quality. This factor contributes to absent or falsely low readings.
8. Applying a sensor to the extremity with an automatic blood pressure cuff will interfere with the instrument's ability to detect a pulse when the cuff inflates. This will activate unwanted alarms.
9. Bright lights can be detected by the photosensor and affect the readings. The probe can be shielded with a cloth to prevent this problem.
10. Dark nail polish may cause false results. Nail polish should be removed. If this is not possible, the probe can be placed sideways.
11. Some dyes used during procedures, such as methylene blue, indiocyanine green, and indiocarmine, can produce false readings. The half-life of these substances should be noted (Philips Medical Systems, 2003).

TABLE 21-2 Terms to Know for ABGs

ABG: Arterial blood gas.
Acidemia: An acid–base disturbance that indicates an excess amount of acid in the blood.
Alkalemia: An acid–base disturbance that indicates an excess amount of base in the blood.
PaO$_2$: The partial pressure of arterial oxygen.
FiO$_2$: The fraction of inspired oxygen.

the FiO$_2$, mode of administration, respiratory rate, and patient's temperature at the time the blood was obtained should accompany the specimen.

Obtaining arterial specimens has several limitations: The procedure can be painful; it can cause damage to the vessel; it compromises blood flow distal to the puncture; and, if not followed by pressure on the site for an adequate amount of time, bleeding can occur. Unfortunately, an ABG does not provide immediate or continuous information. If frequent ABG monitoring is anticipated, an arterial line should be inserted. An arterial line allows the nurse to have a continuous source for drawing ABG specimens while receiving information on the patient's arterial pressure.

Continuous intravascular blood gas monitoring has been studied in some ICUs for a select group of patients requiring repeated blood gas measurements for at least 48 to 72 hours. In this type of monitoring, PO_2, PCO_2, and pH can be measured with electrochemical and photochemical/optical sensors in the radial artery. This technique provides for continuous data but has the disadvantage of yielding unreliable data due to motion, vasospasms, or decreased blood flow. Because of its high costs and minimal benefits, this monitoring device continues to be evaluated in exploratory studies (Ganter & Zollinger, 2003).

Ninety-seven percent of the blood's oxygen is attached to hemoglobin. The remaining 3% is dissolved in the plasma and is measured in the ABG as PaO_2. The greater the partial pressure of oxygen in the blood, the more oxygen that is maintained on the hemoglobin. The normal value is 80 to 100 mm Hg, with 60 mm Hg as the critical value indicative of hypoxemia and mandating use of supplemental oxygen. A value of 45 mm Hg represents a threat to life. The oxyhemoglobin dissociation curve (**Figure 21-1**) shows the percentage of SaO_2 at different partial pressures (Berry & Pinard, 2002).

The oxygen saturation does not change significantly until the partial pressure of oxygen reaches 60 mm Hg (represented by the flat portion of the curve). Then, very little change in partial pressure causes a rapid decline in the oxygen saturation (Berry & Pinard, 2002).

This curve can move either to the right or to the left due to different factors. When the curve shifts to the right, the hemoglobin has less affinity for oxygen and O_2 is released to the cells easily. Conditions that cause a shift to the right include decreased pH, increased pCO_2, hyperthermia, and increased 2,3-DPG (2,3-diphosphoglycerate), a product of glycolysis. A shift to the left indicates that the hemoglobin has a greater affinity for oxygen, making it more difficult to release oxygen to the cells. Conditions that cause a shift to the left include increased pH, decreased CO_2, hypothermia, and less 2,3-DPG. Banked blood does not contain 2,3-DPG and shifts the curve to the left. Monitoring these conditions is important because they influence oxygenation at the cellular level (Berry & Pinard, 2002).

The purpose of respiration is not only to provide oxygenation to the cells but also to help maintain the body's acid–base balance by eliminating or retaining carbon dioxide. Through both of these roles, the cells of the body remain viable. Acid–base balance is monitored by ABG analysis. **Table 21-3** lists the components of the blood gases and their normal values.

pH

An acid donates hydrogen ions, and a base accepts them. A measurement of H^+ ions in a solution is pH. When the H^+ concentration increases in the body, the pH falls; when the H^+ concentration decreases, the pH rises. A pH of 7 is considered neutral. The body's pH is normally between 7.35 and 7.45, so the body is slightly alkaline. With a pH value of less than 7.35, acidosis occurs; a pH greater than 7.45 is called alkalosis.

PaCO$_2$

The lungs regulate $PaCO_2$. This parameter's normal value is 35 to 45 mm Hg. $PaCO_2$ in solution is called carbonic acid. An excess in $PaCO_2$ ($>$ 45 mm Hg) results in respiratory acidosis. Too little $PaCO_2$ ($<$ 35 mm Hg) causes respiratory alkalosis. Conditions that cause respiratory acidosis include:

- Hypoventilation
- CNS disturbances that damage the respiratory center in the medulla
- Medications that depress the respiratory center

FIGURE 21-1 Oxyhemoglobin Dissociation Curve

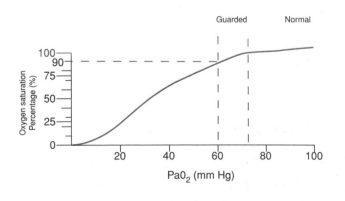

Source: Illustrated by James R. Perron.

TABLE 21-3 Arterial Blood Gas Normal Values

Component	Normal Values	Comments
pH	7.35–7.45	A scale that measures acidity or alkalinity
PaCO$_2$	35–45 mm Hg	Partial pressure of arterial carbon dioxide
PaO$_2$	80–100 mm Hg	Partial pressure of arterial oxygen
HCO$_3$	22–26 mEq/L	Bicarbonate ion
SaO$_2$	95%–100%	Arterial saturation of oxygen
BE	−2 to +2	Base excess

- Pulmonary disease that affects diffusion (chronic obstructive pulmonary disease [COPD], pneumonia, pulmonary edema)
- Airway obstruction

Conditions that cause respiratory alkalosis include:

- Hyperventilation
- Anxiety reactions
- CNS disturbances that stimulate the respiratory center in the medulla, such as some brain tumors, meningitis, and encephalitis
- Hyperthyroidism

HCO_3

The kidneys regulate HCO_3. The normal value of HCO_3 is in the range of 22 to 26 mEq/L. HCO_3 represents the metabolic component of the blood gas. Too little HCO_3 (< 22 mEq/L) is metabolic acidosis. Too much HCO_3 (> 26 mEq/L) is metabolic alkalosis. The following conditions cause metabolic acidosis:

- Diabetes
- Starvation
- Anaerobic metabolism
- Chronic diarrhea

The following conditions cause metabolic alkalosis:

- Vomiting
- Gastric suction
- Hypokalemia
- Excessive use of antacids

COMPENSATION

The body attempts to maintain a ratio of 20:1 bicarbonate to acid, which equates to a pH of 7.40. This balancing act is called compensation. Respiratory compensation occurs in seconds to minutes; in contrast, it takes the kidneys hours or days to compensate. The respiratory center in the medulla responds to changes in pH. When metabolic acidosis occurs (HCO_3 < 22 mEq/L), the respiratory center is stimulated and hyperventilation occurs in an effort to blow off acid and return the acid–base ratio to normal. When metabolic alkalosis occurs (HCO_3 > 26 mEq/L), the respiratory center is depressed. In an attempt to hold on to acid, the rate and depth of respiration decrease. The renal tubules respond to the pH level. When respiratory acidosis occurs, the kidneys will excrete H^+ ions and hold on to HCO_3. When respiratory alkalosis occurs, the kidneys will hold on to the H+ ions and excrete HCO_3. If the pH is returned to 7.35–7.45, compensation has taken place. An attempt to reach this pH is called partial compensation (Pruitt & Jacobs, 2004).

When compensation occurs, looking at the variation from the normal pH of 7.40 identifies the primary disturbance. If the value is less than 7.40, acidosis is the primary disturbance. If the value is greater than 7.40, alkalosis is the primary disturbance.

BASE EXCESS

Base excess is the amount of HCO_3 needed to return the pH to normal. This calculated value is not related to a respiratory component of the acid–base balance. The following examples will guide you through the steps for interpreting blood gases.

Questions Asked to Analyze Arterial Blood Gases

1. Is it acidic or alkaline?
2. What is the cause?
3. Is there compensation?

Example 1

Mrs. B. is being admitted to the ICU following emergency gallbladder surgery for monitoring due to a recent history of myocardial infarction (MI). Prior to her transfer from the postanesthesia care unit (PACU), she was extubated. She is able to be aroused but remains sedated. Her post-extubation ABG levels are pH 7.32; $PaCO_2$ 57.8; and HCO_3 26.1.

1. Is it acidic or alkaline? 7.32 = acidic.
2. What is the cause? Acidosis is caused by a high $PaCO_2$ or a low HCO_3. The $PaCO_2$ is high, making the primary disturbance respiratory.
3. Is there compensation? The HCO_3 is normal and the pH is abnormal, so compensation has not taken place.

This patient has an uncompensated respiratory acidosis. Due to the sedation, she is hypoventilating and is unable to eliminate CO_2.

Example 2

Mr. R. is admitted from the emergency department (ED) to the ICU due to uncontrolled diabetes. He has rapid and deep respirations and a fruity smell to his breath. He has poor skin turgor and dry mucous membranes. His ABG levels are pH 7.36; $PaCO_2$ 28; and HCO_3 20.

1. Is it acidic or alkaline? 7.36 is on the acid side of normal.
2. What is the cause? Acidosis is caused by a high $PaCO_2$ or a low HCO_3. The HCO_3 is low, making the primary disturbance metabolic.
3. Is there compensation? The pH is normal and the $PaCO_2$ is low, so compensation has taken place.

This patient has compensated metabolic acidosis. His blood sugar is 400 mg/dL. Due to insulin deficiency, he is unable to metabolize sugar and is utilizing his protein stores for energy. A byproduct of protein metabolism is ketones, which are acids. Mr. R. is blowing off carbon dioxide to compensate for the acidosis (Kussmaul respirations).

$EtCO_2$ MONITORING

$EtCO_2$ (see **Table 21-4**) is a noninvasive method for measuring the amount of CO_2 at end-expiration. It approximates the $PaCO_2$ in healthy individuals, with $EtCO_2$ having a gradient of 2 to 5 mm Hg lower than that for $PaCO_2$. Changes in $EtCO_2$ can be detected much earlier than changes in SpO_2, and supplemental oxygen has been shown to keep SpO_2 levels high with periods of apnea even when CO_2 values reach dangerous levels (Carroll, 2002).

One method commonly used to detect CO_2 is to pass exhaled air through a sample chamber that exposes it to infrared light. The capnometer measures the amount of infrared light absorbed by CO_2 as compared to the amount of light absorbed by a control sample that does not contain CO_2. Another method measures the molecular weight of expired CO_2.

Two methods for the analysis of CO_2 are mainstream and sidestream. Mainstream analysis utilizes a chamber to the air circuit closest to an endotracheal or tracheotomy tube where the sensor analyzes the exhaled air. The advantage of mainstream analysis is that measurements are immediate (Anderson & Breen, 2000). Sidestream analysis entrains exhaled air into a tube connected to a chamber containing the sensor. The advantage of sidestream analysis is that it can be used on both intubated and nonintubated patients. There is a slight delay in the analysis, however. When the patient is spontaneously breathing, the capnometer is attached to a nasal cannula-type device. Any air leak from the patient to the chamber will lead to erroneous values. The numeric value representing the amount of exhaled CO_2 can be displayed as a percentage of the total gas or as a partial pressure.

The disadvantages associated with $EtCO_2$ equipment contribute to a continuing controversy around the usefulness of capnometry in the ICU. The equipment is often bulky. Secretions, humidity, and condensation may incapacitate the system. Calibration is needed with a high FiO_2. Newer models, however, claim to have resolved these issues.

In the ICU, continuous capnography is usually implemented as a component of either the cardiac monitoring system or the ventilator. The pattern obtained with a capnogram reflects the amount of CO_2 detected throughout the respiratory cycle.

Causes of some variations in the capnography pattern are described in **Box 21-2**. By analyzing these patterns, the patient's disease entity (COPD) or treatment (e.g., paralytic agent or mechanical ventilation) can be monitored. This monitoring, however, occurs routinely in the ICU using a respiratory component of the cardiac monitor system and the ventilator display. Why, then, is another piece of equipment needed?

TABLE 21-4 Terms to Know for $EtCO_2$ Monitoring

$EtCO_2$: End-tidal carbon dioxide; the amount of carbon dioxide detected at end-expiration.

$PaCO_2$: Partial pressure of arterial CO_2.

$PACO_2$: Partial pressure of alveolar CO_2.

Capnometer: A device that measures the amount of carbon dioxide in the airway.

Capnometry: A numeric value of the concentration of CO_2.

Capnography: A continuous visual recording of the amount of CO_2 produced throughout the respiratory cycle.

Deadspace: Air that does not participate in the exchange of gases.

V/Q mismatch: Unequal ventilation to perfusion.

Box 21-2

Causes of Variations in the Capnogram

- Obstructive airway disease when exhalation is longer and the plateau sloped upward
- Inappropriate sensing of the patient's respiratory effort while receiving mechanical ventilation, noted by a slight deflection during the plateau produced by the inspiratory effort made by the patient
- Spontaneous respiratory effort in a patient receiving paralytic agents, leading to a recording of the inspiratory effort as a slight deflection (cleft)
- Rebreathing of carbon dioxide, revealed in an increasing baseline
- Rounded waveforms, indicating a kinked endotracheal tube
- Variation in respiratory patterns (e.g., apnea when the baseline is prolonged and no CO_2 is detected)
- Ventilator disconnect, leading to a flat line

Sources: Frakes, 2001; Good, 2001.

Ventilatory insufficiency due to an increase in shunting (the percentage of blood going from the right heart to the left heart without being oxygenated) is common to ICU patients. With ventilation/perfusion mismatch, there is an increase in deadspace. (Deadspace refers to the areas of the respiratory tract that do not participate in gas exchange.) With increases in deadspace, the gradient between aveolar and CO_2 levels become larger. This gradient is not reflective of $PaCO_2$. Thus, in critically ill patients, capnometry is an unreliable indicator of $PaCO_2$. Advocates of $EtCO_2$ monitoring will argue that they can identify trends by knowing the gradient between the $PACO_2$ and the $PaCO_2$. Research has not established trending as being reliable with critically ill patients. How, therefore, can $EtCO_2$ help to monitor the critically ill patient?

The purpose of $EtCO_2$ monitoring is to detect the presence of CO_2. CO_2 is a waste product of cellular metabolism; it is carried by the blood to the lungs to be diffused through the alveolar capillary membrane and removed during expiration. Blood flow must be present for CO_2 to diffuse across the alveolar capillary membrane. A sudden drop in $EtCO_2$ can reveal an interruption in perfusion caused by a pulmonary embolism or decreased cardiac output due to hypovolemia, positive end-expiratory pressure (PEEP), heart failure, or cardiac arrest. Monitoring the $PACO_2$–$PaCO_2$ gradient can reveal deadspace changes (Frakes, 2001).

$EtCO_2$ monitoring in critical care appears to be quite beneficial during a cardiopulmonary arrest. The literature, recommends, however, that more research be conducted to prove its efficacy (Frakes, 2001; Harris, 2005; St. John, 2003). CO_2 detection, nevertheless, has been well established as one modality to confirm placement of an endotracheal tube. Directly after intubation, an immediate verification of placement is needed. This confirmation entails the use of a colorimetric detector. A colorimetric detector contains a pH-sensitive filter paper. The detector also has an adapter that fits onto an endotracheal tube and the bag-valve device. As the patient is ventilated, the detector will change color if it is exposed to CO_2, confirming tracheal placement of the tube. In general, if the filter remains purple, this indicates an esophageal intubation. If the filter paper turns yellow, this indicates a tracheal intubation (Remember: purple means poor; yellow means yes). The device is then discarded.

Errors can be made when CO_2 detection alone is used for confirmation of the tube placement, for two reasons. First, if the patient has ingested antacids or carbonated beverages prior to the intubation, CO_2 will be detected in an esophageal intubation (false positive). Second, if there is no perfusion during a code, there is no CO_2 diffusion and, therefore, no change in color even though the placement might be correct (false negative). During intubation, some CO_2 may enter the esophagus. It is essential to use a manual resuscitator and administer six breaths via the endotracheal tube after the intubation but before using the colorimetric detector to confirm tube placement. These six breaths will eliminate any CO_2 that entered the esophagus and rule out a false-positive finding (Frakes, 2001). $EtCO_2$ detectors can be damaged by mucus, vomitus, intratracheal epinephrine, or exposure to humidity for 15 to 20 minutes (Anderson & Breen, 2000). Continuous $EtCO_2$ can also monitor for endotracheal tube dislodgement (International Consensus on Science, 2000).

An increase in $EtCO_2$ during a code situation can also be used to monitor the effectiveness of compressions and, when compressions are stopped, can detect the reestablishment of circulation before a pulse is detected. Many authorities use $EtCO_2$ as a predictor of outcome in a cardiopulmonary arrest. An $EtCO_2$ level of lower than 10 mm Hg for 20 minutes has a mortality rate of 100% (Ahrens, 2003).

PATIENT OUTCOMES

Nurses can help ensure obtainment of optimal patient outcomes such as those listed in **Box 21-3**, through the use of evidence-based interventions for patients receiving respiratory monitoring.

SUMMARY

Respiratory monitoring provides tools to assist with assessing and managing patients. These tools are most effectively used when they are correlated with the patient's status. Clinical judgment is enhanced by taking advantage of a variety of monitoring and diagnostic methods. Nursing interventions often take the form of selecting various monitoring modalities or evaluating data from monitoring devices to ensure vigilance in assessing changes in patient status.

Box 21-3
Optimal Patient Outcomes

- Oxygen saturation will be within expected range
- $EtCO_2$ will be within expected range
- Acid-base balance is present

CASE STUDY

Mr. J., an 81-year-old retired college professor, was admitted from the ED to the MICU; he was intubated, alert, and only occasionally triggering the ventilator. His medical record revealed a history of COPD, hypertension, and coronary artery disease. In the ED, Mr. J. reported that he had a cold for about a week and came to the hospital because of his increasing shortness of breath. His condition rapidly deteriorated, and he was intubated.

Mr. J. lives in a first-floor apartment located close to a market and, although frequently short of breath, he is able to attend to his basic needs (shopping, cooking, and cleaning) independently. He enjoys reading and watching documentaries on television. His daughter lives nearby and visits him often, assisting him when needed but allowing him to remain independent.

At the hospital, the patient's O_2 saturation was 96%. He was on a FiO_2 of 50%. His post-intubation ABG results were as follows:

pH   7.46
$PaCO_2$ 44
PaO_2 77
Bicarbonate 31

CRITICAL THINKING QUESTIONS

1. Is it acidic or alkaline?
2. What is the cause?
3. Is there compensation?
4. Do the ABG data correlate with the clinical picture?

The nurse collaborates with the physician and the respiratory therapist, and sedation is ordered to promote rest. Mr. J. is treated with antibiotics for pneumonia, is successfully weaned from the ventilator, and upon discharge is able to resume his normal lifestyle.

Mr. J. lives with a high degree of vulnerability. His PaO_2 is normally in the 60s—on the steep portion of the oxyhemoglobin dissociation curve—and any degree of respiratory compromise will cause him to desaturate. His ability to compensate shows some degree of resiliency. Due to his advanced disease, however, he will be back in the hospital with a good degree of predictability. With the resources available to him, with the support of his daughter, and his willingness to participate in his own care responsibly, he may be able to remain stable for a period of time.

5. Which disciplines should be consulted to work with this patient?
6. How would you modify your plan of care for patients of diverse backgrounds?
7. What type of issues may require you to act as an advocate or moral agent for this patient?
8. How will you implement your role as a facilitator of learning for this patient?

Using the Synergy Model to Develop a Plan of Care

	Patient Characteristics	Subjective and Objective Data	Evidence-based Interventions	Outcomes
SYNERGY MODEL	Resiliency			
	Vulnerability			
	Stability			
	Complexity			
	Resource availability			
	Participation in care			
	Participation in decision making			
	Predictability			

CRITICAL THINKING QUESTIONS

1. Write a case example from the clinical setting highlighting one patient characteristic. Explain how this characteristic was observed through subjective and objective data for a respiratory patient.
2. Utilize the form to write up a plan of care for one client in the clinical setting with a respiratory problem.
3. Take one patient outcome for a patient and list evidence based interventions found in a literature review for this patient.
4. Design a teaching brochure for teaching the staff nurses about end-tidal CO_2 monitoring.

Online Resources

Capnography in Critical Care: www.capnography.com/

Comprehensive site from the MESA Community College Nursing Objects Library (everything from anatomy and physiology and assessment of the respiratory system to ABG analysis): www.mc.maricopa.edu/dept/d31/nur/learning_objects/_systems/Respiratory.html

REFERENCES

Ahrens, T. (2003). Capnography application in acute and critical care. *AACN Clinical Issues, 14*(2), 122–132.

Anderson, C. T., & Breen, P. H. (2000). Carbon dioxide kinetic and capnography during critical care. *Critical Care, 4*(4), 207–215.

Berry, B. E., & Pinard, A. E. (2002). Assessing tissue oxygenation. *Critical Care Nurse, 22*(3), 22–40.

Carroll, P. (2003a). Pitfalls, perils, and pearls of pulse oximetry. *RT*. Retrieved July 6, 2005, from www.rtmagazine.com/Articles.ASP?articleid=R0304F07

Carroll, P. (2003b). Pulse oximetry—in context. *RN Web*. Retrieved July 6, 2005, from http://rnweb.com/rnweb/article/

Carroll, P. (2002). Procedural sedation: Capnography's heightened role. *RN, 65*(10), 54–62.

Church, V. (2001). Managing the risk of DVT and PE. *Nursing 2001*. Retrieved October 16, 2005, from www.Nursingcenter.com/library/JournalArticle.Asp?Article_ID=101068

Frakes, M. A. (2001). Measuring end-tidal carbon dioxide: Clinical applications and usefulness. *Critical Care Nurse, 21*(5), 23–35.

Ganter, M., & Zollinger, A. (2003). Continuous intravascular blood gas monitoring: Development, current techniques, and clinical use of a commercial device. *British Journal of Anaesthesia, 91*(3), 397–407.

Giuliana, K. K., & Higgins, T. L. (2004). New generation pulse oximetry in the care of critically ill patients. *American Journal of Critical Care, 13*(6), 1–8.

Good, V. S. (2001). Continuous end-tidal carbon monoxide monitoring. In D. J. Lynn-McHale & K. K. Carlson (Eds.), *AACN procedure manual for critical care* (pp. 64–70). Philadelphia: Saunders.

Grap, M. J. (2002). Protocols for practice: Pulse oximetry. *Critical Care Nurse, 22*(3), 69–74.

Harris, C. R. (April 15, 2005). ACLS update 2005.org. Retrieved September 6, 2005, from www.americanheart.org/presenter.jhtml?identifier=3012156

International Consensus on Science. (2000). *Guidelines 2000 for Cardiopulmonary Resuscitation and Emergency Cardiovascular Care*. American Heart Association in Collaboration with the International Liaison Committee on Resuscitation (ILCOR).

Philips Medical Systems. (2003). *Understanding Pulse Oximetry: SpO$_2$ Monitoring* [brochure].

Pruitt, W. C., & Jacobs, M. (2004). Interpreting arterial blood gases: Easy as ABC. *Nursing 2004, 34*(8), 50–53.

Schutz, S. L. (2001). Oxygen saturation monitoring by pulse oximetry. In D. J. Lynn-McHale & K. K. Carlson (Eds.), *AACN procedure manual for critical care* (pp. 77–82). Philadelphia: Saunders.

St. John, R. E. (2003). Protocols for practice: End-tidal carbon dioxide monitoring. *Critical Care Nurse, 23*(4), 83–85.

CHAPTER 22

Select Respiratory Disorders, Airway Adjuncts, and Noninvasive Ventilation

Leslie Golden   Roberta Kaplow   Dianne Earnhardt

LEARNING OBJECTIVES

Upon completion of this chapter, the reader will be able to:

1. Distinguish ventilation problems from perfusion problems.
2. Explain the pathophysiology of ventilation and perfusion problems.
3. Describe the management of ventilation and perfusion problems.
4. Discuss the rationale and insertion techniques for oropharyngeal and nasopharyngeal airways.
5. Compare modes of noninvasive ventilation.
6. List optimal patient outcomes that may be achieved through evidence-based management of respiratory disorders.

A vast number of diseases can cause respiratory distress or respiratory failure. Such respiratory conditions will require respiratory interventions. This chapter examines some of the more common respiratory conditions that will likely require intubation and mechanical ventilation. These illnesses and injuries vary in terms of their severity. Each one addressed in the context of critical care must be assumed to be at the more severe end of the spectrum. These conditions can be subdivided into vascular (a form of ventilation/perfusion [V/Q] mismatch), restrictive (another form of V/Q mismatch), and obstructive. Acute respiratory distress syndrome (ARDS) and other respiratory conditions are discussed in Chapters 24 and 25.

VASCULAR CAUSES OF RESPIRATORY FAILURE: VENTILATION/PERFUSION MISMATCH (DEADSPACE)

Because the functions of the heart and lungs are interrelated, even down to the capillary alveolar membrane, it comes as no surprise that intravascular emboli could interfere with the entire process of diffusion of oxygen into the bloodstream. Most of the respiratory system, from the nares down to the smallest of terminal bronchioles, serves only as a conduit for inhaled gases. In terms of ventilation, only the alveolus is thin enough to allow diffusion of oxygen and carbon dioxide; in terms of perfusion, only the capillary membrane is thin enough as well. The entire respiratory tree is, in terms of diffusion of gases, *deadspace*.

Deadspace is defined as an area in the respiratory tree where gases flow (ventilation), but where circulation is inadequate for gas exchange (perfusion). This does not mean that the nose, mouth, throat, trachea, bronchi, and bronchioles lack blood flow; rather, it simply means that they do not participate in gas exchange as the alveoli do. Deadspace is normal from the nares to the terminal bronchioles, but whenever an embolus of any type cuts off circulation to an alveolus, there is an area of functional deadspace. The patient breathes perfectly well and can even be given 100% oxygen, but the capillaries surrounding these alveoli remain blocked. This situation produces an abnormal increase in deadspace, one type of V/Q mismatch. The greater the area of nonperfused lung, the greater the client's respiratory distress. Supplemental oxygen and even mechanical ventilation may help symptoms and even preserve life, but therapy is directed toward improving perfusion to the affected alveoli. The most common cause is pulmonary embolism (PE) due to thrombus, but fat and amniotic fluid emboli are other known sources of V/Q mismatch.

Pulmonary Embolism

PE is usually the result of a deep vein thrombosis (DVT). A PE is more common in venous stasis states (e.g., surgery, pregnancy), abnormalities of vessel walls (e.g., varicose veins), hypercoagulable states (e.g., from oral contraceptives, coagulation abnormalities), morbid obesity, and advanced age. Most initial symptoms are due to a sudden increase in deadspace (e.g., dyspnea and tachypnea), but subsequent symptoms of restrictive (e.g., pulmonary edema) and obstructive (e.g., bronchospasm) lung disease may develop as well. The constellation of symptoms may mimic pneumonia, asthma, aortic dissection, myocardial infarction, or many other cardiac and respiratory illnesses. They may even appear to be due to a severe panic or anxiety attack. Diagnosis is usually made via a V/Q scan. See **Table 22-1**.

Treatment of PE includes respiratory support and cardiac support as needed, along with heparinization. If the embolus is massive, heparinization may be inadequate and pulmonary artery embolectomy under cardiopulmonary bypass (CPB) may be necessary. Patients who are experiencing chest pain must be carefully medicated so as to prevent respiratory or cardiac depression. After initial recovery, the patient is maintained on anticoagulant therapy for at least six months and observed for the development of pulmonary hypertension, a potentially life-shortening complication. Finally, a cause for the initial embolus should be sought.

TABLE 22-1 Signs and Symptoms of Pulmonary Embolism

Sign/Symptom	Incidence
Cyanosis	19%
Tachypnea (> 20 breaths/min)	96%
S_3 or S_4 gallop	34%
Rales	58%
Tachycardia (> 100 beats/min)	44%
Fever (38–39 °C)	43%
Diaphoresis	36%

Source: Feied & Handler, 2004.

Fat Embolism

Emboli of fatty particles most often occurs 12 to 72 hours after long bone fracture, especially of the femur or tibia, as bone marrow enters the circulation. It may also occur in acute pancreatitis, CPB, parenteral infusion of lipids, or liposuction. The usual symptoms are acute hypoxemia; mental confusion; and petechiae over the palate, face, anterior neck, shoulders, and chest. This syndrome can be immediately fatal if severe; it may also progress to ARDS. Treatment is supportive (Papagelopoulos, 2003).

Amniotic Fluid Embolism

Emboli of amniotic fluid can occur during cesarean section or normal spontaneous vaginal delivery, when amniotic fluid and fetal cells enter the maternal circulation. Symptoms are similar to those of massive PE and are fatal more often than not. If the mother survives the initial insult, treatment is supportive (Perozzi, 2004).

RESTRICTIVE LUNG DISEASE: VENTILATION/PERFUSION MISMATCH (SHUNT)

More often, the difficulty in V/Q lies not in the capillaries surrounding the alveoli, but rather in the alveoli themselves. If gas cannot enter the alveoli, the V/Q mismatch is on the ventilation side. This scenario is referred to as *shunt*. Such a V/Q mismatch occurs when inhaled gas is prevented or restricted from entering the alveoli. Restrictive lung disease may be intrinsic (i.e., within the lung tissue itself) or extrinsic (i.e., due to external compression), as in space-occupying conditions that prevent full expansion of the lungs (McLean, 2001).

The restriction of gas flow can occur at the alveolar level (e.g., atelectasis, pneumonia, pulmonary edema), throughout the lung tissue from alveoli to bronchioles to bronchi at a microscopic level (e.g., pulmonary fibrosis), or affecting an entire normal lung from external compression (e.g., pleural effusion, pneumothorax, hemothorax, flail chest). Other examples of extrinsic restrictive lung disease affecting normal lungs include neuromuscular diseases such as muscular dystrophy or morbid obesity. Both of these conditions restrict the patient from full chest excursion and prevent effective breathing.

Atelectasis (Acute Process)

Atelectasis involves collapse of the alveoli, usually due to accumulation of mucus in the alveoli or bronchioles. Small, scattered areas of alveolar collapse may occur, or an entire lobe (usually a dependent one) could be affected. The patient usually experiences only a mild decrease in oxygenation, as compensatory mechanisms decrease blood flow to the collapsed alveoli (hypoxic pulmonary vasoconstriction). The patient often develops fever (an inflammatory response), without infection. This response is very common in the bedridden patient or in the patient with cystic fibrosis. Treatment usually includes ambulation, change in position, chest physiotherapy, incentive spirometry, coughing and deep breathing, and adequate hydration to liquefy viscous secretions in the alveoli. The intubated patient will be limited in some of these aspects and will also need suctioning to clear the endotracheal tube (McAlister, 2005).

Pneumonia (Acute Process)

Pneumonia may be viral, bacterial, or caused by other organisms. Although these organisms exist everywhere in the community, pneumonia usually develops in those individuals with weakened immune systems, such as the elderly, chronically ill, transplant patients, or those with acquired immune deficiency syndrome (AIDS). In any of these cases, pneumonia may be so severe that respiratory support becomes necessary.

Pneumonia may also develop in hospitalized patients, especially those who are bedridden or immobile as a *nosocomial* (hospital-acquired) infection. These organisms find a particularly favorable environment in the atelectatic areas of the lung, so atelectasis in the hospitalized patient almost always precedes a hospital-acquired pneumonia. The intubated patient is at even greater risk for pneumonia. This infection develops because the normal protections from infection (ciliated mucous membranes, sneeze and cough reflexes) are bypassed or suppressed. In addition, contaminated foreign bodies such as suction catheters may introduce organisms into the normally sterile tracheobronchial tree. Virulent organisms thrive in the hospital environment, such as methicillin-resistant *Staphylococcus aureus* (MRSA) and vancomycin-resistant *Enterococcus* (VRE).

Pneumonia also involves an inflammatory reaction in affected areas of the lung. Symptoms are very similar to those of atelectasis, but are much more severe and long-lasting because they arise from a true infection of lung tissue, not just inflammation. In addition, the patient has a productive cough and may develop bronchospasm (a form of obstructive lung disease). The treatment is similar to that of atelectasis, but also includes antibiotic therapy, cultures, serial chest radiographs, and lab tests (e.g., arterial blood gases) to evaluate for improvement. Even after all apparent trace of pneumonia is resolved, lung function in affected areas may not be fully normal for an additional 6 to 8 weeks. It should also be noted that infections such as sepsis and pneumonia are often a cause of death in critically ill patients who might otherwise have survived their original illness (Menéndez & NEUMOFAIL Group, 2005).

Pulmonary Edema (Acute Process)

Pulmonary edema is usually an acute process that arises from leakage of intravascular fluid into the interstitial spaces of the lungs and into the alveoli. It has three possible causes: (1) volume: too much fluid is presented to the delicate pulmonary capillaries; (2) pressure: the pulmonary capillaries constrict to such a degree that (a normal amount of) fluid is forced across the capillary into the alveolus; or (3) capillary injury: the pulmonary capillary membrane itself leaks even with a normal amount of blood flow under normal pressure. **Table 22-2** summarizes the various causes and forms of pulmonary edema.

In all cases, the patient will be dyspneic and tachypneic, and some degree of sympathetic nervous system (SNS) stimulation will occur. The SNS-induced tachycardia, hypertension, pallor, and diaphoresis are especially pronounced in the patient with cardiogenic, neurogenic, and cocaine-induced pulmonary edema because of more pronounced SNS stimulation.

TABLE 22-2 Pulmonary Edema

Causes	Examples
Excessive blood volume	Excessive IV fluid administration Renal failure Chronic heart failure (CHF) Cocaine-induced acute myocardial ischemia/infarction
Abnormal pulmonary capillary pressure (normal volume)	Neurogenic pulmonary edema Cocaine-induced pulmonary vasoconstriction High-altitude pulmonary edema Negative-pressure pulmonary edema (caused by extreme negative intrathoracic pressure created when trying to inhale against a totally obstructed airway)
Pulmonary capillary membrane injury (normal volume, normal pressure)	ARDS Post-traumatic multiple-system organ failure Aspiration pneumonitis Rapid-reexpansion of a collapsed lung Drug-induced (opioid or cocaine overdose) pulmonary edema

Note the effects of cocaine on all forms of pulmonary edema.
Note: ARDS = acute respiratory distress syndrome
Source: Hauser, 2005.

Treatment includes the use of supplemental oxygen and resolution of the underlying cause. Diuretics are often useful in cases of excessive blood volume. In some cases, positive-end expiratory pressure (PEEP) may be the only way to drive oxygen across the alveolar capillary interface; it may also serve to limit the exudation of pink, frothy fluid into the alveoli sometimes seen in severe pulmonary edema. No amount of suctioning will clear the lungs of the blood-tinged, frothy fluid. In fact, the brief removal of PEEP allows more fluid to pour into the alveoli. Suctioning should be limited to a reasonable amount to prevent occlusion of the endotracheal tube, usually every 2 to 4 hours (Bixby, 2005).

Pulmonary Fibrosis (Chronic Process)

In pulmonary fibrosis, lung tissue is replaced by scar tissue in response to chronic inflammation. The most common causes are sarcoidosis, hypersensitivity pneumonitis, eosiniphilic granuloma, pulmonary alveolar proteinosis, and lymphan-

giomyomatosis. **Table 22-3** delineates the most common findings in these more chronic pulmonary restrictive diseases.

Inflammation and destruction of pulmonary interstitial tissue are often associated with inflammation of the pulmonary vasculature. This process may precipitate the development of pulmonary hypertension and cor pulmonale (Karnani, 2005).

Skeletal Deformities (Chronic Process)

The bony skeleton housing the thorax can affect the expansion of the lungs. The most commonly seen thoracic skeletal defects are sternal abnormalities, kyphosis, and scoliosis. Pectus carinatum is an outward bowing of the sternum, often called "pigeon breast," and is primarily a cosmetic concern. Pectus excavatum is an inward bowing of the sternum. Unless severe, it usually causes no cardiopulmonary decompensation. Surgical repair of the sternum is indicated for those patients with restrictive pulmonary disease or cardiovascular compromise.

TABLE 22-3 Chronic Intrinsic Restrictive Disease

Disease	Cause	Other	Treatment
Sarcoidosis	Sarcoid granulomas infiltrate tissues throughout the body; most prominent in the thoracic lymph nodes and lungs.	Also affects larynx, heart, liver, spleen; hypercalcemia may also be seen.	Respiratory support and steroids to decrease inflammation.
Hypersensitivity pneumonitis	Diffuse inflammation (granuloma formation in interstitial tissue) 4–6 hours after inhalation of dust with fungi, spores, or animal or vegetable matter.	Acute onset of dyspnea, cough, hypoxemia; may cause pulmonary fibrosis after repeated episodes.	Respiratory support.
Eosinophilic granuloma	Probably an allergic reaction to inhaled antigens, usually cigarette smoke; alveoli are replaced by granulomas.	Rare, but most common in 20- to 40-year-olds; frequent bronchospasm.	Smoking cessation; steroids, if extensive fibrosis has not yet developed.
Pulmonary alveolar proteinosis	Deposition of lipid-rich proteinaceous material in alveoli; cause unknown. May occur without a "trigger."	Also seen with AIDS, chemotherapy, or inhalation of mineral dust.	Respiratory support; if no spontaneous remission, bronchial lavage.
Lymphangiomyomatosis	Proliferation of smooth muscle in abdominal and thoracic lymphatics, veins, and bronchioles; seen most frequently in females of reproductive age.	Presents as progressive dyspnea, hemoptysis, recurrent pneumothoraces, and ascites.	Respiratory support including treatment of bronchospasm (obstructive as well); death in 4 years.

Source: Sharma, 2004.

Kyphosis is an anterior posterior curve in the vertebral column. The typical "dowager's hump" of old age is an example of isolated kyphosis. Kyphosis in adolescents and young adults is usually associated with scoliosis. Scoliosis is an "S"-shaped curve, usually most obvious at the lumbar spine. This component of the curve usually causes back pain and difficulties with ambulation. As if to balance the lumbar curve, there is usually a compensatory curve in the thoracic vertebrae. If the curve is severe, both chest excursion and lung expansion are restricted and pulmonary vasculature in the involved lung is compressed. Chronic hypoventilation ensues; chronic hypoxemia is common and causes a chronic elevation of hemoglobin and hematocrit. All of these factors combine to precipitate the development of pulmonary hypertension and cor pulmonale. Pneumonia is a very common development in this population, further diminishing lung function (Markström, 2002).

Neuromuscular Disorders (Chronic Process)

Muscles control and coordinate breathing, from the small muscles controlling airway reflexes (sneeze, cough, and gag) to the accessory muscles of the thorax to the largest muscle, the diaphragm. Neuromuscular diseases can affect the function of any or all of these muscles, restricting the flow of air to the alveoli. Some of the more common neuromuscular diseases are listed in **Table 22-4**.

Pleural Effusion (Acute Process)

The pleura are paired membranes that line both the inner chest wall and the surface of the lung. The pleura normally secrete a small amount of fluid, just enough to lubricate the membranes so as to permit smooth movement of the lung within the chest. The small amount of normal pleural fluid also helps the pleura adhere to each other, helping to create the negative pressure necessary for normal inspiration. Any accumulation of fluid between these two membranes (the pleural space) restricts normal lung expansion.

Several types of fluids may accumulate in the pleural space. Serous fluid (hydrothorax) accumulates in severe congestive heart failure (CHF) because pulmonary edema is so severe that it involves the alveoli, affects the interstitial space, and finally extends to the pleura. Infections such as bronchitis can trigger a generalized inflammatory response in the pleura, leading to collection of serous fluid in the pleural space. This condition, which is sometimes called "pleurisy," can persist even after the pulmonary infection is resolved. Bloody inflammatory pleural effusions are often seen in malignant disease, while pure blood (hemothorax) is seen with chest trauma. Hemothorax in chest trauma may be rapidly progressive and life-threatening. It not only restricts lung expansion and may cause mediastinal shift, but may also indicate direct lung injury or tears in the great vessels (aorta, pulmonary

---

TABLE 22-4 Neuromuscular Diseases and Pulmonary Effects

Disease	Comments
Spinal cord (C3 or higher)	Phrenic nerve is at the C3 level; it controls the diaphragm even if diaphragm innervation is preserved. Loss of intercostal and abdominal muscle function limits cough and breathing. May breathe poorly if supine.
Guillain-Barré syndrome	An ascending paralysis that may stop at any level, from weak feet and ankles to total paralysis. Usually occurs after a viral illness and is associated with extreme heart rate and blood pressure instability. Usually resolves spontaneously after 2 months, although some have persistent weakness.
Amyotrophic lateralizing sclerosis (ALS; Lou Gehrig's disease)	Degenerative disease of the motor ganglia (nerve) in the spinal cord and spinal pyramidal tracts (brain). Usually affects men 40–60 years of age. Begins in hands and eventually affects all but eye muscles. High risk for aspiration. Eventual respiratory failure as well as tachycardia, labile blood pressure, and emotional lability. No treatment. Death in 6 years.
Myasthenia gravis	Chronic autoimmune disease that usually affects women ages 20–40 or men older than 60. Caused by destruction of the neuromuscular junction. Usually starts with diplopia, ptosis, and dysphagia with high risk for aspiration; may involve other muscles. Waxes and wanes in severity. Treated with drugs to improve nerve transmission and immunosuppressants.
Muscular dystrophies	Most common type is Duchenne's. Progressive weakness of all muscles with associated respiratory failure; may develop kyphoscoliosis (further restricts). Duchenne's type also involves cardiac muscle. Death at age 15–25 years due to CHF or pneumonia.

Source: Hauser, 2005.

artery) or great veins (vena cavae, pulmonary veins). Disruption of the lymphatic system in the chest may cause collections of milky white lymphatic fluid called chyle (chylothorax). Finally, collections of pus (empyema) may develop in the pleural space in intrathoracic infections.

Symptoms depend on the size of the pleural effusion and the rapidity of its development. Small effusions, or even moderate but slowly accumulating effusions, may go unnoticed in an otherwise healthy person. Pleural effusions of increasing size, however, are associated with increasing degrees of respiratory distress. If left untreated, these effusions may compress and therefore restrict air flow in the ipsilateral lung. As effusions progress, they can cause mediastinal shift and compromise cardiac function, and they may even begin to affect the contralateral lung.

Treatment includes respiratory support and resolution of the underlying cause of the pleural effusion. Hydrothorax caused by CHF may diminish with cardiac medications, especially diuretics. Hydrothorax due to inflammatory response may respond to diuretics and anti-inflammatory agents. If these conditions do not resolve or if the hydrothorax is large, fluid may have to be drained by *thoracentesis*. Hemothorax, chylothorax, and empyema must be drained. Reaccumulation of the pleural effusion may require placement of chest tubes (Wing, 2004).

Pneumothorax (Acute Process)

Pneumothorax occurs when air accumulates in the pleural space. It may occur externally in penetrating chest trauma or internally due to a tear in the lung parenchyma. The internal tears can be due to blunt chest trauma and pulmonary contusion without penetration, rib fracture without penetration to the skin and muscle, use of excessive positive pressure for ventilation, or idiopathic and spontaneous causes. When intrapleural air can escape, there is some degree of respiratory distress. In nonpenetrating injuries, however, air often cannot escape. It then accumulates under increasing pressure, first compressing the ipsilateral lung (on the same side), then the mediastinum, and finally the contralateral lung (on the opposite side). The result is called tension pneumothorax.

Symptoms depend on the size of the pneumothorax and the rapidity of its development. Even small pneumothoraces cause severe dyspnea and chest pain; hypoxemia and hypotension are common. Small pneumothoraces can be observed for spontaneous resolution, but the rest require needle aspiration of accumulating air or placement of a chest tube to allow exit (without reentry) of air from the pleural space (Ryan, 2005).

Flail Chest (Acute Process)

In flail chest, several sections of the ribs are fractured in such a way that they become "unhinged" from the chest wall and respond in a paradoxical way to normal inspiration. Instead of expanding the thoracic cavity on inspiration, the destabilized portion collapses inward. On expiration, the same section of destabilized rib moves outward. This causes restriction to air entry. Treatment consists of positive-pressure ventilation, which serves to splint the chest wall until it is healed or until the chest wall can be stabilized (Goss, 2004).

OBSTRUCTIVE CAUSES OF RESPIRATORY FAILURE

In obstructive lung disease, both perfusion to the alveoli and inspiration of inhaled gases are normal, but *expiration* of exhaled gases is obstructed. This condition may be a reversible process, as seen in bronchospasm and asthma, but obstruction to expiration is fixed in chronic obstructive pulmonary disease (COPD).

Bronchospasm (Acute Process)

The bronchi and bronchioles contain a layer of smooth muscle that can constrict the bronchi in response to irritants such as foreign bodies, dust, or fumes. This would seem to be a protective reflex, because bronchospasm could protect the lower airways from further inhalation of irritants. Usually bronchospasm becomes counterproductive when inhaled gases cannot be exhaled through acutely narrowed airways. At this point, the patient may begin to wheeze. The wheezing reflects the turbulence caused as exhaled air is forced out across narrowed airways. The patient may also cough, which is a form of forced expiration. The patient will become dyspneic, feel anxious, and may feel "crampy" pain or pressure in the general area of the bronchospasm. Many patients describe this sensation as feeling "tight." Patients feel that they cannot inhale; the reality is that they cannot exhale (and therefore inhalation is next to impossible without ever-increasing air trapping) (Kallstrom, 2005).

Anxiety stimulates the SNS. The patient hyperventilates, causing carbon dioxide levels to fall (hypocarbia and respiratory alkalosis). This degree of hyperventilation is disproportionate to the degree of anxiety; rather, it reflects neural reflexes in the lungs. The patient can hyperventilate to the point of dizziness and fainting. If bronchospasm does not resolve, oxygen levels will eventually plummet and carbon dioxide levels will rise (respiratory acidosis) (Kallstrom, 2005).

Bronchospasm can resolve spontaneously, because bronchodilation is part of the normal SNS (fight or flight) response. If it does not resolve, inhaled bronchodilators such as albuterol (Proventil®) may help break the bronchospasm. Of course, the irritant stimulus should be removed as well.

Asthma (Chronic Process with Episodes of Acute Exacerbation)

The pathophysiology of asthma is a two-fold disease. The more insidious component is that of chronic airway inflammation, which is characterized by increased secretions and edema. Over time, this chronic inflammation can damage the airways. The more obvious component is bronchial hyperreactivity with reversible airway obstruction, which is characterized by the tendency to wheeze, cough, and trap air in the alveoli. Triggers to bronchospasm in the asthmatic include bronchial infection, allergens, aspirin, occupational chemicals (e.g., chlorine gas, ammonia fumes, latex), exercise, and nocturnal asthma (worsens at night). All triggers relate to hypersensitivity reactions or to an imbalance in the parasympathetic and sympathetic nervous systems.

Airway inflammation and expiratory obstruction (bronchospasm) tend to be more severe and persistent in the person with asthma than in the patient with isolated bronchospasm. The avoidance of triggers and suppression of the inflammatory response achieve prevention of both components with membrane stabilizers (sodium cromolyn), leukotriene inhibitors, and/or inhaled steroids. These are all preventative medications; they are ineffective in acute asthma attacks. Acute asthma attacks can be fatal. Treatment centers on removing triggers, providing hydration to liquefy viscous secretions, giving intravenous (IV) steroids for suppression of the hyperactive immune response, and administering inhaled or IV bronchodilators. If these measures prove ineffective, the patient is said to be in *status asthmaticus*. Unremitting bronchospasm is fatal, so these patients may be intubated and may be placed under general anesthesia for several days to interrupt the process of continuous bronchospasm (Tsai, 2005). This more serious form of asthma, status asthmaticus, is discussed in Chapter 24.

Chronic Obstructive Pulmonary Disease (Chronic Process)

COPD is a progressive disease characterized by *irreversible* expiratory air flow obstruction. (There is often a small component of reversible expiratory air flow obstruction as well that is very similar to asthma.) COPD has two components: chronic bronchitis and pulmonary emphysema. Most patients have a combination of both conditions. Both chronic bronchitis and pulmonary emphysema develop after years of cigarette smoking or secondhand smoke. Patients may be admitted to the intensive care unit (ICU) with an acute exacerbation of COPD.

These individuals usually present with very high levels of carbon dioxide and lower levels of oxygen. **Table 22-5** delineates the comparative features of the two disease processes.

Treatment focuses on relief of symptoms and slowing the progression of the disease. Therapies include smoking cessation, oxygen therapy, bronchodilators, and nasal continuous positive airway pressure (CPAP). Occasionally, patients with severe emphysema may benefit from lung reduction surgery (McAllister, 2005).

AIRWAY ADJUNCTS

Two common adjuncts used in the ICU to enhance airway patency are oropharyngeal and nasopharyngeal airways. Correct selection and proper placement are essential skills for the ICU nurse.

Oropharyngeal Airways

An oropharyngeal airway is used to maintain the airway in a patient who is unconscious. This device, which is made of hard plastic, is intended to prevent the patient's tongue from slipping to the back of the throat and obstructing the airway (see **Figure 22-1**).

Oropharyngeal airways are available in a variety of sizes, so the correct size must be selected for the individual patient. The correct method to measure an oropharyngeal airway is to place the flat end of the airway at the tip of the patient's mouth. The other end of the airway should reach the tip of the jaw (see **Figure 22-2**). If the oropharyngeal airway inserted is too large, the patient's airway may become obstructed or the patient may gag. If the airway is too small (**Figure 22-3**), it will not protect the patency of the airway, because the tongue will not be prevented from slipping to the back of the throat.

TABLE 22-5 Comparison of Chronic Bronchitis and Pulmonary Emphysema

Abnormality	Chronic Bronchitis	Pulmonary Emphysema
Injury	Inflammation of airways	Destruction of lung parenchyma
Airway obstruction	Narrowing, increased mucus	Loss of elastic recoil; development of bullae
Symptoms	Chronic, daily cough; moderate dyspnea	Severe dyspnea
$PaCO_2$	Increased	Normal to decreased
PaO_2	Marked decrease ("blue bloater")	Mild decrease ("pink puffer")
Hemoglobin	Increased	Normal to decreased
Cor pulmonale	Severe	Mild decrease ("pink puffer")
Prognosis	Poor	Good

Source: McAllister, 2005.

FIGURE 22-1 Oropharyngeal Airway

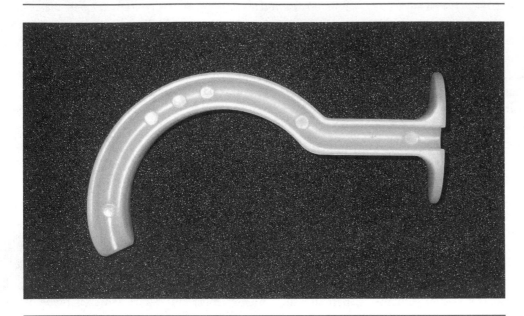

Source: Photo by James R. Perron.

Once the correct size of oropharyngeal airway has been selected for the patient, the device can be inserted by one of two
methods. First, a tongue blade may be used to hold the tongue
forward and the airway inserted following the natural curvature
of the mouth. Second, the airway may be inserted with the tip facing up toward the back of the patient's mouth. When the airway
is at the back of the tongue, it is rotated 180 degrees so the tip
points down, following the natu-
ral curvature of the mouth.

An oropharyngeal airway
may remain in place as long as
the patient is unconscious. Once
the patient is conscious, it is removed because the patient may
gag and vomit, which can result
in aspiration.

Nasopharyngeal Airways

A nasopharyngeal airway, also
known as a nasal trumpet, is
made of soft rubber and is better
tolerated in a conscious patient.
An opening throughout the tube
allows the patient to breathe
through the nostril and facilitates suctioning.

Like oropharnyngeal air-
ways, nasopharyngeal airways

come in a variety of sizes, so the
correct size must be selected for
the individual patient. The size
is based on the internal diameter of the tube. Tubes with larger
internal diameters are longer. In
general, a size 6 or 7 is used on a
small adult, a size 7 or 8 is used
on a medium-sized adult, and a
size 8 or 9 is used on a large
adult. To determine the correct
size for the patient, measure
from the tip of the nose. If the
end of the nasopharyngeal airway reaches the tip of the earlobe, it is the correct size (see
Figure 22-4).

To insert a nasopharyngeal
airway, lubricate it first with a
water-soluble lubricant. The
airway is then inserted into the
nostril following the natural
curvature of the nasopharynx. If resistance is felt during insertion, the airway may be twisted as it is inserted. If resistance persists, the other nostril or a smaller-size airway may
be attempted. Once in place, air can be felt from the opening of the airway. Complications of nasopharyngeal airway
insertion include nosebleeds, laryngospasm, gagging, and
vomiting.

FIGURE 22-2 Measuring Oropharyngeal Airway (Correct Size)

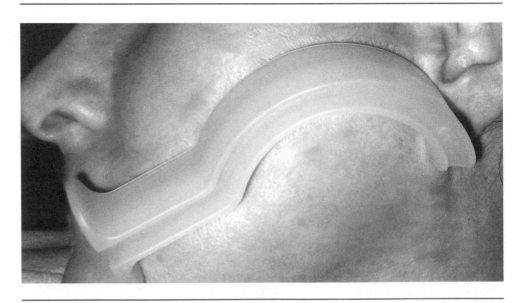

Source: Photo by James R. Perron.

NONINVASIVE VENTILATION

If a patient experiences a critical event related to a respiratory disorder, such as any one of those discussed in this chapter or those described in Chapter 24, intubation and mechanical ventilation may be indicated. One way to avert this invasive measure along with its associated complications (e.g., infection) is with the implementation of noninvasive ventilation (NIV) techniques (Focus on ALS, 2005).

NIV is the delivery of mechanical ventilation with a nasal or face mask (Friolet, Liaudet, & Eckert, 2004). Two NIV techniques include CPAP and bilevel positive airway pressure (BiPAP). As their names suggest, machines are used for both of these techniques to deliver positive pressure. The techniques are considered noninvasive because an endotracheal tube is not inserted into the trachea.

FIGURE 22-3 Measuring Oropharyngeal Airway (Too Short)

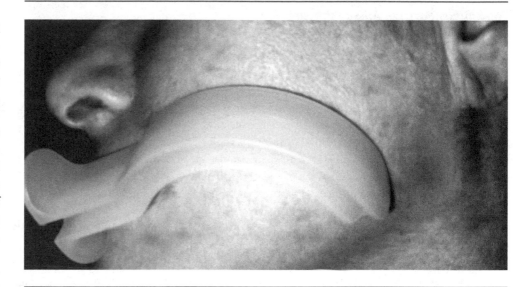

Source: Photo by James R. Perron.

Benefits of NIV

In addition to preventing intubation, NIV techniques reportedly decrease mortality of some patients with acute respiratory failure (Brochard et al., 1995; Friolet et al., 2004; Poponick, Renston, Bennett, & Emerman, 1999). Data suggest the need for intubation may be decreased by as much as 44%, and mortality may be decreased by 50% in patients with acute respiratory failure (Plant, Owen, & Elliott, 2000). There is also a reported decrease in both of these variables in patients with severe acute respiratory syndrome (SARS) (Yam et al., 2005).

NIV methods are effective in enhancing alveolar ventilation (Preston, 2001). They also decrease the work of breathing and improve gas exchange (Friolet et al., 2004). NIV decreases the incidence of nosocomial pneumonia, enhances patient comfort, decreases length of stay, and decreases costs (Sharma, 2005).

Indications for NIV

NIV may be an alternative to intubation for patients with COPD exacerbations who are admitted to the hospital with respiratory failure (Balami, 2005; Chapman & Davies, 2003; Plant, Owen, Parrott, & Elliott, 2003). In addition to its adoption in patients with respiratory failure with hypercarbia, NIV is being used in patients with acute respiratory failure with acute hypoxemia (Layfield, 2002). It may also be useful in some patients with asthma (Pagani, Oddo, & Schaller, 2004).

FIGURE 22-4 Measuring Nasopharyngeal Airway (Correct Size)

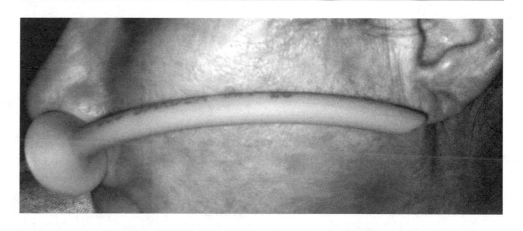

Source: Photo by James R. Perron.

Methods of NIV

Continuous Positive Airway Pressure

With CPAP, air is delivered to the lungs through a tight-fitting mask. The mask fits over the patient's nose or nose and mouth, and is connected to a pump. The pump provides a constant positive pressure through the mask. This positive pressure is delivered to the patient with each breath, is used to keep alveoli open, and increases the amount of air breathed in. The constant pressure keeps alveoli open during inhalation and exhalation. Despite the fact that the individual must exhale against pressure, CPAP does not increase the work of breathing. The patient must be able to continuously breathe spontaneously, because the mask and pump do not provide any breaths for the patient (ImpactED, 2005; Medline Plus, 2005). The usual range of CPAP is 5 to 15 cm H_2O (Lung Cancer Frontiers, 2005).

Use of CPAP has been shown to enhance the management of patients with chronic heart failure. Symptom relief, improved left ventricular function, and enhanced oxygenation have been reported. Patients who receive CPAP with pulmonary edema have demonstrated improvement in their hemodynamic status, symptoms, and oxygenation (Nadar, Prasad, Taylor, & Lip, 2005).

Bilevel Positive Airway Pressure

BiPAP is considered a refinement of CPAP. It provides positive airway pressure at the end of exhalation as well as a higher positive airway pressure during inhalation (pressure support), which enhances oxygenation and ventilation (Lung Cancer Frontiers, 2005). With BiPAP, two different pressures are set and separately adjusted. One pressure is for inspiration to assist the patient to inhale; the other is to help the patient exhale. The higher pressure is for inhalation (IPAP), while the lower pressure is for exhalation (EPAP). These pressures are pressure support and CPAP, respectively. The preset pressure is delivered with each breath.

When the patient begins to inhale, the machine senses a decrease in air flow within the circuit and delivers higher pressure (IPAP) to support the patient's inspiratory effort. This change augments the patient's tidal volume. As the patient completes inhalation, the device senses a decrease in inspiratory flow; the patient is allowed to exhale and the pressure returns to the CPAP (or EPAP) level. The net effect of BiPAP is increased delivery of air with less work of breathing. It has been suggested that the independent pressures might lead to lower airway pressures than with CPAP alone (Focus on ALS, 2005).

In BiPAP, the IPAP is higher than the EPAP. IPAP is usually set at 5 to 10 cm H_2O. EPAP is usually set at 3 to 5 cm H_2O. EPAP is titrated upward in 3- to 5-cm H_2O increments if clinically indicated (ImpactED, 2005). Initial settings may be IPAP 10 cm and EPAP 4 cm (Lung Cancer Frontiers, 2005).

With BiPAP, CPAP is delivered at a high flow. The machine cycles between high positive pressure and low positive pressure (Sharma, 2005).

Newer BiPAP machines have an added feature, spontaneous/timed mode delivery. With this feature, if the patient does not spontaneously breathe within a specified period, the BiPAP machine will initiate a breath for the patient. A predetermined number of breaths can be set to be delivered to the patient (Focus on ALS, 2005).

The oxygen source is complicated with BiPAP, because the machine usually does not have an oxygen control. The oxygen must be added to the mask or circuit through a flow valve by a respiratory therapist trained in setting up the equipment.

Nursing Management of the Patient Receiving NIV

For NIV to be successful, the mask must be adequately sealed to the patient's face (Babu & Chauhan, 2003). Leaks from the mask may occur (Sharma, 2005).

Because of the complexity of the oxygen setup, it is essential for the ICU nurse to monitor the patient's oxygenation status via pulse oximetry (ImpactED, 2005; Schwartz, Kacmarek, & Hess, 2004). Patients receiving NIV must be monitored for comfort, respiratory status (e.g., observation for dyspnea, respiratory rate, and SpO_2), level of consciousness, and hemodynamic status. Other nursing interventions are listed in **Table 22-6**.

Complications of NIV

Few complications have been reported with NIV. Those reported include facial skin breakdown from the pressure of the mask and straps on the face, gastric distention, eye irritation, and sinus pain or congestion. Hypotension and decreased preload may occur (Sharma, 2005). Other possible complications are described in Table 22-6.

PATIENT OUTCOMES

Nurses can help ensure obtainment of optimal patient outcomes such as those listed in **Box 22-1**, through the use of evidence-based interventions for patients with respiratory

---

Box 22-1
Optimal Patient Outcomes

- Patent airway
- No ventilation/perfusion mismatch
- Absence of complication related to non-invasive ventilation
- Oxygen saturation within expected range
- Acid-base status within expected range

TABLE 22-6 Complications of NIV

Complication	Cause	Intervention
Claustrophobia	Mask fitting too tightly on face to minimize leakage	Patients must be reassured and assessed for comfort. Anxiolytics may be warranted.
Pressure areas around the face	Mask and straps fitting tightly on face	Placement of a piece of a hydrocolloid dressing in pressure-prone places (e.g., bridge of nose).
Dryness of lips and nasal passages	Delivery of dry air under high pressure	Apply lip balm or use nasal spray.
Gastric distention	Swallowing air	Nasogastric tube insertion is not needed.
Aspiration	Gastric distention	Check for presence of nausea, increased abdominal girth, and tympany upon percussion. Administer antiemetics, as needed.
Corneal irritation	Air blowing continuously in the eyes	Ensure adequate mask seal on face. Keep eyes moist with drops or ophthalmic ointment.
Hypoventilation	Air leak	Ensure adequate mask seal on face.

Source: ImpactED, 2005.

disorders or with airway adjuncts or receiving noninvasive ventilation.

SUMMARY

Patients with respiratory conditions who have large amounts of secretions, are unable to clear their secretions, have impaired mental status, are uncooperative, are hemodynamically unstable, need airway protection, or are in need of continuous ventilatory support should not be considered for NIV (Sharma, 2005). However, in patients with acute respiratory failure who do not have any of these contraindications, NIV may decrease length of hospital stay, number of complications, and mortality rates (Antonelli et al., 1998; Brochard et al., 1995).

CASE STUDY 1

You receive a report on your patient, a 23-year-old man who was involved in a motor vehicle crash. He was in apparent good health until he grazed a guardrail while driving at 95 miles per hour. His car spun out of control and crashed against another car, killing a passenger in the other car. Your patient was wearing a seat belt but sustained a closed head injury, left-sided rib fractures with pulmonary contusion, flail chest, and hemo/pneumothorax. There were no intra-abdominal injuries, but he did sustain a left femur fracture. His drug screen was positive for cocaine, marijuana, and alcohol.

The patient had a ventricular drain placed for intracranial pressure (ICP) monitoring. He was intubated with an 8.0 endotracheal tube (ETT) taped at 23 cm, and ventilated on FiO_2 .60, PEEP 5 cm, Vt 800 mL, and rate 12 breaths per minute. He has a left pleural chest tube to water seal. He is medically paralyzed on a vecuronium bromide (Norcuron®) drip and sedated with morphine and midazolam (Versed®) prn. His oxygen saturation is 100% and $EtCO_2$ is 33. The patient is hyperventilated to decrease ICP. Heart rate (HR) ranges from 96 to 110 beats per minute; blood pressure ranges from 110/75 to 140/95, even with sedation. His last blood gas results were as follows:

pH	7.42
$PaCO_2$	30 mm Hg
PaO_2	176 mm Hg
HCO_3^-	22
BE	−4

Several hours into your shift you notice that your patient's oxygen saturation has decreased from 100% to 98% but $EtCO_2$ is unchanged.

CRITICAL THINKING QUESTIONS

1. Is this change significant or can it be observed for a more dramatic change? Why or why not?

The ETT is secured at 23 cm. A repeat chest radiograph confirms appropriate ETT placement. After 30 minutes, oxygen saturation is again 100% and you draw an arterial blood gas. The results are as follows:

pH	7.41
$PaCO_2$	32 mm Hg
PaO_2	104 mm Hg
HCO_3^-	22
BE	−4

2. Why is the PaO_2 still decreased?
3. After chest PT and suctioning, the patient begins coughing. ICP spikes repeatedly to the mid-30s. What can be done to interrupt this process and to prevent its recurrence? (May need to refer to Chapter 27 for help with this question.)
4. After several hours of relative stability, oxygen saturation drops to 85%, $EtCO_2$ drops to 23, HR increases to 145, and BP soars to 170/110. ICP is 25. The patient has developed petechiae on the face and upper chest. What has happened and what should you do?
5. Which disciplines should be consulted to work with this client?
6. What type of issues may require you to act as an advocate or moral agent for this patient?
7. How will you implement your role as a facilitator of learning for this patient?
8. Utilize the form to write up data and a plan of care for a patient with one of the respiratory disorders described in this chapter who is in the clinical setting. Rate the patient as a level 1, 3, or 5 on each characteristic. Identify the level of nurse characteristics needed in the care of this patient.
9. Take one patient outcome for a patient and list evidence-based interventions found in a literature review for this patient.

Using the Synergy Model to Develop a Plan of Care

	Patient Characteristics	Subjective and Objective Data	Evidence-based Interventions	Outcomes
SYNERGY MODEL	Resiliency			
	Vulnerability			
	Stability			
	Complexity			
	Resource availability			
	Participation in care			
	Participation in decision making			
	Predictability			

CASE STUDY 2

T.U. is a 67-year-old patient with a history of COPD. He was a two-pack-per-day tobacco smoker for 25 years. He has had multiple admissions to the hospital with acute exacerbations of COPD in the past, including two extended courses of intubation and mechanical ventilation. Over the past day, T.U. had become progressively dyspneic and lethargic. His wife brought him to the ED because he "wasn't getting any better." Upon recovery from his last exacerbation, T.U. discussed with his wife his wishes not to be intubated again.

Upon admission to the ED, T.U. was drowsy but easily arousable, tachypneic at 36 breaths per minute, and in mild distress. Arterial blood gas results were as follows:

pH   7.24
$PaCO_2$ 70
PaO_2 51
SaO_2 79%
HCO_3 32

Based on his expressed wishes, T.U. was admitted to the ICU and was not intubated. The decision was made to initiate BiPAP with IPAP 12 cm H_2O and EPAP 3 cm H_2O. T.U.'s condition improved over the course of the next few days, and he was transferred out of the ICU and eventually discharged to home.

CRITICAL THINKING QUESTIONS

1. Interpret the arterial blood gas results for T.U.
2. Describe the pressure settings used in BiPAP.
3. Why was BiPAP the appropriate choice of therapy for T.U.?
4. Describe your course of action if the ICU physician decided to intubate the patient.

Online Resources

American Lung Association, Lung Volume Reduction Surgery Fact Sheet:
www.lungus.org/site/pp.asp?c=dvLUK90oEbb=992745

Clinical evidence: www.clinicalevidence.com/ceweb/conditions/rda.rda.jsp

FSU College of Medicine, general respiratory disorders patient/family resources:
http://fsumed-dl.slis.ua.edu/patientinfo/pulmonology/general.htm

University of Maryland Medical Center, Respiratory Disease: www.umm.edu/respiratory/

REFERENCES

Antonelli, M., Conti, G., Rocco, M., Bufi, M., DeBlasi, R. A., Vivino, G., et al. (1998). A comparison of non-invasive positive-pressure ventilation and conventional mechanical ventilation in patients with acute respiratory failure. *New England Journal of Medicine, 339,* 429–435.

Babu, K. S., & Chauhan, A. J. (2003). Non-invasive ventilation in chronic obstructive pulmonary disease: Effective in exacerbations with hypercapnic respiratory failure. *British Medical Journal, 326*(7382), 177–178.

Balami, J. (2005). Non-invasive ventilation in older people. *Geriatric Medicine, 35*(6), 61–64.

Bixby, M. (2005). Turn back the tide of cardiogenic pulmonary edema. *Nursing 2005, 35*(5), 56–61.

Brochard, L., Mancebo, J., Wysocki, M., Lofaso, F., Conti, G., Rauss, A., et al. (1995). Non-invasive ventilation for acute exacerbations of COPD. *New England Journal of Medicine, 33,* 817–822.

Chapman, S. J., & Davies, C. W. (2003). Non-invasive positive pressure ventilation in acute respiratory failure. *Care of the Critically Ill, 19*(5), 145–149.

Feied, C., & Handler, J. A. (2004). Pulmonary embolism. Retrieved November 12, 2005, from www.emedicine.com/emerg/topic490.htm

Focus on ALS. (2005). Retrieved October 20, 2005, from www.focusonals.com/cpap_and_a_bipap.htm

Friolet, R., Liaudet, L., & Eckert, P. (2004). Value of non-invasive ventilation in intensive care. *Revue Medicale de la Suisse Romande, 124*(6), 337–340.

Goss, J. F. (2004). Complexities of blunt chest trauma: Prehospital assessment and management of rib fractures, flail chest, pulmonary contusions, pneumothorax, hemothorax, traumatic asphyxia and diaphragmatic rupture. *Journal of Emergency Medical Services, 29*(11), 44–46, 48–57.

Hauser, S. L. (2005). Dyspnea and pulmonary edema. In *Harrison's principles of internal medicine* (16th ed.). New York: McGraw-Hill.

ImpactED. (2005). Retrieved October 20, 2005, from www.impactednurse.com/nutsandbolts/BiPAP.html

Kallstrom, T. J. (2005). Focus on allergies and asthma. Treating bronchospasm associated with asthma and COPD. *American Association of Respiratory Care Times, 29*(6), 4, 6–7.

Karnani, N. G. (2005). Evaluation of chronic dyspnea. *American Family Physician, 71*(8), 1529–1538, 1473–1475, 1612 passim.

Layfield, C. (2002). Non-invasive BiPAP—implementation of a new service. *Intensive and Critical Care Nursing, 18*(6), 310–319.

Lung Cancer Frontiers. Retrieved October 20, 2005, from www.lungcancerfrontiers.org/books/pul_pro/mechanical-ventilatory.html

Markström, A. (2002). Quality-of-life evaluation of patients with neuromuscular and skeletal diseases treated with noninvasive and invasive home mechanical ventilation. *Chest, 122*(5), 1695–1700.

McAlister, F. A. (2005). Incidence of and risk factors for pulmonary complications after nonthoracic surgery. *American Journal of Respiratory and Critical Care Medicine, 171*(5), 514–517.

McAllister, M. (2005). Promoting physiologic-physical adaptation in chronic obstructive pulmonary disease: Pharmacotherapeutic evidence-based research and guidelines. *Home Healthcare Nurse, 23*(8), 523–533.

McLean, B. (2001). Rotational kinetic therapy for ventilation/perfusion mismatch. *Connect: The World of Critical Care Nursing, 1*(4), 113–114, 116–118.

Medline Plus. (2005). CPAP. Retrieved October 20, 2005, from www.nlm.nih.gov/medlineplus/ency/article/001916.htm

Menéndez, R., & NEUMOFAIL Group. (2005). Guidelines for the treatment of community-acquired pneumonia: Predictors of adherence and outcome. *American Journal of Respiratory and Critical Care Medicine, 172*(6), 757–762.

Nadar, S., Prasad, N., Taylor, R. S., & Lip, G. Y. (2005). Positive pressure ventilation in the management of acute and chronic cardiac failure: A systematic review and meta-analysis. *International Journal of Cardiology, 99*(2), 171–185.

Pagani, J. L., Oddo, M., & Schaller, M. D. (2004). Severe acute asthma. *Revue Medicale de la Suisse Romande, 124*(6), 333–336.

Papagelopoulos, P. J. (2003). Pulmonary fat embolism after total hip and total knee arthroplasty. *Orthopedics, 26*(5), 523–529.

Perozzi, K. J. (2004). Amniotic fluid embolism: An obstetric emergency. *Critical Care Nurse, 24*(4), 54–61.

Plant, P. K., Owen, J. L., & Elliott, M. W. (2000). Early use of non-invasive ventilation for acute exacerbations of chronic obstructive pulmonary disease on general respiratory wards: A multicentre randomised controlled trial. *Lancet, 355*, 1931–1935.

Plant, P. K., Owen, J. L., Parrott, S., & Elliott, M. W. (2003). Cost effectiveness of ward based non-invasive ventilation for acute exacerbations of chronic obstructive pulmonary disease: Economic analysis of randomized controlled trial. *British Medical Journal, 326*(7396), 956.

Poponick, J. M., Renston, J. P., Bennett, R. P., & Emerman, C. L. (1999). Use of a ventilatory support system (BiPAP) for acute respiratory failure in the emergency department. *Chest, 116*, 166–171.

Preston, R. (2001). Introducing non-invasive positive pressure ventilation. *Nursing Standard, 15*(26), 42–45.

Ryan, B. (2005). Pneumothorax: Assessment and diagnostic testing. *Journal of Cardiovascular Nursing, 20*(4), 251–253.

Schwartz, A. R., Kacmarek, R. M., & Hess, D. R. (2004). Factors affecting oxygen delivery with bi-level positive airway pressure. *Respiratory Care, 49*(3), 270–275.

Sharma, S. (2004). Restrictive lung disease. Retrieved November 12, 2005, from emedicine.com/med/topic201.htm

Sharma, S. (2005). Noninvasive positive-pressure ventilation. Ventilation, non-invasive. Retrieved October 20, 2005, from www.emedicine.com/med/topic3371/htm

Tsai, A. C. (2005). A meta-analysis of interventions to improve care for chronic illnesses. *American Journal of Managed Care, 11*(8), 478–488.

Wing, S. (2004). Pleural effusion: Nursing care challenge in the elderly. *Geriatric Nursing, 25*(6), 348–354.

Yam, L. Y., Chan, A. Y., Cheung, T. M., Tsui, E. L., Chan, J. C., & Wong, V. C. (2005). Non-invasive versus invasive ventilation for respiratory failure in severe acute respiratory syndrome. *Chinese Medical Journal, 118*(17), 1413–1421.

CHAPTER 23

Mechanical Ventilation

Suzanne M. Burns

LEARNING OBJECTIVES

Upon completion of this chapter, the reader will be able to:

1. Explain the main indications for mechanical ventilation.

2. Compare the modes and parameters of mechanical ventilation.

3. Discuss complications related to mechanical ventilation and associated nursing interventions.

4. Describe how to wean a patient from mechanical ventilation.

5. List optimal patient outcomes that may be achieved through evidence-based management of the ventilated patient.

Mechanical ventilation through an artificial airway, often referred to as invasive ventilation, is a commonly required therapy for critically ill patients. Reasons for its use include apnea, respiratory failure, impending respiratory failure, severe oxygenation problems, and respiratory muscle fatigue. In each of these cases, the selection of the ventilator modes depends on the disease or condition of the patient, the effectiveness of the modes in relation to the patient's condition, and the type of ventilator and modes available. In addition, the preferences of the clinicians managing the ventilator play a part in selection. For patients to be cared for optimally by the intensive care unit (ICU) nurse, the reasons for mechanical ventilation, ventilator parameters, modes (both traditional and new), potential complications of mechanical ventilation, and the process of weaning patients from the ventilator must be understood.

CONCEPTS OF POSITIVE-PRESSURE VENTILATION

Reasons for Mechanical Ventilation

Apnea, such as is present with some neuromuscular conditions or with cardiopulmonary collapse, is an obvious reason for mechanical ventilation to be instituted. So, too, is the need to intubate and ventilate patients who require anesthesia for surgery. Other reasons, which may not be as readily understood, include acute ventilatory failure, impending ventilatory failure, severe hypoxemia, and respiratory muscle fatigue (see **Box 23-1**).

Negative- Versus Positive-Pressure Ventilation

Normal breathing is referred to as negative-pressure ventilation. When we initiate a breath, the pressure in the pleural space becomes negative as the muscles of respiration contract and the chest wall moves outward. A vacuum is created in the pleural space, and the negative pressure is transmitted through the thorax. Air moves from higher (atmosphere) to lower pressure (the lungs), and a breath is completed as the pressures equalize. Some negative pressure ventilators, such as the iron lung, still exist and are used in rare cases. However, the vast majority of mechanical ventilation today is done with positive-pressure modes of ventilation. With positive-pressure ventilation, each breath is delivered into the lungs under pressure (i.e., above atmospheric pressure). Positive-pressure ventilation is further broken down into volume or pressure ventilation.

Box 23-1

Definitions

Acute Ventilatory Failure

Acute ventilatory failure can occur with any condition. It is defined as a pH of 7.25 or less, with an arterial partial pressure of carbon dioxide ($PaCO_2$) of 50 mm Hg or higher.

Impending Ventilatory Failure

Impending ventilatory failure is less definitive than acute ventilatory failure. In this case, the patient may have a series of arterial blood gases (ABGs) that show progressive deterioration of the pH and $PaCO_2$. Alternatively, physical signs and symptoms may suggest impending failure. An example is in the case of a severe asthmatic who may not be able to say a whole sentence and is diaphoretic, tachycardic, and confused. In this case, intubation and ventilation are indicated.

Severe Hypoxemia

An arterial partial pressure of oxygen (PaO_2) of 50 mm Hg or less on room air indicates a critical level of oxygen in the blood. Although oxygen delivery devices may be used before intubation, the refractory nature of the shunt (air passing from the right side to the left side of the heart without getting oxygenated) may require intubation and ventilation.

Respiratory Muscle Fatigue

All muscles can become fatigued if the workload is too high. Fatigue occurs when the muscles' energy stores become depleted. Weakness, hypermetabolic states, and chronic lung disease are examples of conditions in which patients are especially prone to fatigue. Once fatigue occurs, the muscles no longer contract optimally and hypercarbia results. Signs and symptoms of fatigue or impending fatigue include dyspnea, tachypnea, chest-abdominal asynchrony, and elevations in CO_2 (a late sign). Mechanical ventilation can restore the respiratory muscles by decreasing or eliminating the workload (Roussos & Koutsoukou, 2003).

Volume Versus Pressure Ventilation

With volume ventilation (also known as volume-targeted ventilation), a predetermined volume is delivered to the patient with every breath. However, the pressure it takes to deliver the breath varies depending on the level of lung compliance (i.e., the ease with which the lungs distend) or airways resistance (i.e., the resistance to flow through the airways).

Pressure ventilation (also known as pressure-targeted ventilation) requires that the clinician select a pressure; with each breath, that pressure is maintained throughout inspiration. With pressure ventilation, volume varies with changes in compliance and resistance. Despite the fact that volume is not ensured with most pressure modes (some exceptions are described later in this chapter), other attributes of pressure ventilation have contributed to its popularity (Pierce, 2000). The flow pattern of gas with this mode is felt to provide a better distribution of gas than volume-targeted ventilation does (Burns, 2005).

VENTILATOR PARAMETERS AND MODES

Ventilator Parameters

For the various volume and pressure modes of ventilation to be understood and applied correctly, an understanding of how ventilator breaths are delivered is necessary. Referred to as "ventilator parameters," these parameters include tidal volume (Vt), respiratory rate or frequency, minute ventilation (MV), inspiratory pressure level (IPL), inspiratory time (Ti), inspiratory to expiratory (I:E) ratio, sensitivity, positive end expiratory pressure (PEEP), and fraction of inspired oxygen (FiO_2). Not all parameters are used with each mode. All of the parameters are summarized in **Table 23-1**.

Tidal Volume (Vt)

Vt is the amount of gas set to be delivered with each breath. This parameter is set between 8 and 12 mL/kg in the adult. However, in patients with acute respiratory distress syndrome (ARDS), much smaller Vts are required. In these patients, research has demonstrated that a Vt of 6 mL/kg is necessary to protect the noncompliant (i.e., stiff) alveoli from injury (Acute Respiratory Distress Syndrome Network, 2000). This type of acute lung injury is called volu-trauma and is described in the section on complications.

Respiratory Rate (RR) or Frequency

The RR is the number of breaths set to be delivered to the patient each minute. It is set between 10 and 20 breaths/min and

TABLE 23-1 Common Ventilator Settings

Setting	Definition	Usual Range
Tidal volume	The amount of gas set to be delivered with each breath	6–12 mL/kg body weight.
Respiratory rate	The number of breaths delivered each minute	Variable, based on patient need. Usual range is 10–20/min.
Minute ventilation	The amount of gas exchanged in one minute	Normal minute ventilation is 5–10 L/min. Tidal volume and respiratory rate are usually set to achieve this range.
Inspiratory pressure limit	The maximum amount of pressure that will be exerted on the lungs to allow for delivery of tidal volume	Based on patient's condition.
Inspiratory time	The amount of time allotted for inspiration of each breath	0.7–1.0 sec.
I:E ratio	The ratio of time between inspiration and exhalation for each breath	1:2 is most common, but can vary based on the patient's condition. For example, longer times for exhalation are necessary for complete emptying with bronchoconstriction.
Sensitivity	How easy it is for the patient to initiate or trigger a spontaneous breath	-1 to -2 cm H_2O
PEEP	Pressure exerted to keep alveoli open at the end of exhalation	3–5 cm H_2O is considered "physiologic." Higher levels are common in critically ill patients.
FiO_2	The percentage of oxygen delivered to the patient	21–100% (i.e., .21–1.00).

is based on the patient's condition, arterial blood gas (ABG) results, pulse oximetry, and end-tidal CO_2.

Minute Ventilation (MV)

MV is the amount of gas exchanged in one minute and is the product of Vt and RR. In normal adults, an MV of 5 to 10 L is adequate for maintenance of gas exchange. Unfortunately, critically ill patients often require much higher MVs. A high MV is indicative of inefficient gas exchange. Some ventilators allow the clinician to select a desired MV as a mode option.

Inspiratory Pressure Level (IPL)

Pressure modes of ventilation require that a pressure level be selected. This pressure level is determined by the clinical goal of therapy. If the goal is to maintain a target Vt, then the pressure level is adjusted to attain that Vt (recall that the volume varies from breath to breath, but an acceptable range is the goal). If the patient has a very noncompliant lung condition such as ARDS, however, the clinical goal may be to limit the pressure. IPL may be called by different names depending on the mode or make of the ventilator.

Inspiratory Time (Ti) and Inspiratory to Expiratory Ratio (I:E Ratio)

Each breath consists of two phases: inspiration and expiration. The ventilator requires only that inspiration be set; expiration is passive. In most adults, Ti is set between 0.7 and 1.0 second and is determined by the flow rate (how quickly the gas is delivered). The higher the flow, the shorter the Ti, and vice versa. The I:E ratio is generally 1:2 or 1:3 but may vary depending on the clinical goal. For example, in a patient with asthma, bronchoconstriction may limit the complete emptying of the lung during exhalation. To ensure that the Vt is completely exhaled, the I:E may be set to 1:3 or 1:4. Inverse I:E ratios of 1:1, 2:1, 3:1, and 4:1 are also possible with some modes used for ARDS.

Sensitivity

Sensitivity ("trigger sensitivity") refers to how easy it is for the patient to initiate or trigger a spontaneous breath. Two types of sensitivity exist: pressure and flow triggering. With pressure triggering, the clinician sets the sensitivity pressure to a negative number (e.g., −1 or −2 cm H_2O); the more negative the number, the harder the work of the patient. When the patient initiates a breath, a negative pressure is created and a breath, or additional flow, is delivered. With flow triggering, the ventilator senses a drop in flow with the patient's spontaneous effort. The drop in flow triggers the delivery of a breath (Squadrone, Gregoretti, & Ranieri, 2005).

Positive End Expiratory Pressure (PEEP)

In many restrictive disease conditions such as ARDS, pulmonary edema, pneumonia, and atelectasis, the volume of air normally present in the lungs at the end of a resting exhalation, called functional residual capacity (FRC), is lost. Loss of FRC contributes to shunt and hypoxemia. PEEP is used to restore the FRC and decrease the shunt. While a PEEP level of 3 to 5 cm H_2O is considered "physiologic," higher levels are common in critically ill patients with high oxygen requirements. Addition of PEEP keeps alveoli open at the end of exhalation.

A parameter related to PEEP is continuous positive airway pressure (CPAP). Because it is also called a mode and is commonly used as a last step in the weaning process, CPAP is discussed in the section on modes of ventilation.

Fraction of Inspired Oxygen (FiO$_2$)

FiO_2 is the percentage of oxygen delivered to the patient; it varies from .21 to 1.00. If levels of 50% or greater are required to maintain adequate oxygenation, increases in PEEP may be considered to enhance alveolar opening and subsequently augment oxygenation.

Volume Modes

Control Mode

With control mode, the ventilator provides all of the patient's MV. The clinician sets the Vt, RR, Ti, sensitivity (this is always set even with the control mode so that a patient is not "locked out" and can initiate a breath), PEEP, and FiO_2. Generally, the term "control mode" is used to describe situations in which the patient is chemically relaxed or is paralyzed from a spinal cord or neuromuscular disease and is, therefore, unable to initiate spontaneous breaths. The ventilator mode setting may be set on controlled mandatory ventilation, control ventilation, assist/control, or synchronized intermittent mandatory ventilation (SIMV)—all of these options provide volume breaths at the clinician-selected rate.

Assist/Control or Assisted Mandatory Ventilation   This option requires that Vt, RR, Ti, sensitivity, PEEP, and FiO_2 be set for the patient. When the patient initiates a spontaneous breath between control breaths, a full-volume breath is delivered.

Intermittent Mandatory Ventilation and Synchronized Intermittent Mandatory Ventilation (SIMV)   This mode requires

that Vt, RR, Ti, sensitivity, FiO_2 and PEEP be set. In between "mandatory breaths," patients can spontaneously breathe at their own rate and depth. With SIMV, the ventilator synchronizes the mandatory breaths with the patient's own inspirations. While this mode was commonly used in the past to wean patients, it is selected less frequently today.

Pressure Modes of Ventilation

Pressure Support Ventilation (PSV)   The PSV mode is used with patients who are breathing spontaneously. The patient's inspiratory effort is augmented with a preselected pressure level. Pressure support offers assistance to overcome resistance of the artificial airway (endotracheal tube [ETT]), ventilator circuits, and ventilator demand valves. With PSV, the clinician selects an IPL (sometimes labeled PS level), sensitivity, FiO_2, and PEEP. When the patient initiates a breath, a high flow of gas is delivered to the preselected pressure level, and this pressure is maintained throughout inspiration. The patient determines the parameters of Vt, RR, and Ti. The advantage of this mode is that it provides for decreased work of breathing for the patient, although this is a function of the selected pressure level.

Pressure Control (PC) and Pressure Control/Inverse Ratio Ventilation (PC/IRV)   PC is a control mode and requires that the clinician select IPL, RR, Ti, sensitivity, FiO_2, and PEEP. PC/IRV combines pressure-limited ventilation with an inverse ratio of inspiration to expiration. The clinician selects the IPL, RR, Ti (to ensure an inverse I:E ratio of 1:1, 2:1, 3:1, or 4:1), FiO_2, and PEEP level. With the prolonged inspiratory times, auto-PEEP may result. Auto-PEEP, the result of not providing adequate time for exhalation, may be a desirable outcome of the inverse ratios. This mode is often used for patients with ARDS. The disadvantage of this mode is that Vt will be affected with changes in compliance and resistance. For example, patients with stiffer lungs will receive less tidal volume.

Continuous Positive Airway Pressure (CPAP)   This ventilatory option is similar to PEEP in that it is designed to restore functional residual capacity. Unlike PEEP, however, it is provided without positive-pressure ventilator breaths. CPAP is referred to as a spontaneous breathing mode because all breaths are patient initiated. Settings are sensitivity, PEEP, and FiO_2. CPAP is a popular mode choice for spontaneous-breathing weaning trials. Short-duration trials (i.e., 30 minutes to 2 hours) of CPAP are interspersed with rest using modes that provide more complete ventilatory support.

Newer Pressure Mode Options

PSV, PC, and PC/IRV are among the traditional pressure options available on most ventilators. Some newer ventilators offer additional modes as well. Some of these mode options are described briefly in this section.

Volume-guaranteed pressure (VGP) modes combine PSV (decelerating flow pattern) with guaranteed volume delivery. A variety of options are available depending on the manufacturer. These modes were developed to ventilate patients using pressure while ensuring that Vt and MV are maintained (Bear Medical Systems, 2005; Marquette Critical Care, 2005; Puritan Bennett, 2005; Respironics, 2005). The following are a sample of VGP options available on ventilators; they are a mix of control (i.e., RR and Ti selected) and spontaneous breathing options:

- Pressure Augmentation (Bear 1000, Bear Medical Systems, Palm Springs, California)
- Volume Support (VS) (Siemens-Marquette Critical Care Bridgewater and Puritan Bennett 840, Pleasanton, California)
- Pressure Regulated Volume Control (PRVC) (Siemens-Marquette Critical Care Bridgewater, New Jersey)
- Volume Ventilation Plus (Puritan Bennett 840, Pleasanton, California)

Parameters that are set for VGP options include Vt, FiO_2, PEEP, sensitivity (all), and RR and Ti (only for the control modes).

An example of a VGP option for spontaneously breathing patients is VS ventilation. With this mode, the clinician selects the desired Vt, and the ventilator then adjusts the pressure support level (in 3-cm H_2O increments) on a breath-to-breath basis to provide this volume. Thus all the breaths are pressure breaths. Advantages of this mode include a guarantee that a minimal Vt is being delivered with each breath, use of the lowest amount of required pressure support, and easier weaning and greater comfort. The disadvantages are that the patient must be breathing spontaneously, the Vt must be set appropriately, and a backup mode must be available in the event the patient develops apnea (Sottiaux, 2001).

An example of a VGP option for controlled ventilation is Pressure Regulated Volume Control (PRVC). The RR, Ti, Vt, FiO_2, PEEP, and sensitivity (so the patient can take breaths) are preset. The ventilator adjusts the pressure level, as described in the VS option, to ensure the desired Vt. A pressure limit is set to prevent high airway pressures and complications such as pneumothorax.

Airway pressure release ventilation (APRV) and bilevel positive airway pressure (BiPAP) (Puritan Bennett 840, Pleasanton, California) are two other new options. APRV allows for spontaneous breathing on a preset (relatively high) CPAP level, which is interrupted by a short (one-second) release for further expiration. This mode is designed for the pa-

tient with ARDS. The brief releases allow for improved emptying of alveolar units while preventing complete lung deflation. With ARPV, the ventilator cycles between the selected CPAP level and the baseline (usually zero). The pressure release allows for CO_2 to be eliminated. This mode has been shown to decrease the need for paralysis and sedation, increase cardiac performance, decrease vasopressor use, and decrease airway pressures (Kaplan, Bailey, & Formosa, 2001).

BiPAP allows for spontaneous breathing during both inspiratory and expiratory cycles of respiration. Two levels of pressure are set: high PEEP and low PEEP. These levels are somewhat comparable to the IPL and PEEP levels set with PC. BiPAP mode is considered appropriate in patients with ARDS, individuals with noncompliant lungs, and patients in whom the use of paralytic agents is undesirable.

NURSING MANAGEMENT OF THE PATIENT ON MECHANICAL VENTILATION

Meticulous nursing care of the patient on mechanical ventilation is essential to optimize patient outcomes and to prevent complications. A combination of clinical judgment, caring practices, clinical inquiry, and acting as a facilitator of learning competencies is essential.

Troubleshooting Ventilator Alarms

When the ventilator is set up, a number of alarm parameters are set to alert clinicians of possible changes in the patient's condition. A troubleshooting guide for ventilator alarms appears in Table 23-2.

Sedation

Intubated and ventilated patients may require the administration of sedatives and sometimes paralytic agents to promote comfort, decrease the work of breathing, and promote patient ventilator synchrony (Kong & Bion, 2003). Common sedatives used for these purposes include propofol (Diprivan®), a very-short-acting agent for intravenous infusion use only; lorazepam (Ativan®), an intermediate-acting benzodiazepine that may be given orally, intramuscularly, or intravenously; and midazolam (Versed®), a short-acting benzodiazepine that may be given intramuscularly or intravenously. Regardless of the agent used, it is essential that sedation infusions be interrupted until the patient is awake at least daily to ensure that oversedation does not occur.

Avoiding Complications of Mechanical Ventilation: Applying the Science

Mechanical ventilation for more than three consecutive days is considered long term and is associated with increased

TABLE 23-2 Common Ventilator Alarms

Alarm	Possible Causes	Actions
High pressure limit	Patient requires suctioning. Kinking of ventilator tubing. Coughing. Biting on endotracheal tube. Water in ventilator tubing. Patient ventilator dyssynchrony (breathing against the ventilator) from agitation, pain, anxiety, or changes in physical status such as pneumothorax. Increased lung stiffness from disease progression (e.g., ARDS, pneumonia, pneumothorax). Increased airway resistance (e.g., bronchospasm). Tube migration into the right mainstem bronchus. Other conditions that impair breathing, such as ascites or late pregnancy.	Auscultate breath sounds bilaterally to check for the presence of equality and for adventitious sounds. Determine whether the patient requires suctioning. Check for the presence of any of the other causes. Insert bite block if indicated. Administer analgesics, sedation, or anxiolytics, as indicated. Provide psychosocial support and a calm environment. Reassure the patient as needed.
High respiratory rate	Patient is breathing faster than the preset rate. May indicate pain or anxiety or that the patient is awakening from sedation or anesthesia. May indicate changing compliance (e.g., pulmonary edema, pneumothorax), resistance (e.g., bronchospasm), or pulmonary embolus.	Explore potential reasons. Administer pain medication or sedation if clinically indicated. Seek consultation from a seasoned clinician or respiratory therapist.
Low inspiratory pressure	Leak or disconnect somewhere in the system. Endotracheal tube cuff may need more air.	Check for a leak or disconnect. If unable to locate the problem and alarm persists, call respiratory therapy. Follow institutional policy for reinflating endotracheal tube cuffs, as indicated. If unable to quickly identify and remedy the cause of the alarm, initiate manual ventilation and call for help.
Low minute volume	Leak or disconnect somewhere in the system.	Check for a leak or disconnect. If unable to quickly identify and remedy the cause of the alarm, initiate manual ventilation and call for help.
Low exhaled tidal volume	Leak or disconnect somewhere in the system. Leak in the endotracheal tube cuff. The patient may have become disconnected from the ventilator. The patient is taking shallow breaths at a volume less than the preset volume on the alarm, depending on the mode of ventilation in use. Lungs are less compliant, so less air can be delivered to the patient. Air leaking out of the chest tube if one is present.	Check whether the patient is disconnected from the ventilator; reconnect if disconnected. Check for a leak or disconnect. Reinflate the cuff according to institutional policy and procedure if the cuff is deflating. If the patient has a chest tube, check the water seal chamber for presence of an air leak. If unable to quickly identify and remedy the cause of the alarm, initiate manual ventilation and call for help.
Low PEEP/CPAP	Leak or disconnect somewhere in the system.	Check for a leak or disconnect. If unable to quickly identify and remedy the cause of the alarm, initiate manual ventilation and call for help.
Apnea	The patient did not take a breath within the preset time interval.	Assess if the patient is breathing on own. If no breathing is present, call for help, begin manual resuscitation immediately, and notify the physician and respiratory therapy.

TABLE 23-2 Common Ventilator Alarms

Alarm	Possible Causes	Actions
Low oxygen pressure	There is a malfunction with the oxygen delivery to the ventilator.	Remove the patient from the ventilator. Use a bag-valve device to ventilate patient via the ETT. If unable to quickly identify and remedy the cause of the alarm, initiate manual ventilation and call for help.

complications and poor outcomes (e.g., increased lengths of stay, death) (Douglas, Daly, Gordon, & Brennan, 2002). Complications such as ventilator-associated pneumonia (VAP), immobility, urinary tract infections, deep vein thrombosis, gastrointestinal bleeding, barotrauma, volu-trauma, and critical illness myopathies and neuropathies are common (Tablan, Anderson, Besser, Bridges, & Hajjeh, 2003). Complications not discussed in other chapters of this book will be described.

Ventilator-Associated Pneumonia

A common complication and cause of significant morbidity and mortality in ventilated patients is VAP. As a result, organizations such as the Centers for Disease Control and Prevention and the Institute for Healthcare Improvement have made recommendations for healthcare institutions to decrease the occurrence of this complication. One of the most important recommendations is that the head-of-bed elevation be at least 30° to minimize the risk of aspiration of gastric contents. Other recommendations (which have varying levels of evidence supporting them) include strategies such as continuous subglottic suctioning, in-line suction catheters, and mouth care. Further illustrating the magnitude of the importance of VAP, the Joint Commission on Accreditation of Healthcare Organizations (JCAHO) has included VAP prevention in its 2005 National Patient Safety Goals (JCAHO, 2006).

Barotrauma

Barotrauma refers to damage created by pressure. The resultant injury allows for the passage of air into a space in which it is abnormal. Also referred to as air leak disease, barotrauma is seen in many forms, such as pneumothorax, pneumomediastinum (air in the mediastinum or thoracic cavity), and pneumoperitineum (air in the peritoneal cavity). However, pneumothorax is a major—and dreaded—complication of mechanical ventilation. It is especially feared when the pneumothorax is under tension. With a tension pneumothorax, air moves from the lung into the pleural space, resulting in lung collapse. Subsequent positive-pressure breaths result in in-

creased intrathoracic pressure and cardiac tamponade. Signs and symptoms include dyspnea, tachypnea, tachycardia (early), elevated blood pressure (early), elevated chest on the affected side, tracheal deviation to the opposite side, and tympanic percussion sounds. As the pneumothorax continues to compress the heart, hypotension, bradycardia, and death ensue. For these reasons, early detection and treatment are essential. Treatment consists of the placement of a large-bore needle into the second intercostal space, mid-clavicular line, to rapidly decompress the pneumothorax.

While all ventilated patients—especially those with severe illnesses—are at risk for pneumothorax, attention to the pressures associated with mechanical ventilation is essential if barotrauma is to be avoided. In the patient with acute asthma, for example, bronchoconstriction of the airways results in dynamic hyperinflation (overinflated lungs) (Corbridge & Corbridge, 2005). The overdistention increases the pressure in the lungs and may result in barotrauma and hemodynamic compromise. Hypotension results because the lungs of the asthmatic patient are compliant; lung overdistention is transmitted to the pulmonary capillary bed, compressing the capillaries and decreasing venous return. In this example, mechanical ventilation interventions are aimed at decreasing the variables that contribute to the high distending pressures. These measures include decreasing the rate, shortening the inspiratory time, and decreasing the Vt (Corbridge & Corbridge).

Volu-trauma

A separate but related phenomenon to barotrauma is volu-trauma. This complication of mechanical ventilation refers to acute lung injury associated with the mechanical ventilation of ARDS patients' lungs. As noted earlier (and discussed in detail in Chapter 25), ARDS lungs are very noncompliant (stiff). To distend them, high pressures are necessary. In human studies, investigators have found that ventilating the lung at small Vts (i.e., 6 mL/kg) improved the mortality of patients with ARDS (Acute Respiratory Distress Syndrome Network, 2000). To that end, ventilation of patients with ARDS may include using low-targeted Vts (Acute Respiratory Distress Syndrome Network).

Critical Illness Myopathies and Neuropathies

Ventilated patients often require sedatives and narcotics to ensure their comfort and tolerance of the therapy. Even when high doses of sedatives and narcotics are given, however, patient–ventilator synchrony sometimes is not possible. In such cases, paralytic agents are necessary. Even though their use may be lifesaving, the associated complications are of concern to all caregivers and point to the importance of limiting these agents' use when possible. The use of paralytic agents alone or in combination with steroids may result in critical illness myopathies or neuropathies (and often a combination of the two) (Murray et al., 2002). The result is profound weakness, prolonged duration of ventilation, and increased length of stay. Weaning from mechanical ventilation is gradual, and physical rehabilitation is frequently necessary. Some modes of ventilation may obviate the need for paralytic agents and should be considered.

Other Nursing Interventions

Patients requiring mechanical ventilation are assessed on an ongoing basis to evaluate them for ventilator tolerance. Changes in cardiac output, gas exchange, breathing pattern, and use of accessory muscles are monitored especially closely with ventilator changes and during weaning. With any adverse changes in the patient's condition, the nurse assesses potential causes, in addition to confirming that the ventilator mode and settings are as anticipated. Whenever the patient is distressed and the immediate cause cannot be identified and remedied, the nurse should seek help immediately.

The ETT must be well secured to prevent inadvertent extubation. This may be accomplished with tape or a commercially available device. In addition, the location of the tube (in cm) is noted (e.g., generally 21 to 22 cm at the lip) to ensure that the tube has not migrated (down or up). The use of restraints is determined by hospital policy, and they should rarely be used to prevent self-extubation unless other interventions are unsuccessful.

To prevent lip necrosis, the ETT can be moved daily from one side of the mouth to the other. Cuff inflation pressures (generally no higher than 20 mm Hg) are carefully monitored to prevent overinflation and complications such as tracheo-esophageal fistulas, tracheal stenosis, or tracheal malacia.

Being intubated and receiving mechanical ventilation can be stressful for the patient. Sources of stress include pain, fear, anxiety, sleep disturbances, tenseness, inability to speak/communicate, lack of control, nightmares, and loneliness (Rotondi et al., 2002). Nursing measures are incorporated into the care of the patient to ameliorate or minimize these stressors. Providing a mechanism for patients to communicate and giving anxiolytics judiciously are helpful. Methods to assist with sleep disturbances are described in Chapter 5. Spending time with the patient and allowing for frequent family visitation may minimize loneliness.

The ICU nurse can also act as a facilitator of learning for the patient and family. Helping the family understand the rationale for use of the ventilator, the reason their loved one is unable to vocalize, and what to expect goes a long way toward decreasing anxiety and fear and building trust. Teaching how the weaning process is variable is also important, so that expectations are realistic. (Weaning is discussed in the next section.) Timing of teaching is critical and varies with the individual. Finally, the provision of requested information in understandable terms and psychosocial support of the family are essential components of ICU nursing.

WEANING FROM THE VENTILATOR

Weaning from mechanical ventilation, also called ventilator liberation, refers to the process of the patient assuming more and more of the work of breathing and finally demonstrating that ventilator support is no longer required. Weaning can be accomplished with an ETT or a tracheostomy tube in place. In the case of the ETT, the final step in the process is the removal of the tube (extubation). With a tracheostomy, the final step may be the ability to breath spontaneously for a designated period of time with the tube in place.

Weaning Assessment

Once the patient is no longer in the critical stage of illness, plans for weaning are initiated. The first step is to determine whether the patient is ready to begin the process. It starts by ensuring that the reason for mechanical ventilation has resolved or improved and that sedatives, if used in the acute stage of illness, are appropriately decreased (Kress et al., 2003; Kress, Pohlman, O'Connor, & Hall, 2000; MacIntyre et al., 2001). Numerous tests and measurements are performed, including arterial blood gases, oxygen saturation, end-tidal carbon dioxide monitoring, respiratory waveform monitoring, and physical signs and symptoms. In addition, weaning indices have been used in the past to attempt to predict the outcome of weaning trials (Burns, Burns, & Truwit, 1994; Goodnough-Hanneman, 1994). To date, none have proven to be a strong predictor of wean trial outcome (MacIntyre et al.). However, comprehensive, systematic assessments appear to keep care planning on target, decrease variation in the processes of care, and improve outcomes (Burns et al., 1998). An example of one such weaning assessment tool is seen in **Figure 23-1**.

FIGURE 23-1 Burns Weaning Assessment Program©

Patient _____

Not
Yes No assessed   **GENERAL ASSESSMENT**

__ __ __ 1. Hemodynamically stable (pulse rate, cardiac output)?
__ __ __ 2. Free from factors that increase or decrease metabolic rate (seizures, temperature, sepsis, bacteremia, hypo/hyperthyroid)?
__ __ __ 3. Hematocrit >25% (or baseline)?
__ __ __ 4. Systemically hydrated (weight at or near baseline, balanced intake and output)?
__ __ __ 5. Nourished (albumin >2.5, parenteral/enteral feeding maximized)? (If albumin is low and anasarca or third spacing
      is present, score for hydration should be No.)
__ __ __ 6. Electrolytes within normal limits? (including Ca^{++}, Mg^+, PO_4).
      *Correct Ca^{++} for albumin level.
__ __ __ 7. Pain controlled? (subjective determination)
__ __ __ 8. Adequate sleep/rest? (subjective determination)
__ __ __ 9. Appropriate level of anxiety and nervousness? (subjective determination)
__ __ __ 10. Absence of bowel problems (diarrhea, constipation, ileus)?
__ __ __ 11. Improved general body strength/endurance (i.e., out of bed in chair, progressive activity program)?
__ __ __ 12. Chest roentgenogram improving?

Respiratory Assessment
Gas flow and work of breathing

__ __ __ 13. Eupneic respiratory rate and pattern (spontaneous respiratory rate <25, without dyspnea, absence of accessory
      muscle use).
      *This is assessed off the ventilator while measuring #20–23.
__ __ __ 14. Absence of adventitious breath sounds (rhonchi, rales, wheezing)?
__ __ __ 15. Secretions thin and minimal?
__ __ __ 16. Absence of neuromuscular disease/deformity?
__ __ __ 17. Absence of abdominal distention/obesity/ascites?
__ __ __ 18. Oral endotracheal tube ≥ 7.5 or trach ≥ 6.5

Airway clearance

__ __ __ 19. Cough and swallow reflexes adequate?

Strength

__ __ __ 20. Negative inspiratory pressure <−20 cm H2O
__ __ __ 21. Positive expiratory pressure >+30 cm H2O

Endurance

__ __ __ 22. Spontaneous tidal volume >5 mL/kg?
__ __ __ 23. Vital capacity >10 to 15 mL/kg?

Arterial blood gases

__ __ __ 24. pH between 7.30–7.45
__ __ __ 25. $PaCO_2$ approximately 40 mm Hg (or baseline) with minute ventilation <10 L/min (evaluated while on ventilator)
__ __ __ 26. PaO_2 >60 on FiO_2 <40%

To score the BWAP: divide the number of "yes" responses by 26

Source: Reprinted with permission from Suzanne Burns: © Burns.

Weaning Trial Protocols

Studies have demonstrated that the use of multidisciplinary weaning protocols improves outcomes—specifically, ventilator duration and lengths of stay in the hospital (Grap et al., 2003; MacIntyre et al., 2001; Marelich et al., 2000; Vitacca et al., 2001). The protocols consist of a "wean screen" (i.e., when to "go" criteria), the protocol (i.e., mode and duration of the trial), and criteria defining wean trial intolerance (i.e., when to "stop"). Most of the protocols also define how to provide ventilatory rest between trials. An example of a weaning protocol is seen in **Figure 23-2**. Today, most trials of weaning are done using a spontaneous breathing mode method such as "blow-by/T-piece," CPAP, and PS.

Blow-by/T-Piece and CPAP Trials

The terms "blow-by" and "T-piece" are used interchangeably. These methods provide a continuous flow of humidified gases at a predetermined FiO_2 to the patient (i.e., the gases "blow by"). While the methods generally are delivered by means of a humidifier separate from the ventilator, some ventilators provide a similar method and do not require additional equipment. "T-piece" refers to the adaptor sometimes used with this method, which is shaped like a "T". In contrast to the blow-by/T-piece methods, CPAP is a positive-pressure mode. All of these methods, however, require that the patient breathe spontaneously. Trials using these methods require a high degree of patient work, and fatigue may result if the trials are unduly long in duration. Studies have shown that short-duration trials (30 minutes to 2 hours, once or twice per day) using these methods are best. Between trials, a support mode of ventilation is used to "rest" the patient.

PSV Trials

PSV provides positive pressure with spontaneous inspiration, thereby augmenting or assisting inspiration. Workload, then, is dependent on the pressure level. Spontaneous breathing trials using PSV can be gradually and gently managed. The PSV level can be decreased in stages, so that abrupt increases in patient workload are avoided.

Other Modes of Weaning

Many combinations of modes and methods are used in clinical practice. However, few have demonstrated superiority over the spontaneous breathing trials described previously. In any event, the most important aspects of successful ventilator liberation include correcting physiologic and psychological factors that might impede weaning, aggressively testing for readiness, and initiating early but appropriate spontaneous

breathing trials. Protocols that clearly define "when to go" and "when to stop" decrease variation and help move the weaning process forward.

Multidisciplinary Approaches to Weaning

Multidisciplinary system approaches to weaning appear to result in positive outcomes (Burns et al., 1998; Henneman, Dracup, Ganz, Molayeme, & Cooper, 2002; Smyrnios et al., 2002) and are to be encouraged. These approaches incorporate numerous evidence-based aspects of care, such as protocols for sedation management and weaning trials, prophylaxis guidelines (e.g., deep vein thrombosis, sinusitis, gastrointestinal bleeding), timing of tracheostomy, nutrition interventions, and mobility plans. A key aspect of these initiatives is the use of an advanced practice nurse to guide and manage the process (Burns et al.). Much as with protocols, such initiatives are in large part successful because they decrease variations in care processes and encourage the development of a multidisciplinary team approach to weaning.

PATIENT OUTCOMES

Nurses can help ensure obtainment of optimal patient outcomes such as those listed in **Box 23-2**, through the use of evidence-based interventions for patients receiving mechanical ventilation.

SUMMARY

Mechanical ventilation is a modality used to help deliver oxygen and eliminate CO_2. There are many modes of ventilation available. When placing a patient on a ventilator, several decisions are made about appropriate settings. These decisions are based on the patient's clinical condition, physiological parameters, and goals of ventilation. A multidisciplinary approach to care is essential to help ensure weaning and other optimal patient outcomes.

Box 23-2
Optimal Patient Outcomes

- Spontaneous breathing without an artificial airway
- Adequate ventilation within expected range
- Patient ventilator synchrony
- Improvement or resolution of underlying disease process
- Improved nutritional status
- Decreased length of time on the ventilator

FIGURE 23-2 Weaning Protocols

Weaning Trial Screen: assessed daily.

1. Hemodynamic stability (no dysrhythmias, HR≤120, absence of vasopressors - - low dose dopamine and dobutamine are exceptions)
2. FiO$_2$ ≤ 50%
3. Positive End Expiratory Pressure ≤ 8 cm H$_2$0
4. BWAP > 45% (in patients ventilated less than 3 days, a BWAP assessment is not necessary)
5. *If the patient meets all these criteria a **wean trial protocol** is initiated following discussion with multidisiplinary team.*

Wean Trial Protocol: Continuous Positive Airway Pressure (CPAP) *(1 trial - 1 hour duration)*

1. One trial of CPAP is attempted daily. The trial may last no more than 1 hour total unless previously negotiated with health care team.
2. With any signs of intolerance (see definition below), the trial is discontinued and the patient is returned to a resting mode until the next trial.
3. When the complete trial is sustained without signs of intolerance, the team is approached and extubation is discussed.
4. Full respiratory muscle rest is provided between trials and at night.

OR

Wean Trial Protocol: Pressure Support Ventilation (PSV) (2 trials - 4 hrs duration)

1. Start at PSV max level (level to attain RR ≤ 20 with Vt of 8 - 10 ml/kg)
2. Decrease PSV by 5 cm H$_2$0.
3. If no signs of intolerance are evident during the first four hour trial, the PSV is decreased by another 5 cm H$_2$0 for the 2nd trial.
4. With any signs of intolerance during trials, the patient is returned to previous level for the next 4 hour trial.
5. If unable to tolerate, the patient is fully rested until the next day when the process begins again.
6. Once the patient is able to sustain 5 - 6 cm PSV without signs of intolerance (for 4 hours) the team is approached and extubation is discussed.

Intolerance for either protocol is defined as any of the following (3-5 minutes sustained):

1. RR ≥ 35 for 5 mm
2. O$_2$ sat ≤ 90% or a decrease of 4%
3. HR ≥ 140 and/or a 20% sustained change of HR in either direction
4. Systolic BP ≥ 180, ≤ 90 mm Hg
5. Excessive anxiety or agitation
6. Diaphoresis

Rest for either Protocol:

1. PSV max: PSV max is that pressure level required to attain a RR or 20 or less and a Vt of 8-10 ml/kg. Respiratory pattern should be synchronous and there should be no accessory muscle use.
2. Other modes: With volume modes such as Assist Control (A/C) or Intermittent Mandatory Ventilation (IMV), respiratory muscle rest is not assured unless there is cessation of respiratory muscle activity. Therefore, rest is considered that level of support required to prevent patient initiated breaths. When IMV is used, PSV may be added for protection (i.e., as a "safety"). Regardless, the goal is cessation of spontaneous effort.

Source: Adapted from University of Virginia Health System MICU weaning protocol (© 2002 by the Rector and Board of Visitors of the University of Virginia).

CASE STUDY

A 62-year-old patient in the medical ICU with sepsis and ARDS is intubated and ventilated through a size 7.5 oral endotracheal tube. The settings on the ventilator are $FiO_2 = 0.8$, A/C mode with a respiratory rate of 20, Ti = 1 sec, Vt = 800 mL, and PEEP = 5 cm H_2O. The patient is agitated and thrashing, breathes a total of 40 times per minute, and has the following ABG: pH = 7.32, $PaCO_2 = 34$ mm Hg, $PaO_2 = 52$ mm Hg, $HCO_3 = 20$ mEq/mL.

CRITICAL THINKING QUESTIONS

1. What are your thoughts about how the patient is tolerating the ventilator?

2. What can be done to ensure that complications such as barotrauma and volu-trauma do not occur?

3. How should weaning progress?

The nurse and the respiratory therapist monitor the O_2 saturation while the two parameters (PEEP and FiO_2 are decreased). First the FiO_2 is decreased to 45%. The O_2 saturation is 97% after 30 minutes on the setting, so the PEEP is then decreased to 8 cm H_2O. With this intervention, the saturation drops to 95%; RR and Vt are 20 beats/min and 400 mL, respectively. Because the patient now meets the wean screen criteria, a CPAP trial on 8 cm H_2O is initiated. Unfortunately, the patient does not tolerate the trial. RR increases to 42 beats/min, and saturation decreases to 89%. The patient is tachycardic and diaphoretic. He is placed back on PSV and rested overnight. A CPAP trial is provided early the next day, and the patient tolerates a 30-minute CPAP trial without signs of intolerance. After obtaining an ABG (pH = 7.42, $PaCO_2 = 39$, $PaO_2 = 80$) on CPAP, the team decides to extubate the patient. The extubation is successful and the patient is transferred to the floor later that evening.

4. Why was the weaning trial outcome unsuccessful one day yet successful the very next day?

CRITICAL THINKING QUESTIONS

1. Use the form to write up a plan of care for one client in the clinical setting on mechanical ventilation. Rate the patient as a level 1, 3, or 5 on each characteristic. Identify the level of nurse characteristics needed in the care of this patient.
2. Take one patient outcome for a patient and list evidence-based interventions found in a literature review for this patient.

Using the Synergy Model to Develop a Plan of Care

Patient Characteristics	Level (1, 3, 5)	Subjective and Objective Data	Evidence-based Interventions	Outcomes
Resiliency				
Vulnerability				
Stability				
Complexity				
Resource availability				
Participation in care				
Participation in decision making				
Predictability				

Online Resources

Critical Care Medicine Tutorials, mechanical ventilators: www.ccmtutorials.com/rs/mv/page3.htm

Ventilator System Check—AARC Clinical Practice Guideline: www.rcjournal.com/online_resources

Patient education: www.patienteducation.upmc.com/pdf/ventilatorbooklet.pdf

Ventilator: www.meded.ucsd.edu/isp/2001;sicu/vent.html

Ventilator management: www.emedicine.com/emerg

REFERENCES

Acute Respiratory Distress Syndrome Network. (2000). Ventilation with lower tidal volumes as compared with traditional tidal volumes for acute lung injury and the acute respiratory distress syndrome. *New England Journal of Medicine, 342*, 1301–1307.

Bear Medical Systems. (2005). Retrieved July 1, 2005, from www.bearmedical.com

Burns, S. M. (2005). Mechanical ventilation of patients with acute respiratory distress syndrome and patients requiring weaning. The evidence guiding practice. *Critical Care Nurse, 25*(4), 14–16, 18, 20–24.

Burns, S. M., Burns, J. E., & Truwit, J. D. (1994). Comparison of five clinical weaning indices. *American Journal of Critical Care, 3*, 342–352.

Burns, S. M., Marshall, M., Burns, J. E., Ryan, B., Nilmoth, D., Carpenter, R., et al. (1998). Design, testing, and results of an outcomes-managed approach to patients requiring prolonged mechanical ventilation. *American Journal of Critical Care, 7*, 45–57.

Corbridge, T., & Corbridge, S. J. (2005). Severe asthma exacerbation. In M. Fink, E. Abraham, J-L. Vincent, & P. M. Kochanek, *Textbook of critical care* (5th ed., pp. 587–597). Philadelphia: Saunders.

Douglas, S. L., Daly, B. J., Gordon, N., & Brennan, P. F. (2002). Survival and quality of life: Short-term versus long-term ventilator patients. *Critical Care Medicine, 30*, 2655–2662.

Goodnough-Hanneman, S. K. (1994). Multidimensional predictors of success or failure with early weaning from mechanical ventilation after cardiac surgery. *Nursing Research, 43*, 4–10.

Grap, M. J., Strickland, D., Tormey, L., Keane, K., Lubin, S., & Emerson, J. (2003). Collaborative practice: Development, implementation and evaluation of a weaning protocol for patients receiving mechanical ventilation. *American Journal of Critical Care, 12*, 454–460.

Henneman, E., Dracup, K., Ganz, T., Molayeme, O., & Cooper, C. B. (2002). Using a collaborative weaning plan to decrease duration of mechanical ventilation and length of stay in the intensive care unit for patients receiving long-term mechanical ventilation. *American Journal of Critical Care, 11*, 132–140.

Joint Commission on Accreditation of Healthcare Organizations. (2006). Retrieved January 6, 2006, from www.jcaho.org

Kaplan, L., Bailey, H., & Formosa, V. (2001). Airway pressure release ventilation increases cardiac performance in patients with acute lung injury/adult respiratory distress syndrome. *Critical Care, 5*, 221–226.

Kong, K. L., & Bion, J. F. (2003). Sedating patients undergoing mechanical ventilation in the intensive care unit—winds of change? *British Journal of Anaesthesia, 90*(3), 267–269.

Kress, J. P., Gehlbach, B., Lacy, M., Pliskin, N., Pohlman, A. S., & Hall, J. B. (2003). The long-term psychological effects of daily sedative interruption on critically ill patients. *American Journal of Respiratory and Critical Care Medicine, 168*(20), 1457–1461.

Kress, J. P., Pohlman, A. S., O'Connor, M. F., & Hall, J. B. (2000). Daily interruption of sedative infusions in critically ill patients undergoing mechanical ventilation. *New England Journal of Medicine, 342*, 1471–1477.

MacIntyre, N. R., Cook, D. J., Ely, E. W. Jr, Epstein, S. K., Fink, J. B., Heffner, J. E., et al. (2001). Evidence-based guidelines for weaning and discontinuing ventilatory support: A collective task force facilitated by the American College of Chest Physicians; the American Association for Respiratory Care; and the American College of Critical Care Medicine. *Chest, 120*(6 Suppl), 375S–395S.

Marelich, G. P., Murin, S., Battistella, F., Inciardi, J., Vierra, T., & Roby, M. (2000). Protocol weaning of mechanical ventilation in medical and surgical patients by respiratory care practitioners and nurses: Effect on weaning time and incidence of ventilator associated pneumonia. *Chest, 118*, 459–467.

Marquette Critical Care. (2005). Retrieved July 26, 2005, from http://www.marquette.com/criticalcare

Murray, M. J., Cowen, J., DeBlock, H., Erstad, B., Gray, A. W., Tescher, A. N., et al. (2002). Clinical practice guidelines for sustained neuromuscular blockade in the adult critically ill patient. *Critical Care Medicine, 30*(1), 142–156.

Pierce, L. N. (2000). Traditional and non-traditional modes of mechanical ventilation. *Critical Care Nurse, 20*(1), 81–84.

Puritan Bennett. (2005). Retrieved July 26, 2005, from http://www.puritanbennett.com

Respironics. (2005). Retrieved July 26, 2005, from http://www.respironics.com

Rotondi, A. J., Celluri, L., Sirio, C., Mendelsohn, A., Schulz, R., Belle, S., et al. (2002). Patients' recollections of stressful experiences while receiving prolonged mechanical ventilation in an intensive care unit. *Critical Care Medicine, 30*(4), 746–752.

Roussos, C., & Koutsoukou, A. (2003). Respiratory failure. *European Respiratory Journal, 22*(Suppl. 47), 3S–14S.

Smyrnios, N. A., Connolly, A., Wilson, M. M., Curley, F. J., French, C. T., Heard, S. O., et al. (2002). Effects of a multifaceted, multidisciplinary, hospital-wide quality improvement program on weaning from mechanical ventilation. *Critical Care Medicine, 30*, 1224–1230.

Sottiaux, T. M. (2001). Patient–ventilator interactions during volume-support ventilation: Asynchronized and tidal volume instability—a report of three cases. *Respiratory Care, 46*(3), 255–262.

Squadrone, V., Gregoretti, C., & Ranieri, V. M. (2005). Patient–ventilator interaction. In M. P. Fink, E. Abraham, J-L. Vincent, & P. M. Kochanek, *Textbook of critical care* (5th ed., pp. 505–510). Philadelphia: Saunders.

Tablan, O. C., Anderson, L. J., Besser, R., Bridges, C., & Hajjeh, R. (2003). Guidelines for preventing health-care–associated pneumonia; recommendations of CDC and the Healthcare Infection Control Practices Advisory Committee. *Morbidity and Mortality Weekly Report, 53*(RRO3), 1–36.

Vitacca, M., Vianello, A., Colombo, D., Clini, E., Porta, R., Bianchi, L., et al. (2001). Comparison of two methods for weaning COPD patients requiring mechanical ventilation for more than 15 days. *American Journal of Respiratory and Critical Care Medicine, 164*, 225–230.

CHAPTER 24

Common Respiratory Disorders

Michael Day

LEARNING OBJECTIVES

Upon completion of this chapter, the reader will be able to:

1. Differentiate between common respiratory disorders seen in adult patients.
2. Describe clinical manifestations of common respiratory disorders.
3. Discuss treatment options for common respiratory disorders seen in the adult patient.
4. Identify appropriate evidence-based interventions based on clinical judgment for the adult patient experiencing common respiratory disorders.
5. Utilize clinical inquiry in identifying educational resources for the patient with a respiratory disorder.
6. List optimal patient outcomes that may be achieved through evidence-based management of common respiratory disorders.

Patients are commonly hospitalized for respiratory disorders. These disorders can range from the ordinary, such as pneumonia, to the extraordinary, such as avian influenza. Having a basic understanding of respiratory disorders will allow the intensive care unit (ICU) nurse to influence how patients recover from, and even survive, their hospitalization.

This chapter is divided into two sections. The first section discusses respiratory infections. The second section discusses alterations in gas exchange and ventilation. The basic pathophysiology of each disorder, along with its signs and symptoms, is presented. Evidence-based treatment options are then reviewed, followed by patient and family education considerations. By understanding these processes, the ICU nurse will be able to assist patients in their recovery and enhance their level of comfort.

INFLUENZA

Pathophysiology

Influenza is caused by a viral infection that usually simultaneously affects both the upper and lower respiratory tracts. Although influenza is usually benign, it has caused pandemics that have literally killed millions of people—most recently during World War I. Most influenza deaths are caused by either pneumonia or exacerbations of pre-existing diseases, such as heart or respiratory conditions, in conjunction with the influenza. There are two distinct types of influenza: type A and type B, with type A being the most common. The viruses that cause influenza frequently mutate or shift their surface antigens to create new strains (Porth, 2002a), leading to the requirement of yearly vaccinations for the most current strain of influenza. Respiratory syncytial virus (RSV), a disease that has primarily been thought of as a pediatric disease, has been recognized as an important disease in the elderly and high-risk populations; it carries a high mortality rate and is associated with use of healthcare resources similar to that of influenza (Falsey, Hennessey, Formica, Cox, & Walsh, 2005).

Of major concern for the future is the evolution of an *avian* strain of influenza that has crossed over into the human population from birds. The first cases were discovered in 1997 in Hong Kong, and new cases have since emerged in several Asian countries and Europe. This new variant of influenza carries mortality rates as high as 50%. Even though epidemics of this strain have been contained by the fact that it is transmitted primarily from birds to humans, along with the implementation of rigorous public health measures, the world public health community is extremely concerned about the possibility of the strain becoming transmissible *between* humans, which has already occurred in isolated cases. Humans have no innate immunity to this strain of influenza and could be subjected to a pandemic of major portions (Centers for Disease Control [CDC], 2005a).

Influenza can take three distinct forms of infection: simple rhinotracheitis; a viral respiratory infection, which sets the stage for a bacterial infection; and a frank viral pneumonia. The form of infection may be directly related to the mode of transmission. If a patient is infected with large droplets or by hand–respiratory tract contact, the infection initially remains limited to the upper respiratory tract. This initial infection allows the patient's immune system to develop antibodies to the infection and usually prevents disease progression into viral pneumonia. If the patient is exposed to small droplets, they may bypass the upper respiratory tract and infect the lower respiratory tract before the patient's body has time to develop antibodies to the infection. The rapid infection of the lower respiratory tract is responsible for the progression of viral pneumonia from onset of symptoms to significant hypoxemia and even death, over the course of a few days.

When infecting the respiratory tract, the virus produces a patchy destruction of the serous cells and the cilia lining of the respiratory tract. This damage allows extracellular fluid to escape through the basement membrane into the respiratory tract, causing accumulation of secretions. As the respiratory tract heals, the serous cells heal more quickly than the cilia. Although secretions are produced, because the cilia remain damaged, the secretions may not be moved up the respiratory tract where they can be coughed out. The accumulation of secretions provides an ideal medium for an overlaying bacterial infection (Porth, 2002a).

Signs and Symptoms

Symptoms typically associated with influenza include rapid onset, chills and fever, rhinorrhea, nonproductive cough, sore throat, malaise, and muscle aching. Unfortunately, the initial symptoms are difficult to distinguish from those of other respiratory viral infections. Antigen detection tests can confirm most influenza, though such tests are not currently available for avian flu (CDC, 2005a). Rapid identification of influenza is helpful both to establish viral treatment and to prevent the inappropriate use of antibiotics, which have no effect on viral diseases.

Treatment

Treatment is primarily directed toward symptom relief and consists of rest, keeping warm, and drinking large amounts of fluids. Rest decreases oxygen demand and may help keep the infection from spreading from the upper to the lower respiratory tract. Maintaining warmth may inhibit the virus's replication, which is optimal at a temperature of 95 °F (35 °C). Ingesting fluids prevents dehydration, which can affect the lining of the respiratory tract.

The advent of antiviral drugs has had a significant impact on both symptom relief and survival of patients suffering from influenza. The first-generation drugs [amantadine hydrochloride (Endantadine®) and rimantadine hydrochloride (Flumadine®)] prevent replication of the viral RNA by interfering with its uncoating within the host cell. They are effective only against type A and have seen significant increases in resistance as the viruses are more widely exposed to them. Zanamivir (Relenza®) and oseltamivir (Tamiflu®) represent the second generation of drugs and prevent viral RNA replication. All four antiviral medications must be started within 48 hours of symptom onset to be effective in stopping viral replication.

Patients with preexisting comorbidities such as chronic obstructive pulmonary disease (COPD) or diabetes have the potential for admission to the ICU if they contract influenza. Patients with COPD may develop respiratory distress; patients with diabetes may develop alterations in glucose metabolism. Patients, especially elderly ones, may develop dehydration and electrolyte imbalances, necessitating ICU management.

Patient and Family Education

The patient and family must receive instruction regarding the spread of influenza and the need for consistent and effective handwashing technique. The main issue for patient education revolves around symptom management and the maintenance of rest, warmth, and hydration. If the patient's condition becomes such that intubation and ventilation are required, further education for the patient and family will be needed regarding the endotracheal (ET) tube and ventilator.

Yearly influenza vaccination is an important aspect of patient education, especially for those patients considered to be at high risk: the elderly, patients with chronic medical problems, and patients with compromised immune systems. Immunizations should also be considered for the caregivers of such patients, to reduce the patients' exposure (Porth, 2002a).

PNEUMONIA

Pathophysiology

Inflammation of the lung parenchyma is the pathophysiologic hallmark of pneumonia. Microorganisms that penetrate into the lower airways are usually destroyed and/or moved up and out of the respiratory tract by ciliary action and so will not cause pneumonia. However, if a large amount of microorganisms is aspirated, if the pathogens are extremely virulent, or if the patient is immunocompromised, pneumonia will be more likely to develop. Typically, pneumonia is caused by the inhalation of microorganisms or from colonized areas of the upper respiratory tract. Patients with nasogastric (NG) or ET tubes in place are more vulnerable to pneumonia because the normal upper respiratory protective mechanisms are disrupted by the NG tube and secretions have a tendency to accumulate above the ET tube balloon. In addition, the ET tube bypasses the protective mechanisms of the epiglottis and the vocal cords, making aspiration more likely. Inhalation of gastric contents or other noxious elements establishes an inflammatory response that causes the accumulation of secretions in the alveoli, setting the stage for a bacterial overgrowth. Other conditions may also predispose the patient to development of pneumonia (see **Table 24-1**). Pneumonia may also be caused by microorganisms migrating from other infected sites within the lung or from other parts of the body via the bloodstream (Porth, 2002a).

Pneumonias have evolved to be classified as either community acquired or hospital acquired. The definitions reflect when the infection was identified and where the patient was prior to the identification of the infection. A pneumonia is considered community acquired if it was present when the patient was admitted to the hospital or developed within 48 hours of admission. If the pneumonia develops more than 48 hours after an admission into a hospital, it is deemed hospital acquired. If the patient had been in long-term care for 14 days or more prior to his or her admission to the hospital, pneumonia would be considered hospital-acquired (Porth, 2002a). The distinctions between community- and hospital-acquired pneumonias are important, because hospital-acquired pneumonias are more likely to be bacterial and, due to antibiotic resistance, are more difficult to treat.

Community-acquired pneumonia is most commonly caused by *Streptococcus pneumoniae* and less commonly by *Haemophilus influenzae, Staphylococcus aureus, Legionella pneumonphila*, gram-negative bacilli, and a variety of other bacteria. In the past, bacterial pneumonias have been referred to as typical pneumonias. Various mycoplasma and viral causes of community-acquired pneumonia have been identified, including influenza, RSV, adenovirus, measles, herpes simplex, varicella, and parainfluenza. Pneumonias caused by microorganisms other than bacteria have been referred to as atypical pneumonias. Dysphagia has been identified as a risk factor in the elderly population, especially nursing home patients; in contrast, patients without a spleen may succumb to an *S. pneumoniae* infection (Cunha, 2004; File, 2003; Marik & Kaplan, 2003). Mortality for community-acquired pneumonia ranges from 1% to 2% for patients younger than age 60 with no comorbidity to as high as 50% in those patients requiring treatment in an ICU (Halm & Teirstein, 2002).

Hospital-acquired pneumonias are almost always caused by bacteria that are commonly found in healthcare facilities. The types of bacteria most commonly responsible are *Pseudomonas aeruginosa, S. aureus, Escheria coli, Serratia, Enterobacter,* and *Klebsiella* species. Because of

TABLE 24-1 Respiratory Defense Mechanisms and Conditions That Impair Their Effectiveness

Defense Mechanism	Function	Factors That Impair Effectiveness
Nasopharyngeal defenses	Remove particles from the air; contact with surface lysosomes and immunoglobulins (IgA) protects against infection	IgA deficiency state, hay fever, common cold, trauma to the nose
Glottic and cough reflexes	Protect against aspiration into tracheobronchial tree	Loss of cough reflex due to stroke or neural lesion, neuromuscular disease, abdominal or chest surgery, depression of the cough reflex due to sedation or anesthesia, presence of a nasogastric tube
Mucociliary blanket	Removes secretions, microorganisms, and particles from the respiratory tract	Smoking, viral diseases, chilling, inhalation of irritating substances
Pulmonary macrophages	Removes microorganisms and foreign particles from the lung	Chilling, alcohol intoxication, smoking, anoxia

Source: Porth, 2002a.

their long-term presence within healthcare facilities, these bacteria have evolved to become resistant to multiple antibiotics, making them more difficult to treat. Hospital-acquired pneumonias have a mortality rate of 20% to 50% (Porth, 2002a). Patients who are particularly at risk for hospital-acquired pneumonias include those who have chronic lung conditions, have an artificial airway (ET or tracheostomy tube), are immunocompromised, have supine head positioning, or are receiving enteral feedings (Kollef, 2004).

Bacterial pneumonia results in an infection within the alveolar space, where the bacteria multiply and cause a subsequent inflammation. The inflammation then leads to the collection of fluid in the alveoli. In contrast, viral pneumonias are confined to the alveolar septum.

Immunocompromised patients are at significant risk for developing pneumonia, because their immune systems are unable to cope with a sustained assault of microorganisms confronted daily. Microorganisms involved may include bacteria, viruses, protozoa, fungi, or mycobacteria. Patients with compromised immune systems include those who are taking corticosteroids or other immunosuppressing drugs, patients with solid-organ or hematologic cancers, transplant recipients, and individuals who are positive for human immunodeficiency virus (HIV) or with acquired immunodeficiency syndrome (AIDS). One of the more significant causes of pneumonia in the immunocompromised patient population is *Pneumocystis carinii*.

P. carinii occurs so frequently in patients with AIDS that it is considered a criterion for diagnosis. *P. carinii* is a parasite of unknown classification, although it was recently reclassified as a fungus and does not cause disease in healthy patients. Once the parasite is inhaled by an immunocompromised patient, it attaches to the alveolar membrane, where it feeds and reproduces, causing alveolar membrane edema and collection of fluid in the alveoli (Thomas & Limper, 2004).

A variety of conditions may mimic pneumonia, including bronchiolitis obliterans and organizing pneumonia (BOOP), bronchial neoplasms, and systemic lupus erythematosis (Rome, Murali, & Lippmann, 2001).

Signs and Symptoms

Pneumonia may present in a number of ways, depending on the type and virility of the microorganism, the comorbidities of the patient, the amount of microorganisms that reach the lower respiratory tract, and other factors (see Table 24-1). Typically, patients present with fever, cough, general malaise, and chest tightness or discomfort. Some patients may present with life-threatening hypoxia or respiratory failure.

Patients with bacterial pneumonia will usually have a more rapid onset and may present with fever as high as 106 °F (41.1 °C), chest pain, and a watery sputum that becomes bloody or rust-tinged and purulent over time. Tachycardia and tachypnea will usually be present. Inspiratory and expiratory crackles, with decreased breath sounds, will usually be heard over the area involved. Pulse oximetry (SpO_2) will usually show some degree of hypoxia (Porth, 2002a).

A variety of procedures are used to diagnose the disease and identify the particular bacterium responsible. Chest radiographs are routinely completed to gauge the extent of the disease and its response to treatment. Initial chest radiographs may show patchy or consolidated infiltrates. Patchy or scattered infiltrates usually represent bronchopneumonia, whereas lobar pneumonia is demonstrated by consolidation in one lobe. Sputum analysis is utilized to identify the specific bacterium. In patients who are unable to cough effectively so as to produce a sample, sputum may be obtained using nebulizer treatments with a variety of medications or saline. Should these techniques prove unsuccessful, careful nasotracheal suctioning or use of a flexible bronchoscope may produce a sputum specimen. The nasotracheal suctioning usually is not deep enough to obtain samples, but it stimulates the patient to cough and bring the sputum up to the suction catheter, where it is collected in a sterile trap. Washings obtained with a bronchoscope are often referred to as bronchial alveolar lavage (BAL).

In patients with viral pneumonia, the onset of symptoms typically occurs more gradually and is somewhat different from that associated with bacterial pneumonia. Patients usually have a low-grade fever, muscle pains, headache, and a dry, nonproductive cough. Chest radiographs usually reveal diffuse infiltrates because the inflammation is in the alveolar epithelium rather than in the alveoli as with bacterial pneumonia. While sputum cultures are used to diagnose viral pneumonia, it is often difficult to obtain samples because of the small amount of sputum produced. One of the major concerns with viral pneumonia is that it predisposes the patient to the development of an overlaying bacterial pneumonia by affecting the patient's respiratory tract defenses. In addition, some viruses, (e.g., herpes simplex, varicella) can cause acute inflammation and necrosis of the alveolar epithelium.

Immunocompromised patients with pneumonia will exhibit symptoms related to the type and amount of infective organism present, their immune status, and their comorbid conditions, if any. The onset of *P. carinii* pneumonia is usually abrupt, with tachypnea, shortness of breath, a mild nonproductive cough, high fever, intercostal retractions, and patchy involvement throughout the lungs. As the disease rapidly spreads, gas exchange is compromised and the patient may require ET intubation and mechanical ventilation. Diagnosis is confirmed by stains that identify the cysts in sputum.

Treatment

Community-acquired pneumonia may be treated with empiric antibiotics, based on knowledge of the predominate bacterial causes. Once the specific bacterium causing the pneumonia is identified, appropriate antibiotics are begun. Although empiric therapy has been extensively used in the past, and to some extent is still used today for community-acquired pneumonias, antibiotics for hospital-acquired pneumonias are usually ordered based on the results of sputum or BAL cultures. Identifying the specific pathogen is necessary to prevent unnecessary use of inappropriate antibiotics, which can lead to increasing bacterial resistance. Other factors to consider in ordering antibiotics are the patient's age, preexisting medical conditions, and the severity and location of the infection.

Treatment for patients with both bacterial and viral pneumonia focuses on maintaining adequate oxygenation and ventilation. While oxygen therapy may be as simple as a nasal cannula, it may extend across the spectrum to mechanical ventilation with 100% oxygen. Additional ventilation therapies that may be used in patients with pneumonia include continuous positive airway pressure(CPAP) or bilevel positive airway pressure (BiPAP), though these measures are usually reserved for less severely ill patients in an attempt to prevent intubation. These modalities are discussed in Chapter 23.

Mucolytics, such as N-acetylcysteine, may be utilized to help the patient mobilize and cough out the secretions. Adequate hydration is important to maintain the liquidity of the secretions. If the patient is unable to orally ingest adequate amounts of fluid, intravenous (IV) fluid therapy may be necessary. Adequate nutrition is important to provide energy for breathing, while rest is often prescribed to decrease O_2 demand and CO_2 production.

Patient and Family Education

Both the patient and family will need information regarding the type of pneumonia and the therapies involved in treatment. This information allows them to cooperate more fully in the patient's care and understand the limitations the patient will have until the pneumonia clears. The importance of maintaining oxygen devices in place, the need for adequate fluid and nutrition intake, limitations on the patient's activity, and the need to take the antibiotic as prescribed must be stressed.

TUBERCULOSIS

Pathophysiology

Once thought to be almost eradicated in the United States due to the increased use of antibiotics starting in the 1950s, tuberculosis (TB) has become more common in the past two decades. However, with more funding and attention, the number of TB cases has decreased in recent years. The incidence of TB increased with the emergence of HIV infections and growth of the population with compromised immune systems (CDC, 2005b). The incidence of TB is higher in immigrants from other countries, with the case rate among foreign-born persons being eight times higher than among U.S.-born patients (CDC, 2004). A high prevalence of the disease is found in facilities where the inhabitants are closely comingled or overcrowded, such as prisons, drug treatment facilities, migrant farm camps, and homeless shelters (CDC, 2005b).

The organism that causes TB, *Mycobacterium tuberculosis*, has a unique outer waxy capsule that makes it more resistant to antibiotics than other bacteria. This waxy coating provides the bacteria with the ability to persist in old lesions and then reanimate, causing a new round of the disease.

TB is spread by airborne droplets. Patients with primary TB may spread droplet nuclei into the air by coughing, sneezing, or talking. The moisture carrying the droplet nuclei evaporates, leaving it suspended in the air. Another person then inhales the droplets. The droplet nuclei are so small that they may bypass the normal mucocillary upper respiratory tract defense mechanisms and be deposited in the terminal bronchiole or alveoli. Although the bacilli do not illicit an early immunoglobulin response, once established in the lower respiratory tract, they are engulfed by macrophages. In the macrophages, the bacteria divide every 25 to 32 hours. When the macrophage successfully destroys some of the bacilli, the released antigens stimulate the T lymphocytes to initiate a cell-mediated immune response and hypersensitivity. The bacilli continue to multiply slowly until they cause a cellular immune response that walls off the bacilli and activate immune cells into a lesion, usually from 2 to 12 weeks after the initial exposure. The bacilli may also invade the tracheobronchial lymph nodes, producing further lesions there (Porth, 2002a).

The hypersensitivity immune response is important in limiting further bacilli replication and provides additional protection if more bacilli are inhaled. Over time, the necrotic lesions are surrounded by scar tissue that will usually calcify, leading to the characteristic radiograph patterns associated with primary TB. Until the lesions are walled off, the patient may spread the bacilli by coughing or sneezing them into the air from where they have migrated into the bronchioles.

Progressive primary TB may occur, in a reactivated form, in patients with a history of previous exposure to the bacilli whose immune function has become compromised. It may also appear as a new infection in an immunocompromised patient. The bacilli may spread to multiple areas of the lungs through the bronchial tree. Because of the hypersensitivity immune response, multiple cavitations develop over time, causing extensive damage to the lungs (Porth, 2002a).

Signs and Symptoms

Primary TB usually causes no signs or symptoms. Patients often do not realize that they have been exposed. The presence of primary TB is often identified by a positive tuberculin skin test, the Mantoux test.

A newer test, the QuantiFERON®-TB Gold, mixes the patient's blood with TB proteins. It is less subject to reader error and bias than the Mantoux skin test and should be used to screen for those individuals considered to be at increased risk for TB exposure, including susceptible populations and healthcare workers (Mazurek & Villarino, 2003). However, this test has not been readily adopted by all public health departments (CDC, 2005b).

A patient with progressive active TB will often have a constellation of symptoms, including night sweats, low-grade fever, weight loss, anorexia, and fatigue. A dry, nonproductive cough occurs early but will gradually become productive with purulent sputum that may be occasionally blood-tinged. Dyspnea, initially exertional and then on resting, will gradually develop (CDC, 2005b).

While the Mantoux skin test, QuantiFERON®-TB Gold, and chest radiograph are used to screen for TB, definitive diagnosis is established with the identification of *M. tuberculosis* bacilli in the sputum (CDC, 2005b). Obtaining sputum may pose quite a challenge. If the patient is unable to cough up an adequate sputum specimen, nebulized normal saline may provide the necessary moisture. Sputum specimens may also be obtained directly via bronchoscopy or with BAL. Because sputum is often swallowed, gastric samples may also yield the bacilli. Typically, early-morning specimens are collected over several days to determine the presence of the bacilli.

Treatment

Developed in 1921, the bacille Calmette-Guérin vaccine is a modified strain of the *M. tuberculosis* bovine type that is given only to those patients who have a negative tuberculin skin test. The vaccine will cause a positive tuberculin skin test for about 10 years and is administered to populations with a high exposure risk, such as children who are chronically exposed to the bacilli or healthcare workers providing care to high-risk populations (Porth, 2002a). The vaccine is not commonly used in the United States, but is often given to infants and children in countries where TB is endemic (CDC, 2005b).

While a culture provides a definitive diagnosis of TB, antibiotic therapy may be started based on clinical findings and positive Acid–Fast Bacillus results (American Thoracic Society,

CDC, & Infectious Diseases Society of America, 2003). Because of its ability to mutate quickly, remain in a dormant state, and grow slowly, an active *M. tuberculosis* infection may be treated with multiple antibiotics for as long as six months. However, in patients with HIV, with multidrug-resistant strains or who interrupt treatment, therapy may be longer. The standard treatment for active TB is a combination of antibiotics, primarily isoniazid used in combination with rifampin (Rifadin®), pyrazinamide (Tebrazid®), or ethambutol (Myambutol®), usually given in oral form. Streptomyocin sulfate, the first antibiotic used for active TB, is less useful because of increasing resistance to the drug (American Thoracic Society, CDC, & Infectious Diseases Society of America). The success of the treatment, and prevention of inadequate doses fostering the development of resistant strains, depends on the patient regularly taking the medications for the time prescribed (American Thoracic Society, CDC, & Infectious Diseases Society of America). Prophylactic treatment is recommended for specific populations who do not have active TB, with isoniazid (see **Table 24-2**).

Relapse is defined as the situation in which the patient becomes culture negative while receiving therapy but, at some time after completion of therapy, becomes culture positive or shows chest radiograph evidence of active TB. Most relapses occur within 6 to 12 months of therapy. Drug-resistant strains

---

TABLE 24-2 Patients Needing Prophylactic Treatment for Tuberculosis

Positive skin test with close exposure to those with active tuberculosis

Conversion from a negative to positive tuberculin skin test within two years

History of untreated or inadequately treated tuberculosis

Chest x-ray evidence of tuberculosis, with no positive bacteriologic evidence

Positive HIV test or have AIDS

Younger than 35 years of age with a positive tuberculin skin test of unknown duration

Patients with special risk factors
- Silicosis
- Diabetes mellitus
- Prolonged corticosteroid therapy
- Immunosuppression therapy
- End-stage renal disease
- Chronic malnutrition
- Hematologic or reticuloendothelial cancers

Source: Porth, 2002a.

are more likely when the patient was allowed to self-administer the medications or used a non-rifamycin regimen (American Thoracic Society, CDC, & Infectious Diseases Society of America, 2003).

Patients with TB may be admitted to the ICU with respiratory insufficiency. In the case of immunocompromised patients, admission may be related to super-infection. Patients with TB in the ICU are placed in a negative-pressure room or one with a high-efficiency particulate air (HEPA) filter to remove TB particles, thereby decreasing the circulating volume of bacilli (CDC, 2005b). Healthcare providers and visitors are required to wear an N-95 respiratory mask while in the patient's room. Providers are required to be fit-tested for the mask on an annual basis. Special respiratory precautions are observed.

Patient and Family Education

Education primarily focuses on complying with the medication schedule, which may be difficult because it may last for up to a year. Because of the length of the medication course, it is very important to impress on the patient and the family the need to take the medication, even though the patient may feel better within a few weeks of starting the medications (American Thoracic Society, CDC, & Infectious Diseases Society of America, 2003; CDC, 2005b). After taking medications for approximately three weeks, the patient is usually no longer infectious. Family members of patients with TB should be counseled on the need to be tested for TB.

Good nutrition and adequate rest are vital to the recovery of the TB patient. Nutritional counseling may provide additional support and information to maintain weight. Nutritional support for ICU patients is further discussed in Chapter 33.

ASTHMA

Pathophysiology

Smooth muscles control the diameter of the terminal bronchioles by constricting and relaxing in response to a variety of normal physiology demands. The smooth muscles are controlled by the autonomic nervous system, with parasympathetic stimulation causing constriction of the bronchioles and sympathetic stimulation causing dilation. For example, when a person exercises, the smooth muscles relax, increasing the diameter of the bronchioles, allowing for more air movement into the alveoli. In asthma, the bronchioles are hypersensitive to a variety of stimuli, which leads to sporadic episodes of narrowing of the airways. However, asthma often evolves into a chronic disease that significantly decreases respiratory function over time. In addition, the smooth muscles will constrict in response to a local inflammatory response, most commonly in response to exposure to some allergen.

Asthma has been diagnosed in more than 26 million Americans, with approximately one-third of those being children. Asthma is essentially a hypersensitivity response to a variety of stimuli (see **Table 24-3**). Because of previous exposures and the development of an antigenic response, repeated exposure to such stimuli causes inflammation, which in turn leads to both constriction of the bronchial smooth muscle and a hypersensitivity to stimuli. An asthma attack can be best described as usually occurring in two distinct phases: the acute or early phase and the late phase (Porth, 2002b).

In the acute phase of an asthma attack, when a stimulus is inhaled, mast cells lining the bronchiole create an antigen response. The antigen response from the mast cells causes a rapid bronchiole constriction, usually within 10 to 20 minutes. In addition, mast cells are stimulated to increase mucus production, further occluding the already constricted airway. Increased vascular permeability causes more mucosal edema formation, while parasympathetic stimulation increases bronchoconstriction. The combination of mucosal edema and bronchoconstriction is usually responsive to bronchodilators.

The late phase of an asthma attack usually develops from four to eight hours after exposure to a stimulus and may last for hours to weeks after the initial attack. The late phase is characterized by inflammation and increased airway responsiveness to subsequent triggers and is initiated by the inflammatory

TABLE 24-3 Factors Contributing to an Asthma Attack

- Allergens
- Dust mites
- Unprotected exposure to cold air
- Drugs
- Hormonal changes
- Airborne pollutants
- Nonsteroidal anti-inflammatory drugs (NSAIDs)
- Organic dusts (wood, grains)
- Perfumes and colognes
- Cockroach allergen
- Respiratory tract infections
- Animal dander
- Hyperventilation
- Exercise
- Smoke
- Chemicals and/or gases
- Tobacco smoke (direct or secondhand)
- Emotional upsets
- Gastroesophageal reflux
- Fungus and molds

Source: Porth, 2002b.

mediators released by the mast cells, macrophages, and damaged epithelial cells. These mediators attract other inflammatory cells, such as neutrophils, basophils, and eosinophils, which exacerbate existing edema and airway responsiveness. In addition, inflammation decreases the ability of the mucociliary system to move secretions to the upper bronchioles where they may be expectorated. The late phase can create a cyclical process in which exacerbations continue and may, over time, create a chronic inflammatory state that leads to chronic limitations in air flow through the bronchioles (Porth, 2002b).

One unique feature of asthma is air trapping. As the patient inhales, the inflamed and edematous bronchioles dilate and allow air into the alveoli. However, when the patient exhales, the bronchioles close and prevent the air from passively escaping from the alveoli. The repeated breaths cause the alveoli to distend and "trap" the air within. Over time, the entrapped air allows for increasingly smaller volumes of air to be exchanged within the alveoli. In addition, the entrapped air within the alveoli decreases the effectiveness of any attempts at coughing.

Signs and Symptoms

A patient experiencing an asthma attack may experience a wide range of symptoms, from mild wheezing and chest tightness to complete respiratory failure. The triggers for an asthma attack are varied and may be additive. Attacks are often worse at night because of a late response to an allergen inhaled during the evening hours.

The typical symptoms associated with an asthma attack include chest tightness, wheezing, and an increased respiratory rate, associated with prolonged expiration. A cough may be initially present. As the severity of the attack increases, accessory muscle use is noted, along with loud (often audible) wheezing and an increasingly ineffective cough. Breath sounds become distant because of air trapping and are usually present with air hunger. Dyspnea may initially be mild, but may reach the point where the patient may be able to speak only one or two words at a time, between breaths. As the attack progresses, air flow is markedly decreased, breath sounds may become inaudible ("silent chest"), and wheezing may diminish. At this point, complete respiratory failure is imminent (Porth, 2002b).

Establishing a diagnosis of asthma is usually accomplished by a careful evaluation of the patient's history, physical examination, laboratory tests (complete blood count with differential, sputum analysis), and pulmonary function tests (PFTs). A "challenge" test may be conducted to assess airway responsiveness by exposing the patient to a variety of triggers and assessing the response. PFTs provide useful information in the non-acute setting and can help determine the level and course of treatment. The main components for a PFT for an asthma patient are the forced expiratory volume (FEV_1), which measures the volume of air that is forcibly exhaled in one second, and the peak expiratory flow (PEF), defined as the maximum flow rate at the outset of forced expiration. Both parameters are measured in liters per second and can be directly related to the severity of the disease or attack (see **Table 24-4**). PFTs are seldom used during an acute attack, but may be conducted after the patient is stabilized to assess response to therapy. Arterial blood gases (ABGs) may be drawn during an acute attack, with a carbon dioxide level (PCO_2) greater than 70 mm Hg (respiratory acidosis) indicating impending respiratory failure.

Treatment

Prevention of an acute attack is the first line of defense for patients with asthma and typically revolves around avoidance of known triggers. Identifying the various triggers may be accomplished by obtaining a careful history, by desensitization to known triggers, by using skin injections that block immunoglobulin E (IgE) response to those triggers, and by teaching the patient to employ controlled breathing and relaxation techniques. Medications used to prevent acute attacks include systemic corticosteroids, which are usually inhaled on a regular basis to prevent the systemic effects of oral or injectable steroids and are more effective than short-acting bronchodilators in reducing exacerbations (Sin, Man, Sharpe, Gan, & Man,

TABLE 24-4 Classification of Asthma Severity

Severity	Day Symptoms	Night Symptoms	FEV_1	PEF Variability
Mild intermittent	< 2 day/week	< 2 night/month	≥ 80%	< 20%
Mild persistent	> 2/week but < 1/day	> 2 night/month	≥ 80%	20–30%
Moderate persistent	Daily	> 1 night/week	> 60% but < 80%	> 30%
Severe persistent	Continual	Frequent	≤ 60%	> 30%

FEV_1: forced expiratory volume in 1 second.
PEF: peak expiratory flow.
Source: Adapted from National Asthma Education and Prevention Program, 2002, p. 5.

2004). Short-acting bronchodilators may be used when exposure to a known trigger has been identified by the patient.

The panic and anxiety of an acute attack can exacerbate the attack but may be reduced by portraying a calm and reassuring manner on the part of all caregivers. Although oxygen is typically required, the presence of an oxygen mask over the face may cause further panic. One technique that works well is to allow the patient to hold the mask near the mouth.

Pharmacology for an acute attack usually begins with inhaling short-acting, β_2-adrenergic agonist bronchodilators [albuterol (Proventil®), formoterol fumarate (Foradil Aerosolizer®), levalbuterol (Xofenex®), metaproterenol (Alupent®), pirbuterol (Maxair®), terbutaline (Brethine®)] delivered by metered-dose inhalers (MDIs) or nebulizer to reverse bronchospasms. The β_2-adrenergic agonist bronchodilators relax the bronchial smooth muscles, usually within 30 minutes. While the β_2-adrenergic agonist bronchodilators are important for the short-term treatment of acute asthma, they should not be used too frequently (National Asthma Education and Prevention Program, 2002).

A second type of medication that may be inhaled comprises the acetylcholine receptor antagonists [ipratropium (Atrovent®), tiotropium bromide (Spiriva®)], which block the vagal nerve pathways that cause bronchospasm, especially in the larger airways. Because these medications work on different causes of the bronchospasm, they may be given together or found together in a combination medication. Short-course systemic corticosteroids may be used in moderate or severe attacks to decrease the inflammation associated with an acute attack and to prevent it from progressing to the late phase.

In the unusual situation where a patient with asthma develops respiratory failure, intubation and mechanical ventilation may be necessary. Mechanical ventilation is generally used only as a last resort because of the possibility of causing further bronchial spasms and the threat of hospital-acquired pneumonia. However, it may be needed to maintain oxygenation and ventilation until the various medications break the inflammation and spasm cycles (Porth, 2002b).

A variety of long-term medications are used to prevent acute attacks and control persistent symptoms. Inhaled corticosteroids decrease both inflammation in the bronchial tissue and airway sensitivity to triggers. They are delivered via an MDI to prevent the systemic effects associated with oral or parental administration. Medications in this class include beclomethasone (Beclovent®), flunisolide (AeroBid®), fluticasone proprionate (Flonase®), mometasone furoate monohydrate (Nasonex®), and triamcinolone (Aristocort®). These agents are more effective in improving airway function and inflammation than β_2-adrenergic agonist bronchodilators (Larj & Bleecker, 2004).

A number of other medications affect the initiation of inflammation in a variety of ways. Leukotriene inhibitors such as montelukast (Singulair®) and zafirlukast (Acculate®) prevent leukotriene activation. Cromolyn (NasalCrom®) and nedocromil (Tilade®) stabilize mast cells, while omalizumab (Xolair®) inhibits IgE binding to mast cells. The end result of using these medications is to prevent inflammation from occurring. Long-acting β_2-adrenergic agonist bronchodilators are used to keep the bronchial smooth muscles relaxed; they are often given in conjunction with anti-inflammatory medications and may be inhaled [salmeterol (Serevent®)] or taken orally (albuterol). Combination therapy, involving both inhaled steroids and long-acting β_2-adrenergic agonist bronchodilators, has been shown to improve lung function and decrease the need for short-acting β_2-adrenergic agonist bronchodilators (Donohue, 2004; National Asthma Education and Prevention Program, 2002). Theophylline, whose exact mechanism of action is unknown, represents an alternative to other long-term medications. Because of the wide variability in its elimination pattern, blood levels must be regularly drawn to prevent toxicity. Theophylline is not commonly used for the treatment of asthma.

Antibiotics may be indicated for comorbidities such as bacterial pneumonia or sinusitis. However, they are not recommended routinely for treatment of asthma (National Asthma Education and Prevention Program, 2002). Antibiotics would be recommended if patients exhibited fever and purulent sputum, evidence of pneumonia, or suspected bacterial sinusitis.

Status Asthmaticus

Status asthmaticus (SA) is an emergent complication of asthma in which symptom management does not respond to initial bronchodilator therapy. Patients may be admitted to the ICU with respiratory failure requiring intubation and mechanical ventilation, bronchodilator therapy, and IV fluids (Keresmer, 2000).

Beta agonists and corticosteroids are the basis of treatment of SA. Steroids, in addition to exerting their anti-inflammatory action, decrease mucus production and help improve oxygenation. Patients receiving corticosteroids and beta agonists should be monitored for hypokalemia.

Several studies have been conducted evaluating management strategies of SA. Carmargo, Spooner, and Rowe (2003) compared continuous and intermittent administration of beta agonists. They concluded that continuous administration resulted in fewer hospital admissions and a small but significant improvement in PFTs.

Magnesium sulfate administration was studied by Alter, Koepsell, and Hilty (2000). Magnesium acts as a smooth muscle relaxant by altering the influx of calcium into cells; it also has anti-inflammatory properties. The researchers concluded that magnesium boluses were beneficial in improving airway function and recommended it in patients experiencing severe bronchospasm.

Because patients with SA often develop metabolic acidosis, a study on the use of sodium bicarbonate was undertaken in pediatric patients with SA. In this sample of patients, six received bicarbonate. Results suggested a decrease in respiratory distress and a significant decrease in CO_2 levels. No side effects related to bicarbonate therapy were noted (Buysse & de Hong, 2002).

Intubation with mechanical ventilation is generally used as a last resort because it is associated with several complications. Indications identified for intubation include increasing fatigue, persistent or increasing elevations in CO_2 levels, and decreased respiratory rate. Patients who are intubated and receiving mechanical ventilation are at risk for developing a pneumothorax because the narrow airways and increased lung volumes lead to high airway pressures. If patients with SA require intubation, use of the largest ET tube is suggested (size 8 or above, if possible) to minimize airway resistance and to facilitate suctioning (Boushey & Venhayya, 2005).

Patient and Family Education

Patient and family education focuses on identification and avoidance of known triggers of asthma attack. Avoidance of identified or suspected allergens, such as tobacco smoke, perfumes, and chemicals, may prevent many acute asthma attacks. Exercise-induced asthma is thought to be caused by the loss of heat and water from the bronchial tree (Porth, 2002b) and is often exacerbated by cold.

One aspect of education that may have a positive effect on outcomes is the use of a written action plan. Such plans have led to reductions in emergency room visits and hospitalizations as well as improvements in lung function (National Asthma Education and Prevention Program, 2002).

Awareness of the signs and symptoms of an attack are important, because the attack may be dealt with by administering short-acting β_2-adrenergic agonist bronchodilators. By gaining control of the attack as quickly as possible, the patient may be able to prevent progression to a late-phase attack.

CHRONIC OBSTRUCTIVE PULMONARY DISEASE

Pathophysiology

COPD refers to two related respiratory diseases: chronic bronchitis and emphysema. While in the past they were considered separate disease entities, chronic bronchitis and emphysema are almost always seen together in the same patient, although the contributions of each disease to symptom presentation and clinical course vary from patient to patient. "Based on current knowledge, a working definition of COPD is a disease state that is characterized by airflow limitation that is not fully reversible. The airflow limitation is both progressive and associated with an abnormal inflammatory response of the lungs to noxious particles or gases" (Global Initiative for Chronic Obstructive Lung Disease, 2005, p. 6). When referring to COPD, the discussion will focus on both chronic bronchitis and emphysema.

The most common cause of COPD is smoking. The hazards of smoking have been well documented, particularly since the U.S. Surgeon General's report on the health hazards of smoking in 1964. "The common statement that only 15–20% of smokers develop clinically significant COPD is misleading. A much higher proportion develops abnormal lung function at some point if they continue to smoke" (Global Initiative for Chronic Obstructive Lung Disease, 2005, p. 8). While smoking is the single greatest cause of COPD, it has wide-ranging effects on the respiratory tract.

The irritation caused by smoking initiates an inflammatory response in the lungs that leads to fibrosis of the bronchial walls, excessive secretion of mucus, and destruction of the elastic portions of the peripheral airways (bronchi and bronchioles less than 2 mm in diameter) and alveoli tissues. The fibrosis causes hypertrophy of the peripheral airways, which in turn decreases the diameter of the lumen. The increased mucus production fills the narrowed peripheral airway lumen, further decreasing its diameter. Elastic tissue in the peripheral airway that normally keeps the bronchioles open and prevents them from collapsing is lost. In addition, an imbalance of proteinases and antiproteinases and the oxidative stress caused by the inflammatory damage tend to perpetuate the ongoing destruction of lung tissue (Respiratory Disorders, 2002).

Chronic bronchitis involves inflammation of the bronchi with excessive mucus production. The greater mucus production, along with the associated inflammation, narrows the lumen of the bronchi and promotes air trapping. The excess mucus also hinders the ability of the cilia to move secretions into the upper airways, where they may be coughed out. While bacterial and viral infections commonly occur in patients with chronic bronchitis, they are considered a result—rather than a cause—of the disease (Porth, 2002b).

By far, the major cause of emphysema has been identified as smoking, with a much smaller number of patients having a genetic deficiency of a protease inhibitor, α_1-antitrypsin (Petty, 2005). As many as 15% of patients diagnosed with COPD have never smoked, however, but rather may have had other exposures or childhood chest infections (Petty). Other, unidentified genetic factors may also predispose a person to develop emphysema.

Smoking causes an inflammatory response in the lungs that leads to the release of proteases, enzymes that hydrolize (break) polypeptide chains in lung tissue. Normally, a variety of protease inhibitors (e.g., α_1-antitrypsin) counteract the proteases. In the lungs of a smoker, the protease inhibitors are insufficient to counteract the effects of the inflammation, resulting in damage to the elastic tissue in the lungs. A genetic deficiency of α_1-antitrypsin promotes the appearance of emphysema in a small number of patients, most of whom are younger than 40 years of age. Smoking and repeated respiratory infections will also increase the risk of emphysema in this subgroup of patients.

Emphysema causes an irreversible enlargement of the alveolar wall, with a subsequent decrease in the elastic recoil needed for exhalation. The diminished recoil lowers the internal pressure in the bronchiole, allowing it to collapse before all of the air is expelled from the alveoli and thereby limiting exhalation. In addition, the enlarged alveoli compress the adjacent capillaries, decreasing perfusion and ventilation in the same affected areas of the lung. Over time, the continued hyperinflation will trap air, decrease the amount of air expelled with each breath, and cause the alveoli to merge and form bullae (air spaces > 1 cm), which are usually located in the peripheral areas of the lung (Respiratory Disorders, 2002).

Signs and Symptoms

Patients with bronchitis typically present with shortness of breath and a decrease in exercise tolerance, which often will have been present in some form for more than 10 years. The pervasive cough is usually more productive in the morning. Dyspnea, with an associated increase in expiratory time, gradually increases, until it may be present even at rest. The bronchial secretions and narrowing airways cause a mismatch of ventilation and perfusion, with some areas of the lung being well perfused but lacking adequate ventilation. Patients with bronchitis are unable to increase their ventilation and overcome the mismatch. The result is a patient who develops both hypoxemia and cyanosis.

Patients with bronchitis will have dyspnea and tachypnea that is more pronounced with exercise, but may be present at rest. Produced sputum may be gray, white, or yellow, or may become purulent when an acute infection is present. A prolonged expiratory phase, with expiratory crackles and wheezes, will usually be present along with cyanosis. Clubbing of the fingertips may be also found. ABG values will show hypoxemia (PaO_2 < 80 mm Hg) and hypercapnia ($PaCO_2$ > 45 mm Hg). The lack of oxygen in the blood will often stimulate the overproduction of red blood cells (RBCs), a condition referred to as compensatory polycythemia, with RBCs > 6.0×10^6. If the condition has persisted long enough, pulmonary hypertension, along with right ventricular hypertrophy (cor pulmonale) and right ventricular failure, will develop, causing peripheral edema from the back pressure. Other complications of chronic bronchitis may include pneumonia, respiratory failure, and dysrhythmias (Porth, 2002b).

A diagnosis of bronchitis is made when the previously described findings are coupled with the results of a variety of procedures and tests. Chest radiograph, electrocardiogram, and sputum analysis are utilized to rule out other disease processes, such as TB, pneumonia, and cardiovascular disease. PFTs typically demonstrate an increase in forced vital capacity (FVC) time, which is the volume forcibly exhaled after a maximal inhalation over time. FEV_1 is decreased. The GOLD Global Strategy for the Diagnosis, Management, and Prevention of Chronic Obstructive Pulmonary Disease (Global Initiative for Chronic Obstructive Lung Disease, 2005) has created a simplified system for identifying the severity of COPD that does not distinguish between chronic bronchitis and emphysema (see **Table 24-5**).

TABLE 24-5 Classification of Severity of COPD

Stage	Characteristics
0: At risk	• Normal spirometry • Chronic symptoms (cough, sputum production)
I: Mild COPD	• FEV_1/FVC < 70% • $FEV_1 \geq$ 80% predicted • With or without chronic symptoms (cough, sputum production)
II: Moderate COPD	• FEV_1/FVC < 70% • 50% $\leq FEV_1$ < 80% predicted • With or without chronic symptoms (cough, sputum production)
III: Severe COPD	• FEV_1/FVC < 70% • 30% $\leq FEV_1$ < 50% predicted • With or without chronic symptoms (cough, sputum production)
IV: Very Severe COPD	• FEV_1/FVC < 70% • FEV_1 < 30% predicted or FEV_1 < 50% predicted plus chronic respiratory failure

Classification based on post-bronchodilator FEV_1.
FEV_1: forced expiratory volume in one second.
FVC: forced vital capacity.
Respiratory failure: arterial partial pressure of oxygen (PaO_2) less than 8.0 kPa (60 mm Hg) with or without arterial partial pressure of CO_2 ($PaCO_2$) greater than 6.7 kPa (50 mm Hg) while breathing at sea level.
Source: Global Initiative for Chronic Obstructive Lung Disease, 2005, p. 7.

Because of the loss of both ventilation and perfusion, patients with emphysema are able to somewhat compensate for the hypoxemia by hyperventilating. The hyperventilation, using accessory muscles, will usually maintain relatively normal blood gas levels until late in the disease. Exhalation is prolonged due to trapping of air. Patients with emphysema will often develop "pursed lip" breathing, whereby they exhale through taut lips, increasing the airway pressure and thereby keeping the airways open and allowing for more effective exhalation. As the work of breathing increases further, inadequate food intake can become an issue, often with significant weight loss.

Upon examination, patients with advanced emphysema typically have a "barrel" chest, with a protruding abdomen and tachypnea and dyspnea on exertion. Crackles and inspiratory wheezes, along with decreased breath sounds, are often found. Clubbing of the fingertips may be also found. ABG values will show hypoxemia ($PO_2 < 80$ mm Hg) and hypercapnia ($PCO_2 > 45$ mm Hg) only late in the disease process. Polycythemia (hematocrit $> 55\%$) may develop due to arterial hypoxemia. Right ventricular hypertrophy (cor pulmonale) and right ventricular failure may develop, though they tend to cause peripheral edema only late in the disease process. PFT results are similar to those patients with chronic bronchitis (Global Initiative for Chronic Obstructive Lung Disease, 2005).

Treatment

A variety of therapies are used to treat patients with COPD; these measures are primarily directed toward relief of symptoms, because none will reverse the long-term decline in lung function. Treatment is characterized by a stepwise increase, depending on the severity of the disease. The first drugs given are the short-acting β_2-adrenergic agonist bronchodilators (albuterol, formoterol, levalbuterol, metaproterenol, pirbuterol, terbutaline). Inhaled long-acting β_2-adrenergic agonist bronchodilators (salmeterol) may be even more effective, because they also decrease the incidence of bacteria adhering to epithelial cells. Ipratropium, an inhaled anticholinergic bronchodilator, blocks the vagal nerve pathways causing bronchospasm, especially in the larger airways; it also decreases the volume of sputum produced. While most inhaled corticosteroids do not affect the inflammation in chronic COPD, a combination of fluticasone and salmeterol is used for chronic bronchitis. Corticosteroids are useful in acute exacerbations of COPD or when the disease coexists with asthma; these agents can have an important impact on morbidity and mortality (Mapel, 2004). Theophylline is used to treat patients who do not respond well to inhaled bronchodilators. Theophylline is thought to have several effects on the respiratory system, including improvement of respiratory muscle function and central ventilatory drive and increased clearance of mucus. Blood levels must be regularly drawn to prevent toxicity, because the majority of this drug's benefits occur at near-toxic doses.

Oxygen therapy is typically used when patients exhibit significant hypoxemia (arterial $PO_2 < 55$ mm Hg). Oxygen, usually in the form of a nasal cannula, is delivered to keep the arterial PO_2 between 55 and 65 mm Hg, or a saturation of approximately 90%. At this level, both dyspnea and pulmonary hypertension are decreased. If requirements increase over time, O_2 may be delivered by transtracheal catheter (Porth, 2002b).

Bullectomy, in which the large bullae are surgically removed, may be of benefit for some patients, especially when the bullae occupy more than 50% of the hemithorax and compress nearby functioning lung tissue. Lung reduction surgery has been demonstrated to be effective in increasing survival and function in upper lobe emphysema, but not lower lobe emphysema [National Emphysema Treatment Trial (NETT), 2003]. In addition, the benefits of lung reduction surgery in patients with α_1-antitrypsin deficiency have been found to be less significant than the benefits seen with the NETT protocol (Tutic et al., 2004). Further research is continuing regarding a variety of new approaches for lung reduction surgery, including the use of sealants, banding, and valves (Brenner et al., 2004). Lung transplantation may be appropriate for selected patients with advanced COPD and secondary pulmonary hypertension; this surgery may improve quality of life and functional status but does not increase survival over two years (Global Initiative for Chronic Obstructive Lung Disease, 2005).

Patient and Family Education

Because smoking is the major cause of COPD, significant efforts should be directed toward its cessation. In fact, stopping smoking can increase lung function by as much as 30% in as little as two to three months. Nicotine replacement therapy is very effective in helping patients quit smoking, especially if it is paired with changes in behavior, such as a "stop smoking" program. Nicotine, which reduces the physical cravings of tobacco, comes in many forms (lozenges, gum, transdermal patches, nasal sprays, and inhalers). Bupropion (Wellbutrin®), a selective serotonin reuptake inhibitor, has been shown to help 49% of smokers who used it to quit for one month. When combined with a nicotine patch, the percentage of those who quit increased to 58% (American Cancer Society, 2003). Other methods that have been used to help patients quit smoking include hypnosis, acupuncture, aversion therapy, and adopting a "health belief model" of thinking. Often multiple methods are employed at the same time to increase the chances of success. No single program will be successful for every person, but with repeated attempts, success can be achieved.

Instruction and continual review of the use of MDIs (including the use of "spacers") is of vital importance to ensure the proper delivery of inhaled medications. Such instruction and review should be provided both in written format and with the return demonstration of the necessary skills to confirm the patient's understanding.

Pulmonary rehabilitation can increase patients' ability to manage their own disease while decreasing hospitalizations (Wouters, 2004). Physical conditioning leads to better physical endurance. Breathing exercises can recondition the diaphragm and improve gas exchange. Energy conservation and work simplification strategies to minimize dyspnea can also help make the patient's life more manageable. Airway irritants, such as tobacco smoke, must be avoided as much as possible. If patients live in a cold environment, they should wear a mask to prevent bronchospasm associated with inhaling cold air.

Because an acute infection may cause an exacerbation of COPD and be life-threatening, the patient and family must remain vigilant. Contact with others who have respiratory illnesses, such as influenza, should be avoided. Hand washing has been shown to be an effective way to prevent the spread of diseases (National Center for Infectious Diseases, 2000). Annual immunizations for the current strain of influenza can reduce the frequency, virility, and length of subsequent infections. Vaccines for pneumococcal pneumonia may be appropriate, but the data supporting their routine use are unclear (Global Initiative for Chronic Obstructive Lung Disease, 2005). Patient and family awareness of changes in sputum color, consistency, and/or quantity may help identify the early onset of an acute respiratory infection and allow for an earlier start of a course of appropriate antibiotics. Antibiotics are not routinely given for COPD but rather are reserved for patients with an acute infection. When an infection is identified by worsening dyspnea an increase in sputum volume and purulence, the antibiotic should provide coverage for *S. pneumoniae*, *H. influenzae*, and *M. cararrhalis* (Gronkiewicz & Brokgren-Okonek, 2004).

Because it may be difficult for patients with COPD to breathe and eat at the same time, malnutrition may reduce respiratory muscle function and may adversely affect mortality in this population. Significant emphasis should be directed toward appropriate nutrition management, with a consultation with a nutrition support dietitian who has experience working with patients with COPD (Wouters, 2004). While consumption of carbohydrates may increase CO_2 production, it becomes an issue only when the patient routinely follows a high-carbohydrate diet. Small meals, spaced throughout the day, may provide less pressure on the diaphragm, allowing less interference with breathing (Gronkiewicz & Brokgren-Okonek, 2004; Porth, 2002b). In addition, dental conditions may have a negative effect on nutrition intake (Global Initiative for Chronic Obstructive Lung Disease, 2005).

The chronic and debilitating nature of COPD has a profound influence on patients' psychological condition (Gronkiewicz & Brokgren-Okonek, 2004; Wouters, 2004). Mental health disorders may have a significant effect on the medical outcome of treatment. Many patients may benefit from treatment for anxiety and depression (Gronkiewicz & Brokgren-Okonek).

PATIENT OUTCOMES

Nurses can help ensure obtainment of optimal patient outcomes such as those listed in **Box 24-1** through the use of evidence-based interventions for patients with respiratory disorders.

SUMMARY

Common respiratory diseases present as some of the most frequently encountered entities in the ICU setting. The severity of these diseases may range from patients who require very simple assessment and interventions, such as nasal cannula for an immediate postoperative patient with asthma, to the highly complex, such as a patient with end-stage COPD who is intubated and mechanically ventilated. An understanding of the pathophysiology, assessment, and treatment options will provide the ICU nurse with the most appropriate techniques for making a substantial difference in the course of the patient's hospitalization.

Box 24-1
Optimal Patient Outcomes

- Oxygen saturation within expected range
- Acid-base status within expected range
- No use of accessory muscles
- Dyspnea is minimized
- Absence of activity intolerance
- Ability to perform activities of daily living
- Coping with chronic illness

CASE STUDY

A 42-year-old patient was admitted to the ICU from the ED with a diagnosis of status asthmaticus. The patient presented with a report of chest tightness, shortness of breath, and a dry cough; stated that he had a cold a few days ago. Physical exam revealed a patient in moderate distress, using accessory muscles to breathe. Breath sounds were diminished bilaterally, with expiratory wheezing noted. The patient was tachypneic at 38 breaths/min and had a SpO_2 of 90% on room air. He was given oxygen via nasal cannula, oral steroids, and nebulized β-agonists with minimal improvement. He was transferred to the ICU for respiratory management.

In the ICU, the patient received frequent bronchodilator treatments via nebulizer and continued to receive nasal oxygen and corticosteroids. ABG results revealed a mild respiratory alkalosis with compensatory metabolic acidosis. The patient received intravenous fluids with 0.9% normal saline at 125 mL/h. His condition stabilized, and he did not require mechanical ventilation. He was discharged from the ICU in less than 36 hours.

CRITICAL THINKING QUESTIONS

1. What is the etiology for the ABG results?

2. Why did the patient require intravenous fluids?

3. If the patient required mechanical ventilation, what complication would he be primarily at risk for, and why?

4. Which disciplines should be consulted to work with this client?

5. What types of issues may require you to act as an advocate or moral agent for this patient?

6. How will you implement your role as a facilitator of learning for this patient?

7. Write a case example from the clinical setting highlighting one patient characteristic. Explain how the characteristic was observed through subjective and objective data.

8. Utilize the form to write up a plan of care for one client in the clinical setting with a common respiratory disorder.

9. Write a case example from the clinical setting. Rate the patient as a level 1, 3, or 5 on each characteristic. Identify the level of nurse characteristics needed in the care of this patient.

10. Take one outcome for a patient and list evidence-based interventions found in a literature review.

Using the Synergy Model to Develop a Plan of Care

	Patient Characteristics	Level (1, 3, 5)	Subjective and Objective Data	Evidence-based Interventions	Outcomes
SYNERGY MODEL	Resiliency				
	Vulnerability				
	Stability				
	Complexity				
	Resource availability				
	Participation in care				
	Participation in decision making				
	Predictability				

Online Resources

Centers for Disease Control and Prevention: www.cdc.gov/asthma/faqs.htm

Cleveland Clinic. (2001). Nutritional guidelines for people with COPD: www.clevelandclinic.org/health/health-info/docs/2400/2411.asp?index=9451

Influenza Pandemics of the 20th Century: www.cdc.gov/ncidod/EID/vol7eno01/05-1254.htm/

Mechanical ventilation in adults with status asthmaticus: http://patients.uptodate.com/topicasp?file=asthma/9160.

REFERENCES

Alter, H. J., Koepsell, T. D., & Hilty, W. M. (2000). Intravenous magnesium as adjuvant in acute bronchospasm: A meta-analysis. *Annals of Emergency Medicine, 36*(3), 191–197.

American Cancer Society. (2003). Guide for quitting smoking. Retrieved September 11, 2005, from www.cancer.org/docroot/ped/content/ped_10_13x_quitting_smoking.asp?sitearea=ped

American Thoracic Society, Centers for Disease Control and Prevention, & Infectious Diseases Society of America. (2003). Treatment of tuberculosis. *Morbidity and Mortality Weekly Report, 52*(RR-11), 1–77.

Boushey, H. A., & Venkayya, R. (2005). Mechanical ventilation in adults with status asthmaticus. Retrieved September 29, 2005, from http://patientsuptodate.com/topcasp?file=asthma/9160

Brenner, M., Hanna, N. M., Mina-Araghi, R., Gelb, A. F., McKenna, R. J., & Colt, H. (2004). Innovative approaches to lung volume reduction for emphysema. *Chest, 126*, 238–248.

Buysse, C. M., & de Hong, M. (2002). Treatment of status asthmaticus in children: Is there a place for sodium bicarbonate. *Critical Care, 6*(Suppl. 1), 25.

Carmargo, C. A., Spooner, C. H., & Rowe, B. H. (2003). Continuous versus intermittent beta-agonist in the treatment of acute asthma. *Cochrane Database System Review, 4*:CD001115.

Centers for Disease Control and Prevention (CDC). (2004). Reported tuberculosis in the United States, 2003. Retrieved August 22, 2005, from www.cdc.gov/nchstp/tb/surv/surv2003/default.htm

Centers for Disease Control and Prevention (CDC). (2005a). Information about avian influenza (bird flu) and avian influenza A (H5N1) virus. Retrieved August 13, 2005, from http://www.cdc.gov/flu/avian/gen-info/facts.htm

Centers for Disease Control and Prevention (CDC). (2005b). Questions and answers about TB—2005. Retrieved August 22, 2005, from http://www.cdc.gov/nchstp/tb/faqs/qa.htm

Cunha, B. A. (2004). Empiric therapy for community-acquired pneumonia. *Chest, 125*, 1913–1919.

Donohue, J. F. (2004). Therapeutic responses in asthma and COPD: Bronchodilators. *Chest, 126*, 125S–137S.

Falsey, A. R., Hennessey, P. A., Formica, M. A., Cox, C., & Walsh, E. E. (2005). Respiratory syncytial virus infection in elderly and high-risk patients. *New England Journal of Medicine, 352*, 1749–1759.

File, T. M. (2003). Community-acquired pneumonia. *Lancet, 362*, 1991–2001.

Global Initiative for Chronic Obstructive Lung Disease. (2005). Global Strategy for the Diagnosis, Management, and Prevention of Chronic

Obstructive Pulmonary Disease. Retrieved September 28, 2005, from http://www.goldcopd.com/GuidelinesResources.asp?l1=2&l2=0

Gronkiewicz, C., & Brokgren-Okonek, M. (2004). Acute exacerbation of COPD: Nursing application of evidence-based guidelines. *Critical Care Nursing Quarterly, 27,* 336–352.

Halm, E. A., & Teirstein, A. S. (2002). Management of community-acquired pneumonia. *New England Journal of Medicine, 347,* 2039–2045.

Kercsmer, C. M. (2000). Acute inpatient care of status asthmaticus. *Respiratory Care Clinics of North America, 6*(1), 155–170.

Kollef, M. H. (2004). Prevention of hospital-associated pneumonia and ventilator-associated pneumonia. *Critical Care Medicine, 32,* 1396–1405.

Larj, M. J., & Bleecker, E. R. (2004). Therapeutic responses in asthma and COPD: Corticosteroids. *Chest, 126,* 138S–149S.

Mapel, D. W. (2004). Treatment implications of morbidity and mortality in COPD. *Chest, 126,* 150S–158S.

Marik, P. E., & Kaplan, D. (2003). Aspiration pneumonia and dysphagia in the elderly. *Chest, 124,* 328–336.

Mazurek, G. H., & Villarino, M. E. (2003). Guidelines for using the QuantiFERON-TB test for diagnosing latent *Mycobacterium tuberculosis* infection. *Morbidity and Mortality Weekly Report, 52*(RR-2), 15–18.

National Asthma Education and Prevention Program. (2002). Expert panel report: Guidelines for the diagnosis and management of asthma—update on selected topics 2002. National Institutes of Health Publication no. 02-5075. Retrieved September 9, 2005, from www.nhlbi.nih.gov/guidelines/asthma/execsumm.pdf

National Center for Infectious Diseases. (2000). An ounce of prevention: Keeps the germs away. Retrieved September 11, 2005, from http://www.cdc.gov/ncidod/op/handwashing.htm

National Emphysema Treatment Trial (NETT). (2003). Evaluation of lung reduction surgery for emphysema. Retrieved September 11, 2005, from http://www.nhlbi.nih.gov/health/prof/lung/nett/lvrsweb.htm

Petty, T. L. (2005). Commentary: Addressing the growing menace of COPD. *Postgraduate Medicine, 117*(3), 13–16.

Porth, C. M. (2002a). Alterations in respiratory function: Respiratory tract infections, neoplasms, and childhood disorders. In C. M. Porth, *Pathophysiology: Concepts of altered health states* (pp. 605–632). Philadelphia: Lippincott Williams & Wilkins.

Porth, C. M. (2002b). Alterations in respiration: Alterations in ventilation and gas exchange. In C. M. Porth, *Pathophysiology: Concepts of altered health states* (pp. 633–670). Philadelphia: Lippincott Williams & Wilkins.

Respiratory disorders. (2002). In *Atlas of pathophysiology* (pp. 78–110). Springhouse, PA: Springhouse.

Rome, L., Murali, G., & Lippmann, M. (2001). Nonresolving pneumonia and mimics of pneumonia. *Medical Clinics of North America, 85,* 1511–1530.

Sin, D. D., Man, J., Sharpe, H., Gan, W. Q., & Man, S. F. (2004). Pharmacological management to reduce exacerbations in adults with asthma. *Journal of the American Medical Association, 292*(3), 367–376.

Thomas, C. F., & Limper, A. H. (2004). Medical progress: *Pneumocystis* pneumonia. *New England Journal of Medicine, 350,* 2487–2498.

Tutic, M., Bloch, K. E., Lardinois, D., Brack, T., Russi, E. W., & Weder, W. (2004). Long-term results after lung volume reduction surgery in patients with {alpha}1-antitrypsin deficiency. *Journal of Thoracic and Cardiovascular Surgery, 128,* 408–413.

Wouters, E. F. (2004). Management of severe COPD. *Lancet, 364,* 883–895.

CHAPTER 25

Acute Respiratory Distress Syndrome

Kelly Brennan-Paddock   M. Dave Hanson

LEARNING OBJECTIVES

Upon completion of this chapter, the reader will be able to:

1. Explain the predisposing direct and indirect factors associated with the development of ARDS.

2. Describe the pathophysiology and clinical manifestations of ARDS.

3. Identify evidence-based interventions and investigational therapies to treat ARDS.

4. Design a staff education plan for ventilator-associated pneumonia.

5. Describe the clinical findings that indicate ARDS is resolving.

6. List optimal patient outcomes that may be achieved through evidence-based management of ARDS.

Acute respiratory distress syndrome (ARDS) is a progressive form of acute respiratory failure. It is a result of either indirect or direct insult, which leads to alveolar capillary inflammation and damage. **Table 25-1** lists the predisposing direct and indirect factors associated with the development of ARDS. In ARDS, interstitial edema forms and prevents normal gas exchange. This edema formation leads to respiratory distress, refractory hypoxemia, pulmonary infiltrates, and reduced lung compliance (Davies & Hoffman, 2000). ARDS can often be a challenge to diagnosis because this syndrome can mimic other lung conditions.

In the United States alone, approximately 150,000 cases of ARDS are reported each year. Many believe that the true incidence is underestimated and that many more cases go undiagnosed (Howard, Courtney-Shapiro, Kelso, Gotz, & Morris, 2004). ARDS has a mortality rate of about 40%, with death usually resulting from multiple organ failure and complications rather than from lung failure alone. However, even this mortality rate represents a huge improvement over previous years, when ARDS had a 70% mortality rate. Increased awareness, better understanding of the disease process, and improved medical management have all contributed to the increased survival rate (ARDS Foundation, 2005).

DEFINITION AND ETIOLOGY

ARDS is a pulmonary disorder of critically ill patients of any age that typically occurs following an acute injury to the body. The term *acute lung injury* is sometimes used in the same setting as ARDS, but includes less severe instances of generalized, acute lung injury.

The insult that leads to the development of ARDS is believed to either directly (e.g., aspiration of highly acidic gastric contents or the inhalation of toxic gases) or indirectly (e.g., release of chemical mediators in response to systemic disorders such as sepsis, trauma, or pancreatitis) injure the lung and surrounding pulmonary tissue. The precipitating event produces alveolocapillary membrane damage, overwhelming lung inflammation, noncardiogenic pulmonary edema, shunting, and hypoxemia. Shunt refers to the percentage of blood that goes from the right side to the left side of the heart without being oxygenated. It occurs when blood passes by an alveolus but does not pick

TABLE 25-1 Predisposing Factors Associated with the Development of ARDS

- Sepsis
- Trauma
- Pneumonia (primary bacterial or viral)
- Aspiration of gastric contents
- Shock (prolonged or profound)
- Burns
- Inhalation of smoke or noxious gases
- Cardiopulmonary bypass surgery
- Fat emboli
- Massive blood transfusions
- Pancreatitis
- Drug overdose
- High concentrations of supplemental oxygen
- Near drowning
- Radiation therapy
- Disseminated intravascular coagulation (DIC)

Source: Mortelliti & Manning, 2002.

up oxygen. The lung of a patient with ARDS can primarily be characterized by a combination of atelectasis, surfactant dysfunction, and alveolar flooding caused by protein-rich pulmonary edema and interstitial inflammation (Hubmayr, 2002).

PATHOPHYSIOLOGY

The pathophysiology of ARDS is extremely complex and involves numerous inflammatory mediators, toxic oxygen radicals, and alterations of the surfactant system (Mortelliti & Manning, 2002). The normal process of breathing is interrupted in the patient with injury to the alveolocapillary membrane. The pathologic hallmark of ARDS is diffuse alveolar damage that results in loss of integrity of the alveolar–capillary barrier, escape of protein-rich fluid from blood vessels, pulmonary edema, and hypoxemia from intrapulmonary shunting. The development of ARDS can be divided into three distinct phases (Conrad, 2005). **Table 25-2** describes the characteristics of each phase of ARDS.

In the beginning, the damage to the pulmonary capillary endothelium activates the complement cascade and inflammatory response. In addition, damage to the endothelial tissue promotes platelet aggregation, which then leads to intravascular thrombus formation. The release of platelets in ARDS is problematic because the platelets are responsible for the activation of neutrophils. The presence of neutrophils, in turn, is responsible for the release of several inflammatory mediators that injure cells, promote inflammation and fibrosis, and alter the tone of the bronchi. These inflammatory mediators bring

about overwhelming damage and increased membrane permeability to the alveolocapillary bed. The inflammatory mediators involved in this destructive process include the following substances:

- Proteolytic enzymes (protease and serrapepetase)
- Toxic oxygen products (superoxide radical, hydroxyl radical, and hydrogen peroxide)
- Arachidonic acid metabolites (prostaglandins, thromboxanes, and leukotrienes)
- Other mediators (platelet-activating factor, tumor necrosis factor, and interleukins)

The increased permeability of the alveolocapillary membrane causes fluid, proteins, plasma, and blood to leak into the interstitial and intra-alveolar spaces. This movement of substances from the capillary bed into the pulmonary interstitium results in gross pulmonary edema and hemorrhage that quickly leads to alveolar flooding and atelectasis (collapsed alveoli). The resulting atelectasis is due in part to reduced surfactant activity because the alveoli and respiratory bronchioles have either become saturated with fluid or completely collapsed. These pathologic changes lead to dramatically low lung compliance (decreased ability of the lungs to stretch and inflate), decreased functional residual capacity (amount of air in the lung after a normal exhalation), ventilation/perfusion (V/Q) imbalances (pulmonary blood is shunted from the right to left side of the heart), increased deadspace (the part of the airways that does not participate in gas exchange), profound hypoxemia, increased work of breathing, and pulmonary hypertension.

Within two to three days, interstitial and bronchoalveolar inflammation begins to develop, and epithelial and interstitial

TABLE 25-2 Phases of ARDS

Phase	Characteristics/Description
Exudative phase	Injury to the endothelium and epithelium results in inflammation and leakage of fluid into the alveoli.
Fibroproliferative phase	Fibroblasts reproduce and flow into the lung tissue. Injury can improve or persist.
Fibrosis phase	Pulmonary fibrosis develops at varying levels depending on the resolution of inflammation.

Source: Conrad, 2005.

cells multiply. Hyaline membranes then begin to form and collagen accumulates rapidly, which results in severe interstitial fibrosis that damages lung tissue (Mortelliti & Manning, 2002). The inflammation, endothelial damage, and capillary permeability associated with ARDS eventually result in a systemic inflammatory response syndrome (SIRS), possible multiple-organ dysfunction syndrome (MODS), and even death. SIRS is discussed in more depth in Chapter 51.

CLINICAL MANIFESTATIONS

Generally, ARDS develops within 24 to 48 hours after the initial injury or illness and progresses over time. **Box 25-1** describe the classic clinical presentation of ARDS.

The actual diagnosis of ARDS is based on the physical examination, analysis of arterial blood gases (ABGs), and radiological findings. Early diagnosis requires a high index of suspicion with the onset of dyspnea in settings that predispose patients to ARDS. A presumptive diagnosis can be made with ABG analysis and chest radiograph. The ABG analysis initially

Box 25-1
Clinical Manifestations of ARDS

*Marked dyspnea (early)
*Refractory hypoxemia (unresponsive to oxygen therapy)
*Diffuse alveolar infiltrates evident on chest radiograph
*Pulmonary artery occlusive pressure (PAOP) < 18 mm Hg
Rapid, shallow respirations with intercostal and suprasternal retractions observed on inspiration (early)
Crackles, rhonchi, or wheezes upon auscultation of lung fields (early/intermediate)
Respiratory alkalosis (early; becomes acidosis in advanced stage)
Decreased lung compliance (intermediate)
Skin may appear cyanotic or mottled; may not improve with oxygen administration (intermediate)
Hypotension (late)
Decreased cardiac output (late)

*Most common signs and symptoms.
Source: Mortelliti & Manning, 2002.

yields results indicative of acute respiratory alkalosis: very low PaO_2, normal or low $PaCO_2$, and elevated pH. (Chapter 21 described ABG analysis in detail.) The extremely low PaO_2 often persists despite high concentrations of oxygen, indicating that pulmonary shunting is taking place. It occurs because oxygen cannot travel through collapsed and consolidated lung tissue, which is a classic finding in ARDS.

It is important to appreciate that radiographic changes often lag many hours behind functional changes, but eventually this diagnostic tool shows diffuse bilateral alveolar infiltrates. The presentation of these pulmonary infiltrates is similar to that of acute pulmonary edema of cardiac origin; with the ARDS patient, however, the cardiac silhouette is often normal.

Because the diffuse alveolar infiltrates that appear on chest radiographs can resemble pulmonary edema associated with heart failure or disease, a pulmonary artery catheter may be useful. Pulmonary artery catheters are discussed in Chapter 11. Typically, pulmonary arterial occlusive pressure (PAOP) is low (< 18 mm Hg) in ARDS and high (> 20 mm Hg) in heart failure.

Pulmonary embolism (PE) can mimic ARDS. Therefore, if PE is considered likely, pulmonary angiography should be performed to confirm the diagnosis of ARDS once the patient is stabilized. *Pneumocystis carinii* pneumonia and occasionally other primary lung infections may also mimic ARDS and should be considered, especially in immunocompromised patients.

MEDICAL MANAGEMENT

Patients diagnosed with ARDS require a multidisciplinary approach to care to effectively manage the syndrome and its potential complications. Registered nurses, registered dietitians, pharmacists, pulmonologists, intensivists, and other specialists are all integral to providing optimal care to these critically ill patients.

The ARDS patient requires mechanical ventilation and continuous hemodynamic monitoring. A pulmonary artery catheter may be used for obtaining pulmonary artery pressures, central venous pressure, and wedge pressure, and for determining a complete cardiac profile. Central lines are usually needed for medication and fluid administration. Urinary catheters with a urimeter can help to accurately measure hourly intake and output.

Mechanical Ventilation

The ARDS patient almost always requires endotracheal intubation to promote better gas exchange. Depending on the severity of the disease, mechanical intubation can last anywhere from two weeks to two months. The aim of mechanical ventilation is to promote gas exchange while protecting the lung (Gattinoni,

Eleonaora, & Caironi, 2005). After much research, the ARDS Network has found that low tidal volume and higher positive-end and expiratory pressure (PEEP) ventilation significantly increases the survival rate and reduces mortality by 22% (ARDS Network, 2000). A more in-depth explanation of the modes of ventilation appears in Chapter 23. Patients treated with traditional ventilation, which entails higher tidal volumes and lower PEEP, had significantly more days of nonpulmonary organ dysfunction compared with patients treated with higher PEEP and lower tidal volumes (Hough et al., 2005). The ARDS Network developed a protocol that has become standard of care for all ARDS patients; since the protocol became available in 2000, mortality in these patients has declined by 20% (Kallet et al., 2005).

According to the ARDSNet protocol, a ventilator mode of assist control with a high respiratory rate and a tidal volume goal of 6 mL/kg of predicted body weight (PBW) should be used on ARDS patients. The plateau pressure (the pressure that is maintained during part of inspiration, or Pplats) should be kept at 30 cm H_2O or less. The oxygenation goal is to maintain PaO_2 of 55 mm Hg to 80 mm Hg or a SpO_2 of 88% to 95%. Weaning FiO_2 to maintain these goals should be started immediately to prevent oxygen toxicity. Incremental FiO_2/PEEP combinations should be used. The protocol also includes pH management and steps for weaning (ARDS Clinical Network, 2004).

PEEP is an extremely important intervention for ARDS patients. PEEP prevents the continuous opening and closing of the alveoli, which results in more inflammation and edema formation in the lungs itself (Gattinoni et al., 2005). It also causes more inflammatory cell mediators to be systemically released, which contributes to circulatory failure, coagulation problems, and renal failure. Although PEEP can be increased up to 24 cm H_2O per the protocol, most patients cannot tolerate some of the side effects of PEEP, such as decreased venous return (the amount of blood returning to the right heart) and hence decreased cardiac output (the amount of blood ejected by the heart each minute).

Inversing the inspiratory to expiratory ratio can also help oxygenate ARDS patients, because it allows more time on inspiration than expiration, theoretically improving oxygenation. Since this regimen is not physiologically normal, patients must be sedated and paralyzed when it is employed. Although inverse ratio ventilation is not recommended by the ARDSNet protocol, it may be used as a rescue maneuver. This ventilator mode is a pressure-controlled inverse ratio, unlike the volume-driven traditional ventilator therapy. Its benefits include less lung stretching, better hemodynamic tolerance with improved preload/venous return, and improved oxygenation at lower FiO_2 settings. This mode causes the patient to auto-PEEP, enhancing alveoli recruitment related to the shorter expiration time.

Kinetic Therapy

Kinetic therapy, by definition, is the continuous side-to-side turning ranging from 30° to 62° by the use of specialty beds. The average healthy person has a major change in body position on average of every 11.6 minutes. In contrast, the intubated and sedated patient may be turned on average every 2 hours. Kinetic therapy has been shown to improve V/Q match and distribution of pleural pressures, mobilize static fluid and lymphatic drainage, and improve oxygenation (Sebat, Henry, Musthafa, & Johnson, 2004). Some studies show a 50% reduction in ventilator-associated pneumonia (VAP) and a 38% reduction in atelectasis with this strategy. Besides providing pulmonary benefits, kinetic therapy can decrease skin breakdown and urinary tract infections (Ahrens, Kollef, Stewart, & Shannon, 2004). To achieve the maximum benefit, early intervention is key.

Placing the patient in a prone position is a more aggressive form of kinetic therapy. Manual proning is difficult to perform, is labor-intensive, and is most often used as a rescue intervention (Sebat et al., 2004). Since the recent introduction of the proning bed, physicians are now using this form of kinetic therapy for patients with severe ARDS or for patients who do not respond to traditional 62° rotation. Besides the benefits associated with traditional rotation therapy, proning helps recruit dorsal consolidated lung, decrease pleural effusions, and enhance rapid secretion mobilization (Sebat et al.). Although studies involving small samples have shown promising results, more research needs to be done on the mortality rates of proning.

One problem commonly encountered with kinetic therapy is the unstable patient's inability to tolerate turning. In this case, the patient may be acclimated to turning. The degree of rotation is started at 10° to 20° and gradually increased per physician order. Also, it is important to understand that kinetic therapy may not be initiated on everyone. This therapy is contraindicated in patients receiving hemodialysis and in patients who have open sternums or abdomen, head injuries with high intracranial pressure, or an unstable pelvis or spine. Patients must be adequately sedated during continuous kinetic therapy.

Fluid Balance

Fluid balance maintenance can be challenging in patients with ARDS. These patients have increased capillary permeability so fluid tends to leak into the lung tissue. At the same time, patients might be intravascularly dry and susceptible to hypotension, especially if they are receiving high levels of PEEP. Therefore, fluid resuscitation may be required to help maintain adequate blood pressure. There is great debate over whether crystalloids or colloids should be used to resuscitate the patient. Most agree that it depends on the patient population (surgical versus trauma) and physician preference. After fluid status has been normalized, diuretics and mild fluid restrictions may be implemented to relieve pulmonary congestion and to improve oxygenation. Daily weight, intake and output, vital signs, and hemodynamic values are monitored as well to help balance fluid status (Davies & Hoffman, 2000).

Investigational Therapies

Surfactant Administration

Unfortunately, numerous studies have not found any differences in mortality rates between groups that have received surfactant administration compared with those that received placebos (Bosma, Fanelli, & Ranieri, 2005). Although components of surfactant have been identified, the exact pathophysiology of surfactant in ARDS patients remains unclear. Many believe that the destruction and structural alteration of surfactant are caused by inflammation, cell debris, and the protein-rich edema in the alveoli. The concept of delivering this local therapy sounds interesting, and researchers continue to investigate it (Baudouin, 2004).

Drotrecogin Alfa (Activated)

Drotrecogin Alfa (activated) (Xigris®) has anti-inflammatory, antithrombotic, and profibrinolytic properties. In 2001, the U.S. Food and Drug Administration approved this drug as a treatment for severe sepsis. Clinical trials have shown that Xigris® effectively reduces the mortality of septic patients. The exact mechanism of action remains unknown, however, and more trials are underway (Rice & Bernard, 2004). Given that inflammation and microthrombi are also present in ARDS, the question of whether Xigris® might work in ARDS has been recently proposed, but remains largely unstudied. Few studies have used Xigris® in noninfectious/inhalation injury ARDS patients and obtained promising results, but many questions remain unanswered. Until more studies are conducted, Xigris® is not considered standard in treating ARDS.

Inhaled Nitric Oxide

Inhaled nitric oxide (inhaled NO or iNO) is a local pulmonary vasodilator that is primarily used to treat pulmonary hypertension. It has no systemic effects because iNO is inactivated immediately when it comes in contact with hemoglobin, which results in the formation of methemoglobin (Klein, Blackbourne, & Barquist, 2004). Due to its pulmonary vasodilatation properties, iNO helps redistribute blood flow, thereby improving oxygenation. Given that ARDS is characterized by pulmonary

shunting and hypoxemia, it was thought that iNO might improve V/Q mismatch and oxygenation, resulting in decreased ventilator days and mortality (Kaisers, Busch, Deja, Donaubauer, & Falke, 2003). Unfortunately, multiple studies have found that although there is a significant increase in PaO_2 with iNO compared with placebo in the first 48 hours, the ventilator days and mortality rate remained the same (Taylor et al., 2004). Furthermore, iNO therapy costs thousands of dollars per day. Because of the high costs and current study results, iNO is not routinely used in the management and treatment of ARDS (Klein et al.).

Glucocorticoids

Some researchers had suggested that steroids might decrease the inflammation in the acute (exudative) phase of ARDS and, therefore, increase the survival rate. Current data do not support this use, and early steroid treatment is rarely initiated. Whether steroids might be effective in the late (fibrotic) stage of ARDS is still being debated, although the general consensus is that it is not indicated (Bosma et al., 2005). However, patients with ARDS may benefit from steroid therapy if they have adrenal insufficiency or if they are not responding to conventional treatment (Thompson, 2003). Studies are still being conducted to determine whether late-phase, low-dose steroids might decrease morbidity and mortality rates of ARDS.

Extracorporeal Membrane Oxygenation

While extracorporeal membrane oxygenation (ECMO) has been used successfully in pediatric patients, in whom it produced a survival rate of 70% to 90%, it has not been proven to be consistently effective in adult ARDS patients. Few studies have shown survival rates greater than 50%. In addition, adult ECMO is costly and requires the services of a skilled and dedicated staff. Although successful cases have been documented, ECMO is not considered standard ARDS therapy and is used primarily as a rescue intervention (Hemmila et al., 2004; Klein et al., 2004). While more studies need to be conducted, a few institutions have found ECMO to be a realistic treatment modality for ARDS.

COMPLICATIONS AND NURSING INTERVENTIONS

Complications may result either from ARDS itself or from its treatment. **Table 25-3** outlines the common complications associated with ARDS. Because ARDS is usually the result of sepsis, MODS is the most common complication and has the largest impact on mortality. Treatment for MODS is supportive until organ function can be restored.

TABLE 25-3 Complications Commonly Associated with ARDS

Infection	Gastrointestinal
VAP	Stress ulcer
Central line infections	GI bleeding
Sepsis	Ileus
Urinary tract infections	**Renal**
Respiratory	Acute renal failure
Pulmonary embolism	Permanent renal damage
Barotrauma	**Other**
O_2 toxicity	Skin breakdown
Pulmonary fibrosis	Anemia
Prolonged mechanical	Hyperglycemia
ventilation	MODS
Prolonged weaning	Coagulation dysfunction
Cardiac	
Decreased cardiac output	
Arrhythmias	

VAP = ventilator-associated pneumonia; GI = gastrointestinal; MODS = multiple-organ dysfunction syndrome.
Source: Ware & Matthay, 2000.

ARDS occurs suddenly, is often difficult to diagnose, has numerous complications, and is considered life-threatening. As a consequence, the role intensive care unit (ICU) nurses play is paramount in achieving high-quality outcomes. The plan of care is an excellent means of communicating the appropriate nursing diagnoses, interventions, and patient-specific goals. **Table 25-4** lists some common problems that may arise while caring for the patient experiencing ARDS.

TABLE 25-4 Care-Related Problems Associated with ARDS

- Impaired gas exchange
- Ineffective airway clearance
- Ineffective breathing pattern
- Risk for aspiration
- Altered nutrition: less than body requirements
- Risk for infection
- Altered tissue perfusion

Source: Conrad, 2005.

Ventilator-Associated Pneumonia

VAP is a frequent complication in intubated mechanically ventilated patients. Risk factors include an impaired or weakened immune system, prolonged intubation, aspiration from gastric contents or oral mucosa, traumatic intubation, and contaminated medical equipment. Although kinetic therapy significantly reduces VAP, the best treatment for VAP is prevention (Ahrens et al., 2004). A number of nursing interventions can be implemented to prevent VAP, including handwashing before and after each patient contact, elevating the head of the bed at 30° or more unless contraindicated, using a reverse Trendelenburg position in specialty beds, using a closed endotracheal suctioning system or sterile technique, and providing oral hygiene at least every four hours with chlorohexidine rinse. A more in-depth discussion of VAP appears in Chapter 23.

Stress Ulcers

Any critically ill patient is at high risk for stress ulcers. Bleeding from the ulcer site occurs about 30% of the time in ARDS patients (Davies & Hoffman, 2000). Prevention is essential and should be initiated immediately with the mechanically ventilated patient. Starting enteral nutrition and prescribing prophylactic H_2-receptor blockers or proton pump inhibitors are just some of the ways to prevent stress ulcers. Conditions such as infections, shock, acidosis, and hypotension should also be managed aggressively (Davies & Hoffman).

Skin Breakdown

Many factors can attribute to skin breakdown in ARDS patients, including immobility due to sedatives or paralytics, medical equipment such as endotracheal tubes and kinetic specialty beds, malnutrition and catabolic states, incontinence, shock, and high doses of vasopressors. Once again, prevention is imperative. Frequent skin assessment and evaluation of current treatment should be a top priority. The institution's skin and wound team should be consulted for appropriate interventions and treatment plans. Other interventions include, but are not limited to, turning patients every two hours and using pressure-relieving devices, repositioning endotracheal tubes every eight hours or more frequently if necessary, using barrier and medicated ointments, and using incontinence collection devices.

Barotrauma

Barotrauma is the result of overdistention and rupture of alveoli during mechanical ventilation. Air then is found in areas where it should not be, which can produce a pneumothorax, pneumomediastinum, subcutaneous air, and subcutaneous emphysema (Davies & Hoffman, 2000). Using low tidal volume ventilation or following the ARDSNet protocol can prove helpful in preventing barotrauma. Barotrauma is primarily a result of the overdistention seen with high levels of PEEP and high Pplat readings; it often results in chest tube placement.

PATIENT OUTCOMES

Nurses can help ensure obtainment of optimal patient outcomes such as those listed in **Box 25-2**, through the use of evidence-based interventions for patients with acute respiratory distress syndrome.

SUMMARY

Since the first clinical presentation of ARDS, there has been great controversy surrounding this syndrome's incidence, natural history, and mortality. Despite this debate, substantial progress has been made in the understanding of acute lung injury. ICU nurses play a pivotal role in improving the health care of critically ill patients suffering from ARDS. Because ARDS can result from many different causes, and because its symptoms may vary, there is even greater need for skilled critical care clinicians to provide vigilant nursing care to these highly vulnerable, unstable, and complex patients.

Box 25-2
Optimal Patient Outcomes

- Oxygen saturation within expected range
- Absence of complications related to PEEP therapy
- Cardiac output within expected range
- Chest radiographs return to baseline
- Hemodynamic status stable
- Activity tolerance in expected range
- Family coping with acute illness

CASE STUDY

A healthy 27-year-old male weighing 80 kg sustained a crushing injury to both lower extremities. After being stabilized in the emergency department, he was transferred to the operating room for an open-reduction external fixation. He was admitted post-operatively for close observation and monitoring to the ICU with 0.9% normal saline infusing at 125 mL/hr. The next morning his vital signs were stable and his lungs were clear, so the 0.9% normal saline was decreased to 50 mL/hr. Later that same day, he was transferred to the surgical floor in stable condition. At 0900 on post-op day 3, he began experiencing sudden shortness of breath with SpO_2 of 90% on room air. The nurse placed him on 3 L of oxygen via nasal cannula, and the physician was immediately notified. At 1200, his oxygen saturation remained low and his oxygen was increased to 50% face mask. The physician was again notified, and additional orders were received for a STAT ABG and portable chest radiograph. ABG results revealed the following: pH 7.50; pCO_2 36; pO_2 58; HCO_3 24; and SaO_2 85%. Chest radiograph revealed diffuse bilateral infiltrates. Subsequently, the physician was notified of both the ABG and chest x-ray results. By 1600, the patient was diaphoretic, tachypneic, and experiencing intercostal retractions. His vital signs were as follows: BP 140/85; HR 110; RR 40; and SpO_2 83%. He was becoming more difficult to arouse, so the Rapid Assessment Team was called to come and evaluate the patient. Upon arrival of the Rapid Assessment Team, the patient was orally intubated and transferred back to the ICU. Upon auscultation of the patient's lungs, coarse rhonchi were heard bilaterally. He was placed on the ventilator with the following settings: AC, rate 20; FiO_2 70; Vt 450; and PEEP 10 cm H_2O. Thirty minutes later, an ABG showed the following results: pH 7.54; pCO_2 38; pO_2 46; HCO_3 22; and SpO_2 78%. The intensivist was notified, and additional changes were made to the ventilator.

Over the course of the next 24 hours, the patient's condition continued to deteriorate and a pulmonary artery catheter was placed. His PAOP is now 10 mm Hg, and there is no evidence of left atrial hypertension. The most recent chest radiograph showed worsening diffuse bilateral alveolar infiltrates, but the cardiac silhouette appeared normal.

CRITICAL THINKING QUESTIONS

1. What physiological process has occurred to cause the change in the condition of this patient?
2. What were the predisposing factors associated with the development of this particular medical condition?
3. What are the priority nursing diagnoses for this patient?
4. Which interventions do you anticipate while caring for this patient, and why?
5. Is this patient at risk for developing any complications? If so, which ones?
6. Which other healthcare disciplines need to be involved in planning care, and why?
7. What is the mortality rate associated with this patient's medical condition? Explain the primary cause of death related to ARDS.
8. How can you support the patient's family members and friends?
9. Which medical intervention has been proven to decrease morbidity and increase the survival rate in ARDS?
10. What are the main components of the ARDSNet protocol?
11. What is kinetic therapy, and when is it appropriate to use?
12. What are some common complications of ARDS, and why do they occur?
13. Which nursing interventions might help decrease complications associated with ARDS?
14. Which assessment findings and diagnostic tools should be utilized to monitor the progression or resolution of ARDS?
15. What are the systemic benefits of lower tidal volumes and higher PEEP compared with traditional ventilation?
16. How will you implement your role as a facilitator of learning for this patient and family?
17. Utilize the form to write up a plan of care for a client with ARDS in the clinical setting. Rate the patient as a level 1, 3, or 5 on each characteristic.

Using the Synergy Model to Develop a Plan of Care

	Patient Characteristics	Level (1, 3, 5)	Subjective and Objective Data	Evidence-based Interventions	Outcomes
SYNERGY MODEL	Resiliency				
	Vulnerability				
	Stability				
	Complexity				
	Resource availability				
	Participation in care				
	Participation in decision making				
	Predictability				

Online Resources

American Association of Critical-Care Nurses, Ventilator-Associated Pneumonia Practice Alert:
www.aacn.org/aacn/practicealertnsf/vwdoc/practicealertmain

ARDS Network: www.ardsnet.org

ARDS Support Center: www.ards.org

Understanding ARDS—Acute Respiratory Distress Syndrome and Its Effect on Victims and Loved Ones:
www.ards.org/learnaboutards/whatisards/brochure/

REFERENCES

Acute Respiratory Distress Syndrome Network. (2000). Ventilation with lower tidal volumes as compared with traditional tidal volumes for acute lung injury and the acute respiratory distress syndrome. *New England Journal of Medicine, 342*(18), 1301–1308.

Ahrens, T., Kollef, M., Stewart, J., & Shannon, W. (2004). Effect of kinetic therapy on pulmonary complications. *American Journal of Critical Care, 13,* 376–382.

ARDS Clinical Network. (2004). Mechanical ventilation protocol summary. Retrieved July 3, 2004, from www.ardsnet.org

ARDS Foundation. (2005). Facts about ARDS. Retrieved July 2, 2005, from www.ardsfoundationil.com/facts.htm

Baudouin, S. (2004). Exogenous surfactant replacement in ARDS—one day, someday or never. *New England Journal of Medicine, 351,* 853–855.

Bosma, K., Fanelli, V., & Ranieri, V. M. (2005). Acute respiratory distress syndrome: Update on the latest developments in basic and clinical research. *Current Opinion in Anesthesiology, 18*(2), 137–145.

Conrad, S. A. (2005). Adult respiratory distress syndrome. *eMedicine Instant Access to the Minds of Medicine.* Retrieved June 18, 2005, from www.emedicine.com/EMERG/topic503.htm

Davies, P. J., & Hoffman, L. (2000). Respiratory failure. In S. M. Lewis, M. H. Heitkemper, & S. R. Dirksen, *Medical-Surgical nursing assessment: Assessment and management of clinical problems* (5th ed., pp. 1910–1911). St. Louis, MO: Mosby.

Gattinoni, L., Eleonaora, C., & Caironi, P. (2005). Monitoring of pulmonary mechanics in acute respiratory distress syndrome to titrate therapy. *Current Opinions in Critical Care, 11*(3), 252–258.

Hemmila, M., Rowe, S., Boules, T., Miskulin, J., McGillicuddy, J. W., Schuerer, D. J., et al. (2004). Extracorporeal life support for severe acute respiratory distress syndrome in adults. *Transactions of the Meeting of the American Surgical Association,* CXXII, 193–205.

Hough, C. L., Kallet, R. H., Ranieri, V. M., Rubenfeld, G., Luce, J. M., & Hudson, L. (2005). Intrinsic positive end-expiratory pressure in acute respiratory distress syndrome network subjects. *Critical Care Medicine, 33*(3), 527–532.

Howard, A., Courtney-Shapiro, C., Kelso, L., Goltz, M., & Morris, P. (2004). Comparison of three methods of detecting acute respiratory distress syndrome: Clinical screening, chart review and diagnostic coding. *American Journal of Critical Care, 13,* 59–64.

Hubmayr, R. D. (2002). Perspective on lung injury and recruitment. A skeptical look at the opening and collapse story. *American Journal of Respiratory Critical Care Medicine, 165,* 1647–1653.

Kaisers, U., Busch, T., Deja, M., Donaubauer, B., & Falke, K. J. (2003). Selective pulmonary vasodilation in acute respiratory distress syndrome. *Critical Care Medicine, 31*(4), S337–S342.

Kallet, R. H., Jasmer, R. M., Pittet, J., Tang, J., Campbell, A. R., Dicker, R., et al. (2005). Clinical implementation of the ARDS Network protocol is associated with reduced hospital mortality compared with historical controls. *Critical Care Medicine, 33*(5), 925–929.

Klein, Y., Blackbourne, L., & Barquist, E. S. (2004). Non-ventilatory based strategies in the management of acute respiratory distress syndrome. *Journal of Trauma, 57*(4), 915–924.

Mortelliti, M. P., & Manning, H. L. (2002). Acute respiratory distress syndrome. *American Family Physician, 65*(9), 1823–1830.

Rice, T., & Bernard, G. R. (2004). Drotrecogin alfa (activated) for the treatment of severe sepsis and septic shock. *American Journal of Medical Sciences, 328*(4), 205–214.

Sebat, F., Henry, K., Musthafa, A., & Johnson, D. (2004). The utility of an automated proning and kinetic therapy bed and its effect on lung recruitment, ventilator days and mortality in patients with acute lung injury. *American College of Chest Physicians.* Retrieved June 15, 2005, from http://metting.chestjournal.org

Taylor, R., Zimmerman, J., Dellinger, R. P., Straube, R. C., Criner, G., Davis, K., et al. (2004). Low-dose inhaled nitric oxide in patients with acute lung injury: A randomized controlled trial. *Journal of the American Medical Association, 291*(13), 1603–1609.

Thompson, B. T. (2003). Glucocorticoids and acute lung injury. *Critical Care Medicine, 31*(4), S253–S257.

Ware, L. B., & Matthay, M. A. (2000). The acute respiratory distress syndrome. *New England Journal of Medicine, 342*(18), 1334–1349.

Neurology

CHAPTER 26

Neurologic Anatomy, Physiology, and Assessment

Joyce King

LEARNING OBJECTIVES

Upon completion of this chapter, the reader will be able to:

1. Review the neurological physiology.

2. Discuss the anatomy and physiology of the central and peripheral nervous systems.

3. List the techniques that are used for assessing the nervous system.

4. Identify the difference between abnormal and normal neurological findings.

This chapter focuses on one of the major control systems of the body—the nervous system. It provides an overview of the anatomy and physiology of the central nervous system (CNS) and the peripheral nervous system (PNS) as well as describes the assessment of the nervous system.

As changes occur in the external and internal environments of the body, the nerve cells receive this information and transmit it to other cells. The nervous system exerts primary control over the body's muscular and glandular activities, with the goal of maintaining homeostasis. This system is organized into the CNS, which is composed of the brain and spinal cord, and the PNS, which consists of nerve fibers that carry information between the CNS and other parts of the body.

The PNS is further subdivided into the afferent and efferent divisions. The afferent nervous system carries sensory or visceral information to the CNS, while the efferent nervous system transmits information from the CNS to the muscles or glands to bring about a desired effect. The efferent nervous system is also subdivided into the somatic nervous system, which innervates skeletal muscle, and the autonomic nervous system, which innervates smooth muscle, cardiac muscle, and glands.

To make things even more complicated, the autonomic nervous system is further divided into the sympathetic nervous system (SNS) and the parasympathetic nervous system. Both systems innervate the same organs, but generally act in opposition to each other. For example, the sympathetic system increases the heart rate; the parasympathetic system slows it down.

Three classes of neurons make up the nervous system:

- The *afferent neuron* has at its peripheral ending a sensory receptor that generates action potentials in response to a particular type of stimulus. It consists of a long peripheral axon that propagates the action potential to the cell body, which is located adjacent to the spinal cord, and a short central axon, which passes from the cell body into the spinal cord where it synapses with other neurons within the spinal cord.

- The *efferent neuron's* cell body originates in the CNS. Efferent axons carry information from the CNS to the effector organs.

- *Interneurons* lie within the CNS between the afferent and efferent neurons. They are important in the integration of peripheral responses to peripheral information (e.g., hot object, pull your hand away). They are also responsible for the abstract phenomena associated with the "mind" (e.g., thoughts, emotions, memory, and motivation).

OVERVIEW OF NEUROLOGIC ANATOMY AND PHYSIOLOGY

The neuron is the functional unit of the nervous system. Humans have about 100 billion neurons in their brain alone. All neurons have three parts. *Dendrites* receive information from another cell and transmit the message to the cell body. The *cell body* contains the nucleus, mitochondria, and other organelles. The *axon* conducts messages away from the cell body (see **Figure 26-1**). Some axons are wrapped in an insulating myelin sheath. In the CNS, oligodendrocytes are the myelin-forming cells, whereas Schwann cells perform this function in the PNS. Some exposed areas of the axonal membrane are not covered by the myelin sheath, known as the nodes of Ranvier.

All cell membranes, including neurons, have an unequal distribution of ions (i.e., sodium and potassium ions) and electrical charges between the two sides of the membrane, which creates the membrane potential. Sodium ions (Na^+) are concentrated on the outside of the membrane, giving the outside a positive charge. Potassium ions (K^+) are concentrated inside the membrane, giving the inside a negative charge. This charge difference, which is known as the resting potential, is measured in millivolts (mV). The resting potential of a typical nerve cell is -70 mV. Nerve and muscle are excitable tissues; that is, they are capable of changing their membrane potential and producing electrical signals when stimulated. Muscle cells use these electrical signals to turn on specialized contractile processes (Sherwood, 2004).

In nerve cells, these fluctuations in membrane potential produce two types of signals: (1) graded potentials and (2) action potentials. Graded potentials are local changes in membrane potential that occur in varying degrees of magnitude: The stronger the triggering event, the larger the graded potential. Each potential is produced by a specific triggering event that causes gated ion channels to open. Graded potentials serve as short-distance signals within the neuron but can initiate an action potential. During an action potential, the membrane potential rapidly reverses (becomes more positive) as a result of rapid changes in the membrane permeability of sodium and potassium, which permits rapid fluxes of these ions in and out of the cell (see **Figure 26-2**). The rising phase of the action potential (depolarization) is due to sodium channels opening, allowing the positively charged sodium ions to flow into the cell so that the inside of the membrane temporarily becomes more positive than the outside. The falling phase (repolarization) is brought about by potassium channels opening, allowing the positively charged potassium ions to flow out of the cell, resulting in the inside of the cell again having a negative charge; simultaneously, there is an inactivation or closing of the sodium channels. Once initiated, action potentials are propagated throughout an excitable cell. It is the task of the sodium–potassium (Na^+-K^+) pump, a protein located in the cell membrane that actively transports

FIGURE 26-1 Anatomy of a Neuron

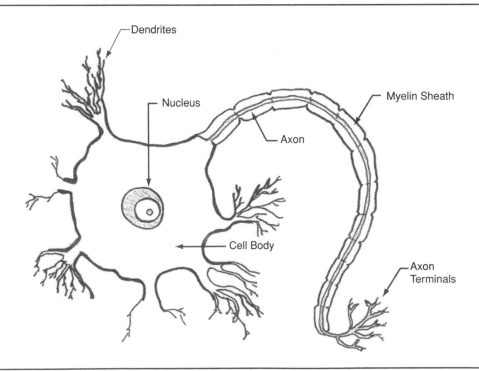

Source: Illustrated by James R. Perron.

FIGURE 26-2 Schematic of an Action Potential

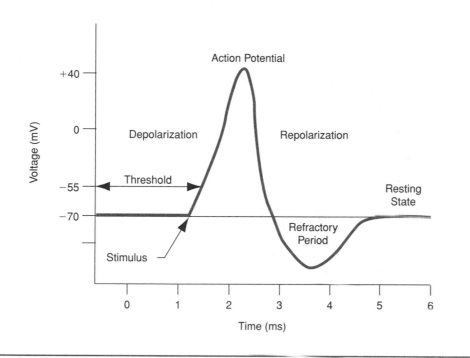

Source: Illustrated by James R. Perron.

ions against their concentration gradients, to restore the ions to their original locations.

An action potential is self-propagating. Once started, it will continue moving down the axon in only one direction, like the falling of dominos. Action potentials are propagated either by local current flow (called contiguous conduction) in nonmyelinated fibers or by saltatory conduction in myelinated fibers. With contiguous conduction, local current flow between an active area and an adjacent inactive area brings the inactive area to the threshold, triggering another action potential in the inactive area. With saltatory conduction, the impulse jumps over the myelinated region from one node of Ranvier to the next. Myelinated fibers conduct impulses about 50 times faster than do unmyelinated fibers of comparable diameter. Destruction of the myelin occurs in the disease known as multiple sclerosis, resulting in impaired nerve function and symptoms such as muscular weakness and paralysis.

A junction between a nerve cell and another cell, such as another neuron or a muscle cell, is called a synapse. A neuron-to-neuron synapse involves the axon terminal of a presynaptic neuron and the dendrites of a postsynaptic neuron. The space between the presynaptic and postsynaptic membrane is called the synaptic cleft. Action potentials in the presynaptic

neuron influence the membrane potential in the postsynaptic neuron. Neurotransmitters (e.g., acetylcholine), which are stored in small synaptic vesicles clustered in the axon terminal, carry the signal from the presynaptic neuron, across the synaptic cleft, to the postsynaptic neuron (see **Figure 26-3**). Arrival of the action potential causes some of the vesicles to release their neurotransmitter load via the process of exocytosis. As the neurotransmitter diffuses across the synaptic cleft, it binds to specific receptors on the postsynaptic cell's membrane, causing ion channels on that cell to open. Some neurotransmitters excite the postsynaptic neuron, whereas others inhibit it. After the neurotransmitter relays its message, it is rapidly removed from the synaptic cleft either by undergoing enzymatic degradation or by actively being taken back up into the axon terminal, where it can be stored and released at another time.

Both drugs and diseases can modify synaptic transmission. For example, cocaine blocks the reuptake of the neurotransmitter dopamine at presynaptic terminals. The result is prolonged activation of neural pathways that use this chemical as a neurotransmitter. With myasthenia gravis, a disease characterized by muscular weakness, the body produces antibodies against the acetylcholine receptor. As a result, not all of the released acetylcholine can find a receptor with which to bind, decreasing synaptic transmission.

THE CENTRAL NERVOUS SYSTEM

The CNS serves as the control center of the body. As mentioned earlier, it consists of the brain and the spinal cord. The majority of the cells within the CNS are not neurons, but rather glial cells. Glial cells support the interneurons physically, metabolically, and functionally. They include astrocytes, oligodendrocytes, ependymal cells, and microglia cells.

The delicate central nervous tissue is well protected. The major structures that help guard the CNS from damage are the skull and vertebral column, the meninges (the dura mater,

FIGURE 26-3 Synaptic Structure and Function

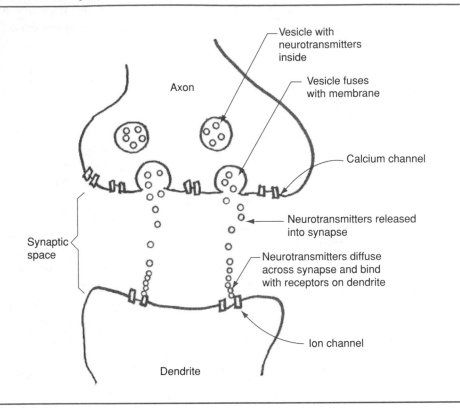

Source: Illustrated by James R. Perron.

arachnoid mater, and pia mater), the cerebral spinal fluid, and the highly selective blood–brain barrier, which limits access of blood-borne materials into the brain tissue.

The major components of the brain are the cerebral cortex, the cerebellum, the brain stem, and subcortical structures, including the basal nuclei, thalamus, and hypothalamus (see **Figure 26-4**). The cerebral cortex is the site of initiation of all voluntary motor output, final perceptual processing of all sensory input, and integration of most higher neural activity. This integration is important for even a simple task, such as picking a flower: Vision of the flower takes place in one area of the cortex, response to the fragrance takes place in another area, and movement is initiated by yet another area. The cerebellum is important in balance as well as in planning and execution of voluntary movement. The brain stem, a vital link between the spinal cord and higher brain regions, consists of the medulla, pons, and midbrain. The basal nuclei play an important role in the control of movement and are especially crucial for the muscle contractions involved in posture and support. The thalamus is a sensory relay station. It screens out insignificant signals and routes the important sensory impulses to appropriate areas of the cortex, as well as to other regions of

the brain. The thalamus also reinforces voluntary muscle activity initiated by the cortex. The hypothalamus regulates many homeostatic functions (e.g., body temperature, thirst, food intake, anterior pituitary hormone secretion).

The spinal cord serves as the neuronal link between the brain and the PNS. It extends through the vertebral canal and is connected to the spinal nerves. The spinal nerves consist of 8 pairs of cervical nerves, 12 pairs of thoracic nerves, 5 pairs of lumbar nerves, 5 pairs of sacral nerves, and 1 coccygeal nerve.

The spinal cord comprises both white matter and gray matter. The gray matter forms a butterfly-shaped region on the inside of the spinal cord that is surrounded by the outer white matter. The gray matter consists primarily of neuronal cell bodies and their dendrites, the short interneurons, and glial cells. Each half of the gray matter is divided into a dorsal horn, a ventral horn, and lateral horn. Spinal nerves connect with each side of the spinal cord through a dorsal root, where afferent fibers carrying incoming signals enter the spinal cord, and a ventral root, where efferent fibers carrying outgoing signals leave the spinal cord.

The white matter is organized into tracts or bundles of nerve fibers with similar function. The tracts are grouped into columns that extend along the length of the spinal cord. Each tract begins or ends within a particular area of the brain, and each carries a specific type of information. All communication up and down the spinal cord takes place in either the ascending or descending tracts. The ascending tract or afferent tract carries sensory information to the CNS. The descending tract relays information from the brain to the efferent neurons.

The spinal cord is also responsible for the integration of many basic reflexes. A reflex is any response that occurs automatically without conscious effort. Two types of reflexes are distinguished: (1) basic reflexes, which are built-in reflexes, such as pulling the hand away from a hot object; and (2) acquired reflexes, which are the result of practice and learning,

FIGURE 26-4 The Components of the Brain

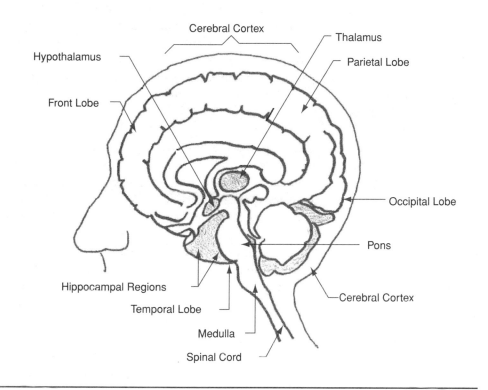

Source: Illustrated by James R. Perron.

such as typing at the computer. The neural pathway involved in accomplishing reflex activity is known as a reflex arc.

THE PERIPHERAL NERVOUS SYSTEM

The PNS is responsible for picking up any change in the internal and external environment, transmitting that information to the CNS, and then responding appropriately. This ability of the organism to deal with changes in the environment is necessary for the maintenance of homeostasis. The PNS can be separated into two divisions: the sensory (afferent) division and the motor (efferent) division.

Afferent Division

For the purposes of this chapter, we will limit our discussion of the afferent division to receptor physiology, somatosensory pathways, and acuity. The details of the physiology of vision, hearing, taste, and smell are beyond the scope of this discussion.

The major role of the afferent division is to detect, encode, and transmit information. Receptors are the detectors of this system. At their peripheral endings, afferent neurons have receptors that detect changes in both the internal and external environments. They are then able to encode that infor-

mation into action potentials that are transmitted by the afferent neurons to the CNS. Six types of receptors exist: photoreceptors, mechanoreceptors, thermoreceptors, osmoreceptors, chemoreceptors, and nociceptors or pain receptors. Each type is specialized so that it responds more readily to one type of stimulus. For example, the receptors in the eye respond to light, and the receptors in the ear respond to sound waves. Some receptors have the ability to respond weakly to other than their major stimulus but still give rise to the same sensation. For instance, the light receptors in the eye can also respond to pressure, resulting in the person "seeing stars." Two general types of receptors are distinguished: specialized endings of the afferent neuron and separate cells that are closely associated with the peripheral ending of the neuron. When these receptors are stimulated, they promote nonselective opening of ion channels; this activity alters the membrane permeability of the receptor, resulting in a graded receptor potential. The magnitude of the receptor potential depends on the strength of the stimulus and the rate of application or removal of the stimulus. The receptor potential is converted to action potentials by the opening of Na^+ channels in the afferent neuron membrane adjacent to the receptor. A large receptor potential induces more rapid firing of action potentials. Similarly, stimulus strength reflects the size of the area stimulated.

On reaching the spinal cord, afferent information can go in one of two directions: It can participate in a reflex arc or it can be relayed to the brain for further processing. All information is propagated via somatosensory pathways to the CNS through the same type of signal, the action potential. The brain can decode the type and location of the stimulus by noting the type and location of the activated receptor and the specific pathway over which the information was transmitted to a particular area of the cerebral cortex.

Acuity refers to the discriminative ability. Both the receptive field size and the density of receptors influence acuity. The smaller the receptive field and the greater the density of the receptors, the greater the acuity or discriminative ability of the sensory neuron. For example, an estimated 17,000 tactile mechanoreceptors are present in the fingertips and palm of each hand; in contrast, the skin of the calf of the leg has relatively few sensory endings with larger receptive fields.

Efferent Division

The CNS controls the activities of effector organs (muscles and glands) by transmitting signals to these organs through the efferent division of the PNS. The involuntary branch of the PNS division—the autonomic nervous system—innervates cardiac muscle, smooth muscle, most exocrine glands, and some endocrine glands. The voluntary branch of the efferent division—the somatic nervous system—innervates skeletal muscle.

The autonomic nervous system consists of a two-neuron chain (see Figure 26-4). The cell body of the first neuron is located in the CNS. The axon or pre-ganglionic fiber synapses with the cell body of the second neuron. The cell body of this second neuron lies within a ganglion outside the CNS. The axon or post-ganglionic fiber innervates the effector organ. Recall that this system is subdivided into the SNS and the parasympathetic nervous system (PNS). The sympathetic nerve fibers originate in the thoracic and lumbar regions of the spinal cord. Most pre-ganglionic fibers of this system are short and synapse with cell bodies of post-ganglionic neurons within the ganglia that lie in a sympathetic ganglion chain. The parasympathetic nerve fibers arise from the cranial and sacral areas of the CNS. These pre-ganglionic fibers are long, finally ending when they reach the terminal ganglia that lie in or near the effector organ. Very short post-ganglionic fibers terminate on the cells of an organ itself.

The nerve fibers involved in the autonomic nervous system communicate via neurotransmitters. Pre-ganglionic fibers of both the SNS and PNS release the neurotransmitter acetylcholine. However, the neurotransmitters released from the post-ganglionic nerve fibers differ between the SNS and PNS. The PNS releases acetylcholine (called cholinergic fibers), whereas the SNS releases norepinephrine (called adrenergic fibers). Both the SNS and PNS innervate most visceral organs, exerting opposite effects in a particular organ. This dual innervation allows precise control over the organ's activity.

The somatic nervous system consists of motor neurons that innervate skeletal muscle. Acetylcholine is the neurotransmitter that links the electrical activity in motor neurons with the electrical activity in skeletal muscle cells. Each axon terminal of a motor neuron forms a neuromuscular junction with a single muscle cell. An action potential in the motor neuron results in the release of acetylcholine, which in turn binds to receptors on the motor end plate. As a result, ion channels open in the motor end plate and the motor end plate depolarizes. This potential change is known as the end-plate potential. Local current flow between the depolarized end plate and adjacent membrane initiates an action potential, which propagates throughout the muscle fiber and ultimately results in the muscle fiber contracting. Acetylcholinesterase, an enzyme located in the muscle cell membrane, inactivates acetylcholine, terminating the muscle cell's response.

NEUROLOGICAL ASSESSMENT

Unlike many other disorders in which the signs of the disease are visible (e.g., a rash) or palpable (e.g., a mass), neurological conditions may be detected only by specific examination techniques. Even though highly advanced neuroimaging techniques are now available, the neurological examination still provides the clinician with the most important and relevant information about a patient's diagnosis. The neurological examination includes evaluation of mental status, the cranial nerves, the sensory and motor systems, the reflexes, and cerebellar function, including gait. Tools required for a thorough exam include an ophthalmoscope, a reflex hammer, a tuning fork, a tongue blade, cotton balls, and a supply of safety pins.

The mental status evaluation consists of asking the patient a series of questions that assess orientation to time, place, and person; short- and long-term memory; and various abilities, such as thinking abstractly, following instructions, using language, and solving math problems (Bickley & Szilagyi, 2003).

Glasgow Coma Scale

The Glasgow Coma Scale (GCS) is a scoring system used in the intensive care unit (ICU) to assess the neurological status of a patient. It is relatively simple, has consistent inter-rater reliability, and allows the nurse to trend neurological status over time (Bateman, 2001). **Box 26-1** shows the elements of the GCS. The nurse scores the patient on three categories: eye opening, motor response, and verbal response. A score is calculated by adding up the numbers from each category, with the maximum score possible being 15. A score of 9 to 12 suggests a moderate neurological deficit, and a score of 8 or less is considered a severe deficit (Bateman). The motor response on the GCS takes into consideration the posturing status of the patient. If the patient demonstrates decorticate rigidity (abnormal flexion), a score of 3 is given. Decorticate rigidity occurs when the patient flexes only the arms at the elbow and wrist in response to a painful stimuli. If the patient shows decerebrate rigidity, a score of 2 is given. Decerebrate rigidity (abnormal extension) occurs when the patient extends the arms in response to painful stimuli. **Figure 26-5** illustrates both types of posturing.

Box 26-1
Glasgow Coma Scale

Eye Opening (4)
Spontaneous	4
To sound	3
To pain	2
Never	1

Motor Response (6)
Obeys commands	6
Localizes pain	5
Normal flexion (withdrawal)	4
Abnormal flexion	3
Extension	2
No response	1

Verbal Response (5)
Oriented	5
Confused conversation	4
Inappropriate words	3
Incomprehensible sounds	2
None	1

Most ICU nursing documentation flow sheets have a section to document the GCS every shift and whenever a change occurs. Even though the GCS is widely utilized, the nurse's first indication of an alteration in neurological status is the patient's

FIGURE 26-5 Posturing

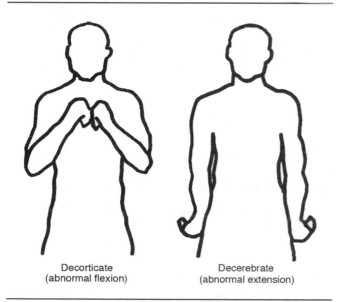

Decorticate (abnormal flexion)

Decerebrate (abnormal extension)

Source: Illustrated by James R. Perron.

level of consciousness. A change in the level of consciousness can be as slight as a complaint of a headache or as severe as slurred speech. The nurse should assess for changes or new onset of headaches, restlessness, irritability, slurred speech, disorientation, inability to follow commands, or altered thought processes.

Cranial Nerves and Sensory System

Twelve pairs of cranial nerves lead directly from the brain to various parts of the head and neck. Not all cranial nerves are generally tested in a routine physical examination. If a cranial nerve disorder is suspected, the function of that specific nerve is tested (see **Table 26-1**).

The sensory system is tested by evaluating the surface of the body for loss or change in sensation. Usually the clinician concentrates on the area where the patient feels numbness, tingling, or pain. Light touch, pain, heat, cold, and vibration sensations may be used to assess sensory function. To test position sense, the clinician has the patient close the eyes; the clinician then moves the finger or toe up or down and asks the patient to describe its position. To test for stereognosis, a familiar object (e.g., coin) is placed in the patient's hand while his or her eyes are closed and the patient is asked to identify the object.

Weakness or paralysis of a muscle may indicate damage to a motor nerve. Clinicians first evaluate the patient for muscle atrophy, which results when a motor neuron is not stimulating the muscle, and then test for weakness in various muscles by asking the person to push or pull against resistance.

Evaluation of reflexes determines whether the sensory nerve to the spinal cord, the nerve connections in the spinal cord, and the motor nerves back to the muscle are all functioning. The reflexes most commonly tested are the biceps, brachioradialis, triceps, patellar, and ankle jerks. A test for the plantar reflex (Babinski's sign) is performed by firmly stroking the lateral aspect of the sole of the foot with a sharp object such as a key. The normal response is plantar flexion of the great toe, which is considered an absent or negative Babinski sign. Dorsiflexion of the great toe, a positive Babinski sign, suggests an upper motor neuron dysfunction (Lower, 2002).

The cerebellum is primarily responsible for coordination of movement. Dysfunction results in a variety of signs such as ataxia, difficulty in maintaining an upright posture, intention tremors, and slurred speech. A variety of tests are used to assess cerebellar function:

- Walk heel-to-toe.
- Stand still with both feet together and the eyes closed (Romberg test).

TABLE 26-1 Testing the Cranial Nerves

Cranial Nerve	Name	Function	Test
I	Olfactory	Smell	Identify items with specific odors (e.g., coffee, cloves); test each nostril separately.
II	Optic	Vision; detection of light by the pupil	Eye chart; visual fields; funduscopic exam.
III	Oculomotor	Upward and downward eye movement; pupillary constriction or dilation in response to light	Extraocular movement is tested by following a moving object; pupillary reaction to light; pupillary accommodation.
IV	Trochlear	Downward and inward eye movement	Extraocular movement.
V	Trigeminal	Facial sensation and chewing	Sensation is tested using a safety pin and a wisp of cotton. Test the blink reflex by touching the cornea with a cotton wisp. Muscles of mastication are tested by asking the patient to clench the teeth and to open the jaw against resistance.
VI	Abducens	Lateral eye movement	Extraocular movement.
VII	Facial	Facial expression; taste in the front two-thirds of tongue	Have patient smile, open mouth and show the teeth, and close the eyes tightly. Taste is tested using substances that are sweet (sugar), sour (lemon juice), salty (salt), and bitter (aspirin, quinine, or aloe).
VIII	Acoustic	Hearing and balance	Hearing is tested with a tuning fork. To test balance, have the patient walk a straight line.
IX	Glossopharyngeal	Swallowing, gag reflex, and speech	Because cranial nerves IX and X control similar functions, they are tested together. Have the patient swallow and say "ah-h-h" to check the movement of the palate and uvula. To evoke the gag reflex, touch the back of the throat with a tongue blade.
X	Vagus	Swallowing, gag reflex, and speech	Same as for cranial nerve IX.
XI	Accessory	Range of motion of neck and shoulder shrugging	Turn head and shrug the shoulders against resistance.
XII	Hypoglossal	Tongue movement	Stick out tongue—note any deviation.

- Have the patient use the forefinger to reach out and touch the clinician's finger and then the patient's own nose; repeat these actions rapidly.
- Supinate and pronate the hands rapidly while tapping on the thigh.

Orthostatic hypotension, reduction or absence of sweating, or difficulty initiating or maintaining an erection indicate autonomic nervous system dysfunction. To evaluate the arteries going to the brain, the clinician places a stethoscope on the neck and listens for characteristic sounds caused by turbulent blood flow through a narrowed area (bruits). However, procedures such as color Doppler ultrasonography, magnetic reso- nance angiography [also referred to as magnetic resonance imaging], or cerebral angiography are needed for an accurate evaluation of narrowed arteries.

Pupil Assessment and Eye Movement

Pupils are assessed using a light (typically a penlight) reflected in the eyes. This technique allows the nurse to detect a deficit in cranial nerve III, the oculomotor nerve. Pupil response is a function of the autonomic nervous system. Pupils should be equal in size and should react equally and accommodate to light reflected in the eye. In this instance, the nurse would document the client as having pupils that are equally round, reactive to light and accommodation. Accommodation is assessed when you shine the light in one eye and look at the opposite eye to ensure that the reaction is the same in a dimly lit room. Pupils should react briskly. A sluggish response of a pupil should be reported, because it could be due to cerebral edema. Pupillary change is usually a late sign in the physiological processes occurring in the brain, however. An abnormal finding, such as a dilated or nonreactive pupil, would indicate compression of the oculomotor nerve. A pinpoint pupil indicates an injury to the lower brain stem. Medications can sometimes affect pupillary response—for example, atropine can cause dilation, and narcotic overdose can cause pinpoint pupils (Lower, 2002).

Eye movement is controlled by cranial nerves III, IV, and VI. These nerves allow the eyes to look in six different directions, collectively known as the field of vision. To test these nerves, the nurse has the conscious patient follow a pen in six directions, observing for symmetry of eye movement. The nurse will document whether extraocular movements are normal or abnormal. A normal response is when the patient is able to follow the pen with a gaze in all six directions. Abnormal findings are noted when the patient cannot look in any or all of the directions.

If a patient is unconscious, then the oculocephalic reflex (doll's eyes reflex) or the oculovestibular reflex is tested (Malik & Hess, 2002). The oculocephalic reflex should not be tested until cervical trauma is ruled out, because this test requires the nurse to briskly turn the patient's head from side to side. The reflex is intact if the eyes deviate in the opposite direction from the side on which the head is turned. The reflex is not intact if the eyes move in the direction that the head is turned, remain midline, or move in opposite direction from one another. Documenting what is observed when testing this reflex is important to ensure a clear understanding among all healthcare providers. The results of this test are often misunderstood and poorly documented, and terms such as "positive" or "negative" are used when the nurse should document whether the reflex is "intact" or "not intact" (Malik & Hess).

The oculovestibular reflex is known as the cold caloric test. This nurse will assist with this test, while the physician or mid-level provider performs the test on an unconscious patient. Cold, iced water is drawn up in a syringe and injected into the ear canal. A normal response will result in a rapid deviation of the eyes toward the irrigated ear. If the eye does not move in this direction, chart an abnormal response and exactly what was observed (Malik & Hess, 2002). **Table 26-2** summarizes common neurological procedures.

SUMMARY

Neurological assessments should be performed at baseline and every shift. More frequent assessments should be conducted upon the orders given by the physician, according to facility policy, or if the nurse suspects a change associated with a neurological condition. ICU nurses will have a critical care flow sheet on which to document their assessment findings. The level of detail provided by the neurological assessment will depend on the circumstances. A strong knowledge base of the anatomy and physiology of the neurologic system will lay a solid foundation for a comprehensive assessment and can lead to optimal patient outcomes.

TABLE 26-2 Neurological Procedures

Doppler ultrasonography	An ultrasound examines the blood flow in the major arteries and veins in the arms and legs to diagnose alterations, such as a blood clot, venous insufficiency, arterial occlusion, or narrowing.
Magnetic resonance angiography/magnetic resonance imaging	A two-dimensional or three-dimensional image of the blood vessels is produced through the use of magnetic fields and radio waves to diagnose aneurysms, congenital heart disorders, renal artery stenosis, vasculitis, and atherosclerosis.
Cerebral angiography	Contrast material is injected into one or both of the carotid and/or vertebral arteries that are in the neck.
Electroencephalography	This procedure records the electrical activity of the brain.
Lumbar puncture	A needle is used to draw spinal fluid from the lumbar subarachnoid space. Spinal fluid can be examined for infection, blood, and increased pressure. The patient should be placed in a knee-chest position by the nurse. Post-procedure care requires keeping the patient flat to prevent spinal headache and monitoring for fever.

CRITICAL THINKING QUESTIONS

1. What is the difference between two stimuli of different strengths if both bring the membrane potential to threshold, generating an action potential?

2. What is meant when an individual is referred as "left-brain" or "right-brain"?

3. How does the central nervous system cooperate with the autonomic nervous system to maintain body temperature?

4. How would you assess cranial nerves XI and XII?

5. Which procedure requires the nurse to place the patient in a knee-chest position?

6. Which cranial nerves control eye movement?

7. What Glasgow Coma Scale score would you assign to a patient who presented with eye opening to sound, has movement localized to pain, and makes incomprehensible sounds?

8. If a patient is exhibiting decorticate posturing, how would you describe the movement of the patient in your nursing notes?

9. Design four questions that could be utilized to assess a patient's mentation.

10. When would a nurse never assess the oculocephalic reflex?

Online Resources

Online tutorial: http://lessons.HarveyProject.org/development/nervous_system/index.html

Neuroscience tutorial: http://thalamus.wustl.edu/course

Layperson's view of brain chemistry: www.maui.net/~jms/brainuse.html

Thorough ANS review: www.jdaross.mcmail.com/Autonomic/ANS4.htm

Fun ANS Web site: http://faculty.washington.edu/chudler/auto.html

REFERENCES

Bateman, D. E. (2001). Neurological assessment of coma. *Journal of Neurology, Neurosurgery and Psychiatry, 71*(Suppl. 1), i13–i17.

Bickley, L. S., & Szilagyi, P. G. (2003). *Bates' guide to physical examination and history taking* (8th ed.). Philadelphia: Lippincott Williams & Wilkins.

Lower, J. (2002). Facing neuro assessment fearlessly. *Nursing, 32*(2), 58–65.

Malik, K., & Hess, D. C. (2002). Evaluating the comatose patient. Rapid neurologic assessment is key to appropriate management. *Postgraduate Medicine, 111*(2), 38–40, 43–46, 49–50.

Sherwood, L. (2004*). Human physiology: From cells to systems* (3rd ed.). Cincinnati, OH: Wadsworth.

CHAPTER 27

Multimodal Neurological Monitoring

DaiWai M. Olson

LEARNING OBJECTIVES

Upon completion of this chapter, the reader will be able to:

1. Describe methods to monitor intracranial pressure.

2. Calculate cerebral perfusion pressure.

3. Describe invasive brain monitoring techniques.

4. List optimal patient outcomes that may be achieved through evidence-based management of the neuro ICU patient.

Imagine yourself traveling to a foreign country. You check in at your hotel and try to relax by watching a little television. When the TV set comes to life, you find that the sound is turned off. Too tired to hunt for the remote control, you try to understand the show. How will you interpret the actions? It is quite likely that you can determine whether the show is a mystery, comedy, or action-adventure, but will you understand the plot? Now you figure out how to turn the sound on. The words are in a foreign language, but you can still identify more components of the show. Are the actors shouting, laughing, or threatening? This additional mode of monitoring provides new information—cues that add to your understanding of the show. Finally, you discover how to add subtitles. You can now read the dialogue. This third mode of input provides an even clearer understanding of the television show. Using all three of these modes of information (observing action, hearing tone, and reading dialogue) to provide cues to the events that are unfolding, you are able to develop a more comprehensive understanding of the plot.

Multimodal monitoring is not a new concept in healthcare. For example, multimodal monitoring of the cardiovascular system is used extensively in critical care. Nurses monitor the electrical rhythm of the heart, observe and record the pulse rate, take the blood pressure, and, in some cases, rely on invasive monitoring to assess cardiac output. Thus there are multiple sources of cues from which to draw conclusions about the heart.

Until fairly recently, neurological monitoring has been somewhat less sophisticated, often relying solely on subjective clinical assessment tools such as the Glasgow Coma Scale (GCS) to provide cues about changes in the patient's condition. Rapidly evolving technology now allows us to look at the brain from multiple vantage points and provides us with new cues. In this chapter, we explore various aspects of multimodal neurological monitoring, which involves continuous monitoring of more than one parameter, using two or more techniques.

THE PHYSICAL NEUROLOGICAL EXAMINATION

The neurological examination has been, and will likely remain, the first and primary mode of coming to know the neurologically injured patient. The physical examination of the patient may take place at any time. This examination is not limited in style or depth, but generally consists of assessing the patient's level of consciousness, ability to respond, the presence of any sensory or motor impairment, and some aspects of cranial nerve function. The physical neurological examination is discussed at length in Chapter 26.

INVASIVE BRAIN MONITORING

Intracranial Pressure Monitoring

There is no doubt that the ability to monitor intracranial pressure (ICP) has revolutionized the care of the neuro-intensive care unit (ICU) patient. Because the brain is contained within an inflexible skull, any change in volume is reflected as a change in pressure. With the advent of ICP monitoring, we have a strong modality for monitoring the brain. We can observe changes in ICP and thereby gain an understanding of what is happening inside the skull on a minute-to-minute basis. Today, ICP monitoring remains the fundamental cornerstone of multimodal neurological monitoring. It is recommended that all patients with a severe brain injury as evidenced by physical exam (GCS score < 9) or radiographic finding [computerized tomography (CT) of the brain] receive some form of ICP monitoring (Greenberg, 2001).

The concept of ICP monitoring via an intraventricular catheter (IVC) was first introduced using models in 1951 (Guillaume & Janny, 1951). Nine years later, Lundberg (1960) described the different physiology of waveforms that can be observed. ICP can be measured in cm H_2O, but is most commonly measured in mm Hg. Although normal ICP varies with age, it is generally agreed that the range of normal values is from 0 to 15 mm Hg. Treatment guidelines recommend an upper threshold for treatment of 20 to 25 mm Hg (Greenberg, 2001).

Because ICP can change suddenly and drastically, it is monitored continuously. The documentation guidelines for recording ICP values vary within each institution and are directed by the institutional policy. Typically, values are recorded once every 15 minutes. These values may represent an average ICP or a single ICP value observed at the end of a 15-minute time frame, however, so they may not reflect the dynamic state of the brain (Feldman & Narayan, 2000). Therefore, treatment is based on trends and sustained elevations.

Infection remains the primary complication of ICP monitoring. In 1995, Bader, Littlejohns, and Palmer published a paper reporting a 0% infection rate. They recommended that all intraventricular ICP monitoring devices be placed in the operating room; dressing changes adhere to strict aseptic technique; and prophylactic antibiotics be used. Other authors suggest that the routine use of prophylactic antibiotics is not indicated, however, and that other factors, such as length of ICP monitoring

and cerebrospinal fluid (CSF) leak, are more likely to lead to infection (Rebuck, Murry, Rhoney, Michael, & Coplin, 2000).

Types of Monitors

Several types of ICP monitoring systems are commercially available and currently being marketed to the ICU. While each device may have subtle differences, there are essentially only two forms of ICP monitoring systems: fluid-filled and transducer-tipped (fiberoptic). The term *ventriculostomy* is often misused and refers to the location of the catheter, not to the type of monitor. A ventriculostomy catheter may use either fiber-optic or fluid-filled pressure monitoring, but is always placed into one of the ventricles within the brain (**Table 27-1**).

These two technologies offer specific advantages and disadvantages. Hence, the determination of which device to use is an art, determined by the goal of monitoring, location of the injury, familiarity with each ICP monitor, and therapeutic goals. For example, if a patient has hydrocephalus (confirmed by brain CT), the logical choice is to place an intraventricular fluid-filled catheter capable of draining CSF. Later in this chapter, we will discuss the concept of monitoring the penumbra, the area of tissue surrounding the primary injury. In the case of monitoring a specific region of the brain, a transducer-tipped monitoring system is preferred because fluid-filled catheters are placed into the ventricular space and reflect global changes in ICP, whereas a transducer-tipped system will provide more information about a specific area of the brain.

Hydrostatic Systems (External Strain Gauge) To monitor ICP using a fluid-filled pressure transducer, a catheter is placed such that the terminal end of the catheter lies within either of the lateral ventricles of the brain. To accomplish this, a thin,

---

TABLE 27-1 Cranial Access

Insertion of any intracranial monitoring device requires gaining cranial access. Generally, these steps are followed:

1. Obtain informed consent.
2. Prep and drape the patient.
3. Prepare the insertion site—antibacterial scrub, clip hair (optional) and numb the site with local anesthetic.
4. Make a small incision (incision extends to the depth of the exterior skull).
5. Drill a hole in the skull (a hand-operated drill is commonly used).
6. Puncture the dura mater, which allows for instrumentation to be passed into the brain tissue.
7. Insert the monitoring device (catheter or bolt-system).
8. Secure the device (including occlusive dressings).

hollow catheter is passed through the skull and dura and into the fluid-filled spaces (ventricles) within the brain; it is then connected to a strain gauge transducer (Greenberg, 2001). Upon insertion, the catheter is filled with CSF. The remaining space in the tubing that leads to the external transducer is flushed with preservative-free 0.9% saline so that a continuous column of fluid exists from the intraventricular space through to the transducer. This continuous column of fluid allows each pulsatile wave to be carried along the length of the tubing to the transducer.

To ensure accuracy, the transducer must be zero-calibrated and level with the foramen of Monro. The process for zero-calibrating the transducer varies depending on the equipment used. The foramen of Monro is generally considered to be the optimal reference point because it aligns most closely with the center of the head. Externally, the foramen of Monro can be roughly determined by drawing an imaginary line between the two external auditory meati (EAM); see **Figure 27-1**.

After the transducer has been zero-calibrated and leveled to the foramen of Monro, the transducer will provide a reflection of the intraventricular pressure. It must be cautioned that several problems may occur and result in erroneous readings. For example, any breaks or interruptions in the continuous fluid column (e.g., air bubbles, tissue, blood clots) may create

artifact and impede the accuracy of the waveform and pressure readings.

Poiseuille's law discusses fluid dynamics and helps to explain why blood, blood clots, or brain matter may cause a dampened waveform and reflect an inaccurate ICP reading. The essential components of Poiseuille's law state that flow depends on the viscosity of the fluid, the driving pressure, the radius of the system (artery, capillary, tubing) through which it flows, and the length of the vessel or tubing (Perez, 2002).

Ensuring that the transducer is level to the foramen of Monro is crucial to interpreting the accuracy of any obtained values. Patients may change position or the head of bed may be raised or lowered. Even a change of a few centimeters will affect the accuracy of the readings. The term "leveling" is used by ICU nurses to refer to the process of ensuring that the pressure transducer is at an equal level to the foramen of Monro. Most frequently, this is accomplished by using a string level from the patient's EAM to the zero reference on the transducer. More recently, practitioners have begun to use laser-guided levels. Simply put, if the transducer is not level, it is not accurate.

Fluid-filled transducer systems require very little additional equipment for continuous monitoring; this feature coupled with the decreased cost of monitoring has made this system very popular. Another major advantage to a fluid-filled column is the ability to drain CSF when the ICP is elevated. Finally, because risk of infection is inherent in any invasive procedure, the ability to tunnel the catheter under the scalp becomes an advantage in reducing the risk of infection (Bader et al., 1995). The fact that the pressure within the ventricles is a reflection of the global pressure within the cranial vault is both an advantage and a disadvantage. On the one hand, it provides some information about the "big picture" of what is happening inside the skull. On the other hand, regional, focal, or compartmentalized changes in pressure may not be readily apparent.

FIGURE 27-1 Placement of Fluid-Filled Intraventricular Catheter

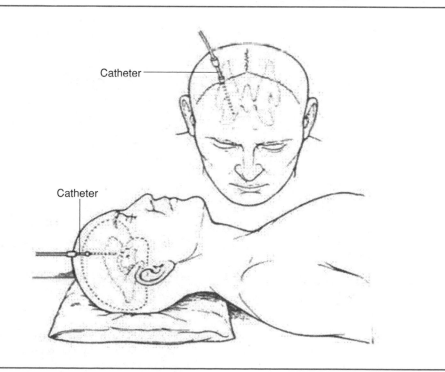

Catheter

Catheter

Source: Permission for use of illustration obtained from Integra Neurosciences.

Transducer-Tipped Systems (Fiberoptic)   A transducer-tipped pressure monitoring system enables the ICU team to monitor the pressure in a specific area of the brain. The ability to place the transducer at the tip of the catheter is accomplished through the use of fiber-optic technology. A small fiber-optic cable passes through the housing of the catheter and transmits changes in pressure sensed at the tip of the catheter along the length of the cable to a signal converter, from which a digital value and waveform may be displayed. This system, like fluid-filled systems, has both advantages and disadvantages.

The disadvantage of transducer-tipped systems is that they must be zero-calibrated prior to insertion and cannot be recalibrated after insertion. Thus, if the fiber-optic cable breaks, the system must be replaced. Additionally, specialized monitoring equipment is required to transform the signal carried by the fiber-optic cable, whereas most fluid-filled columns can be connected to a standard pressure transducer. When patients are transferred from one hospital to another, the systems may be incompatible.

The advantages of the transducer-tipped system are related to the dynamic response of the brain to injury. Unlike fluid-filled systems, transducer-tipped systems may be placed into any region of the brain. This flexibility enables the ICU team to place the catheter into that area of the brain most at risk for secondary injury. Furthermore, because the pressure sensor is located within the skull, it is not necessary to continuously re-level the transducer. As the patient changes position or the bed is raised and lowered, the transducer will continue to provide reliable data. Finally, the pressure values from transducer-tipped catheters are considered to be more accurate over time (Trauma.org, 2000).

Hybrids: The Next Wave in Monitoring   Recently, ICP monitoring devices have begun to incorporate the positive aspects of both transducer-tipped and fluid-filled systems. These devices typically have a hollow catheter through which fluid may pass; this setup allows for the drainage of CSF and permits an external transducer to be used to monitor the fluid column pressure. Additionally, a fiber-optic cable runs the length of the catheter and transmits pressure readings from the tip of the catheter. Additional features of these hybrid-type systems include the ability to monitor brain temperature, pH, and CO_2.

Location, Location, Location

The name of each ICP monitoring device holds clues to the location of the monitor as well as indicates its strengths and limitations. The three primary spaces to which an ICP monitor may be placed are the subarachnoid, intraparenchymal, and intraventricular. As such, an understanding of the terms used to describe basic cerebral anatomy is essential.

Subarachnoid   A subarachnoid bolt (also called a subarachnoid screw), pictured in **Figure 27-2**, penetrates the scalp and cranium, with the tip of the catheter terminating in the subarachnoid space. This monitor does not penetrate into the brain, so it can be quickly and easily placed. Unfortunately, cerebral edema may occlude the transducer and result in false readings when ICP is elevated. The lack of direct association with brain tissue may also lead to falsely lowered ICP readings. As a consequence, this system is less frequently used.

FIGURE 27-2 Placement of Two ICP Monitors

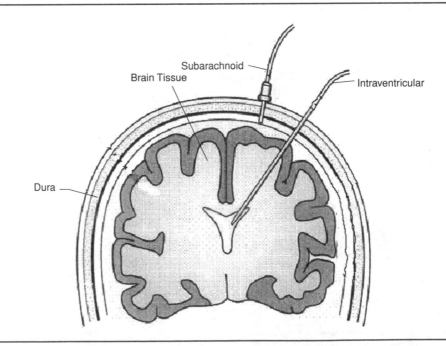

Note: In this view, the subarachnoid bolt does not penetrate the pia mater as would an intraparenchymal ICP monitor. Also, the tip of the intraventricular catheter is shown clearly in the lateral ventricle.
Source: Permission for use of illustration obtained from Integra Neurosciences.

Intraparenchymal An intraparenchymal monitor is very similar to a subarachnoid monitor except that the intraparenchymal monitor terminates in brain tissue. This transducer-tipped system has a fiber-optic catheter that is placed just below the dura, arachnoid, and pia mater. A frequent goal in intraparenchymal monitoring is to place the catheter into, or very near, the penumbra (see **Box 27-1**). The intraparenchymal space may or may not reflect global cerebral edema because subdivisions within the brain, such as the falx cerebri and the tentorium, serve to compartmentalize some of the areas of the brain.

Intraventricular The ventricles are a series of connected spaces within the brain. Although four ventricles exist, typically the lateral ventricles get all the attention. Figure 27-2 shows an IVC passing through the skull, dura, and brain tissue and ultimately terminating in the intraventricular space. The lateral ventricles may vary in size depending on the amount of CSF or cerebral edema present. A CT scan of the brain is always indicated to guide insertion of an IVC.

Intraventricular Monitoring

The primary indication for ICP monitoring is to provide the ICU team with information about the dynamics within the skull. This information offers cues that the patient may be experiencing cerebral edema and is at risk for secondary brain injury. ICP is an expression of the pressure exerted against the inside of the skull by the combination of blood, CSF, and brain tissue (Littlejohns, Bader, & March, 2003). Fluctuations in ICP are the result of an increase or decrease in one or more of these volumes without a corresponding change in one or more of the other volumes (Greenberg, 2001).

Box 27-1
The Penumbra

The penumbra is the area of the brain that surrounds the focal area of injury or infarct. The penumbra is therefore not the same for each patient, but rather is described in reference to an individual patient's injury. It is generally considered to be the brain tissue that is at highest risk for secondary brain injury. The medical team may elect to monitor brain pressures in the penumbra to monitor the effectiveness of treatments aimed at sparing the penumbra.

Normal ICP is generally considered to be less than 15 mm Hg; and intracranial hypertension is generally classified as a pressure greater than 20 mm Hg (Arbour, 2004; Greenberg, 2001). Episodes of intracranial hypertension are associated with an increased risk of secondary brain damage (Wong, 2000). Procedures that directly reduce ICP include active CSF drainage, osmotic therapy, and positioning (March, 2000; Marik, Varon, & Trask, 2002). Currently, no gold standard for the minimum value at which ICP treatment should be initiated exists, but a value of 20 to 25 mm Hg is reported as the upper limit at which treatment should be initiated (Bullock et al., 2000; Greenberg). Episodes of ICP elevation greater than 25 mm Hg can be life-threatening (Hickey, 2002). **Figure 27-3** reveals a sagittal view of the ventricles within the brain.

Physical Interventions to Manage Elevated ICP Why is an elevation in ICP considered life-threatening? What really goes on? To understand this process, we need to understand the formula **CPP = MAP − ICP**. ICP reflects the total pressure within the skull; normal ICP is 0 to 15 mm Hg. CPP stands for cerebral perfusion pressure; normal CPP is 70 to 80 mm Hg. MAP, mean arterial pressure, is the driving force that gets oxygen-enriched blood into the skull. The blood pressure (MAP) must be high enough to overcome the resistance in ICP such that an adequate amount of brain tissue is perfused. Consider two examples. In the first example, the ICP is 12 mm Hg, and the blood pressure is 120/80 mm Hg with a MAP of 93. The CPP is 88 mm Hg, and the brain is receiving an adequate supply of oxygen-enriched blood. In the second example, the blood pressure is still 120/80 mm Hg with a MAP of 93, but the ICP has risen drastically to 45 mm Hg and the CPP has fallen to 55 mm Hg. A CPP less than 60 mm Hg will not provide an adequate supply of blood to the brain (Robertson, 2001).

The positive effects from proper positioning cannot be overemphasized. The management and treatment of increased ICP must begin with proper alignment of the head and neck. General guidelines indicate that the head of the bed should be elevated at 30° (Hickey, 2002). This positioning promotes a decrease in ICP, but the nurse should be careful to monitor for any potential decrease in brain perfusion that may also result from head elevation (AANN, 2004). While some controversy has emerged regarding how high and when to elevate the head of the bed, the need to ensure that the head is properly aligned is a fundamental nursing task (Robertson, 2001). The head should be in a physiologically neutral position to promote the passive flow of venous blood from the cranial vault through the jugular veins (Blumenfeld, 2002).

FIGURE 27-3 The Ventricles within the Brain (the ventricles, shown in gray in this sagittal view, are interconnected deep within the brain)

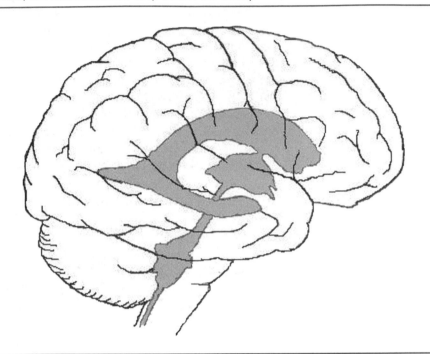

Source: Illustrated by James R. Perron.

In the average adult, CSF is produced in the arachnoid villi at the rate of approximately 20 mL/hr or about 500 mL/day. Placing an IVC allows the ICU nurse to passively drain CSF from the ventricles. As CSF is drained off, the pressure should decrease accordingly. There is a risk for upward herniation caused by decompression of the ventricles; to decrease this risk, no more than 30 mL of CSF should be drained at any one time (Greenberg, 2001).

Currently, CSF drainage is a process of passively allowing CSF flow from the ventricles, through an externalized catheter (shunt), and into a collection device. The rate and volume of CSF may be controlled by the nurse. A stopcock valve is typically placed near the external strain gauge transducer and opened intermittently to permit the flow of CSF. To prevent episodes of excessive drainage, caution must be exercised to ensure that the stopcock valve does not remain open when unattended. Because the CSF drains against the pressure of gravity, it is possible to raise or lower the drainage chamber and partially control the threshold for CSF drainage. However, episodes such as patient coughing, endotracheal suctioning, and position changes can drastically alter the balance of pressure.

In a case of extreme cerebral edema that is unresponsive to conventional therapy, surgical intervention may be indicated. The two surgical procedures associated with directly decreasing ICP are partial lobectomy and hemicraniectomy. Partial lobectomy is the surgical removal of a portion of the brain tissue. Here the Monroe-Kellie doctrine comes into play: A direct decrease in brain volume corresponds to a direct decrease in ICP. Lobectomy surgeries typically remove that portion of brain that is most injured and least likely to recover. Hemicraniectomy is the removal of a large portion of the skull. This surgical procedure allows for expansion of the brain beyond its normal boundaries. Early hemicraniectomy has been linked to improved outcomes in some brain-injured patients (Patterson, Bloom, Coyle, Mouradjian, & Wilensky, 2005).

Pharmacotherapy to Manage Elevated ICP Recall the Monroe-Kellie doctrine: An increase in ICP means that blood or brain or CSF has increased, and we need to reduce the amount of one of these. But how do we reduce the amount of brain? We could remove a portion of the brain tissue (partial lobectomy), which carries not only the risks associated with surgery, but also the risk of removing an important part of the brain that may leave the patient worse off than before. We can, however, decrease the amount of brain using a few different medications.

Mannitol (Osmitrol®) is an osmotic diuretic. When it is administered, the blood circulating through the brain has a high affinity for water. Mannitol does not cross the blood–brain barrier, so water moves passively out of the brain cells and into the bloodstream, where it is excreted as urine. Essentially, this medication decreases ICP by decreasing brain volume (Hickey, 2002).

Intravenous (IV) hypertonic saline is defined as any solution that is greater than 0.9% NaCl. Common solutions have NaCl concentrations of 1.8%, 3%, or 7.5% (Suarez, 2004). The primary mechanism of action of hypertonic saline is similar to that of Mannitol: It draws water from the brain, thereby reducing the brain volume (Johnson & Criddle, 2004).

The guidelines for the treatment of brain injury suggest that patients with a GCS score of less than 9 should be endotracheally intubated and mechanically ventilated. This treatment allows for two things to happen. First, the endotracheal tube protects the airway. Second, mechanical ventilation allows for some control of arterial oxygen and carbon dioxide levels. Because carbon dioxide is a powerful vasodilator, an increase in carbon dioxide ($PaCO_2$) will result in increased blood flow (Hickey, 2002). Increased oxygen is measured as an increase in the partial pressure of oxygen (PaO_2) and is associated with vasoconstriction. Inadequate oxygenation of cerebral tissues is associated with increased cell death and further mitochondrial dysfunction (Zauner, Daugherty, Bullock, & Warner, 2002).

Continuous IV sedation is a common treatment for patients with acute neurological injury. Sedation is indicated for injury prevention, facilitation of medical therapies, or humanitarian reasons (Murdoch & Cohen, 2000; Young, Knudsen, Hilton, & Reves, 2000). Control of ICP often requires sedation during the acute and early subacute phases of brain injury (Jacobi et al., 2002). IV sedation facilitates mechanical ventilation, permits the patient to remain in a more calm state, and improves end-organ perfusion (Burchardi, 2004; Dennis & Mayer, 2001). In some cases, neuromuscular blockade is indicated to prevent increased ICP secondary to increased muscle tone, avoid inadvertent Valsalva maneuver associated with endotracheal intubation, and decrease the cerebral metabolic demand (Hickey, 2002).

Corticosteroids are no longer indicated for the routine treatment of cerebral edema. Once a mainstay of ICP reduction therapy, corticosteroids have not been demonstrated to reduce ICP in patients with traumatic brain injury or brain injury secondary to cerebral infarction. These agents are, however, currently used in the management of vasogenic edema (most commonly noted with brain tumor resection) (Bullock et al., 2000).

Brain Oxygen Monitoring

As the understanding of the critical role that oxygen plays in the recovery of brain injury has grown, so has the desire to understand oxygen levels in the brain (Zauner et al., 2002). Most recently, many neuro ICUs have begun to examine the role of oxygen and oxygen pressure monitoring within the brain in the setting of acute neurological injury. Central to the following discussion on brain oxygen monitoring is a quick review of cerebral anatomy and physiology.

Blood supply comes to the brain anteriorly through the carotid arteries and posteriorly via the vertebral-basilar system (Blumenfeld, 2002). These vessels join at the Circle-of-Willis, and blood is distributed to the cerebral cortex via the anterior-, middle-, and posterior-cerebral arteries. Because the brain does not store oxygen, it requires a constant fresh supply of oxygenated blood to flow through these vessels.

Decreases in the amount of oxygen available to the brain are associated with an increased risk of cerebral ischemia (Meixensberger et al., 2003). As such, recent developments in technology have focused on efforts to measure parameters associated with brain oxygenation (Bader, Littlejohns, & March, 2003).

Jugular Venous Oxygen Saturation

Jugular bulb monitoring provides a measure of the blood oxygen saturation in the venous jugular vein ($SjvO_2$). Anatomically, the jugular bulb is located approximately level with the foramen of Monro (AANN, 2004). Jugular bulb monitoring entails the use of a fiber-optic (oximetric) catheter and monitoring system. The catheter is usually placed into the jugular bulb on the side of the primary injury (Hickey, 2002). Because the jugular bulb receives blood from the brain, changes in $SjvO_2$ are considered to reflect global changes in brain oxygen consumption. Normal $SjvO_2$ is 60% to 80%, and values less than 50% are considered to equate with episodes of cerebral hypoxia (Kiening, Unterberg, Bardt, Schneider, & Lanksch, 1996). Aside from infection, the primary complications of this therapy stem from the difficulty of obtaining and ensuring proper placement of the catheter tip into the jugular venous bulb. The risks include venous thrombosis, carotid artery puncture, and catheter migration resulting in false or misleading data. The difficulty in obtaining equipment and ensuring accurate placement of the oximetric catheter creates limitations on the reliability of the data obtained from $SjvO_2$ catheters and, thereby, the practice itself.

Brain Tissue Oxygen Monitoring

Currently, most studies of direct brain oxygen monitoring have focused on the partial pressure of brain tissue oxygen ($PbtO_2$) as measured in the intraparenchymal tissue (Littlejohns et al., 2003). The Licox Catheter (Integra Neurosciences, Plainsboro, New Jersey) is an intraparenchymal monitor that is placed in the penumbra of the brain (Littlejohns et al.). The Licox catheter measures $PbtO_2$. Normal values for $PbtO_2$ are considered to be greater than 25 mm Hg. Values less than 20 mm Hg are generally of concern and represent the upper threshold for treatment. A decrease in the $PbtO_2$ measured in the penumbra of an injury is a reflection of regional cerebral hypoxia and may represent ongoing secondary injury (AANN, 2004). **Box 27-2** describes another technology for monitoring blood oxygen.

Treatment goals are aimed at improving microperfusion. This is usually accomplished by noting the various elements that affect tissue perfusion. An increase in oxygen tension (PaO_2) in the arterial circulation may increase the driving force

Box 27-2

INVOS Cerebral Oximeter System

Regional changes in brain oxygen may also be measured using a noninvasive monitor. One such monitor, the INVOS Cerebral Oximeter system, consists of a monitor and cables that can be connected to sensors placed on the patient's forehead. The central concept of the INVOS system relies on detecting changes in the oxygen saturation by measuring refracted near-infrared light photons that have been transmitted into the skull. This technology is conceptually similar to the use of pulse oximetry for measuring arterial oxygen saturation. These changes are thought to reflect regional changes in cerebral perfusion and provide a noninvasive method of monitoring for acute changes in the brain.

of oxygen, thereby increasing perfusion. Often, decreases in $PbtO_2$ are reflective of other changes in the brain, such as increased ICP or cerebral hyperthermia. Treatment goals should focus on alleviating these causative factors and increasing blood supply to the at-risk tissue.

Brain Temperature Monitoring

Temperature monitoring is not new to nursing. However, recent advances in technology have provided a means to directly monitor brain temperature. This, in turn, has resulted in research that correlates changes in brain temperature with changes in brain function (Dietrich, 2001; Soukup et al., 2002). Typically, an invasive thermistor (temperature-sensing device) is used as part of another monitoring system. Brain temperature is generally 0.5 to 1. 0°C higher than the core body temperature. Therapeutic hypothermia is currently being used as a treatment modality following sudden cardiac arrest as a means of preserving brain function. It is also being explored as a treatment in early brain injury recovery to prevent secondary brain injury. While therapeutic hypothermia is considered to be experimental, aggressive efforts to maintain normal temperature are indicated in the treatment of brain injury (Marion, 2004).

NONINVASIVE BRAIN MONITORING

Seizure Monitoring

Electroencephalography monitoring provides a graphical representation of the physiological activity in the brain. All activity generates some form of energy, and these changes in energy in turn generate an electrical signal (Rampil, 1998). Electrical activity results from the movement of ions across membranes (Martin, 2000). In the brain, this is a relatively unstable state because various parts of the brain are stimulated during different activities. The electrical signals that we read from the scalp as an electroencephalogram (EEG) assist with the assessment of cerebral function (Arbour, 2003). In particular, the electrical signal generated by brain activity has specific characteristics that have been identified and linked to specific neurological conditions and brain-state changes.

Perhaps the most common use of EEG pattern recognition is the identification and monitoring of seizure activity. Each seizure is a potentially life-threatening event, so it is important to note the seizure's time of onset, duration, and physical characteristics (see Chapter 28). If the seizure is prolonged, or if questions remain about the patient's condition, an EEG may be performed to look for the presence of epileptiform waves (Hickey, 2002).

Sedation Monitoring

Observational Sedation Assessment

The Ramsay Scale   The Ramsay Scale was first described in a 1974 publication as a component of a study examining a sample of 30 patients receiving a steroid anesthetic (Ramsay, Savege, Simpson, & Goodwin, 1974). Six levels of sedation were formulated as a means to examine the effects of a single sedating agent. The Ramsay Scale is a subjective assessment tool in which the rater makes a "best guess" determination of the patient's current level of sedation. The assessment is essentially composed of two questions: (1) Is the patient awake? and (2) How does the patient respond?

Sedation assessment with the Ramsay Scale begins with passive observation of the patient. The determination must first be made of whether the patient is awake. Patients who are deemed to be awake will be given a score of 1, 2, or 3; patients who are asleep will be given a score of 4, 5, or 6. If an awake score is indicated, the assessor next grades the patient's responsiveness. Awake patients who respond to stimuli in an agitated manner are scored 1, awake patients who require verbal stimuli to produce a response are scored 3, and all other awake patients are scored 2. If the patient is deemed to be asleep, the assessor administers verbal and tactile stimulation. A loud auditory stimulus, such as calling the patient's name, and a glabellar tap (tapping the forehead) are used as stimuli for sleeping patients. Hence, the score for patients who are asleep is based on a brisk (4), sluggish (5), or lack of response (6) to these stimuli.

There is a great deal of subjective interpretation within the application of the Ramsay Scale in both the clinical and research settings. Hansen-Flaschen, Cowen, and Polomano (1994) have argued that the levels of sedation described in this scale are neither clearly defined nor mutually exclusive. It is possible, for example, to observe a patient who is responding to commands only (level 3), yet remains cooperative, oriented, and tranquil (level 2). The definitions for terms such as "brisk response" and "sluggish response" are not evident. Furthermore, the scale gives no indication of how to score a patient who has neither a brisk nor a sluggish response. Questions arise when examples are given: How is a patient scored if there is no response to a loud auditory stimulus, but a brisk response to a light glabellar tap? Some authors have elected to modify the Ramsay Scale, often omitting portions of the description of levels (Hall et al., 2001).

The Sedation-Agitation Scale

The Sedation-Agitation Score (SAS) has been prospectively tested and found to be reliable and valid for use in the critical care setting (Yukioka, 2001). The SAS is a single-item, 7-point scale. Scores range from a low of 1, which indicates the lowest level of responsiveness (deep sedation), to a high of 7, which represents the severe agitation. The SAS uses a combination of passively observable and response-generated behaviors to characterize activity in seven categories ranging from unarousable to dangerous agitation (Jacobi et al., 2002).

The Richmond Agitation-Sedation Scale

The Richmond Agitation-Sedation Scale (RASS) has also been tested for reliability. It was concluded that the tool has good inter-rater reliability and correlates well with both the Ramsay and SAS sedation scales (Ely et al., 2003; Sessler et al., 2002). The RASS is also a single-item scale, but has 10 levels of response, ranging from −4 to +5. Because the RASS was developed by a multidisciplinary team including nurses, the tool has good clinical utility (Olson, Cheek, & Morgenlander, 2004). Additionally, because the RASS requires the nurse to assess multiple factors for each level, the tool may

result in a higher degree of inter-rater reliability than scales such as the SAS, which focuses on a single assessment parameter. These scales all look at the patient's condition as it exists at a single moment in time.

Physiological Assessment of Sedation

Bispectral Index Monitoring The BIS monitor (**Figure 27-4**) was developed by Aspect Medical (Newton, MA) through an 11-year validation and utility testing phase (Olson, Chioffi, Macy, Meek, & Cook, 2003). The BIS software uses power spectral and bispectral analysis technology to examine EEG features that are clinically linked to states of increased and decreased cortical arousal. Since 2002, the BIS monitor has been marketed to the ICU setting as a tool for sedation monitoring (Olson et al., 2004). It has been shown to provide clinically relevant information in the titration of sedating medications (Arbour, 2000; Gilbert, Wagner, Halukurike, Paz, & Garland, 2001).

BIS monitoring is noninvasive. A single self-adhesive sensor is placed across the forehead, extending downward to the

FIGURE 27-4 BIS Monitor

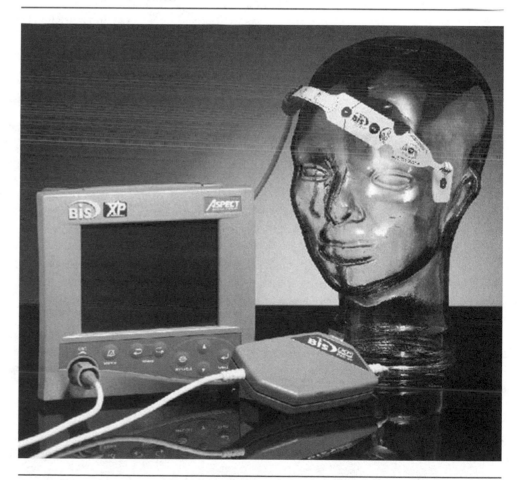

Source: Permission obtained from Aspect Medical Systems, Newton, MA.

space between the outer canthus of the eye and the hairline. This sensor detects EEG signals from the brain, which are carried to a digital signal converter and processed via spectral analysis. The converted signal is displayed as a whole number between 0 and 100. BIS values have been shown to provide a reliable index of the degree of sedation in patients receiving mechanical ventilation and sedative agents after surgery, trauma, or medical illness (Gilbert et al., 2001). The BIS score is continuously updated and is interpreted along a continuum, representing a measure of cerebral cortical activity (Yamaguchi et al., 2002). The lowest value, 0, corresponds to isoelectric activity (a flat EEG waveform). Scores between 90 and 100 correlate with an awake state, 70's to 80's with moderate (conscious) sedation, 60's to 70's with deep sedation, and 40's to 60's with general anesthesia (Olson et al., 2003). Variability in scores is related to the individual response of the patient.

The BIS monitor provides not only the current BIS score but several other important parameters. For example, single-channel raw EEG tracing may be continuously displayed on the lower half of the screen, and the Signal Quality Index (SQI) bar, an indication of the reliability of the signal, displayed near the top of the screen. Higher SQI values indicate a more reliable signal and hence a greater chance that the BIS value is a reliable indication of the patient's current level of consciousness. The electromyographic (EMG) bar indicates the degree of EMG activity. EMG activity may be associated with any activity that increases muscle tone, such as seizure, tension, and eye movement. Poor electrode contact will also increase the EMG signal.

Neuromuscular Monitoring

A variety of patient conditions may lead to prolonged periods of neuromuscular blockade or chemical paralysis. Conditions such as status epilepticus and severe brain injury with refractory intracranial hypertension are two examples. Agents such as vecuronium (Norcuron®) and pancuronium (Pavulon®) are administered to block the transmission of the nerve impulse before it is transmitted to the skeletal muscle (Hickey, 2002). Neuromuscular blockade monitoring is a vital component of monitoring the chemically paralyzed patient. The use of a peripheral nerve stimulator, also called a twitch monitor or train-of-four monitor, is advocated for any patient receiving a neuromuscular-blocking agent (Arbour, 2003). The peripheral nerve stimulator supplies a series of four low-voltage electrical impulses to a muscle (typically the ulnar muscle). The ICU nurse notes the number of muscle responses (finger twitches) during each train-of-four event. Complete neuromuscular blockade, for example, would be reflected as a response rate of 0 out of 4.

Transcranial Doppler Studies

Transcranial Doppler (TCD) studies are a noninvasive means of assessing the intra-arterial velocities of blood flow through the cerebral arteries (AANN, 2004). Increases in velocities have been linked to cerebral artery vasospasm (Gupta et al., 2004). If vasospasm is left untreated, blood flow may become occluded and the patient may experience a stroke event. The accuracy of TCD studies is operator-dependent. TCDs are performed using ultrasound probes that are used to view the cerebral vessels through a series of bone windows. Technicians generally begin a study by finding the middle cerebral artery. Factors such as prior surgery, bone density, age, brain atrophy, and calcification will all affect the ability of the operator to accurately obtain readings.

Radiography

Computerized Tomography

CT, also called computerized axial tomography (CAT), provides a radiographic image of the axial plane of various tissues in the body—a sharp contrast to the flat plate provided by standard radiographic studies. In the brain, these images reveal marked differentiation between bone, gray matter, white matter, extravascular blood, and CSF within the ventricles. CT scanning without the use of IV contrast is a relatively quick study and can be completed in only a few minutes.

Magnetic Resonance Imaging

Magnetic resonance imaging (MRI) has an advantage over CT in that the former technology does not involve radiation and offers greater image detail. New functional techniques may even provide temporal (time-related) resolution that can be used to explore how the brain works. However, current MRI scanners are much larger and less comfortable than CT scanners. When the physical restrictions of MRI are combined with the more extensive length of time required to complete each study, the benefits of MRI versus CT must be critically evaluated to determine the best option for each patient.

PATIENT OUTCOMES

Nurses can help ensure obtainment of optimal patient outcomes such as those listed in **Box 27-3**, through the use of evidence-based interventions for patients receiving multimodal neurological monitoring.

SUMMARY

Patients in the ICU are increasingly dependent on technology to maintain life. Organ-specific monitoring—a new and rapidly evolving science—provides the opportunity to better understand how therapeutic interventions may benefit our patients. Neurological monitoring, which incorporates analysis of aspects of both the peripheral and central nervous systems, is one example of organ-specific monitoring.

Think back to the vignette presented at the beginning of this chapter. While watching a foreign TV show, you realized the benefits of having multiple sources of information. Each additional mode of monitoring the TV show improved your understanding of the events. Likewise, multimodal neurological monitoring provides different modes of understanding how medical therapies affect the brain and nervous system. Only through developing a comprehensive understanding of the limitations and benefits of each component will you be able to fully understand how these tools allow you to know your patient.

Box 27-3
Optimal Patient Outcomes

- Intracranial hemodynamic status stable
- Improved neurological functioning
- Reduced secondary brain tissue ischemia
- ICP within normal range
- CPP within normal range
- MAP within normal range
- Absence of infection due to intracranial monitoring

CRITICAL THINKING QUESTIONS

1. Multimodal neurological monitoring provides the nurse with the opportunity to see the patient's brain through a variety of lenses. With the increasing use of technology to virtually *see* what is happening inside the patient's skull, how do we ensure that ICU nurses do not lose sight of the patient as a holistic being?

2. The greatest risk comes from placing too much faith in any one mode of monitoring. In the example of a foreign TV show, what would you deduce if your only mode of monitoring was a short snippet of sound, and you heard a gunshot and then a scream? How accurate would you be in determining which show you are watching? What possible false conclusions might you draw? How could you test your assumptions?

3. You are working in a busy neuro-ICU. You notice that each time the family of the 23-year-old trauma patient enters the room, they point at the monitor. The father of your patient tells you, "The brain temperature is 37.2 degrees. That's good, because now we know she'll be okay." How do you respond to this family? Do you think it is a good thing or a bad thing that the father observes the brain temperature?

CASE STUDY

During your critical care rotation as a student nurse, you are working with Mary, an ICU nurse with 10 years of experience in the neuro-ICU. Together, you prepare for a new admission. Mary explains that you will soon be receiving a patient who is being transferred from a local hospital for more specialized care. She explains that the patient, Ms. Nguyen, is a 37-year-old female who awoke with the worst headache of her life. Her husband called 911, and she was quickly transported to the emergency department. While undergoing a brain CT, she experienced a seizure and was emergently intubated. Her CT scan confirmed diagnosis of a right temporal subarachnoid hemorrhage (SAH).

> SAH can be graded using several scales. Ms. Nguyen has a Fisher grade 3 and a Hunt and Hess grade 3 SAH. A cerebral angiography done at your facility will later confirm the presence of ruptured middle cerebral artery (MCA) aneurysm.

Immediately upon her arrival, you move Ms. Nguyen to a hospital bed. Mary places a pulse oximetry probe on Ms. Nguyen's finger as she receives the following report from the flight nurse: "She was pretty sedated when we got to the outside hospital and I didn't get much of an exam. We had some trouble—she became combative in-flight so we increased the propofol (Diprivan®) infusion to 45 mcg/kg/min. I also gave her 25 mcg of fentanyl (Sublimaze®) IV about 30 minutes ago. Her heart rate and blood pressure are stable, and we have her on a portable ventilator at 1.00 FiO$_2$, with 10 cm H$_2$0 of pressure support and 5 cm H$_2$0 of PEEP (positive end expiratory pressure)."

Mary turns the propofol infusion off to perform her baseline neurological exam. By stopping the propofol, Mary is able to evaluate Ms. Nguyen's best level of function. Ms. Nguyen is not able to follow commands and opens her eyes only to deep painful stimulus. She has no response to central pain on her left side, but does reach to grab the endotracheal tube with her right hand. Her pupils are 3 mm in size with sluggish response. Because the patient has an unprotected aneurysm, Mary is quick and decisive. She consults the medical team and resumes the propofol infusion as she places a BIS sensor across Ms. Nguyen's forehead: "They want to keep her sedated until she goes to surgery. We'll keep the BIS below 60 for now." Mary completes the remainder of her physical exam, and within the hour Ms. Nguyen is taken to the operating room where a clip is placed across the neck of her aneurysm.

Following a successful surgery, the patient returns to the ICU with an indwelling ventriculostomy on her left side, and a PbtO$_2$ monitor on the right side of her skull. Over the next two weeks, nursing care focuses on preventing secondary brain injury that could result from cerebral edema and cerebral vasospasm. Ultimately, Ms. Nguyen is transferred to a rehabilitation facility with left-sided weakness. Her ICU stay was marked by multiple episodes of intracranial hypertension treated primarily with mannitol and CSF drainage.

Her single most critical event occurred four days after her surgery. The nursing staff responded to an alarm indicating a sudden drop in Ms. Nguyen's brain temperature. This was immediately followed by a decrease in her PbtO$_2$ and an eventual increase in her ICP. Despite nonfocal pupillary findings, these observations combined to support a picture of brain herniation syndrome. The ICU nurse, alert to this risk, called a neuro-code, and an emergency brain CT scan was performed simultaneously with the administration of mannitol. The scan confirmed an increase in cerebral edema. Following the mannitol dose, the brain temperature returned to baseline, but an ICP of 33 mm Hg and only a slight improvement in PbtO$_2$ values led the medical team to order a single dose of hypertonic saline (30 mL of 23.4% NaCl to be given over 15 minutes). This medication resolved Ms. Nguyen's intracranial hypertension and cerebral hypoxia.

CRITICAL THINKING QUESTIONS

1. Describe how the nursing staff was able to incorporate and act upon multiple sources of information.
2. Which disciplines should be consulted to work with this patient? Develop an agenda for a team conference with the disciplines identified. Use the following table.

Discipline	Potential Contribution to Optimal Patient Care

3. What types of issues might require you to act as an advocate or moral agent for this patient?
4. How will you implement your role as a facilitator of learning for this patient?
5. Utilize the form to write up a plan of care for one client in the clinical setting.

	Patient Characteristics	Subjective and Objective Data	Evidence-based Interventions	Outcomes
SYNERGY MODEL	Resiliency			
	Vulnerability			
	Stability			
	Complexity			
	Resource availability			
	Participation in care			
	Participation in decision making			
	Predictability			

6. What level of nursing characteristics was displayed in this case? Rate the nurse as a level 1, 3, or 5 on each characteristic in the following table.

Nurse Characteristics	Level (1, 3, 5)	Qualities Displayed by the Nurse in the Case	Actions the Nurse Can Take to Demonstrate Characteristic
Clinical judgment			
Advocacy/moral agency			
Caring practices			
Collaboration			
Systems thinking			
Response to diversity			
Facilitator of learning			
Clinical inquiry			

SYNERGY MODEL

Online Resources

Glasgow Coma Scale: www.trauma.org/swres/gcs.html

Train-of-Four Monitoring: http://pedsccm.wustl.edu/CLINICAL/NMB_monitoring.html

ICP Monitoring and Monro-Kellie doctrine: http://www.trauma.org/neuro/icp.html

REFERENCES

AANN. (2004). *AANN core curriculum for neuroscience nursing* (4th ed.). St. Louis, MO: Saunders.

Arbour, R. B. (2004). Intracranial hypertension: Monitoring and nursing assessment. *Critical Care Nurse, 24*(5), 19–20, 22–16, 28–32.

Arbour, R. B. (2003). Continuous nervous system monitoring, EEG, the bispectral index, and neuromuscular transmission. *AACN Clinical Issues, 14*(2), 185–207.

Arbour, R. B. (2000). Using the bispectral index to assess arousal response in a patient with neuromuscular blockade. *American Journal of Critical Care, 9*(6), 383–387.

Bader, M. K., Littlejohns, L. R., & March, K. (2003). Brain tissue oxygen monitoring in severe brain injury, II. Implications for critical care teams and case study. *Critical Care Nurse, 23*(4), 29–38, 40–42, 44.

Bader, M. K., Littlejohns, L., & Palmer, S. (1995). Ventriculostomy and intracranial pressure monitoring: In search of a 0% infection rate. *Heart & Lung, 24*(2), 166–172.

Blumenfeld, H. (2002). *Neuroanatomy through clinical cases.* Sunderland, MA: Sinauer.

Bullock, M. R., Chesnut, R. M., Clifton, G. L., Ghajar, J., Marion, D. W., Narayan, R., et al. (2000). *Management and prognosis of severe traumatic brain injury.* New York: Brain Trauma Foundation.

Burchardi, H. (2004). Aims of sedation/analgesia. *Minerva Anesthesiology, 70*(4), 137–143.

Dennis, L. J., & Mayer, S. A. (2001). Diagnosis and management of increased intracranial pressure. *Neurology India, 49*(Suppl. 1), S37–S50.

Dietrich, W. (2001). Temperature changes and ischemic stroke. In M. Fisher & J. Bogousslavsky (Eds.), *Current review of cerebrovascular disease* (4th ed., pp. 45–55). Philadelphia: Current Medicine.

Ely, E. W., Truman, B., Shintani, A., Thomason, J. W., Wheeler, A. P., Gordon, S., et al. (2003). Monitoring sedation status over time in ICU patients: Reliability and validity of the Richmond Agitation-Sedation Scale (RASS). *Journal of the American Medical Association, 289*(22), 2983–2991.

Feldman, Z., & Narayan, R. K. (2000). Intracranial pressure monitoring: Techniques and pitfalls. In P. R. Cooper & J. G. Golfinos, *Head injury* (4th ed., pp. 265–292). New York: McGraw-Hill.

Gilbert, T. T., Wagner, M. R., Halukurike, V., Paz, H. L., & Garland, A. (2001). Use of bispectral electroencephalogram monitoring to assess neurologic status in unsedated, critically ill patients. *Critical Care Medicine, 29*(10), 1996–2000.

Greenberg, M. S. (2001). *Handbook of neurosurgery* (5th ed.). Lakeland, FL: Thieme.

Guillaume, J., & Janny, P. (1951). Continuous intracranial manometry; importance of the method and first results. *Presse Medicale, 84*(2), 131–142.

Gupta, C., Husain, M., Kumar, M., Kohli, N., Tiwari, V., Vatsal, D. K., et al. (2004). Transcranial Doppler sonography evaluation in patients with vasospasm following subarachnoid haemorrhage. *Journal of the Indian Medical Association, 102*(4), 191–192, 194, 196.

Hall, R. I., Sandham, D., Cardinal, P., Tweeddale, M., Moher, D., Wang, X., et al. (2001). Propofol vs midazolam for ICU sedation: A Canadian multicenter randomized trial. *Chest, 119*(4), 1151–1159.

Hansen-Flaschen, J., Cowen, J., & Polomano, R. C. (1994). Beyond the Ramsay Scale: Need for a validated measure of sedating drug efficacy in the intensive care unit. *Critical Care Medicine, 22*(5), 732–733.

Hickey, J. V. (2002). *The clinical practice of neurological and neurosurgical nursing* (5th ed.). Philadelphia: Lippincott.

Jacobi, J., Fraser, G. L., Coursin, D. B., Riker, R., Fontaine, D., Wittbrodt, E. T., et al. (2002). Clinical practice guidelines for the sustained use of sedatives and analgesics in the critically ill adult. *Critical Care Medicine, 30*(1), 119–141.

Johnson, A. L., & Criddle, L. M. (2004). Pass the salt: Indications for and implications of using hypertonic saline. *Critical Care Nurse, 24*(5), 36–38, 40–44, 46.

Kiening, K. L., Unterberg, A. W., Bardt, T. F., Schneider, G. H., & Lanksch, W. R. (1996). Monitoring of cerebral oxygenation in patients with severe head injuries: Brain tissue PO_2 versus jugular vein oxygen saturation. *Journal of Neurosurgery, 85*(5), 751–757.

Littlejohns, L. R., Bader, M. K., & March, K. (2003). Brain tissue oxygen monitoring in severe brain injury, I. Research and usefulness in critical care. *Critical Care Nurse, 23*(4), 17–25.

Lundberg, N. (1960). Continuous recording and control of ventricular fluid pressure in neurosurgical practice. *Acta Psychiatrica Scandinavica, 36*(Suppl. 149), 1–193.

March, K. (2000). Intracranial pressure monitoring and assessing intracranial compliance in brain injury. *Critical Care Nursing Clinics of North America, 12*(4), 429–436.

Marik, P. E., Varon, J., & Trask, T. (2002). Management of head trauma. *Chest, 122*(2), 699–711.

Marion, D. W. (2004). Controlled normothermia in neurologic intensive care. *Critical Care Medicine, 32*(2 Suppl.), S43–S45.

Martin, J. H. (2000). The collective electrical behavior of cortical neurons: The electroencephalogram and the mechanisms of epilepsy. In E. R. Kandel, J. H. Schwartz, & T. M. Jessell (Eds.), *Principles of neural science* (4th ed., pp. 777–791). New York: McGraw-Hill, Health Professions Division.

Meixensberger, J., Vath, A., Jaeger, M., Kunze, E., Dings, J., & Roosen, K. (2003). Monitoring of brain tissue oxygenation following severe subarachnoid hemorrhage. *Neurological Research, 25*(5), 445–450.

Murdoch, S., & Cohen, A. (2000). Intensive care sedation: A review of current British practice. *Intensive Care Medicine, 26*(7), 922–928.

Olson, D. M., Cheek, D. J., & Morgenlander, J. C. (2004). The impact of bispectral index monitoring on rates of propofol administration. *AACN Clinical Issues, 15*(1), 63–73.

Olson, D. M., Chioffi, S. M., Macy, G. E., Meek, L. G., & Cook, H. A. (2003). Potential benefits of bispectral index monitoring in critical care. A case study. *Critical Care Nurse, 23*(4), 45–52.

Patterson, J., Bloom, S. A., Coyle, B., Mouradjian, D., & Wilensky, E. M. (2005). Successful outcome in severe traumatic brain injury: A case study. *Journal of Neuroscience Nursing, 37*(5), 236–242.

Perez, R. J. (2002). *Design of medical electronic devices.* San Diego, CA: Academic Press.

Ramsay, M. A., Savege, T. M., Simpson, B. R., & Goodwin, R. (1974). Controlled sedation with alphaxalone-alphadolone. *British Medical Journal, 2*(920), 656–659.

Rampil, I. J. (1998). A primer for EEG signal processing in anesthesia. *Anesthesiology, 89*(4), 980–1002.

Rebuck, J. A., Murry, K. R., Rhoney, D. H., Michael, D. B., & Coplin, W. M. (2000). Infection related to intracranial pressure monitors in adults: Analysis of risk factors and antibiotic prophylaxis. *Journal of Neurology, Neurosurgery, and Psychiatry, 69*(3), 381–384.

Robertson, C. S. (2001). Management of cerebral perfusion pressure after traumatic brain injury. *Anesthesiology, 95*(6), 1513–1517.

Sessler, C. N., Gosnell, M. S., Grap, M. J., Brophy, G. M., O'Neal, P. V., Keane, K. A., et al. (2002). The Richmond Agitation-Sedation Scale: Validity and reliability in adult intensive care unit patients. *American Journal of Respiratory and Critical Care Medicine, 166*(10), 1338–1344.

Soukup, J., Zauner, A., Doppenberg, E. M., Menzel, M., Gilman, C., Bullock, R., et al. (2002). Relationship between brain temperature, brain chemistry and oxygen delivery after severe human head injury: The effect of mild hypothermia. *Neurological Research, 24*(2), 161–168.

Suarez, J. I. (2004). Hypertonic saline for cerebral edema and elevated intracranial pressure. *Cleveland Clinic Journal of Medicine, 71*(Suppl. 1), S9–S13.

Trauma.org. (2000). Neuromonitoring for traumatic brain injury. Retrieved February 10, 2006, from www.trauma.org/neuro/neuromonitor.html

Wong, F. W. (2000). Prevention of secondary brain injury. *Critical Care Nurse, 20*(5), 18–27.

Yamaguchi, F., Oi, Y., Aoki, W., Nakamura, R., Igarashi, A., Kubota, M., et al. (2002). BIS monitoring is useful for reliable intraoperative cortical mapping during brain tumor operations. *Neurological Surgery, 30*(11), 1181–1188.

Young, C., Knudsen, N., Hilton, A., & Reves, J. G. (2000). Sedation in the intensive care unit. *Critical Care Medicine, 28*(3), 854–866.

Yukioka, H. (2001). More accurate Sedation Agitation Scale grading. *Critical Care Medicine, 29*(3), 698.

Zauner, A., Daugherty, W. P., Bullock, M. R., & Warner, D. S. (2002). Brain oxygenation and energy metabolism: Part I—biological function and pathophysiology. *Neurosurgery, 51*(2), 289–301.

Common Neurologic Disorders

Krista M. Garner

LEARNING OBJECTIVES

Upon completion of this chapter, the reader will be able to:

1. Discuss the cerebral vascular circulation.
2. Outline the sensory and muscular spinal nerves.
3. Summarize the pathology of common neurologic disorders.
4. Identify evidence-based interventions for common neurologic disorders.
5. List optimal outcomes that may be achieved through evidence-based management of common neurologic disorders.

Neuroscience nursing has emerged as one of the fastest-growing areas of specialty practice (Hickey, 2003). Advancements in both neuroscience research and clinical practice are providing new and exciting roles for registered and advanced practice nurses. Healthcare trends have encouraged the specialty practice of neurocritical care collaborative teams based on favorable patient and financial outcome results in current literature (Suarez et al., 2004; Varelas et al., 2004). With the assumption of new roles in practice come greater responsibilities and accountability for providing the highest level of care for the neurologic patient. To achieve these goals, the neuroscience critical care nurse must have a strong neuroscience knowledge base from which to grow in complexity, as the ever-changing evidence-based research drives the practice trends to higher levels of reasoning and decision making.

This chapter begins by providing a brief overview covering spinal nerve roots and cerebrovascular circulation. Understanding the complex anatomy of the cerebrovasculature is essential when caring for the critically ill neurologic patient. Complications involved with the blood supply of the brain are generally most prevalent in neurocritical care, accounting for a large percentage of poor neurologic outcomes.

Cerebral circulation is the responsibility of two pairs of arteries: the two internal carotid arteries, accounting for anterior circulation, and the two vertebral arteries, accounting for posterior circulation. Each area of circulation includes distal branches as well as communicating penetrators responsible for a constant and well-networked blood supply. **Table 28-1** and **Table 28-2** describe the major cerebral branches and the areas they supply.

The spinal cord is an elongated mass of nerve tissue from which 31 pairs of spinal nerves exit: 8 cervical, 12 thoracic, 5 lumbar, 5 sacral, and 1 coccygeal. Each spinal nerve has a dorsal root by which afferent impulses enter the cord and a ventral root by which efferent impulses leave. The dorsal roots convey sensory input from specific areas of the body known as dermatomes. The ventral roots convey motor impulses, known as myotomes, from the spinal cord to the body (**Table 28-3**).

MANAGING ELEVATED INTRACRANIAL PRESSURE

Elevated intracranial pressure (ICP) is one of the major deteriorating factors in patients with intracerebral lesions (Forster & Engelhard, 2004). Because the cranium is rigid and

TABLE 28-1 Major Internal Carotid Arterial Branches

Artery	Area Supplied
Ophthalmic	Orbits and optic nerves
Posterior communicating (Pcom)	Connects the carotid circulation with the vertebrobasilar circulation
Anterior choroidal	Part of choroid plexuses of lateral ventricles; hippocampal formation; portions of globus pallidus; part of internal capsule; part of amygdaloid nucleus; part of caudate nucleus; part of putamen
Anterior cerebral (ACA)	Medial surfaces of frontal and parietal lobes; part of cingulated gyrus and "leg area" of precentral gyrus
Recurrent artery of Heubner	Special branch of ACA; penetrates the anterior perforated substances to supply part of the basal ganglia and genu of internal capsule (also called medial striate artery)
Middle cerebral (MCA)	Entire lateral surfaces of the hemisphere except for the occipital pole and the inferolateral surface of the hemisphere (supplied by posterior cerebral artery)
Lenticulostriate (from MCA)	Part of basal ganglia and internal capsule
Anterior communicating (Acom)	Connects the two ACAs

Source: Reprinted with permission from Emory University.

noncompliant, any increase in cerebral volume will, in turn, elevate cranial pressure (**Figure 28-1**). The major pathophysiologic problems associated with increased ICP are ischemia and herniation (Josephson, 2004).

The normal range of ICP is 0 to 15 cm H_2O. Elevations beyond these levels can rapidly lead to brain damage. Cerebral perfusion pressure (CPP) is mean arterial pressure (MAP) minus ICP. Global ischemic injury results from a critical reduction of CPP, and thus of cerebral blood flow (CBF). Mechanical compression and herniation of brain tissue—the second mechanism of injury—occurs with space-occupying mass lesions and compartment syndrome of brain contents (Josephson, 2004).

TABLE 28-2 Major Vertebral Arterial Branches and the Cerebral Areas They Innervate

Artery	Area Supplied
Vertebral Branches	
Anterior spinal	Anterior two-thirds of spinal cord
Posterior spinal	Posterior one-third of spinal cord
Posterior inferior cerebellar (PICA)	Undersurface of the cerebellum, medulla, and choroid plexuses of fourth ventricle
Basilar Artery Branches	
Posterior cerebral (PCA)	Occipital lobes, medial and inferior surfaces of the temporal lobes, midbrain, and choroid plexuses of third and lateral ventricle
Posterior choroidals (from PCA)	
Medial posterior choroidal	Tectum, choroid plexus of third ventricle, and superior and medial surfaces of the thalamus
Lateral posterior choroidal	Penetrates the choroidal fissures and anastomosing with branches of the anterior choroidal arteries
Anterior inferior cerebellar artery (AICA)	Undersurface of the cerebellum and lateral surface of the pons
Superior cerebellar artery (SCA)	Upper surface of the cerebellum and midbrain
Pontine	Pons

Source: Reprinted with permission from Emory University.

TABLE 28-3 Sensory Nerve Roots (Dermatome) and Motor Nerve Roots (Myotomes) and the Areas They Innervate

Spinal Nerves	Dermatome (Sensory Nerve Roots)	Muscles (Motor Nerve Roots)
C-2	Back of head	Neck
C-3	Neck	Neck
C-4	Neck and upper shoulder	Neck, diaphragm
C-5	Lateral aspect of shoulder	Neck, diaphragm
C-6	Thumb; radial aspect of arm	Diaphragm, shoulder, elbow
C-7	Middle finger; middle palm; back of hand	Forward thrust of shoulder
C-8	Ring and little finger; ulnar forearm	Adduction/extension of arm, wrist
T-1, T-2	Inner aspect of the arm; shoulder blade	Control of thoracic, abdominal, and back muscles (T-1 to T-12)
T-4	Nipple line	
T-7	Lower costal margin	
T-10	Umbilical region	
T-12, L-1	Groin region	
L-2	Anterior thigh and upper buttocks	Flexion of hip
L-3, L-4	Anterior knee and lower leg	Extension of leg
L-5	Dorsum of foot; great toe	Flexion of foot
S-1, S-2, S-3	Foot, toes, medial thigh	Perineal area and sphincters
S-4, S-5	Genitals area	

Sources: Hickey, 2003; Wijdicks, 2003.

Following is a list of the most current options in the literature today for the treatment of increased ICP. Chapter 27 discusses ICP monitoring in more detail.

Head and Body Position

Because cerebral venous outflow is obstructed, ICP increases when the head is in a non-neutral position (Forster & Engelhard, 2004). Durward, Amacher, and DelMaestro (1983) have shown that elevation of the head to 15 to 30 degrees produces a consistent reduction of ICP.

Osmotic Agents

In osmotic drug therapy, an osmotic pressure difference is induced between the blood and the brain, thereby causing extraction of water from the cerebrum into the intravascular space (Josephson, 2004). Two osmotic drugs are most commonly used in this manner: mannitol (Osmitrol®) and hypertonic saline. Both are extremely effective initial treatment modalities when bolused for the reduction of ICP.

Anesthetic and Paralytic Agents

Sedation using hypnotic, narcotic, and paralytic agents is performed to reduce stress and to control ICP (Forster & Engelhard, 2004). The drugs are chosen to achieve the effects of decreased cerebral metabolic rate and reduced CBF and cerebral blood volume (CBV).

Ventilation

The respiratory alkalosis caused by induced mechanical hyperventilation can quickly and effectively lower ICP by causing cerebral vasoconstriction and reduced CBV (Josephson, 2004). Hyperventilation is conducted to get the PCO_2 at a level between 30 and 35 mm Hg. Even though it is an effective acute intervention for increased ICP, prolonged hyperventilation should be avoided due to the increased risk of cerebral ischemia with excessive vasoconstriction (Steiner et al., 2005).

Other treatment modalities for the treatment of increased ICP drawing interest in the literature include induced hypothermia (Commichau, Scarmeas, & Mayer, 2003; Shiozaki et al., 2003) and early surgical decompression via craniectomy (Albanese, Leone, & Alliez, 2003; Cho, Chen, & Lee, 2003).

COMMON NEUROLOGIC DISORDERS AND EVIDENCE-BASED INTERVENTIONS

Neurologic dysfunction can be a result of a multitude of differential diagnoses and, when severe enough, will require intensive critical care with specific, timely, and well-organized nursing care. Critical care management is not always standard procedure, but rather varies depending on the case and the patient. Thus it allows room for interpretation and intervention based on research, experience, and advanced knowledge.

FIGURE 28-1 ICP Waveform Pulsatility—Cerebral Hyperemia; Increased Blood Volume; Increased Brain Volume; Raised ICP

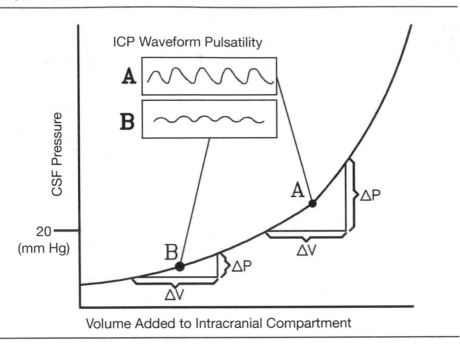

Source: Reprinted with permission from Marshall & Mayer (1997) *On Call: Neurology* (p. 159).

The following are some of the most common neurologic diagnoses and current evidence-based interventions for care relevant to the intensive care unit (ICU) nurse.

Cerebrovascular Complications

Hemorrhagic and ischemic stroke are two of the principal complications of the cerebral vasculature. Of those patients suffering from strokes in the United States each year, approximately 80% to 85% experience ischemic stroke, while 15% to 20% undergo hemorrhagic stroke.

Ischemic Stroke

An ischemic stroke results from the acute interruption of blood flow to a volume of brain tissue supplied by an artery (Singh, 2004). It is, therefore, a central cause of brain damage in neurologic patients, making prevention a primary mission for the medical community. The term "time is brain" rings true for the intensive care patient, because prolonged reduction or absence of blood flow to a certain area of the brain results in irreversible neuronal injury. Goals for managing the patient with acute ischemic stroke are twofold: (1) enhancement of CBF and (2) neuroprotection, with the aim to reduce the intrinsic vulnerability of brain tissue to ischemia (Singh) (**Box 28-1**).

Hemorrhagic Stroke

There are two types of hemorrhagic stroke: intracranial hemorrhage (ICH), which occurs with bleeding into the brain tissue, and subarachnoid hemorrhage (SAH), which occurs with bleeding into the subarachnoid space beneath the arachnoid mater of the meninges. Clinically, ICH provokes the same effect on the brain as space-occupying lesions and is often related to contusions from traumatic brain injury. If unable to be surgically evacuated, ICH is often associated with a poor outcome and increased mortality, secondary to increased ICP with potential for brain herniation.

SAH is most often the result of a ruptured cerebral aneurysm. Typically, the patient presents acutely, without warning, with what is described as "the worst headache" of the patient's life. After aneurysmal rupture, 10% of patients die suddenly, before ever receiving medical attention. Of the patients who reach the emergency department or neuroscience ICU, 20% to 30% arrive comatose and die within three months (Wijdicks, 2003).

The primary step in the management of SAH is aneurysmal repair, either by surgically clipping the neck of the aneurysm or by occluding the sac by endovascular coiling technique. Whether the aneurysm is repaired or not, intensive neurologic monitoring is required due to the high prevalence of secondary complications imposed by the initial traumatic event (**Box 28-2**).

SAH is graded on a scale from grade I (asymptomatic or minimal headache) to grade V (presenting in a deep coma). The Hunt and Hess grading scale was developed in 1958 to classify cerebral aneurysms. Several complications are associated with an SAH: rebleeding, cerebral vasospasm, and volume and osmolar disturbances, such as hypernatremia. Management of patients with an SAH includes blood pressure control and aneurysm precautions: a quiet, dark room with minimal stimulation; elevation of the head of the bed to 30 degrees; blood pressure control; and pain control for headache. To prevent vasospasms, triple-H therapy is utilized: hypervolemia, hemodilution, and hypertensive ther-

Box 28-1

Treatment Interventions for Managing the Patient with Ischemic Stroke

Thrombolytic Therapy (tPA)

- Supported through research
- Reopen occluded vessels with IV medications such as tPA
- Narrow time window (3–6 hours)
- Strict inclusion/exclusion criteria

Data from National Institute of Neurological Disorders and Stroke rt-PA Stroke Study Group, 1995.

Anticoagulant/Antiplatelet Therapy

- Controversial
- Prevents progression or reoccurrence of stroke using IV or low-molecular-weight heparin

Data from Caplan, 2004.

Management of Increased ICP and Cerebral Edema

- Mannitol, 3% saline
- Hyperventilation
- Sedation
- Decompressive surgery

Data from Caplan, 2004; National Institute of Neurological Disorders and Stroke rt-PA Stroke Study Group, 1995.

Blood Pressure Management

- Controversial
- Some trials suggest lowering BP can have adverse effects
- Lowering BP usually deferred unless end-organ damage is present or MAP >130 mm Hg or SBP > 220 mm Hg

Data from Adams, Brott, & Cromwell, 1994; Ahmed, Nasman, & Wahlgren, 2000.

Strict Glycemic Control

- Associated with improved outcome in stroke patients
- Goal is to maintain blood glucose 80–110 mg/dL with IV insulin

Data from Juvela, Siironen, & Kuhmonen, 2005; Paolino & Garner, 2005.

Fever Control/Induced Hypothermia

- Shown to improve cerebral ischemic injury especially in cardiac arrest patients
- Neuroprotective strategy

Sources: Commichau, Scarmeas, & Mayer, 2003.

apy. The first goal of therapy is to keep the patient's central venous pressure (CVP) reading at 10 to 12 mm Hg and pulmonary artery occlusive pressure (PAOP) at 15 to 18 mm Hg through the use of volume expanders such as colloids or crystalloids. The second goal is to maintain a patient's hematocrit between 33% and 38% by administering blood transfusions or performing phlebotomy treatment on polycythemic patients. The third goal

with triple-H therapy is to manage hypertension by maintaining a systolic blood pressure between 110 and 160 mm Hg.

Status Epilepticus

Status epilepticus (SE), or continuous seizure activity, is a medical emergency that requires rapid and vigorous treatment to prevent neuronal damage and systemic complications.

Box 28-2

Secondary Complications as a Result of Aneurysmal SAH

Rebleeding of Unrepaired Aneurysm

- Highest percentage within the first 24 hours of the initial bleed
- 30% risk in the first month

Data from Ohkuma, Tsurutani, & Suzuki, 2001.

Acute Hydrocephalus

- Occurs as a result of blood obstructing the reabsorption process from the subarachnoid space
- Many times relieved with the placement of a ventricular drain
- Dangerous elevation in ICP if CSF is not diverted via external shunting

Respiratory Failure

- Mainly a product of decreased level of consciousness with an inability to protect the airway
- Requires intubation through acute phase of illness

Neurogenic Cardiac Stunning

- Transient ischemic injury to the myocardium
- Produces inefficient cardiac function

Vasospasm

- Delayed cerebral ischemia occurring in 70% of patients with aneurysmal SAH
- May lead to symptomatic brain ischemia or infarct in 36% of all patients
- Classically occurs during post initial bleed days 4–15
- Treatment options include: triple-H therapy (hemodilution, hypertension, and hypervolemia), cerebral angiogram with angioplasty, and systemic or intra-arterial calcium channel blockers

Sources: Liu-Deryke & Rhoney, 2006; Sen & Albon, 2003.

Management of the patient with SE should focus on termination of seizures, prevention of seizure recurrence once status is controlled, management of precipitating causes of SE, and management of complications (Chapman, Smith, & Hirsch, 2001). Along with clinical correlation, electroencephalographic confirmation of SE should be accomplished as early as possible so that treatment strategies (**Box 28-3**) can quickly be implemented. Cerebral metabolic decompensation occurs after approximately 30 minutes of uncontrolled convulsive activity (Chapman et al., 2001).

Four types of seizures may occur: focal motor, generalized tonic-clonic, complex partial, and nonconvulsive status. A focal motor seizure involves the face or limb and often moves from distal to proximal. A generalized tonic-clonic seizure results in a convulsion with tongue biting followed by a postictal period of altered sensorium and urinary loss. A complex partial seizure manifests with an aura that can be followed by a tonic-clonic seizure. With a nonconvulsive status seizure, there is a loss of consciousness or altered sensorium with minimal face or limb movement.

Infections of the Nervous System

A multitude of infectious etiologies affect the nervous system. The two most common that are addressed in the neuroscience ICU are bacterial meningitis and viral encephalitis. Both types of infections can be extremely toxic, imposing life-threatening complications to the acutely ill patient.

Bacterial Meningitis

Bacterial meningitis is a pyogenic, or purulent, infection that involves the pia-arachnoid layers of the meninges, the subarachnoid space, and the cerebral spinal fluid (CSF) (Hickey, 2003). This type of infection primarily occurs in one of three ways: (1) bacteria gain access either via blood or through the spread of nearby infections, such as sinusitis oritis; (2) CSF is contaminated through surgical procedures or by penetration

Box 28-3

Emergency Medical Management for Status Epilepticus

1. Standard ABCs of Life Support
   - Support airway (most likely requires intubation)
   - Maintain blood pressure
   - Support circulation
2. Pharmacologic Management
   - Recommended initial first-line therapy is a benzodiazepine; lorazepam (Ativan®) 0.1 mg/kg at < 2 mg/min
   - Act as agonists at GABAa receptors and promote inhibition of neuronal firing
   If seizure activity persists
   - Second-line therapy is hydantoins, phenytoin (Dilantin®) 20 mg/kg at < 50 mg/min, fosphenytoin (Cerebyx®) 20 mg/kg at 150 mg/min
   - Followed by scheduled daily dosing
   If seizure activity persists
   - Midazolam (Versed®) 0.1–0.3 mg/kg followed by continuous IV infusion of 0.05–2.0 mg/kg/hr
   - Shown to rapidly control seizures that have not responded to traditional first- and second-line agents
   If seizure activity persists
   - Propofol (Diprivan®) initial dose 3–5 mg/kg followed by continuous IV infusion of 1–15 mg/kg/hr
   If seizure activity persists
   - Phenobarbital (Luminal®) 10–20 mg/kg at < 50 mg/min or pentobarbital (Nembutal®) 5–12 mg/kg followed by continuous infusion of 1–10 mg/kg/hr
   - Goal of therapy is to achieve a comatose state with a "burst suppression" pattern on EEG
3. Once there is a cessation of seizure activity for over 12 to 24 hours, a slow taper of continuous IV infusions should begin with the goal of treating complications and preventing recurrent seizure activity.

Sources: Bassin, Smith, & Bleck, 2002; Chapman, Smith, & Hirsch, 2001.

---

of invasive catheters that reside in the brain; or (3) bacteria invade the meninges through the skull or other dural defects. Community-acquired bacterial meningitis is typically caused by such organisms as *Streptococcus pneumoniae, Haemophilus ylococcus influenzae,* and *Neisseria meningitides,* whereas hospital-acquired meningitis is usually caused by *Staphylococcus aureus, Streptococcus* A and B, *Escherichia coli, Klebsiella, Proteus,* and *Pseudomonas.* Both community- and hospital-acquired meningitis produce similar classic signs and symptoms, including fever, headache, nuchal rigidity, altered level of consciousness (LOC), and photophobia.

The gold standard for the diagnosis of meningitis is direct CSF evaluation via lumbar puncture or aspiration of CSF from ventricular tubing. Treatment measures should be immediate, with initial interventions including general supportive treatments for complications such as septic shock, seizures, and increased ICP. Drug therapy should begin immediately, using broad-spectrum antibiotic coverage until the causative organism is identified. In most cases, intravenous antibiotics are warranted for many weeks to ensure complete irradication of the infectious organism. Highly resistant organisms, such as methicillin-resistant *staphylococcus aureus,* may require direct antimicrobial contact through the intrathecal route in conjunction with intravenous therapies.

Viral Encephalitis

Viral encephalitis is of sporadic or epidemic occurrence and can be caused by a multitude of atypical viruses, including herpes simplex virus, Epstein-Barr virus, and mosquito-transmitted organisms (malaria, West Nile, Eastern equine, Western equine, and St. Louis). The severity depends on the virus type. Viral encephalitis can produce rapid deterioration in a patient's neurologic status. Its many signs and symptoms vary according to the invading organism and the area of the brain involved (Hickey, 2003). Basic symptoms, such as fever, headache, stiff neck, and change in LOC, are similar to those exhibited with bacterial meningitis. More severe symptoms progress to seizure activity, coma, and paralysis.

Viral encephalitis is diagnosed by serological and CSF analysis, as well as through the patient's clinical exam. There is no definitive treatment for viral encephalitis and, in most cases, a specific viral etiology is never identified. Supportive care measures for secondary complications focus on the usual standard of care and can last weeks or months, depending on the severity of symptoms and the rate of neurologic improvement (**Box 28-4**).

Herpes simplex encephalitis type 1, which is associated with the common cold sore, is a particularly severe form of encephalitis with a very high morbidity and mortality rate. Intravenous acyclovir (Zovirax®), given prior to the onset of coma, is the standard of treatment.

Brain Death

Brain death is defined as a total loss of brain function, meaning life has come to an end and the patient has passed away (Wijdicks, 2003). Life support is futile, but is continued briefly to make organ donation possible. Brain death in adults is frequently a consequence of severe traumatic brain injury or of compartment syndrome of the brain from a massive hemorrhage causing cerebral herniation. The task of declaring brain death, which includes a precise clinical examination, interpretation of diagnostic findings, ruling out conditions that mimic brain death, and proper execution of brain death determination practices, is extremely complicated for the neuroscience specialist. Complete destruction of the brainstem, where most autonomic reflex function is controlled, is required to confirm brain death. **Box 28-5** describes the clinical criteria for determining brain death in adults.

> **Box 28-5**
> # Clinical Criteria for Brain Death in Adults
>
> - Coma—no eye opening to a painful stimulus
> - Absence of motor response to a painful stimulus
> - Absence of pupillary response to light—pupils midposition and dilated 4–6 mm (CNs II, III)
> - Absence of corneal reflexes—reflexive eyelid closure with corneal stimulus (CNs V, VII)
> - Absence of caloric response—reflexive eye deviation toward cold stimulus injected directly into the inner ear (CNs VIII, III, VI)
> - Absence of a gag and cough reflex in response to deep suctioning (CNs IX, X)
> - Positive apnea test—absence of a respiratory drive at a partial pressure of arterial carbon dioxide (PCO_2) that is 60 mm Hg or 20 mm Hg above normal baseline values
>
> The clinical examination and apnea testing are generally performed by two separate physicians 6 hours apart although requirements vary per institution.
>
> *Sources:* Wijdicks, 2001; Wood, Becker, McCartney, D'Alessandro, & Coursin, 2004.

> **Box 28-4**
> # Common Supportive Care Measures for Viral Encephalitis
>
> - Steroids to control malignant cerebral edema
> - Mechanical ventilation for respiratory support
> - Anticonvulsants/EEG monitoring for seizure prevention
> - Continuous or frequent analgesics for pain control
> - Sedatives for anxiety and to decrease cerebral metabolic demand
> - Antipyretics/endovascular cooling to control hyperthermia

In addition to the clinical exam, confirmatory diagnostic testing may be used at the physician's discretion, or if situations such as hypothermia, sedation, or metabolic derangements cloud the diagnosis of brain death. To document cessation of blood flow through the cerebrovascular system, bedside testing is preferred.

Once brain death is confirmed, organ procurement is an option if vital functions are artificially maintained, the family requests or agrees to donation, the patient fits donation criteria, and the patient's organs are not irreversibly damaged. The Federal Conditions of Participation of the Centers for Medicare and Medicaid Services require hospitals to notify their local organ-procurement organization in a timely manner of impending death. "Timely" means notification prior to brain death or before the withdrawal of life support. Potential donors must be ruled in or out based on exclusion criteria. Once a potential donor is identified, discussions regarding donation can be initiated with the family (Wood, Becker, McCartney,

D'Alessandro, & Coursin, 2004). Chapter 59 provides more detail on organ donation.

PATIENT OUTCOMES

Nurses can help ensure attainment of optimal patient outcomes such as those listed in **Box 28-6** through the use of evidence-based interventions.

SUMMARY

Being an ICU nurse in the care of a neurologically compromised patient is challenging and requires high levels of clinical judgment in the management of symptoms. Collaborative care teams have shown to improve morbidity and mortality in this critically ill population. The medical and nursing community can continue to improve this trend by practicing under evidence-based guidelines and moving toward greater achievements in research through data collection and continuing ed-

ucation. Knowledgeable ICU nurses are extremely vital practitioners to the team, striving to accomplish the primary goal of quality, cost-efficiency, and compassionate care.

Box 28-6
Optimal Patient Outcomes

- Intracranial pressure in expected range
- Neurologic findings in expected range
- Patient safety maintained during seizure activity
- Absence of signs and symptoms of infection
- Family uses effective coping strategies
- Patient/family expresses readiness for death

CASE STUDY

B.H. is a 36-year-old female who was brought into the emergency department with a history of being confused during the morning hours. Her confusion was apparent when she went to the bank and could not remember how to drive herself back home. She stopped to ask for directions and ultimately asked someone to call her husband, who came to take her to the hospital. She complained of having the "worst headache" of her life.

Physical Examination

The patient had a Glasgow Coma Scale score of 14, intact cranial nerves, headache with a score of 10 on a scale of 1 to 10, neck stiffness, photophobia, and low back pain. Her blood pressure was 178/92 with heart rate of 88. The monitor displayed a normal ECG. She was afebrile.

Diagnostic Tests

CT scan of the head revealed a small subarachnoid hemorrhage indicating a grade I SAH. The patient had a CT angiography and then an intra-arterial digital subtraction angiography with three-dimensional imaging. A decision was made to proceed with microsurgical treatment. Microsurgical treatment involved clipping the aneurysm using nonmagnetic titanium clips.

Postoperative Management

The patient was monitored and treated for several days in the ICU by a team of nurses, physicians, and other healthcare professionals. The patient was transferred to a neuro stepdown unit for several days prior to being discharged to a rehabilitation unit.

CRITICAL THINKING QUESTIONS

1. What are three symptoms of cerebral aneurysm?
2. What are the components of triple-H therapy?
3. List five aneurysm precautions for the preoperative patient.
4. Design a teaching plan for the family of an SAH patient.

5. Use the form to write up data and a plan of care for a patient with SAH in the clinical setting. Rate the patient as a level 1, 3, or 5 on each characteristic. Identify the level of nurse characteristics needed in the care of this patient.

6. Take one patient outcome for a patient and list evidence-based interventions found in a literature review for this patient.

Using the Synergy Model to Develop a Plan of Care

	Patient Characteristics	Subjective and Objective Data	Evidence-based Interventions	Outcomes
SYNERGY MODEL	Resiliency			
	Vulnerability			
	Stability			
	Complexity			
	Resource availability			
	Participation in care			
	Participation in decision making			
	Predictability			

Online Resources

American Stroke Association: www.strokeassociation.org/presenter.jhtml?identifier=1200037

National Stroke Association: http://www.stroke.org/site/PageServer?pagename=HOME

National Institute of Neurological Disorders and Stroke: www.ninds.nih.gov/

American Heart Association Stroke Guidelines: www.americanheart.org/presenter.jhtml?identifier=3004586

Stroke Coding Guide of the American Academy of Neurology: www.stroke-site.org/guidelines/stroke_coding.html

Epilepsy information: www.epilepsy.com/

Meningitis Research Foundation: www.meningitis.org/

The Brain Aneurysm Foundation: http://www.bafound.org/info/subarachnoid.php

REFERENCES

Adams, H. P., Brott, T. G., & Cromwell, R. M. (1994). Guidelines for the management of patients with acute ischemic stroke: A statement for healthcare professionals from a special writing group of the Stroke Council, American Heart Association. *Stroke, 25,* 1901–1914.

Ahmed, N., Nasman, P., & Wahlgren, N. G. (2000). Effect of intravenous nimlodipine on blood pressure and outcome after acute stroke. *Stroke, 31,* 1250–1255.

Albanese, J., Leone, M., & Alliez, J. R. (2003). Decompressive craniectomy for severe traumatic brain injury: Evaluation of the effects at one year. *Critical Care Medicine, 31,* 2535–2538.

Bassin, S., Smith, T. L., & Bleck, T. P. (2002). Clinical review: Status epilepticus. *Critical Care, 6*(2), 137–142.

Caplan, L. R. (2004). Thrombolysis 2004: The good, the bad, and the ugly. *Review of Neurological Disease, 1*(1), 16–26.

Chapman, M. G., Smith, M., & Hirsch, N. P. (2001). Status epilepticus. *Anaesthesia, 56*(7), 648–659.

Cho, D. Y., Chen, T. C., & Lee, H. C. (2003). Ultra-early decompressive craniectomy for malignant middle cerebral artery infarction. *Surgical Neurology, 60,* 227–232.

Commichau, C., Scarmeas, N., & Mayer, S. (2003). Risk factors for fever in the neurologic intensive care unit. *Neurology, 60*(5), 837–841.

Durward, Q. J., Amacher, A. L., & DelMaestro, R. F. (1983). Cerebral and cardiovascular responses to head elevation in patients with intracranial hypertension. *Journal of Neurosurgery, 59,* 938–944.

Forster, N., & Engelhard, K. (2004). Managing elevated intracranial pressure. *Current Opinion in Anaesthesiology, 17*(5), 371–376.

Hickey, J. V. (2003). *The clinical practice of neurological and neurosurgical nursing* (5th ed.). Philadelphia: Lippincott Williams & Wilkins.

Josephson, L. (2004). Management of increased intracranial pressure. *Dimensions of Critical Care Nursing, 23*(5), 194–207.

Juvela, S., Siironen, J., & Kuhmonen, J. (2005). Hyperglycemia, excess weight, and history of hypertension as risk factors for poor outcome and cerebral infarction after aneurysmal subarachnoid hemorrhage. *Journal of Neurosurgery, 102*(6), 998–1003.

Liu-Deryke, X., & Rhoney, D. H. (2006). Cerebral vasospasm after aneurysmal subarachnoid hemorrhage: An overview of pharmacologic management. *Pharmacotherapy, 26*(2), 182–203.

National Institute of Neurological Disorders and Stroke rt-PA Stroke Study Group. (1995). Tissue plasminogen activator for acute ischemic stroke. *New England Journal of Medicine, 333,* 1581–1587.

Ohkuma, H., Tsurutani, H., & Suzuki, S. (2001). Incidence and significance of early aneurysmal rebleeding before neurosurgical or neurological management. *Stroke, 32*(5), 1176–1180.

Paolino, A. S., & Garner, K. M. (2005). Effects of hyperglycemia on neurologic outcome in stroke patients. *Journal of Neuroscience Nursing, 37*(3), 130–135.

Sen, J., & Albon, B. A. (2003). Triple-H therapy in the management of aneurysmal subarachnoid haemorrhage. *Lancet Neurolinquist, 2,* 614–621.

Shiozaki, T., Nakajima, Y., Taneda, M., Tasaki, O., Inoue, Y., Ikegawa, H., et al. (2003). Efficacy of moderate hypothermia in patients with severe head injury and intracranial hypertension refractory to mild hypothermia. *Journal of Neurosurgery, 99*(1), 47–51.

Singh, V. (2004). Critical care assessment and management of acute ischemic stroke. *Journal of Vascular and Interventional Radiology, 15*(1, Part 2), S21–S27.

Steiner, L. A., Balestreri, M., Johnston, A. J., Coles, J. P., Smielewski, P., Pickard, J. D., et al. (2005). Predicting the response of intracranial pressure to moderate hyperventilation. *Acta Neurochirurgica, 147*(5), 477–483.

Suarez, J. I., Osama, O., Suri, M., Feen, E. S., Lynch, G., Hickman, J., et al. (2004). Length of stay and mortality in neurocritically ill patients: Impact of a specialized neurocritical care team. *Critical Care Medicine, 32*(11), 2311–2317.

Varelas, P. N., Conti, M. M., Spanaki, M. V., Potts, E., Bradford, D., Sunstrom, C., et al. (2004). The impact of a neurointensivist-led team on a semiclosed neurosciences intensive care unit. *Critical Care Medicine, 32*(11), 2191–2198.

Wijdicks, E. F. (2003). *The clinical practice of critical care neurology* (2nd ed.). New York: Oxford University Press.

Wijdicks, E. F. (2001). Current concepts: The diagnosis of brain death. *New England Journal of Medicine, 344*(16), 1215–1221.

Wood, K. E., Becker, B. N., McCartney, J. G., D'Alessandro, A. M., & Coursin, D. B. (2004). Current concepts: Care of the potential organ donor. *New England Journal of Medicine, 351*(26), 2730–2739.

Neurologic Injuries

Kelly Nadeau

"I have a neuro patient?!" Sometimes those words strike fear in the most experienced nurse, so it is understandable that a nursing student or a new nurse might have a moment of pause when receiving that assignment. It is unclear why neuro patients are so unsettling to so many nurses, but here's one theory. For each system, there is a "gold standard" for diagnosis. For example, all patients with suspected myocardial infarctions have trending of their cardiac enzymes, especially troponin. This allows for a reasonably certain diagnosis that is based on laboratory or radiology findings. Unfortunately, there really isn't a defining test like that for neurologically compromised patients. Although radiology and technological advances have progressed, the most reliable indication for neurologically compromised patients remains the trending of neurologic assessment findings and the critical thinking skills of the nurse.

PATHOPHYSIOLOGY

When a cell is injured, the cell membrane permeability changes. This allows the normally extracellular sodium to rush into the cell. As the sodium enters, water follows it, causing the cell to swell. The sodium–potassium pump kicks into action, trying to rid the cell of the excess sodium. The water that followed the sodium into the cell puts pressure on the mitochondria. (Recall that the mitochondria are the source of energy for the cell.) If the mitochondria are under pressure, they cannot produce the normal amount of energy. The energy from the mitochondria is what fuels the sodium–potassium pump; without energy, the sodium–potassium pump is not efficient and edema continues to accumulate within the cell. The other result of not having the mitochondria as the energy source is that the cell changes from aerobic to anaerobic metabolism, producing lactic acid and free oxygen radicals as by-products.

The next step is critical: Either the source of injury to the cell is removed at this point, allowing the cell to regain aerobic metabolism, rid itself of excess sodium and water, and return to normal functioning, or the cell may rupture. If the cell bursts, the intracellular contents are released, which include lysosomes. These enzymes clean up the debris from the ruptured cell, but also irritate the surrounding cells, causing injury to them, and the process begins again. Although cells can be injured by thermal, mechanical, or toxic sources, the most common cause of cellular injury is hypoxia (Jacobs & Hoyt, 2000).

What does cellular pathophysiology have to do with neurologic injuries? Everything! Once a cell ruptures and dies, new cells will be formed—except in the central nervous system and heart. We do not regenerate cells in the brain or spinal cord at this time, so as cells are lost, so is function. It is imperative to retain as many functioning neurologic cells as possible.

The actual mechanism that causes the neurologic injury is called the primary injury. Except for injury prevention tactics, such as wearing helmets and seatbelts, it isn't possible to eliminate the primary injury as we care for the patient. For example, a primary injury would occur if the patient has a mechanical injury to a cranial vessel from a fragment of fractured skull, causing a hemorrhage. Secondary injury occurs when the cells distal to the injured vessel become hypoxic. The goal in caring for patients with neurologic injuries is to minimize secondary injury.

INTRACRANIAL PRESSURE AND CEREBRAL PERFUSION PRESSURE

The other critical concepts to understanding head injuries are intracranial pressure (ICP) and cerebral perfusion pressure (CPP). The skull is a closed box with one opening, the foramen magnum. The contents of the skull are brain tissue, blood, and cerebrospinal fluid (CSF). As the amount of one component increases, something else has to decrease. For example, if a patient has cerebral edema causing an increase in the space occupied by brain tissue, blood and/or CSF will be shunted away from the cranial vault to accommodate the swollen tissue. The pressure exerted by the three components within the skull is ICP. If there is an increase in one of the components, the ICP will rise.

Because a continual supply of oxygenated blood is critical for brain cells to function, it is important to maintain a CPP between 60 and 70 mm Hg. Calculation of CPP is described in Chapter 27. Calculation of mean arterial pressure (MAP) is explained in **Box 29-1**.

Box 29-1

Calculation of Mean Arterial Pressure

$$\frac{\text{Systolic Pressure} + \text{Diastolic Pressure} (\times 2)}{3}$$

Example: A patient has a blood pressure of 110/65. To calculate the MAP:

Diastolic pressure $\times 2 = 65 \times 2 = 130$

Systolic pressure $= 110$

$130 + 110 = 240$

$240/3 = \textbf{80}$ mm Hg

HEAD INJURIES

The most common mechanism of injury for head trauma is motor vehicle crashes. Falls, assaults, and penetration-like gunshot wounds are also frequently seen causes. Head injuries also occur with sports or recreational activities, where the risk of injury increases when the appropriate protective equipment is not used—for example, helmets in football or skateboarding.

Concussion

The most common closed head injury is a concussion. This condition occurs when the brain is jostled inside the cranial vault. Symptoms will vary depending on which part of the brain is affected. The frontal lobe is often the victim; the symptoms of an injury to this area of the brain are classically repetitive questioning and amnesia of the event since the frontal lobe controls short-term memory. The victim may or may not have a loss of consciousness, nausea, and slight visual disturbances. Headache is a frequent complaint. The computerized tomography (CT) scan will be normal, and symptoms usually clear within 24 hours (Brain Trauma Foundation, 2000; McQuillan & Mitchell, 2002).

Contusions

Contusions range in severity, depending on which lobe or lobes of the brain are involved. Contusions are bruised areas of brain tissue that become damaged as the brain bounces off ridges of bone inside the skull during a motor vehicle crash or fall, for example. Just as with any bruise, they look worse before they begin to improve, so they will require serial CT scans over several days to watch the contusion "blossom" and then resolve. Reviewing the functions of the lobes of the brain will help guide the assessment of the patient as described in Chapter 26. For example, a patient with an occipital lobe contusion from a backward fall down the stairs will need special monitoring for visual acuity and visual interpretation (Brain Trauma Foundation, 2000; McQuillan & Mitchell, 2002).

Diffuse Axonal Injury

Diffuse axonal injury is the most severe type of closed head injury. It occurs when the neurons are stretched or sheared so that they can no longer synapse with the next neuron. This type of damage is seen after a deceleration injury, such as a motor vehicle crash or a fall. The patient is usually immediately unresponsive and requires assistance with ventilation. The CT scan may show some slight diffuse edema on presentation, but then appears normal. Complete supportive care is required. Although it is not clear how the mechanism of the recovery works, if the patient is going to arouse and make some type of recovery, that response usually occurs in the first three months after the injury.

There are exceptions to this observation, of course, but the three-month window is a very common guideline (Brain Trauma Foundation, 2000; McQuillan & Mitchell, 2002).

Fractures

Skull fractures may be linear, depressed, or compound. Linear skull fractures look like a cracked egg shell. They are visible on plain skull films or on CT scan. The danger with linear fractures is that they may have nicked a blood vessel that lies just under the skull itself.

Depressed skull fractures occur when a section or more of bone fragment becomes embedded in the brain tissue. This patient usually requires surgery to debride that section of underlying brain and elevate the skull fragments (Samii & Tatagiba, 2002).

Compound skull fractures are open fractures with communication between the brain and the environment. These are of concern because if the dura is interrupted, the patient has a greater risk for infection because the blood–brain barrier is violated. Gunshot wounds cause compound skull fractures and then enter into the brain tissue itself.

A basilar skull fracture is a linear fracture at the base of the skull that is associated with a dural tear. Signs and symptoms include spinal fluid leakage from the nose or ears, raccoon's eyes (periorbital ecchymosis), and Battle's sign (bruising on the mastoid bone, behind the ear). Drainage from the nose or ear should be tested for glucose levels using a bedside glucometer. If the glucose of the fluid is greater than 200 mg/dL, it is indicative of CSF. Another technique to test for CSF is to test the leakage on filter paper. The blood will separate from the CSF and leave a halo or ring sign on the paper. However, the presence of a ring sign is not exclusive to CSF. A highly sensitive test for CSF measures beta-2 transferrin, which requires as little as 1/50th of a drop of fluid for analysis (Meco, Oberascher, Arrer, Moser, & Albegger, 2003). Management of basilar skull fracture includes observation for meningitis or encephalitis and for signs of an epidural hematoma. While administration of prophylactic antibiotics is commonplace, data suggest that they are not effective in preventing the development of meningitis in patients with a basilar skull fracture (Ratilal, Costa, & Sampaio, 2006).

Intracranial Hemorrhage

Epidural Hematoma

An epidural hemorrhage or bleed is a collection of blood between the skull and the dura. The most common cause is a linear fracture of the temporal bone that nicks the middle meningeal artery, causing a hemorrhage. Patients with epidural hematomas often exhibit a classic symptom pattern. Immediately post-injury, they will experience a brief loss of consciousness. This often occurs before prehospital personnel arrive, so patients may be unaware they have experienced a loss of consciousness. A period of lucidity follows, which usually coincides with emergency prehospital care. Patients are brought to the emergency department with a Glasgow Coma Scale score of 14 or 15 and equal, reactive pupils. Later during their evaluation, they experience a decline in level of consciousness from increasing ICP. Additionally, their pupils become unequal. The pupil on the side of the hemorrhage will become dilated and nonreactive to light. The other side will still have a round, reactive pupil. This effect is caused by the hemorrhage putting pressure on cranial nerve III (CN III), which controls whether pupils can react to light. With CN III pinched from pressure, it can no longer signal the pupil to constrict to light (Cushman et al., 2001).

Epidural hematomas require immediate surgical intervention to remove the clot. While the risk of infection is always a concern postoperatively, these patients do not have an elevated risk because the meninges and the blood–brain barrier remain intact. With prompt diagnosis and treatment, these patients usually have a good prognosis (Cushman et al., 2001).

Subdural Hematoma

Subdural hematomas usually have a venous origin and are caused by tears in the bridging veins that connect various hemispheres and lobes of the brain. They vary in terms of their severity and symptoms depending on the size of the vein that is bleeding. Large venous collections may produce lateralizing symptoms of a unilateral fixed and dilated pupil and require immediate surgical intervention. Smaller collections may have more subtle findings. If the patient has a small subdural hematoma that is not producing lateralizing symptoms, the treatment may be close observation with serial CT scans over the next hours to days. These patients have a higher infection risk postoperatively because the meninges must be violated to evacuate the clot (Cushman et al., 2001).

Subarachnoid Hematoma

A subarachnoid hemorrhage is caused by the rupture of capillaries, usually from shearing injuries that bleed into the subarachnoid space. The blood mixes with the CSF that normally circulates in that space and disperses over the brain. These fluids cause a more global ICP increase. This kind of hemorrhage is considered inoperable because it is spread throughout the entire subarachnoid space in the central nervous system. Blood mixed with the CSF also impairs the reabsorption of CSF through the arachnoid villa, because they may be coated in blood. This can further increase ICP if the CSF begins to accumulate (Cushman et al., 2001).

Intracranial Hemorrhage

Intracranial hemorrhage within the brain tissue varies in severity depending on its location and the number of areas of hemorrhage. **Box 29-2** and **Box 29-3** detail drug therapy and nursing management for head injuries, respectively.

SPINAL CORD INJURIES

The same principles of cellular response to injury, primary injury, and secondary injury noted with head injury also apply to spinal cord injury. The goal of treatment is to minimize secondary injury and prevent complications. Secondary damage to the spinal cord can also occur from hypovolemic shock, resulting in hypoperfusion to the spinal cord (Jacobs & Hoyt, 2000).

Common mechanisms of spinal cord injury include motor vehicle crashes, falls, and diving accidents. Take the time to review the motor and sensory functions associated with the various levels of the spinal cord. For example, the cervical area is the most frequently damaged because it is the most mobile. This area controls the phrenic nerve, which exits the spinal cord around C4–C5. The phrenic nerve controls the function of the diaphragm. If this nerve is involved, the patient will experience breathing difficulties, which could be life-threatening and require immediate intervention (Jacobs & Hoyt, 2000).

VERTEBRAL FRACTURES

Vertebral fractures may occur in any portion of the spinal column and may involve different portions of the vertebrae. Fractures are classified as stable or unstable. Stable fractures have no potential to impinge upon the cord. Unstable fractures may have already caused cord damage or have the potential to cause damage. Patients with such injuries must remain immobilized until the vertebral fracture can be repaired.

Concussion

The spinal cord may sustain a concussion, similar to the brain in a closed head injury. In such a case, there is a temporary alteration in motor and/or sensory function with return to full function.

Contusion

Cord contusion may occur from a vertebral fracture that bruises the cord or from the cord impacting intact vertebrae in a deceleration injury (from abrupt stopping after high speed). Severity and symptoms depend on the location of the contusion, other physiologic conditions such as hemorrhage, and the amount of cell death.

Transection

Cord transections may be complete or incomplete. Complete cord transections at the time of the injury cause a total loss of motor and sensory function below the level of the injury. Incomplete transections are much more common and vary in terms of their severity and symptoms. Some common types of incomplete transections are described here:

- Anterior cord syndrome from acute anterior cord compression—exhibits loss of motor function, loss of pain, temperature, crude touch, and pressure. Proprioception, fine touch, fine pressure, and vibration are intact.
- Posterior cord syndrome from acute posterior cord compression—proprioception, vibration, fine touch, and fine pressure are lost. Motor function, pain, temperature, crude touch, and pressure are intact.
- Central cord syndrome from swelling in the center of the cord—loss of motor and sensory function below the level of the lesion with greater loss in the arms than in the legs.
- Brown-Sequard Syndrome from transverse hemisection of the cord—usually caused by a penetrating injury. It results in loss of motor function on the same side as the injury and loss of sensory function on the opposite side.

Remember the principles of cellular injury: What may have started as an incomplete transection may become complete with cellular swelling and rupture. Additionally, a cord

Box 29-2
Drug Therapy

Class	Drug	Indications
Diuretics	mannitol, furosemide	Decreases intracranial pressure
Steroids	dexamethasone, methylprednisolone	Decreases inflammation
Anticonvulsants	phenytoin, fosphenytoin, diazepam, lorazepam, phenobarbital sodium	Inhibits seizures

---

Box 29-3
Nursing Management of Head Injury

Interventions	Rationale
Assess neurological status	Changes may indicate worsening condition
Monitor ICP	Changes may indicate worsening condition
Maintain airway	Hypoxia can cause cerebral vasodilation
Hyperventilation	Maintains PCO_2 at 35 mm Hg to cause vasoconstriction
Minimize stimuli	Decreases ICP
Head of bed elevated	Decreases ICP
Implement early nutrition	Positive nitrogen balance
Emotional support	Provides communication
Education	Provides knowledge of patient condition and treatment

---

injury at C6, for example, may seem to progress upward to C5 because of the progressive cellular edema post injury. These patients must be reevaluated frequently and consistently to observe for changes in symptoms.

Neurogenic Shock and Spinal Shock

Neurogenic shock and spinal shock are frequently seen immediately post-incident in the patient with a spinal cord injury. Neurogenic shock is actually shock that causes cellular ischemia. The mechanism of injury in this case is that sympathetic tracts in the spinal column become damaged and may block sympathetic transmission, leaving parasympathetic symptoms. Patients will exhibit heart rates that are normal to bradycardic, blood pressures that are normal to hypotensive, slowed respiratory rates, and skin that is warm with pink mucous membranes and good capillary refill because veins are dilated and filled with blood. These symptoms are counter to the typical "shock" picture of hypotensive, tachycardic, cool, clammy, and pale and may fool the inexperienced nurse into thinking this patient is compensating well, when actually the blood volume is in the periphery and not perfusing the vital organs of heart, lungs, brain and injured area. This situation can actually lead to increased organ damage due to the enhanced ischemia. The treatment for neurogenic shock is not more fluids; the patient already has blood volume, but it needs to be diverted back to the areas of concern. This type of patient may actually receive a vasoconstrictor to force blood out of the venous storage.

Spinal shock is really a misnomer: It isn't "shock" at all, in the classic definition of inadequate cellular perfusion. When the spinal cord is injured, regardless of the degree of injury, it seems to shut down to assess the damage. During this time,

all motor, sensory, and deep tendon reflexes are lost below the level of the injury. Because the patient then presents to the emergency department immediately post-injury, there may be flaccidity and total loss of sensation noted. It is impossible to actually know the full extent of the injuries until the spinal shock resolves. This may take hours to days to weeks and will be determined when deep tendon reflexes return. In planning the care of this patient and the family, remember that waiting is difficult. Actual rehabilitation and future planning depend on knowing the extent of injury.

Care of the Patient with a Spinal Cord Injury

The priorities of care for injured patients remain the same regardless of the mechanism of injury. The primary survey for injured patients consists of the ABCDs:

A—airway with cervical spine control

B—breathing, with particular attention to the cervical area and intercostal muscles

C—circulation, which includes checking pulses, stopping external bleeding, and obtaining intravenous (IV) access

D—disability; a quick neurologic exam for responsiveness and pupil checks

After the primary survey is completed and the necessary interventions have been made (e.g., intubation, ventilation, and starting IV fluids), the patient must be assessed thoroughly to identify all other injuries (Moore, Feliciano, & Mattox, 2004).

Immediately post-injury, the patient will require immobilization with a long spine board during assessment of the injury. Spine boards are very hard and cause pressure areas on

Box 29-4
Nursing Management of Spinal Cord Injury

Interventions	Rationale
Assess neurologic status (loss of consciousness, motor, and sensory)	Changes may indicate worsening condition
Maintain alignment	Decreases risk of cord compression
Assess respiratory status	Early identification of respiratory dysfunction
Assess for autonomic dysreflexia	Removes stimuli causing dysreflexia
Provide nutrition	Balances nitrogen state
Skin care protocol	Prevents skin breakdown
Monitor bowel movement	Prevents impaction
Emotional support	Provides communication and support
Education	Provides knowledge of patient condition and treatment

the posterior surface from the occiput to the heels. Minimize the amount of time the patient is on the board as much as possible, and begin skin care early (Russo-McCourt, 2002). **Box 29-4** describes additional nursing management that is required for this patient.

Steroid Use after Spinal Cord Injury

Steroid administration is a controversial issue in the treatment of spinal cord injuries. Steroids stabilize cell membranes, which limits cord edema and ischemia in some patients. They are potentially useful in blunt trauma. The initial dose of steroids must be given within the first eight hours of injury.

Areas of Research

Scientists and other members of the healthcare community are aggressively researching methods to minimize the effects of spinal cord injury. Much attention was gained for this cause due to the efforts of the Christopher Reeve Foundation after his injury. Currently, an ongoing study called Procord is seeking to determine the effects of taking the patient's own macrophages (a type of white blood cell), treating them in a proprietary process, and then injecting them into the injured area of the patient's spinal cord. This research has produced positive early results in clinical trials. For more information, see www.proneuron.com.

PATIENT OUTCOMES

Nurses can help ensure attainment of optimal patient outcomes such as those listed in **Box 29-5** through the use of evidence-based interventions for neurologic injuries.

SUMMARY

Nurses working in the intensive care unit (ICU) may encounter a number of patients with a neurologic injury. An understanding of the risk factors, pathophysiologic changes, and management is essential for optimal patient outcomes to occur. One of the pivotal competencies that an ICU nurse must demonstrate when caring for this patient population is advocacy/moral agency. This is in light of the high morbidity and mortality rates reported.

Box 29-5
Optimal Patient Outcomes

- Uses effective coping strategies
- Cerebral perfusion pressure in expected range
- Mean arterial pressure in expected range
- Intracranial pressure in expected range
- Airway remains patent
- Physical comfort in expected range
- Modifies lifestyle as needed

CASE STUDY

A 28-year-old male patient arrives at a trauma center following a fall from his roof. He has an open tibia fracture, a bruise to his left lower chest, and a tender left upper quadrant. He presents with a Glasgow Coma Scale score of 8 and is moving all extremities. His right pupil is fixed and dilated, and his left pupil is normal size and reactive to light. Even without an ICP monitor, it can be safely assumed that his ICP is elevated. His blood pressure on admission is 90/60, so his MAP is 70 mm Hg. A MAP of 70 mm Hg, after subtracting an elevated ICP, drops the CPP to below 60 mm Hg and is not allowing for adequate perfusion, which will increase the amount of secondary brain injury.

CRITICAL THINKING QUESTIONS

1. Which disciplines should be consulted to work with this client?
2. What types of issues may require you to act as an advocate or moral agent for this patient?
3. How will you implement your role as a facilitator of learning for this patient?
4. Write a case example from the clinical setting, highlighting one patient characteristic. Explain how the characteristic was observed through subjective and objective data.
5. Utilize the form to write up a plan of care for one client in the clinical setting.
6. Write a case example from the clinical setting. Rate the patient as a level 1, 3, or 5 on each characteristic. Identify the level of nurse characteristics needed in the care of this patient.
7. Take one patient outcome for a patient and list evidence-based interventions found in a literature review for this patient.

Using the Synergy Model to Develop a Plan of Care

	Patient Characteristics	Subjective and Objective Data	Evidence-based Interventions	Outcomes
SYNERGY MODEL	Resiliency			
	Vulnerability			
	Stability			
	Complexity			
	Resource availability			
	Participation in care			
	Participation in decision making			
	Predictability			

Online Resources

Proneuron Technologies: www.proneuron.com

Steroids for Spinal Cord Injury: www.trauma.org/spine/steroid.html

National Spinal Cord Injury Association: www.spinalcord.org

Spinal Cord Injury Resource Center: www.spinalinjury.net

Brain Injury Resource Center: www.headinjury.com

REFERENCES

Brain Trauma Foundation. (2000). Management and prognosis of severe traumatic brain injury. Retrieved July 26, 2005, from www2.braintrauma.org/guidelines/index.php

Cushman, J., Agarwal, N., Fabian, T. Garcia, V., Nagy, K., Pasquale, M., et al. (2001). Practice management guidelines for the management of mild traumatic brain injury. *The Eastern Association of the Surgery of Trauma Practice Management Guidelines Work Group.* Retrieved July 26, 2005, from www.east.org

Jacobs, B., & Hoyt, K. S. (Eds.). (2000). *Trauma nursing core course provider manual* (5th ed). Chicago: Emergency Nurses Association.

McQuillan, K., & Mitchell, P. (2002). Traumatic brain injuries. In K. McQuillan, K. VonReuden, R. Hartsock, M. Flynn, & E. Whalen (Eds.), *Trauma nursing: From resuscitation through rehabilitation* (pp. 393–451). Philadelphia: Saunders.

Meco, C., Oberascher, G., Arrer, E., Moser, G., & Albegger, K. (2003). Beta-trace protein test: New guidelines for the reliable diagnosis of cerebrospinal fluid fistula. *Otolaryngology Head Neck Surgery, 129*(5), 508–517.

Moore, E., Feliciano, D., & Mattox, K. (Eds.). (2004). *Trauma* (5th ed.). New York: McGraw-Hill.

Ratilal, B., Costa, J., & Sampaio, C. (2006). Antibiotic prophylaxis for preventing meningitis in patients with basilar skull fractures. *Cochrane Database of Systematic Reviews,* (1), CD004884.

Russo-McCourt, T. (2002). Spinal cord injuries. In K. McQuillan, K. VonReuden, R. Hartsock, M. Flynn, & E. Whalen (Eds.), *Trauma nursing: From resuscitation through rehabilitation* (pp. 393–451). Philadelphia: Saunders.

Samii, M., & Tatagiba, M. (2002). Skull base trauma: Diagnosis and management. *Neurological Research, 24*(2), 147–156.

Cerebrovascular Disorders

Susan Yeager

Arteriovenous malformations (AVM) and cerebral aneurysms can cause subarachnoid and intracranial hemorrhage with devastating results. Prompt diagnosis and treatment by practitioners educated in cerebral vascular care are pivotal to providing appropriate interventions to optimize outcomes. This chapter will describe the incidence, pathophysiology, diagnosis, and treatment of AVMs and cerebral aneurysms.

ARTERIOVENOUS MALFORMATIONS

AVM Incidence

Since only 12% of AVMs cause symptoms, the incidence of AVM in the United States is not fully known. The incidence is thought to be around 1 per 100,000, equaling 300,000 cases. As technology advances and early detection increases, these numbers may rise. The average age of AVM diagnosis is 33 years, with 64% being identified before age 40 (Greenburg, 2001).

Untreated AVMs represent a threat to patients, because they have an annual major hemorrhage rate of anywhere from 2% to 17% (Bollet et al., 2004). AVMs account for 8.6% of all subarachnoid hemorrhages (SAHs) (Hickey & Buckley, 2003). The average rate of hemorrhage increases by 3% annually in unruptured vessels. This risk increases to 6% to 18% the first year after hemorrhage but has been shown to decrease to 4% annually thereafter (Greenburg, 2001; Greene et al., 1995). Although ruptured AVMs cause only 2% of all hemorrhagic strokes, the results can be devastating (Choi & Mohr, 2005). Lethal results from intracerebral AVM hemorrhages have been reported in as many as 29% of cases (Bollet et al.). Fortunately, thanks to advances in technology, twice as many AVMs are being identified before rupture than in years past (Choi & Mohr).

Pathophysiology

Normal cerebral vasculature includes arteries connecting to capillary systems that diminish the intravascular pressure before reconnecting to the veins. With AVMs, high-flow arterial blood shunts directly into low-resistance venous vessels. This tangled bundle of abnormal vessels possesses characteristics of thin or irregular muscularis and elastica, endothelial thickening, and islands of sclerotic tissue (Choi & Mohr, 2005). An AVM has three morphologic components: the feeding arteries, the nidus, and the draining veins. The feeding arteries supply blood flow to the AVM. The nidus is the main tangle of connecting arterial and venous vessels. Dilated veins drain blood flow away from the AVM. Due to the vascular change from a high-flow system to a low-flow system, intravascular pressure is increased, predisposing the vessels to rupture.

The second effect of impaired perfusion is shunting of blood away from the surrounding brain tissue. Little to no functioning brain tissue within the lesion has been found, which leads to the assumption that functional displacement is pushed to the margins of the malformation (Choi & Mohr, 2005). The diversion of vascular blood to the AVM is called the "steal phenomenon." Theoretically, when blood flow into the AVM shunts blood away from surrounding brain tissue, it results in underperfusion and possibly ischemic brain in tissue beneath and around the AVM (Choi & Mohr; Iwama, Hayashida, Takahashi, Nagata, & Hashimoto, 2002).

AVMs are assumed to arise during fetal development. Vessels noted in utero suggest that their course may span over several decades, with some progressing, others remaining static, and a few regressing. AVMs are rarely familial (Choi & Mohr, 2005). Ninety percent of AVMs are supratentorially located, with 15% affecting deep locations (basal ganglia, brain stem, and corpus collosum).

Presentation

Eighty percent of AVM patients who present with symptoms do so between 20 and 40 years of age. The remaining 20% develop symptoms before age 20 (Hickey & Buckley, 2003). The most common clinical presentation for AVMs is intracerebral hemorrhage, which occurs in 50% to 60% of cases (Cockroft, Hwang, & Rosenwasser, 2005). Depending on the lesion's location and its angioarchitecture, the hemorrhage can be parenchymal, subarachnoid, intraventricular, or a combination of these. In patients presenting with hemorrhage, 30% are subarachnoid, 23% are intraparenchymal, 16% are intraventricular, and 31% are combined (Choi & Mohr, 2005). Seizure activity is seen in 30% of symptomatic patients (Cockroft et al.), with headache reported in 11% to 14% (Choi & Mohr). In rare cases, evolving focal neurologic deficits are seen as presenting symptoms. The onset and progression of symptoms has been proposed to be the result of "steal phenomenon" effects or local compression of tissue from the growing lesion. Direct compression of brain matter from the expanding AVM is also theorized to cause areas of localized ischemia (Choi & Mohr).

Diagnosis

Evaluation of these symptoms usually begins with neuroimaging studies. A computerized tomography (CT) scan of the head with and without contrast can reveal bleeding sites and brain tissue abnormalities, often with calcifications. More comprehensive analysis of the tangled blood vessels can be obtained via the injection of radioactive reagents into the bloodstream, followed by a magnetic resonance imaging (MRI) technique. This study can be used to further identify AVM location in comparison to surrounding brain structures. The gold standard for AVM imaging is four-vessel angiography. This invasive procedure involves threading a wire through a femoral artery catheter into the origin of the cranial vessels. A contrast reagent is then delivered close to the AVM site and examined under fluoroscopy imaging. Flow into and out of the vessels can be observed. Three-dimensional angiography is the latest technology in AVM diagnosis, which provides a 360-degree view of the feeder arteries, nidus, and venous outflow vessels. At present, no international standards or diagnostic algorithms for AVM detection exist (Choi & Mohr, 2005).

Treatment

The decision regarding whether and how to treat an evolving AVM depends on a variety of factors. These factors include the patient's age, medical condition, symptoms, AVM size, AVM location, and type of venous drainage (Nakaji & Spetzler, 2005). Additionally, the natural history of AVMs in general should be considered. Research data suggest that the hemorrhage rate of unruptured AVMs is approximately 3% per year (Nakaji & Spetzler). After hemorrhage, rebleed rates have been noted to increase (Cockroft et al., 2005). Mortality rates associated with episodes of bleeding are 10%, with an average neurologic morbidity of 20% (Nakaji & Spetzler). Given the relatively high morbidity and mortality associated with hemorrhage, elimination of AVMs is usually considered desirable.

Options for treatment currently fall into three categories: surgical resection, endovascular embolization, and radiosurgery. While surgical resection is a mainstay, AVM management generally requires multiple modalities and a team approach. Long-term risk versus immediate risk of various treatment options should be considered. Collaborative discussions with the patient among the neurosurgeon, interventional radiologist, and radiation oncologist, coupled with the underlying knowledge of practitioner skill and experience with lesions, will further guide treatment choices.

Surgical Resection

Research regarding optimal treatment for AVMs is ongoing. Currently, it is thought that the best candidates of surgical resection are patients with a good life expectancy, angiographic or clinical risk factors, small to medium-size AVMs (see **Table 30-1**) (Cockroft et al., 2005), good medical condition, positive symptoms, and AVMs anatomically located in surgically ac-

TABLE 30-1 Spetzler–Martin Surgical Grading Scale for Cerebral Arteriovenous Malformations

Category		Point Value
Size (maximal dimension)		
	< 3 cm	1
	3–6 cm	2
	> 6 cm	3
Location		
	Noneloquent brain	0
	Eloquent brain	1
Venous drainage		
	Superficial only	0
	Deep	1

Source: Greenburg, 2001.

cessible parts of the brain. Additional reasons to choose surgery are the AVM's association with aneurysms or venous outflow obstruction and a patient who has failed endovascular therapy or radiotherapy (Nakaji & Spetzler, 2005). An advantage of surgical treatment is the possible complete removal of the malformation in one operation. Surgical risks include perioperative hemorrhage, infection, brain edema, stroke, and death (Choi & Mohr, 2005).

If chosen, surgical treatment may begin with an MRI with fiducial placement. Fiducials are circular discs that are placed on the patient's scalp prior to the MRI (see **Figure 30-1**). The location of the fiducials is processed by a stealth navigator computer, which calculates the three-dimensional location of the AVM. This image is then used at the time of surgery to help locate the malformation precisely, thus minimizing injury to the surrounding brain and maximizing lesion removal. Access to the AVM occurs via craniotomy bone removal. Once visualization occurs, excision of lesions using standard microsurgical techniques generally begins

with the arterial feeders. Arterial feeder removal is then followed by excision of the nidus and resection of the draining veins. Intraoperative and/or postoperative angiogram is used to determine the presence of residual lesions. If present, residual lesions should be immediately resected or treated, utilizing alternative therapy to prevent vessel rupture.

Endovascular Treatment

The goal of endovascular therapy is to obliterate the feeding arteries and the vessels at the site of the nidus (Choi & Mohr, 2005). The first endovascular treatment of a cerebral arteriovenous malformation was performed in 1960 by injecting silastic spheres through surgically exposing the cervical carotid artery (Howington, Kerber, & Nelson, 2005). Due to the inadvertent occlusion of normal vessels and neurologic injury with this agent, assessment of various occlusion strategies to advance techniques continued. In 1974, Serbinenko succeeded in accessing cerebral arteries by using a detachable balloon mounted on a floating catheter (Hoelper, Hofmann, Sporleder, Soldner, & Behr, 2003; Serbinenko, 1974). While it offered improved results, this technique was not vessel-specific because the balloon was carried distally within the vessel with the most flow, and the balloon size precluded its entrance into the nidus (Howington et al.).

The use of particles as embolic agents for AVM treatment began in the 1970s. Since that time, embolic endovascular

FIGURE 30-1 Fiducial Placement

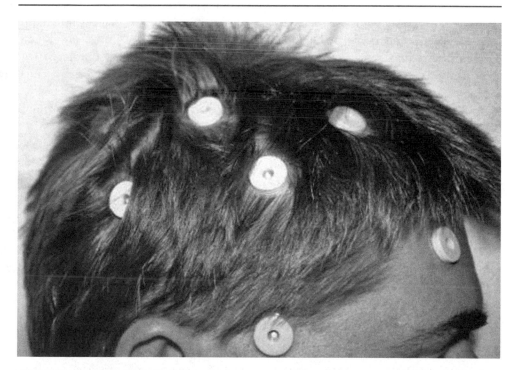

therapy has continued to evolve. Current agents include N-butylcyanoacrylate (NBCA), detachable coils, or Onyx® liquid polymer (Choi & Mohr, 2005). NBCA (Trufill®) is the most popular liquid agent and is the only "glue" approved by the U.S. Food and Drug Administration for use in cerebral AVMs. NBCA is a clear, colorless, radiolucent liquid that begins polymerization upon contact with blood saline and ionic contrast media (Cockroft et al., 2005). Onyx, a nonthrombogenic, liquid alcohol polymer, is another embolic agent currently being evaluated for efficacy in obliteration of AVMs. Coil therapy will be discussed under aneurysm treatment but also may be used in endovascular occlusion.

To achieve the goal of endovascular therapy, staged procedures over several days or weeks may be necessary to facilitate the gradual adjustment of vessels to pressure changes. Total embolization of AVMs occurs in 13% to 40% of patients (Choi & Mohr, 2005; Hartmann et al., 2002). Morphological characteristics of the AVM may cause embolization to be done as an adjunct to surgery or radiosurgery with the focus not being obliteration but rather reduction in the AVM size and bleeding risk (Choi & Mohr). Preoperative embolization should be done 24 to 48 hours prior to surgical intervention, because development of collateral flow into the nidus can occur within two days (Buckmiller, 2004).

Complications of intravascular AVM treatment can be characterized as ischemic, hemorrhagic, or groin related. Ischemic events occur due to glue emboli or catheter-induced dissection or vascular occlusion. Hemorrhagic complications can occur due to vessel rupture or inadvertent occlusion of the draining veins, which may result in too rapid an alteration in nidus hemodynamics and ultimately bleeding. Potential groin complications include infection and pseudoaneurysms. Mortality and morbidity rates of patients endovascularly treated for AVMs since 1990 are 1% and 8%, respectively (Cockroft et al., 2005).

Radiosurgery

The principle underlying radiosurgery is the use of focused radiation beams into selective tissue for ionization. Radiosurgery began in 1949 with the use of proton particles to irradiate brain tumor lesions. The "gamma knife" followed in 1968 and used cobalt-60 within a helmet device to direct gamma radiation to a specific area. Another type of radiosurgery called the LinAc was introduced in the mid-1980s. This device differs from the gamma knife in that radiation is emitted by a single source that rotates slowly around the patient's head. Ionization produces inorganic ions, which are deleterious to cells, secondary to the formation of free radicals that are harmful to cell and nuclear membranes. Irreparable damage

ensues, resulting in permanent thickening of vascular channels, thrombosis, and cell death (Hickey & Buckley, 2003).

Due to limited studies demonstrating data on survival, quality of life, and neurologic progression-free survival, the efficacy of AVM treatment utilizing radiosurgery remains controversial (Bollet et al., 2004). Some have proposed observation of inoperable AVMs rather than nonsurgical treatment. The current opinion is that stereotactic radiosurgery may be a preferred treatment for patients with an AVM located in deep structures or eloquent cortex (i.e., motor strip) lesions.

AVM treatment invariably requires a multidisciplinary approach to care and treatment, and many factors need to be considered to determine the appropriate treatment in each case. One such factor evaluated when considering radiosurgery is AVM size. Cure rates after stereotactic radiosurgery decrease as the AVM volume increases. Reduction of AVM volume to less than 10 cm has been associated in case studies with higher cure rates. In these situations, endovascular embolization or surgical techniques may be used to reduce the AVM size or eliminate certain angiographic features such as intranidal aneurysms (Cockroft et al., 2005). Aside from size, common risk factors for radiosurgery complications reported in the literature include location, previous hemorrhage, and irradiated volume (Bollet et al., 2004).

Concerns associated with radiosurgery include lag time between treatment and results (AVMs take one to three years for maximal shrinkage) and effects of radiation on healthy brain tissue. The appropriateness of radiation, total radiation dosage, and type of radiation delivered are determined through collaborative discussions between the neurosurgeon and the radiation oncologist. During these discussions, consideration is given to these potential concerns related to AVM size, location, age, and general health of the patient (Kemeny, Radatz, Rowe, Walton, & Hampshire, 2004).

Nursing Care

Admission of AVM patients into the intensive care unit (ICU) begins with an accurate report of presenting events and baseline neurologic function. Ongoing monitoring of neurologic changes occurs via frequent neurologic assessments. Hemorrhage prevention and symptom management—especially blood pressure control—are the focus of AVM nursing treatment. Whether or not the lesion was detected after an initial bleed, preventing bleeding focuses on seizure control, lifestyle modifications, and prevention of hypertension.

Blood pressure control can be achieved through medication administration as well as environmental control. Antihypertensives are ordered with a target systolic or mean arterial pressure listed as the focus of therapy. The postoperative period can cause a phenomenon called "normal-pressure perfusion breakthrough." The theory is that changes in blood pressure and flow can cause postoperative swelling or hemorrhage due to loss of autoregulation (Greenburg, 2001). Minimizing pain through administration of narcotic or alternative treatments and controlling stress-inducing situations will also assist in blood pressure reduction.

Prophylactic antiseizure medication administration can occur but may be reserved until seizure activity is noted. Lifestyle modifications include smoking cessation and limitation of exertion until the lesion is controlled.

CEREBRAL ANEURYSMS

Aneurysm Incidence

The incidence of aneurysms is difficult to estimate. However, data suggest an incidence of 5% (Greenburg, 2001). Aneurysms can be classified as ruptured or unruptured. The unruptured to ruptured ratio is 5:6 to 5:3, equivalent to an approximate 50% rupture rate (Ogilvy & Carter, 2003). The incidence of ruptured cerebral aneurysms ranges from 6 to 16 per 100,000 (Khandelwal, Kato, Sano, Yoneda, & Kanno, 2005; Manno, 2004; Linn, Rinkel, & van Gijn, 1996), or approximately 25,000 to 30,000 SAHs from aneurysms annually in the United States (Khandelwal et al.; Menghini, Brown, Sicks, O'Fallon, & Wiebers, 1998).

Morbidity and mortality from ruptured aneurysms remain significant. Mortality from ruptured aneurysms has been reported as high as 50% (Khandelwal et al., 2005; van Gijn & Rinkel, 2001). Prehospital death is thought to be related to direct neural destruction and increased intracranial pressure from exceeding reasonable limits of blood, and sudden death from ventricular arrhythmias (Khandelwal et al.). Of patients who make it to institutions to receive care, 25% die within two weeks of their admission (Khandelwal et al.; Satoh, Nakamura, Kobayashi, Miyata, & Matsutani, 2005). Of the survivors, 20% to 30% live with significant neurologic deficits (Khandelwal et al.; Rosenorn et al., 1987). Therefore, a thorough understanding of aneurysm pathology, diagnosis, and management are necessary to minimize the impact of these events on patients' lives.

Pathophysiology

The exact mechanism of aneurysm formation is controversial. Cranial vessels are known to be less elastic and have less musculature. Additionally, larger cerebral vessels are located in the subarachnoid space with little connective support, which may predispose them to the development of aneurysms (Hop, Rinkel, Algra, & van Ginj, 1998). What is known is that aneurysms tend to arise from areas of vessel bifurcation. One

theory is that hemodynamic stress over time causes degeneration of the vasculature (Hickey & Buckley, 2003). Atherosclerosis or hypertension may therefore predispose individuals to develop aneurysms. Consistent risk factors cited for aneurysmal SAH include hypertension, smoking, and alcohol consumption. If two first-degree relatives have aneurysms, the incidence of additional family members having aneurysms is 15% (Ogilvy et al., 2001). Increased risk of aneurysm development is also noted in first-degree relatives of persons with known lesions. Second-degree relative risk, however, is equal to that of the general public (Greenburg, 2001; Ogilvy et al.). Gender and ethnicity also play roles: Incidence seems to increase in females, and African Americans are twice as likely as whites to develop aneurysms (Hickey & Buckley).

Location of aneurysms may vary, with 85% occurring within the anterior circulation. The three most common locations are the anterior communicating artery (Acom; 30%), the posterior communicating artery (Pcom; 25%), and the middle cerebral artery (20%). Posterior circulation aneurysm can also occur, with 10% being located on the basilar artery and 5% occurring in the posterior inferior cerebral artery or vertebral artery. Multiple aneurysms are noted in 20% to 30% of the patient population (Zipfel, Bradshaw, Bova, & Friedman, 2004). **Figure 30-2** identifies the location of aneurysms.

Cerebral aneurysms evolve into a variety of sizes and shapes. **Table 30-2** classifies these aneurysms by size. The most common aneurysmal shapes are berry or fusiform. Berry or saccular aneurysms are the most common type. These aneurysms have a neck or stem with a balloon-like outpouching. Berry aneurysms are most likely to be found at vessel bifurcations. Fusiform aneurysms are typically found in the vertebrobasilar system and are an outpouching without a stem.

Presentation

Presentation of patients with aneurysms can be separated into unruptured and ruptured cases. Most patients with unruptured aneurysms are completely asymptomatic. In approximately 40% of these cases, warning signs may be present. These localized symptoms may result from aneurysmal growth and compression on structures or intermittent, small leakage of blood (sentinel hemorrhage). Symptoms may include headache, third nerve palsies (i.e., dilated pupils, ptosis), extraoccular motor deficits (cranial nerves III, IV, and VI), vision changes, pain above and behind the eye, localized headaches, nuchal rigidity (neck pain with flexion), seizures, and photophobia (Greenburg, 2001).

Aneurysm patient presentation usually occurs as a result of hemorrhage. Usually this bleeding is subarachnoid, but it can also result in intracerebral hemorrhage (20–40%), intra-

FIGURE 30-2 Aneurysm Location on the Circle of Willis

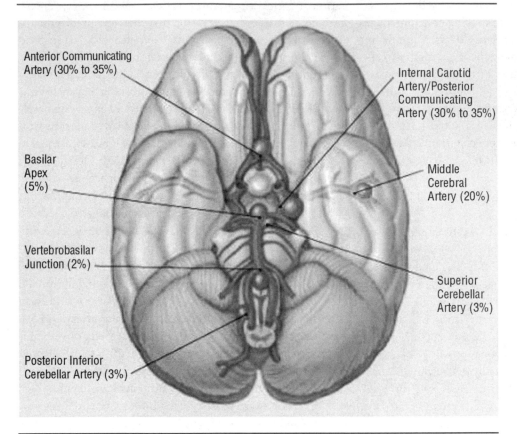

Anterior Communicating
Artery (30% to 35%)

Internal Carotid
Artery/Posterior
Communicating
Artery (30% to 35%)

Basilar
Apex
(5%)

Middle
Cerebral
Artery (20%)

Vertebrobasilar
Junction (2%)

Superior
Cerebellar
Artery (3%)

Posterior Inferior
Cerebellar Artery (3%)

Source: Reprinted with permission from Boston Scientific at www.bostonscientific.com

ventricular hemorrhage (13–28%), or subdural blood (2–5%) (Weir, Disney, & Karrison, 2002). The severity of presenting symptoms may correlate with the bleeding amount, but typical descriptions include thunderclap headache ("worst headache of my life") and nausea and vomiting with or without loss of consciousness. Additional symptoms may include cranial nerve deficits, stiff neck/neck pain, blurred vision, seizures, hypertension, bradycardia, and, depending on the area of cortex involved in the hemorrhage, localized motor weakness (Linn et al., 1996).

TABLE 30-2 Aneurysm Classification by Size

Small	≤ 10 mm
Medium	10–15 mm
Large	15–25 mm
Giant	25–50 mm
Super-giant	> 50 mm

Source: Greenburg, 2001.

Diagnosis

Evaluation of patients begins with a thorough patient history and a comprehensive neurologic exam. Once those data are obtained, diagnostic evaluation usually begins with a cerebral CT scan. For purposes of bleeding/aneurysm diagnosis, no contrast is needed. Because etiology is usually unknown upon presentation, initial evaluation will likely include CT scan with and without contrast. CT scans have been reported to have a 93% to 100% diagnostic sensitivity for identifying subarachnoid blood, but sensitivities have been found to correlate with the timing of CT obtainment relative to headache onset (Edlow & Caplan, 2000; Linn et al., 1996).

If CT findings are negative for blood and increased intracranial pressure is not suspected, lumbar puncture may be used to determine the presence of subclinical red blood cells (RBCs) and xanthrochromia (representing bile in the cerebrospinal fluid [CSF]). Discovery of RBCs in the CSF at times presents diagnostic difficulties, because "traumatic" lumbar punctures resulting in spillage of blood into the catheter and fluid occur in approximately 20% of cases (Linn et al., 1996). When this problem occurs, differentiation may be based on the presence or absence of xanthrochromia. Xanthrochromia develops in approximately 12 hours and generally takes two weeks to clear following an SAH (Linn et al.). If the diagnosis is still unclear, additional studies are warranted and may include CT angiography (CTA), MRI/angiography, and angiograms.

Early CT scan techniques were insensitive to aneurysm detection. With the advances in spatial resolution and CTA, however, sensitivity to aneuryms has improved (Boesiger & Shiber, 2005). CTA utilizes a vein-injected contrast agent. An automatic injector machine is used to control the timing and rate of injection. After the injection, a rotating detector creates a fan-shaped beam of x-rays that is captured on film. With the advent of spiral CT technology, three-dimensional "casts" of the blood vessels are possible. Advantages of CTA include being minimally invasive and offering a relatively quick turnaround time. Disadvantages include a lack of detection of smaller vessel abnormalities, potential allergic reactions, and nephrotoxicity from contrast agents.

MRI was introduced into clinical practice in the mid-1970s. MRI utilizes radio waves in a strong magnetic field. The magnetic field lines up protons, which are then spun by radiofrequency waves and produce signals. These signals are processed by the computer and ultimately result in sharp, detailed images. Contrast is generally used to highlight the vessel structures. Though it is thought to be more sensitive than CT in aneurysm detection (Mitchell, Gholkar, Vindlacheruvu, & Mendelow, 2004), MRI cannot be used in patients with implanted metal such as pacemakers or metallic ear transplants. In addition, given that MRI technology generally requires patients to tolerate confined spaces, patient size or claustrophobia may limit its use. Additionally, MRI will not detect small aneurysms (4 mm or less).

Cerebral angiography was introduced in 1927 (Boesiger & Shiber, 2005). The technology has advanced since then, such that the 360-degree angiogram represents the current gold standard for aneurysm detection. In this technique, the patient is usually sedated and may be intubated and anesthetized to minimize movement. Groin arteries are accessed utilizing a large-bore catheter. After arterial access is obtained, the neurologic radiologist threads a thin, flexible wire into the carotid-vertebral artery system. Contrast agents are then injected into the vessel, while images of contrast flow are monitored utilizing fluoroscopic techniques. The sensitivity and specificity of angiography are high and represent the standard against which other tests are judged.

Treatment

Aneurysm treatment includes measures taken both before and after definitive treatment by surgical and endovascular means. Before an aneurysm has been definitively treated, blood pressure control and symptom management are key. Target systolic and mean arterial pressure goals vary among institutions, physicians, and individual patients, with no evidence-based standard having been documented as yet. Hypertension avoidance is achieved through antihypertensive agents given intermittently or via continuous drip.

Symptom control begins with airway management, which may include mechanical intubation. Patients with a Glasgow Coma Scale score less than 8 should be electively intubated to prevent aspiration pneumonia. Lidocaine may be used prior to intubation to depress the cough reflex and thus avoid increases in intracranial pressure. Circulation and hemodynamic stabilization are achieved with fluid therapy. Pain and nausea control through narcotic and antiemetic administration may be needed. In these circumstances, care should be taken to avoid oversedation to support continued neurologic assessment.

Seizure management is controversial but is usually recommended after a known seizure. Proponents of prophylactic management suggest that seizure onset may result in increased intracranial pressure and possible rebleeding.

Hydrocephalus occurs in approximately 20% of ruptured aneurysms as subarachnoid, intraventricular, or intracranial blood prevents CSF flow through the ventricular system (White, Teasdale, Wardlaw, & Easton, 2001). This complication may occur upon presentation or evolve within hours to days. Treatment requires placement of an intraventricular catheter for both CSF drainage and intracranial pressure monitoring. Lumbar drains may serve the same purpose but require further clinical evaluation before they can be recommended for all patients.

Admission electrocardiogram (ECG), chest radiograph, serum electrolytes, hematology panel, coagulation parameters, and type and cross matching are also included in the admission workup and preparation for potential diagnostic intervention and definitive treatment. Definitive treatment can be separated into surgical and endovascular modalities.

Surgical Techniques

Direct surgical clipping of intracranial aneurysms was first attempted in the 1930s, but mortality at that time was high (Boesiger & Shiber, 2005; White, Wardlaw, & Easton, 2000). Surgical clipping of aneurysms did not gain favor until the mid-1970s. Based on the scientific foundation from an international, randomized trial, surgically treated patients had a 6.5-year total mortality of 37% compared to 55% for the then standardized regulated bedrest group and 39.6% for the regulated bedrest with hypotension group (Boesiger & Shiber). Incremental reductions in surgical risk for ruptured intracranial aneurysms have since been achieved through enhanced microsurgical instruments and techniques, advances in intensive and anesthesia care, improved diagnostics, and the development of neurosurgery as a subspecialty (Molyneux et al., 2005).

Intracranial clipping is achieved through a craniotomy. Microdissection down to the aneurysmal lesion may be aided by the placement of a lumbar drain or a ventricular catheter. The drain may be placed to evacuate CSF to aid in microdissection. Once visualized, the neurosurgeon places a surgical clip at the neck of the aneurysm or feeding artery if the aneurysm itself is unclipable and the risk of permanent neurologic impairment is absent or considered to be less than the risk of re-rupture. When clipping is not possible due to aneurysmal anatomy, surgical wrapping using fibrin glue, Teflon®, or other polymers may occur (Greenburg, 2001).

The benefits of surgical techniques include direct access in case of aneurysm rupture and definitive resolution of the aneurysm. Permanent aneurysm eradication utilizing surgical techniques occurs in more than 90% of patients, with morbidity and mortality of surgical treatment estimated at 5% to 15% (Wijdicks, Kallmes, Manno, Fulgham, & Piepgras, 2005). **Figure 30-3** displays the surgical clipping of an aneurysm. Due to its relatively low complication rate and its ability to promote clot evacuation, microsurgery has been established as the gold standard for aneurysm treatment.

Timing of surgery remains controversial, however. In patients with a Hunt–Hess Grade of 4 to 5 (**Table 30-3**), a period of stabilization (usually more than 10 to 14 days post SAH) is recommended. The argument for delay in such cases revolves around the presence of a solid clot (which is more difficult to remove), brain edema (which would require more brain manipulation to obtain aneurysm access), potentially increased risk of aneurysm rupture, and possibly increased vasospasm risk following surgery secondary to vessel manipulation (Greenburg, 2001). Factors supporting delayed surgery include poor medical condition, poor neurologic condition (Hunt–Hess Grade 4 or greater), significant cerebral edema, active vasospasm, and difficult-to-clip aneurysms (Greenburg). Proponents of early treatment for patients who present with SAH believe that this approach eliminates subsequent bleeding, facilitates vasospasm treatment, and enables cerebral lavage

TABLE 30-3 Hunt–Hess Subarachnoid Hemorrhage Classification

Grade	Description
0	Unruptured aneurysm
1a	No acute meningeal/brain reaction but fixed neurologic deficit
1	Asymptomatic, or mild headache or slight nuchal rigidity
2	Cranial nerve palsy (i.e., III, VI), moderate to severe headache, nuchal rigidity
3	Mild focal deficit, lethargy, or confusion
4	Stupor, moderate to severe hemiparesis, early decerebrate rigidity
5	Deep coma, decerebrate rigidity, moribund appearance

Source: Greenburg, 2001.

to enhance elimination of potential vasospasmotic agents (Le Roux et al., 1995). Factors that favor choosing early intervention include good medical and neurologic condition, large amounts of SAH that increase the likelihood of subsequent vasospasm development, and large amount of clot with effacement of tissue (Greenburg).

Endovascular Techniques

Due to the invasive nature of cranial surgery and advancement of endovascular technology, debate regarding the optimal aneurysm treatment continues. The results of the International Subarachnoid Aneurysm Trial added more fuel to this debate. This study demonstrated that 23.7% of endovascularly treated patients were dependent or dead at one year versus 30.6% of surgical patients (Molyneux et al., 2005).

The introduction of the Guglielmi detachable coil in 1991 revolutionized cranial intravascular treatment. Continued enhancements such as the advent of soft and three-dimensional (3-D) coil technology and cranial stents have made coiling possible in lesions previously considered beyond the realm of intervention (Wiebers et al., 2003). **Figure 30-4** shows the use of coiling in an aneurysm.

When treating the aneurysm, patients are anesthetized to minimize motion during the delicate portions of coil placement or vessel sacrifice via balloon occlusion. If continuous neurologic evaluation is needed, a patient may be awakened and given sedative and analgesic agents. Access of the groin occurs, utilizing a femoral sheath. A guide catheter is then placed

FIGURE 30-3 Surgical Clipping of an Aneurysm

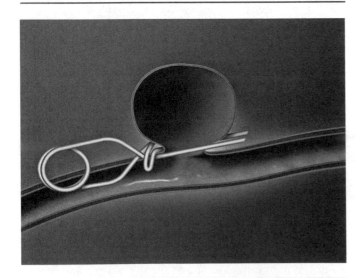

Source: Reprinted with permission from Boston Scientific at www. bostonscientific.com

FIGURE 30-4 Staged Endovascular Coiling Utilizing 3-D Coils

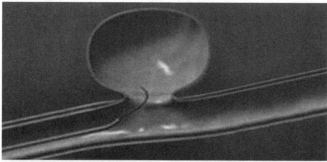

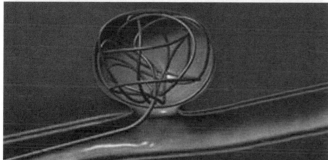

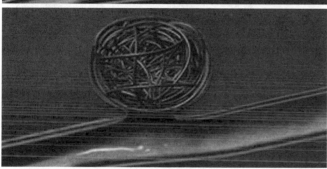

in the target vessel, with care being taken to avoid contact with the aneurysm wall. After matching the aneurysm diameter and coil properties, device selection occurs. Coil systems generally consist of a thin, spiral-woven, platinum, helix-shaped wire soldered to a stainless steel delivery system. Inside the delivery system, coils are straight; due to circular memory, however, they will resume the helix shape once deployed into the aneurysm. More elaborate coils include two-diameter, complex 3-D configuration, Dacron fibers, and bioactive technologies. The purpose of each coil is to enhance placement and promote thrombus occlusion of the aneurysm. Multiple coils are needed to pack the aneurysm and achieve occlusion.

Stent-assisted coiling is a relatively new technique that serves as a buttress to the coil. The balloon-expanded or self-

expandable stent is placed outside the aneurysm neck and supports the implanted coils from slipping into the vessel. (See **Figure 30-5**.) Concerns regarding stent usage include induction of intimal hyperplasia or occlusion of small side branches. To minimize vessel occlusion, patients who are coiled with or without stenting are generally placed on aspirin with or without clopidogrel (Plavix®) once the aneurysm has been occluded. This is true even if the patient orginally presented with bleeding. Liquid embolic agents (i.e., Onyx®) may also be used for aneurysm occlusion, though coiling remains the gold standard.

Benefits of coiling include its less invasive nature, decreased system stress, and decreased length of stay. Ongoing analysis of the permanency of coiled aneurysm is needed, however. Complications of coiling include ischemic events secondary to coil herniation with thrombus formation or with distal embolization, aneurysm rupture or perforation, and groin complications. To prevent or minimize catastrophic consequences of intervention, care should be delivered in centers that focus on neurologic intervention to enable prompt management by skilled practitioners (Wiebers et al., 2003).

Patient selection for intervention versus surgical treatment requires a collaborative discussion between the neurosurgeon and the interventional radiologist. Characteristics considered in the decision-making process include aneurysm size, dome-to-neck ratio, Hunt–Hess grading, patient age, comorbidities, surgical accessibility, and practitioner skill.

FIGURE 30-5 Endovascular Stenting Prior to Aneurysm Coiling

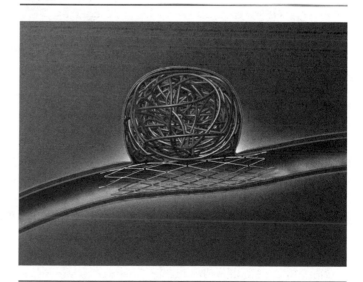

Nursing Care

Once treatment is provided, patient care focuses on early identification and prevention of neurologic sequelae. In non-hemorrhagic aneurysm patients, care consists of frequent cranial nerve and motor strength evaluations in the neurologic ICU. Post-procedure angiography may occur the following morning or during a follow-up visit several months to weeks after the procedure. Timing of subsequent angiograms is not standardized, but intraoperative angiograms are a current trend (Wiebers et al., 2003). If no neurologic changes occur, patient activity can progress with patient discharge occurring within several days of admission. Education related to wound care (groin or cranial), signs of neurologic dysfunction, lifestyle changes, and activity limitation should occur. Blood pressure management may also need to be monitored or treated in the outpatient arena.

Hemorrhagic aneurysmal patients are at risk for a variety of complications, including vasospasm, hyponatremia, neurogenic pulmonary edema, cardiac dysfunction, and chronic hydrocephalus. Each of these sequelae is associated with its own set of treatment strategies.

Vasospasm

Cerebral vasospasm has been described as sustained arterial contraction that is unresponsive to vasodilator medications (Oyama & Criddle, 2004). Vasospasm-induced narrowing has been estimated to occur in 70% to 90% of SAH patients. Symptomatic vasospasm occurs in only 30% of cases (Brislstra, Algra, & Rinkel, 2002; Hanel, Demetrius, & Wehman, 2005) and has an associated mortality of 7% (Levati, Solaini, & Boselli, 1998; Rosen, Sekhar, & Duong, 2000); severe deficits are noted in an additional 7% of cases (Sen et al., 2003). Vessel narrowing is defined as radiographic or clinical (symptomatic). Radiographic vasospasm occurs when visible narrowing utilizing contrast injection under angiographic observation is noted. Clinical or symptomatic narrowing develops accompanied by functional manifestations dependent upon the cerebral area affected and the degree of ischemia. Symptomatic vasospasm assessment findings range from headache, lethargy, and intermittent disorientation to hemiparesis and permanent disability (Rosen et al., 2000).

Vasospasm pathology is poorly understood. The process is self-limited. It generally begins no sooner than 3 days after SAH and resolves within 21 days. Despite our currently limited understanding of its pathology, vasospasm development can be predicted based on a variety of factors—namely, the amount and location of blood, with a higher incidence seen in Fisher Group 3 (see **Table 30-4**), increasing patient age, and history of tobacco use (Greenburg, 2001).

TABLE 30-4 Fisher Subarachnoid Hemorrhage Classification

Group	Description
1	No detectable blood on CT
2	Diffuse or vertical blood layers < 1 mm thick that do not appear dense enough to represent a large, thick homogeneous clot
3	Localized clot greater than 1 mm thick in vertical plane or greater than 5 × 3 mm in longitudinal and transverse dimensions in the horizontal plane
4	Intracerebral or intraventricular clots, but with only diffuse blood or no blood in basal cisterns

Source: Greenburg, 2001.

Diagnosis of vasospasm begins by ruling out other potential causes, such as hydrocephalus, cerebral edema, seizure activity, hyponatremia, hypoxia, and sepsis. Onset generally occurs between 4 and 14 days post SAH. Although the gold standard of testing is cerebral angiogram, large-vessel spasm may also be detected utilizing transcranial Doppler (TCD). TCD is a noninvasive cerebral artery velocity evaluation. Utilization of hand-held Doppler technology through temporal bone windows enables monitoring of large cerebral vessels. Because major vessels are the only arteries assessible with this technology, TCD should be used as a screening tool and angiograms employed as the definitive form of evaluation.

Once diagnosed, or if increased risk is suspected, several treatment options can be implemented to prevent or minimize sequelae from vasospasm. An initial prevention strategy is the use of nimodipine (Nimotop®). This calcium channel blocker is the only pharmacologic agent found useful in vasospasm treatment (Kassell et al., 1990). The dose is 60 mg orally every four hours; if hypotension occurs, 30 mg every two hours may be given for 21 days.

Hyperdynamic or triple-H therapy is another vasospasm treatment option. The use of hypertensive therapy as a treatment against vessel narrowing was first noted in 1951. Further evaluation of this concept was not achieved until the late 1960s, when the use of volume expanders and vasopressors to raise blood pressure were noted to reverse or minimize neurologic symptoms (Molyneux et al., 2005). More widespread use of triple-H therapy began with the "early treatment of aneurysm" trend. In the late 1970s, a small cohort of patients with symptomatic vasospasm was treated with colloids and phenylephrine (Neosynephrine®) to induce hypertension, and their neurologic deficits were successfully reversed. In 1982, the concept of hemodilution as a vasospasm treatment was introduced (Rosen et al., 2000). This theory proposed that by utilizing colloids, blood viscosity could be lowered and cerebrovascular resistance thereby decreased, with resultant blood flow increase. Balancing the oxygen carrying capacity with improved flow, a hematocrit of 30% was proposed as ideal. Evidence to support this theory has yet to be obtained, making this treatment controversial.

After definitive aneurysm treatment, benefit has been demonstrated with systemic blood pressure elevation using volume expansion and ongoing blood pressure support (Greenburg, 2001). Target blood pressures are controversial, because the patient's baseline pressure needs to be taken into account (Rosen et al., 2000).

Several risk factors from triple-H therapy warrant consideration when initiating care. Approximately 10% to 20% of patients with SAH will develop pulmonary edema, especially when they are given crystalloid volume expansion (Rosen et al., 2000). Dilutional hyponatremia of less than 135 mEq/L is seen in 3% of patients and myocardial infarction in 2%; catheter-related complications from pulmonary artery catheters (sepsis, 13%; subclavian vein thrombosis, 1.3%; and pneumothorax, 1%) are also seen (Rosen et al.). Therefore, care should be taken when initiating therapy, although no specific standards related to timing or appropriateness of interventions currently exist.

Once vasospasm is detected, additional pharmacologic and mechanical treatment options are available. Intra-arterial papaverine (Para Time® SR) or verapamil hydrochloride (Calan®) may be given during an angiogram to provide short-term vasospasm relief. Because effects last for only a few hours, the patient may require multiple interventions over several days despite the risk of the invasive procedure. In addition to pharmacologic treatment, mechanical options are available.

Percutaneous balloon angioplasty may be needed in severe vasospasm. Similar to cardiac angioplasty, this technology involves threading a flexible catheter through the arterial system into the position of spasm. Once placed, the pressure-controlled balloon can be inflated with resultant displacement of previously narrowed vessel walls. Procedural risks include arterial occlusion, rupture, or dissection. Use of this technology requires large cerebral vessels and the services of an interventional radiologist trained in cerebral procedures (Greenburg, 2001).

The current strategies of calcium channel blockers and triple-H therapy have reduced mortality and morbidity rates of vasospasm from 20% in the 1980s to the current rate of 5% to 10% (Corsten et al., 2001). Advances in technology and pharmacology continue to be explored in an effort to further decrease the incidence of clinically significant vasospasm.

Additional therapies requiring more study include the use of microdialysis, mild hypothermia (32–34°C) (Rosen et al., 2000), high-dose (4–5.5 mg/dL) magnesium sulfate therapy, transcranial cerebral oximetry, and molecular biology. All have demonstrated promise for vasospasm diagnosis or treatment (Nagao, Irie, & Kawai, 2003).

Hyponatremia

Hyponatremia affects 10% to 40% of patients with SAH. This condition is defined as a sodium level of less than 135 mEq/L for at least a day. Signs of hyponatremia include fever, headache, nausea and vomiting, muscle cramps, weakness, and confusion. As values drop below 110 mEq/L, stupor, seizures, and coma may occur. Several theories have been suggested to explain the link between SAH and hyponatremia. One proposes a transient release of antidiuretic hormone, which results in Syndrome of Inappropriate Antidiuretic Hormone secretion, and a dilutional drop in sodium. Another theory, which is more widely accepted, is based on the fact that atrial natriuretic factor rises and stimulates urinary loss of sodium (cerebral salt wasting). Neurologic dysfunction may occur, with hyponatremic patients having three times the incidence of delayed cerebral infarction after SAH than normonatremic patients (Gasser, Khan, & Yonekawa, 2003). Factors that increase the likelihood of hyponatremia include congestive heart failure (CHF), cirrhosis, adrenal insufficiency, diabetes, and the use of nonsteroidal inflammatory drugs (NSAIDs), acetaminophen, narcotics, and thiazide diuretics (Veyna, Seyfried, & Burke, 2002).

Treatment of SAH-related hyponatremia differs from that provided to the general population. Fluid restriction (a usual treatment) in this population may result in increased blood viscosity and may result in ischemia from vasospasm (Gasser et al., 2003). Instead, treatment with normal or hypertonic saline, sodium tablets, or fludrocortisone acetate should be used.

Regardless of the cause, hyponatremia should be corrected slowly. If done too rapidly, the patient can be placed at risk for rebound cerebral edema. To prevent this complication, correction should not exceed a rate of 1.3 mEq/L/hr or more than 10 mEq/L in 24 hours. Frequent monitoring of chemistry values is also necessary to react to complications in a timely manner.

Neurogenic Pulmonary Edema

Massive sympathetic outflow may mediate the development of extravasation of plasma proteins across the pulmonary parenchyma (Linn et al., 1996). This results in an acute form of pulmonary edema, which may occur at the moment of SAH or within several days of injury. Reversal of this phenomenon occurs by itself, but ventilatory support is generally needed in the short term (Linn et al.).

Cardiac Dysfunction

Cardiac abnormalities with acute ECG changes are noted in almost half of patients with SAH. Presentation can occur at the time of SAH or as long as two weeks into the clinical course (Linn et al., 1996). Abnormalities can present as inverted T waves, any variety of dysrhythmias, or lethal variations that may result in sudden death. Cardiac enzyme elevation may occur and is frequently associated with myocardial dysfunction and subendocardial ischemia.

Echocardiogram analysis may demonstrate significantly lowered ejection fractions with myocardial motionlessness. This dysfunction may present much like heart failure or respiratory distress syndrome. Unlike the cardiac ischemic changes seen in coronary artery disease, this "stunned myocardium" is usually reversible (Linn et al., 1996). Support for the patient experiencing this complication may include inotropic therapy, pulmonary artery monitoring, and ventilatory support as needed.

Hydrocephalus

Due to variations in definitions, the stated incidence of acute hydrocephalus ranges from 20% to 60%, with a more commonly stated range of 15% to 20% (Greenburg, 2001). Fortunately, 30% to 60% of these patients demonstrate no alteration in consciousness. Acute hydrocephalus may convert to chronic hydrocephalus when arachnoid granulations develop adhesions or permanent impairment. While not all patients convert to chronic hydrocephalus, the phenomenon does occur in 50% of SAH patients. In such a case, CSF diversion devices should be placed after post-hemorrhage protein and RBC counts decrease to avoid catheter occlusion.

General Care

Due to the generalized total body stress associated with SAH, gastric ulcer stress prophylaxis should be undertaken in all these patients. Additionally, nutrition in some form should be initiated as soon as clinically possible. Patients' relative immobility should make constipation and deep venous thrombosis (DVT) prophylaxis a standard of care. Stool softeners should be given to all patients, with constant surveillance of bowel activity. A minimum of sequential compression devices should occur. Controversy exists regarding the use of unfractionated or low-molecular-weight heparin products in this population, but anticoagulation is generally avoided. Activity progression should occur when the patient is clinically able. Collaborative involvement of disciplines such as physical, occupational, and

speech therapy may be required, depending on the degree of neurologic impairment.

Familial Education

Family education should be ongoing throughout the patient's hospitalization. Due to the acute nature of most patient admissions, nurses can expect to have to repeat instructions and explanations of the plan of care multiple times. Compassionate inclusion of family members will minimize stress.

PATIENT OUTCOMES

Nurses can help ensure attainment of optimal patient outcomes such as those listed in **Box 30-1** through the use of evidence-based interventions for cerebrovascular disorders.

SUMMARY

The outcome of AVM or aneurysm rupture can range from life-changing to death. Minimization of the impact of vascular malformations on patients' lives can occur with prompt diagnosis and treatment. A multidisciplinary approach to treatment includes a variety of informed clinicians, including ICU nurses, neurosurgeons, neuroradiologists, and radiation oncologists, in institutions where the latest advances in treatment can be offered. Future research will continue to focus on refinement of treatment options from surgical techniques, interventional occlusion catheters and devices, and radiosurgery techniques.

Early diagnosis and obliteration of cerebral vascular malformations in tertiary centers that focus on their treatment are needed to minimize neurologic consequences. Collaborative care between neurosurgeons, neuroradiologists, critical care nurses, and multidisciplinary team members will assist the patient and family in achieving their new level of wellness. To collaborate fully, ongoing research and awareness of AVM and aneurysm treatment are necessary.

Box 30-1
Optimal Patient Outcomes

- Cognitive status in expected range
- Patient and family participate in planning/providing care
- Physical comfort in expected range
- Decreased frequency of vasospasm
- Remains calm and tranquil
- Family uses stress reduction strategies

CASE STUDY

After having surgery to repair a torn knee ligament, T.F., a 32-year-old male, started experiencing global headaches. Because T.F.'s only history was asthma related to smoking, the original diagnosis was spinal headache from the spinal block he received for knee surgery.

The patient's headache persisted for several months, with an exacerbation prompting his visit to the Emergency Department. Because he lived alone, T.F. was driven to the hospital by his parents. His head CT scan was negative for blood but demonstrated calcified lesions in his left parietal region. Admission vital signs were T 98.4°F, HR 88, BP 168/90, RR 16, and SpO$_2$ 94% on room air. He rated his global headache as 8/10.

T.F. was admitted to the neurologic critical care (NCC) unit for hourly vital sign and neurologic observation, and for pain and blood pressure control. A cranial MRI with and without contrast demonstrated what appeared to be an AVM. A four-vessel cerebral angiogram done later in the day verified the diagnosis. T.F. was then prepped for a follow-up angiogram for occlusion of the AVM. The following day, T.F. underwent Black Onyx occlusion of his AVM with 90% occlusion. Despite being educated on the smell omitted from Black Onyx, T.F. was nervous about the potential reactions of others to the odor.

Post-procedure care included frequent neurologic and sheath/groin checks, pain control, and vital sign management. The sheath remained intact for intraoperative usage to complete the AVM occlusion.

On the morning of surgery, T.F. received a stereotactic localizing MRI with fiducials. Utilizing the stereotactic navigational system, the neurosurgeon obtained access through a cranial incision. After complete resection of the AVM confirmed by an intraoperative angiogram, T.F. returned to the NCC. Hourly vital sign and neurologic checks and groin care occurred throughout the night.

The next morning, T.F. was doing well. His postoperative cranial wrap was removed, demonstrating an incision that was clean, dry, and intact with staples. His IV was saline locked, and the urinary catheter and arterial line discontinued. T.F. moved to the floor with vital signs being taken every four hours. He was evaluated and released and returned to his home on the second postoperative day. His home instructions included smoking cessation, pain medication, incisional care, activity progression, and follow-up instructions with the neurosurgeon and neurologic interventionalist.

CRITICAL THINKING QUESTIONS

1. As the nurse caring for this patient, what information would you give the family when they state, "We have never heard of an AVM. What is this?"
2. The family asks how an AVM is treated. What would be the best response?
3. After receiving Black Onyx to partially occlude an AVM, the patient complains of a headache without focal neurologic signs. What is the probable source of his headache?
4. What postoperative problems should you be assessing for with a patient who has undergone surgery for an AVM?
5. Prior to discharge, how would you plan to transition the patient to a neuro step-down unit?
6. Which disciplines should be consulted to work with this client?
7. How would you modify your plan of care for patients of diverse backgrounds?
8. What type of issues may require you to act as an advocate or moral agent for this patient?
9. How will you implement your role as a facilitator of learning for this patient?
10. Use the form to write up a plan of care for one client in the clinical setting with a cerebral aneurysm or AVM. Rate the patient as a level 1, 3, or 5 on each characteristic. Identify the level of nurse characteristics needed in the care of this patient.
11. Take one patient outcome for a patient and list evidence-based interventions.

Using the Synergy Model to Develop a Plan of Care

	Patient Characteristics	Level (1, 3, 5)	Subjective and Objective Data	Evidence-based Interventions	Outcomes
SYNERGY MODEL	Resiliency				
	Vulnerability				
	Stability				
	Complexity				
	Resource availability				
	Participation in care				
	Participation in decision making				
	Predictability				

Online Resources

National Organization of Vascular Anomalies: www.novanews.org/vascularmalformations.htm

Brain, arteriovenous malformation: www.emedicine.com/radio/topic93.htm

Timing of surgery for aneurysmal subarachnoid haemorrhage (Cochrane Review):
www.cochrane.org/cochrane/revabstr/ab001697.htm

Calcium antagonists for aneurysmal subarachnoid haemorrhage (Cochrane Review):
www.cochrane.org/cochrane/revabstr/ab000277.htm

Subarachnoid hemorrhage: www.emedicine.com/neuro/topic357.htm

REFERENCES

Boesiger, B. M., & Shiber, J. R. (2005). Subarachnoid hemorrhage diagnosis by computed tomography and lumbar puncture: Are fifth generation CT scanners better at identifying subarachnoid hemorrhage? *Journal of Emergency Medicine, 29*(1), 23–27.

Bollet, M. A., Anxionnat, R., Buchheit, I., Bey, P., Cordebar, A., Jay, N., et al. (2004). Efficacy and morbidity of arc-therapy radiosurgery for cerebral arteriovenous malformations: A comparison with the natural history. *International Journal Radiation Oncology Biology Physics, 58*(5), 1353–1363.

Brilstra, E., Algra, A., & Rinkel, G. (2002). Effectiveness of neurosurgical clip application in patients with aneurysmal subarachnoid hemorrhage. *Journal of Neurosurgery, 97*, 1036–1041.

Buckmiller, L. (2004). Update on hemangiomas and vascular malformations. *Current Opinion in Otolaryngology and Head and Neck Surgery, 12*(6), 476–487.

Choi, J., & Mohr, J. (2005). Brain arteriovenous malformations in adults. *Lancet Neurology, 4*(5), 299–308.

Cockroft, K., Hwang, S., & Rosenwasser, R. (2005). Endovascular treatment of cerebral arteriovenous malformations: Indications, techniques, outcome and complications. *Neurosurgery Clinic in North America, 16*, 367–380.

Corsten, L., Raja, A., Guppy, K., Roitberg, B., Misra, M., Alp, M. S., et al. (2001). Contemporary management of subarachnoid haemorrhage. *Surgical Neurology, 56*(3), 140–150.

Edlow, J., & Caplan, L. (2000). Avoiding pitfalls in the diagnosis of subarachnoid hemorrhage. *New England Journal of Medicine, 342*, 29–36.

Gasser, S., Khan, N., & Yonekawa, Y. (2003). Long term hypothermia in patients with severe brain edema after poor grade subarachnoid haemorrhage. *Journal of Neurosurgery Anesthesiology, 15*, 240–248.

Greenburg, M. (2001). SAH and aneurysms. *Handbook of neurosurgery* (5th ed., pp. 754–791). Lakeland, FL: Thieme Greenburg Graphics Inc.

Greene, K. A., Jacobowitz, R., Marciano, F. F., Johnson, B. A., Spetzler, R. F., & Harrington, T. R. (1995). Impact of traumatic subarachnoid hemorrhage on outcome in nonpenetrating head injury. Part I: A proposed computerized tomography grading scale. *Journal of Neurosurgery, 83*(3), 445–452.

Hanel, R., Demetrius, K., & Wehman, J. (2005). Endovascular treatment of intracranial aneurysms and vasospasm after aneurysmal subarachnoid hemorrhage. *Neurosurgical Clinics of North America, 16*, 317–353.

Hartmann, A., Pile-Spellman, J., Stapf, C., Sciacca, R. R., Faulstich, A., Mohr, J. P., et al. (2002). Risk of endovascular treatment of brain arteriovenous malformations. *Stroke, 33*(7), 1816–1820.

Hickey, J., & Buckley, D. (2003). Arteriovenous malformations and other cerebrovascular anomalies. In J. Hickey (Ed.), *The clinical practice of neurological and neurosurgical nursing* (pp. 549–558). Philadelphia: Lippincott Williams & Wilkins.

Hoelper, B. M., Hofmann, E., Sporleder, R., Soldner, F., & Behr, R. (2003). Transluminal balloon angioplasty improves brain tissue oxygenation and metabolism in severe vasospasm after aneurysmal subarachnoid hemorrhage: Case report. *Neurosurgery, 52*(4), 970–974.

Hop, J., Rinkel, G., Algra, A., & van Gijn, J. (1998). Quality of life in patients and partners after aneurysmal subarachnoid hemorrhage. *Stroke, 29*, 798–804.

Howington, J., Kerber, C., & Nelson, L. (2005). Liquid embolic agents in the treatment of intracranial arteriovenous malformations. *Neurosurgery Clinic in North America, 16*, 355–363.

Iwama, T., Hayashida, K., Takahashi, J. C., Nagata, I., & Hashimoto, N. (2002). Cerebral hemodynamics and metabolism in patients with cerebral arteriovenous malformations: An evaluation using positron emission tomography scanning. *Journal of Neurosurgery, 97*(6), 1314–1321.

Kassell, N. F., Torner, J. C., Haley, E. C., Jane, J. A., Adams, H. P., & Kongable, G. L. (1990). The international cooperative study on the timing of aneurysm surgery, part 1: Overall management results. *Journal of Neurosurgery, 73*(1), 18–36.

Kemeny, A. A., Radatz, M. W., Rowe, J. G., Walton, L., & Hampshire, A. (2004). Gamma knife radiosurgery for cerebral arteriovenous malformations. *Acta Neurochirurgica Supplement, 91*, 55–63.

Khandelwal, P., Kato, Y., Sano, H., Yoneda, M., & Kanno, T. (2005). Treatment of ruptured intracranial aneurysms: Our approach. *Minimal Invasive Neurosurgery, 48*(6), 325–329.

Le Roux, P. D., Elliott, J. P., Downey, L., Newell, D. W., Grady, M. S., Mayberg, M. R., et al. (1995). Improved outcome after rupture of anterior circulation aneurysms: A retrospective 10-year review of 224 good-grade patients. *Journal of Neurosurgery, 83*, 394–402.

Levati, A., Solaini, C., & Boselli, L. (1998). Prevention and treatment of vasospasm. *Journal of Neurosurgical Sciences, 42*(Suppl. 1), 27–31.

Linn, F., Rinkel, G., & van Gijn, J. (1996). Incidence of subarachnoid hemorrhage: Role of region, year, and rate of computed tomography: A meta-analysis. *Stroke, 27*, 625–629.

Manno, E. (2004). Subarachnoid hemorrhage. *Neurological Clinics of North America, 22*, 347–366.

Menghini, V. V., Brown, R. D., Sicks, J. D., O'Fallon, W. M., & Wiebers, D. O. (1998). Incidence and prevalence of intracranial aneurysms and hemorrhage in Olmstead County, Minnesota, 1965–1995. *Neurology, 51*(2), 405–411.

Mitchell, P., Gholkar, A., Vindlacheruvu, R., & Mendelow, A. (2004). Unruptured intracranial aneurysms: Benign curiosity or ticking bomb? *Lancet Neurology, 3*, 85–92.

Molyneux, A. J., Kerr, R. S., Yu, L. M., Clarke, M., Sneade, M., Yarnold, J. A., et al. (2005). International subarachnoid aneurysm trial of neurosurgical clipping versus endovascular coiling in 2143 patients with ruptured intracranial aneurysm: A randomized trial. *Lancet, 360*(9488), 1267–1274.

Nagao, S., Irie, K., & Kawai, N. (2003). The use of mild hypothermia for patients with severe cerebral vasospasm: A preliminary report. *Journal of Clinical Neuroscience, 10*, 208–210.

Nakaji, P., & Spetzler, R. (2005). Indications for surgical treatment of arteriovenous malformations. *Neurosurgery Clinic in North America, 16*, 365–366.

Ogilvy, C. S., & Carter, B. S. (2003). Stratification of outcome for surgically treated unruptured intracranial aneurysms. *Neurosurgery, 52*(1), 82–87.

Ogilvy, C. S., Stieg, P. E., Awad, I., Brown, R. D., Kondziolka, D., Rosenwasser, R., et al. (2001). American Heart Association scientific statement: Recommendations for the management of intracranial arteriovenous malformations: A statement from health care professionals from a special writing group of the Stroke Council, American Stroke Association. *Stroke, 32*(6), 1458–1471.

Oyama, K., & Criddle, L. (2004). Vasospasm after aneurysmal subarachnoid hemorrhage. *Critical Care Nurse, 24*(5), 58–67.

Rosen, C. L., Sekhar, L. N., & Duong, D. H. (2000). Use of intra-aortic balloon pump counterpulsation for refractory symptomatic vasospasm. *Acta Neurochirurgica, 142*(1), 25–32.

Rosenorn, J., Eskesen, V., Schmidt, K., Espersen, J. O., Haase, J., Harmsen, A., et al. (1987). Clinical features and outcome in 1076 patients with ruptured intracranial saccular aneurysms: A prospective consecutive study. *British Journal of Neurosurgery, 7*, 33–45.

Satoh, A., Nakamura, H., Kobayashi, S., Miyata, A., & Matsutani, M. (2005). Management of severe subarachnoid hemorrhage: Significance of assessment of both neurological and systemic insults at acute stage. *Acta Neurochirurgica Supplement, 94*, 59–63.

Sen, J., Belli, A., Albon, H., Morgan, L., Petzold, A., & Kitchen, N. (2003). Triple-H therapy in the management of aneurysmal subarachnoid haemorrhage. *Lancet Neurology, 2*(10), 614–621.

Serbinenko, F. (1974). Balloon catheterization and occlusion of major cerebral vessels. *Journal of Neurosurgery, 41*(2), 125–145.

Van Gijn, J., & Rinkel, G. (2001). Subarachnoid hemorrhage: Diagnosis, causes and management. *Brain, 124*, 249–278.

Veyna, R., Seyfried, D., & Burke, D. (2002). Magnesium sulfate therapy after aneurysmal subarachnoid hemorrhage. *Journal of Neurosurgery, 96*(3), 1–11.

Weir, B., Disney, L., & Karrison, T. (2002). Sizes of ruptured and unruptured aneurysms in relation to their sites and the ages of patients. *Journal of Neurosurgery, 96*(1), 64–70.

White, P., Teasdale, E., Wardlaw, J., & Easton, V. (2001). Intracranial aneurysms: CT angiography and MR angiography for detection prospective blinded comparison in a large patient cohort. *Radiology, 219*, 739–749.

White, P., Wardlaw, J., & Easton, V. (2000). Can noninvasive imaging accurately depict intracranial aneurysms? A systematic review. *Radiology, 217*, 361–370.

Wiebers, D. O., Whisnant, J. P., Huston, J., Meissner, I., Brown, R. D., Piepgras, D. G., et al. (2003). Unruptured intracranial aneurysms: Natural history, clinical outcomes, and risks of surgical and endovascular treatment. *Lancet, 362*(9378), 103–110.

Wijdicks, E., Kallmes, D., Manno, E., Fulgham, J., & Piepgras, D. (2005). Subarachnoid hemorrhage: Neurointensive care and aneurysm repair. *Mayo Clinical Procedure, 80*(4), 550–559.

Zipfel, G. J., Bradshaw, P., Bova, F. J., & Friedman, W. A. (2004). Do the morphological characteristics of arteriovenous malformations affect the results of radiosurgery? *Journal of Neurosurgery, 101*(3), 393–401.

ACKNOWLEDGMENT

The author acknowledges Gregory Balturshot, MD, neurosurgeon; Ronald Budzig, MD, neurologic interventional radiologist; and Boston Scientific for their assistance with the creation of this chapter.

Gastrointestinal

Gastrointestinal Anatomy, Physiology, and Assessment

Joyce King

LEARNING OBJECTIVES

Upon completion of this chapter, the reader will be able to:

1. Describe the organs of the digestive tract and the basic digestive process.

2. Discuss the general mechanisms of regulating digestive function.

3. Identify the roles of enzymes and gastrointestinal hormones in the digestive process.

4. List the techniques that are used for assessing the gastrointestinal system.

5. Identify the difference between abnormal and normal gastrointestinal assessment findings.

Cells need nutrients, vitamins, and minerals to survive. The digestive system meets these cellular needs by removing the substances from the external environment (the digestive tract) and presenting them to the cells in a form that they can utilize. This process is another important step in maintaining homeostasis. This chapter briefly discusses the basic digestive processes: motility, secretion, digestion, and absorption. It also reviews the anatomy of the digestive tract and discusses techniques used in the assessment of the gastrointestinal (GI) system.

BASIC DIGESTIVE PROCESSES

Motility is the process whereby muscular contractions mix and move the contents of the digestive tract forward. The smooth muscle of the digestive tract maintains a constant low level of contraction known as tone. Tone maintains a steady pressure on the digestive tract contents and prevents permanent stretching. Propulsive movements (peristalsis) push the contents forward through the digestive tract at varying speeds. Mixing movements promote digestion by mixing food with the digestive juices and facilitate absorption by increasing contact of intestinal contents with the absorbing surfaces of the digestive tract (Clark, 2005).

Secretion involves the release of digestive juices (e.g., hydrochloric acid, enzymes) into the lumen of the digestive tract; these juices aid in digestion and absorption of food. This process is under neural and/or hormonal regulation.

Digestion refers to the breakdown of food structure by enzymes produced within the digestive system so that the nutrients locked in the complex foods become available for absorption and use. For instance, a carbohydrate molecule is too large to be able to be absorbed into the circulation. Enzymes will first break down this large molecule into smaller molecules called monosaccharides. The monosaccharides are then able to be absorbed across the epithelial cells and into circulation. Proteins are degraded into amino acids and small polypeptides, and fats are degraded into monoglycerides and free fatty acids. Unless an individual has a malabsorption problem, 100% of food digested is absorbed; therefore, caloric intake is regulated at the level of ingestion.

Absorption refers to the process whereby the products that result from digestion are transferred from the digestive tract lumen into the blood or lymph. Most absorption takes place in the small intestines. Villi, microvilli, and mucosal folds increase the absorptive surface area of the small intestine. During the process of absorption, nutrient molecules must cross the mucus layer, the epithelium, the interstitial space, and the capillary wall (Martini & Bartholomew, 2000). The specific processes involved in crossing these layers will be discussed later in this chapter.

REGULATION OF THE DIGESTIVE TRACT

Four factors affect the regulation of digestive system function: (1) autonomous smooth muscle function, (2) intrinsic nerve plexi, (3) extrinsic nerves, and (4) gastrointestinal hormones.

The autonomous smooth muscle function consists of self-induced electrical activity in the smooth muscle, referred to as the basic electrical rhythm (BER) or pacesetter potential. Pacesetter cells do not have a constant resting potential, but rather display rhythmic variations in the membrane potential that cyclically bring the membrane closer to or farther from the threshold value. The membrane potential may eventually reach the threshold, triggering a volley of action potentials resulting in repeated, rhythmical muscle contractions. The rate of rhythmic digestive contractile activities, such as peristalsis, depends on the rate of action potentials triggered by these pacesetter cells (Clark, 2005).

The second factor involved in the regulation of digestive tract function is the intrinsic nerve plexi. This interconnecting network of nerve cells (i.e., myenteric plexus and submucous plexus) is located within the digestive tract wall and allows for a considerable degree of self-regulation. These cells are primarily responsible for coordinating local activity within the digestive tract, such as motility and secretion of enzymes and hormones (Clark, 2005).

The third factor is the extrinsic nerves that originate outside the digestive tract and innervate the various digestive organs (i.e., sympathetic and parasympathetic nervous systems). These nerves help to coordinate activity between different regions of the gastrointestinal tract (Clark, 2005). For example, the act of chewing not only results in an increase in salivary secretions in the mouth but, via input from the vagus nerve, also increases secretions from the stomach, pancreas, and liver in anticipation of the arrival of food.

The fourth factor involved in regulation of digestive function is the gastrointestinal hormones, which are released primarily in response to specific local changes in the luminal contents. These hormones can exert either excitatory or inhibitory influences on smooth muscle and exocrine gland cells (i.e., enzyme-producing cells). The wall of the digestive tract contains three types of sensory receptors that respond to these local changes: (1) chemoreceptors, (2) mechanoreceptors, and (3) osmoreceptors. Chemoreceptors are sensitive to the chemical components of the chyme (i.e., the amount of fat present). Mechanoreceptors (pressure receptors) are sensitive to the stretch or tension within the wall of the digestive tract. The osmoreceptors are sensitive to the osmolarity of the luminal contents (Clark, 2005).

Clearly, regulation of gastrointestinal function is highly complex. As noted here, several synergistic and overlapping pathways influence the processes of digestion and absorption.

COMPONENTS OF THE DIGESTIVE SYSTEM

This section examines the four basic digestive processes—motility, secretion, digestion, and absorption—at each organ along the digestive tract. The digestive tract, also called the alimentary canal, is a series of hollow organs joined in a long tube running from the mouth to the anus (**Figure 31-1**).

Mouth

In the *mouth*, the first step in the digestive process is chewing. Chewing breaks food into smaller pieces to facilitate swallowing, mixes food with saliva, and stimulates the taste buds. Saliva—the secretion associated with the mouth—is produced by three pairs of salivary glands and is composed primarily of water, mucus, and enzymes. Saliva initiates digestion of carbohydrate through the action of salivary amylase (Martini & Bartholomew, 2000). Note that no absorption of nutrients occurs in the mouth, although some medications can be absorbed by the oral mucosa [e.g., nitroglycerin (Nitrostat®)].

Esophagus

The esophagus is primarily involved with swallowing, the process of moving food from the mouth to the stomach. The esophagus secretes mucus to protect the mucosal membranes from any sharp edges of the food products as well as from any acid or enzymes in the gastric juice if gastric reflux should occur. No digestion or absorption occurs in the esophagus.

At either end of the esophagus are *sphincters*. The upper sphincter is the pharyngoesophageal sphincter. This sphincter remains closed except during swallowing and prevents large volumes of air from entering the digestive tract. The lower sphincter, the gastroesophageal sphincter, prevents reflux of gastric contents (Martini & Bartholomew, 2000).

Stomach

The stomach is a J-shaped saclike chamber that is divided into three sections: the fundus, body, and antrum. At the distal end of the stomach is the pyloric sphincter, which acts as a barrier between the stomach and the small intestine. Major functions of the stomach are to store food and then to empty the partially

FIGURE 31-1 The Digestive Tract

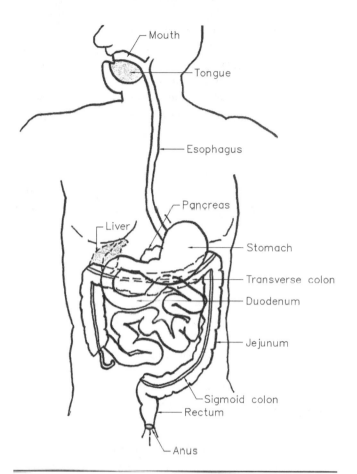

Source: Illustrated by James R. Perron.

digested food into the duodenum at a rate that does not exceed the small intestine's capacity to handle it. Another important function is to secrete hydrochloric acid (HCl) and enzymes that initiate protein digestion. In the stomach, strong peristaltic contractions mix the food with HCl and the digestive enzymes, producing chyme. In the antrum (lower stomach), peristaltic contractions are responsible for gastric emptying. The main factor that influences the strength of the contractions is the amount of chyme in the stomach. Factors in the duodenum are also of primary importance in controlling the rate of gastric emptying. These factors include the amount of fat and/or acid in the chyme, the osmolarity of the chyme, and duodenal distention.

The cells responsible for gastric secretion are located in the gastric mucosa in what are called gastric pits (Martini & Bartholomew, 2000). Three types of secretory cells are found in the walls of the pits. The *mucous neck cells* secrete thin, watery mucus that provides a mucosal barrier, protecting the stomach

lining from gastric secretions. The *chief cells* secrete the enzyme precursor pepsinogen. The *parietal cells* secrete HCl and intrinsic factor; intrinsic factor is essential for intestinal absorption of vitamin B_{12}. These secretions are all released into the lumen of the stomach (Martini & Bartholomew).

Endocrine cells, called *G cells*, which are located in the pyloric region of the stomach, secrete the hormone gastrin into the blood. Gastrin, in turn, stimulates both the parietal cells and chief cells to increase secretion of HCl and pepsinogen. HCl is not actively involved in the digestion of food but rather is responsible for activating the enzyme precursor pepsinogen so that it becomes the active enzyme pepsin. Pepsin then initiates the digestion of protein. No food or water is absorbed into the blood from the stomach, although alcohol and aspirin are absorbed from this site (Martini & Bartholomew, 2000).

Control of gastric secretion involves three phases: the cephalic phase, the gastric phase, and the intestinal phase. The cephalic phase refers to the increase in secretion of HCl and pepsinogen that occurs when a person thinks about, smells, or tastes food. The gastric phase occurs when food actually reaches the stomach. Distention of the stomach and the chemical content of food are responsible for increasing gastric secretions during this phase. The intestinal phase of gastric secretion encompasses factors originating in the small intestine that influence gastric secretion. While the other phases are excitatory, this phase is inhibitory, helping to shut off gastric secretions as the chyme begins to be emptied into the small intestine (Martini & Bartholomew, 2000).

Pancreas

The pancreas has both exocrine and endocrine functions. The exocrine portion consists of acinar cells, which secrete three types of enzymes, and duct cells, which secrete an alkaline secretion that is rich in sodium bicarbonate. The three types of pancreatic enzymes are proteolytic enzymes (e.g., trypsin), which are involved in protein digestion; pancreatic amylase, which continues the carbohydrate digestion that was initiated in the mouth; and pancreatic lipase, the major enzyme involved in fat digestion. The proteolytic enzymes are secreted in an inactive state and become activated only when they reach the lumen of the small intestine, although both amylase and lipase are secreted in the active state. Pancreatic enzymes are most effective at breaking down their specific nutrients in a neutral or slightly alkaline environment; therefore the alkaline fluid secreted from the duct cells serves the important function of neutralizing the acidic chyme.

The exocrine secretions are regulated primarily by two hormones, secretin and cholecystokinin (CCK). Both of these hormones are released from the duodenal mucosa. Secretin is released in response to the presence of acid in the duodenum, which in turn stimulates the pancreatic duct cells to secrete sodium bicarbonate. CCK is released in response to the presence of fat in the chyme, which results in the stimulation of pancreatic enzyme secretion (Clark, 2005).

Liver

The liver performs a wide variety of functions and, in fact, is the most important metabolic organ in the body. The only function that will be discussed in this chapter is the role that the liver plays in the digestive process—specifically, in biosynthesis and secretion of bile. Bile is secreted by the liver and is concentrated and stored in the gallbladder between meals. CCK stimulates contraction of the gallbladder, which in turn results in the release of bile, via the common bile duct, into the duodenum. Bile then facilitates both fat digestion, by the emulsification of large fat droplets, and fat absorption, through micellar formation. *Micelles* transport the water-insoluble products of fat digestion to the intestinal wall where they can be absorbed (Sherwood, 2004).

Small Intestine

The small intestine is the site where most digestion and absorption take place. This 6-meter tube extends between the stomach and the large intestine and has three subdivisions: the duodenum, the jejunum, and the ileum. Special anatomical features greatly increase the surface area for absorption—namely, the circular folds of the inner surface of the intestine, villi, and microvilli or brush border. Altogether, the folds, villi, and microvilli increase the surface of the small intestine 600 times more than if the tube were lined by a flat surface (Clark, 2005).

The cells of the brush border contain three types of enzymes:

- Enterokinase activates trypsinogen.
- Disaccharidases complete carbohydrate digestion with the end-product being monosaccharides (e.g., glucose, lactose).
- Aminopeptidases complete protein digestion with the end-product being amino acids.

Very little peristalsis occurs in the small intestine. Instead, motility consists primarily of segmentation that both mixes the nutrients with digestive juices secreted into the small intestine lumen and slowly propels the chyme forward (Clark, 2005).

Large Intestine

The horseshoe-shaped large intestine begins at the end of the ileum and ends at the anus. It consists of the colon, cecum, appendix, and rectum. The large intestine is primarily a drying and storage organ whose major function is the reabsorp-

tion of water. Approximately 500 mL of chyme enter the large intestine from the ileum; of this amount, about 350 mL are absorbed, leaving only about 150 mL to be expelled as feces. No digestion and minimal absorption occur in the large intestine. In addition to water and sodium being absorbed, vitamin K, which is synthesized by bacteria in the lumen of the colon, is absorbed as well (Martini & Bartholomew, 2000).

Organs that help with digestion, but are not part of the digestive tract, include the tongue and the salivary glands.

Tongue

The tongue is composed of voluntary skeletal muscle and is important in guiding food within the mouth during chewing and swallowing. Another important function of the tongue is taste; taste buds are embedded in the surface of the tongue.

Salivary Glands

The salivary glands produce saliva. The most important salivary proteins are the enzyme amylase, which initiates carbohydrate digestion; mucus, which facilitates swallowing by providing lubrication; and lysozyme, an enzyme that destroys bacteria within the mouth (Clark, 2005).

ASSESSMENT OF THE GASTROINTESTINAL SYSTEM

Gastrointestinal complaints are common problems in clinical practice. The first step in the assessment process is a careful and detailed interview. Frequently, the interview will lead you to the underlying disorder. Gastrointestinal symptoms that are commonly reported include indigestion, anorexia, nausea, vomiting, hematemesis, abdominal pain, dysphagia (difficulty swallowing), jaundice, and change in bowel function, including constipation, diarrhea, and bleeding. It is important to focus on descriptive characteristics for each of the patient's symptoms, such as their timing (onset, frequency, duration), their location (**Figure 31-2**), their severity, aggravating or alleviating factors, associated symptoms, and the patient's thoughts on what precipitated or caused the problem (Bickley & Hoekelman, 2003). "How has your appetite been?" may be a good initial question that may lead to identification of problems such as indigestion, nausea and vomiting, anorexia, excessive belching, and changes in the patient's weight. A thorough medical history should include questions regarding previous procedures (both diagnostic and surgical), illnesses, hospitalizations, immunizations (e.g., hepatitis A or B), medications (including prescription, over-the-counter, and herbal remedies), and allergies. A family history of gastrointestinal problems, such as Crohn's disease, may be helpful in the assessment of your patient.

FIGURE 31-2 Four Quadrants of the Abdomen

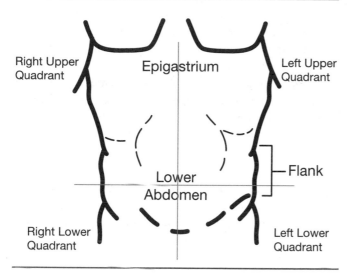

Source: Illustrated by James R. Perron.

Many exogenous factors can contribute to GI symptoms and diseases, including infectious diseases (e.g., hepatitis and travel-acquired intestinal organisms), toxic chemicals, and stress (Bickley & Hoekelman, 2003). It is important to remember that the bowel is often a sounding board for our emotions.

PHYSICAL ASSESSMENT

The physical examination of the abdomen includes inspection, auscultation, percussion, and palpation. The patient's bladder should be emptied prior to the exam. Place the patient in the supine position with a pillow under the head and with the knees slightly bent. Having the patient place arms folded across the chest helps to relax the abdominal muscles. As you examine the abdomen, imagine lines drawn vertically and horizontally through the umbilicus that divide it into four quadrants (see Figure 31-2): right upper quadrant, left upper quadrant, right lower quadrant, and left lower quadrant. Visualize the organs in each quadrant as you proceed with the examination. When referring to any findings, describe them using the appropriate quadrant (Bickley & Hoekelman, 2003).

Begin the examination with a thorough inspection, noting the abdominal contour and symmetry. Abdominal asymmetry may be caused by obesity, organomegaly, or fluid and/or gas distention. Carefully observe the skin for color, texture, turgor, hair distribution, presence of veins, striae, or scars. Silvery-white striae are common findings and are caused by rapid stretching of the skin as occurs with pregnancy; purple-blue striae may be indicative of Cushing's syndrome (Bickley & Hoekelman, 2003). Ecchymosis around the umbilicus

(Cullen's sign) occurs in intraperitoneal hemorrhage. Normal aortic pulsation is frequently visible in the epigastric area (see Figure 31-2).

Auscultation of the abdomen provides information regarding bowel motility. Both percussion and palpation can have an effect on bowel motility; therefore, it is important to auscultate before percussing or palpating the abdomen. Using the stethoscope's diaphragm placed lightly against the patient's skin, listen for bowel sounds in each of the four quadrants. Normal bowel sounds vary, but they generally sound gurgly and occur anywhere from 5 to 30 times per minute. Bowel sounds may be altered in diarrhea, intestinal obstruction, peritonitis, or with laxative use. Using the bell of the stethoscope, listen in the epigastrium and in each of the upper quadrants for bruits. Bruits are vascular sounds that resemble heart murmurs and may be heard when there is turbulent blood flow caused by either constriction or dilation of the blood vessels (Bickley & Hoekelman, 2003). This part of the examination is especially important with hypertensive patients. You may also auscultate over the iliac arteries if you suspect arterial insufficiency in the legs (**Figure 31-3**). Auscultate over the liver and spleen to detect any peritoneal friction rubs that may be present with infection, tumors, or infarcts.

Percussion, or tapping against the patient's skin, helps to assess the amount of fluid or gas in the abdomen, locate and estimate the size of a mass, and estimate both liver and spleen size. To perform percussion, place the distal joint of your middle finger of your nondominant hand on the patient's ab-

FIGURE 31-3 Listening Points for Abdominal Bruits

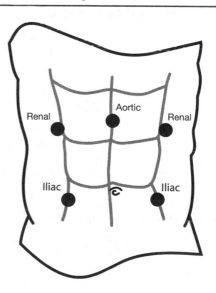

Source: Illustrated by James R. Perron.

domen. Make sure that no other part of your hand is touching the abdomen. With a quick, sharp, bent, relaxed wrist motion, strike your finger with the tip of the middle finger of your dominant hand. With practice, you will discern subtle sound differences: Dullness is a muffled, thud-like sound that is heard over the liver, spleen, or tumors; tympany is a drum-like sound that is heard over gas-filled organs such as the stomach and intestines. Percuss in each quadrant as well as over the liver and spleen. The normal liver is 6 to 12 cm at the right midclavicular line; the normal spleen is less than 7 cm at the left midaxillary line. It is important to note that a full stomach or intestine can cause a dull sound (Bickley & Hoekelman, 2003).

Percussion can also be useful for assessing possible ascites. Because fluid characteristically moves to dependent areas of the abdomen, a patient with ascites most likely will have a tympanic sound with percussion in the mid-abdominal area and a dull sound in the flank areas (Bickley & Hoekelman, 2003). Remember that percussion gives only a gross estimate of the size, location, and presence of fluid. The definitive test for abnormal findings is an abdominal ultrasound.

Palpation, or feeling the abdomen, helps to determine the presence of muscle spasms, fluid, and masses, and assesses any tenderness. Each quadrant is palpated using both light and deep palpation techniques. Note any tenderness, pain, or rigidity. Involuntary rigidity or muscle spasm may indicate peritoneal inflammation. Light palpation is helpful in identifying abdominal tenderness; deeper palpation is useful for assessing organs such as the liver, spleen, and kidneys and detecting masses. Rebound tenderness is associated with peritoneal inflamma-

tion. To assess for rebound tenderness, press your fingers slowly and deeply, and then quickly withdraw your fingers (Bickley & Hoekelman, 2003). Pain that is induced or worsens with quick release is a reliable test for peritoneal inflammation.

Assessment findings can indicate many pathological conditions. Clustering symptoms together can lead the nurse to hypothesize about possible causes of assessment data. **Table 31-1** lists some abnormal findings and possible causes for them.

The following common diagnostic procedures may be useful in assessing gastrointestinal conditions:

* *Barium studies.* This test involves the patient swallowing barium or having a barium enema prior to diagnostic imaging studies. A barium swallow allows diagnosis of inflammatory, neoplastic, and motility disorders and of lesions that cause stenosis or obstruction. Typical indications for barium enemas include symptoms of colon carcinoma, diverticular disease, and inflammatory bowel disease. Use of barium is discouraged because it interferes with other tests being performed later (e.g., colonoscopy or angiogram) (Holzman, Schirmer, & Nasraway, 2005).
* *Flexible sigmoidoscopy.* This direct visualization of the distal colon is used to evaluate rectal bleeding, new-onset or persistent diarrhea or constipation, mass on digital examination, and left lower quadrant abdominal pain and cramping (National Digestive Diseases Information Clearinghouse, 2006).
* *Colonoscopy.* This test is similar to sigmoidoscopy, except that a colonoscopy allows the practitioner to visualize

TABLE 31-1 Abnormal Assessment Data

Data	Possible Cause
Asymmetry in the upper quadrant	Tumor, pancreatic cyst, gastric dilatation
Asymmetry in the lower quadrant	Ovarian tumors, fibroid tumors, pregnancy, bladder distention
Ecchymosis around umbilicus (Cullen's sign)	Intraperitoneal hemorrhage
Jaundice	Altered liver function
Diminished or absent bowel sounds	Postoperative, peritonitis, paralytic ileus, late bowel obstruction
Increased bowel sounds	Diarrhea, gastroenteritis, complete intestinal obstruction, bleeding ulcers
Bruit over vessels	Aneurysm
Friction rub over spleen or liver	Splenic infarct, hepatic tumor
Continuous venous hum over periumbilical	Hepatitic cirrhosis
Dullness percussed over midaxillary line	Enlarged spleen
Pain on palpation	Peritoneal inflammation
Abdominal distention	Trapped air or fluid in the abdomen

Sources: Bickley & Hoekelman, 2003; Bickley & Szilagyi, 2003.

the entire large bowel and not just the sigmoid or lower portion of the colon (Tham & Collins, 2000).

- *Ultrasound.* This test is used to detect gallbladder stones and to evaluate the liver and spleen. A disadvantage of ultrasound is its inability to penetrate gas-filled structures, such as the colon and stomach (Valley & Fly, 2006).
- *Urea breath test.* This test is used to diagnose *Helicobacter pylori* infection of the stomach, the major etiologic factor for patients with active peptic ulcer disease (National Guideline Clearinghouse, 2006).
- *Abdominal paracentesis.* This test is used for diagnosing the cause of ascites. It is also used to remove large amounts of fluid in patients where the increased intra-abdominal pressure (IAP) is causing respiratory distress (Nissl, 2006).

- *Intra-abdominal pressure monitoring.* This test identifies intra-abdominal hypertension through a urinary catheter. Measuring the pressure in the bladder indicates the IAP. Increased IAP leads to respiratory compromise, organ hypoperfusion, and a high mortality rate. Intra-abdominal hypertension has been defined as a pressure reading greater than 20 mm Hg (Brooks, Simpson, Delbridge, Beckingham, & Girling, 2005). At high pressures (> 25 mm Hg) surgical decompression is mandatory (Malbrain, 2005).

SUMMARY

Assessment of the gastrointestinal system can be challenging. It is important to remember that a timely and accurate assessment can help in making the correct diagnosis of the patient's problem and may alter the patient's outcome.

CRITICAL THINKING QUESTIONS

1. Why does a partial gastrectomy frequently lead to pernicious anemia?
2. How is the stomach lining protected from damage from the strong hydrochloric acid secretions? What effect do nonsteroidal anti-inflammatory drugs have on the lining of the stomach?
3. List signs and symptoms that arise when the gastrointestinal system is hypoperfused.
4. Which diagnostic test should be ordered to measure intra-abdominal hypertension?
5. What are the implications for alkalizing the gut with either H_2 blockers or antacids?

Online Resources

Abdominal Compartment Syndrome: www.trauma.org/resus/DCSacs.html

Society of Gastrointestinal Nurses and Associates: www.sgna.org

GI system tutorial: www.le.ac.uk/pathology/teach/va/anatomy/case6/frmst6.html

Digestive System Learning Resources and Animations: www.innerbody.com/image

REFERENCES

Bickley, L. S., & Hoekelman, R. A. (2003). *Bates' guide to examination and history taking* (8th ed.). Philadelphia: Lippincott Williams & Wilkins.

Bickley, L. S., & Szilagyi, P. G. (2003). *Cecil textbook of medicine* (22nd ed.). Philadelphia: Saunders.

Brooks, A. J., Simpson, A., Delbridge, M., Beckingham, I. J., & Girling, K. J. (2005). Validation of direct intraabdominal pressure measurement using a continuous indwelling compartment pressure monitor. *Journal of Trauma-Injury Infection and Critical Care, 58*(4), 830–832.

Clark, R. K. (2005). *Anatomy and physiology: Understanding the human body.* Boston: Jones and Bartlett.

Holzman, N. L., Schirmer, C. M., & Nasraway, S. A. (2005). Gastrointestinal hemorrhage. In M. P. Fink, E. Abraham, J. L. Vincent, & P. M. Kochanek (Eds.), *Textbook of critical care* (5th ed., pp. 973–982). Philadelphia: Saunders.

Malbrain, M. (2005). Incidence of intra-abdominal hypertension in the intensive care unit. *Critical Care Medicine, 33*(9), 2150–2153.

Martini, F. H., & Bartholomew, E. F. (2000). *Essentials of anatomy and physiology* (2nd ed.). Upper Saddle River, NJ: Prentice-Hall.

National Digestive Diseases Information Clearinghouse. (2006). Flexible sigmoidoscopy. Retrieved January 6, 2006, from http://digestive.niddc.nih.gov/ddiseases/pubs/sigmoidoscopy/index.htm

National Guideline Clearinghouse. (2006). Procedure guideline for C-14 urea breath test. Retrieved January 6, 2006, from www.guideline.gov/summary/summary.aspx?doc_id=2947

Nissl, J. (2006). Paracentesis. Retrieved January 6, 2006, from www.webmd.com/hw/brain_nervous_system/hw198220.asp

Sherwood, L. (2004). *Human physiology: From cells to systems* (3rd ed.). Cincinnati, OH: Wadsworth.

Tham, T., & Collins, J. (2000). *Gastrointestinal emergencies.* London: BMJ Books.

Valley, V. T., & Fly, C. A. (2006). Ultrasonography, abdominal. Retrieved January 6, 2006, from www.emedicine.com/emerg/topic621.htm

CHAPTER 32

Gastrointestinal Interventions

Pat Ostergaard   Roberta Kaplow

LEARNING OBJECTIVES

Upon completion of this chapter, the reader will be able to:

1. Explain the indications for GI procedures.

2. Describe the complications associated with a GI procedure.

3. Develop a plan of care for the patient undergoing a GI procedure.

4. Demonstrate appropriate patient teaching prior to a patient undergoing a GI procedure.

5. List optimal outcomes that may be achieved through evidence-based management of patients undergoing GI interventions.

Admissions to the intensive care unit (ICU) with gastrointestinal (GI) problems are most often attributed to bleeding (see Chapter 34). The most common sources are ulcer erosions and/or perforations, Mallory-Weiss syndrome, and varices. Although treatment options for these patients vary, most will require a diagnostic test and/or procedure. This chapter describes specific diagnostic and therapeutic GI procedures that may take place in the ICU or in the treatment of critically ill adults.

GASTRIC LAVAGE

Gastric lavage is the procedure of instilling large volumes of tap water or normal saline into the abdomen by inserting a large-bore tube (e.g., Ewald®, Levine®, Argyl®, or nasogastric tube) through the nose or mouth, down the esophagus, and into the stomach. A topical anesthetic may be sprayed into the back of the throat or placed on the tube before its insertion so as to minimize irritation and gagging as the tube is being placed. Once the fluid is instilled into the abdominal cavity, it is then drained back out by suction or gravity drainage, depending on institutional procedures. This procedure may be intermittent or continuous, depending on the patient's condition.

Frequently, the purpose is to localize the site of upper GI bleeding; evaluate the severity of bleeding; cleanse the stomach of clots; prevent aspiration of clots; or prevent nitrogenous load absorption (from red blood cell death). Less frequently, gastric lavage can be used to remove drugs ingested by overdose. Recently, however, gastric emptying has fallen out of favor in the case of overdose because of complications and the lack of evidence for clinical benefit. Position statements have stated that gastric lavage should be used in restricted settings (Eddleston, Juszczak, & Buckley, 2003). According to one poison control center specialist, gastric lavage is indicated for life-threatening overdose or poisoning. When the ingestion occurred less than one hour previously, lavage is beneficial. Gastric lavage is also used with drugs having a delayed absorption, such as with enteric-coated, long-acting, or sustained-release drugs. Gastric lavage may be beneficial when "handfuls" of drugs have been ingested, when bowel sounds are absent or hypoactive, or when liquid medications or poisons in toxic amounts have been ingested. Data suggest that lavage is only 10% to 60% effective (Blazys, 2000).

Regardless of the purpose of the gastric lavage, extreme caution must be taken if used for patients with esophageal varices or history of recent GI surgeries (Thomas, 2001). Lavage should not be used with patients who have central nervous system depression. Other contraindications include patients at risk for hemorrhage or GI perforation, and patients who have ingested hydrocarbons or corrosive substances.

Complications identified with gastric lavage include esophageal or gastric perforation, endotracheal intubation with lavage tube, aspiration, and hypothermia. The latter complication is more common in elderly patients. In the case of overdose, a common complication of gastric lavage is that substances are forced beyond the pyloric sphincter into the small bowel (Eddleston et al., 2003). Oral, nasal, or pharyngeal injuries may occur during lavage tube insertion. As a consequence, the patient's airway should always be protected during the procedure. Vagal stimulation can cause bradycardia. The use of warm water for lavage decreases the risk of hypothermia (Blazys, 2000).

Patient preparation for gastric lavage will include patient/family education. The patient will be placed on cardiac monitor, automatic blood pressure cuff, oxygen by nasal cannula or mask, and pulse oximeter. An IV line will be started, oral airway inserted, and suction set up; the patient will also be positioned in left lateral or in high Fowler's position. If the patient does not have an intact gag reflex, endotracheal intubation may be necessary. Emergency equipment (e.g., bag-valve-mask, emergency cart, suction equipment) must be at the bedside during the procedure.

The post-procedure assessment by the ICU nurse will include measurement of blood volume loss, vital signs, lab values as ordered, fluid status, cardiac rhythm, and head-to-toe physical assessment. If the purpose of the lavage was to lower toxic levels of an ingested drug, the nurse must also monitor the patient's neurological status. The ICU nurse should monitor for complications such as aspiration, displacement of the tube, and a clogged tube, which may require reinsertion (Thomas, 2001).

ENDOSCOPIC PROCEDURES

Upper GI Endoscopy

An esophagogastroduodenoscopy (EGD) is a procedure performed to evaluate the lining of the esophagus, the stomach, and the upper portion of the duodenum. A thin, flexible, lighted tube with a camera is inserted into the mouth and then advanced into the esophagus. A small instrument may be passed through this scope to take a sample of tissue for biopsy. The primary indication for an upper endoscopy is to view the inner lining of the esophagus, the entire stomach, and approx-

imately five inches of the upper small bowel to identify ulcers and abnormalities (Zuckerman & Lotsoff, 2003). EGD is the diagnostic procedure of choice for all cases of upper GI bleeding (Manning-Dimmitt, Dimmitt, & Wilson, 2005) and is preferred to diagnose stomach cancer (Layke & Lopez, 2004). This procedure is also the best way to evaluate suspected complications of gastroesophageal reflux disease (GERD) (Szarka, DeVault, & Murray, 2001).

Complications of an upper endoscopy are rare but may include esophageal perforation and bleeding. In one study of patients who underwent GI procedures, a small percentage (4.2%) developed a bacteremia after EGD (Nelson, 2003).

Patient preparation for an upper endoscopy entails taking nothing by mouth (NPO) for six hours prior to procedure to decrease the risk for aspiration. An IV catheter will be inserted so that IV sedation can be administered during the procedure (Zuckerman & Lotsoff, 2003). Patients undergoing procedures such as EGD or colonoscopy (discussed later in this chapter) are often anxious. High levels of anxiety may result in more difficult and painful procedures. In one study, patients who listened to music reduced their anxiety score statistically more than patients who did not. Music is a noninvasive nursing intervention that can decrease anxiety before GI procedures (Hayes, Buffum, Lanier, Rodahl, & Sasso, 2003). More information on the use of music therapy can be found in Chapters 3 and 9.

Post procedure, the ICU nurse should monitor vital signs, oxygen saturation, and for return of the gag reflex. Assessment for signs and symptoms of bleeding and respiratory distress should be performed as well. The patient should be positioned with the head of the bed elevated for aspiration precautions until fully awake (Zuckerman & Lotsoff, 2003).

Flexible Sigmoidoscopy

A flexible sigmoidoscopy is an examination of the lining of the rectum and sigmoid colon, and may include evaluation of part of the descending colon (American Medical Association [AMA], 2002). In this procedure, a thin, short, flexible, lighted tube (sigmoidoscope) is inserted into the rectum. This scope transmits an image via a tiny camera to a screen that allows the physician to carefully examine the lining of the large intestines from the rectum to the sigmoid (descending) colon. This tube may also instill air to distend the bowel for better visualization. If a polyp or inflamed tissue is visualized, the physician can insert a tiny instrument into the tube to remove the polyp or take a piece of tissue for biopsy (Kuric, 2004).

Indications for a flexible sigmoidoscopy may include diarrhea, abdominal pain, and constipation. Identification of bleeding and inflammation as well as visualization of abnormal growths and ulcers in the descending colon and rectum are other indications. Diagnosis of irritable bowel syndrome in patients older than age 50 may require flexible sigmoidoscopy or colonoscopy (Hyams, 2001). This test may also detect early signs of cancer. Flexible sigmoidoscopy procedures do not visualize the transverse or ascending colon, however. In extreme cases, flexible sigmoidoscopy can provide an immediate diagnosis of patients with diarrhea who are suspected of having *Clostridium difficile* infection (Schroeder, 2005). Potential complications include bleeding and puncture of the colon.

Patient preparation ideally would include a thorough cleansing of the bowel with enemas and/or laxatives and a clear liquid diet for 12 to 24 hours before the procedure. However, in the ICU, this is not always appropriate.

One study compared three forms of bowel preparation for flexible sigmoidoscopy. In this study, patients were given one of three colon preparations: two Fleet® enemas; magnesium citrate orally the evening before, clear liquid diet, and two bisacodyl (Dulcolax®) suppositories the day of the exam; or magnesium citrate orally the evening before, clear liquid the day of the exam, and two Fleet® enemas one hour before the procedure. Results showed that the magnesium citrate and Fleet® enema preparation were well tolerated and acceptable for 70% of patients (Herman, Shaw, & Loewen, 2001). The use of these preps is based on the evaluation of the ICU patient's condition.

To perform the procedure, the patient is placed on the left side. An IV line is started, oxygen is applied, and baseline vital signs are obtained.

Following the procedure, the patient will be monitored for signs and symptoms of bleeding and possible perforation. Other complications of a flexible sigmoidoscopy that have been reported include pain, infection, vasovagal response, and abdominal distention (AMA, 2002). Nelson (2003) reported a post-flexible sigmoidoscopy bacteremia rate of 0.5%. Vital signs are to be obtained, and oxygen saturations are to be monitored as per institutional protocol (Kuric, 2004).

Colonoscopy

In a colonoscopy, a long, flexible, lighted tube is inserted into the rectum and slowly guided into the colon to permit visualization of the entire colon from the rectum to the lower end of the small intestines. The scope bends to allow the physician to move it around the curves in the bowel. A biopsy can be taken through a tiny instrument passed through the scope. The physician may also pass a laser, heater probe, or electrical probe or inject medication through the scope to stop bleeding. Indications for a colonoscopy include detection of early signs of cancer and diagnosis of the cause of unexplained changes in bowel habits, inflammation, growths, ulcers, and sources of bleeding. Colonoscopy is the diagnostic procedure of choice for acute lower GI bleeding (Manning-Dimmitt et al., 2005). Again, diagnosis of irritable bowel syndrome in patients older than age 50 may require colonoscopy or sigmoidoscopy (Hyams, 2001).

Computerized tomographic (CT) colonography, also called virtual colonoscopy, is an evolving technology being evaluated for colorectal cancer screening. According to the findings of a meta-analysis, its performance has varied widely across studies. The reasons for the variability in findings are poorly defined. Because a CT colonography does not accurately detect polyps smaller than 10 mm, it may not be preferred over colonoscopy. These issues must be resolved before CT colonography can be advocated for generalized screening for colorectal cancer (Mulhall, Veerappan, & Jackson, 2005; Zakowski, Seibert, & VanEyck, 2004). At present, CT colonography may be useful in patients with obstructing tumors and in patients in whom colonoscopy is incomplete for other reasons (Cotton et al., 2004).

Preparation for a colonoscopy usually involves three days of a clear liquid diet and a laxative the night before the procedure. The patient is positioned on the left side. An IV line is started, oxygen is applied, and baseline vital signs are obtained.

As with patients who undergo EGD, patients who undergo colonoscopy may have high levels of anxiety. In one study, although conducted on patients having colonoscopy as an ambulatory procedure, listening to music during the procedure decreased the level of anxiety without other anxiolytic methods (Andrada et al., 2004).

Post-procedure assessment includes monitoring for signs and symptoms of bleeding/hemorrhage and possible perforation. Vital signs are obtained, and oxygen saturation is monitored as per institutional protocol (Gastroenterology Consultants Ltd, 2005). A 2.2% bacteremia rate was reported in one study of patients who underwent colonoscopy (Nelson, 2003). Aspiration should be observed for, because 43% of patients in one recent study who received sedation or topical anesthesia developed respiratory complications (Livett, 2005).

Scleral Endoscopic Therapy

Sclerotherapy entails the direct injection of a sclerosing agent into a visible vein. The solution irritates, dehydrates, changes surface tension, or destroys the endothelial cells to produce initially a small thrombosis and then permanent fibrosis of the vein (Marting, 2000). A fiber-optic endoscope is passed through the esophagus, through the stomach, and into the duodenum. A sclerosing agent may then be injected through a special port on the scope into the vessel that is bleeding. This procedure should be done using moderate sedation. Indications for this procedure are to locate the source of bleeding and to control or prevent bleeding from varices, gastric ulcers, or duodenal ulcers (Vlavianos & Westaby, 2001).

Emergency sclerotherapy is widely used as a first-line therapy for variceal bleeding in cirrhosis, although pharmacological treatment with vasopressors may stop bleeding in the majority of patients. Agents used in one extensive literature review included vasopressin (Pitressin®), terlipressin (Novapressin®), somatostatin (Aminopan®), and octreotide (Sandostatin®) (D'Amico, Pagliaro, Pietrosi, & Tarantino, 2005). Results from one study suggested that prophylactic sclerotherapy for esophageal varices might be more effective in prolonging long-term survival of patients with liver cirrhosis in the absence of hepatocellular carcinoma, compared with emergency sclerotherapy (Ogusu et al., 2003).

Possible complications with scleral endoscopic therapy include aspiration, perforation of esophagus, atelectasis, bradyarrhythmias, respiratory depression (due to sedation), and sepsis. The bacteremia rate found in one study of patients who underwent scleral endoscopic therapy was 15.4% (Nelson, 2003).

To prepare the patient for scleral endoscopy, the ICU nurse will apply oxygen, pulse oximetry, and a blood pressure cuff and connect the patient to a cardiac monitor. Baseline vital signs and IV access will be obtained. Suction will be set up. Atropine is kept at the bedside in the event of vagal stimulation.

Post-procedure assessment will include vital signs, evaluation of airway and respiratory status, and return of the gag reflex. The ICU nurse will monitor for dysrhythmias and interpret coagulation lab study results. The patient is positioned on the left side with the head elevated until the cough, gag, and swallow reflexes return (Vlavianos & Westaby, 2001).

Variceal Banding

Variceal banding is an endoscopic procedure during which small elastic "O" rings are placed around varices to cause strangulation and sloughing of tissue. This tissue is then replaced by fibrous tissue (Zuckerman & Lotsoff, 2003). Variceal banding is the treatment of choice for bleeding varices. A 50% reduction in rebleeding has been reported with this procedure (Lin, Bilir, & Powis, 2000; Vlavianos & Westaby, 2001). Pre- and post-procedure patient care is the same as for patients who receive scleral endoscopic therapy.

Endoscopic Retrograde Cholangiopancreatography

Endoscopic retrograde cholangiopancreatography (ERCP) combines the use of a scope and radiographs to visualize the pancreatic and bile ducts. The endoscope is passed into the stomach and duodenum (as with the EGD) to visualize the lining of these organs. The scope is passed until it reaches the area of the duodenum where the biliary tree and pancreas open into the duo-

denum. A small tube is placed through the scope, and dye is injected to the bile duct. X-rays are taken immediately to identify obstructions by gallstones or narrowing of the bile ducts. An instrument can be inserted into the scope to remove obstructions and take tissue for a biopsy (Andriulli et al., 2003).

The primary indications for ERCP are to diagnose chronic pancreatitis and conditions affecting the gallbladder and bile ducts; other conditions of the liver and pancreas may be detected as well. ERCP is the gold standard for treatment of obstructive jaundice, placement of biliary stents, and drainage of pseudocysts. However, a relatively new technique—therapeutic ultrasonography—has proven effective in cases where ERCP has been unsuccessful (Cipolletta, Bianco, Rotondano, & Marmo, 2000; Giovannini, 2004).

Pancreatitis is the most frequent complication of ERCP. The incidence of clinically significant pancreatitis following an ERCP ranges from 1% to 13.5% (Pande & Thuluvath, 2003). Administration of pharmacological agents to prevent or limit this complication has been the topic of several recent studies. Other, less frequent complications include infection, bleeding, and perforation of the duodenum (Andriulli et al., 2003; Demols & Deviere, 2003; Testoni, 2004). The bacteremia rate in one study of patients who underwent ERCP was 11% (Nelson, 2003).

In a study of 45 patients, with a mean age of 58 years, who underwent ERCP, preoperative education and explanation of how to communicate during the procedure enhanced patient cooperation and patient satisfaction (Ratanalert, Soontrapornchai, & Ovartlarnporn, 2003). The nurse should expect the patient to exhibit irritability, hyperexcitability, and poor cooperation during an ERCP. Educating the patient before the procedure takes place can help to keep the patient relaxed and self-confident during the ERCP. Information giving should focus on details of the procedure and feelings such as discomfort or pain that might occur during the procedure (Ratanalert et al., 2003).

SURGICAL PROCEDURES

Percutaneous Transjugular Intrahepatic Portosystemic Shunt

Percutaneous transjugular intrahepatic portosystemic shunt (TIPS) is the procedure of choice when surgery is indicated for varices. This interventional treatment results in decompression of the portal system (Ochs, 2005). The purpose of a TIPS is to decompress the portal venous system and therefore prevent rebleeding from varices or stop or reduce the formation of ascites (Boyer & Haskal, 2005). It is also useful in the treatment of complications of portal hypertension, bleeding varices, and ascites. TIPS is an accepted procedure indicated for patients who do not respond to sclerotherapy, variceal banding, or pharmacologic intervention, or who have problematic ascites (Brigham, 1998). The procedure involves placement of a metal stent to create an opening in the intrahepatic tract. Pre-procedure laboratory tests should include serum electrolytes, blood count, coagulation profile, liver function, and renal function (Boyer & Haskal, 2005).

Potential complications include puncture of the hepatic artery or biliary tree, rupture of the portal vein or liver capsule, or stent thrombosis or migration (Maciel et al., 2003). Other reported disadvantages of TIPS include the induction of hepatic encephalopathy, infection, renal failure, migration into the portal vein or right atrium, and shunt dysfunction (Siewert, Salzmann, Purucker, Schurmann, & Matern, 2005). Complications of TIPS that have been reported include thrombosis, occlusion/stenosis, transcapsular puncture, intraperitoneal bleed, hepatic infarction, fistulae, sepsis, infection, hemolysis, encephalopathy, and stent migration or placement in the inferior vena cava (Boyer & Haskal, 2005).

Ten percent of patients with cirrhosis develop refractory ascites, which has significant morbidity and a one-year survival of less than 50%. Patients with refractory ascites may benefit from TIPS. An extensive literature review was conducted to compare TIPS and paracentesis in these patients with regard to overall short- and long-term survival, effectiveness, and complications. Results suggested that TIPS removed ascites more effectively than did paracentesis (discussed later in this chapter). After one year, the beneficial effects of TIPS on ascites were still evident. Mortality, GI bleeding, septicemia/infection, acute renal failure, and disseminated intravascular coagulation did not differ significantly between the two groups. However, hepatic encephalopathy occurred significantly more often in the TIPS group (Saab, Nieto, Ly, & Runyon, 2005).

A portal caval shunt, although rarely done, may be considered for some patients. This surgical procedure involves connecting the portal vein to the inferior vena cava in an attempt to decrease portal pressure. Recipients of liver transplant often have portal caval shunts for portal hypertension (Nosaka et al., 2003). Potential complications of this procedure include encephalopathy and formation of peptic ulcers. Postoperatively, the nurse must assess carefully for signs and symptoms of encephalopathy, septic shock, renal failure, bleeding, and intravascular hemolysis (Bernard, Hagihara, Burke, & Kugelmas, 2001).

Other Procedures

Esophagogastric tamponade tubes may be inserted to provide direct pressure as a temporary means of controlling active bleeding from gastric or esophageal varices (Day, 2001). The most common types of esophagogastric tubes are listed in **Table 32-1**.

Emergency equipment listed in **Table 32-2** must be available at the bedside of any patient being treated with an esophagogastric tamponade tube. Maximum time of therapy is 36 hours for the esophageal balloon and 72 hours for the gastric balloon (Day, 2001).

Patient care entails positioning the patient in high Fowler's position (if alert) or on the left side (if unconscious). Provision of oral care every two hours and frequent oral suctioning are important. Nares care should be provided if the patient is nasally intubated. Monitoring for airway patency and signs of distress (e.g., tachypnea, stridor, cough) is essential. Gastric and esophageal output should be monitored and measured. Institutional policy should be followed for specific care of each port on the tube.

Tamponade for treatment of esophageal varices may be accompanied by several complications, some of which may be life-threatening. Therefore, extreme caution should be used when performing the insertion of an esophagogastric tamponade tube. While hemostasis is not achievable by tamponade in 8% to 50% of patients, and 50% of the patients experience rebleeding, use of tamponade may achieve stabilization of a patient so that sclerotherapy or surgery becomes a treatment option (Greenwald, 2004).

LIVER BIOPSY

A liver biopsy is a procedure that extracts liver tissue to be sent for analysis by a pathologist. Liver biopsy, while formerly used only for diagnostic purposes, has additional purposes such as assessment of disease progression, response to therapy, and diagnosis of transplant rejection (Looi, 2005). Several methods are used to perform a liver biopsy:

TABLE 32-1 Common Esophagogastric Tubes

Tube	Port
Minnesota (four lumen)	Esophageal and gastric balloon
	Esophageal and gastric lavage/suction
Sengstaken-Blakemore tube (three lumen)	Gastric and esophageal balloon
	Gastric suction/lavage

Source: Day, 2001.

TABLE 32-2 Required Equipment at Patient Bedside for Esophagogastric Tamponade Tube

Equipment	Rationale
Sphygmomanometer	To measure balloon pressures
Four rubber-tipped clamps	For clamping balloon ports
Adhesive tape	For securing tubes
Two suction setups	One for esophageal, one for gastric
Nasogastric tubes	One for Minnesota, two for Sengstaken-Blakemore
Normal saline	For irrigation
Emergency intubation equipment	To manage airway during emergency
Bite block	To prevent biting on tube
Atropine	To manage vagal bradycardias
Scissors	To cut tubes in emergency for airway management

Source: Day, 2001.

- *Percutaneous liver biopsy.* The skin is numbed with a local anesthetic where a small incision may or may not be made, depending on type of needle used. A special needle is then passed through the skin into the liver, at an intercostal space anterior to the mid-axillary line. The liver is located by percussion and tapping by the physician.
- *Percutaneous image-guided liver biopsy.* The needle insertion is guided by CT scan or ultrasound images.
- *Laparoscopic liver biopsy.* A small incision is made into the abdomen and a laparoscope is inserted. A laparoscope is a telescope that magnifies the objects it sees and sends images to a monitor. The physician watches the monitor and uses instruments to remove the sample. Ultrasound may be used in conjunction with the laparoscope.
- *Transvenous biopsy.* A catheter is inserted into the right internal jugular vein, through the right atrium, and into the superior vena cava and hepatic vein; it is then guided into the liver. A biopsy needle is inserted into the catheter and into the liver. This procedure may be used when the patient has clotting problems or ascites (Maciel et al., 2003; National Digestive Disease Information Clearinghouse [NDDIC], 2005).
- *Open surgical liver biopsy.* This method is rarely used except as a part of another surgical procedure. An aspirating needle or a wedge section will be done. Indications for this procedure include diagnosing and staging disease of the liver (Spycher, Zimmerman, & Reichen, 2001).

In preparation for a liver biopsy, the patient may not take aspirin, aspirin-containing products, ibuprofen, or anticoagulants. The patient should be NPO for eight hours. IV fluids, sedative drugs, pain medication, antibiotics, antiemetics, and supplemental oxygen will be provided. The patient must be instructed to lie completely still and maintain expiration during the procedure.

Post-procedure care entails keeping the patient on the right side for 1 to 2 hours (or as directed by the physician), bedrest for 8 to 12 hours, assessment and treatment of pain and any complications, and monitoring of vital signs, urinary output, intake and output, and hemoglobin and hematocrit. In a study of positioning of patients following liver biopsy, it was found that right-sided and supine positioning were best tolerated (Hyun & Beutel, 2005).

Potential complications of liver biopsy include infection, fever, pain, swelling, drainage, redness at the insertion site, shortness of breath, pneumothorax, puncture of gallbladder, bleeding, abdominal swelling or bloating, worsening abdominal pain, and nausea or vomiting. Pain may be referred to the shoulder. Bleeding may occur up to 15 days post-procedure (NDDIC, 2005).

PARACENTESIS

During a paracentesis, a needle is inserted through the abdominal wall and into the peritoneum to remove fluid for diagnostic or therapeutic purposes. Indications include evaluation of an abdominal injury; removal of ascites, which is causing difficulty breathing, pain, or affecting the function of the kidneys or bowel; prevention of peritoneal rupture; and diagnosis of infections in the peritoneal fluid or certain types of cancer (Huether, 2002).

Complications of paracentesis include bowel perforation, bladder perforation, bleeding, intravascular volume loss, infection at the insertion site, hypotension, and needle puncture of the abdominal blood vessels (Rushing, 2005).

Patient preparation for a paracentesis includes obtaining baseline assessment of fluid and electrolyte status. A urinary catheter is inserted if patients are unable to empty their bladder. Abdominal girth is measured. The patient is positioned supine or may tilt toward the side of the procedure. Prior to the procedure, the patient should be assessed for any bleeding or problems with clotting. A patent IV is needed. During and following the procedure, the ICU nurse should observe for signs and symptoms that may indicate hypovolemia, such as pallor, diaphoresis, hypotension, and tachycardia (Rushing, 2005).

Post-procedure care entails measurement of abdominal girth so that a pre-post measurement is documented. Girth measurement is best performed by the same person to ensure consistency. The amount of fluid removed is documented, as well as color and clarity of the fluid. Intake and output are monitored. The insertion site is assessed for drainage or signs of infection. The patient is assessed for hematuria, hypotension, fever, severe abdominal pain, bleeding from the needle insertion site, change in bowel sounds, and tachycardia (Huether, 2002; Rushing, 2005).

PATIENT OUTCOMES

Nurses can help ensure attainment of optimal patient outcomes such as those listed in **Box 32-1** for patients undergoing GI interventions.

SUMMARY

The GI tract is the largest endocrine system of the body and has a complex relationship with the accessory organs (pancreas, liver, and gallbladder) of the body. Each component both affects and depends on the others. ICU nurses must be familiar with the physiology of this system so that they can understand the multitude of GI problems the critically ill patient faces. Included in this knowledge are the many diagnostic and therapeutic exams the critically ill patient may undergo. The nurse is required to understand and support the patient through these procedures to ensure the best possible outcome for each patient.

Box 32-1
Optimal Patient Outcomes

- Airway remains patent
- Physical comfort in expected range
- Hemoglobin and hematocrit in expected range
- Restoration of gag reflex (post-procedure)
- Knowledge of follow-up care
- Return of vital signs to pre-procedure level

CASE STUDY

S.G. is a 57-year-old patient with a history of alcoholism, mild cirrhosis, and hypertension. He was admitted to the ICU from the Emergency Department with mental status changes, abdominal distention, and abdominal pain.

His wife reports that he has been more sleepy than usual over the past few days and his "beer belly" has been getting bigger. She reported that the patient said he had been "putting on a few pounds" and was going to cut down to only two six-packs per day. Today, the patient was barely arousable, so she called for an ambulance to bring him to the hospital.

The patient has no significant surgical history. His wife denies use of tobacco or recreational drugs.

S.G was admitted to the ICU. Upon admission physical exam, the following observations were noted: stuporous, but responsive to painful stimuli; makes purposeful movements; PERL; sclera non-icteric. The patient was intubated for airway control and placed on a T-piece with 40% oxygen. The abdominal exam suggested the presence of ascites.

Vital signs: B/P 92/60; T 37.2°C; HR 106; RR 28

General: slightly jaundiced

HEENT: sclera non-icteric

Neurological: stuporous, but responsive to painful stimuli, made purposeful movements, PERL and 3 mm dilated

Heart: NSR on cardiac monitor with no ectopy; no murmurs, rubs, or gallops

Lungs: coarse breath sounds, diminished at bases, decreased chest excursion

Abdomen: distended with ascites; liver and spleen were not palpable

Laboratory Data upon ICU Admission

Na 137 mEq/L

K 5.3 mEq/L

Cl 97 mEq/L

CO_2 11 mEq/L

Glucose 198 mg/dL

BUN 31 mg/dL

Creatinine 2.1 mg/dL

pH 7.32

$PaCO_2$ 18 mm Hg

PaO_2 81 mm Hg

SaO_2 91%

HCO_3 16 mEq/L

Serum lactate 9.4 mg/dL

AST 522 IU/L

ALT 178 IU/L

Total bilirubin 9.8 mg/dL

PT 29.8 sec

PTT 92.3 sec

INR 5.8

Total protein 4.5 Gm/dL

Albumin 1.9 Gm/dL

Ammonia 147 μmol/L

WBC 12.8/mm^3

Hgb 9.7 Gm/dL

Hct 28.9%

Platelets 177 $\times 10^3$

S.G. was started on lactulose (Cephulac®) via nasogastric tube. A paracentesis was performed, and 500 mL of fluid were removed. Fluid removal was stopped at that point because S.G.'s chest expansion increased and SpO_2 increased to 95%.

CRITICAL THINKING QUESTIONS

1. What is the most likely cause of this patient's ascites and liver dysfunction?

2. Why were only 500 mL of ascitic fluid removed?

3. What complications should the ICU nurse assess for after paracentesis?

4. What signs and symptoms would you anticipate assessing if the patient sustained a bowel perforation from the paracentesis?

5. Which disciplines should be consulted to work with this client?

6. What type of issues may require you to act as an advocate or moral agent for this patient?

7. How will you implement your role as a facilitator of learning for this patient?

8. Use the form to write up a plan of care for one client requiring a GI procedure in the clinical setting. Rate the patient as a level 1, 3, or 5 on each characteristic. Identify the level of nurse characteristics needed in the care of this patient.

9. Take one patient outcome and list evidence-based interventions for this patient.

Using the Synergy Model to Develop a Plan of Care

	Patient Characteristics	Level (1, 3, 5)	Subjective and Objective Data	Evidence-based Interventions	Outcomes
SYNERGY MODEL	Resiliency				
	Vulnerability				
	Stability				
	Complexity				
	Resource availability				
	Participation in care				
	Participation in decision making				
	Predictability				

Online Resources

The Atlas of Gastrointestinal Endoscopy: www.endoatlas.com

Practice guideline for the creation of a transjugular intrahepatic portosystemic shunt: www.acr.org/s_acr/bin.asp?CID=1076& DID=12295&DOC=FILE.PDF

National Digestive Disease Information Clearinghouse: http://digestive.niddk.nih.gov/diseases/pubs/liverbiopsy

Society of Gastroenterology Nurses and Associates: www.sgna.org

REFERENCES

American Medical Association (AMA). (2002). *Current procedural terminology: CPT 2002.* Chicago: AMA Press.

Andrada, M. J., Vidal, A. A., Aguilar-Tablada, T. C., Reina, I. G., Silva, L., Guinaldo, A. R., et al. (2004). Anxiety during the performance of colonoscopies: Modification using music therapy. *European Journal of Gastroenterology and Hepatology, 16*(12), 1381–1386.

Andriulli, A., Caruso, N., Quitadamo, M., Forlano, R., Gioacchino, L., Spirito, F., et al. (2003). Antisecretory vs. antiproteasic drugs in the prevention of post-ERCP pancreatitis: The evidence-based medicine derived from a meta-analysis study. *Journal of the Pancreas, 4*(1), 41–48.

Bernard, A. C., Hagihara, P. F., Burke, V. J., & Kugelmas, M. (2001). Endoscopic localization and management of colonic bleeding in patients with portal hypertension. *Surgical Laparoscopy, Endoscopy and Percutaneous Techniques, 11*(3), 195–198.

Blazys, D. (2000). Use of lavage in treating overdose. *Journal of Emergency Nursing, 26*(4), 343–344.

Boyer, T. D., & Haskal, Z. J. (2005). American Association for the Study of Liver Diseases practice guidelines: The role of transjugular intrahepatic portosystemic shunt creation in the management of portal hypertension. *Journal of Vascular and Interventional Radiology, 16*(5), 615–629.

Brigham, L. E. (1998). Transjugular intrahepatic portosystemic shunt (TIPS). *Gastroenterology Nursing, 21*(6), 243–246.

Cipolletta, L., Bianco, M. A., Rotondano, G., & Marmo, R. (2000). Pancreatic head mass: What can be done? Diagnosis: ERCP and EUS. *Journal of the Pancreas, 1*(3), 108–110.

Cotton, P. B., Durkalski, V. L., Pineau, B. C., Palesch, Y. Y., Mauldin, P. D., Hoffman, B., et al. (2004). Computed tomographic colonography (virtual colonoscopy): A multicenter comparison with standard colonoscopy for detection of colorectal neoplasia. *Journal of the American Medical Association, 291*(14), 1713–1719.

D'Amico, G., Pagliaro, L. L., Pietrosi, G. G., & Tarantino, I. I. (2005). Emergency sclerotherapy versus medical interventions for bleeding oesophageal varices in cirrhotic patients. *The Cochrane Library (Oxford), 3* (ID #CD002233).

Day, M. W. (2001). Esophagogastric tamponade tube. In D. Lynn-McHale & K. Carlson (Eds.), *AACN procedure manual for critical care* (4th ed., pp. 655–663). Philadelphia: Saunders.

Demols, A., & Deviere, J. (2003). New frontiers in the pharmacological prevention of post-ERCP pancreatitis: The cytokines. *Journal of the Pancreas, 4*(1), 49–57.

Eddleston, M., Juszczak, E., & Buckley, N. (2003). Does gastric lavage really push poisons beyond the pylorus? A systematic review of the evidence. *Annals of Emergency Surgery, 42*(3), 359–364.

Gastroenterology Consultants, Ltd. (2005). Gastroenterology Consultants. Retrieved October 21, 2005, from www.giconsultant.com/gastro-desc.asp

Giovannini, M. (2004). Therapeutic ultrasonography in pancreatic malignancy. Is the ERCP passe? *Journal of the Pancreas, 5*(4), 304–307.

Greenwald, B. (2004). The Minnesota tube: Its use and care in bleeding esophageal and gastric varices. *Gastroenterology Nursing, 27*(5), 212–219.

Hayes, A., Buffum, M., Lanier, E., Rodahl, E., & Sasso, C. (2003). A music intervention to reduce anxiety prior to gastrointestinal procedures. *Gastroenterology Nursing, 26*(4), 145–149.

Herman, M., Shaw, M., & Loewen, B. (2001). Comparison of three forms of bowel preparations for screening flexible sigmoidoscopy. *Gastroenterology Nursing, 24*(4), 178–181.

Huether, S. (2002). Alteration in digestive functions. In K. McCance & S. Huether (Eds.), *Pathophysiology: The biological basis for disease in adults and children* (4th ed., pp. 1261–1298). St. Louis, MO: Mosby.

Hyams, J. S. (2001). Diarrhea/constipation/pain: When is it irritable bowel syndrome? *Consultant, 41*(8), 1089–1091.

Hyun, C. B., & Beutel, V. J. (2005). Prospective randomized trial of post-liver biopsy recovery positions: Does positioning really matter? *Journal of Clinical Gastroenterology, 39*(4), 328–332.

Kuric, J. (2004). Gastrointestinal tract bleeding. In S. Melander (Ed.), *Case studies in critical care nursing* (3rd ed., pp. 256–264). Philadelphia: Saunders.

Layke, J. C., & Lopez, P. P. (2004). Gastric cancer: Diagnosis and treatment options. *American Family Physician, 69*(5), 1133–1140, 1145–1146.

Lin, T. C., Bilir, M., & Powis, M. (2000). Endoscopic placement of Sengstaken-Blakemore tube. *Journal of Clinical Gastroenterology, 3*(1), 29–32.

Livett, H. (2005). Pulmonary aspiration related to conscious sedation in endoscopy. *Gastrointestinal Nursing, 3*(6), 33–39.

Looi, L. M. (2005). Hepatobiliary practical: How to get the best out of a liver biopsy. *Medical Journal of Malaysia, 60*(Suppl. B), 144–145.

Maciel, A., Marchiori, E., Silva De Barros, S., Cerski, T., Tarasconi, D., & Ilha, D. (2003). Transjugular liver biopsy: Histological diagnosis success comparing the trucut to the modified aspiration Ross needle. Retrieved October 14, 2005, from www.scielo.br/scielo.php?script=sci-arttext&pid=S0004-28032003000200004

Manning-Dimmitt, L. L., Dimmitt, S. G., & Wilson, G. R. (2005). Diagnosis of gastrointestinal bleeding in adults. *American Family Physician, 71*(7), 1339–1346.

Marting, B. (2000). Continuing education. Understanding sclerotherapy. *Plastic Surgical Nursing, 20*(4), 209–215, 229.

Mulhall, B. P., Veerappan, G. R., & Jackson, J. L. (2005). Meta-analysis: Computed tomographic colonography. *Annals of Internal Medicine, 142*(8), 635–650.

National Digestive Disease Information Clearinghouse. (2005). Retrieved October 30, 2005, from http://digestive.niddk.nih.gov/diseases/pubs/liverbiopsy

Nelson, D. B. (2003). Infection control during gastrointestinal endoscopy. *Journal of Laboratory and Clinical Medicine, 141*(3), 159–167.

Nosaka, T., Teramoto, K., Tanaka, Y., Igari, T., Takamatsu, S., Kawamura, T., et al. (2003). Varicose bleeding after liver transplantation in a patient with severe portosystemic shunts. *Journal of Gastroenterology, 38*(7), 700–703.

Ochs, A. (2005). Transjugular intrahepatic portosystemic shunt. *Digestive Diseases, 23*(1), 56–64.

Ogusu, T., Iwakiri, R., Sakata, H., Matsunaga, K., Shimoda, R., Oda, K., et al. (2003). Endoscopic injection sclerotherapy for esophageal varices in cirrhotic patients without hepatocellular carcinoma: A comparison of longterm survival between prophylactic therapy and emergency therapy. *Journal of Gastroenterology, 38*(4), 361–364.

Pande, H., & Thuluvath, P. J. (2003). Pharmacological prevention of post-endoscopic retrograde cholangiopancreatography pancreatitis. *Drugs, 63*(17), 1799–1812.

Ratanalert, S., Soontrapornchai, P., & Ovartlarnporn, B. (2003). Preoperative education improves quality of patient care for endoscopic retrograde cholangiopancreatography. *Gastroenterology Nursing, 26*(1), 21–25.

Rushing, J. (2005). Protect your patient during abdominal paracentesis. *Nursing, 35*(8), 14.

Saab, S., Nieto, J. M., Ly, D., & Runyon, B. A. (2005). TIPS versus paracentesis for cirrhotic patients with refractory ascites. *Cochrane Database of Systematic Reviews, 3* (CD004889).

Schroeder, M. S. (2005). *Clostridium difficile*–associated diarrhea. *American Family Physician, 71*(5), 921–928.

Siewert, E., Salzmann, J., Purucker, E., Schurmann, K., & Matern, S. (2005). Recurrent thrombotic occlusion of a transjugular intrahepatic portosystemic stent-shunt due to activated protein C resistance. *World Journal of Gastroenterology, 11*(32), 5064–5067.

Spycher, C., Zimmerman, A., & Reichen, J. (2001). The diagnostic value of liver biopsy. Retrieved October 14, 2005, from www.biomedcentral.com/1471-230x/1/12

Szarka, L. A., DeVault, K. R., & Murray, J. A. (2001). Diagnosing gastroesophageal reflux disease. *Mayo Clinic Proceedings, 76*(1), 97–101.

Testoni, P. A. (2004). Pharmacological prevention of post-ERCP pancreatitis: The facts and the fiction. *Journal of the Pancreas, 5*(4), 171–178.

Thomas, R. H. (2001). Gastric lavage in hemorrhage and in overdose. In D. Lynn-McHale & K. Carlson (Eds.), *AACN procedure manual for critical care* (4th ed., pp. 664–673). Philadelphia: Saunders.

Vlavianos, P., & Westaby, D. (2001). Management of acute variceal haemorrhage. *European Journal of Gastroenterology and Hepatology, 13*(4), 335–342.

White, A. (2004). Acute pancreatitis. In S. Melander (Ed.), *Case studies in critical care nursing* (3rd ed., pp. 265–284). Philadelphia: Saunders.

Zakowski, L., Seibert, C., & VanEyck, S. (2004). Evidence-based medicine: Answering questions of diagnosis. *Clinical Medicine and Research, 2*(1), 63–69.

Zuckerman, G. R., & Lotsoff, D. S. (2003). Upper and lower gastrointestinal bleeding: Principles of diagnosis and management. In R. S. Irwin, J. M. Rippe, & H. Goodgeart (Eds.), *Irwin & Rippe's intensive care medicine* (5th ed., pp. 1089–1092). Philadelphia: Lippincott Williams & Wilkins.

CHAPTER 33

Nutrition Concepts for Clinical Practice in the Critically Ill Adult

Linda DeStefano

LEARNING OBJECTIVES

Upon completion of this chapter, the reader will be able to:

1. Describe methods to evaluate the nutritional status and metabolic needs of critically ill adults.

2. Describe the importance of timely initiation of nutritional support.

3. Discuss how to select the most appropriate method of delivery of nutrition.

4. List potential risks with providing nutritional support and relative prevention strategies.

5. Describe patient safety issues related to administration of various types of nutritional support.

6. List optimal patient outcomes that may be achieved through evidence-based management of nutrition.

Nutrition is a key component of health maintenance, preservation, and restoration. Contrary to outdated beliefs that many hospitalized patients are "too sick to be fed," we now know that appropriate and timely nutritional interventions can improve patient recovery and survival, decrease complication rates, and decrease costs. Many patients who are critically ill are unable to take food orally for various reasons, indicating a need for specialized nutritional support. In this situation, strong evidence supports using enteral—rather than parenteral—feeding in absence of any true contraindication. This preference is reflected in published guidelines from leading national organizations such as the American Society of Parenteral and Enteral Nutrition (ASPEN), the American College of Chest Physicians, the British Society of Gastroenterology, and Canadian Clinical Practice Guidelines. The rationale and benefits favoring enteral over parenteral nutrition will be addressed in this chapter, along with other evidence-based best practice issues related to safe delivery and providing optimal nutritional support to the hospitalized/critically ill patient.

REVIEW OF THE LITERATURE

The incidence of malnutrition in critically ill patients is extremely high. Rates are reported to be 25% to 50% on admission, and an additional 25% to 30% of patients may develop malnutrition during their hospital stay (Barton, 2004). Malnutrition can have a cascade of negative effects on patient outcomes. An increasing nutrition deficit during a long intensive care unit (ICU) stay is associated with increased morbidity (Fung, 2000).

There are as many definitions of malnutrition as there are sources for it. Many patients enter the hospital in a malnourished state or develop it from starvation resulting in protein and/or calorie malnutrition, specific nutrient deficiencies, or hypermetabolism resulting from a disease process and the extreme catabolic state of major illness. Regardless of the cause of the malnutrition, the goal upon admission is to develop a plan of care focused on achieving and maintaining anabolic status.

STARVATION VERSUS STRESS HYPERMETABOLISM

Starvation develops when nutrient or caloric intake is inadequate to meet demands; it is characterized by a specific adaptive response aimed at *preserving lean body mass*.

Stress hypermetabolism is the metabolic response to critical illness, which is usually associated with some degree of perfusion deficit (shock) and resultant microcirculatory injury. Also referred to as the "injury stress response," stress hypermetabolism differs from chronic starvation but can also lead to malnutrition and breakdown of lean body mass for energy. Critically ill patients are at risk for a combination of starvation and physiologic stress due to nothing by mouth (NPO) orders, decreased intake, and hypermetabolism resulting from injury, burns, trauma, major surgery, sepsis, or other illness. The profound effect of the stress response heightens the metabolic rate, which in turn leads to increased oxygen consumption and neurohumoral activation. This central nervous system–mediated endocrine response produces an increase in circulating counterregulatory hormones such as catecholamines, glucocorticoids and mineralcorticoids (e.g., cortisol and aldosterone), and glucagon, among others. Inflammatory mediators such as interleukins may be involved in this process, though the exact mechanisms involved remain poorly understood.

The injury stress response can vary in severity, depending on the diagnosis or degree of insult to the patient. Some severe burn patients, for example, may double their energy consumption and metabolic demand as a result of the injury stress response, creating vicious cycles of glucose storage depletion leading to breakdown of lean body mass for energy production. Because of this process (which is known as catabolism), the patient with severe injury stress response will require higher amounts of protein intake in an effort to minimize erosion of lean body mass and mobilization of valuable muscle protein. Despite efforts to provide protein intake and keep the patient in nitrogen balance, we are usually not able to control this protein turnover. Thus muscle wasting and depletion of serum proteins, such as albumin, continue to occur.

Many vital organs are involved in the process of muscle breakdown. Combined protein and calorie deficiencies may result in delayed weaning from mechanical ventilation, undesirable structural effects on the heart (among other detriments to major body organ functions), and compromise of the immune system. Wound healing is also impaired, which predisposes the patient to infection, increased length of hospital stay, and requirement of a higher level of care. Providing optimal nutrition support can be a complex process, and clinical education for the specialized needs of the hospitalized patient population is frequently inadequate. Furthermore, the failure to follow standardized guidelines may be another reason patients receive less than optimal nutrition therapy. In 2002, ASPEN published evidence-based guidelines and recommendations for the administration of specialized nutrition support (ASPEN, 2002a, 2002b).

Further challenges may emerge in the metabolically stressed patient or the critically ill patient as we attempt to determine when to begin feeding, what type of nutrition, and how to deliver nutrition. Following a comprehensive patient assessment, the goal should be to select the safest, most physiologic, cost-effective method of delivery. A multidisciplinary approach including collaboration with dietitians and nutrition support specialists is the key to achieving optimal patient outcomes.

BEST PRACTICES

Patient Evaluation: Components of Nutritional Assessment

Subjective and Objective Assessment

A *subjective global assessment* includes collection of complex data such as dietary history, pertinent health history, medications, and weight loss, which can be the strongest indicator of nutritional status or predictor of mortality. *Objective data* include the results of a physical exam focusing on general appearance, signs of muscle and fat wasting, cachexia, obesity, presence of wounds, fluid balance abnormalities, ascites, or edema. Body measurements and body mass index (BMI) are mainly used in the outpatient setting. **Box 33-1** describes calculation of the BMI. **Box 33-2** categorizes a patient based on BMI.

Despite the recognized use of BMI to define obesity by the Centers for Disease Control and Prevention (CDC), new findings suggest that the waist-to-hip ratio is actually a better measure of obesity. The waist-to-hip ratio is also the best obesity measure for assessing a person's risk of heart attack. By utilizing this ratio, the proportion of people deemed to be at risk of heart attack increases threefold (Yusuf et al., 2005).

Box 33-1

Calculation of Body Mass Index (BMI)

BMI = Weight (in kg)/height (in meters)^2
Normal = 20–25 kg/m^2

1. Convert weight in pounds to kilograms by dividing the weight by 2.2.
2. Convert height in inches to meters by multiplying by 0.0254.
3. Square that number.
4. Divide height by that squared number.

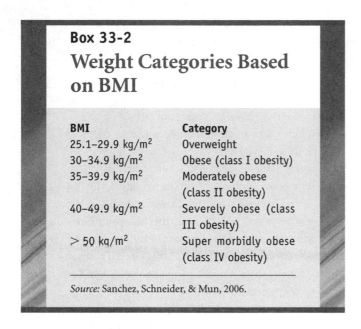

Box 33-2

Weight Categories Based on BMI

BMI	Category
25.1–29.9 kg/m²	Overweight
30–34.9 kg/m²	Obese (class I obesity)
35–39.9 kg/m²	Moderately obese (class II obesity)
40–49.9 kg/m²	Severely obese (class III obesity)
> 50 kg/m²	Super morbidly obese (class IV obesity)

Source: Sanchez, Schneider, & Mun, 2006.

Biochemical (Laboratory) Data

Biochemical (laboratory) data may include protein and micronutrient (vitamin or mineral) levels if clinical evidence suggests possible deficiencies. Protein markers such as serum albumin, prealbumin, and others should not be used to reflect adequacy of nourishment in the sick patient, however (Seres, 2005). Albumin levels, for example, are affected by conditions such as dehydration, sepsis, and liver dysfunction, experienced by the critically ill patient. Instead, the literature suggests use of a functional assessment (i.e., medical history, physical exam, and assessment of organ and muscle function) in conjunction with laboratory data to evaluate a critically ill patient's nutritional status (Bellini, 2006).

Estimating Caloric Needs and Nutrient Requirements

Several methods are currently available for estimating energy expenditure (EE). The problem is that most tools are predictive in only about 50% of patients and results may vary up to 500 kcal/day, which can represent a 20% to 30% variation from their actual needs.

Formulas and Equations

Although complex formulas are available, controversy exists regarding their accuracy in obese or severely malnourished individuals (Krenitsky, 2005). The easiest method is the simplified predictive formula, which uses a standard amount of 20 to 30 kilocalories per kilogram of body weight (average = 25 kcal/kg). Patient requirements also vary depending on the severity of their illness and changes in their clinical status. Some experts recommend using lower requirements during periods of clinical instability (e.g., hypotension requiring vasopressors or high respiratory demands) and higher requirements (up to 40 kcal/kg) in some extremely stressed states.

Indirect Calorimetry

Some experts consider indirect calorimetry to be the "gold standard" for determining energy requirements and estimating caloric needs. The procedure uses a *metabolic cart* to evaluate the resting energy expenditure (REE) and the respiratory quotient (RQ), which is calculated from the carbon dioxide production divided by the oxygen consumption. This calculation may be useful in determining which fuel source (i.e., fat, carbohydrate, or protein) the patient is most utilizing for energy, but it certainly has considerable limitations. Proper calibration of the equipment is essential, and many sources of error exist, including FiO_2 greater than 60%, dialysis or chronic renal failure, respiratory rate greater than 35, system leak, chest tube air leak, or fistula. In addition, results are unreliable in an agitated, restless patient. The procedure is usually performed by a respiratory therapist. Some hand-held devices are available, but their clinical validity is controversial.

Selecting a Method of Delivery

If an oral diet is contraindicated, NPO may be ordered for patients who are not alert, who are unconscious or neurologically impaired, who have swallowing or gag difficulties, who have complicated gastrointestinal (GI) issues, or during the perioperative/procedure period. Rest of the GI tract may be warranted following abdominal and other surgeries when persistent postoperative ileus is present. In the uncomplicated surgical patient, small bowel function does return early, which makes the small intestine the best site for early postoperative enteral tube feeding even in the absence of bowel sounds. Passage of flatus commonly indicates the end of a postoperative ileus. Factors that can prolong an ileus and depress GI function include sympathetic activity from stress or pain, abdominal distention, intraperitoneal irritation, electrolyte imbalances, autonomic drugs or vasopressors, narcotics (especially morphine), propofol (Diprivan®), and some disease processes.

Administration of tube feeding in critically ill patients can be complex, but its benefits far outweigh the associated risks. We tend to think of the gut as a digestive and absorptive organ; in reality, it is involved in many other systemic processes. First, providing food in the GI tract helps maintain normal metabolic pathways in which nutrients are absorbed and then go to the liver via the portal system for intermediary metabolism. Nutrients are then prepared for use on a cellular level before being released into systemic circulation. In contrast, when we feed intravenously, the nutrients go to systemic circulation *first*, and only then to the liver, bypassing the gatekeeper, protein synthesis, and detoxifying functions. Total parenteral nutrition (TPN) is really not total or complete as the commonly used name implies; it lacks fiber, intact protein, iron, glutamine, and some other components. Enteral nutrition also causes the gallbladder to contract from the release of cholecystokinin. As a consequence, in patients receiving enteral (or parenteral) nutrition, cholestasis and gallbladder sludge contribute to the development of acalculous cholecystitis and cholelithiasis, a complication of not using the GI tract. To avoid this complication, patients may receive slow infusion of tube feeding, usually 10 to 20 mL/hr while receiving parenteral nutrition to help maintain these physiologic processes.

Enteral nutrition also helps maintain normal intestinal pH and flora, thereby preventing bacterial overgrowth and slowing the invasion of opportunistic organisms such as *clostridium difficile*. During critical illness, especially in the sepsis patient, the gut has increased permeability and bacterial translocation may occur.

The gut is considered the largest immune organ in the body and may become pro-inflammatory if not fed. The GI tract has major contributions to the immune system: 70% to 80% of the body's immune cells are derived from the gut-associated lymph tissue (GALT), which may be preserved by the administration of tube feeding. As a protective mechanism, lymphocytes produced within the gut travel through the lymphatics and migrate to help the defenses of other organs, thereby preventing infection.

In contrast, the dysfunctional gut is now believed to be the reservoir for pathogens, contributing to the spread of multisystem organ failure–associated infections (SCCM/ACCP, 2002). It is only within recent years that experts have recognized the importance of maintaining GI function as a means to preserve immune function and promote healing. Data suggest that enteral feeding is superior to parenteral nutrition for maintaining gut structure and function (Grant & Martin, 2000). The presence of nutrients in the gut helps to maintain the functional structures of the intestine, known as villi. These fingerlike projections located along the lumen of the intestine are responsible for the absorption of nutrients and food. Cells in the GI tract turn over about every three to five days and require stimulation to maintain their function. Otherwise, the villi atrophy, leading to decreasing surface area of the intestine where nutrients are absorbed, which can cause feeding intolerance and malabsorption problems.

PRACTICAL INFORMATION FOR OPTIMAL DELIVERY: PARENTERAL NUTRITION

Some experts say that administering parenteral nutrition without true contraindication to using the GI tract is delivery of substandard care. Opinion varies regarding the absolute contraindications to enteral feeding. Most of these involve true GI tract malfunctions:

- Intestinal obstruction or perforation
- Prolonged ileus
- Severe GI bleeding or hemorrhage
- High-output enterocutaneous fistula
- Diffuse peritonitis
- Intractable vomiting or severe diarrhea
- Hypoperfusion/acute decompensating shock (unstable hemodynamic status requiring vasopressors) not perfusing the bowel, which can further compromise blood pressure and increase O_2 demand of the gut, causing ischemia
- Severe acute pancreatitis during initial resuscitation
- Some cases of short bowel syndrome and severe malabsorption
- No GI access available

Options for parenteral nutrition include TPN or peripheral parenteral nutrition (PPN), depending on the location of the tip of the vascular access device. The difference between TPN and PPN lies in the concentration and osmolarity of the solution. Concentrated formulations in standard TPN solutions should be used only following radiographic confirmation of true central catheter position to avoid phlebitis and vascular damage. Ideally, the catheter tip should be placed in the superior vena cava (SVC), just above the right atrium where maximal blood flow occurs, for optimal dilution of the infused solution. Properly placed peripherally inserted central catheters (PICCs) may be used similar to central lines. Although the site of catheter entry is in an extremity, the tip of the catheter is in the central location. The CDC has published guidelines for many catheter-related issues.

Glucose control may be more difficult with parenteral nutrition as compared to enteral nutrition. Insulin requirements have been reported to be as much as 26% greater with parenteral nutrition. Higher blood glucose levels have been correlated to a higher incidence of complications in the critically ill patient (van den Berghe et al., 2003). For prevention of catheter-related bloodstream infection, it is important to maintain tight glycemic control and select the most appropriate access device based on the duration of therapy and risk of insertion complication (CDC, 2002).

PRACTICAL INFORMATION FOR OPTIMAL DELIVERY: ENTERAL NUTRITION

Selecting the Right Enteral Route

Gastric or small bowel access needs to be established by a nasal, oral, or percutaneous method. Gastric access can be achieved either by the nasogastric (NG) or orogastric (OG) route for short-term enteral nutrition, or percutaneous endoscopic gastrostomy (PEG) if greater than 30 days of enteral nutrition are predicted. Small bowel access can be established by nasal (nasal-jejunostomy tube [NJT]), surgical, or percutaneous methods (percutaneous endoscopic jejunostomy [PEJ]).

Gastric Feeding

Gastric feeding is generally well tolerated. However, during critical illness, GI motility often slows, causing delayed gastric emptying and high gastric residual volumes (GRVs). Other conditions and patient populations that also have increased incidence of feeding intolerance include diabetic (especially if blood sugar is not controlled), hypokalemic, neurologically impaired, and postoperative patients. Furthermore, many medications commonly given to the hospitalized patient may suppress GI motility, such as narcotics, sedatives, neuromuscular-blocking agents, and vasopressors. Decisions regarding access for enteral nutrition should be made after considering the effectiveness of gastric emptying, GI anatomy, and aspiration risk. In the event that gastric feeding is not tolerated, as evidenced by repeated high GRV, small bowel feeding (SBF) may be indicated to prevent risk of aspiration, although this practice remains controversial. Initial management of high GRV may entail either decreasing the rate of infusion or stopping feedings for a few hours. Both interventions require reassessment.

Small Bowel Feeding

SBF may be indicated in patients when goal rates with gastric feeding are not met and underfeeding is problematic. SBF is an excellent alternative to the initiation of parenteral nutrition whenever reasonable. Patients with severe acute pancreatitis can safely be fed enterally following initial resuscitation (after being stabilized) using a nasojejunal tube inserted past the ligament of Treitz. Feeding into the jejunum will bypass the stimulation of pancreatic enzymes. Studies comparing enteral to parenteral nutrition in this patient population have demonstrated decreased infectious complications, organ failures, and mortality when such individuals are enterally fed (Nathens et al., 2004). Other patient populations where SBF may be indicated include patients who require supine, prone, or modified Trendelenburg positioning and patients who are having multiple procedures, which often contributes to inadequate feeding due to repeated stopping and starting. Repeated interruptions of enteral feedings result in significant underfeeding in critically ill patients (O'Leary-Kelley et al., 2005). Patients with persistent high gastric outputs can also be enterally fed with a post-pyloric feeding tube and NG tube attached to suction for gastric decompression. Some PEJ tubes have two lumens—one gastric port and one distal port for feeding—to accommodate this situation.

Nutrition Timing: Early Versus Late

The definition of "early" in terms of nutritional support varies from 6 to 72 hours, with an average of 24 to 48 hours, considering the hemodynamic stability of the patient. Early feeding is indicated when patients are admitted to the hospital already compromised or in a hypermetabolic state. "Trickle feeds" or trophic feeds within 24 to 48 hours have demonstrated the best outcomes in mechanically ventilated, critically ill patients (i.e., mortality reduction and fewer infectious complications) (Heyland et al., 2003). Waiting as long as five to seven days to initiate nutritional support may be acceptable in the stable, noncompromised patient who entered the hospital in a well-nourished state (e.g., an uncomplicated elective surgery patient).

Rate of Delivery

In acutely ill patients, continuous feeding using a volumetric infusion pump is most common; however, it is also reasonable to initiate bolus feedings prior to discharge for gastric methods such as NG and PEG in an effort to establish a home regimen. SBF should *always* be administered continuously because the small bowel is not a reservoir like the stomach. Patients can develop diarrhea and dumping syndrome from bolus feeding into the small bowel; for this reason, this practice is not recommended.

When selecting an initial rate, the general rule is to start slowly and titrate up. Full-strength formula is most commonly used. Many published protocols start at 10 to 25 mL/hr and increase by 10 to 25 mL/hr every 4 to 6 hours until the goal rate is achieved. Increasing the rate too quickly can create signs of intolerance such as bloating, dumping syndrome, diarrhea, abdominal pain, or more serious complications in a hypoperfused bowel. The patient requiring vasopressors for blood pressure support can develop distal bowel necrosis from administering feeding without adequate blood flow in the bowel, creating a clinical picture of sepsis or acute abdomen. As with any clinical practice guideline, clinical judgment should *always* be considered first, keeping a careful view of the patient's overall clinical status and abdominal assessment.

Overfeeding can be as harmful as underfeeding. Overfeeding can cause metabolic complications and excessive CO_2 production, which can delay weaning from mechanical ventilation. Also, many critically ill patients who are mechanically ventilated receive propofol for sedation. This lipid emulsion contains 1.1 kcal of energy, which is a very similar amount of calories per volume to most standard-tube feeding formulations. Thus, when infused simultaneously, the tube feeding rate should be reduced to compensate for the amount of propofol given. For example, if the goal rate of tube feeding is

60 mL/hr while the propofol is infusing at 10 mL/hr, the tube feeding rate should be reduced to 50 mL/hr during that time to avoid overfeeding.

Formula Selection

A standard formula is usually sufficient to meet the patient's energy requirements. Many specialized formulas have not been proven beneficial and are much more expensive. Selection of the appropriate formula should be based on functioning and capacity of the GI tract, the patient's underlying disease status, and patient tolerance. Many formulas are very similar in makeup, with only slight differences in their nutritional content. Specifics vary, and institutions select product lines to meet their general needs. For example, some high-protein formulas contain higher levels of potassium, which may be of concern in hyperkalemic and renal compromised patients. Pulmonary formulas with higher amounts of fat and lower amounts of carbohydrate were previously thought to decrease CO_2 production, which may contribute to ventilator dependence. Avoiding excess caloric intake, in general, will avoid this complication. High-fat formulas are not generally as well tolerated, and many mechanically ventilated patients are receiving propofol for sedation. This combination can create a situation in which patients receive an extremely high percentage of their calories from fat. A fiber formulation is usually recommended for patients with feeding-related diarrhea. Dietitians are an excellent resource for obtaining this information, and consultation with them should be a standard practice for all tube-fed patients.

It is important for the ICU nurse to be knowledgeable of the primary characteristics of enteral feedings. One way to categorize tube feedings is based on their protein forms—either polymeric (blenderized), elemental, or free amino acids. **Table 33-1** lists several formula characteristics and patient indications.

It is necessary to give free water to tube-fed patients. The amount is generally 30 to 35 mL/kg of body weight, subtracting the estimated water content of the feeding (usually about 83% in standard 1 kcal/mL formulas) and any intravenous (IV) fluids, and adding any abnormal losses. For example, in a 58-kg woman, 35 mL/hr would translate to about 2,000 mL/day. If her tube feeding intake was 1,300 mL/day (1,300 × 0.83 = 1,080 mL free water) and she had about 600 mL IV antibiotic per day, her free water requirement would be about 320 mL/day. High gastric output, diarrhea, or other excessive

TABLE 33-1 Enteral Formulas

Formula	Characteristics	Indications
Standard	Isotonic May or may not contain fiber 1.0 kcal/mL (approximate)	Most patient populations as tolerated
High protein	Protein > 15% total kcal Isotonic 1.0 kcal/mL or more	Patients with wounds, burns, trauma Hypermetabolic, septic patients Malnourished patients
Fiber containing	Fiber 5–14 Gm/L 1.0 kcal/mL	Most patients unless gastrointestinal contraindication Can help decrease diarrhea Caution with hypoperfused bowel
Concentrated	1.5–2.0 kcal/mL High caloric density High osmolality	Fluid restricted
Renal specific	Protein content variable Low electrolyte content High caloric density (2.0 per mL)	Renal failure Usually nondialysis patient *Not* indicated in CRRT patients
Glucose intolerance specific	Low carbohydrate content High fat content 1.0 kcal/mL (approximate)	Difficult glycemic control
Elemental	Pre-digested Partially or completely hydrolyzed protein Osmolality varies, usually hyperosmolar 1.0 kcal/mL or more	Rarely indicated Short bowel, malabsorption Severe acute pancreatitis if not tolerating standard formula
Immune enhancing or stress formulas	May contain glutamine, argentine, omega-3 fatty acids, nucleotides	Varies depending on substrate Benefits are not generalizable May be harmful in some patient populations
	Others	Controversy regarding use

losses should be added to that amount requiring replacement. It is very important to consider the patient's electrolyte status and fluid balance while closely observing for evidence of heart failure, fluid overload, or syndrome of inappropriate antidiuretic hormone secretion, which are conditions that generally require fluid restriction.

MANAGEMENT AND SAFETY ISSUES RELATED TO ENTERAL FEEDING

Tolerance

Methods to assess tolerance include clinical exam (particularly abdominal and respiratory exam) and GRV assessment.

The concept of assessing the GRV is the subject of much debate in the literature. Limitations of using GRV as a marker of intolerance include its lack of sensitivity to detect true aspiration of feeding. For example, some studies have found a high percentage of patients with documented residual of 5 mL or less who were positive for tracheal aspiration (McClave et al., 2005).

An important consideration related to obtaining accurate GRV is the diameter of the feeding tube. Aspirates from small-bore tubes less than 10 French may be unreliable due to the tubing collapsing from pressure created during aspiration. When aspirating for GRV from narrow feeding tubes, the nurse may obtain small or no GRV. This may result in inaccurate interpretation of findings (Thomas, 2001). Inserting 20 to 30 mL of air in small-bore tubes prior to aspiration may help to decrease this error.

Another potential source of error is malposition of the tube. If the tip of the tube is not in the level of fluid or is looped around in the stomach, no aspirates will be obtained, even if they are truly present. The tube may be inadvertently pulled back 10 to 20 cm from the last radiograph, which commonly occurs with patient manipulation and self-rotating beds. This may leave the tip in the distal esophagus; therefore no residuals will be obtained. For this reason, it is extremely important to check the tube-securing device and to document the depth of feeding tubes every shift or according to hospital policy. Many tubes have centimeter markings on them; otherwise, the length of tube remaining outside the body can be measured and documented. A few facilities perform daily radiographs to verify tube placement, but malposition could still be missed between daily films.

Keeping these points in mind, it is clear that gastric residual amounts should be assessed. Various amounts of residual end points are described in the literature. GRV greater than 200 mL on repeated attempts generally indicates that gastric feeding is not tolerated. The Canadian guidelines use a residual amount of 250 mL to determine gastric intolerance, at which time a prokinetic agent such as metoclopramide (Reglan®) is added to the treatment plan for 24 hours. If GRV remains more than 250 mL and four doses of metoclopramide have been given, then post-pyloric feeding is indicated (Greenwood & the Critical Care Practice Guidelines Council, 2003). Erythromycin 250 mg twice daily via NG tube is another effective prokinetic agent administered to stimulate GI motility and decrease residual volumes, although there are issues with emerging antibiotic resistance to consider with its use.

Assessing residual volumes in the small bowel is not usually required. Because the bowel is not a reservoir like the stomach, residuals there should be less than 20 to 30 mL. However, if residuals of 50 to 100 mL are obtained in SBF, it may indicate migration of the tube back into the stomach or a distal bowel obstruction. Some facilities incorporate this assessment into hospital policy every shift in an effort to identify this potential complication.

Complications of Enteral Feeding

Complications of enteral feeding can be classified as mechanical, GI, metabolic, infectious, or a combination of factors.

Mechanical: Tube Malposition

Pleural tube placement is common among even the most skilled practitioners and can cause acute respiratory compromise or pneumothorax. Empyema and bronchopleural fistula have also been reported (Thomas, 2001). Larger-bore stiff tubes and tubes with stylets are most likely to cause perforation. Intracranial placement has been reported as well (Metheny, 2002). Some facilities have formed nutrition support teams so as to decrease the number of nurses inserting tubes in an effort to improve competence and decrease the number of negative outcomes. Generally, for tubes with centimeter markings, accidental lung placement can usually be detected if resistance is encountered upon insertion at the 30- to 45-cm marking. Patients who have a decreased level of consciousness and altered gag reflex may not exhibit any clinical signs of misplacement, however. Some facilities incorporate a mandatory radiograph at 30 to 40 cm of insertion to detect possible bronchial placement before further advancement of the tube is allowed. Radiographic confirmation should *always* be performed after blind insertion prior to administration of any feeding or medication. Air insufflation with auscultation has been proven to be an unreliable technique to assess proper tube placement (American Association of Critical-Care Nurses, 2005a; Thomas, 2001).

Mechanical: Tube Clogging

Improper medication administration techniques are highly responsible for tube occlusions, especially in smaller-bore tubes, which are more likely to clog. If multiple medications are to be administered through the feeding tube, a PEG may be more practical if long-term therapy is anticipated. A size 10 French or smaller tube may provide more comfort to the patient, but administering medications and accuracy of checking GRV may be compromised. PEJ tubes usually have a small bore, and administering medications through them is challenging to prevent clogging; therefore, when these tubes are surgically placed, many surgeons discourage this practice.

Medications in pill form need to be crushed thoroughly, dissolved completely, and given separately, flushing with at least 20 mL of warm water in between each medication, whenever feeding is interrupted, and routinely every four hours. Of note, not all pills can be crushed for instillation through an NG tube. Elixirs need to be diluted well and have a tendency to clog tubes, especially sorbitol-based liquids with inadequate flushing. Proteins can cause clogging in the presence of an acidic environment. For example, high-protein formulas are highly likely to clog tubes. Acidic substances such as cola or cranberry juice are no longer recommended for declogging feeding tubes for this reason. Pancreatic enzymes may be effective for declogging, although flushing with warm water is overall the best and easiest method.

Mechanical and Gastrointestinal: Aspiration

Aspiration is the leading cause of pneumonia in the ICU and the most serious complication of enteral tube feeding (McClave et al., 2002). There is much debate regarding true aspiration in the tube-fed patient. True incidence has been difficult to determine in the past because of vague definitions, poor assessment monitors, and varying levels of clinical recognition. Most aspiration pneumonia is caused by oral secretions in patients with altered swallowing capabilities or subglottic secretions in mechanically ventilated patients rather than tube feeding in the airway. As many as 45% of normal individuals aspirate during sleep (McClave et al., 2002). Blue food coloring should not be used due to reports of severe adverse events including gastric bacterial colonization, systemic dye absorption, and death (American Association of Critical-Care Nurses, 2005b; McClave et al., 2005). Elevation of the head of bed to 30 to 45 degrees and maintaining good oral hygiene to minimize oral bacterial colonization are the best preventive measures and should be a part of standard evidence-based care.

Gastrointestinal: Nausea, Vomiting, Diarrhea

Nausea or vomiting can occur with enteral feeding—primarily gastric feeding—and can usually be managed by adding a prokinetic agent to stimulate motility (e.g., metoclopramide) or an antiemetic. Diarrhea is the most frequently reported GI complication, and usually has an osmotic or infectious etiology. Osmotic diarrhea occurs when a non-absorbable substance in the bowel pulls in excess water. Many liquid medications are sorbitol-based, which can cause this effect, as can some tube-feeding formulations. Lactose intolerance is also a cause of osmotic diarrhea, although commercial formulas are lactose-free. Infectious diarrhea is most commonly caused by *Clostridium difficile* or cytomegalovirus in acute care settings (Eisenberg, 2002). A stool culture should be sent if this etiology is suspected or in the event of recent antibiotic usage. Consultation with the clinical pharmacist regarding the medication regime for possible contributors, the dietitian or nutritional specialist, and the physician is a multidisciplinary approach that can determine the optimal plan of care.

Metabolic: Refeeding Syndrome

Starved or severely malnourished patients can undergo life-threatening fluid and electrolyte shifts following the initiation of aggressive nutritional support therapies. This phenomenon, which is known as the "refeeding syndrome," occurs more frequently in parenteral than enteral support. Monitoring of electrolytes upon initiation of therapy is critical, especially in high-risk patients. Dietitians routinely assess for this complication.

Metabolic: Hyperglycemia

Glucose control is more difficult with parenteral nutrition but can occur with caloric or steroid administration. Insulin resistance is common in the critically ill, and maintaining strict glycemic control has demonstrated the best outcomes (van den Berghe et al., 2003).

Contamination

Aseptic technique should be maintained at all times when handling all enteral nutrition products. Published guidelines recommend changing volumetric pump tubing and solution every 24 hours or more frequently to prevent bacterial growth. Plastic bottle systems that are ready to spike, prime, and hang are gaining popularity in many facilities both for their convenience and for their ability to reduce microbial risk. Some of these closed systems are designed to remain aseptic for 24 to 48 hours. Always check the manufacturer's guidelines. Supplements should not be added to tube feeding formula because of potential risk of contamination.

PATIENT OUTCOMES

Nurses can help ensure attainment of optimal patient outcomes such as those listed in **Box 33-3** for patients receiving nutritional support.

Box 33-3
Optimal Patient Outcomes

- Nutrition biochemical measures not compromised
- Gastric residual volume in expected range
- Weight in expected range
- No evidence of aspiration of enteral feedings
- Tolerance to enteral feedings
- Knowledge of rationale for enteral or parenteral feedings
- Absence of complications of enteral or parenteral feedings

SUMMARY

Nutrition is a key component of patient recovery and reduction of complications during an episode of illness. Providing safe and effective nutritional support can best be accomplished using a multidisciplinary team approach combined with skilled nursing practice and critical thinking.

Delivery of effective nutritional support to critically ill patients requires an understanding of the energy needs of each patient. Many disease processes lead to increased caloric requirements. In contrast, some therapies decrease the metabolic response. Both underfeeding and overfeeding a critically ill patient may prolong hospitalization and increase morbidity and mortality (Fung, 2000).

CASE STUDY

S.D. is a 77-year-old who was admitted to the ICU with community-acquired pneumonia. Pertinent medical history includes diabetes, chronic obstructive pulmonary disease, and transient ischemic attacks. Arterial blood gas results in the Emergency Department reflected poor oxygenation and respiratory failure. Subsequently, S.D. was intubated, placed on mechanical ventilation, and given propofol (Diprivan®) for sedation. Due to hemodynamic instability, her blood pressure was maintained on a norepinepherine infusion and fluid resuscitation was provided. A nasogastric (NG) tube was inserted for medication administration, and 500 mL of greenish aspirate was obtained. The NG tube at this time was connected to low intermittent suction.

Approximately 24 hours later, the patient was more hemodynamically stable and the decision was made to begin nutrition support. NG output for the last 12 hours was slightly less than 200 mL. Blood sugars have been mostly in the 180 to 220 mg/dL range, with current sliding-scale insulin coverage.

CRITICAL THINKING QUESTIONS

1. Should enteral or parenteral nutrition be considered?
2. Describe key issues related to selecting the most appropriate method of delivery.
3. What are two methods that can be used to evaluate the nutritional status and metabolic needs of this patient?

Other Patient Information

Height: 5 ft, 6 in
Weight: 62 kg
Following consultation with the dietitian, standard tube feeding (1.0 kcal/mL) was started at 20 mL/hr with orders to titrate up conservatively by 10 mL every 8 hours until the "goal rate" was reached, considering concurrent propofol infusion (1.1 kcal/mL).

CRITICAL THINKING QUESTIONS

4. Calculate the patient's BMI.
5. Estimate the amount of daily kilocalories required.
6. Calculate the goal rate with propofol infusion at 5 mL/hr.
7. Estimate the amount of free water the patient should receive daily.
8. What are two important clinical practice issues related to enteral feeding?
9. Describe two patient safety issues related to enteral feeding.

The following morning, the gastric residual volume (GRV) was found to be 240 mL. The feeding was placed on hold at this time. Two hours later, the GRV was 160 mL and the feeding was resumed. By the end of the next day, the goal rate was achieved. Erythromycin 250 mg BID for six doses via NG tube was initiated to stimulate gastric motility.

CRITICAL THINKING QUESTIONS

10. What are some of the factors contributing to feeding intolerance in this patient?
11. When are prokinetic agents indicated to enhance motility?
12. Describe a scenario in which small bowel feeding would be indicated.
13. Use the form to write up a plan of care for a patient receiving enteral or parenteral nutrition in the clinical setting. Rate the patient as a level 1, 3, or 5 on each characteristic.
14. Take one patient outcome for a patient and list evidence-based interventions found in a literature review for this patient.

Using the Synergy Model to Develop a Plan of Care

	Patient Characteristics	Level (1, 3, 5)	Subjective and Objective Data	Evidence-based Interventions	Outcomes
SYNERGY MODEL	Resiliency				
	Vulnerability				
	Stability				
	Complexity				
	Resource availability				
	Participation in care				
	Participation in decision making				
	Predictability				

Online Resources

American College of Chest Physicians: www.accp.org

American Society of Parenteral and Enteral Nutrition: www.clinnutr.org

British Society of Parenteral and Enteral Nutrition: www.BAPEN.org.uk

Canadian Nutrition Clinical Practice Guidelines: www.criticalcarenutrition.com

Centers for Disease Control and Prevention: www.cdc.gov

National Guideline Clearinghouse: www.guideline.gov

REFERENCES

American Association of Critical-Care Nurses. (2005a). Practice alert: Dye in enteral feeding. *AACN News.* Retrieved October 5, 2005, from www.aacn.org/AACN/aacnnews.nsf/GetArticle/Articlethree224

American Association of Critical-Care Nurses. (2005b). Practice alert: Verification of feeding tube placement. *AACN News.* Retrieved October 5, 2005, from www.aacn.org/AACN/aacnnews.nsf/GetArticle/Articlethree225

American Society of Parenteral and Enteral Nutrition. (2002a). Guidelines for the use of parenteral and enteral nutrition in adult and pediatric patients. *Journal of Parenteral and Enteral Nutrition, 26*(Suppl.), 18–21.

American Society of Parenteral and Enteral Nutrition. (2002b). Guidelines for the use of parenteral and enteral nutrition in adult and pediatric patients. *Journal of Parenteral and Enteral Nutrition, 26*(Suppl.), 33–41.

Barton, R. G. (2004). Proceedings of the Society of Critical Care Medicine Board Review Course. Phoenix, AZ.

Bellini, L. M. (2006). Assessment of nutrition in the critically ill. Retrieved on August 28, 2006, from www.utdol.com/utd/content/topic.do?topickey=cc_medi/17912

Centers for Disease Control and Prevention (CDC). (2002). Guidelines for the prevention of intravascular catheter related infections. *Morbidity and Mortality Weekly Report, 51*, RR-10.

Eisenberg, P. (2002). An overview of diarrhea in the patients receiving enteral nutrition. *Gastroenterology Nursing, 25*(3), 95–104.

Fung, E. B. (2000). Estimating energy expenditure in critically ill adults and children. *AACN Clinical Issues, 11*(4), 480–497.

Grant, M. J., & Martin, S. (2000). Delivery of enteral nutrition. *AACN Clinical Issues, 11*(4), 507–516.

Greenwood, J., & the Critical Care Practice Guidelines Council. (2003). Enteral nutrition feeding guideline. Retrieved October 5, 2005, from www.criticalcarenutrition.com

Heyland, D., Rupinder, D., Drover, J., Gramlich, L., Dodek, P., & the Canadian Critical Care Clinical Practice Guidelines Committee. (2003). Canadian clinical practice guidelines for nutrition support in mechanically ventilated, critically ill adult patients. *Journal of Parenteral and Enteral Nutrition, 27*(5), 355–373.

Krenitsky, J. (2005). Adjusted body weight, pro: Evidence to support the use of adjusted body weight in calculating calorie requirements. *Nutrition in Clinical Practice, 20*(4), 468–473.

McClave, S. A., DeMeo, M. T., DeLegge, M. H., DiSario, J. A., Heyland, D. K., Maloney, J. P., et al. (2002). North American summit on aspiration in the critically ill patient: Consensus statement. *Journal of Parenteral and Enteral Nutrition, 26*(6), S80–S85.

McClave, S. A., Lukan, J. K., Stefater, J. A., Lowen, C. C., Looney, S. W., Matheson, P. J., et al. (2005). Poor validity of residual volumes as a marker for risk of aspiration in critically ill patients. *Critical Care Medicine, 33*(2), 324–330.

Metheny, N. A. (2002). Inadvertent intracranial nasogastric tube placement. *American Journal of Nursing, 102*(8), 25–27.

Nathens, A. B., Curtis, R., Beale, R., Cook, D., Moreno, R., Romand, J. A., et al. (2004). Management of the critically ill patient with severe acute pancreatitis. *Critical Care Medicine, 32*(12), 2524–2533.

O'Leary-Kelley, C. M., Puntillo, K. A., Barr, J., Stotts, N., Douglas, M. K., et al. (2005). Nutritional adequacy in patients receiving mechanical ventilation who are fed enterally. *American Journal of Critical Care, 14*(3), 222–231.

Sanchez, V. M., Schneider, B. E., & Mun, E. C. (2006). Surgical management of severe obesity. Retrieved June 14, 2006, from www.utdol.com/utd/content/topic.do?topic_key=gi_dis/32649&type=A&selectedTitle=3~14

Seres, D. (2005). Surrogate nutrition markers, malnutrition, and adequacy of nutritional support. *Nutrition in Clinical Practice, 20*, 308–313.

Society of Critical Care Medicine/American College of Chest Physicians (SCCM/ACCP). (2002). *Combined Critical Care Course.* Chicago: Society of Critical Care Medicine.

Thomas, D. R. (2001). Annals of long term care: Clinical care and aging. *A Complete Primer on Enteral Feeding, 9*(1), 41–48.

Van den Berghe, G., Wouters, P. J., Boullion, R., Weekers, F., Verwaest, C., Schetz, M., et al. (2003). Outcome benefit of intensive insulin therapy in the critically ill: Insulin dose versus glycemic control. *Critical Care Medicine, 31*, 359–366.

Yusuf, S., Hawken, S., Ounpuu, S., Bautista, L., Franzosi, M. G., Commerford, P., et al. (2005). Obesity and the risk of myocardial infarction in 27,000 participants from 52 countries: A case-control study. *Lancet, 366*(9497), 1640–1649.

Gastrointestinal Bleeding

LEARNING OBJECTIVES

Celeste Smith

Upon completion of this chapter, the reader will be able to:

1. Define GI bleeding.
2. Identify signs and symptoms of GI bleeding.
3. Develop a plan of care for the GI bleed patient.
4. Monitor the GI bleed patient for complications.
5. Educate the patient regarding diagnosis, etiology, and treatment options.
6. List optimal patient outcomes that may be achieved through evidence-based management of GI bleeding.

Gastrointestinal (GI) bleeding is defined as any bleeding that originates in the GI tract. The incidence of acute, massive upper GI bleeding is 40 to 150 occurrences per 100,000 people. The mortality rate is 6% to 10% (Manning-Dimmitt, Dimmit, & Wilson, 2005; Urden, Stacy, & Lough, 2002). While these figures have been relatively unchanged for the last 50 years, a recent study found that GI bleeding was a contributory factor in many patients, although actual GI bleeding deaths occurred in only a small percentage of patients (Gopalswamy et al., 2004).

The amount of bleeding can range from microscopic to life-threatening. Whether the bleeding is microscopic or massive, both can indicate significant disease processes and are therefore equally important to detect. It is essential to note the amount of bleeding and the location of the bleeding to determine which treatment should be initiated. Although the bleeding may originate from any site along the GI tract, the causes and treatment modalities for the upper and lower tract may vary.

The *upper* GI tract stretches from the mouth to the upper part of the small intestines. Bleeding in this area often involves only small amounts of blood and may not be obvious because the blood is moving slowly through the intestines and is partially digested. The person who presents with an upper GI bleed could have coffee-ground emesis, hematemesis (vomiting blood), melena (black, tarry, and foul-smelling stools), or, occasionally, hematochezia (red or maroon-colored stools) (Urden et al., 2002). Black stools are due to the blood oxidizing when exposed to air. When considering an upper GI bleed, the person who presents vomiting blood will usually be the most unstable and will require emergent intervention.

The *lower* GI tract includes the small intestines, colon, and anus. Bleeding from this area can also range from microscopic to massive hematochezia. The person with large-volume hematochezia represents a serious lower GI bleed and will usually require hospitalization. Surgery is indicated for patients who require more than 4 to 6 units of blood in 24 hours or more than 10 units in total (Papadakis & McPhee, 2005). The incidence of acute, emergent lower GI bleeding is 20 to 27 cases per 100,000 people annually; the mortality rate is 4 % to 10% (Manning-Dimmitt et al., 2005).

ETIOLOGY

The most common cause of upper GI bleeding, accounting for approximately 50% of all cases (Urden et al., 2002), is a peptic ulcer. A peptic ulcer usually results from chronic irritation of the stomach lining or gastritis. In the past, ulcers were mainly thought to be caused by stress. It is now believed that the two major causes of duodenal and gastric ulcers are infection with the bacterium *Helicobacter pylori* and the use of non-steroidal anti-inflammatory drugs (NSAIDs). These pain medications include common products such as aspirin, ibuprofen (Advil®), naproxen sodium (Aleve®), and ketoprofen (Orudis®) (American College of Gastroenterology, 2005). Smoking and increased age are also risk factors for upper GI bleeding (Stone, 2003).

The majority of causes for upper GI bleeding seen in the intensive care unit (ICU) are related to peptic ulcers, stress-related erosive syndrome (stress ulcers or hemorrhagic gastritis), and esophageal varices (engorged and distended blood vessels within the esophagus, usually secondary to portal hypertension and liver cirrhosis). Other causes include Mallory-Weiss tear (a tear where the esophagus meets the stomach, usually after vomiting), esophagitis, neoplasm, aortoenteric fistula (abnormal connection between the aortic graft and the bowel mucosa), and angiodysplasia (abnormal dilation or weakened mucosal vessels) (Stone, 2003; Urden et al., 2002).

The most common causes of lower GI bleeding are infectious colitis, anorectal disease (abnormalities of the anal opening), and inflammatory bowel disease in patients younger than age 50. In patients older than age 50, the most common causes include diverticulosis (small pouches that bulge outward in the colon through weak spots), neoplasms, solitary rectal ulcer, use of NSAIDs, and colonic varices. Diverticulosis accounts for 50% of all major lower GI bleed cases in these older patients (Papadakis & McPhee, 2005). The majority of people older than age 80 and half of all people age 60 to 80 have diverticulosis (Medical College of Wisconsin, 2003). Other causes include vascular ectasias or angiodysplasias as well as ischemic colitis (lack of blood supply to the colon) (Cagir & Cirincione, 2004; Papadakis & McPhee). Lower GI bleeding is more common in males, and its incidence increases significantly with age (Papadakis & McPhee). Mallory-Weiss tear occurs as a result of pressure of excessive vomiting. Esophageal varices are discussed in Chapter 35.

ASSESSMENT

The presentation of GI bleeding will vary depending on the severity and length of bleeding. Prolonged bleeding that is microscopic in nature can lead to iron loss and anemia (Stone, 2003). The person may exhibit symptoms of lethargy, pallor, shortness of breath, and possibly chest pain due to a decrease in oxygen carrying capacity secondary to anemia. The person may not have even been aware of any GI bleeding; it may be discovered by the healthcare provider. When a patient presents in the ICU, it is imperative that a detailed GI history be obtained. The nursing admission is helpful in obtaining a generalized health history, but asking specific questions will help in the diagnosis and treatment plan for the GI patient (see **Table 34-1**) (Stone). Ongoing assessment is necessary to identify early blood loss, which will be apparent as a decrease in blood pressure and an increase in heart rate and respiration (due to hypoxia). The frequency of assessment is based on the unit policy but is typically hourly.

One of the main assessment tools for an upper or lower GI bleed is the color of the stool and any emesis. This information can be obtained from the patient, but it is important to obtain a stool specimen or smear to verify the color, because this observation will be very helpful in the diagnosis (see **Table 34-2**). A stool guaiac (hemoccult) is a simple test that may be required to detect the presence of occult (hidden) blood in the stool. In a critically ill patient, the blood is usually obvious in the stool or emesis. It is important to recognize these symptoms to help locate the source of the bleed. Other lab studies that should alert the nurse to bleeding are decreased hemoglobin and hematocrit and a decreased oxygen level on the arterial blood gases.

DIAGNOSTIC TESTING

Diagnostic testing for GI bleeding will depend on the location and severity of the bleed. The physician decides which pro-

---

TABLE 34-1 Nursing Assessment Questions

- What brought you to the hospital?
- What is your age?
- How long have you noticed the symptoms?
- Have they been continuous or intermittent?
- Are your stools black or tarry, maroon or bright red?
- Have you vomited blood or a coffee-ground-looking material?
- Do you have a history of any other stomach problems or ulcers?
- Have you recently had any trauma?
- Are these symptoms new?
- What other symptoms have you been experiencing (e.g., dizziness, passing out)?
- Did you associate anything else with the bleeding?
- Do you take any medications, especially aspirin, NSAIDs, Coumadin®, steroids, or Cox-2 inhibitors?
- What is your daily alcohol intake?

Source: Urden, Stacy, & Lough, 2002.

TABLE 34-2 Locations of Gastrointestinal Bleeding

Location	Signs and Symptoms	Causes
Esophagus	Bright red emesis, coffee-ground emesis, black stools	Esophageal varices, Mallory-Weiss tear, ulcers, liver disorders
Gastric/stomach	Bright red emesis, coffee-ground emesis, black stools	Gastric ulcers, gastritis
Small intestine	Maroon or bright red stools	Ulcer, neoplasms, AV malformations
Colon/large intestine	Bright red stool	Diverticulosis, neoplasm
Anus	Streaked blood or brown stool	Anorectal disorder, hemorrhoid

Sources: American College of Gastroenterology, 2005; Papadakis & McPhee, 2005.

cedure is necessary based on the individual case and symptoms. The nurse should be familiar with the following procedures:

- *Esophagogastroduodenoscopy* (EGD) provides direct visualization of the GI tract via a small flexible scope that is passed orally into the esophagus, stomach, and duodenum. It can be used for diagnosis, biopsy, and treatment interventions. To allow for adequate gastric emptying, if possible, the patient should have nothing by mouth (NPO) for at least six hours prior to the procedure. Moderate sedation is generally used, so intravenous (IV) access and critical care monitoring (frequent vital signs, pulse oximetry, and telemetry) are required. Although it is a relatively low-risk procedure, a thorough history and physical are needed to ensure that EGD is appropriate for the patient (Yusuf & Wofford, 2002).

- *Colonoscopy* provides direct visualization of the lower GI tract via a small flexible scope. The physician can diagnose and treat diverticular bleeding or angiodysplasia by coagulating or injecting the bleeding vessel (Tham & Collins, 2000). One disadvantage of this exam is that it requires bowel preparation with Fleet® phosphosoda, polyethylene glycol, or another form of laxative, as well as receiving NPO. Moderate sedation is used for this exam and requires the same monitoring as an EGD.

- *Enteroscopy* utilizes a longer scope than the EGD, so it can reach the small intestines to visualize bleeding sites or abnormalities. This procedure requires the same monitoring as the EGD. A new tool being used is capsule enteroscopy. With this procedure, the patient swallows a small pill-shaped camera that allows for visualization of the small bowel. Only a few studies have been com-

pleted so far, but capsule enteroscopy has shown promising results as a better diagnostic tool than the push enteroscopy (Manning-Dimmitt et al., 2005).

- In *anoscopy* and *sigmoidoscopy*, a shorter scope is used to visualize the anorectal and sigmoid colon (lower third of the colon).

- *Gastrointestinal bleeding scan* is used to identify an active GI bleed and the location of the bleed, and to determine whether an arteriogram would be helpful. This nuclear medicine exam is primarily used to detect slow rates of bleeding, and the bleeding must be active at the time of the test (Urden et al., 2002).

- *Angiography* is performed by an interventional radiologist to examine the arteries and veins for bleeding. It is used to find a cause of lower GI bleeding. Complications of this procedure may include hematoma, vessel dissection, thrombosis, transient ischemic attack, and renal toxicity from the dye used during the procedure (Holzman, Schirmer, & Nasraway, 2005).

- An *abdominal radiograph* may show free air, representing a perforation. This film is not usually helpful in a critically ill patient (Urden et al., 2002).

- *Transvenous intrahepatic portosystemic shunt* (TIPS) involves placement of a shunt between the portal and hepatic veins to decrease portal vein pressures and relieve acute esophageal variceal bleeding. A stent is placed to keep the shunt patent (Bajwa & Marik, 2005). This procedure is used when endoscopic therapy has failed.

- An *upper GI series* uses barium contrast to show problems such as ulcers in the esophagus, stomach, and duodenum. These films are not useful in acute GI bleeding.

- With a *barium enema*, films are taken after rectal instillation of barium to examine the large intestines. This test is useful in patients who are positive for occult blood. Use of barium is discouraged because it interferes with other tests being performed later (e.g., colonoscopy or angiogram) (Holzman et al., 2005). Gastrointestinal interventions are discussed in depth in Chapter 32.

MEDICAL MANAGEMENT

Regardless of the type of bleeding, the most common presentation of a person with an acute GI bleed will be hypovolemic shock (Urden et al., 2002). Hypovolemic shock involves inadequate perfusion secondary to rapid blood and fluid loss, which can result in multiple organ failure (Kolecki & Menckhoff, 2004). Signs and symptoms of hypovolemic shock may include hypotension, tachycardia, shortness of breath, low urinary output, lightheadedness, fainting, weakness, pallor, and altered mental status. The patient may present with one or more of these symptoms. A more detailed discussion of hypovolemic shock appears in Chapter 18.

Initial resuscitation will be the same for either an upper or lower GI case. The basic ABCs—airway, breathing, and circulation—should be addressed as part of the initial management. Then, immediate stabilization with IV fluids is essential (Casestecker, 2002). Fluids will restore the circulating blood volume to a level that will prevent further shock (Urden et al., 2002). One or more large-gauge IV cannulae should be started in anticipation of the administration of multiple fluids and blood products. Normal saline is the fluid of choice. If the patient is hypotensive, pressure bags may be placed around a bag of IV fluids to promote rapid administration. A volume expander or colloid may also be considered. The rate of the infusion will depend on the severity of symptoms. A general rule is to replace each milliliter of blood loss with 3 mL of crystalloid fluid (Casestecker; Logan, 2002). A central venous pressure line or pulmonary artery (PA) catheter may be needed to monitor the amount of fluids required in patients with known cardiovascular disease. The use of a PA catheter or central line aids in prevention of over- or under-hydration (Tham & Collins, 2000). Use of PA catheters and central venous catheters is discussed in more detail in Chapter 11.

If it is required and when cross-matched blood is available, packed red blood cells should be transfused. If the patient is unstable and there is no time to cross-match blood, O-negative blood should be transfused (Tham & Collins, 2000). Blood transfusions should be given until the systolic blood pressure is greater than 80 mm Hg, the heart rate is less than 100 beats/min, hematocrit is greater than 25%, and, if monitored, central venous pressure is greater than 2 mm Hg. Use of a blood warmer should be considered to administer blood, because this technique avoids complications such as hypothermia. Fresh frozen plasma may be needed to correct coagulopathies associated with massive transfusion with packed red blood cells (Tham & Collins).

Initial blood work should include a complete blood count, coagulation screen, chemistries, liver function tests, and a type and cross match with at least two units held in reserve. The hemoglobin and hematocrit levels can be poor indicators of blood loss, because it can take approximately 72 hours after bleeding for the hemoglobin and hematocrit to drop (Urden et al., 2002). A blood urea nitrogen-to-creatinine ratio greater than 36, in a patient without renal insufficiency, is indicative of a bleed (Casestecker, 2002).

Other interventions may include insertion of a urinary catheter to monitor intake and output, a nasogastric tube to lavage the stomach and prepare for endoscopy, and possibly endotracheal intubation (Urden et al., 2002). If the stomach contains bile but no blood, an upper GI bleed is less likely, although a duodenal site of bleeding could still be possible. Nasogastric aspirate findings are 93% predictive of an upper GI source of bleeding (Casestecker, 2002).

The goal after immediate resuscitation is to perform endoscopy in an attempt to identify the source of bleeding, provide information, and institute appropriate intervention. Early endoscopy within the first 24 hours of an acute bleed is associated with decreased length of hospital stay, a lower rate of recurrent bleeding, and less need for emergent surgical intervention (Casestecker, 2002). Although a range of endoscopic treatments can be used, an injection combined with a thermal method is usually the best treatment. Epinephrine, sclerosants, and clot-producing materials such as fibrin glue are injected into and around the bleeding lesion. Thermal therapy includes isolating the bleeding vessel, then exerting direct pressure with electrocoagulation or a heater-probe. Another option is laser phototherapy, which uses heat and direct vessel coagulation; it is generally not as effective as thermal therapy (Casestecker).

For variceal bleeding, intravariceal injection of a sclerosant is usually attempted, but esophageal band ligation is more efficient and is associated with fewer complications. A balloon tamponade, such as the Sengstaken-Blakemore tube or the Minnesota tube (a tube that is inserted like a nasogastric tube into the stomach and inflated with air to put pressure against the bleeding veins), can be used for massive hemorrhage. Although their use has decreased with the advances in endoscopic interventions, balloon tamponades may still be used temporaily in uncontrolled variceal bleeding.

A Minnesota tube has four lumens (openings). Suction setup is required for two of the lumens, the gastric and esophageal lumens. Each of these lumens has a balloon holding the tube in place in the stomach and esophagus. A manometer is attached to each of the other two lumens to measure pressure in the balloons. A 1-pound weight is attached to the tube, and traction is applied to put tension on the system. The traction should be checked every few hours to ascertain that there is tension on the system. Hospital policies vary with regard to the frequency with which the ICU nurse should obtain balloon pressure readings. The esophageal balloon pressure should not exceed 45 mm Hg. A pair of scissors must be readily available at the patient's bedside to cut the balloons in the event of airway occlusion. Such a problem can occur if the balloons become deflated and migrate up and out of the esophagus. The ICU nurse should also monitor the location of the tube by examining centimeter markings on the tube. A chest radiograph is obtained upon insertion to verify placement. All medications are instilled through the gastric lumen. Because the patient is unable to swallow secretions, frequent oral care is required.

A Sengstaken-Blakemore tube has three lumens. If the patient has this tube inserted, a nasogastric tube must also be placed to remove gastric contents. Principles and care of the patient are the same as for the patient with a Minnesota tube. Once the patient has been stabilized, the balloons are deflated and the tube is left in place for an additional 24 hours to monitor for active bleeding (Greenwald, 2004).

A longer-term solution may be the TIPS procedure, which was discussed earlier in this chapter.

Although endoscopic interventions are effective, rebleeding does occur in 15% to 20% of cases (Casestecker, 2002). If the patient remains hemodynamically unstable, surgery is the most effective way to stop the bleeding (Logan, 2002). Emergency surgical intervention is necessary in 3% to 15% of upper GI bleeding cases and approximately 10% of lower GI bleeding cases (Cagir & Cirincione, 2004; Casestecker).

NURSING MANAGEMENT

Nursing management starts with emergency interventions:

- Assessing the ABCs
- Inserting IV lines
- Administering fluids and blood
- Keeping the patient NPO
- Placing a nasogastric tube
- Obtaining frequent vital signs
- Telemetry monitoring
- Documenting intake and output
- Observing for signs of shock (e.g., tachycardia, hypotension, low urine output, increased respiratory rate, a change in mental status)

Gastric lavage may be required to clear the blood from the stomach, reduce bleeding, and allow for visualization during an endoscopy. After placement of a large-bore nasogastric tube, the stomach is irrigated with 2 to 3 L of tap water. Strict intake and output records should be maintained during this procedure. If the drainage continues to be bloody, imminent treatment is required (Urden et al., 2002).

Pharmacological therapy will be initiated depending on the etiology of the bleed. If the bleed was caused by NSAIDs or other medications, these medications should be discontinued immediately. In most cases, histamine blockers or proton pump inhibitors will be started via infusion or IV boluses. Numerous GI medications may be started based on the bleeding etiology (see **Table 34-3**). A recent study showed that gastric ulcer heal-

ing could be improved by the administration of a combination of proton pump inhibitors and mucosal protective agents (Si, Cao, & Wu, 2005).

If the patient presents with esophageal varices, an octreotide (Sandostatin®) infusion is the drug of choice. It will reduce portal pressure and splanchnic and hepatic blood flow, thereby reducing bleeding (Papadikis & McPhee, 2005).

Vasopressin can be used to control the bleeding by vasoconstriction, but it has many serious side effects. If the patient was positive for the *H. pylori* infection, many different medication regimens may be implemented to eradicate the bacteria. These regimens may include a combination of bismuth subsalicylate (Pepto-Bismol®), metronidazole (Flagyl®), and tetracycline (Tetracyn®) and a H_2 blocker; omeprazole (Prilosec®) and clarithromycin (Azithromycin®) for two weeks, then omeprazole for two weeks; ranitidine bismuth citrate (Tritec®) (RBC) and clarithromycin for two weeks, the RBC for two weeks; Lansoprazole (Prevacid®); amoxicillin (Actimox®) and Clarithromycin for ten days; or omeprazole, clarithromycin and amoxicillin for 10 days (CDC, 2006).

Patient education is an extremely important nursing responsibility and should be initiated as soon as possible. Initially, an explanation regarding GI bleeding, its diagnosis, and treatments should be provided. An endoscopy, in addition to other possible diagnostic tests or surgical intervention, should be discussed, if appropriate. Education will continue throughout the hospitalization. In addition, the patient and significant others will need preparation for discharge and home care. **Table 34-4** identifies some important concepts that should be discussed.

Once the bleeding is under control, routine nursing care should include continued monitoring for signs and symptoms of rebleeding, serial blood counts, hydration, advance diet as tolerated, daily weights, and continued patient education to prepare for discharge. The plan of care should be based on the individual needs and history of the specific patient (see **Table 34-5**).

PATIENT OUTCOMES

Nurses can help ensure attainment of optimal patient outcomes such as those listed in **Box 34-1** for the patient with a GI bleed.

SUMMARY

GI bleeding accounts for approximately 300,000 hospital admissions annually. Nearly all GI hemorrhage patients will require care in the ICU setting (Urden et al., 2002). The ICU nurse's most important role is to prevent multiple organ dysfunction syndrome by preventing sustained hypovolemic shock. This is accomplished by understanding the risk factors, etiology, and interventions of the GI bleed patient. Once hemo-

TABLE 34-3 Drugs Used in Gastrointestinal Disorders/Bleeding

Classification	Indications	Advantages	Disadvantages
Antacids Aluminum hydroxide and magnesium carbonate (Maalox®, Gaviscon®) Aluminum hydroxide, magnesium hydroxide, and simethicone (Mylanta®) Calcium carbonate (Tums®) Magaldrate (Riopan®) Dihydroxyaluminum sodium carbonate (Rolaids®)	Neutralize stomach acid; simethicone breaks down gas bubbles; foaming agents keep stomach juices from coming in contact with the esophagus	Simple and inexpensive; take effect within 1 hour; calcium carbonate may also help boost calcium intake in women	Effects usually last only a short time; sodium bicarbonate is not recommended for people who must reduce salt in their diet; calcium can stimulate acid rebound and kidney stones; magnesium can cause diarrhea; aluminum can cause constipation; patient may require an NGT/feeding tube if unable to take oral medication
Anticholinergics Atropine sulfate (Atropine®) Glycopyrolate (Robinul®) Propantheline (Pro-Banthine®) Scopolamine (Transderm-Scop®)	Decrease gastric secretions by inhibiting acetylcholine	Can be given intravenously or transdermally	Cause dry mouth in a patient who is probably NPO; tachycardia and drowsiness; must use caution with patients with known heart disease
Histamine-Receptor (H$_2$) Antagonists Cimetidine (Tagamet®) Famotidine (Pepcid®) Nizatidine (Axid®) Ranitidine (Zantac®)	Decrease hydrochloric acid by blocking the receptors that control that secretion	No known serious side effects; much less expensive than proton pump inhibitors	Some H$_2$ blockers interact with other medications; 50% of patients with erosive esophagitis will not get relief or healing of their esophagus on the usual doses
Proton Pump Inhibitors Esomeprazole (Nexium®) Lansoprazole (Prevacid®) Omeprazole (Prilosec®) Pantoprazole (Protonix®) Rabeprazole (Aciphex®)	Stop acid secretion by disabling the acid pump	More effective in healing erosive esophagitis and gastric ulcers as compared to the H$_2$ blockers; can give in continuous infusion; advantage of once-daily dosing; serious side effects are very rare	More expensive when compared to standard doses of H$_2$ blockers; must give IV Protonix with filter
Mucosal Protective Agents Sucralfate (Carafate®)	Protect the stomach's mucous lining from the damage of the acid	Serious side effects are very rare	Should be administered separately from other drugs due to the potential to alter the absorption; patient may require an NGT/feeding tube if unable to take oral medication; if on tube feedings, must stop feedings for 1 hour before and 1 hour after dose due to absorption issues
Prostaglandin Analogues Misoprostol (Cytotec®)	Protect the stomach mucosa by mimicking the action of prostaglandin E$_1$ in the body	Side effects are rare; diarrhea is most common but is usually controlled by taking with food	Cytotec should not be used in women of childbearing potential unless the patient requires NSAID therapy and is at high risk of GI complications; can cause induction of labor in pregnant women

TABLE 34-3 Drugs Used in Gastrointestinal Disorders/Bleeding (continued)

Classification	Indications	Advantages	Disadvantages
Somatostatin Analogues Octreotide acetate (Sandostatin®)	Reduce portal hypertension in acute variceal bleed patients	As effective as vasopressin, but have fewer side effects; can be used in addition to endoscopic therapy of esophageal varices, or alone if endoscopy is unavailable or unsuccessful	May lower blood sugar levels
Pituitary Hormones Vasopressin (Pitressin®)	Reduce bleeding by causing vasoconstriction in the splanchnic bed	Can be given via selective arterial infusion or via a central venous line	Serious side effects such as myocardial or mesenteric ischemia and infarction; use great caution in patients with underlying coronary artery disease or vascular disease; rarely used due to the effectiveness of octreotide acetate

Sources: Cagir & Cirincione, 2004; www.barrettsinfo.com, 2004.

dynamically stable, close observation is essential to monitor for complications and rebleeding. As with any disorder, thorough education is essential to ease anxiety and prevent further admissions.

TABLE 34-4 Patient Education for Acute Gastrointestinal Bleeding

- Orientation to the ICU environment
- Causes and treatments for GI bleed
- Acute interventions/treatment regimens to decrease anxiety and knowledge deficits
- Pain control
- Instructions on signs and symptoms of GI bleeding
- When to call the physician or return to the hospital if GI bleeding symptoms reappear
- New medications and their doses, interactions, and side effects
- Lifestyle changes/modifications of risk factors (e.g., smoking or alcohol cessation, dietary changes, stress management)
- Allow time for discussion and questions and to ensure that the information was clearly understood
- Include family in discussion as appropriate

Sources: Nettina, 2001; Urden, Stacy, & Lough, 2002.

TABLE 34-5 Problem List for Acute Gastrointestinal Bleed

- Hypovolemia
- Decreased cardiac output
- Diarrhea
- Vomiting
- Altered nutrition
- Pain
- Possible aspiration
- Possible infection
- Knowledge deficit
- Anxiety
- Impaired family coping
- Powerlessness

Source: Urden, Stacy, & Lough, 2002.

Box 34-1
Optimal Patient Outcomes

- Vital signs in expected range
- Hemoglobin and hematocrit in expected range
- Physical comfort in expected range
- Intake and output balanced
- Confidence in ability to manage care to avert future bleeding episodes
- Describes strategies to eliminate unhealthy behavior

CASE STUDY

A 45-year-old female presented to the Emergency Department (ED) with complaints of syncope, lightheadedness, and diaphoresis. Her only history was a recent sinus infection for which she was taking azithromycin (Zithromycin®). Her hemoglobin and hematocrit levels were 10.2 (normal for women is 12–16 Gm/dL) and 30.1 (normal for women is 36–48 Gm/dL), respectively. She was diagnosed with dehydration, given 1 L of IV fluids, and discharged home.

The patient returned to the ED 24 hours later with the same symptoms, now with exertional shortness of breath, one episode of hemataemesis, and melena. Her hemoglobin and hematocrit levels were 6.4 and 18.5, respectively. Her electrolytes, platelet count, and liver enzymes were normal. Exam showed no abdominal tenderness or pain. Blood pressure was 98/64, pulse was 110, respiratory rate was 24/min, and temperature was 99.0°F. After a more thorough history was taken, she admitted to taking four to eight aspirins a day over seven days for sinus headaches. She was admitted to the ICU for observation and stabilization with a diagnosis of upper GI bleed secondary to large-dose aspirin use.

CRITICAL THINKING QUESTIONS

1. What should be the *initial* treatment in the emergency department?

2. After two units of packed red blood cells were transfused, an EGD was performed in this patient. The results showed a small antral gastric ulcer with no active bleeding. The area was injected with epinephrine. What would be the best treatment for this patient?

3. Which disciplines should be consulted to work with this client?

4. How would you modify your plan of care for patients of diverse backgrounds (e.g., Jehovah's Witness)?

5. What types of issues may require you to act as an advocate or moral agent for this patient?

6. How will you implement your role as a facilitator of learning for this patient?

7. Use the form to write up the data and a plan of care for a patient with GI bleeding in the clinical setting. Rate the patient as a level 1, 3, or 5 on each characteristic. Identify the level of nurse characteristics needed in the care of this patient.

8. Take one patient outcome for a patient and list evidence-based interventions found in a literature review for this patient.

Using the Synergy Model to Develop a Plan of Care

	Patient Characteristics	Level (1, 3, 5)	Subjective and Objective Data	Evidence-based Interventions	Outcomes
SYNERGY MODEL	Resiliency				
	Vulnerability				
	Stability				
	Complexity				
	Resource availability				
	Participation in care				
	Participation in decision making				
	Predictability				

Online Resources

American College of Gastroenterology: www.acg.gi.org/index.asp

American Gastroenterological Association: www.gastro.org/

Gastroenterology Nursing: www.gastroenterologynursing.com

Society of Gastroenterology Nurses and Associates: www.sgna.org/resources/journal.cfm

REFERENCES

American College of Gastroenterology. (2005). Understanding GI bleeding. Retrieved June 20, 2005, from www.acg.gi.org/patients/gibleeding/ index.asp

Bajwa, O., & Marik, P. E. (2005). The management of gastrointestinal bleeding. In M. P. Fink, E. Abraham, J-L. Vincent, & P. M. Kochanek (Eds.), *Textbook of critical care* (5th ed., pp. 101–108). Philadelphia: Saunders.

Barretts Info.com. (2004). Medical treatment of GERD. Retrieved June 14, 2005, from www.barrettsinfo.com/content/info_2b4_medical.htm

Cagir, B., & Cirincione, E. (2004). Lower gastrointestinal bleeding: Surgical perspective. Retrieved June 10, 2005, from www.emedicine.com/med/topic2818.htm

Casestecker, J. (2002). Upper gastrointestinal bleeding: Surgical perspective. Retrieved June 20, 2005, from www.emedicine.com/med/topic3566.htm

Centers for Disease Control and Prevention (CDC). (2006). Helicobacter pylori and peptic ulcer disease. Retrieved on August 29, 2006, from www.cdc.gov/ulcer/md/htm#Sda

Gopalswamy, N., Malhotra, V., Reddy, N., Singh, B., Markert, R., Sangal, S., et al. (2004). Long-term mortality of patients admitted to the intensive care unit for gastrointestinal bleeding. *Southern Medical Journal, 97*, 955–958.

Greenwald, B. (2004). The Minnesota tube: Its use and care in bleeding esophageal and gastric varices. *Gastroenterology Nursing, 27*(5), 212–217.

Holzman, N. L., Schirmer, C. M., & Nasraway, S. A. (2005). Gastrointestinal hemorrhage. In M. P. Fink, E. Abraham, J-L. Vincent, & P. M. Kochanek (Eds.), *Textbook of critical care* (5th ed., pp. 973–982). Philadelphia: Saunders.

Kolecki, P., & Menckhoff, C. (2004). Shock, hypovolemic. Retrieved June 28, 2005, from www.emedicine.com/emerg/topic532.htm

Logan, R. (2002). *ABC of the upper gastrointestinal tract.* London: BMJ Books.

Manning-Dimmitt, L., Dimmitt, S., & Wilson, G. (2005). Diagnosis of gastrointestinal bleeding in adults. *American Family Physician, 71*, 1339–1346.

Medical College of Wisconsin. (2003). Causes, symptoms and diagnosis of diverticulosis and diverticulitis. Retrieved June 28, 2005, from http://healthlink.mcw.edu/article/930605239.html

Nettina, S. M. (2001). *Lippincott manual of nursing practice* (7th ed.). Philadelphia: Lippincott Williams & Wilkins.

Papadakis, M. A., & McPhee, S. J. (2005). *Current consult medicine.* New York: Lange Medical Books/McGraw-Hill.

Si, J., Cao, Q., & Wu, J. (2005). Quality of gastric ulcer healing evaluated by endoscopic ultrasonography. *World Journal of Gastroenterology, 11*(22), 3461–3464.

Stone, C. (2003). Gastrointestinal bleeding. Retrieved June 14, 2005, from www.nlm.nih.gov/medlineplus/ency/article/003133.htm

Tham, T., & Collins, J. (2000). *Gastrointestinal emergencies.* London: BMJ Books.

Urden, L., Stacy, K., & Lough, M. (2002). *Thelan's critical care nursing: Diagnosis and management* (4th ed.). St. Louis, MO: Mosby.

Yusuf, T., & Wofford, S. (2002). Esophagogastroduodenoscopy. Retrieved June 28, 2005, from www.emedicine.com/med/topic2965.htm

CHAPTER 35

Hepatic Failure

Marian S. Altman

LEARNING OBJECTIVES

Upon completion of this chapter, the reader will be able to:

1. List the etiologies of hepatic failure.

2. Describe the pathophysiology and clinical manifestations of hepatic disease.

3. Discuss current nursing and medical treatment strategies and future treatment options.

4. List optimal outcomes that may be achieved through evidence-based management of the patient with hepatic failure.

Hepatic failure (also known as liver failure) is defined as a loss of 60% of the hepatocytes (cells in the liver that synthesize, degrade, and store substances and secrete bile). It is a clinical syndrome characterized by massive necrosis resulting in the clinical manifestations of liver disease. Hepatic failure can occur suddenly in the event of acute liver injury, or it can have an insidious onset in the case of chronic liver disease. Symptoms of hepatic failure are usually noted after 75% of hepatocyte function is lost.

ETIOLOGY

Acute hepatic failure may be the result of viral, infection, chemical, metabolic, or ischemic etiologies (see **Table 35-1**). The most common causes of acute hepatic failure are viral hepatitis and drug-induced liver injury (Richardson, 2002). Causes of chronic liver disease include cirrhosis, chronic cholestatic disease, chronic viral hepatitis, excessive alcohol consumption, malnutrition, diabetes mellitus, alpha-1 antitrypsin deficiency, Wilson's disease, hemochromatosis, repeated toxin exposure, and malignancies such as hepatocellular carcinoma and cholangiocarcinoma.

Acute Hepatic Failure

Acute hepatic failure refers to fulminant hepatic failure (FHF) and subfulminant hepatic failure (or late-onset hepatic failure) (Sood & Jones, 2006). FHF is defined as "the rapid development of severe acute liver injury with impaired synthetic function and encephalopathy in a person who previously had a normal liver or had well-compensated liver disease" (Goldberg & Chopra, 2006). It is the result of sudden massive necrosis of liver cells, which is itself commonly due to viral infection or exposure to hepatotoxins. This life-threatening form of liver disease is associated with signs and symptoms of encephalopathy and coagulopathy. Acute hepatic failure can develop in less than eight weeks from the onset of illness in a patient without preexisting liver disease. Diagnosis is based on the symptoms of acute liver disease, and hepatic encephalopathy. Acute hepatic failure may also be defined as either hyperacute, acute, or subacute (see **Table 35-2**).

TABLE 35-1 Causes of Acute Hepatic Failure

Viral
Viral hepatitis (A, B, C, D, E)

Viral Infections in Immunosuppressed Patients
Cytomegalovirus, herpes simplex, Epstein-Barr virus, yellow
  fever, *Coxiella burretti*, adenovirus, varicella zoster

Chemical
Hepatotoxic drugs: isoniazide, rifampicin (Rifampin®)
Chemotherapy
Acetaminophen (Tylenol®)
Antibiotics: tetracycline, penicillin, sulfonamides, quinolones
Valproate sodium (Depakene®)
Phosphorus
Monoamine oxidase inhibitors
Alpha methyldopa (Aldomet®)
Nonsteroidal anti-inflammatory drugs: ibuprofen (Advil®)
Anesthetic agents: halothane
Phenytoin (Dilantin®)
Allopurinol
Antihyperglycemics
Acute alcoholic hepatitis

Toxins
Carbon tetrachloride, industrial solvents, herbal medicines,
  herbicides, yellow phosphorus, *Amanita phalloides* mushroom species

Metabolic
Fatty liver of pregnancy, Wilson's disease, Reye's syndrome

Miscellaneous
Unknown, Budd-Chiari syndrome, acute right-sided heart
  failure, cardiac tamponade

Source: Gill & Sterling, 2001.

TABLE 35-2 Types of Acute Hepatic Failure

Hyperacute
Encephalopathy within 7 days of jaundice development. High
  incidence of cerebral edema.

Acute
Encephalopathy within 8 to 28 days of jaundice development.
  Significant cerebral edema. Outcome poor without
  transplantation.

Subacute
Encephalopathy within 4 to 12 weeks of jaundice development.
  Characterized by a high mortality. Low incidence of cerebral
  edema.

Source: Rahman & Hodgson, 2001.

etiologic factors cannot always be identified (Goldberg & Chopra, 2006). Symptoms of FHF include ascites, jaundice, light-colored stools, easy bruising, fever, abdominal pain, itching, dark urine, nausea, anorexia, weakness, and fatigue. As FHF evolves, toxins build up, affecting the brain and causing confusion, inconsistent behavior, and encephalopathy. Patients with FHF are admitted to the intensive care unit (ICU) for monitoring and management of possible complications. These complications include encephalopathy, cerebral edema, sepsis, renal failure, circulatory dysfunction, coagulopathy, GI bleeding, and metabolic derangements such as metabolic acidosis, hypoglycemia, and hypophosphatemia (Goldberg & Chopra).

Cirrhosis

Cirrhosis and end-stage hepatic failure are synonymous. Cirrhosis can interrupt the functioning of healthy liver tissue (National AIDS Treatment Advocacy Project, 2006). It is described as fibrous tissue changes or scarring secondary to several years of injury (Bonis & Chopra, 2006). While liver tissue is usually able to regenerate after injury, chronic injury is characterized by irreversible fibrous scarring and the formation of regeneration nodules. These problems cause irreparable functional damage, resulting in chronic hepatic insufficiency and failure. Any chronic disease of the liver may result in cirrhosis.

The clinical manifestations of cirrhosis are caused by portal hypertension, the loss of metabolic storage, and synthetic function of the liver. The clinical presentation varies widely depending on the amount of functional liver mass and the severity of complications. Symptoms may include itching, jaundice of the skin and eyes (scleral icterus) due to obstruc-

Despite advances in management, mortality ranges from 40% to 80%, related to complications such as cerebral edema, sepsis, hypoglycemia, gastrointestinal (GI) bleed, and acute renal failure (Gill & Sterling, 2001). Treatment is symptomatic and supportive. The hepatocytes can regenerate in four to five weeks if the function of the liver can be supported and no further damage occurs. Chronic hepatitis leads to inflammation, necrosis, and fibrosis. Cirrhosis may result.

PATHOPHYSIOLOGY AND CLINICAL MANIFESTATIONS

Fulminant Hepatic Failure

The pathophysiology of FHF usually begins with exposure of a susceptible person to an agent capable of producing severe hepatic injury. The exact mechanism is not clearly understood and

tion of bile ducts, and fatigue. Other symptoms of cirrhosis are related to the liver's inability to perform its normal functions. For example, the scarring associated with cirrhosis makes it difficult for blood to flow through the liver. As a result, veins outside the liver become engorged (varices). If the pressure in the varices reaches a certain level, they may burst, causing massive bleeding. Bleeding esophageal varices is discussed in more detail in Chapter 34. The cirrhotic liver may also be unable to produce albumin. This effect may result in development of third spacing, especially in the legs (edema), abdomen (ascites), or lungs (pleural effusion). Ascites can lead to the development of peritonitis (Bonis & Chopra, 2006).

Patients with cirrhosis may also develop bleeding problems. This bleeding is related to thrombocytopenia and depletion of clotting factors. A patient with cirrhosis has impaired immune function, which can lead to the development of infections and sepsis. Malnutrition is also common in patients with cirrhosis (Bonis & Chopra, 2006).

Hepatic Encephalopathy

Hepatic encephalopathy is a broad term used to describe the neurological changes caused by hepatic failure. The pathophysiology of hepatic encephalopathy is not clearly understood, but is believed to be related to increased production of ammonia from nitrogenous substances within the gut lumen (Goldberg & Chopra, 2006). The liver metabolizes amino acids for immediate energy or storage. During this process, carbon dioxide (CO_2) and ammonia (NH_3) are released as by-products. Ammonia can also form from the degradation of protein or metabolism of

blood by the natural flora of the gut. As blood is shunted away from the diseased liver, ammonia is not converted to water-soluble urea (which is excreted by the kidneys), so ammonia levels rise. Ammonia crosses the blood–brain barrier, causing a deterioration of brain function. The stage of encephalopathy does not correlate with the ammonia level.

Since the cirrhotic liver also cannot filter toxins adequately, hepatic encephalopathy can result. Hepatic encephalopathy is manifested as monotonous speech, drowsiness, confusion, delirium, or coma (Bonis & Chopra, 2006). Patients with hepatic encephalopathy develop a distinctive breath odor called fetor hepaticus. The sweet fecal breath is a result of mercaptan (a metabolite formed from sulfur-containing amino acids) excretion through respirations instead of through liver detoxification. Mercaptans are neurotoxic and can potentiate ammonia toxicity.

Asterixis—a sudden, brief, nonrhythmic flexion of the hands and fingers when a patient extends an arm and dorsiflexes the wrist—is a warning sign (Whiteman & McCormick, 2005). Hepatic encephalopathy is graded on a scale of 1 to 4 (see Table 35-3).

Cerebral Edema

Cerebral edema develops in 75% to 80% of patients with grade IV encephalopathy. The exact reason for its development is not completely understood, but may be related to such factors as changes in cellular metabolism and alterations in cerebral blood flow (Blei, 2005). Cerebral edema is discussed in more detail in Chapter 27.

TABLE 35-3 Stages of Encephalopathy

Stage	Mental Status Changes	Physical Exam	EEG
1	Confused, altered mood Slowed mentation Disturbed sleep	Mild asterixis Normal tone/reflexes	None/normal
2	Inappropriate behavior Increasingly drowsy	Asterixis Agitated	Generalized slowing Abnormal
3	Stuporous, but arousable Confused, agitated behavior Marked confusion	Asterixis	Abnormal
4	May or may not respond to pain Coma possible	Asterixis absent Unresponsive to painful stimuli	Abnormal

Key: EEG = electroencephalogram

Source: Gill & Sterling, 2001.

Portal Hypertension

The major sequelae of cirrhosis include portal hypertension, hepatic failure, ascites, hepatorenal syndrome, and encephalopathy. The normal liver offers little resistance to blood flow and is known as a low-pressure system. Portal hypertension is an increase in portal venous pressure with vasoconstriction. The increase in pressure hinders blood flow into the liver (Andrew, 2001). As the liver fails, blood flow is reduced. Cirrhosis also impedes blood flow, which in turn increases pressure in the portal system. The ultimate outcome is significant congestion and dilation of the veins in the portal system and shunting of blood away from the liver. A backward flow is created away from the liver, and to the spleen, stomach, and esophagus, in an effort to maintain venous return to the heart. Collateral channels may develop in the gastric fundus, esophagus, abdominal wall, and rectum, shunting blood away from the high-pressure portal system to areas of lower pressure in the GI tract. Bleeding of esophageal varices is a major complication of portal hypertension (Hegab & Luketic, 2001). As the low-pressure veins become distended with blood, the vessels enlarge and varices develop. The dilated, thin-walled veins of the esophagus and GI tract are easily traumatized and therefore may rupture and bleed easily. The risk of bleeding increases as portal pressure increases.

Immunologic Alterations

Portal hypertension decreases blood flow to the liver. As the blood flow through the liver decreases or stagnates, patients have difficulty mounting a response to infection. Seventy percent of the body's macrophages reside in the liver, so the body's ability to fight infection decreases as liver cells are destroyed. Portal hypertension also causes spleen enlargement, which causes destruction of white blood cells, red blood cells, and platelets. Neutrophil malfunction further complicates the problem (Krumberger, 2002).

Fluid Alterations

Portal hypertension causes increased hydrostatic pressure, which forces fluid out of the vessels and into the peritoneal cavity. As this protein-rich fluid shifts its position, peripheral edema in dependent areas and ascites occur. As fluid moves from the vascular space, there is a decrease in circulating volume, hypotension, and lowered renal perfusion.

Ascites

Ascites—excess fluid in the peritoneal cavity—is seen with both acute and chronic hepatic failure. Factors causing ascites are altered plasma oncotic pressure related to decreased albumin synthesis and increased portal venous pressure. As ascites develops, fluid is drawn from the intravascular space to the peritoneal cavity, causing a decrease in circulating volume. The production of aldosterone and antidiuretic hormone (ADH) is stimulated, which causes sodium and water to be reabsorbed in the renal tubules in an effort to increase intravascular volume.

Alterations in Hormone Metabolism

When blood is shunted away from the liver, substances normally detoxified and metabolized by the liver, such as hormones, chemicals, and drugs, never reach their destination. In such a case, glucocorticoids (e.g., cortisol) and mineralocorticoids (e.g., aldosterone and ADH) are not inactivated by the liver. When the diseased liver does not deactivate endocrine hormones, the patient may experience weight gain; a rounded, edematous face; scant body hair; gynecomastia; and impotence (Tayek, 2005).

Alterations in Fat Metabolism

Bile, which consists of bile salts, bile pigments, and cholesterol, decreases the surface tension of fat in the gut by agitating it and making fatty acids more soluble. This allows fat and fat-soluble vitamins (A, D, E, and K) to be absorbed. Bile salts are produced by the hepatocytes from cholesterol in a 1:1 relationship. However, not all of the cholesterol is used when making bile salts. As the liver fails, fat metabolism becomes increasingly more ineffective. The production of bile salts is decreased, causing as much as 40% of lipids to be lost in the stool. This causes steatorrhea—fatty, greasy, foul-smelling stools. Serum cholesterol levels rise, which may cause gallstones. Malnutrition may result from decreased absorption of fat, fat-soluble vitamins, and minerals. **Table 35-4** lists the side effects of decreased absorption of fat-soluble vitamins.

TABLE 35-4 Fat-Soluble Vitamin Deficiency Effects

Vitamin A
  Night blindness, abnormal dryness of eye membranes.

Vitamin D
  Rickets, decreased serum calcium absorption in the gut, which leads to calcium resorption from bone. Bone demineralization may lead to osteomalacia, kyphosis, and fractures.

Vitamin K
  Coagulopathies, hemorrhagic disease.

Source: Uptodate.com, 2006.

OTHER SEQUELAE OF HEPATIC FAILURE

Alteration in Bilirubin Metabolism

Hepatic failure leads to a decreased ability to conjugate bilirubin, the by-product of red blood cell metabolism. As the red blood cell is destroyed, the heme molecule attaches to albumin, creating unconjugated or indirect bilirubin. This type of bilirubin is not soluble and cannot be excreted. Bilirubin is made soluble or conjugated by the liver and is excreted in the bile, urine, and feces, giving them their characteristic colors. As unconjugated bilirubin levels increase to greater than 0.8 mg/dL, the patient appears jaundiced (Krumberger, 2002).

Metabolic Alterations

Metabolic functions of the liver include the metabolism of carbohydrates, fats, and proteins. Carbohydrates arrive in the liver as simple sugars. The liver then metabolizes carbohydrates to energy for immediate use. Any extra carbohydrate in the liver is stored as glycogen (glycogenesis) and can be released when the body needs glucose but other sources are unavailable (glycogenolysis). The liver converts excess carbohydrates to triglycerides, which are then stored. Triglycerides are metabolized to glycerol and fatty acids when needed for energy production. Fatty acids are broken down further into ketones, which are converted to meet cellular energy needs. If glycogen stores become depleted, the liver is able to convert amino acids and fatty acids to glucose in a process called gluconeogenesis. Hepatic failure causes an inability to store glycogen or make glucose out of fat or protein (Krumberger, 2002).

Alteration in Protein Metabolism

The liver synthesizes 90% of all plasma proteins. The major proteins metabolized by the liver are albumin, globulin, and fibrinogen. As the liver fails, protein synthesis decreases (Gheorghe, Iacob, Vadan, Iacob, & Gheorghe, 2005) and less fibrinogen and clotting factors are made. Extrinsic clotting cascade factors II, V, VII, IX, and X become deficient. All of the factors listed except Factor V are vitamin K dependent. Vitamin K is lipid soluble and therefore depends on bile salts for its intestinal absorption. Bile salt secretion failure leads to a deficiency of vitamin-K-dependent clotting factors. An elevated prothrombin time (PT) and partial thromboplastin time (PTT) result, putting the patient at risk for bleeding due to deficiency of clotting factors (Kerr, 2003).

The liver is also unable to remove activated clotting factors, a development that leads to the formation of microthrombi and consumption of platelets and fibrinogen. As these clots break down, fibrin split products are released; these substances are anticoagulants. The liver is unable to synthesize more clotting factors and bleeding results. Eventually, the patient may experience disseminated intravascular coagulation (DIC) (see Chapter 50).

Hepatorenal Syndrome

Renal failure develops in approximately 55% of patients with acute hepatic failure (Richardson, 2002). Its etiologies include toxicity, hypovolemia, sepsis, nephrotoxic drugs, and hepatorenal syndrome. Renal failure without an obvious cause that develops concurrently in a patient with hepatic failure is termed hepatorenal syndrome. The kidneys are structurally normal and may recover if the underlying liver disease is treated (Richardson). Treatment focuses on identifying patients at risk, avoiding nephrotoxic drugs, maintaining circulating volume, monitoring urine output and daily weight, and preventing an accumulation of substances normally inactivated by the liver. Continuous renal replacement therapies may be indicated. Vasodilator effects of low-dose dopamine (Intropin®) may maintain renal perfusion.

Assessment

The clinical manifestations of hepatic failure are directly related to the failure of normal physiologic functions performed exclusively by the liver. The clinical findings of liver failure, pathophysiology involved, and body systems affected are listed in **Table 35-5** and described in the pathophysiology section. Clinical findings vary in relation to the timing of the physical exam and the progression of the disease process. Clinical findings associated with acute hepatic failure may occur in less than two weeks. Examination of the patient reveals a tender enlarged liver and decreased hepatic dullness to percussion.

Collaborative Management

A collaborative, multidisciplinary approach to patient management is essential to obtaining a favorable outcome. There is no specific medical therapy for hepatic failure. Instead, management focuses on supporting liver function until this organ can regenerate, while protecting other body systems from failure (Gill & Sterling, 2001). Supportive measures include maintaining circulating volume, stabilizing hemodynamics, providing nutritional support, controlling electrolyte balance, frequent glucose monitoring, taking aspiration precautions, and controlling ammonia levels to prevent the progression of encephalopathy and its complications. Treatment also focuses on symptom relief. Alcohol and other liver toxins must be avoided. Patients with acute hepatic failure are critically ill and need intensive care monitoring to detect complications. Patients in

TABLE 35-5 Clinical Findings of Hepatic Failure

Body System	Clinical Findings	Pathophysiology
Cardiovascular	Increased cardiac output, heart rate, bounding pulses, systolic ejection murmur	Hyperkinetic circulation
	Decreased blood pressure and renal blood flow, peripheral edema	Third spacing
	Arrhythmias	Fluid and electrolyte imbalances
General	Weight loss, muscle wasting, malnourished	Ineffective metabolism (carbohydrate, fat, protein)
	Malaise, fatigue	Inability to store vitamins and iron
Immune	Leukopenia	Splenomegaly
	Increased infection risk	Decreased Kupffer cell function
Skin	Jaundice	Inability to conjugate bilirubin
	Palmar erythema, hair loss	Inability to detoxify hormones
	Pruritis, dry skin	Elevated bile salts
	Spider angiomas	Portal hypertension
	Xanthomas	Hyperlipidemia
Endocrine	Peripheral edema, increased weight, moon face, striae, decreased libido, testicular atrophy, gynecomastia, impotence, menstrual abnormalities	Inability to detoxify or inactivate hormones
	Hypoglycemia	Decreased glycogen, decreased carbohydrate metabolism
Gastrointestinal	Anorexia, nausea, vomiting	Elevated methylmercaptan
	Steatorrhea, malnutrition, hyperlipidemia	Decreased fat metabolism
	Hematemesis, melena, hematochezia	Portal hypertension
	Clay-colored stools	Inability to conjugate bilirubin
	Epistaxis, gingival bleeding, heme + stools	Decreased synthesis of clotting factors
	Hepatomegaly	
Hematology	Anemia, nose bleeds, gum bleeds, thrombocytopenia, ecchymosis, bruising, purpura, elevated liver enzymes	Splenomegaly, inability to synthesize clotting factors
Neurologic	Sensory disturbances, peripheral degeneration, paresthesia, foot drop, nystagmus, ptosis	Inability to absorb fat-soluble vitamins
Renal	Decreased urine output, elevated BUN and creatinine	Decreased circulating volume, decreased renal blood flow, decreased glomerular filtration rate
Pulmonary	Diaphragm elevation, shortness of breath, decreased lung expansion, pulmonary edema or effusion	Ascites
	Decreased PaO_2 or SpO_2	Increased 2,3-DPG levels

Source: Gill & Sterling, 2001.

acute hepatic failure will require pulmonary artery pressure monitoring to help manage intravascular volume and optimize oxygenation. Management begins with the ABCs. Elective intubation is recommended to prevent aspiration. Positive inotropes, such as dopamine, are often needed to support blood pressure and maintain cardiac output (Krumberger, 2002).

Cerebral edema develops in 70% to 80% of patients with FHF in stage 4 encephalopathy and is a common cause of death (Gill & Sterling, 2001). Diagnosis and management rely on the use of intracranial pressure (ICP) monitoring. Prompt identification and treatment are essential. Stimuli that increase ICP, such as suctioning and high positive end expiratory pressure, should be avoided. Hypotension, hypoxia, and hypercapnia should be prevented. Patients are positioned with the head of the bed elevated at 20 to 30 degrees. It is important to maintain the cerebral perfusion pressure at more than 50 mm Hg and ICP at less than 30 to 40 mm Hg (Rahman & Hodgson, 2001). Mannitol 0.3–0.4 Gm/kg in a 20% solution may also be given (Marrero, Martinex, & Hyzy, 2003). Thiopentone sodium has been used in mannitol-resistant patients.

GI Bleeding Management

Patients with hepatic failure are at risk for upper GI bleeding. Acid suppression using H_2 antagonists, proton pump inhibitors, or sulcrafate (Carafate®) is recommended. Portal hypertension leads to collateral circulation development to and around the liver. The increased pressure causes these vessels to become distended, such that varices may develop. Varices commonly occur at the esophagus, rectum, and abdomen. Their rupture may cause life-threatening bleeding. Signs and symptoms include bright red blood from the patient's GI tract, hypotension, tachycardia, and cool and clammy skin. The patient may also have bloody or black tarry stools, a condition known as melena (Whiteman & McCormick, 2005). To help reduce the risk of an esophageal variceal bleed, the patient may be placed on a beta-adrenergic blocker such as propranolol (Inderal®), which lowers blood pressure. If a patient experiences a bleed, endoscopy is used to find and treat the bleeding site with the use of sclerotherapy. With sclerotherapy, a strong irritating agent is injected into the area to cause scarring. Heater probe, laser therapy, electrocoagulation, rubber band ligation or banding procedure, or hemoclips may also be used (Krumberger, 2005). Octreotide (Sandostatin®) and vasopressin (Pitressin®) are medications that restrict portal inflow by causing vasoconstriction of the splanchnic arteries; they may also help control GI bleeding. Balloon tamponade may be used if the patient is unstable (Whiteman & McCormick). A more in-depth discussion of GI bleeding appears in Chapter 34.

Surgical Management of GI Bleeding

Medical management with sclerotherapy and pharmacologic agents are implemented initially to treat bleeding varices. If the bleeding is uncontrolled, surgical interventions such as antrectomy, gastrectomy, vagotomy, and combination procedures may be necessary. Portal pressure and esophageal variceal complications can also be addressed with a portal caval shunt. Shunts divert blood flow from the portal to the systemic circulation, which bypasses the liver and thereby decreases portal hypertension. Another procedure to control recurrent variceal bleeding is a transjugular intrahepatic portosystemic shunt (TIPS). In this procedure, a stent is placed in the parenchyma of the liver between the hepatic and portal veins to decrease the pressure in the portal vein and varices. TIPS is discussed in more detail in Chapter 34.

Encephalopathy Management

Identifying and correcting precipitating factors, avoiding hepatotoxic drugs, and limiting ammonia production are all steps to treat encephalopathy. The exact pathogenesis of hepatic encephalopathy is uncertain, but a decrease of nitrogenous products from the gut and circulation is known to be accompanied by clinical improvement. In stage 1 or 2 of hepatic encephalopathy, administration of lactulose (Cephulac®) or oral antibiotics that decrease gut flora, such as metronidazole (Flagyl®), and a low-protein diet are beneficial. Oral neomycin is used if the patient has not responded to lactulose within 48 hours (Ferenci, 2006). These medicines, however, have not been shown to improve survival in patients with more advanced stages of hepatic encephalopathy (Gill & Sterling, 2001).

Neomycin, a nonabsorbable antibiotic, destroys the flora in the GI tract that break down protein and result in ammonia production. Neomycin can be administered by mouth or enema. An enema may not be recommended in some cases because it may cause rectal bleeding in the patient with coagulopathies. The dose is generally 500 mg to 1 Gm every 6 hours or a 200 mL enema of 1% solution. Neomycin can cause ototoxicity and nephrotoxicity. Therefore, lactulose is usually the drug of choice. Lactulose is a non-absorbable dissaccharide that is converted in the bowel to lactate and other acids. Lactulose acidifies the bowel environment and binds the ammonia. The laxative effect of this treatment causes the ammonia to then be excreted in the stool. Side effects of this therapy may include bloating, cramping, nausea, or vomiting. Severe diarrhea may result. The dose is 15 to 30 Gm given three to four times a day, or until the patient has two to four stools. An enema of 300 mL of 50% lactulose and 700 mL of water three times per day can also be used.

It is important to rule out any concurrent process that might cause mental status changes, and to begin treatment of encephalopathy while other causes of mental status changes are ruled out. Frequently monitoring a patient's neurological status, reorienting the patient as needed, protecting the patient from injury, and treating any changes are essential.

Nutrition Management

A patient's nutritional status must be assessed. Every patient needs an adequate intake of protein and calories. However, an increased protein load may worsen hepatic encephalopathy. Patients require enough protein for the liver to regenerate, but not so much that ammonia production increases. Roughly 40 Gm per day are suggested (Krumberger, 2002). The oral or enteral route is preferred to maintain intestinal mucosal integrity and decrease bacterial translocation. Although not proven to decrease hepatic encephalopathy or improve survival, branched-chain amino acids are preferred (Gill & Sterling, 2001). It has been suggested that the three essential amino acids (i.e., branched-chain amino acids or L-leucine, L-isoleucine, and L-valine) may have antihepatic encephalopathy activity. Theoretically, it is thought that branched-chain amino acids reduce the accumulation of false neurotransmitters in the brain. These false neurotransmitters are believed to contribute to hepatic encephalopathy (PDR Health, 2006).

Sodium intake should be restricted to less than 2 Gm per day to prevent fluid alterations. It is important to assess the patient's food preferences. Hepatic failure patients will also need frequent assessment of glucose levels, because they are prone to hypoglycemia.

Acetaminophen Overdose Management

Acetaminophen overdose causes depletion of glutathione, which binds the drug and leads to hepatic failure. The goal of initial management of acetaminophen overdose is to prevent continued drug absorption. Interventions include evacuating the stomach and absorbing acetaminophen with activated charcoal. N-Acetylcysteine (Mucomyst®) replenishes the glutathione and limits hepatic damage. This drug is available as an oral preparation, which is given orally or by nasogastric tube and is most effective when administered within 12 hours of ingestion, but may be given up to 36 hours after overdose (Gill & Sterling, 2001). Intravenous N-acetylcysteine is used in Europe and Canada to treat acetaminophen overdose. However, it is not approved by the Food and Drug Administration (FDA) in the United States (Jeffords, Dribben, Porto, Parrish, & Harkins, 2002). Acetaminophen toxicity is further addressed in Chapter 56.

Ascites Management

Ascites is managed by treating the cause (Marrero et al., 2003). It may also be managed with diuretics and sodium restriction. Diuretics such as Aldactone (Spironolactone®, a potassium-sparing diuretic), thiazide, or loop diuretics may be used. Large-volume paracentesis has been shown to be safe and effective (Marrero et al.). Infusion of 6 to 8 Gm of albumin per liter of fluid removed prevents hemodynamic problems. Refractory ascites may be treated with a TIPS (Marrero et al.).

Fluid and Electrolyte Management

A patient's fluid and electrolyte status may be affected by liver disease as well as by interventions used to treat the disease. It is important to monitor and prevent hyperkalemia and intravascular volume depletion. Frequent vital signs, strict intake and output, and daily weight measurements are essential. Potassium, glucose, urinary sodium, blood urea nitrogen (BUN), and creatinine should be monitored daily. Urine output should be monitored hourly and maintained at greater than 0.5 mL/kg/hr. A patient's volume status is carefully monitored by frequent vital signs and hemodynamic monitoring of the pulmonary artery pressures and cardiac output. If signs and symptoms of volume depletion occur, intravenous fluid volume replacement is indicated and the diuretics should be discontinued. Volume is usually replaced with blood if the patient's hemoglobin is low; otherwise, a combination of colloids and crystalloids is used. The use of albumin is controversial (Rahman & Hodgson, 2001). Lactated Ringer's should be avoided, because the liver chiefly metabolizes lactate. It is important to assess for orthostatic changes.

Coagulopathy Management

Most patients with hepatic failure have significant coagulopathy, but spontaneous hemorrhage is uncommon. Coagulopathy is usually not treated, but, if given, treatment may include administration of vitamin K, fresh frozen plasma (FFP), and platelets. Routine use of FFP is not recommended unless spontaneous bleeding occurs, or in preparation for an invasive procedure (Marrero et al., 2003). Vitamin K 10 mg administered daily for three days may be ordered. Frequent monitoring of PT, PTT, and fibrinogen is needed.

Infection Management

Bacterial and fungal infections are common in patients with acute hepatic failure (Rahman & Hodgson, 2001). Infection is managed by prevention and early detection. Strict aseptic technique is needed. Careful handwashing, avoidance of invasive procedures and lines when possible, venipuncture and wound site assessment, regular pulmonary toilet and routine cultures, and chest radiographs may all help prevent infection. Regular microbial surveillance and aggressive treatment of presumed infections are essential given that prophylactic regimens have been shown to be of little benefit (Richardson, 2002). Antibiotics are given as indicated by culture sensitivities.

Transplantation

Currently, liver transplantation is the only definitive, proven treatment for acute hepatic failure. To qualify for transplant, patients must meet very specific criteria. Transplant centers clearly delineate indications and contraindications for transplant. Indications for liver transplantation may include chronic hepatic failure (e.g., cirrhosis), acute hepatic failure, and primary liver tumors (Conrad, 2006).

Advances in surgical techniques and immunosuppressive therapies have enabled liver transplantation to be performed with a high graft success rate and decreased patient mortality rate (Day & Taylor, 2006). Any patient with acute or fulminant hepatic failure should be referred to a transplant center for evaluation. Unfortunately, organs are a scarce resource and the number of organs available falls far short of the number of potential recipients of organs. This imbalance has led to an ever-growing number of candidates waiting for liver transplantation (Rahman & Hodgson, 2001; Stewart, Kozlowski, Segev, Montgomery, & Klein, 2006).

Post-transplant, the patient may be transferred to the ICU. Potential complications in the immediate transplant period include acute rejection and early graft failure, as well as vascular and biliary complications. Immunosuppressive therapy is administered to decrease the chance of rejection (Conrad, 2006). Despite administration of immunosuppressive therapy, some patients may develop rejection following a transplant. The ICU nurse must monitor for the presence of signs of all potential complications.

Acute rejection is not uncommon for the first three months following transplant and manifests as jaundice, itching, lethargy, weakness, malaise, right upper quadrant tenderness, and possibly fevers. Lab data are significant for an initial increase in bilirubin and alkaline phosphatase. This phenomenon is followed by elevations in alanine aminotransferase (ALT) and aspartate aminotransferase (AST). If the patient develops a post-transplant infection, an intra-abdominal bacterial infection is commonly to blame. In contrast, the incidence of fungal infections increases one to two months after transplant (Conrad, 2006). A detailed description of nursing care for organ transplantation can be found in Chapter 58.

When patients receive immunosuppressive therapy, they are vulnerable to infection from less common opportunistic organisms, including fungi (especially *Candida* species), herpes simplex, herpes zoster, *Pneumocystis carinii*, and *Toxoplasmosis*. Patients may also develop nephrotoxicity from cyclosporine or tacrolimus administration. Hyperkalemia, hypervolemia, and hypertension may occur (Conrad, 2006).

Because of the shortage of donor organs, temporary liver-assisting therapies have been developed (Stockmann, Hiemstra, Marquet, & IJzermans, 2000). Experimental treatments such as extracorporeal albumin dialysis and cell-based liver systems may be used as a bridge to transplantation (Whiteman & McCormick, 2005). Liver-assist devices have been evaluated over the past 10 years using porcine or human liver cells. Data from the first randomized, controlled trial support statistically higher survival in patients with fulminant/subfulminant hepatitic failure who received a bioartificial liver than patients in the control group (Demetriou et al., 2004). Transplant of human hepatocytes into the splenic bed has had some success. Xenotransplant with transgenic pigs also remains under investigation (Gill & Sterling, 2001).

PATIENT OUTCOMES

Nurses can help ensure the obtainment of optimal patient outcomes such as those listed in **Box 35-1** through the use of evidence-based interventions for patients with hepatic failure.

SUMMARY

Caring for a patient with acute or chronic liver disease requires early assessment, precise identification, and prompt treatment by a collaborative healthcare team. It is important that ICU nurses understand the physiology, pathophysiology, clinical presentation, and treatment of patients with liver disease to help avoid complications.

Box 35-1
Optimal Patient Outcomes

- Coagulation status within expected range
- Absence of overt signs of bleeding
- Nutritional status within expected range
- No decline in mental status
- Absence of shortness of breath on exertion due to ascites
- Absence of signs and symptoms of infection

CASE STUDY

Mr. S. is a 45-year-old male with a history of cirrhosis. He had been complaining of feeling weak and a lack of appetite for a week prior to his admission. His wife reports that he was turning yellow over the past week. This morning she found him difficult to arouse and confused. The patient was admitted to the ICU. A pulmonary artery catheter and a urinary catheter were inserted. A pulse oximeter was placed on the patient, and he was connected to the cardiac monitor. Admission lab work was sent. The results were as follows:

Na 130 mEq/L

K 3.1 mEq/L

BUN 22 mg/dL

Creat 1.2 mg/dL

PT 25 sec

aPTT 50 sec

WBC 15,000 mm^3

Hgb 10 Gm/dL

Hct 33%

Albumin 2.5 mg/dL

Ammonia 174 mcg/dL

T bili 4.0 mg/dL

AST 70 IU/L

ALT 130 IU/L

The patient's vital signs were as follows:

BP 80/40

HR 140

RR 20

Temp 101°F

CVP 2

PAS 10

PAD 6

PAOP 5

CO 4

CI 1.8

The patient's assessment revealed minimal peripheral edema and clear breath sounds bilaterally, but decreased in the right lower lobe. His respirations were shallow. Fetor hepaticus (foul-smelling breath) was noted. Jaundice and mucosal bleeding were present. The abdominal examination revealed a distended abdomen with hepatomegaly. Bowel sounds were hypoactive. The urinary catheter was draining dark, foamy urine. The patient was confused and uncooperative.

CRITICAL THINKING QUESTIONS

1. The liver is a dynamic organ with many functions. Discuss three major functions of the liver.
2. Mr. S.'s precipitating cause of hepatic failure was cirrhosis. List three other causes of hepatic failure.
3. Mr. S. has a fever and an elevated white blood cell count. Why does he have an increased susceptibility to infection?
4. Which abnormal laboratory and physical findings noted in Mr. S. are indicative of hepatic failure?

Using the Synergy Model to Develop a Plan of Care

	Patient Characteristics	Level (1, 3, 5)	Subjective and Objective Data	Evidence-based Interventions	Outcomes
SYNERGY MODEL	Resiliency				
	Vulnerability				
	Stability				
	Complexity				
	Resource availability				
	Participation in care				
	Participation in decision making				
	Predictability				

Online Resources

HepNet, The Hepatitis Information Network: www.hepnet.com/liver/disease.html

Liver disease: www.medhelp.org/HealthTopics/Liver_Disease.html

Liver diseases: www.nlm.nih.gov/medlineplus/liverdiseases.html.

REFERENCES

Andrew, A. (2001). Portal hypertension: A review. *Journal of Diagnostic Medical Sonography, 17*(4), 193–202.

Blei, A. T. (2005). The pathophysiology of brain edema in acute liver failure. *Neurochemistry International, 47*(1–2), 71–77.

Bonis, P. A., & Chopra, S. (2006). Patient information: Cirrhosis. Retrieved February 10, 2006, from http://patients.uptodate.com/topic.asp?file=livr_dis/4490

Conrad, S. A. (2006). Transplants, liver. Retrieved February 10, 2006, from www.emedicine.com/emerg/topic605.htm

Day, H. L., & Taylor, R. M. (2006). The liver: Part 6: Liver transplantation. *Nursing Times, 102*(3), 30–32.

Demetriou, A. A., Brown, R. S., Busuttil, R. W., Fair, J., McGuire, B. M., Rosenthal, P., et al. (2004). Prospective multi-center trial of a bioartificial liver in treating acute liver failure. *Annals of Surgery, 239*(5), 660–670.

Ferenci, P. (2006). Treatment of hepatic encephalopathy. Retrieved February 10, 2006, from http://patients.uptodate.com/topic.asp?file=cirrhosis/6577

Gheorghe, L., Iacob, R., Vadan, R., Iacob, S., & Gheorghe, C. (2005). Improvement of hepatic encephalopathy using a modified high-calorie high protein diet. *Romanian Journal of Gastroenterology, 14*(3), 231–238.

Gill, R., & Sterling, R. (2001). Acute liver failure. *Clinical Gastroenterology, 33*(3), 191–198.

Goldberg, E., & Chopra, S. (2006). Fulminant hepatic failure: Definition, etiology, and prognostic indicators. Retrieved February 10, 2006, from http://patients.uptodate.com/topic.asp?file=hep_dis/14112

Hegab, A. M., & Lutetic, V. A. (2001). Bleeding esophageal varices: How to treat this dreaded complication of portal hypertension. Symposium: Second of three articles on cirrhosis. *Postgraduate Medicine, 109*(2), 75–76, 81–86, 89.

Jeffords, B. K., Dribben, W. H., Porto, S. M., Parrish, T. M., & Harkins, T. L. (2002). The stability and microbiology of inhalant N-acetylcysteine used as an intravenous solution for the treatment of acetaminophen poisoning. *Academic Emergency Medicine, 9*(5), 487.

Kerr, R. (2003). New insights into haemostasis in liver failure. *Blood Coagulation and Fibrinolysis, 14*(Suppl. 1), S43–S45.

Krumberger, J. (2002). When the liver fails. *RN, 65*(2), 26–30.

Krumberger, J. (2005). How to manage an acute upper GI bleed. *RN, 68*(3), 34–40.

Marrero, J., Martinex, F., & Hyzy, R. (2003). Advances in critical care hepatology. *American Journal of Respiratory Critical Care Medicine, 168,* 1421–1426.

National AIDS Treatment Advocacy Project. Cirrhosis: Advanced liver disease. Retrieved February 10, 2006, from www.natap.org/2002/Oct/103002_2.htm

PDR Health. (2006). Branched-chain aminoacids (L-leucine, L-isoleucine, L-valine). Retrieved February 10, 2006, from www.pdrhealth.com/drug_info/nmdrugprofiles/nutsupdrugs/bra_0042.shtml

Rahman, T., & Hodgson, H. (2001). Clinical management of acute hepatic failure. *Intensive Care Medicine, 27,* 467–476.

Richardson, P. (2002). Acute liver disease. *Hospital Pharmacist, 9,* 131–137.

Sood, G. K., & Jones, B. A. (2006). Acute liver failure. Retrieved August 8, 2006, from www. emedicine.com/med/topic990.htm

Stewart, Z. A., Kozlowski, T., Segev, D. L., Montgomery, R. A., & Klein, A. S. (2006). Successful transplantation of cadaveric polycystic liver: Case report and review of the literature. *Transplantation, 81*(2), 284–286.

Stockmann, H. B., Hiemstra, C. A., Marquet, R. L., & IJzermans, J. W. (2000). Extracorporeal perfusion for the treatment of acute liver failure. *Annals of Surgery, 231*(4), 460–470.

Tayek, J. A. (2005). Lower cortisol concentrations in patients with liver disease: More adrenal failure or more confusion. *Critical Care Medicine, 33*(6), 1254–1259.

Uptodate.com. (2006). Overview of fat-soluble vitamins. Retrieved February 10, 2006, from http://patients.uptodate.com/topic.asp?file=gi_dis/21728

Whiteman, K., & McCormick, C. (2005). When your patient is in liver failure. *Nursing, 35*(4), 58–63.

Hepatitis

Marian S. Altman

More than 50,000 new cases of viral hepatitis are reported each year in the United States. Thirty-two percent are due to hepatitis A virus (HAV), 43% to hepatitis B virus (HBV), 21% to hepatitis C virus (HCV), and 4% to other unidentified viruses (Holcomb, 2002). HBV infection is the most common liver disease worldwide. HCV infection is the leading cause of blood-borne disease in the United States, the most common cause of cirrhosis, the most common indication for liver transplant, and the most common source of hepatocellular carcinoma (Wilson, 2005).

Viral hepatitis was not known until World War II. At that time, there seemed to be two different viruses capable of causing hepatitis. One viral strain was referred to as infectious hepatitis because it was spread through water contamination. The second viral hepatitis, which was spread by way of blood transfusions, was called serum hepatitis. Blood transfusions were first widely used during World War II, and the discovery of serum hepatitis led to the first published paper on the subject in 1943. However, it was not until 1960 that the cause of serum hepatitis, HBV, was isolated. HAV, the cause of infectious hepatitis, was not isolated until the early 1980s. Hepatitis C was identified in 1989. It was previously an unknown strain labeled non-A, non-B hepatitis. Later in the 1980s, hepatitis D and E were named. Hepatitis F and G are the most recently identified, and there is reason to believe that even more hepatitis strains exist (Holcomb, 2002).

PATHOPHYSIOLOGY

Hepatitis may be defined as acute inflammation of the liver, characterized by lobular necrosis and infiltration of the portal tracts by leukocytes. This multisystem infection has many effects: regional lymphadenopathy, splenomegaly, ulceration of the GI tract, acute pancreatitis, myocarditis, serum sickness, vasculitis, and nephritis. Hepatitis may manifest as an acute, acute fulminant, chronic persistent, or chronic active process.

Acute hepatitis is defined as a sudden onset of infection, which is usually self-limiting. Acute fulminant hepatitis also occurs suddenly, but is associated with severe liver function impairment, massive hepatocellular necrosis, and hepatic encephalopathy. It has a poor prognosis. Its most common causes are viral, acetaminophen toxicity, drugs, and mushroom poisoning. During the asymptomatic carrier state, the antigen persists in serum for at least six months. The infected person is unable to clear the antigen due to ineffective cellular immunity. The carrier is able to transmit the virus to others, but has no liver damage.

During the chronic persistent state, the hepatitis antigen persists in the individual's serum for at least six months. The liver is chronically inflamed. The infected individual is unable to clear the antigen due to ineffective cellular immunity. Viral replication persists in the liver during the chronic active process. Liver damage is progressive and is more common among persons with asymptomatic or mild anicteric cases. This type of hepatitis may evolve into cirrhosis, and it is associated with the development of hepatocellular carcinoma.

ETIOLOGY

Hepatitis has many etiologies. Infectious cases may be viral, bacterial, or parasitic. Medications that may cause hepatitis include halothane, nonsteroidal anti-inflammatory drugs (NSAIDs), sulfonamides, ketoconazole, Dilantin®, Rifampin®, and isoniazid. Other causes include carbon tetrachlorides, mushroom poisoning, alcohol, and ischemia. Autoimmune and congenital causes also exist.

HEPATITIS A

Persons at Risk/Transmission

HAV, an RNA virus, is the most common form of hepatitis in the United States. It is estimated that one-third of Americans have evidence of past infection (Wilson, 2005). Hepatitis A occurs sporadically or endemically. Day-care centers can be a reservoir of infection. In developing countries, most people are infected as children and have a subclinical course. Others at risk include household or sexual contacts with infected persons and institutionalized persons such as those in prisons, hospitals, or nursing homes. Transmission occurs through the fecal/oral route, person-to-person contact, and polluted water and food. Percutaneous transmission is rare. Sexual transmission may occur with unsafe or high-risk sex or handling of soiled condoms. Raw shellfish or bivalve shellfish from polluted water may also be a mode of transmission.

Prevention

HAV may be prevented with administration of the hepatitis A vaccine. This vaccine is recommended to be administered four weeks prior to travel (see **Table 36-1**). It is recommended for persons older than two years of age, travelers to areas at risk, men who have sex with men, drug users, patients with chronic liver disease, military personnel, and children in high-risk states or counties (Fleming, 2002). An immune globulin may provide short-term protection. The immune globulin is given within

TABLE 36-1 HAV Vaccines

Adult Doses
Havrix®: 1440 EL.U. booster given 6–12 months
VAQTA®: 50 U/1.0 mL at 0 and 6 months

Other Vaccines Available in Europe
Twinrix®: hepatitis A and B vaccine; One IM injection at 0, 1, and 6 months
Comvax® and Pediarix®: other vaccines

Immunoglobulin
2-mL dose prevents disease for 3–4 months
5-mL dose prevents disease for up to 6 months
Post-exposure prophylaxis: 0.02 mL/kg ASAP

Source: Holcomb, 2002.

two weeks of contact with HAV to individuals who have not received the HAV vaccination. Hand washing, dish washing, and clean food preparation are other methods of preventing HAV transmission.

Signs and Symptoms/Clinical Course

The incubation period is 28 days, with a 20-to 45-day range. The virus is shed in feces during the last two weeks of the incubation period and may also be found in the blood. Symptoms last 2 to 4 weeks and usually occur abruptly. With HAV, the clinical course is self-limiting with no chronic form. Fifteen percent of patients have prolonged signs and symptoms lasting 6 to 9 months. A relapse may occur in fewer than 20% of patients. Adults have more signs and symptoms than children (see **Table 36-2**).

Fulminant hepatitis is rare with HAV infection (Centers for Disease Control and Prevention, 1999). The risk increases in people older than age 40 and in those with underlying liver disease. Mortality is 0.4%. HAV is not chronic in its nature; once persons have had it, they are immune (Durston, 2004). The virus is communicable for 1 to 2 weeks after signs and symptoms disappear.

Laboratory Values

Hepatitis A is often misdiagnosed as gastroenteritis. The definitive diagnosis of hepatitis A infection is made via serological testing. By the time the liver enzymes aspartate aminotransferase (AST) and alanine aminotransferase (ALT) are elevated, antibodies to the virus are detectable in the serum and fecal shedding has ceased. Antibodies to the virus are detectable within three weeks of exposure. Detectable immunoglobulin M (IgM) and total IgM rise and then wane, while immunoglobulin G (IgG) will rise and stay elevated. Bilirubin values are normal to elevated.

TABLE 36-2 Nonspecific Prodromal Signs and Symptoms

Loss of appetite

Dark urine

Pale stools

Jaundice (rare)

Fatigue

Abdominal pain

Nausea

Diarrhea

Fever

Pruritis

Arthralgia

Myalgia

Hepatomegaly

Source: Durston, 2005.

TABLE 36-3 Persons at Risk for HBV

- Intravenous drug abusers
- People who engage in intercourse with infected persons, people with more than one sexual partner per six-month period
- People who engage in anal intercourse
- Occupational exposure: healthcare workers, public safety workers, long-term correctional facility workers, clients and staff in institutions for developmentally disabled persons
- Recipients of tattoos, ear or body piercing (nonsterile practice), acupuncture
- Travelers to high-risk areas such as Asia, Africa, South America, Eastern and Mediterranean Europe, Alaska, Pacific areas
- People who live with carriers/infected persons
- Infants born to infected mothers
- Hemodialysis patients
- Individuals who share toothbrushes or chewing gum with infected person

Source: Durston, 2004.

Treatment

Treatment for acute HAV is symptomatic (Fleming, 2002). Rest is recommended. Vaccination is the treatment of choice for hepatitis A and is given to those older than two years of age and not pregnant. (The dosages are listed in Table 36-1.) The vaccines are inactive and provide lifelong immunity. Other preventive methods include good sanitation and hand washing. An immunoglobulin also provides short-term protection; it should be given within two weeks of exposure. The immunoglobulin increases an individual's immunity for approximately six weeks (Durston, 2004).

HEPATITIS B

HBV is the world's most common blood-borne viral infection and cause of liver disease. A DNA virus causes HBV. More than 2 billion persons are infected with HBV, and there are 350 million chronic carriers worldwide (Fleming, 2002). In the United States, incidence has declined by 65% since 1990 due to infection control efforts, required vaccination of infants, screening of pregnant women, and increased emphasis on safe sex practices. Twenty-five percent of carriers develop serious liver disease (Fleming). Hepatitis B is a major cause of liver cancer and cirrhosis worldwide (Durston, 2004).

Persons at Risk/Transmission

Persons at risk for the HBV are listed in **Table 36-3**. HBV is transmitted via blood-borne methods such as intravenous drug abuse (IVDA), transfusion of blood or blood products, mosquitoes or other blood-sucking insects, and organ transplants.

Mother-to-neonate transmission occurs as well. In such a case, hepatitis B immunoglobulin (HBIG) is given at birth, then the vaccine series is begun. Transmission may also occur via infected equipment.

Prevention

The hepatitis B vaccine is recommended for people with multiple sex partners, those with recent sexually transmitted disease (STD), men who have sex with men, IVDA, healthcare providers, inmates, and patients with chronic liver disease. Available since 1982, the vaccine is routinely administered to those 0 to 18 years old. The vaccine is safe to administer during pregnancy. Two vaccines are licensed in the United States: Recombivax HB® and Energix-B® (Holcomb, 2002). Other prevention methods are listed in **Table 36-4**.

HBIG may be administered post-exposure. HBIG is made from serum with increased levels of hepatitis B antibodies. It is safe; there is no transmission risk with immunoglobulin administration. HBIG is given prophylactically post-exposure and is 70% to 75% effective in preventing HBV. The immunoglobulin may be administered during pregnancy. Once hepatitis B infection is evident clinically or serologically, HBIG cannot neutralize the virus, but it may modify or ameliorate the infection. The dose is administered within 24 to 48 hours of exposure. A second dose is administered in one month (Fleming, 2002).

TABLE 36-4 HBV Prevention Methods

- Use sexual barriers
- Don't share personal items—razor, toothbrush, needles
- Immune globulin
- Universal precautions
- Use disposable utensils if there is not a dishwasher
- Do not donate blood or organs

Source: Durston, 2004.

TABLE 36-6 Normal Liver Function Test Values

Test	Normal Values
ALT	5–35 IU/L
AST	0–35 IU/L
ALP	30–120 IU/L
Total bilirubin	0.1–1.0 mg/dL
Indirect bilirubin	0.2–0.8 mg/dL
Direct bilirubin	0.1–0.3 mg/dL

Signs and Symptoms/Clinical Course

Incubation occurs within 28 to 160 days. Thirty percent of patients have subclinical or asymptomatic disease (Durston, 2004). The most common symptoms are fever, fatigue, muscle or joint pain, loss of appetite, and nausea and vomiting. Many patients attribute these symptoms to the flu. Other signs and symptoms are listed in **Table 36-5**.

Laboratory Values

Liver enzymes (AST and ALT) are usually greater than 1000 IU/L in case of HBV infection. (See **Table 36-6** for normal liver function test values.) Bilirubin is elevated in acute disease. Hepatitis B surface antigen (HbsAg) is a marker of infectivity; it is positive prior to signs and symptoms developing. HbsAg is used to diagnose acute HBV and to detect a carrier state. Hepatitis B core antibody (anti-Hbc) is positive when the person has been infected with HBV at some point during his or her life. Hepatitis B core antibody IgM (IgM anti-Hbc) is increased at the onset of illness and indicates a recent infection. Hepatitis B core antigen (HbcAg) indicates the person is highly infectious. Hepatitis B surface antibody (anti-Hbs) indicates immunity or recovery (Wilson, 2005). Lab markers are shown in **Table 36-7**.

TABLE 36-5 HBV Signs and Symptoms

Jaundice
Abdominal pain
Loss of appetite
Nausea/vomiting
Arthralgias
Fulminant hepatitis (rare)

Source: Durston, 2004.

Treatment

Treatment for an acute infection is supportive and symptomatic (Fleming, 2002). Bedrest, good nutrition, increasing fluids, practicing safe sex, and stopping hepatotoxic drugs are all advised. The treatment of choice for a chronic infection is interferon alpha (Intron® A) and either lamivudine (Epivir®) or adefovir (Hepsera®). Although interferon alpha is effective in suppressing HBV replication, hepatitis B antigen clearance is achieved in only 20% to 30% of patients. Patients taking interferon typically experience flu-like symptoms such as headache, myalgias, fatigue, rigors, fever, and nausea. Long-term side effects may include alopecia, bone marrow suppression, mood changes, depression, seizures, sepsis, retinopathy, and hearing impairment.

Lamivudine (Epivir), a nucleoside reverse transcriptase inhibitor, is administered for one year. Administration may continue after one year if no seroconversion occurs or if the patient develops tolerance to the drug. Resistance to the drug may develop as well. Adefovir (Hepsera®) is used with resistance to Epivir. Relapse is common with drug stoppage (Wilson, 2005).

Many other antivirals, DNA inhibitors, non-interferon immune enhancers, and non-nucleoside analogues are administered in various stages of clinical trials. Websites listing current clinical trials are identified in the Online Resources section of this chapter.

HEPATITIS D

Hepatitis D virus (HDV) is an incomplete RNA virus that requires HBV for its replication. Hepatitis D infection either occurs simultaneously or occurs in patients with preexisting HBV infection. It is rare in the United States (Wilson, 2005).

Persons at Risk/Transmission

HDV is endemic in certain areas of the world, including the Mediterranean basin, Balkan Peninsula, the former USSR, parts of Africa, the Middle East, and the Amazon basin of South

TABLE 36-7 Hepatitis B Blood Test Interpretation

	HbsAg	HbsAb (anti-Hbs)	HbcAb (anti-Hbc)	IgM anti-Hbc
Not immune (susceptible)	Negative	Negative	Negative	
Immune—vaccine	Negative	Positive	Negative	
Immune—infection	Negative	Positive	Positive	
New infection	Positive	Negative	Positive	Positive
Chronic carrier	Positive	Negative	Positive	Negative
Unclear	Negative	Negative	Positive	

Source: Wilson, 2005.

America. In these areas, the virus is spread by person-to-person contact and through sexual contact. It has also been identified in intravenous drug abusers in North America. Incubation is 20 to 50 days. Transmission occurs parenterally in intravenous drug abusers, and less commonly through unprotected sexual activity.

Prevention

There is no vaccine for HDV. Preventing transmission of HBV by administering the vaccine also prevents HDV. Avoiding parenteral exposure and unprotected sex are other preventative measures.

Signs and Symptoms/Clinical Course

Signs and symptoms vary with coinfection versus superinfection. Symptoms are usually self-limiting, and jaundice may occur. Ninety percent of patients do not have any symptoms (Wilson, 2005).

Laboratory Values

ALT is usually elevated; AST may be within normal limits. HBVIgG and HBVIgM are positive. The hepatitis D antigen is detectable in 25% of patients.

Treatment

Preventing HBV treats hepatitis D. Interferon alpha has been effective in treating HDV. However, relapse occurs when the medication is discontinued (Wilson, 2005).

HEPATITIS C

HCV, an RNA virus, was first identified in 1989. HCV is the most common infectious cause of chronic hepatitis, cirrhosis, and hepatocellular carcinoma in the United States and the most common indication for liver transplantation (Fleming, 2002). The number of new infections has declined in recent decades. From 1982–1989, a mean of 232,000 new HCV infections was reported; from 1990–1999 the mean dropped to 67,000. The estimated number of new cases of HCV in 2001, 2002, 2003, and 2004 are 24,000, 29,000, 28,000, and 26,000 respectively (Centers for Disease Control and Protection, 2006). Six genotypes, with more than 50 known subtypes, have been identified. Subtypes 1a and 1b are the most common in the United States (Wilson, 2005). The most common is subtype 1a; subtype 1b is the most aggressive. Subtype 1b predominates in Japan. Subtypes 2a, 2b, 2c, and 3a are found in Europe and respond best to treatment with interferon. Type 3 is found in Thailand, type 4 in northern Africa, type 5 in southern Africa and the Middle East, and type 6 in Hong Kong. Patients may be infected with more than one genotype (Ellett, 2000).

Persons at Risk/Transmission

Persons at risk are listed in **Table 36-8**. Transmission occurs through direct parenteral exposure of infected blood. Primary causes of transmission are transfusion of blood and blood products, intravenous drug use, sexual contact, organ transplantation, perinatal transmission, and occupational exposure. In 10% of patients, no cause can be identified (Wilson, 2005).

TABLE 36-8 Persons at Risk for HCV

- IV drug users—most common mode of transmission
- Clotting factor recipients prior to 1987 when viral inactivation procedures began
- Hemodialysis patients
- Recipients of solid organs or blood products prior to 1992
- Infants born to infected mothers
- Healthcare providers
- Persons with multiple sex partners/infected partners or who have unprotected sex
- Cocaine users
- Persons who undergo tattoo/body piercing with unclean needles/techniques
- Incarcerated persons

Sources: Bockhold, 2000; Strader, Wright, Thomas, & Seeff, 2004.

Prevention

There is no vaccine or immune globulin available for HCV. Therefore, prevention is aimed at decreasing risk factors.

Signs and Symptoms/Clinical Course

The incubation period is 5 to 26 weeks. As many as 70% of patients have no signs or symptoms (Wilson, 2005). Typical signs and symptoms include jaundice, fatigue, dark urine, abdominal pain, loss of appetite, and nausea. Cirrhosis develops in 5% to 20% of infected persons within 20 to 25 years of onset. One to four percent of patients progress to hepatocellular carcinoma in 20 to 30 years (Iosue, 2002).

Laboratory Values

Liver enzymes (AST and ALT) may be normal or elevated. There is no correlation between laboratory values and disease severity. Instead, disease severity is diagnosed through a liver biopsy. A patient's RNA may test positive for HCV 1 to 3 weeks after exposure. With donated blood, initial testing for hepatitis C screens the blood supply for antibodies using an enzyme immunoassay. A positive result is further tested with a more specific recombinant immunoblot assay (RIBA) or nucleic acid test (Fleming, 2002). HCV RNA polymerase chain reaction assay is a standard test for ambiguous results. This lab test is both sensitive and specific, and it may detect low levels of the virus in the blood.

Treatment

The goals of treatment are to reduce the amount of virus in the blood to undetectable levels, to prevent disease progression, to reduce the incidence of hepatocellular carcinoma, and to reduce the need for liver transplant (Fleming, 2002). The best overall sustained viral response is seen with a combination therapy of weekly pegylated alpha interferon and oral ribavirin given twice a day. The dosage of ribavirin is adjusted based on the patient's weight (Holcomb, 2002). Clinical trials are currently evaluating other medications to treat hepatitis C.

Patients being treated for hepatitis C are advised to avoid alcohol, not to use nonprescribed medications, to practice safe sex, to not share personal items, and to not donate blood, semen, or organs. Hepatitis C patients are also vaccinated against hepatitis A and B viruses. Many patients seek alternative methods of treatment such as herbs.

Combination therapy is given for 24 or 48 weeks based on the genotype. Genotype 1 is typically treated with combination therapy for 48 weeks. Genotypes 2 and 3 may be treated for 24 weeks (Iosue, 2002). The response rate tends to be bet-ter if the viral load is lower at initiation of treatment, but is often less effective in African Americans. Genotype 1 has a 42% to 46% response rate. Genotypes 2 and 3 have a 76% to 82% response rate. Patients with low pretreatment HCV RNA levels, minimal fibrosis, ideal body weight, and no cholestasis or iron overload are more likely to respond to treatment (Wilson, 2005). Efficacy is also greater in patients younger than 40, women, and alcohol abstainers.

Treatment is not indicated for all HCV-positive patients. Characteristics of persons for whom therapy is widely accepted, is currently contraindicated, and should be individualized have been described by Strader and colleagues (2004). Once a patient is diagnosed with hepatitis C infection, suitability for treatment is assessed. Next, the genotype is identified. Once combination therapy is begun, the patient is assessed at frequent intervals to ensure tolerance of the medication regime and to obtain lab work to monitor for adverse side effects.

Adverse effects occur in 42% of patients who receive combination therapy (Woods & Herrera, 2002). Many patients stop therapy as a result of these side effects. Side effects typically associated with interferon alpha include neutropenia, thrombocytopenia, depression, hypothyroidism, hyperthyroidism, irritability, concentration and memory disturbances, visual disturbances, fatigue, muscle aches, headaches, nausea, vomiting, skin irritation, low-grade fever, weight loss, insomnia, hearing loss, tinnitus, interstitial fibrosis, and hair thinning. Side effects typically associated with ribavirin include hemolytic anemia, fatigue, itching, rash, sinusitis, birth defects, and gout (Iosue, 2002). Adverse effects tend to be more severe during the initial weeks of treatment and often can be managed by administering the medications prior to bedtime, and in conjunction with analgesics, NSAIDs, and antidepressants (Strader et al., 2004). Psychiatric side effects such as emotional lability, depression, irritability, insomnia, and suicide ideation are seen in 20% of patients.

HEPATITIS E

An RNA virus causes infection with hepatitis E virus (HEV). HEV was formerly called epidemic non-A, non-B hepatitis or enteric hepatitis. Hepatitis E has an epidemiology and clinical course similar to those of hepatitis A. HEV is the most common cause of acute viral hepatitis worldwide (Ellett, 2000).

Persons at Risk/Transmission

HEV is most prevalent among young adults ages 15–40. It is found in developing countries such as those in Asia, Africa, the Middle East, and Central America. Transmission is attributed to inadequate sanitation. Infants born to infected mothers are also at risk. The mode of transmission is through the fecal-oral route. Contaminated water, stool of infected persons, or animals can also be modes of transmission. In addition, outbreaks are seen in areas with flooding.

Prevention

Avoiding drinking water in high-risk areas prevents transmission of HEV. In these areas, it is recommended to boil water or to drink bottled or chlorinated water. It is also advised to avoid ice cubes, uncooked vegetables and shellfish, and unpeeled fruit. There is no vaccine for HEV.

Signs and Symptoms/Clinical Course

The incubation period for HEV is three to nine weeks. Illness lasts one to four weeks and includes a prodromal phase lasting one week, followed by an icteric phase. There is a high mortality when infection occurs in pregnancy, especially during the third trimester (Wilson, 2005). Other signs and symptoms are listed in **Table 36-9**.

TABLE 36-9 Hepatitis E Virus Signs and Symptoms

Jaundice

Abdominal pain

Anorexia

Nausea

Vomiting

Diarrhea

Arthralgia

Dark urine

Fever

Hepatomegaly

Malaise

Pruritis

Source: Ellett, 2000.

Laboratory Values

The liver enzymes AST and ALT, ALP, and GGT are elevated in cases of HEV infection. Bilirubin is elevated. HEV antibodies IgM and IgG are positive.

Treatment

Treatment consists of supportive care such as a nutritious diet, bedrest, non-impact exercise, and eating high-protein foods in the morning when patients are less nauseous. Patient and family education should focus on strategies to prevent transmission in the household (Ellett, 2000).

PATIENT OUTCOMES

Nurses can help ensure the obtainment of optimal patient outcomes such as those listed in **Box 36-1** through the use of evidence-based interventions for patients with hepatitis.

SUMMARY

Viral hepatitis is a leading cause of chronic liver disease worldwide (Gow & Mutimer, 2001). Six viruses are the major causes of hepatitis. Since 1985, much knowledge has been gathered regarding the etiologies, transmission, and treatment of these viruses. Untreated hepatitis infection may progress to cirrhosis, hepatic failure, and hepatoma (Gow & Mutimer). Healthcare providers need to be knowledgeable of the most common causes of hepatitis, and their prevention and treatment.

Box 36-1
Optimal Patient Outcomes

- Patient and family verbalize methods to avoid transmission
- Patient verbalizes understanding of treatment strategies
- Patient verbalizes alleviation of symptoms
- Coagulation profile is in expected range

CASE STUDY

S.L. is a 36-year-old male who was received at a tertiary center after being seen in a rural hospital for severe hypotension, vomiting, and coagulopathy. His history is significant only for hepatitis 10 years prior to this admission. The type of hepatitis was unknown, and no problems had ever been associated with his hepatitis prior to this episode. The patient denies tobacco, alcohol, or illicit drug use. Family history includes a father with diabetes, a mother with hypertension, and a sister with breast cancer. S.L. is not on any prescribed medications. He has a college degree and is employed as a grant writer for a local Arts Council, which is a nonprofit foundation. He is actively involved in the Seventh Day Adventist Church and is on the board of directors for a homeless women and children shelter.

The patient is admitted to the ICU after going to radiology for a chest x-ray and abdominal ultrasound. The ultrasound revealed an enlarged liver, splenomegaly, and ascites. Lab work showed platelet count 42,000, prothrombin time 55.5 sec, PTT 112 sec, alkaline phosphatase 84 IU/L, AST 133 IU/L, ALT 76 IU/L, and total bilirubin 40.3 mg/dL.

The patient was prepped for a paracentesis that was carried out at the bedside. Specimens were sent to the lab for culture and analysis. His abdomen was obese and distended with shifting dullness. He had 3+ pitting edema to the sacrum. Blood cultures and peritoneal fluid showed the presence of *Staphylococcus aureus*.

S.L.'s hospital course was complicated by hypotension requiring vasopressors, sepsis, respiratory failure requiring intubation, and acute renal failure. The patient was managed with Dopamine® at 18 mcg/kg/min, multiple antibiotic therapy, mechanical ventilation (refer to Chapter 23), and continuous venovenous hemofiltration (refer to Chapter 45).

CRITICAL THINKING QUESTIONS

1. How could this patient have gotten hepatitis?
2. What precautions should the nurse take in caring for this patient?
3. Does the patient need isolation precautions?
4. What post-procedure care should be followed after a paracentesis?
5. Which disciplines should be consulted to work with this client?
6. What types of issues may require you to act as an advocate or moral agent for this patient?
7. How will you implement your role as a facilitator of learning for this patient?
8. Write a case example from the clinical setting highlighting one patient characteristic. Explain how the characteristic was observed through subjective and objective data.
9. Use the form to write up a plan of care for one client in the clinical setting.
10. Write a case example from the clinical setting of a client with hepatitis. Rate the patient as a level 1, 3, or 5 on each characteristic. Identify the level of nurse characteristics needed in the care of this patient.
11. Take one patient outcome for a patient and list evidence-based interventions found in a literature review for this patient.

Using the Synergy Model to Develop a Plan of Care

	Patient Characteristics	Levels (1, 3, 5)	Subjective and Objective Data	Evidence-based Interventions	Outcomes
SYNERGY MODEL	Resiliency				
	Vulnerability				
	Stability				
	Complexity				
	Resource availability				
	Participation in care				
	Participation in decision making				
	Predictability				

Online Resources

Centers for Disease Control and Prevention, Hepatitis: www.cdc.gov/ncidod/diseases/hepatitis

Hepatitis B Foundation: www.Hepb.org/drugwatch

Immunization Action Coalition, Summary of Recommendations for Adult Immunization: www.immunize.org/catg.d

NIH Consensus Statement for Management of Hepatitis C:
http://consensus.nih.gov/2002/2002HepatitisC2002116html.htm

L. Scully, Hepatitis Update (1999): www.hepnet.com/update16.html.

A. Sherker, Hepatitis A, D, E, & G (1999): www.hepnet.com/update14.html

Clinical Trials: www.clinical trials.gov

REFERENCES

Bockhold, K. (2000).Who's afraid of hepatitis C? *American Journal of Nursing, 100*(5), 26–32.

Centers for Disease Control and Prevention. *Morbidity and Mortality Weekly Report* (October 1, 1999): www.cdc.gov/mmwr

Centers for Disease Control and Prevention. (2006). Disease burden from hepatitis A, B, and C in the United States. Retrieved September 6, 2006, from www.cdc.gov/NCIDOD/Diseases/Hepatitis/resource/dz_burden02.htm

Durston, S. (2004). The ABCs and more of hepatitis. *Nursing Made Incredibly Easy, 2*(4), 22–32.

Durston, S. (2005). What you need to know about viral hepatitis. *Nursing 2005, 35*(8), 36–42.

Ellett, M. (2000). Hepatitis C, E, F, G, and non-A-G. *Gasterenterology Nursing, 23*(2), 67–72.

Fleming, J. (2002). Current treatment for hepatitis. *Journal of Infusion Nursing, 25*(6), 379–382.

Gow, P., & Mutimer, D. (2001). Treatment of chronic hepatitis. *British Medicine Journal, 323*(17), 1164–1167.

Holcomb, S. (2002). An update on hepatitis. *Dimensions of Critical Care Nursing, 21*(5), 170–177.

Iosue, K. (2002). Chronic hepatitis C: Latest treatment options. *Nurse Practitioner, 27*(4), 32–33, 37–38, 40–42.

Strader, D., Wright, T., Thomas, D. L., & Seeff, L. B. (2004). Diagnosis, management, and treatment of hepatitis C. *Hepatology, 39*(4), 1147–1170.

Wilson, T. (2005). The ABCs of hepatitis. *The Nurse Practitioner: The American Journal of Primary Health Care, 30*(6), 12–21.

Woods, A., & Herrera, J. (2002). Hepatitis C: Latest treatment guidelines. *Consultant*, 1233–1243.

CHAPTER 37

Pancreatitis

Kelly Brewer

Upon completion of this chapter, the reader will be able to:

1. Describe the etiology and incidence of pancreatitis.

2. List the signs and symptoms of acute pancreatitis.

3. Recognize complications of acute pancreatitis.

4. Describe the management of the patient with pancreatitis.

5. Design an educational plan for the patient with acute pancreatitis.

6. List optimal outcomes that may be achieved through evidence-based management of the patient with pancreatitis.

Acute pancreatitis is inflammation of the pancreas. When encountered in the intensive care unit (ICU) setting, it is an unpredictable and often life-threatening medical condition. Acute pancreatitis is frequently accompanied by devastating systemic manifestations such as acute respiratory distress syndrome (ARDS), sepsis, and multiple organ dysfunction syndrome (MODS). Patients and their families may face protracted stays in the ICU, sometimes as long as 45 to 60 days. Nurses caring for these patients must utilize the qualities of the patient, the healthcare team, and the skills of self synergistically, because early diagnosis, continuous assessment, and timely interventions are critical to decrease pancreatic inflammation and to detect and treat complications promptly.

ETIOLOGY AND INCIDENCE

Acute pancreatitis is a disease whose exact mechanism is unknown. It is associated with varying degrees of regional and systemic inflammatory responses. The pathophysiology of acute pancreatitis varies based on etiologic factors. For example, in patients with gallstones, as the stones pass through the ampulla of Vater, an obstruction of the pancreatic duct allows bile to back into the pancreas, causing an enzymatic reaction. Drugs that have been implicated in the development of acute pancreatitis are thought to produce toxins that injure the pancreas and cause destruction of ductal structures and autodigestion of the pancreas itself. These toxins produce hyperstimulation of the pancreas, resulting in inflammation.

Regardless of the etiology, a common pathway for development of acute pancreatitis has been identified. Ultimately, it results from premature activation of digestive enzymes within the pancreas. Trypsinogen, an inactive proenzyme, converts to its active form, trypsin. This conversion promotes the release of other digestive proenzymes, which ultimately causes the pancreas and surrounding tissues to become damaged. The damage produces third spacing of fluid and can lead to necrosis of the pancreas (see **Figure 37-1**) (Draganov & Forsmark, 2003). If the pancreas becomes necrotic, the patient becomes at risk for systemic inflammatory response syndrome (SIRS). SIRS is discussed in detail in Chapter 51.

Acute pancreatitis is classified as either interstitial or necrotizing. A significant increase in morbidity and mortality is associated with necrotizing pancreatitis, particularly if infection is present. Fortunately, fewer than 10% of patients develop this more life-threatening form of the disease. The incidence of acute pancreatitis in the United States varies in reports from 54 to 238 instances/million population/year (Wrobleski, Barth, & Oyen, 1999). Alcohol-related and gallstone-associated acute pancreatitis account for the majority of all cases. Of the top 100 prescribed medications in the United States, 44 have the potential to cause acute pancreatitis. This is of primary concern for patients who are elderly, are human immunodeficiency virus (HIV) positive, or are immunocompromised (Trivedi & Pitchumoni, 2005). Other possible causes include the following conditions (Khoury et al., 2005; Torpy, 2004):

- Hypertriglyceridemia
- Genetic predisposition
- Hyperthyroidism
- Blunt abdominal trauma
- Surgical trauma
- Medications, such as glucocorticoids, sulfonamides, tetracycline (Sumycin®), furosemide (Lasix®), thiazide diuretics, valproic acid (Depakene®), and nonsteroidal anti-inflammatory medications
- Viral or bacterial infection
- Intestinal parasites
- Endoscopic retrograde cholangiopancreatography procedures (ERCP)
- Abdominal or cardiopulmonary bypass surgery (may insult the pancreas by ischemia)
- Carcinoma of the pancreas
- Abdominal trauma
- Major surgery
- Inherited diseases affecting the pancreas, including cystic fibrosis
- Hypercalcemia (usually due to other medical problems)

CLINICAL PRESENTATION

Clinical manifestations of the patient with acute pancreatitis depend on the extent of inflammation and the involvement of

FIGURE 37-1 Pathway to Acute Pancreatitis

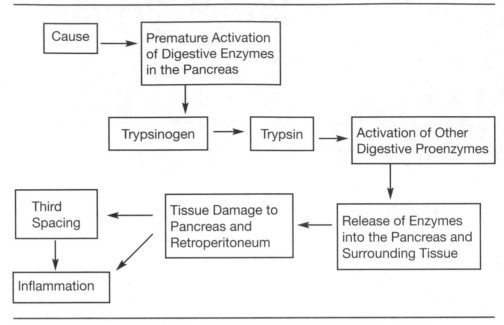

Source: Draganov & Forsmark, 2003.

pancreatic and additional body systems. Thorough physical assessment is imperative to identify this condition. The cardinal symptom of acute pancreatitis is abdominal pain. Most patients will complain of knife-like, mid-epigastric pain that radiates to the back. It may be described as sudden and gnawing in nature. Sitting in a knee-to-chest position may bring relief. Other symptoms may include nausea, vomiting, diaphoresis, weakness, tachycardia, tachypnea, hypotension, and dehydration. Symptoms may become worse after eating.

Physical examination may reveal abdominal tenderness, guarding, and distention (Hemes, 2005). The ICU nurse should assess for bowel sounds, abdominal rigidity, ascites, and rebound tenderness. Jaundice may be present. Careful assessment of pulmonary status is essential, because respirations may be affected by pain, infection, fluid, and hypoxemia. Vital signs must be monitored hourly or according to institutional policy.

The assessment findings for necrotizing pancreatitis are more severe, because fluids can leak into the peritoneum and lead to hypovolemic shock. Ongoing assessment of the patient's level of consciousness and hemodynamic monitoring are essential. The ICU nurse should monitor for hypotension, tachycardia, respiratory distress, decreased urinary output, arterial blood gas values, and skin color over the abdomen. Bruising on the flank area (Grey-Turner sign) and discoloration around the umbilicus (Cullen's sign) should be noted (Hemes, 2005). These signs result from blood-tinged exudates from the pancreas and indicate a severe situation.

PREDICTING SEVERITY OF ACUTE PANCREATITIS

Multiple assessment tools have been developed in an effort to predict which patients are most likely to develop severe manifestations of the disease so as to offer healthcare providers an opportunity to intercede with aggressive treatment, thus reducing complications and mortality. The Ranson's criteria have a greater than 90% accuracy rate in identifying patients who are at high risk; however, the assessment cannot be completed until 48 hours after admission. Three or more signs identified upon admission or during the first 48 hours of hospitalization are predictive of severe acute pancreatitis (see **Table 37-1**).

Lab Values

The serum amylase value is the most important laboratory value in the diagnosis of acute pancreatitis. A level greater than three times normal (normal is 35–115 U/L) is indicative of pancreatitis. Serum amylase levels peak within 24 hours and rapidly fall to normal within 48 to 72 hours. Elevated urinary amylase levels may persist for several days. Serum lipase (2–5 U/L) rises after 48 hours and remains increased for five to seven days. A lipase level greater than 5 U/L is associated with acute pancreatitis. Other lab findings include an elevated white blood cell count, which is associated with the body's stress response, and elevated blood glucose (Hemes, 2005; Wrobleski et al., 1999). High levels of C-reactive protein are associated with pancreatic necrosis (Nathens et al., 2004). There are also high incidences of hyperlipidemia and hypocalcemia with pancreatitis.

TABLE 37-1 Ranson's Criteria for Acute Pancreatitis

Age > 55 years

Leukocyte count > 16,000 mm^3

Serum glucose > 200 mg/dL

LDH > 350 IU/L

AST > 250 IU/L

Evaluate during the Initial 48 Hours

Decrease in hematocrit > 10%

BUN level increase > 5 mg/dL

Serum calcium < 8 mg/dL

Base deficit > 4 mEq/L

Estimated fluid sequestration > 6 L

Arterial PaO$_2$ < 60 mm Hg

Source: Healthcare Freeware, 2005.

Abdominal Imaging

An abdominal flat plate and upright chest films will rule out any other problems that might mimic acute pancreatitis (Wrobleski et al., 1999). Ultrasound of the abdomen will aid in identifying gallstones or a dilated bile duct, as well as assessing the condition of the pancreas. Computerized tomography (CT) scan, however, is diagnostic in nearly all patients with acute pancreatitis. Margins of the pancreas can be appreciated, fluid collections can be identified, and necrotizing pancreatitis can be diagnosed. Patients with necrosis involving more than 30% of the pancreas have a marked increase in mortality (Nathens et al., 2004). If fluid collections are located on the scan, they can subsequently be aspirated through paracentesis (see Chapter 32) and sent for cultures.

Mortality rates from sepsis from pancreatitis have decreased in the past 20 years. "This decrease in mortality has resulted from widespread use of CT scanning, fine needle aspiration of the pancreas, and antimicrobial therapy" (Wrobleski et al., 1999, p. 8).

SYSTEMIC COMPLICATIONS

Massive Hemorrhage and Hypovolemic Shock

Rupture of the pancreatic tissue and bleeding follows necrosis of the tissue, with large volumes of fluid subsequently shifting into the intra-abdominal and intravascular spaces. Vomiting, diarrhea, and fluid loss from nasogastric suctioning may also contribute to hypovolemia. Third spacing of volume may occur due to hypoalbuminemia. Management of fluid status is essential in patients with severe acute pancreatitis, because hypovolemia is a major cause of acute renal failure in these patients. Once the patient's volume status has been normalized, hypotension can be managed with inotropes or vasopressors (Lipsett, 2005).

Pulmonary Complications

Patients with severe acute pancreatitis must have their arterial blood gases monitored for hypoxemia and hypercarbia. Supplemental oxygen therapy is usually required, and intubation and mechanical ventilation may become necessary (Lipsett, 2005). Acute lung injury is a frequent complication of acute pancreatitis. In the early phase, it is associated with SIRS (see Chapter 51). Arterial hypoxemia is common and is a primary criterion for evaluating the prognosis of the disease (Pastor, Matthay, & Frossard, 2003). Of patients with acute pancreatitis, 30% to 60% develop atelectasis, pleural effusions, and diffuse bilateral infiltrates. Respiratory failure develops in 5% to 10% of patients (Wrobleski et al., 1999). When respiratory failure and ARDS occur in patients with necrotizing pancreatitis, many contributing factors are present. (A discussion of

ARDS appears in Chapter 25.) Pleural effusions, ascites, and abdominal distention all limit pulmonary ventilation anatomically. In some cases, a loss of surfactant occurs and the pulmonary endothelium is damaged. Microvascular lung injury can occur in response to the release of inflammatory mediators such as histamine and bradykinin.

Renal Complications

Hypoperfusion of the kidney and thrombosis of the renal artery or vein are primary causes of renal complications for the patient with acute pancreatitis. The patient may have experienced hypovolemia, hypotension, or both, associated with fluid shift or sepsis. In addition, if antimicrobial therapy is part of the treatment plan, renal toxicity may be a side effect of the administration of these drugs.

LOCAL COMPLICATIONS

The local effects of inflammation of the pancreas and fluid surrounding the organ can result in the formation of a pancreatic pseudocyst, abscess, or acute gastrointestinal (GI) bleeding. Pancreatic pseudocysts are accumulations of secretions and debris from the injured pancreas that can rupture and cause bleeding or infection, requiring surgical intervention. An abscess is purulent material within the necrotic pancreas, which can erode through the retroperitoneum into the bowel, pleural space, mediastinum, or pelvis, subsequently leading to sepsis. GI bleeding is the most common complication of acute pancreatitis; it is discussed in detail in Chapter 34.

METABOLIC COMPLICATIONS

Metabolic complications of acute pancreatitis include hypocalcemia and hyperlipidemia related to fat necrosis associated with necrosis of the pancreas. Hyperglycemia may occur as a result of damage to the islet cells. Some suggest that patients with severe acute pancreatitis receive total parenteral nutrition (TPN) in an effort to rest the pancreas and prevent stimulation of pancreatic enzymes associated with enteral feeds (Lipsett, 2005).

PATIENT CARE MANAGEMENT

The cornerstones of management in acute pancreatitis are fluid resuscitation and close monitoring for early signs of organ dysfunction (Nathens et al., 2004). The degree to which the disease progresses and which body systems are affected will determine nursing priorities of care (see **Table 37-2**).

Use of somatostatin (Octreotide®), which was once thought to be useful in the management of acute pancreatitis, is no longer universally recommended (Suc et al., 2004). Some data suggest that deleterious side effects may result with its use

(e.g., increased enzymatic content of the pancreas) (Salem et al., 2003).

SURGICAL MANAGEMENT IN ACUTE PANCREATITIS

Surgical intervention may be indicated for patients with necrotizing pancreatitis, particularly if more than 50% of the organ is involved or in patients with severe disease who are not responding to medical management. Several procedures can be used, including pancreatic resection, various methods for lavage, surgical drainage of abscesses or pseudocysts, and laparotomy to remove a biliary tract obstruction. Open packing may be used with some abdominal wounds (Wrobleski et al., 1999). Nurses must be familiar with these surgical procedures, their implications, the surgical drains used, wound care, and potential complications so as to effectively provide safe care for patients during the postoperative period. Drainage from dressings and all surgical drains must be considered because strict intake and output is calculated for these critically ill patients.

SUMMARY OF KEY RESEARCH

In April 2004, an international consensus conference was held to develop evidence-based recommendations for the management of the critically ill patient with severe acute pancreatitis. A total of 23 recommendations were developed by a panel of 10 persons representing critical care, surgery, and internal medicine after conferring with the literature and experts (see **Table 37-3**). In addition, this group cited the need for well-designed clinical trials to further evaluate several aspects of care, especially in light of the many uncertainties about the pathophysiology of pancreatitis and the promising value of novel therapies in some animal models (e.g., anti-inflammatory mediator therapy) (Nathens et al., 2004).

CHALLENGES FOR THE NURSING STUDENT/FACULTY

Providing care for the critically ill patient can be overwhelming and unnerving for both the nurse caring for the patient and the faculty assigned to guide them through this learning experience. The ICU, with its complex technology and patient care pathways, may seem an uphill struggle. The delivery of care to the patient with acute pancreatitis can be among the most challenging of all cases. Massive fluid shifts and rapid deterioration are not uncommon. The following competencies are essential to care for this patient:

- Skill in monitoring and assessment of vital signs
- Assessment of respiratory status (including pulse oximetry)
- Interpretation of arterial blood gases

TABLE 37-2 Nursing Care Guide for the Patient with Acute Pancreatitis

Care Priority	Nursing Activity	Evidence/Rationale
Aggressive fluid replacement	• Monitor vital signs hourly • Monitor urinary output hourly • Hemodynamic monitoring • Daily weights • Maintain IV access	Goal is to prevent hypovolemia/shock and prevent end-stage shock with associated organ dysfunction. • Recommended to keep PAOP 16–20. • Urine output at least 0.5 mL/kg/hr
Promote oxygenation	• Monitor pulse oximetry • Monitor arterial blood gases PRN • Administration of O_2 PRN • Every 2 hours pulmonary assessments • Assist patient to turn, cough, and deep breathe every 2 hours and PRN • Incentive spirometry every 2 hours • Intensive support with mechanical ventilation	Acute lung injury is a frequent complication of acute pancreatitis. The early identification of hypoxemia through intensive monitoring is essential.
Monitor for early signs of organ dysfunction	• Every 2 hours head-to-toe assessments • Telemetry monitoring	Early identification of complications is essential for obtainment of optimal patient outcomes.
Pain control	• Assess pain using an objective pain scale every 2 hours and PRN • Administer analgesics and monitor patient response • Use nonpharmacological pain management techniques	"Gold standard" opiate of choice has been meperidine (Demerol®). However, unless a stone has been documented in the duct, many advocate use of morphine or fentanyl as the first-line drug. Patient-controlled analgesia (PCA) is recommended whenever possible. Epidural analgesia may also be considered. • Ketorolac (Toradol®) is an excellent adjuvant drug for acute pain.
Maintain electrolyte balance	• Maintain IV access • Administer fluids and electrolytes as ordered • Monitor labs PRN • Monitor for signs and symptoms of hypokalemia, hypocalcemia, and hyperglycemia	Hypocalcemia is often seen in necrotizing pancreatitis. For alcohol-induced pancreatitis, it is important to assess for vitamin deficiencies.
Resting the pancreas	• Maintain NPO status • NG tube to low intermittent suction • Frequent oral care	Results in decreased pancreatic enzyme output. To decrease stomach distention and suppress pancreatic secretions.
Maintain nutritional status	• Administration of enteral feedings or TPN (if unable to tolerate enteral feedings) • Daily weights • Monitor lab values	The goal is to provide adequate calories and protein to meet the patient's metabolic needs without stimulating the pancreas.
Maintain coping strategies	• Assess emotional status • Listen to the patient and the family • Allow for choices when possible • Answer questions in an open and honest manner • Employ coping strategies used in the past	Pancreatitis is a life-threatening and often lengthy illness, which frightens patients and their families. The ICU leaves very little in their control.
Patient/family education	• Prepare patient and family for procedures • Explain the effects of pancreatitis and the implications of complications • Instruct patient and family in discharge teaching, including wound care, dietary restrictions, and medications	Discharge planning begins upon admission to the unit.

Sources: Lipsett, 2005; Reece-Smith, 2005.

TABLE 37-3 Consensus Recommendations for Management of Severe Acute Pancreatitis

1. Recommend ICU admission for patients meeting conventional criteria for admission to a general care unit.
2. Recommend care by an intensivist-led multidisciplinary team with ready access to physicians skilled in endoscopy, ERCP, surgery, and interventional radiology.
3. Recommend close clinical observation regardless of the venue of care.
4. Recommend against the use of markers such as CRP or procalcitonin to guide clinical decision making, predict the clinical outcome of pancreatitis, or triage patients.
5. Recommend a CT scan of the abdomen after adequate fluid resuscitation to confirm the diagnosis of pancreatitis and to rule out alternate diagnosis.
6. Recommend CT to identify local complications be delayed for 48–72 hours when possible, because necrosis might not be visualized earlier.
7. Recommend against the routine use of prophylactic systemic antibacterial or antifungal agents in patients with necrotizing pancreatitis in light of inconclusive evidence and divided expert opinion.
8. Recommend against the routine use of selective decontamination of the digestive tract in the management of necrotizing pancreatitis.
9. Recommend enteral nutrition be used in preference to parenteral nutrition in patients with severe acute pancreatitis. The jejunal route should be used if possible.
10. Recommend parental nutrition be used only when attempts at enteral nutrition have failed after a 5- to 7-day trial.
11. Recommend, when used, parental nutrition be enriched with glutamine.
12. Recommend patients, both enterally and parenterally fed, be managed with protocols ensuring strict glycemic control.
13. Recommend against the routine use of immune-enhancing enteral feed formulas or probiotics.
14. Recommend sonographic or CT-guided fine-needle aspiration with Gram stain and culture of pancreatic or peripancreatic tissue to discriminate between sterile and infected necrosis in patients with radiologic evidence of pancreatic necrosis and clinical features consistent with infection.
15. Recommend against debridement and/or drainage in patients with sterile necrosis.
16. Recommend pancreatic debridement or drainage in patients with infected pancreatic necrosis and/or abscess confirmed by radiological evidence of gas or results of fine-needle aspiration.
17. Recommend operative necrosectomy and/or drainage be delayed by 2–3 weeks to allow for demarcation of the necrotic pancreas.
18. Recommend that gallstone pancreatitis be suspected in all patients with severe acute pancreatitis and, therefore, all patients should have evaluation with sonography and biochemical tests.
19. In the setting of obstructive jaundice and acute pancreatitis due to suspected stones, recommend that ERCP should be performed within 72 hours of onset of symptoms.
20. In the absence of obstructive jaundice, but with acute pancreatitis due to suspected stones, recommend that ERCP be considered within 72 hours of onset of symptoms.
21. General supportive measures used in the critically ill should be employed in patients with severe acute pancreatitis, because these interventions might play an important role in attenuating the inflammatory response. Recommend the use of early volume resuscitation and lung-protective ventilation strategies for patients with acute lung injury.
22. Once the presence of infection is documented or highly suspected and the patient meets the definition of severe sepsis, recommend management according to current sepsis guidelines be initiated. These therapies include the use of activated protein C and low-dose corticosteroids for vasopressor-dependent shock.
23. Recommend against the use of other immune-modulating therapies targeting inflammatory mediators in severe acute pancreatitis.

Source: Nathens et al., 2004.

- Understanding of hemodynamic monitoring
- Assessment skills of strict intake and output
- Monitoring of lab values
- Assessment for signs and symptoms of electrolyte disturbances
- Administration of intravenous fluid
- Administration of mediations for pain control (most frequently patient-controlled analgesia)
- Patient/family support—augmentation of coping strategies
- Delivery of enteral or parenteral feedings

PATIENT OUTCOMES

Nurses can help ensure the obtainment of optimal patient outcomes such as those listed in **Box 37-1** through the use of evidence-based interventions for patients with pancreatitis.

Box 37-1

Optimal Patient Outcomes

- Absence of pain
- Acid-base balance in expected range
- Family demonstrates adequate coping strategies
- Intake and output balanced
- Respiratory rate in expected range
- Nutritional status in expected range

SUMMARY

Acute pancreatitis can be life-threatening and often requires admission to the ICU (Torpy, 2004). These patients are prone to develop several complications, including shock, sepsis, and MODS. Nurses providing care for patients with acute pancreatitis will need to offer emotional support and education to the family, given the extended hospitalization that may be required.

CASE STUDY

B.D. is a 28-year-old male who was admitted to the ICU from the Emergency Department (ED). He reported four days of intermittent abdominal pain that radiated to his back, nausea, and vomiting. The abdominal pain became continuous over the past 12 hours.

B.D. is recently separated from his wife, who was his high school sweetheart. Approximately four months ago, he learned that she was having an extramarital affair and that she was leaving him. Distraught, B.D. began drinking excessively. He admitted to consuming two or three 6-packs of beer and a liter of hard liquor daily over these past four months.

Vital signs in the ED were as follows: B/P 88/62, HR 126, RR 24, temp 100 °F, SpO_2 on room air 89%. B.D. was admitted to the ICU for hemodynamic monitoring and management of systemic inflammatory response syndrome.

On admission to the ICU, B.D. was pale and in obvious discomfort. Physical exam was significant for abdominal tenderness and guarding. Mild distention was noted. He was taken for an abdominal CT scan, which revealed inflammation of the pancreas. Abdominal ultrasound revealed presence of ascites and an enlarged pancreas.

Significant lab data were as follows:

CBC: WBC 17,000 mm^3, Hgb 9.0 Gm/dL, Hct 27%

Amylase 386 IU/L, lipase 30 IU/L

Chemistries: BUN 26 mg/dL, creatinine 1.0 mg/dL, Glucose 243 mg/dL, calcium 7.6 mg/dL

AST: 260 IU/L, LDH 396 IU/L, triglyceride 223 mg/dL

B.D.'s ICU course was complicated by the development of respiratory insufficiency related to bilateral pulmonary infiltrates and atelectasis. He was successfully treated with IV antibiotics. He also developed several pseudocysts over a three-week period, each of which required drainage in the operating room. His nutritional status was maintained with enteral feedings. His condition eventually stabilized, and he was discharged from the ICU.

CRITICAL THINKING QUESTIONS

1. Which disciplines should be consulted to work with this client?
2. What types of issues may require you to act as an advocate or moral agent for this patient?
3. How will you implement your role as a facilitator of learning for this patient?
4. Discuss the pros and cons of using total parenteral nutrition versus enteral feedings in a patient with acute pancreatitis.
5. Write a case example from the clinical setting highlighting one patient characteristic of a patient with acute pancreatitis. Explain how the characteristic was observed through subjective and objective data.

6. Utilize the form to write a plan of care for one client with acute pancreatitis in the clinical setting. Rate the patient as a level 1, 3, or 5 on each characteristic. Identify the level of nurse characteristics needed in the care of this patient.

7. Take one patient outcome for a patient and list evidence-based interventions found in a literature review for this patient.

Using the Synergy Model to Develop a Plan of Care

	Patient Characteristics	Level (1, 3, 5)	Subjective and Objective Data	Evidence-based Interventions	Outcomes
SYNERGY MODEL	Resiliency				
	Vulnerability				
	Stability				
	Complexity				
	Resource availability				
	Participation in care				
	Participation in decision making				
	Predictability				

Online Resources

American Gastroenterological Association: www.gastro.org

National Institute of Diabetes and Digestive and Kidney Diseases: www.niddk.nih.gov

National Pancreas Foundation: www.pancreasfoundation.org

REFERENCES

Draganov, P., & Forsmark, C. (2003). Diseases of the pancreas. Gastroenterology. Retrieved September 30, 2005, from www.acpmedicine.com/sam/pdf/med0405.pdf

Healthcare Freeware. (2005). Retrieved November 12, 2005, from www.healthcarefreeware.com/icu.htm

Hemes, A. R. (2005). Diagnosing acute pancreatitis. *American Journal of Medicine, 18*(2), 109–110.

Khoury, G., Deeba, S., Naradzay, J., Talavera, F., Hardin, E., Halamka, J., et al. (2005). Pancreatitis. Retrieved September 30, 2005, from www.emedicine.com/emerg/topic354.htm

Lipsett, P. A. (2005). Acute pancreatitis. In M. P. Fink, E. Abraham, J. L. Vincent, & P. M. Kochanek, *Textbook of critical care medicine* (5th ed., pp. 1021–1031). Philadelphia: Elsevier Saunders.

Nathens, A. B., Curtis, J. R., Beale, R. J., Cook, D. J., Moreno, R. P., Romand, J. A., et al. (2004). Management of the critically ill patient with severe acute pancreatitis. *Critical Care Medicine, 32*(12), 2524–2536.

Pastor, C. M., Matthay, M. A., & Frossard, J. L. (2003). Pancreatitis-associated acute lung injury: New insights. *Chest, 124*(6), 2341–2351.

Reece-Smith, H. (2005). Management of critically ill patients with severe acute pancreatitis. *Care of the Critically Ill, 21*(2), 35.

Salem, M. Z., Cunha, J. E, Coelho, A. M., Sampietri, S. N., Machado, M. C., Penteado, S., et al. (2003). Effects of octreotide pre-treatment in experimental acute pancreatitis. *Pancreatology, 3*(2), 164–168.

Suc, B., Msika, S., Piccinini, M., Fourtanier, G., Hay, J. M., Flamant, Y., et al. (2004). Octreotide in the prevention of intra-abdominal complications following elective pancreatic resection: A prospective multicenter randomized controlled trial. *Archives of Surgery, 139*(3), 288–294.

Torpy, J. M. (2004). Pancreatitis. *Journal of the American Medical Association, 291*(23), 2902.

Trivedi, C. D., & Pitchumoni, C. S. (2005). Drug-induced pancreatitis: An update. *Journal of Clinical Gastroenterology, 39*(8), 709–716.

Wrobleski, D. M., Barth, M. M., & Oyen, L. J. (1999). Necrotizing pancreatitis: Pathophysiology, diagnosis, and acute care management. *AACN Clinical Issues, 10*(4), 464–477.

Endocrine

CHAPTER 38

Endocrine Anatomy, Physiology, and Assessment

Linda L. Steele

LEARNING OBJECTIVES

Upon completion of this chapter, the reader will be able to:

1. Describe the anatomy and physiology of the endocrine system.

2. Recognize how the endocrine system affects each body system.

3. Accurately assess a patient's endocrine system.

4. Identify diseases that are associated with the endocrine system.

5. Identify laboratory tests that may be performed to assess the endocrine system.

The endocrine system is a complex network found throughout the body that consists of eight glands: the pituitary, thyroid, adrenal, pancreas, gonads (ovaries in females and testes in males), thymus, and pineal glands (see **Figure 38-1**). Nurses and other healthcare providers care for many patients with endocrine-related problems in the intensive care unit (ICU). Systematic assessment of the endocrine system involves knowledge of both the glands that produce the hormones and the actions of the specific hormones secreted by each of these glands.

ANATOMY AND PHYSIOLOGY OF THE ENDOCRINE SYSTEM

Endocrinology encompasses the study of both the endocrine glands and the hormones they produce. The term *endocrine* was coined by Starling to describe the actions of hormones secreted internally as compared to those secreted externally (*exocrine*), such as those found in the gastrointestinal tract. Hormones elicit cellular responses and regulate physiologic processes through a variety of complex feedback mechanisms. **Table 38-1** summarizes the actions of the endocrine glands.

It is not possible to describe and assess the endocrine system based solely on anatomy, because the endocrine glands communicate broadly with other organs (Jameson, 2004).

The interrelatedness of endocrinology with physiologic processes in other specialties is seen with the action of hormones on these systems. Hormones are substances secreted by specialized glands or cells and transported to various receptor sites to elicit a particular response. Hormones have four regulatory purposes: (1) production, use and storage of energy; (2) metabolism of salt and water; (3) growth and development; and (4) reproduction.

An understanding of the physiology of the endocrine system includes knowledge of the actions of hormones and their desired effects on target organs (see **Table 38-2**). For example, hormones play an important role in maintenance of blood pressure, intravascular volume, and peripheral resistance in the cardiovascular system. The peripheral nervous system modulates hormone production in both the adrenal medulla and the pancreatic islet cells (Jameson, 2004).

FIGURE 38-1 Glands of the Endocrine System

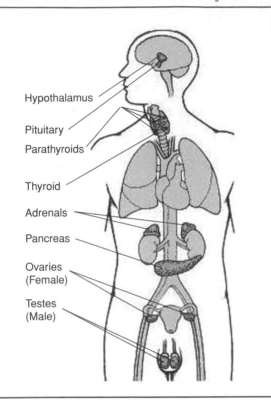

- Hypothalamus
- Pituitary
- Parathyroids
- Thyroid
- Adrenals
- Pancreas
- Ovaries (Female)
- Testes (Male)

Source: Copyright © 2005 John W. Kimball. All rights reserved.

either positive or negative feedback. Positive feedback enables a target cell or organ to produce more of the hormone, whereas negative feedback inhibits the production of the hormone. At times, a more complicated type of negative feedback occurs that allows a backup control system to be activated if an element of the loop fails, as shown in **Figure 38-2**.

Levels of hormones circulating in the blood are also tightly controlled by the following homeostatic mechanisms:

1. When one hormone stimulates the production of a second hormone, the second suppresses the production of the first. For example, when follicle-stimulating hormone (FSH) stimulates the release of estrogens from the ovarian follicle, a high level of estrogen can, in turn, suppress the further production of FSH.
2. Antagonistic pairs of hormones have opposite effects. For example, insulin causes the level of blood glucose to drop when it has risen, whereas glucagons cause glucose to rise when it has fallen.
3. Hormone secretion is increased (or decreased) by the same substance whose level is decreased (or increased) by the hormone. For example, a rising level of calcium in the blood suppresses the production of the parathyroid hormone (PTH). A low level of calcium stimulates production of PTH (Jameson, 2004).

The immune and endocrine systems also work closely together. For example, cortisol, an adrenal glucocorticoid, is a powerful immunosuppressant. A high level of cortisol decreases the body's immune response. Also, cytokines and interleukins affect the functions of the pituitary, adrenal, thyroid, and gonads. Disruption in regulation of immune control can cause common endocrine diseases such as autoimmune thyroid disease and Type 1 diabetes. Less common diseases, such as polyglandular failure, Addison's disease, and lymphocytic hypophysitis, have also been identified as having an immunologic causality (Jameson, 2004).

The endocrine system regulates hormone production by

TABLE 38-1 Actions of the Endocrine Glands

Adrenal glands	Divided into two regions; secrete hormones that influence the body's metabolism, blood chemicals, and body characteristics, as well as influence the part of the nervous system that is involved in the response and defense against stress.
Hypothalamus	Activates and controls the part of the nervous system that controls involuntary body functions, the hormonal system, and many body functions, such as regulating sleep and stimulating appetite.
Ovaries and testicles	Secrete hormones that influence female and male characteristics, respectively.
Pancreas	Secretes insulin that controls the use of glucose by the body.
Parathyroid glands	Secrete a hormone that maintains the calcium level in the blood.
Pineal body	Involved with daily biological cycles.
Pituitary gland	Produces a number of different hormones that influence other endocrine glands.
Thymus gland	Plays a role in the body's immune system.
Thyroid gland	Produces hormones that stimulate body heat production, bone growth, and the body's metabolism.

Source: AMA's Current Procedural Terminology, revised 1998 edition. Copyright 1999 American Medical Association. All rights reserved.

TABLE 38-2 Hormones: Sources, Targets, and Functions

Source	Hormone	Target	Physiologic Effect
Anterior pituitary	Follicle-stimulating hormone (FSH)	Ovary and testes	Growth of ovarian follicles or seminiferous tubules
Anterior pituitary	Luteinizing hormone (LH)	Ovary and testes	Production of estrogen and progesterone or testosterone
Anterior pituitary	Prolactin (LTH)	Ovary and mammary	Stimulates milk production in breast; Maintains secretion of estrogen and progesterone by ovary
Anterior pituitary	Thyroid-stimulating hormone (TSH)	Thyroid	Stimulates secretion of thyroid hormones
Anterior pituitary	Adrenocorticotropic hormone (ACTH)	Adrenal cortex	Stimulates secretion of adrenal cortex hormones
Anterior pituitary	Growth hormone (GH)	General	Stimulates growth
Anterior pituitary	Melanocyte-stimulating hormone (MSH)	Melanocytes	Stimulates dispersal of pigment in chromatophores
Hypothalamus via posterior pituitary	Oxytocin	Uterus and mammary	Stimulates contraction and secretion of milk
Hypothalamus via posterior pituitary	Antidiuretic hormone (ADH)	Kidney	Stimulates reabsorption of water
Thyroid gland	Thyroxin and triiodothyroxine	General	Stimulates metabolism, growth, and development
Thyroid gland	Calcitonin	Bone	Lowers blood calcium level by inhibiting bone breakdown
Parathyroid gland	Parathyroid hormone	Bone, kidney, digestive tract	Increases blood calcium by stimulating bone breakdown
Adrenal cortex	Mineralocorticoids (aldosterone)	Kidney	Maintains sodium and phosphorus balance
Adrenal cortex	Glucocorticoids (cortisol)	General	Raises blood glucose level to adapt to long-term stress
Adrenal cortex	Dehydroepiandrosterone (DHEA)	Ovary and prostate	Stimulates sex drive; Transformation into testosterone and estrogen; Induces labor
Adrenal medulla	Epinephrine (adrenalin)	Muscle, liver	Stimulates glucose release; Short-term coping with stress
Adrenal medulla	Norepinephrine	Blood vessels	Constricts blood vessels; Increases heart rate
Pineal gland	Melatonin	Gonads, pigment cells, other cells	Controls biorhythms; Influences reproduction
Pancreas alpha cells	Glucagon	Liver fatty tissue	Raise blood glucose concentration; Stimulate gluconeogenesis
Pancreas beta cells	Insulin	General	Lower blood glucose concentration; Stimulate glycogen synthesis

continues

TABLE 38-2 Hormones: Sources, Targets, and Functions (continued)

Source	Hormone	Target	Physiologic Effect
Ovary	Estrogen, estradiol	General and uterus	Develops/maintains female characteristics Stimulates growth of uterine lining
Ovary	Progestrogen	Uterus and breast	Stimulates development of uterine lining
Ovary and placenta	Relaxin	Pelvic ligaments	Relaxes pelvic ligaments
Placenta	Chorionic gonadotropin	Anterior pituitary	Stimulates release of FSH and LH
Testes	Testosterone	General and reproductive structures	Develops and maintains male sex characteristics Promotes spermatogenesis
Testes	Inhibin	Anterior lobe of pituitary	Inhibits FSH release
Testes	Testosterone	General and reproductive structures	Develops and maintains male sex characteristics Promotes spermatogenesis
Duodenal mucosa	Secretin	Pancreas	Stimulates secretion of pancreatic juice
Duodenal mucosa	Cholecystokinin	Gallbladder	Stimulates release of bile by gallbladder

Source: Kimball, 2005.

FIGURE 38-2 Hypothalamic-Pituitary-Thyroid Feedback Loop

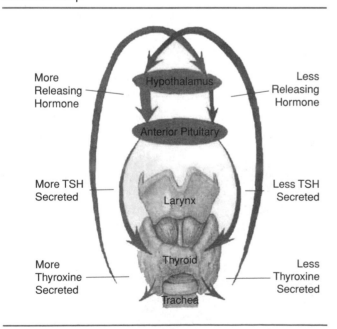

Source: Copyright © 2005. John W. Kimball.

ASSESSMENT OF THE ENDOCRINE SYSTEM

Since the endocrine glands are located throughout the body, assessment of this system is usually included in the overall general examination as well as examinations related to specific body systems. For example, endocrine pathology resulting from overproduction or underproduction of hormones in endocrine glands can be seen in the face, body build, and skin, as well as being evidenced in distinct clinical syndromes affecting specific glands such as the thyroid, parathyroid, adrenal, or pituitary (Epstein, Perkin, Cookson, & de Bono, 2003). Common endocrine disorders may also present with vague symptoms and signs, prompting the healthcare provider to suspect this system when a patient has systemic complaints of fatigue, malaise, or changes in weight (LeBlond, 2004).

History

A thorough history is necessary to begin assessing the endocrine system. The format described in **Table 38-3** should be used to obtain subjective information from the patient as the nurse begins an assessment of the endocrine system.

TABLE 38-3 Subjective Assessment of the Endocrine System

General	Rate status of health in general. Feelings of fatigue, malaise, weakness, lethargy, appetite and/or weight changes, intolerance to heat or cold. Facial changes. Swelling in face or limbs. Polydipsia, polyphagia, polyuria.
Hair and skin	Excessive dryness, coarse or brittle, thinning hair. Dry, coarse skin. Extreme velvety, smooth skin. Sweatiness.
Head and neck	Enlargement of skull, neck swelling, unilateral or bilateral. Difficulty swallowing.
Eyes	Exopthalmos. Dryness. Visual disturbances.
Cardiovascular	Palpitations.
Gastrointestinal	Diarrhea or constipation. Weight gain or loss despite no change in eating habits. Nausea or vomiting. Abdominal pain.
Reproductive	Amenorrhea or menorrhagia. Impotence.
Neurologic	Weakness, paresthesias, headache.
Psychiatric	Change in mental status, irritability, decreased concentration, slowness of thinking, emotional lability, depression.

Source: Jameson, 2004.

TABLE 38-4 Physical Examination Data

General assessment	Height, weight, blood pressure, temperature, pulse pressure, body mass index.
Head and face	Inspect for size, shape, facial expressions, swelling.
Skin	Inspect for color, lesions, pigmentation. Palpate for temperature, texture, turgor.
Hair and nails	Inspect the hair for general distribution. Palpate for texture. Inspect the nails for lesions and cracks.
Neck	Inspect for swelling, pulsations. Palpate the thyroid for symmetry, size, swelling, nodules. Palpate for enlarged lymph nodes.
Mouth	Inspect buccal mucosa for color, pigmentation, hydration, and swelling of the tongue.
Eyes	Inspect for exopthalmos, lid lag, lid spasm, periorbital edema. Check for exudate, hemorrhage, papilledema.
Cardiovascular	Inspect for precordial pulsations. Palpate rate, rhythm, and strength of pulsation. Auscultate for S_1, S_2, extra sounds or murmurs.
Abdomen	Inspect for protuberance, distention, peristalsis. Auscultate for bowel sounds, bruits. Palpate for tenderness, organomegaly.
Female reproductive	Inspect for distribution of pubic hair. Inspect the vagina for color and pigmentation. Palpate the uterus for size, consistency, irregular borders.
Male reproductive	Inspect for distribution of pubic hair. Palpate the testes for shape, size, irregular borders.
Neuromuscular	Inspect for muscle tone and strength. Palpate for paresthesias. Elicit deep tendon reflexes.

Source: Jameson, 2004.

Physical Examination

Since disturbances in the endocrine system may be manifested in a variety of body systems, assessment of the endocrine system involves conducting a complete physical examination. **Table 38-4** identifies data to be assessed for each body system. A thorough physical exam is required.

After obtaining a complete history, physical examination, and findings of laboratory testing, the critical care nurse should develop and prioritize a problem list based on these findings.

DISORDERS OF THE ENDOCRINE SYSTEM

Disorders of the endocrine system include diabetic emergencies (discussed in Chapter 42), and disorders of the thyroid, adrenal, and pituitary (discussed in Chapters 39, 40, and 41, respectively). Other endocrine-related disorders that affect patients who may present in ICU settings are those affecting adrenal function and the parathyroid gland. The primary symptomatology, both objective and subjective, that the ICU nurse should assess in patients is presented in **Table 38-5** and **Table 38-6**.

SUMMARY

Assessment of the endocrine system is complex due to the number of organs and other body systems involved, along with

TABLE 38-5 Cushing's Syndrome and Addison's Disease: Subjective, Objective, and Lab Findings

Corticosteroid Excess: Cushing's Syndrome	Primary Adrenal Insufficiency: Addison's Disease
Subjective	**Subjective**
• Weakness	• Weakness, fatigue, lethargy
• Weight gain	• Nausea and vomiting, diarrhea, weight loss, abdominal pain
• Amenorrhea	• Craving for salt
• Back pain	Symptoms of an Addisonian crisis:
• Depression, mood swings	• Sudden penetrating pain in the lower back, abdomen, or legs
• Increased thirst and urination	• Severe vomiting and diarrhea
	• Dehydration
	• Low blood pressure
	• Loss of consciousness
	Left untreated, an Addisonian crisis can be fatal.
Objective	**Objective**
Hypertension	Reduced growth of hair
Moon face	Mottled skin
Acne	Pigmentation of lips, buccal mucosa, vagina, and rectum
Kyphosis	Orthostatic hypotension
Purple striae on abdomen and thighs	Signs of dehydration
Peripheral edema	
Lab Findings	**Lab Findings**
High white blood count	Poor or no response to adenocorticotropin (ACT H) stimulation
High blood sugar	Decreased to absent levels of blood cortisol with corticotropin-releasing
Low serum potassium	hormone (CRH) stimulation

TABLE 38-6 Hyperparathyroidism and Hypoparathyroidism: Subjective, Objective, and Lab Findings

Hyperparathyroidism	Hypoparathyroidism
Subjective	**Subjective**
Muscle weakness or stiffness	Nervousness
Loss of appetite	Weakness, paresthesias
Weight loss	Muscle stiffness and cramps
Nausea, constipation	Headaches
Polyuria, polydipsia	Abdominal pain
Deafness	
Paresthesias	
Bone pain	
Renal colic	
Objective	**Objective**
Keratitis	Tetany with carpopedal spasm
Hypotonia, muscle weakness	Chvostek and Trousseau signs
Skeletal deformities	Hair loss
Bone fractures	Papilledema
	Cataracts
Lab Findings	**Lab Findings**
Increased blood levels of calcium	Decreased blood levels of calcium
Increased parathyroid hormone	Increased blood levels of phosphorus

Source: www.parathyroid.com.

the actions of hormones on target organs. Critical care nurses and other healthcare providers can enhance their ability to assess the endocrine system through careful, comprehensive history taking; complete physical examination; knowledge of the major organs and systems regulated; and recognition of the signs and symptoms of potential diseases affecting this system. Thus, when patients are admitted to critical care settings, healthcare providers will have the knowledge and competence required to identify and provide optimal care for patients who have disorders related to the endocrine system.

CASE STUDY

The reader may need to refer to Chapter 39 for assistance with this case study.

E.S. is a 76-year-old female who was admitted to the ICU with altered mental status, bradycardia, and hypothermia. She was diagnosed with hypothyroidism 20 years ago and was well controlled on levothyroxine sodium (Synthroid®) until last month, when her condition began to steadily deteriorate. She experienced an acute onset of fever, cough, and chills four weeks ago and thought she had the "flu." During her admission history, she reported being more fatigued than usual, apathetic, and "a little confused." In your nursing assessment you note that she seems more confused and cannot remember what the date is or where she is.

E.S.'s vital signs are as follows: B/P 130/100, HR 62, R 22, T 95.8°F (35.5°C). As you examine her, you note facial puffiness; ptosis; dry, cool, doughy skin; sparse hair; and nonpitting edema of the lower extremities. A tentative diagnosis of myxedema has been made by the physician.

CRITICAL THINKING QUESTIONS

1. Which labs may be ordered? Why? What critical values may be found?
2. What would be the initial IV treatment for E.S.?

The lab values have been called to the unit stat with critical values for Na 109 mEq/l, creatinine 2.4 mg/dL, and CK 90 U/L.

CRITICAL THINKING QUESTIONS

3. Which actions would be taken to correct these abnormal values?
4. Would vasopressors or inotropes be recommended?
5. Should warming blankets be used to correct the hypothermia?

E.S. has received an initial IV T4 dose of 500 mcg.

CRITICAL THINKING QUESTIONS

6. What additional therapy is needed?
7. What signs and symptoms should you closely monitor E.S. for related to this therapy?

E.S. has greatly improved, her vital signs have stabilized, and she is no longer confused. Myxedema coma has a significant mortality rate even with appropriate treatment, so ICU nurses should be alert for the signs and symptoms of myxedema, particularly in elderly women who have an onset of altered mental status during the winter months. An accurate diagnosis of myxedema is difficult because these signs and symptoms may be present in many other diseases. However, suspicion of this disease before progressing to coma should be kept in mind, along with the need for a careful history, physical examination, and laboratory evaluation. The most important elements in treatment of myxedema coma are early recognition, presumptive thyroid hormone replacement, hydrocortisone, and appropriate supportive care (Rhodes, 2000).

CRITICAL THINKING QUESTIONS

8. There are many causes of organic psychosis. Which disorders of the endocrine system may cause your patient to exhibit signs of psychosis? Which signs and symptoms other than psychosis may alert you to suspect a problem with the endocrine system?

9. Altered mental status can be common in older patients. Which specific disorder of the endocrine system is the most common cause of alteration in mental status in the elderly?

10. What are the most common endocrine causes of anovulatory, irregular menstrual bleeding in adolescents?

11. Which disciplines should be consulted to work with this client?

12. What types of issues may require you to act as an advocate or moral agent for this patient?

13. How will you implement your role as a facilitator of learning for this patient?

14. Use the form to write up data and a plan of care for a patient with an endocrine problem in the clinical setting. Rate the patient as a level 1, 3, or 5 on each characteristic. Identify the level of nurse characteristics needed in the care of this patient.

15. Take one patient outcome for a patient and list evidence-based interventions found in a literature review for this patient.

Using the Synergy Model to Develop a Plan of Care

	Patient Characteristics	Level (1, 3, 5)	Subjective and Objective Data	Evidence-based Interventions	Outcomes
SYNERGY MODEL	Resiliency				
	Vulnerability				
	Stability				
	Complexity				
	Resource availability				
	Participation in care				
	Participation in decision making				
	Predictability				

Online Resources

A Tour of the Endocrine System: http://arbl.cvmbs.colostate.edu/hbooks/pathphys/endocrine/

American Autoimmune Related Diseases Association: www.aarda.org/

Cushing's Support and Research Foundation: http://world.std.com/~csrf/

Hypoparathyroidism: www.hypoparathyroidism.org/view_newsletter.php?1998-06

Parathyroid Disease: www.parathyroid.com/parathyroid-disease.htm

Pituitary Foundation: www.pituitary.com/

REFERENCES

American Medical Association. (1999). Current procedural terminology. Retrieved August 1, 2005, from www.ama-assn.org/ama/pub/category/7157.html

Epstein, O., Perkin, G. D., Cookson, J., & de Bono, D. P. (2003). *Clinical examination.* St. Louis, MO: Mosby.

Jameson, L. (2004). Principles of endocrinology. In E. Braunwald (Ed.), *Harrison's principles of internal medicine* (16th ed., pp. 2084–2105). New York: McGraw-Hill.

Kimball, J. W. (2005). Hormones of the human. Retrieved August 1, 2005, from http://users.rcn.com/jkimball.ma.ultranet/BiologyPages/H/Hormones.html

LeBlond, R. (2004). Nonregional systems and diseases. In R. F. LeBlond, R. L. DeGowin, & D. D. Brown (Eds.) *DeGowin's diagnostic examination* (pp. 99–121). New York: McGraw-Hill.

Rhodes, C. (2000). Myxedema coma: Diagnosis and treatment. *American Family Physician, 66,* 2485–2491.

Thyroid Disorders

Cynthia V. Brown

Weighing only 10 to 20 grams normally, the thyroid gland, found at the base of the anterior neck just below the larynx, controls the entire body's metabolic rate and thermoregulation. In the critical care area, minor disturbances of normal function in other organs or systems can cause huge variations in thyroid function and the ability to recover from catastrophic illness. Three disturbances of thyroid function are most likely to be seen in the intensive care unit (ICU): myxedema coma, thyroid storm, and euthyroid sick syndrome. A more rare condition, acute suppurative thyroiditis, is occasionally encountered but will not be discussed in this chapter.

NORMAL THYROID FUNCTION

Thyroid hormones are important regulators of energy production, functional and structural proteins, and the actions of other hormones, such as glucocorticoids, mineralocorticoids, growth factors, and biogenic amines (e.g., catecholamines) (DeGroot, 2005). These hormones affect growth and development, influence the protein that builds muscle, and are largely responsible for regulating temperature, heart rate, mood, alertness, and even the texture and growth of hair and nails. The function of the thyroid gland can affect weight gain or loss because the gland regulates metabolism, which is the rate at which heat (kilocalories) is produced. In the person with a normally functioning thyroid gland, minute-to-minute adjustments are made in the amount of thyroid hormone produced based on how much the body needs at the time.

The thyroid gland produces two thyroid hormones: T4, a relatively weak and inactive hormone, and T3, the biologically active portion of thyroid hormone (Utiger, 2001). Each molecule of T4 contains four iodine atoms. This hormone is stored in the thyroid gland itself, which can hold about a three-month supply (Haynes, 2002). When released, under direction of the pituitary gland (thyroid-stimulating hormone), T4 travels on a protein molecule to the liver and muscles, where it is deiodinated to T3. Again traveling on a protein molecule, T3 goes to the target organs, where it exerts its influence on the function of that particular organ. When this rather delicate balance is upset, either too much thyroid hormone or too little is secreted. In the ICU, the likely scenario of too much thyroid hormone is thyroid storm; too little thyroid hormone may present as myxedema coma. Euthyroid sick syndrome occurs in the setting of either catastrophic illness in a person with otherwise normal thyroid or with chronic illness. Normal thyroid hormone levels are detailed in **Table 39-1**.

THYROID STORM

Thyroid storm, also termed thyrotoxic crisis, is a rarely occurring, severe form of hyperthyroidism leading to systemic decompensation (Hershman, 2002). Thyroid storm occurs most frequently in the setting of Graves' disease, either undiagnosed or undertreated precipitated by a superimposed illness, injury, or surgery.

Cardinal Clinical Signs

- High fever (temperature 102–105°F) with profuse sweating
- Marked tachycardia (pulse 120–140 beats per minute or higher)
- Atrial fibrillation (irregular rhythm; see Chapter 10)
- Heart failure
- Neurological symptoms: confusion, agitation, coma
- Gastrointestinal symptoms: vomiting, profuse diarrhea, hepatomegaly, jaundice

Not all of these signs need be present to diagnose thyroid storm, but many of them will be evident.

Diagnosis

A diagnosis of thyroid storm is made based on clinical signs as well as laboratory studies. Thyroid-stimulating hormone (TSH) will be less than 0.01 mU/L or undetectable, while T3 and T4 levels will be greatly elevated. TSH receptor antibodies help to distinguish Graves' disease from other types of hyperthyroidism. Antibody testing typically takes a week to complete. Treatment of thyroid storm should not be delayed by waiting for the result of an antibody test.

Therapy

Patients with suspected or diagnosed thyroid storm should be managed in the ICU. Treatment has the following goals:

TABLE 39-1 Normal Thyroid Hormone Levels

TSH	0.5–5.0 mU/L
Total T4	4.5–12.5 mcg/dL
Total T3	75–195 ng/dL
Free T4	0.8–2.7 ng/dL
T3 uptake	22–35%

Note: Laboratory results could vary dependent upon equipment.
Sources: Ruggieri & Isaacs, 2004; Wiersinga, 2004.

- Inhibition of thyroid hormone production
- Inhibition of thyroid hormone release from the gland
- Beta-adrenergic blockade
- Supportive therapy for comorbidities
- Identification and treatment of the precipitating event
- Initiation of long-term therapy for the prevention of recurrence

Inhibition of Thyroid Hormone Production

Rapid decrease of hormone production is accomplished with antithyroid medications. Propylthiouracil (PTU) is the preferred antithyroid agent, because this drug prevents the peripheral conversion of T4 to T3. The loading dose of 600 mg and daily doses of 200 mg every four hours will completely block thyroid hormone production. This medication may be administered orally, by nasogastric tube, or rectally. No parenteral preparation of antithyroid hormone is available in the United States.

For patients who cannot take PTU because of a previous allergic response or agranulocytosis, methimazole (Tapazole®) is available. Methimazole is given in 20-mg doses every four hours. Both of these drugs inhibit production of thyroid hormone, but not its release from the gland.

Inhibition of Thyroid Hormone Release

Two or three hours after the loading dose of PTU has been given, thyroid hormone release should be inhibited by administering iodine. Iodine is given after inhibiting hormone production so that it cannot stimulate further hormone production.

1. Lugol's solution: 10 drops, three times per day
   or
2. Supersaturated potassium iodine: 3 drops, three times per day. Administration of iodine precludes radioactive iodine treatment of hyperthyroidism for several weeks. The iodine load must be reduced before radioactive uptake can be obtained for a successful radioactive iodine treatment.
3. Lithium carbonate, 300 mg every 6 hours, can be used in patients with a history of iodine anaphylaxis.

Beta-Adrenergic Blockade

Beta blockade is intended to decrease the signs and symptoms of beta-adrenergic stimulation. These symptoms include tachycardia, restlessness, sweating, tremors, and agitation. Propranolol (Inderal®) is the most widely used agent at an oral dose of 40 to 80 mg every 4 to 6 hours. It may also be given by intravenous (IV) line at a dose of 1 mg every 5 to 10 minutes until heart rate is controlled. Propranolol is contraindicated in patients who have asthma or bronchial spasms or who are in severe heart failure (McDermott, 2002) because it will precipitate further respiratory problems. Esmolol (Brevibloc®) can be given at a rate of 0.25 to 0.50 mg/kg over 1 minute IV, then 0.05 to 0.10 mg/kg/min infusion. Diltiazem (Cardizem®) is another option. It is dosed at 60 to 90 mg every 6 to 8 hours orally, or 0.25 mg/kg over 2 minutes IV, followed by an infusion at a rate of 10 mg/min.

Supportive Therapy

Supportive measures are designed to relieve the symptoms caused by the hyperthyroid state. Stress doses of hydrocortisone are useful due to the high turnover of cortisol during thyroid storm, which renders the patient, in effect, hypoadrenal. In addition, glucocorticoids help to inhibit the peripheral conversion of T4 to T3. The dose for these patients is 100 mg hydrocortisone sodium succinate (Solu-Cortef®) IV every 8 hours. Once the crisis has passed, the dose is tapered to discontinuance over several days.

Fever greater than 102 °F is a hallmark of thyroid storm. To lower body temperature, acetaminophen (Tylenol®) is preferred over salicylates, which displace thyroid hormone from the binding protein and, therefore, may actually increase the level of free thyroid hormone. Cooling blankets and ice packs may also help to decrease fever.

Fluid replacement may be indicated because sweating, diarrhea, and vomiting can lead to significant fluid loss. Dehydration with rhabdomyolitis has been seen as a result. Rhabdomyolitis is a syndrome characterized by myalgia (muscle aches and cramps). In the patient with heart failure, fluid replacement is best accomplished with a pulmonary artery catheter in place to prevent fluid overload. Five percent dextrose with any necessary electrolytes added at a rate of 100 to 200 mL/hr is sometimes required.

Anticoagulation with warfarin (Coumadin®) may be indicated for those patients in atrial fibrillation to avoid embolic events.

Digoxin helps to increase the atrial ventricular conduction time, prolonging the refractory period of the AV node. With this medication, ventricular response to atrial fibrillation is reduced.

Identification of Precipitating Illness or Event

Often, it is easy to identify the precipitating illness or event that leads to thyroid storm (e.g., the patient who ran out of antithyroid medications or the patient with pneumonia). The challenge is those patients who lack a clear history and who cannot reveal any history because they are stuporous, comatose, or too confused. Nonetheless, vigorous efforts to identify the cause are necessary for a successful outcome. Chest radiograph, blood and urine cultures, abdominal radiograph or ultrasound, and computerized tomography (CT) or magnetic resonance imaging (MRI) of the head might be indicated. Further diagnostic studies may be necessary depending on the results of the initial tests.

MYXEDEMA COMA

Myxedema coma is the end point of severe thyroid hormone deficiency in which patients develop multiple organ failure, stupor, and even death. Mortality rate can be as high as 20% to 50%. Myxedema coma occurs more in the winter, in women, in the elderly, and in individuals with a history of hypothyroidism or goiter. Often, as in the case of thyroid storm, there is a precipitating illness or event or, sometimes, over ingestion of sedating medications.

Cardinal Signs

Altered mental status, nonpitting edema, hypotension, hypothermia, hypoventilation, and stupor are some of the signs of myxedema coma. Placed in the context of known hypothyroidism, these signs should lead the clinician to obtain thyroid tests.

Diagnostic Tests

- TSH, free T3 and T4; total T3 and T4
- Cortisol level
- Complete blood count (CBC)
- Biochemical profile that includes liver function, blood urea nitrogen (BUN), and creatinine
- Urinalysis
- Creatine kinase (CK)
- Blood cultures
- Arterial blood gases (ABGs)
- Chest x-ray
- Electrocardiogram (ECG)
- Abdominal ultrasound and CT of the head (if there are signs of intestinal obstruction or neurological deficits)

Significant microcytic anemia suggests a history of menorrhagia or some other bleeding source. Macrocytic anemia suggests a history of malnutrition or, more likely, pernicious anemia, which is a common associated finding in autoimmune disorders.

Therapy

The goal of therapy for myxedema coma is stabilization of vital bodily functions. Patients commonly present with altered mental status, respiratory failure, hypotension, bradyarrhythmia, and a serious precipitating illness.

Respiratory support needs to be initiated early in the course of treatment. Endotracheal intubation is often necessary, especially if the myxedematous tongue has obstructed the upper airway. ABGs should be obtained one hour after intubation and then as clinically indicated to monitor the adequacy of the oxygenation and ventilation.

Medications should be given intravenously because hypotension, ileus, and edema render the absorption of oral or intramuscular medications unreliable. Patients who have developed arrhythmias need cardiac monitoring with dysrhythmia recognition alarms set appropriately. Hypotension will respond better to plasma volume expanders than to adrenergic agents. Bradycardia may require temporary pacing. Pacing can be accomplished with either a transvenous or transcutaneous method.

Electrolyte imbalance usually takes the form of hyponatremia due to a variety of metabolic derangements. This condition may contribute to coma and seizures, which may resolve with administration of hypertonic saline and limited water in the IV fluids. Volume of IV fluids must be monitored carefully via a central venous catheter. Symptoms usually improve when serum sodium levels reach 130 mEq/L.

Patients with anemia may need support with transfusion of packed red blood cells if hematocrit is below 20%. Also, hypothermia may be challenging to measure with conventional thermometers; instead, it is best monitored with core temperature. Warming blankets are not recommended, because they may cause too much peripheral vasodilation and shock. Use of extra blankets is the safest treatment since body temperature will be restored with thyroid hormone replacement.

Hypoglycemia may be a symptom of hypopituitarism or hypoadrenalism. Glucose may be added to the IV infusion early in the treatment, and stress doses of steroids may be given to raise both blood pressure and blood sugar. The nurse should suspect adrenal insufficiency if the cortisol level is inappropriately low for a physically stressed patient. Hydrocortisone sodium succinate (Solu-Cortef®) 100 mg IV every 8 hours is the standard stress dose. Gradual decrease of this dose follows over the next 48 hours, assuming that blood pressure, blood sugar, and electrolytes begin returning to more normal levels.

Thyroid hormone replacement is the specific therapy for myxedema coma. Currently, some controversy persists over the choice of using T4 therapy alone or adding T3 therapy as well. There is consensus that T3 therapy [liothyronine (Thyrolar®)] alone is inappropriate. Loading doses of T4 [levothyroxine (Synthroid®)] are also a subject of much controversy, but accepted to be in the range of 150 to 300 mcg of T4 (or 2 mcg/kg body weight). This dose is given IV over 5 minutes at the beginning of therapy; thereafter, T4 may be given IV 100 mcg every 24 hours. The loading dose of T3 is 10 to 25 mcg IV. The same dose is repeated every 12 hours if indicated. Response to therapy is gauged by patient response—that is, rise of body temperature, pulse, and blood pressure; improvement in mental function and ABGs. When most bodily functions have returned, oral T4 may be started. The usual maintenance dose of T4 is 1.5 mcg/kg.

The need for long-term therapy with T4 should be emphasized to the patient. Indeed, lifelong treatment is necessary. Regular follow-up with the physician every six months is recommended to monitor thyroid levels and to make any necessary adjustment to dosage.

EUTHYROID SICK SYNDROME

Euthyroid sick syndrome refers to a group of changes in serum thyroid hormone and TSH levels that occur in patients with a variety of nonthyroidal illnesses, including infections, trauma, surgery, myocardial infarction, malignancies, inflammatory conditions, and starvation. It is not a primary thyroid disorder, but rather results from changes in the peripheral metabolism and transport of thyroid hormones (Utiger, 2001).

Hormonal Changes

Patients in the ICU will develop low total T3 and free T3 levels, resulting from reduced peripheral conversion of T4 to T3. TSH usually remains in the normal range. The more severe the illness, the lower the T3 levels. Extremely low T3 levels suggest a poor prognosis.

Therapy

The preferred therapy for euthyroid sick syndrome is another area of controversy in thyroid treatment. Currently, there are no data that demonstrate a better recovery or survival rate with treatment versus no treatment. Judgment is often left to the discretion of the consulting endocrinologist. Usually, when the illness resolves, the euthyroid sick syndrome resolves as well.

PATIENT OUTCOMES

Nurses can help ensure the obtainment of optimal patient outcomes such as those listed in **Box 39-1** through the use of evidence-based interventions for patients with thyroid disorders.

SUMMARY

Hyperthyroidism and hypothyroidism are common thyroid disorders, but their respective end points—thyroid storm and myxedema coma—are no longer very common. Nonetheless, ICU nurses need to be aware of the presenting signs and symptoms of each disease entity when faced with a mentally altered, stuporous, or agitated patient. Not only does the hyperthyroid or hypothyroid state require immediate and aggressive treatment, but the precipitating cause of the thyroid imbalance must be found and treated as well.

Those patients who have become ill because they stopped taking their antithyroid medication or thyroid hormone replacement need to be reminded that, with few exceptions, thyroid treatment is lifelong and they must not discontinue their medications for extended periods. Family members also need to be made aware of the importance of maintaining a daily dose of medication, particularly with an elderly family member or one who is forgetful.

Box 39-1

Optimal Patient Outcomes

- Temperature in normal range
- Heart rate in expected range
- Absence of cardiac arrhythmias
- Absence of signs of heart failure
- Absence of gastrointestinal symptoms
- Blood pressure in expected range
- Airway remains patent
- Fluid volume status in expected range
- Hemoglobin and hematocrit within expected range
- Mental status returns to baseline

CASE STUDY

S.T. is a 57-year-old female who was admitted to the ICU from the Emergency Department (ED). Her daughter found her at home in a stuporous state. The daughter reports that the patient had an upper respiratory infection and flu-like symptoms for the past five days. In addition, S.T. told her daughter that she was short of breath with minimal exertion, constipated, more fatigued than usual, and not urinating often. The patient attributed each of these symptoms to having the flu. The patient is a widow who lives alone, but her daughter lives close by and checks on her daily.

In the ED, S.T. experienced a seizure, which lasted 45 seconds. Her vital signs were B/P 132/72, HR 47, RR 24, temp 94.3°F (34.6°C). Her Glasgow Coma Scale score before the seizure was 8. Based on the patient's history and presenting symptoms, thyroid function tests were performed. S.T.'s serum T4 level was below normal levels. A diagnosis of myxedema coma was made. The patient was given 500 mcg of T4 intravenously and was admitted to the ICU for further management.

CRITICAL THINKING QUESTIONS

1. What were the main symptoms that led the healthcare team to suspect myxedema coma in this patient?
2. Discuss thyroid function testing, normal values, and the significance of the abnormal values.
3. Discuss the likely rationale for S.T.'s vital signs.
4. If an arterial blood gas was drawn on S.T., what would you anticipate the findings to be?
5. Name one discipline that should be consulted to work with this patient. Provide a rationale for your choice.
6. What types of issues may require you to act as an advocate or moral agent for this patient?
7. How will you implement your role as a facilitator of learning for this patient?
8. Use the form to write up the data and a plan of care for a patient with a thyroid disorder in the clinical setting. Rate the patient as a level 1, 3, or 5 on each characteristic. Identify the most important nurse characteristics needed in the care of this patient. Provide an explanation of your choice.
9. Take one patient outcome and list evidence-based interventions for this patient.

Using the Synergy Model to Develop a Plan of Care

	Patient Characteristics	Level (1, 3, 5)	Subjective and Objective Data	Evidence-based Interventions	Outcomes
SYNERGY MODEL	Resiliency				
	Vulnerability				
	Stability				
	Complexity				
	Resource availability				
	Participation in care				
	Participation in decision making				
	Predictability				

Online Resources

Common tests to evaluate thyroid gland function: www.endocrineweb.com/tests.html

Euthyroid sick syndrome: www.emedicine.com/med/topic753.htm

Hypothyroidism: www.nlm.nih.gov/medlineplus/ency/article/000353.htm

Myxedema coma: http://patients.uptodate.com/topic.asp?file=thyroid/11535

Myxedema coma: www.thyroidmanager.org/Chapter9/ch_9-4.htm

REFERENCES

DeGroot, L. J. (2005). Graves' disease and the manifestations of thyrotoxicosis. In *The thyroid and its diseases*. Retrieved July 16, 2005, from www.Endotext.com

Haynes, D. F. (2002). Serum chemistries. In M. J. Goolsby, *Nurse practitioner secrets* (p. 41). Philadelphia: Hanley & Belfus.

Hershman, J. M. (2002). Hypothyroidism and hyperthyroidism. In N. Lavin, *Manual of endocrinology and metabolism* (3rd ed., pp. 396–410, 803). Philadelphia: Lippincott Williams & Wilkins.

McDermott, M. T. (2002). Thyroid emergencies. In M. T. McDermott, *Endocrine emergencies* (3rd ed., pp. 302–307). Philadelphia: Hanley & Belfus.

Ruggieri, P., & Isaacs, S. (2004). *A simple guide to thyroid disorders*. Omaha, NE: Addicus Books.

Utiger, R. D. (2001). The thyroid: Physiology, thyrotoxicosis, hypothyroidism, and the painful thyroid. In D. Felig & L. A. Frohman (Eds.), *Endocrinology and metabolism* (4th ed., pp. 259–348). New York: McGraw-Hill.

Wiersinga, W. M. (2004). Adult hypothyroidism. In *The thyroid and its diseases*. Retrieved July 16, 2005, from www.Endotext.com

CHAPTER 40

Adrenal Disorders

Donni Jester

Upon completion of this chapter, the reader will be able to:

1. Explain the function and control of the adrenal glands.

2. Compare and contrast significant disorders of adrenal function.

3. Discuss methods to evaluate adrenal disorders.

4. Describe treatment modalities used for adrenal dysfunction.

5. List optimal outcomes that may be achieved through evidence-based management of the patient with an adrenal disorder.

The intensive care unit (ICU) nurse must have a thorough understanding of the adrenal gland. The adrenal gland is responsible for the secretion of several vital hormones. Therefore, disorders of the adrenal gland can be life threatening.

FUNCTIONAL ANATOMY AND PHYSIOLOGY OF THE ADRENAL GLANDS

There are two adrenal glands located in the retroperitoneal area, closely situated above the kidneys bilaterally. Each gland consists of a capsule, an outer cortex, and an inner medulla. These separate sections act in very different ways.

The adrenal cortex, which is the outer portion of the gland, accounts for 80% of the weight of the gland and is responsible for secretion of glucocorticoids, mineralocorticoids, and adrenal androgens and estrogen. The secretion of glucocorticoids is controlled by the hypothalamus through its release of corticotropin-releasing hormone (CRH), which in turn controls the release of adrenocorticotropic hormone (ACTH) from the pituitary gland. The glucocorticoids function primarily to promote gluconeogenesis in the liver and as anti-inflammatories, immunosuppressants, and growth suppressants. The most important of these glucocorticoids is cortisol. Mineralocorticoids, the most potent of which is aldosterone, act to conserve sodium with a concomitant loss of potassium and hydrogen. The secretion of aldosterone is stimulated by the renin-angiotensin cascade, which in turn is stimulated by sodium and water loss, increased potassium, and decreased intravascular volume.

The adrenal medulla primarily produces catecholamines (epinephrine and norepinephrine), which control the "fight or flight" response. Epinephrine is about ten times more potent than norepinephrine. The secretion of both catecholamines is stimulated by ACTH and the glucocorticoids.

The trigger that causes these systems to begin releasing these hormones is stressors, either emotional or physical. This stress response does not differentiate between the two, and both can set off the response equally well (Kumar, Abbas, & Nelson, 2005).

SIGNIFICANT ADRENAL DISORDERS

Pheochromocytoma

Due to its role in the production of catecholamines and aldosterone, adrenal gland dysfunction must be considered in the setting of acute hypertension. A rare, but frequently suspected cause of hypertension is pheochromocytoma. Pheochromocytomas are found in 0.3% to 1% of patients with sustained hypertension (Palek & Eisenhofer, 2004). This catecholamine-secreting tumor is typically found in the adrenal medulla and may be malignant in 3% to 36% of the cases. Malignancy has been associated with 50% mortality within five years (Palek & Eisenhofer). Norepinephrine secretion is most commonly seen with pheochromocytomas, whereas dopamine is more commonly associated with malignancy. The most common sites for metastasis are regional lymph nodes, liver, bone, lung, and muscle (Asp, 2002a).

The clinical signs and symptoms associated with pheochromocytoma are sustained or paroxysmal hypertension, which occurs in more than 90% of the patients and may be accompanied by alternating postural hypotension. Headache, sweating, palpitations, and pallor are also very common, but flushing is relatively rare. These symptoms last from just a few seconds to hours, and episodes may occur with very irregular frequency. Triggers for these attacks may include diagnostic procedures, anesthesia, drugs, or ingestion of certain foods, such as chocolate (Palek & Eisenhofer, 2004).

Diagnosis of pheochromocytoma depends chiefly on measurement of plasma and urine metanephrines. Measurement of catecholamines by themselves may not yield as accurate a result, because these substances are also secreted by the sympathetic nervous system and are not specific to the adrenal gland. Plasma-free metanephrines are catecholamine metabolites that are produced more constantly and are independent measures of catecholamine release. Fractionated metanephrines will differentiate between normetanephrine and metanephrine. Levels that exceed four times the upper limit of normal confirm the diagnosis. As a second choice, measurement of fractionated urinary metanephrines may be used. For best results, urine should be collected after an episode in which symptoms occurred. To avoid interference with this test, the patient must avoid caffeine, alcohol, acetaminophen, and other drugs (such as tricyclic antidepressants, monomine oxidase inhibitors, and alpha blockers) for three to five days prior to the test. The patient also should not smoke for several hours before the test (Palek & Eisenhofer, 2004).

For nonspecific findings, follow-up tests may include clonidine suppression, in which an oral dose of 0.3 mg/70 kg body weight of clonidine (Catapres®) is administered and levels of norepinephrine are measured in three hours. Failure to suppress levels to either below the upper reference limit or less than 50% of baseline would suggest pheochromocytoma (Palek & Eisenhofer, 2004).

The next step after the metanephrine tests would focus on localization of the tumor. Most tumors are 3 cm or larger, making computerized tomography (CT) or magnetic resonance imaging (MRI) scanning specifically of the adrenal glands and pelvis the most useful initial tool. For maximum specificity, MIBG (scintigraphy after I-131 labeled metaiodobenzylguanidine) may also be performed (Asp, 2002a). For patients with a negative MIBG scan but in whom a high index of suspicion persists, OctreoScan® can be used, although it may be accurate in only 40% to 50% of patients. The newest method for localization is the positron emission tomography (PET) scan, which is an excellent modality for visualization of both primary and metastatic lesions (Palek & Eisenhofer, 2004).

Surgical excision is always the definitive treatment of choice for pheochromocytoma. Pharmacologic blockade prior to surgery is necessary and includes both alpha and beta blockade. Alpha blockade is most commonly accomplished with phenoxybenzamine (Dibenzyline®), and beta blockade is achieved with atenolol (Tenormin®). As hypotension may develop when these agents are administered, postoperative hypotension is minimized by preoperative volume expansion with crystalloids (Asp, 2002a).

If diagnosed early, treatment can result in a cure in 90% of the cases. If left untreated, pheochromocytoma is usually fatal, from arrhythmia, heart attack, or stroke (Palek & Eisenhofer, 2004).

Primary Hyperaldosteronism

Aldosterone is secreted by the adrenal cortex in response to stimulation by angiotensin, ACTH, and elevated potassium levels. Excessive secretion may be found from abnormal adrenal cortex function, usually an adenoma. This condition is referred to as Conn's disease or primary hyperaldosteronism. Secondary hyperaldosteronism is caused by stimulation from the renin-angiotensin system in the kidney. This section focuses on the adrenal disorder of primary hyperaldosteronism.

Excessive secretion of aldosterone from the adrenals may be the cause of approximately 10% of all hypertension cases in the United States (Alexander & Dhuly, 2004). Primary symptoms include hypertension, hypokalemia, and metabolic alkalosis. Excessive fluid volume expansion may occur due to sodium reabsorption but without cardiac or renal failure. Peripheral edema rarely occurs. The oversecretion of aldosterone is usually from a benign, single adrenal adenoma in as many as 90% of the cases. These adenomas are found more commonly in the left adrenal gland but are rarely cancerous. Malignant tumors usually are very large (more than 6 cm) and have generally metastasized by the time of diagnosis (Asp, 2002b). Their metastasis causes excessive renal sodium and water reabsorption and renal secretion of potassium. When chronic, the excessive intravascular volume results in left ventricular hypertrophy and progressive arteriosclerosis with suppressed renin secretion. The resulting hypokalemia causes tetany, paresthesias, skeletal muscle weakness, cardiac arrhythmias, and polyuria (Kumar et al., 2005). The adenomas responsible for this disorder are usually small (less than 2 cm) and are found more in females than males (Alexander & Dhuly). Approximately 30% of the cases of primary hyperaldosteronism derive from idiopathic hyperaldosteronism, which is characterized by bilateral hyperplasia of the adrenal glands. This form is more commonly treated medically (Asp). Additionally, patients with hyperaldosteronism may demonstrate greater left ventricular hypertrophy and myocardial damage than patients with hypertension from other causes (e.g., pheochromocytoma, essential hypertension) (Young, 2003).

The first screening test is a random plasma aldosterone (PA) to plasma renin activity (PRA) ratio. The patient should discontinue use of spironolactone (Aldactone®), an aldosterone antagonist, beta blockers, and eplerenone (Inspra®) two weeks before this test. A ratio greater than 20:1 is suggestive of the disorder, and a ratio greater than 50:1 is virtually diagnostic (Alexander & Dhuly, 2004). Confirmatory tests may include intravenous (IV) isotonic saline loading or a three-day oral salt loading challenge to evaluate whether aldosterone suppression can be achieved. Consideration must be given to the risk of hypokalemia and pulmonary edema in patients with cardiac disease. After the third day of salt loading, a 24-hour urine collection is obtained. Urinary secretion of aldosterone greater than 12 mcg/24 hr is considered strongly indicative of hyperaldosteronism (Young, 2003).

Imaging studies have the common problem of often identifying adrenal "incidentalomas" that are functionally not significant. If imaging is used, thin-sliced spiral CT scanning is preferred. If a single adenoma is found in a patient with the biochemical markers for hyperaldosteronism, especially with a normal appearance to the contralateral gland, no further testing may be needed.

The gold-standard testing for localization of the abnormal gland is adrenal venous sampling. This test is accomplished by inserting catheters into both adrenal veins and the inferior vena cava to directly measure aldosterone output. The ratio between the two glands should be greater than 10:1. However, this procedure is more invasive and risky than the previously discussed tests (Asp, 2002b). Potential complications of adrenal venous sampling include bleeding and adrenal infarction.

Treatment for an isolated adrenal adenoma is usually surgical, with a laparoscopic approach being most favored. Preoperatively, potassium levels should be corrected with an aldosterone antagonist, which should be discontinued postoperatively, and a generous sodium diet allowed, avoiding postoperative hyperkalemia. Eplerenone (Inspra®), a selective aldosterone receptor antagonist (SARA), may be used in place of spironolactone. This relatively new medication is associated with fewer side effects than spironolactone, such as gynecomastia, impotence, and menstrual irregularities. Within a year of surgery, most patients will still be normotensive and potassium levels will be normal (Young, 2003).

Medical management for those patients who have bilateral disease or who are not surgical candidates should consist of aldosterone antagonists (i.e., spironolactone or eplerenone). Alternatively, those intolerant of these drugs can take amiloride hydrochloride (Midamor®) (5 to 15 mg twice daily) to correct hypokalemia with a concomitant antihypertensive, such as a calcium channel blocker or angiotensin-converting enzyme (ACE) inhibitor (Asp, 2002b).

Adrenal Insufficiency

Primary adrenal insufficiency involves destruction or impairment of the adrenal cortex, resulting in inadequate production of cortisol. The primary cause of this damage is an autoimmune adrenalitis called Addison's disease. This relatively uncommon disorder occurs more often in women and typically appears in patients between 30 and 60 years of age. It can also occur as a result of bilateral adrenal hemorrhage, infectious adrenalitis, and, more rarely, bilateral metastatic disease, although the loss of more than 90% of the gland would be necessary before symptoms become evident. Primary adrenal insufficiency results in increased levels of ACTH with an inadequate cortisol response.

Secondary adrenal insufficiency is usually a result of pituitary dysfunction, usually from space-occupying lesions, infiltrative diseases such as sarcoidosis, infectious disease, hemorrhage into a pituitary adenoma (pituitary apoplexy), or severe head trauma. A specific secondary cause is Sheehan's syndrome, which occurs after delivery of a baby due to shock from blood loss (Jones, 2002). In secondary adrenal insufficiency, no increase in ACTH is apparent.

Tertiary adrenal insufficiency is iatrogenic; it results from long-term glucocorticoid use for other causes that result in failure of the adrenals to resume production of cortisol in the absence of exogenous administration. This diagnosis should be considered in anyone who has received more than 20 mg daily of prednisone or glucocorticoid equivalent for more than one month (Jones, 2002).

The primary signs and symptoms associated with adrenal insufficiency are weakness, fatigue, and anorexia with weight loss. Vague abdominal pain, hypoglycemia, and confusion are also common. In patients with primary insufficiency, the increase in ACTH results in hyperpigmentation, or bronzing skin discoloration, which is not seen in secondary insufficiency. Addisonian crisis occurs when a precipitating stressor (such as infection, vomiting, or diarrhea) causes vascular collapse with severe hypotension and shock (Kumar et al., 2005). Laboratory tests will most commonly reveal hyponatremia, hyperkalemia, mild normocytic, normochromic anemia, prerenal azotemia, increased thyroid-stimulating hormone (TSH), and hypercalcemia.

Diagnosis can be made by a low cortisol level (less than 5 mcg/dL) in the setting of the clinical symptoms; a level in excess of 20 mcg/dL rules out the disorder. The physiologic peak production of cortisol occurs in the early morning (between 4 and 8 A.M.). Therefore, testing should occur during that time and should include an ACTH level to assist in differentiating primary from secondary insufficiency. If the patient has low to borderline low levels (i.e., less than 10 mcg/dL), stimulation of adrenal cortisol release can be made by IV or intramuscular (IM) injection of ACTH [cosyntopin (Cortrosyn®)] with measurement of cortisol levels at 30 and 60 minutes after injection. A peak level that is double the baseline level and a minimum level greater than 18 mcg/dL is considered a sufficient response to rule out the disease (Charmandari & Chrousos, 2003).

Treatment of crisis should include the five S's—salt, sugar, steroids, support, and search for precipitating cause (Jones, 2002). Left untreated or insufficiently treated, adrenal crisis is fatal. Large volumes of IV D_5NS with administration of IV dexamethasone (Decadron®) or hydrocortisone (SoluCortef®) are crucial. Hydrocortisone 100 mg may be preferred initially due to its quick response and the dose repeated every eight hours. Dexamethasone 4 mg may also be chosen, because it will not interfere with cortisol measurements. Once the patient is stabilized, the precipitating cause determined and addressed, and the diagnosis confirmed by tests, the dose of steroids may be tapered to a maintenance oral dose in three to four days.

Chronic management will include daily glucocorticoid administration and perhaps mineralocorticoid replacement. If hydrocortisone is used, it has some mineralocorticoid effect, so a separate medication may not be required. The usual dose is 15 to 20 mg in the morning and 5 to 10 mg in the evening. One-half to two-thirds of the total dose is given in the morning, with the remaining being given in the evening; this regimen approximates the normal daily peaks (Arlt, 2004). Longer-acting glucocorticoids, such as prednisone or dexamethasone, should be avoided due to their glucocorticoid ex-

cess signs, such as loss of lean body mass and excessive fat deposition. If a mineralocorticoid is needed to prevent sodium loss, volume depletion, and hyperkalemia, fludrocortisone (Florinef®) as a daily 0.1 mg dose is used (Charmandari & Chrousos, 2003). Mineralocorticoid use is indicated only in case of primary adrenal deficiency, and its use should be monitored by taking blood pressure, sodium, potassium, and serum renin levels. If hypertension develops, a decreased dose should be considered. Some evidence supports the use of DHEA replacement therapy to improve mood and well-being in these patients; trials are currently underway to evaluate this treatment. If used, the dose range for DHEA replacement is 25 to 50 mg every morning (Arlt).

The most important part of chronic management is good patient education. All patients with adrenal insufficiency should wear a Medic-Alert® bracelet. Patients should also know the signs of insufficiency and how to stress-dose for illness or injury. Since the body is incapable of mounting an appropriate stress response with this condition, the patient should know how to compensate for this failure. Stress doses for mild to moderate stressors, such as infections, would be to double or triple the maintenance dose for three days, then taper back down to the usual maintenance doses. Major stressors, such as surgery or severe infections, may require IV doses of 50 to 100 mg of hydrocortisone every eight hours, tapering by half the day after surgery or as the patient stabilizes, and then transitioning back to oral doses over several days. Patients should keep a vial of 100 mg injectable hydrocortisone with instructions in how to administer as an emergency measure (Jones, 2002).

Cushing's Syndrome

The majority (more than 70%) of patients with Cushing's syndrome have Cushing's disease, a pituitary gland defect in which increased ACTH production results in excessive cortisol production. However, this syndrome is seen often enough from other causes to warrant discussion in this section. Other causes of Cushing's syndrome include ectopic ACTH production, usually from oat cell tumors of the lung and pheochromocytomas. Twenty percent of patients will have an actual adrenal adenoma producing the excess cortisol; the syndrome may also be caused by exogenous steroid administration for other disease states, such as asthma and chronic obstructive pulmonary disease (Samuels, 2002).

The presenting signs of Cushing's syndrome are obesity, specifically in the abdominal or truncal area, and supraclavicular fat pads and dorsocervical fat pads, also called a "buffalo" or "dowager's" hump. Another characteristic is the rounding of the face ("moon" face). This can often be best noted by examining photos of the patient from several years back for comparison. Purplish striae on the abdomen or breasts, easy bruising, acne, hirsutism, wasting of the extremities, and a pendulous abdomen are also noted (Kumar et al., 2005).

Clinical symptoms will include hypertension, atherosclerosis, osteopenia or fractures, and abnormal glucose tolerance or outright diabetes. Although increased ACTH levels from the pituitary cause the hypercortisolism, the levels are rarely high enough to cause the bronzing of the skin noted in hypoadrenalism. Patients who do present with this symptom usually have ectopic secretion from a tumor, which carries a particularly grim prognosis. This variation is seen more in men, although 80% of all patients with Cushing's disease are women. Patients with Cushing's disease have a markedly higher mortality rate, usually from cardiovascular disease or infections (Samuels, 2002). Left untreated, the disease is associated with a 50% mortality rate at five years. Patients can also have waxing and waning periods of hypercortisolemia, which means the clinician needs to have a high index of suspicion and test early (Morris & Grossman, 2002).

The gold-standard screening test is the 24-hour urine free cortisol level, ideally using liquid chromatography-mass spectroscopy, which can screen out interfering substances that may skew the results. Although loss of circadian rhythm in production of cortisol occurs in Cushing's disease, serum cortisol levels can be obtained. It is advised to draw the sample during the normal physiologic peak of production between 8 and 10 A.M. and to include ACTH levels to distinguish between pituitary and adrenal disease. An ACTH of less than 10 pg/mL indicates a more likely adrenal or ACTH-independent cause; an ACTH greater than 15 pg/mL is usually a pituitary or ACTH-dependent cause.

Dexamethasone suppression tests, in which a dose of dexamethasone is administered—either the 1 mg overnight dexamethasone suppression test (DST) or the two-day DST using low-dose dexamethasone—may be used to evaluate appropriate suppression of cortisol production. Both tests have their drawbacks, which should be considered when deciding on a method (Nieman, 2004). Both are based on the assumption that exogenous administration of dexamethasone will suppress the hypothalamic-pituitary axis while not interfering with measurements of endogenous cortisol. Simultaneous measurement of dexamethasone levels should be done to confirm adequate dosing of dexamethasone. CRH testing has also been used to distinguish ACTH-independent from ACTH-dependent disease (Morris & Grossman, 2002).

The next step is to determine the site of the defect. If the previous tests have indicated an ACTH-independent source, MRI or CT scanning of the adrenal glands may localize the tumor. A unilateral mass will usually be seen. Bilateral gland hyperplasia with possible nodules is more commonly seen with

ACTH-dependent (pituitary) causes. It is more difficult to distinguish between ectopic ACTH-producing tumors and pituitary tumors. In centers with experienced interventional radiologists, inferior petrosal sinus samplings (IPSS) can measure ACTH levels from the pituitary gland. Since ectopic ACTH production is usually from the lung or thymic region, chest CT or MRI can be used to identify these lesions (Nieman, 2004).

Treatment for Cushing's syndrome entails resection of the adenoma, either through transphenoidal resection of the pituitary adenoma or with radiation therapy if the patient is not a surgical candidate. This therapy will likely result in panhypopituitarism, requiring multiple hormonal replacements. Gammaknife radiosurgery has been used with some success as a second-line choice for patients with Cushing's disease (Morris & Grossman, 2002). Resection of the adrenal adenoma, either unilateral or bilateral, using a laparoscopic approach is the procedure of choice for adrenal adenomas. Ectopic ACTH sources can be resected or, if not located, a bilateral adrenalectomy can be performed. Postoperative management for all of these patients will require steroid replacement, as with adrenal insufficiency, at stress doses with a gradual taper to physiologic doses for maintenance, if indicated (Nieman, 2004).

Medical management can be considered for ectopic ACTH-producing patients or failed surgical patients. **Box 40-1** lists drug therapies.

Box 40-1

Pharmacological Therapies for Ectopic ACTH-Producing Patients

Ketoconazole (Nizoral®)
Aminoglutethamide (Cytadren®)
Mitotane (Lysodren®)
Etomidate (Amidate®)
5-HT$_3$ antagonists
dopamine agonists
Octreotide (Somatostatin®)
Sodium valproate (Depacon®)
Mifepristone (Mifeprex®)

Source: Aniszewski, Young, Thompson, Grant, & van Heerden, 2001.

PATIENT OUTCOMES

Nurses can help ensure the obtainment of optimal patient outcomes such as those listed in **Box 40-2** through the use of evidence-based interventions for patients with adrenal disorders.

SUMMARY

The adrenal gland secretes essential hormones for life. Critical care nurses can enhance patient outcomes by assessing and monitoring patients' adrenal function through identification of alterations. Vigilant monitoring of patients in adrenal crisis is the responsibility of critical care nurses.

Box 40-2

Optimal Patient Outcomes

- Mean arterial pressure within expected range
- Verbalizes comfort
- Absence of postural hypotension
- Electrolytes and acid-base balance within expected range
- Verbalizes knowledge of diagnostic tests
- Blood sugar within expected range
- Verbalizes chronic management strategies of adrenal disorders

CASE STUDY

A 61-year-old female was admitted to the ICU with chest pain and ECG changes consistent with an inferior wall MI (ST-segment elevation in leads 2, 3, and aVF, plus elevated troponin levels). She had been to her primary care physician twice in the past few weeks with flu-like symptoms. Her symptoms were attributed to an upper respiratory infection rather than the flu. Her past medical history is significant for GI bleeding, adrenal insufficiency, one-pack-per-day tobacco smoking, and depression. Her current medications include glucocorticoids and medication for depression. She is five feet two inches tall and weighs 168 pounds. She works in a day-care center with children younger than age 5.

In the ICU, her chest pain was rated 5/10. The patient was started on oxygen given by nasal cannula at 3 L/min, a nitroglycerine infusion at 10 mcg/min, and morphine 4 mg IV. Her IV was 0.9% normal saline at KVO. Her admitting vital signs were B/P 126/52, HR 110, and RR 24, and she was afebrile. Within two hours of admission, vital signs were B/P 80/42, HR 110, and RR 26. She was diaphoretic, was cold and clammy, and had two bouts of nausea and vomiting but her chest pain had resolved. Her lab data were significant for hyponatremia (122 mEq/L) and hyperkalemia (5.5 mEq/L).

CRITICAL THINKING QUESTIONS

1. What symptoms were associated with adrenal insufficiency in this case?
2. Which management strategies would you anticipate for this patient given a diagnosis of adrenal insufficiency?
3. Which presenting symptoms might divert the ICU nurse from focusing on the patient's adrenal insufficiency?
4. Which disciplines should be consulted to work with this client?
5. How will you implement your role as a facilitator of learning for this patient?
6. Use the form to write up a plan of care for one patient with an adrenal disorder in the clinical setting.
7. Rate the patient as a level 1, 3, or 5 on each characteristic. Identify the level of nurse characteristics needed in the care of this patient.

Using the Synergy Model to Develop a Plan of Care

	Patient Characteristics	Level (1, 3, 5)	Subjective and Objective Data	Evidence-based Interventions	Outcomes
SYNERGY MODEL	Resiliency				
	Vulnerability				
	Stability				
	Complexity				
	Resource availability				
	Participation in care				
	Participation in decision making				
	Predictability				

Online Resources

Your Adrenal Glands: www.endocrineweb.com/adrenal.html

National Adrenal Disease Foundation: www.medhelp.org/nadf

Addison's Disease: www.nkddk.nih.gov/health/endo/pubs/addison/addison.htm

The Addison & Cushing International Federation: www.nvacp.nl/page.php?main=5

Pituitary Network Association: www.pituitary.org/disorders/cushings_disease.aspx

REFERENCES

Alexander, E., & Dhuly, R. (2004). Aldosterone excess. Retrieved August 23, 2005, from www.Endotext.org

Aniszewski, J. P., Young, W. F., Thompson, G. B., Grant, C. S., & van Heerden, J. A. (2001). Cushing syndrome due to ectopic adrenocorticotropic hormone secretion. *World Journal of Surgery, 25*(7), 934–940.

Arlt, W. (2004). Management of adrenal insufficiency. *The Endocrine Society's 86th Annual Meeting meet-the-professor handouts* (pp. 171–175). New Orleans, LA: The Endocrine Society.

Asp, A. (2002a). Pheochromocytoma. In M. McDermott (Ed.), *Endocrine secrets* (3rd ed., pp. 247–251). Philadelphia: Hanley & Belfus.

Asp, A. (2002b). Primary aldosteronism. In M. McDermott (Ed.), *Endocrine secrets* (3rd ed., pp. 241–246). Philadelphia: Hanley & Belfus.

Charmandari, E., & Chrousos, G. (2003). Adrenal insufficiency. Retrieved August 26, 2006, from www.Endotext.org

Jones, R. (2002). Adrenal insufficiency. In M. McDermott (Ed.), *Endocrine secrets* (3rd ed., pp. 255–260). Philadelphia: Hanley & Belfus.

Kumar, V., Abbas, A., & Nelson, F. (2005). *Robbins and Cotran pathologic basis of disease* (7th ed.). Philadelphia: Elsevier Saunders.

Morris, D., & Grossman, A. (2002). Cushing's syndrome. Retrieved August 26, 2005, from www.Endotext.org

Nieman, L. (2004). Diagnosis and management of Cushing's syndrome. *The Endocrine Society's 86th Annual Meeting meet-the-professor handouts* (pp. 73–78). New Orleans, LA: The Endocrine Society.

Palek, K., & Eisenhofer, G. (2004). Pheochromocytoma. *The Endocrine Society's 86th Annual Meeting meet-the-professor handouts* (pp. 279–286). New Orleans, LA: The Endocrine Society.

Samuels, M. (2002). Cushing's syndrome. In M. McDermott (Ed.), *Endocrine secrets* (3rd ed., pp. 199–207). Philadelphia: Hanley & Belfus.

Young, W. (2003). Primary aldosteronism: Update on diagnosis and treatment. *Clinical Endocrinology Update 2003 Syllabus* (pp. 131–137). Chevy Chase, MD: The Endocrine Society Press.

CHAPTER 41

Pituitary Disorders

Christopher A. Vreeland

LEARNING OBJECTIVES

Upon completion of this chapter, the reader will be able to:

1. Identify structures of the pituitary gland.

2. Discuss the physiology of the pituitary gland.

3. Identify and discuss the major pituitary hormones, their feedback pathways, and their target organs.

4. Identify signs and symptoms of common pituitary disorders.

5. Recognize and implement appropriate nursing interventions.

6. List optimal outcomes that may be achieved through evidence-based management of the patient with a pituitary disorder.

A thorough understanding of the anatomy and physiology of the pituitary gland is essential to recognize and treat signs and symptoms of the most common pituitary disorders. The hormones produced by the pituitary are necessary for the normal function of all humans. Problems involving the pituitary are frequently difficult to identify. They are very often attributed to other systems, environmental situations, or medical problems. Finally, once one has deciphered the clues and decided the patient has a pituitary disorder, it will be up to the intensive care unit (ICU) nurse to administer proper care.

ANATOMY AND PHYSIOLOGY

The pituitary gland is generally about the size of a pea and sits in a space that is well protected on all sides by bone. This compartment, or sella turcica, is located in the skull between the eyes and well back toward the middle of the brain. It is not actually in direct contact with the brain. It has a small stem, or infundibular stalk, that serves as the link between the hypothalamus, a structure within the brain, and both lobes of the pituitary gland.

The pituitary gland has two parts, or lobes, that perform vastly different functions. The anterior lobe, or adenohypophysis, is the larger of the two lobes. The posterior lobe, or the neurohypophysis, is just behind the adenohypophysis and distributes its hormones through nervelike cells. The anterior portion secretes many of the hormones, sometimes called trophic factors, which regulate day-to-day endocrine function. The posterior lobe stores and ultimately distributes two hormones, oxytocin and antidiuretic hormone (ADH).

The connection of the pituitary gland to the brain is integral to its normal function. The hypothalamus is where much of the stimulus for secretion of pituitary hormone originates. In the case of the anterior pituitary, the hypothalamus secretes releasing factors that find their way downward indirectly. Through a series of small vessels that converge to form a plexus or network, secretory releasing factors collect and then drain down a network of vessels within the infundibular stalk until they reach the anterior pituitary. Once these releasing factors are within the adenohypophysis, they stimulate cells within a secondary plexus to secrete hormones. The pituitary hormone produced in this way empties into this plexus, which ultimately drains into anterohypophyseal veins. From there, hormones are delivered to their target organs.

The secretory mechanism of the posterior pituitary is, however, remarkably different. The neurohypophysis releases fewer hormones and distributes them in a completely different fashion. The two principal hormones released by the posterior pituitary are made outside the gland itself. Cells of the supraoptic nucleus (part of the hypothalamus) synthesize ADH. Oxytocin is made in another section of the hypothalamus, the paraventricular nucleus (Robertson, 2001). Both hormones are transported down to the posterior pituitary, where they are stored. The hypothalamus uses the same neurosecretory cells to stimulate the release of the appropriate hormone.

The anterior pituitary produces more separate hormones and thus exerts greater influence on daily function. Six major hormones are produced: growth hormone (GH), sometimes termed somatotropin; adrenocorticotropic hormone (ACTH), also called corticotrophin; thyroid-stimulating hormone (TSH) or thyrotropin; follicle-stimulating hormone (FSH); luteinizing hormone (LH); and prolactin (PRL) or lactogenic hormone (Snyder, 2001). Two of these products—namely, GH and PRL—are not trophic hormones. That is, they do not directly control the functioning of a specific target organ (Snyder). The other four hormones affect the operation of major endocrine systems in the body.

The trophic hormones of the anterior pituitary have varied effects on the function of the endocrine system as a whole. TSH stimulates the thyroid to synthesize hormones of the thyroid gland and helps to maintain blood flow to the gland. ACTH regulates the production and secretion of adrenal hormones. It, too, helps regulate blood flow to the organ. FSH has slightly different roles in men and women. In men, the target organs are the testes, where FSH regulates the rate of spermatogenesis and causes production of testosterone to increase. In women, FSH affects the ovaries by facilitating the growth of follicles and stimulates synthesis of estrogen and progesterone. LH also acts in the testes to promote synthesis and secretion of testosterone in men. In women, LH is essential for ovulation and the formation of the corpus luteum from a ruptured follicle. FSH is required in men and women for these processes to occur (Molitch, 2001).

As mentioned earlier, PRL and GH are the only two nontrophic hormones secreted by the anterior pituitary (Molitch, 2001). PRL plays a primary role in breast development and lactation. First, it acts in the presence of estrogen to prepare the breast for lactation after the birth of an infant. Then, it promotes lactation both on delivery and when sucking by the baby begins. This hormone is found in males in low levels, but its specific function is unknown. It is the most promi-

nent product of most pituitary tumors in men or women (Molitch).

GH is unique in that it has no specific target organ. Its secretion is controlled by hepatic and hypothalamic releasing factors. Further, differences among races and gender are apparent as to how GH is secreted. Factors such as stress, fitness level, sleep habits, nutritional status, and other hormones (e.g., thyroid hormone, insulin, androgens, and steroids) influence the release of GH (Molitch, 2001). This hormone's effects on the body are as unique as its secretory patterns. First, it acts directly on bone and cartilage to cause growth in both structures. In addition, it promotes an increased rate of protein synthesis. This process, combined with increased RNA transcription within cells due to the activity of GH, causes increased rates of overall growth (Snyder, 2001). Further effects of GH include reduction of sodium and potassium excretion, increased absorption of calcium in the gastrointestinal tract, and catabolism of stored fat cells, sometimes causing hyperglycemia as a result.

The posterior pituitary releases two important hormones: ADH and oxytocin. Recall that both hormones are synthesized outside the pituitary gland. They are transported to the neurohypophysis through neurosecretory cells from the supraoptic nucleus and paraventricular nucleus. Release from storage occurs upon appropriate stimulation by the hypothalamus.

The target organs for ADH are the kidneys. This hormone causes the distal tubules and collecting ducts to be more permeable to water, so it promotes water reabsorption. If ADH is absent, these structures are almost completely impermeable to water and greater quantities of dilute urine are produced. Ethyl alcohol and caffeine, for example, are weak inhibitors of ADH secretion (Molitch, 2001). Consumption of these substances will result in short-term diuresis. The normal secretion of ADH, however, is controlled primarily by the hypothalamus. The hypothalamus monitors both the osmolarity of blood plasma and the circulating vascular volume to regulate release of ADH (Robertson, 2001). Special receptors adapted to these specific functions stimulate the hypothalamus when changes in either index are detected.

Oxytocin affects the quality of contraction in smooth muscle throughout the body. It is most notable for its effects on the pregnant uterus. Oxytocin is secreted in large quantities as labor progresses, causing expulsion of the fetus from the uterus at the appropriate time. It also causes the cells of the alveoli in the nipple to contract, forcing milk into the ducts and lacteal openings to the nipple (Molitch, 2001).

Secretion of hormones from both parts of the pituitary can be influenced by many factors. Environmental stimuli and diurnal patterns play a role in secretion of pituitary hormones.

As noted earlier, some drugs can change the secretion pattern for PRL. Some speculate that oxytocin secretion can be triggered by the physical stimulation of copulation. In fact, it is known that certain hypothalamic and pituitary hormones are secreted cyclically. Secretion of GHs and PRL is greatest just after falling asleep. TSH secretion reaches its peak between the hours of 8 P.M. and midnight. ACTH secretion rises to its maximum between the hours of 2 A.M. and 4 P.M., resulting in maximal cortisol levels at 8 A.M. This is why cortisol levels are most useful for evaluating adrenal function when they are drawn at, or very near, 8 A.M. Evidence of loss of this pattern of secretion can be an important clue to possible pituitary dysfunction or disease (Robertson, 2001).

DISORDERS OF THE PITUITARY

The presentation and diagnosis of pituitary disorders are both subtle and demanding. The symptoms of these disorders can mimic any of a number of common somatic complaints. Correct diagnosis is aided greatly by the vigilant care provider and confirmed with timely magnetic resonance imaging (MRI) of the brain and pituitary gland (National Institutes of Health [NIH], 2004). Proper nursing care can make the course of treatment shorter and much more comfortable for the patient.

The most prevalent pituitary pathology is the presence of an adenoma. Roughly 15% of all tumors found in the skull are those of the pituitary gland. The incidence of pituitary tumors is about 1 in 10,000 people, but these tumors are very rarely malignant (NIH, 2004). Usually, the tumor will secrete pituitary hormones or take up valuable space in the sella turcica, or both conditions may exist. Other causes for pituitary tumors include craniopharyngioma, primary pituitary carcinoma, meningioma, and metastatic carcinoma. By far, the most common cause in clinical practice is the benign pituitary adenoma that secretes one of a few of the pituitary hormones (Vance, 2004). Only 10% to 20% of pituitary adenomas do not produce some type of pituitary hormone. Some tumors produce PRL (the most prevalent clinical presentation), causing galactorrhea (excessive flow of milk during lactation) or gonadal dysfunction (Robertson, 2001). Others produce ACTH (probably the second-most prevalent clinical presentation), which results in Cushing's disease. Still others may produce GH, which can cause gigantism or acromegaly.

Two problems associated with pituitary disease require intervention: hypopituitarism and hyperpituitarism. Both conditions, regardless of their underlying cause, will have detectable physical findings indicating dysfunction of the pituitary gland or a target organ as a result of a congenital or acquired defect (Robertson, 2001). Hypopituitarism may occur as a single hormone deficiency, combination hormone deficiency, or total hormone deficiency. Naturally occurring pathology is generally insidious and is directly related to the size and nature of the cause. Panhypopituitarism refers to a complete failure of pituitary function. More often, this condition is a result of empty-sella syndrome, head trauma, or surgical removal of all or a significant portion of the pituitary gland (Robertson). Evaluation and diagnosis are made through thorough physical exam and measurement of hormone levels. Physical findings include fine wrinkling of the face, loss of sexual function and libido in men, premature aging, loss of axillary and pubic hair, breast and genital atrophy, and amenorrhea in premenopausal women. If panhypopituitarism occurs before puberty, short stature for age will be seen (Geffner, 2002). Reduced visual acuity without obvious concomitant cause or visual field impairment on exam of the cardinal fields of gaze may signal expansion of a pituitary mass (Vance, 2004).

Singular deficiency of any of the primary pituitary hormones has clearly defined signs and symptoms. PRL deficiency is manifested as failure to lactate in the postpartum phase of childbirth. It is most prevalent in Sheehan's syndrome (postpartum pituitary hemorrhage and necrosis), which occurs during the delivery process. Other clinically relevant findings include increased intracranial pressure, headache, visual deficits, stiff neck, papilledema, and convulsions (Snyder, 2001).

Gonadotropin deficiency, or hypogonadism, is the most common pituitary problem in adults. It is caused most often by tumors—namely, craniopharyngiomas, a congenital defect, or certain adenomas. Thyrotropin deficit, sometimes referred to as secondary hypothyroidism, is either hypothalamic or purely pituitary in nature. Isolated low levels of TSH, and often of other pituitary hormones, help to differentiate this disorder from primary hypothyroidism (Vance, 2004).

ACTH deficiency is the most serious problem related to pituitary dysfunction. It rarely occurs in an isolated fashion, which aids in its distinction from primary adrenal failure. Symptoms include nausea, vomiting, hyperthermia, poor response to any kind of stress, and, eventually, total collapse.

Low GH is seen in adults, but its most profound effects are most evident in children. The result of GH deficit is short stature for age, delayed sexual characteristics, normal to exceptional mentality and intellect, and dry, wrinkled skin that appears to be premature aging (Snyder, 2001).

Hyperpituitarism, in contrast to deficiency of hormone, is the overproduction of a pituitary product. It almost always involves only a single hormone. Excess pituitary hormone can result from decreased production of a target gland. In most cases, a pituitary adenoma is present and secretes GH, PRL, or ACTH inappropriately. Overproduction of GH before onset of puberty causes a condition called gigantism, in which the patient grows symmetrically to very large proportions (i.e., up to eight to nine feet tall). This person may be unusually strong, but osteoporosis and muscle weakness are evident in later stages. After puberty, the disorder is termed acromegaly. Most often, somatotrophic adenomas are responsible for acromegaly. Clinical signs and symptoms develop insidiously over years, with hypopituitarism eventually occurring if the tumor is undiscovered and continues to grow. The patient may notice a progressive increase in ring and shoe sizes over the years. Frontal and orbital ridges become more prominent as GH secretion rises. Prognathism, or projection of the mandible, occurs and a characteristic facial appearance emerges.

Inappropriately high levels of PRL result from a PRL-secreting adenoma. In women, elevated PRL can cause galactorrhea, amenorrhea, decreased libido, and, in some cases, hirsuitism with lower estrogens. Men with this tumor will have PRL-induced hypogonadism and a space-occupying lesion of the pituitary (Snyder, 2001). In either case, the lesion is diagnosed through MRI, PRL levels, visual field exam, and thorough history. Care must be taken to evaluate the method used to measure actual PRL levels, because dilution of the specimen can greatly affect the accuracy of the diagnosis (Vance, 2004).

Elevated production of ACTH is termed Cushing's disease. The overproduction of ACTH stimulates excess production of cortisol, resulting in a disorder called Cushing's syndrome. Clinical signs of Cushing's syndrome include easy bruising, thin arms and legs with protuberant abdomen, "buffalo hump" (supraclavicular fat pad), purple striae usually on the abdomen, rounded "moonlike" appearance of the face, unexplained weight gain, and, in women, increased body and facial hair. The diagnosis of this syndrome is made through careful physical examination combined with appropriate laboratory evaluation (ACTH, morning cortisol, 24-hour urine collection for free cortisol) and MRI of the pituitary and brain.

Disorders involving pathology based in the posterior pituitary are far rarer than those of the adenohypophysis. The two clinically relevant disorders are diabetes insipidus (DI) and syndrome of inappropriate antidiuretic hormone (SIADH) secretion. The cause for both disorders usually involves a pathologic process exclusive of the pituitary gland itself. Patients with either of these conditions may be admitted to the ICU for management.

Diabetes insipidus (DI) is the term used to describe a deficiency of ADH release from the neurohypophysis. A lack of ADH results in poor renal reabsorption of water, which in turn leads to production of large amounts of dilute, low-osmolarity urine (Robertson, 2001). Clinical features of DI include polyuria and excessive thirst with accompanying polydipsia. Onset of symptoms is sudden, and urine output can be profound, reaching ten liters or more in a 24-hour period. Laboratory evidence for this syndrome includes hypernatremia and serum hyperosmolarity. Urine specific gravity is low (less than 1.005), and urine osmolality is usually less than 200 mOsm/kg. Underlying causes of DI include severe head trauma, carcinoma, meningitis, infiltrative tuberculosis, abscesses, sarcoidosis, surgical or radiological hypophysectomy or injury, and idiopathic occurrence. Treatment is with ADH administered most often through nasal spray used once daily. Oral agents, such as chlorpropamide (Diabinese®), carbamazepine (Tegretol®), clofibrate (Atromid-S®), thiazide diuretics, and indomethacin (Indocin®), are also available but are less efficacious for most patients (Robertson, 2001).

Syndrome of inappropriate ADH secretion (SIADH) is the excessive release of ADH despite plasma osmolarity or existing volume deficit. The normal inhibition of ADH by the posterior pituitary is absent, resulting in excessive reabsorption of water in the kidneys. Fluid overload, hyponatremia, and hemodilution are the measurable effects of SIADH. Causes of SIADH may include non-endocrine tumors impinging upon posterior pituitary control centers, ADH-secreting tumors, various carcinomas and malignant conditions, central nervous system trauma (e.g., subdural hematoma), stress, pain, and severe hypovolemia. Treatment includes fluid restriction, diuretics, continued assessment of sodium balance and evidence of heart failure, and treatment of any underlying cause of the syndrome. SIADH is discussed in more detail in Chapter 47.

MANAGEMENT OF PITUITARY DISORDERS

Treatment for pituitary tumors depends largely on their function, size, and degree of involvement with adjacent structures. For instance, a prolactinoma of moderate size is treated with medications initially, providing it is relatively small and confined to the sella. A larger lesion, which is diffusely involved in adjacent tissue, requires debulking with the "gamma knife." This procedure uses directed radiation to help shrink or eliminate a diffuse, large pituitary tumor. A fast-growing adenoma that compromises visual function or causes apoplexy is appropriately resected transphenoidally. Radiosurgery is used with relatively stable, slower-growing tumors (Sheehan, Kondziolka, Flickinger, & Lunsford, 2003). In any case, the primary concern is patient safety and comfort.

Nursing considerations for this type of patient relate to the immediate postoperative period. Prior to surgery, the patient is evaluated by a collaborative team consisting of the primary care physician, an endocrinologist, and the neurosurgeon (Vance, 2004). Once the diagnosis is made, surgery is swiftly planned and executed. It is during the immediate postoperative period that effective nursing care is crucial. As with any postoperative patient, frank bleeding, fever, intractable vomiting, or malignant hyperthermia must be reported to the physician and appropriate care must be initiated without delay. This patient should be monitored for copious urinary output for the first 36 to 48 hours after surgery, because it could signal DI. Furthermore, the nurse should immediately begin replacement of corticosteroids to prevent the onset of adrenal crisis. Thyroid and gonadal hormone replacement may begin in this period but are not as critical as adrenal hormone. The patient must be monitored for any changes in visual field or extraocular movements, because either could signal potentially detrimental complications of surgery. Evaluation of laboratory data postoperatively—most notably, the complete blood count and a comprehensive metabolic profile—can identify infection, blood loss, volume depletion/overload, and renal failure before signs or symptoms may become clinically evident.

The ICU nurse should also begin planning for patient discharge. The patient is discharged on corticosteroid replacement, pain medication, and any adjunctive treatment for surgical complications (e.g., swelling, wound drainage, antiembolism devices). Evaluation by an endocrinologist should occur two to four weeks after surgery or sooner if DI becomes evident. At this visit, the endocrinologist evaluates pituitary function, examines the patient for signs and symptoms of postoperative problems, and prescribes appropriate hormone replacement, which will be taken for life (Vance, 2004).

PATIENT OUTCOMES

Nurses can help ensure the obtainment of optimal patient outcomes such as those listed in **Box 41-1** through the use of evidence-based interventions for patients with pituitary disorders.

SUMMARY

Pituitary disorders can be primary (hyposecretion or hypersecretion) or secondary (hypothalamic dysfunction or target cell hyporesponsiveness). Signs and symptoms can vary depending on the specific disorder, the affected region of the pituitary involved, and hormones affected. Critical care nurses face the challenge of understanding the pituitary gland, hormones secreted, hormone replacement therapy, and surgical interventions.

Box 41-1
Optimal Patient Outcomes

- Intake and output balanced
- Serum sodium and potassium within expected range
- Verbalizes knowledge of disease process
- Verbalizes knowledge of symptoms
- Copes with body image changes
- Verbalizes knowledge of treatment modalities
- Complies with water restriction when diagnosed with SIADH

CASE STUDY

D.P. was admitted to the ICU from the general surgical floor. He underwent a lung resection for bronchogenic carcinoma. Since the loss of his wife of 37 years earlier this year, he has had a history of episodes of agitation for which he was receiving haloperidol (Haldol®).

Due to postoperative pain and nausea for which he was medicated, D.P. refused to cooperate with pulmonary toileting procedures; he did not use the incentive spirometer, spent minimal time out of bed ambulating, and did not deep breathe. Earlier in the day, he complained of a headache, for which he received 650 mg of acetaminophen (Tylenol®). His primary nurse found him restless and confused. Vital signs at that time were B/P 136/72, HR 114, RR 28, temp 99 °F, and SpO$_2$ 87% on room air. D.P. was transferred to the ICU with acute respiratory failure, possibly due to pneumonia.

On admission, D.P. was stuporous. Chest radiograph on admission to the ICU confirmed the diagnosis of pneumonia. Significant lab data included Na 119 mEq/L, K 3.2 mEq/L, serum osmolality 240 mOsm/kg, and urinary sodium 42 mEq/L. A diagnosis of SIADH was made. D.P. was started on hypertonic (3%) saline to raise his sodium levels 0.5 to 1 mEq/hr with a maximum of 10 to 12 mEq in the first 24 hours. He was placed on fluid restriction not to exceed 800 mL in 24 hours. He was also given furosemide (Lasix®) and started on demeclocycline (Declomycin®) 150 mg by nasogastric tube QID.

D.P.'s serum sodium normalized over the next few days without incident, and he was transferred back to the general unit.

CRITICAL THINKING QUESTIONS

1. Which factors put D.P. at risk for the development of SIADH?
2. Explain the rationale for fluid restriction, use of hypertonic saline, and diuretics in this scenario.
3. When cognitively appropriate, what type of diet is appropriate for D.P.?
4. How would you implement your role as a facilitator of learning for this patient?
5. Which disciplines should be consulted to work with this client?
6. Write a case example from the clinical setting highlighting one patient characteristic of a patient with a pituitary disorder. Explain how the characteristic was observed through subjective and objective data.
7. Use the form to write up a plan of care for one client with a condition involving the pituitary gland in the clinical setting. Rate the patient as a level 1, 3, or 5 on each characteristic. Identify the level of nurse characteristics needed in the care of this patient.
8. Take one patient outcome and list evidence-based interventions for this patient.

Using the Synergy Model to Develop a Plan of Care

Patient Characteristics	Level (1, 3, 5)	Subjective and Objective Data	Evidence-based Interventions	Outcomes
Resiliency				
Vulnerability				
Stability				
Complexity				
Resource availability				
Participation in care				
Participation in decision making				
Predictability				

Online Resources

Causes of Hyponatremia: http://patients.uptodate.com/topic.asp?file=fldlytes/7034&title=Adrenal+insufficiency

Endocrine Surgeon: www.endocrinesurgeon.co.uk/pituitary/pituitary8.html

Endocrinology Health Guide, The Pituitary Gland: www.umm.edu/endocrin/pitgland.htm

Pituitary Foundation: www.pituitary.org.uk

Pituitary Gland: health.howstuffworks.com/adam-200093.htm

REFERENCES

Geffner, M. E. (2002). Hypopituitarism in childhood. Retrieved August 28, 2005, from www.medscape.com/viewarticle/438527

Molitch, M. E. (2001). Neuroendocrinology. In D. Felig & L. A. Frohman (Eds.), *Endocrinology and metabolism* (4th ed., pp. 109–172). New York: McGraw-Hill.

National Institutes of Health. (2004). Medical encyclopedia: Pituitary tumor. Retrieved August 14, 2005, from www.nlm.nih.gov/medlineplus/ency/article000704.htm

Robertson, G. L. (2001). Posterior pituitary. In D. Felig & L. A. Frohman (Eds.), *Endocrinology and metabolism* (4th ed., pp. 217–258). New York: McGraw-Hill.

Sheehan, J. P., Kondziolka, D., Flickinger, J., & Lunsford, L. D. (2003). Radiosurgery for nonfunctioning pituitary adenoma. Retrieved August 28, 2005, from www.medscape.com/viewarticle/456136

Snyder, P. J. (2001). Diseases of the anterior pituitary. In D. Felig & L. A. Frohman (Eds.), *Endocrinology and metabolism* (4th ed., pp. 173–216). New York: McGraw-Hill.

Vance, M. L. (2004). Treatment of patients with a pituitary adenoma: One clinician's experience. Retrieved August 28, 2005, from www.medscape.com/viewarticle/474897

CHAPTER 42

Diabetic Emergencies

Sarah Freeman

LEARNING OBJECTIVES

At the end of this chapter, the reader will be able to:

1. Describe the etiology of hypoglycemia and hyperglycemia.

2. Explain the alterations in fluid and electrolytes that occur with diabetic emergencies.

3. Differentiate between the hypoglycemic emergencies, DKA, and HHS.

4. Discuss the clinical judgment required in the medical and nursing management of DKA and HHS.

5. Delineate appropriate patient and family teaching strategies for the acutely ill diabetic patient.

6. Recognize resources available to the nursing and healthcare community to further assist in care and education of the diabetic patient and the family.

7. List optimal outcomes that may be achieved through evidence-based management of the acutely ill diabetic patient.

Diabetes mellitus (DM) is one of the most prevalent chronic diseases, with an estimated 17 million persons or about 6% of the population being affected. Its economic impact is estimated at more than $130 billion, and the disease accounts for approximately 10% of total U.S. healthcare expenditures (American Diabetes Association [ADA], 2005a). DM is actually a clinical syndrome or group of metabolic disorders that is characterized by an absolute or relative deficiency of insulin, all leading to hyperglycemia. **Table 42-1** describes the different types of diabetes. Patient self-management along with aggressive medical management is required to prevent complications. If diabetes is not well controlled, it can not only cause long-term complications (**Table 42-2**), but can also present as a medical emergency. Patients with these emergencies (**Table 42-3**) usually present in the Emergency Department (ED) and require hospitalization and admission to an intensive care unit (ICU).

PATHOPHYSIOLOGY

Critically ill patients can present with either Type 1 or Type 2 diabetes. The disease occurs when an increase of glucose in the blood is present and a deficiency of insulin production by the beta cells in the pancreas occurs. The cells need insulin so that they can take in glucose as a source of energy. Without glucose, the cells use fats and proteins as energy sources, initiating a cascade of events that can result in diabetic emergencies of diabetic ketoacidosis (DKA) and hyperosmolar hyperglycemic states (HHS).

Type 1 diabetes is associated with three factors: (1) destruction of pancreatic beta cells by an autoimmune process, (2) genetically susceptible individuals, and (3) an environmental trigger such as a virus (coxsackie B4, retroviruses, rubella, cytomegalovirus, Epstein-Barr), dietary factors (cow's milk has been implicated), or stress. The combination of these three factors seems to underlie the development of Type 1 diabetes (ADA, 2004).

Type 2 diabetes occurs due to insulin resistance and is thought to be related to both genetics and environmental factors. Specifically, the predisposition for Type 2 diabetes is stronger than that for Type 1 disease, and environmental factors such as overeating, obesity, inactivity, malnutrition in utero, age, and ethnicity play a role in the development of Type 2 diabetes. Insulin resistance has now been classified as a syndrome—

TABLE 42-1 Types of Diabetes

Type 1	Autoimmune destruction of the beta cells that leads to absolute insulin deficiency
Type 2	Insulin resistance, impaired insulin secretion, and increased glucose production
Gestational	Glucose intolerance during pregnancy
Other types	Endocrinopathies, drug induced, genetic defects, infection

Source: ADA, 2005b.

TABLE 42-3 Diabetic Emergencies

Hyperglycemia

Hyperglycemia with hyperosmolarity

Ketosis without acidosis

Diabetic ketoacidosis

Hypoglycemia

Source: ADA, 2004.

"the insulin resistance syndrome," which consists of insulin insensitivity and insulin unresponsiveness. This syndrome consists of a clustering of conditions: Type 2 diabetes, central obesity, hypertension, and dyslipidemia (Fletcher & Lamendola, 2004, p. 339). Diabetes can occur due to a number of other reasons, however. **Table 42-4** shows associated etiologies for the development of diabetes.

HYPOGLYCEMIA

Hypoglycemia can be a life-threatening event if left untreated. Seen in both Type 1 and Type 2 diabetes, hypoglycemia comprises an imbalance of insulin and glucose. Glucose is the brain's metabolic fuel. The brain does not synthesize or store large quantities of glucose, so it is therefore dependent on

blood glucose concentration. If this concentration falls below normal levels, the physiological effects to the brain may be profound, leading to coma and ultimately death (Cryer, Davis, & Shamoon, 2003).

In Type 1 diabetes, the onset of the disease is acute and is typically found in younger age groups, often accompanied by a history of polyuria, polydipsia, lethargy, and weight loss over a period of up to two weeks. The majority of patients will present with ketoacidosis and hypoglycemia. Ketoacidosis results in salt and water depletion, loss of skin turgor, tachycardia, hypotension, and deep and sighing breath (Kussmaul respira-

TABLE 42-2 Long-Term Complications of Diabetes Mellitus

Cardiovascular disease	
Retinopathy	Nonproliferative
	Preproliferative
	Proliferative
Nephropathy	Microalbuminuria
	Proteinuria
	Renal insufficiency
	End-stage renal disease
Neuropathy	Distal
	Large fiber
	Autonomic
	• Eye
	• Cardiovascular
	• Gastrointestinal
	• Metabolic
	• Genitourinary and sexual

Source: ADA, 2004.

TABLE 42-4 Etiologies of Diabetes

Diseases of the pancreas	Pancreatitis
	Neoplasia
	Cystic fibrosis
	Hemochromatosis
Endocrinopathies	Acromegaly
	Cushing's syndrome
	Hyperthyroidism
	Pheochromocytoma
Drug/chemical induced	Pentamidine
	Glucocorticoids
	Thiazides
	Dilantin
Infection	Congenital rubella
	Cytomegalovirus
Immune mediated (uncommon)	Stiff-man syndrome
	Anti-insulin receptor antibodies
Genetic syndrome associated with diabetes mellitus	Down's syndrome
	Turner's syndrome
	Freidreich's ataxia
	Huntington's chorea
	Porphyria
	Prader-Willi syndrome

Source: Norman Endocrine Surgery Clinic, 2005.

tions; breath has odor of acetone). Hypoglycemia is a common occurrence, with glucose levels from 50 to 60 mg/dL occurring in about 10% of the patients (Laing et al., 1999). This can lead to chronic asymptomatic hypoglycemia. The patient may then go on to experience symptomatic hypoglycemia at an average of about two episodes per week.

In the Diabetes Control and Complications Trial (DCCT), 65% of the participants reported severe hypoglycemia that required assistance or hospitalization (DCCT, 1998). This severe hypoglycemia constitutes an emergency, because 2% to 4% of the deaths from Type 1 diabetes are attributed to very low blood glucose levels (Cryer et al., 2003).

Type 2 diabetes is typically found in older age groups, obese individuals, and persons who have a history of hypertension. Type 2 diabetes begins with fatigue and malaise before the classic signs of thirst, polyuria, and nocturia occur. Affected individuals have had a long-standing episode of hyperglycemia: Type 2 diabetics, however, have a lower incidence of hypoglycemia. Hypoglycemia in Type 2 diabetes is about one-tenth of that seen with Type 1 diabetes (United Kingdom Prospective Diabetic Study Group, 1995). Patients who are treated with both oral medications and insulin are more likely to experience hypoglycemia (**Table 42-5**) (ADA, 2004).

Hypoglycemia can present as mild, moderate, or severe (**Table 42-6**). Mild to moderate hypoglycemia can usually be handled by the patient and does not require healthcare assistance. Severe hypoglycemia, which causes adrenergic symptoms (sweating, tremor, palpitations, tachycardia, agitation, nervousness, hunger), neurological symptoms (impairment of consciousness, mental concentration, vision, speech, and memory; blurred vision; fatigue; seizures; paralysis; ataxia; loss of consciousness; aggressive behavior), and cognitive impairment, usually requires medical intervention. If severe hypoglycemia is left untreated, coma, brain damage, and even death may occur (Mathur, 2005).

Diagnosis of hypoglycemia is made by correlating the presenting symptoms with a low plasma glucose level as well as the

TABLE 42-6 Symptoms of Hypoglycemia

Mild	Moderate	Severe
Neurogenic	**Neurogenic**	**Neurogenic**
Tremors	Tremors	Tremors
Palpitation	Palpitation	Palpitation
Anxiety	Anxiety	Anxiety
Tachycardia	Tachycardia	Tachycardia
Diaphoresis	Hunger	Hunger
Hunger	Paresthesia	Paresthesia
Paresthesia	Blurred vision	Blurred vision
Neuroglycopenic	**Neuroglycopenic**	**Neuroglycopenic**
Fatigue	Extreme fatigue	Extreme fatigue
	Confusion	Confusion
	Behavioral changes	Behavioral changes
	Difficulty concentrating	Difficulty concentrating
	Somnolence	Somnolence
		Loss of consciousness
		Inability to awaken
		Seizures

Source: Cryer, Davis, & Shamoon, 2003.

fact that resolution of the symptoms is seen when the plasma glucose levels are raised.

Many times patients with hypoglycemia are treated in the ED and may not need to be admitted to the ICU. These patients, because of their mental confusion, need to be treated with parenteral glucose. Glucagon hydrochloride (GlucaGen®), in the form of intramuscular (IM) injection or intravenous (IV) administration, can be used in Type 1 diabetes. Because glucagon also stimulates insulin production, it is less useful in Type 2 diabetes. IV glucose is the medication of choice for severe hypoglycemia in Type 2 diabetics. Repeat glucose infusion is often needed to maintain euglycemia. Since glucagon can restore blood sugar levels within 5 to 10 minutes, blood sugar levels should be rechecked in 15 minutes.

Nursing care of patients with severe hypoglycemia includes close monitoring of vital signs as well as level of consciousness (**Figure 42-1**). Blood glucose levels need to be checked frequently for several hours, because recurrent hypoglycemia is common. As soon as the patient is able, small frequent feeding to help stabilize the glucose level is recommended. It is essential that the blood glucose level is stabilized before discharge and that there is an absence of recurrent hypoglycemia. For this reason, a 24-hour ICU admission may be recommended. When

TABLE 42-5 Percentage of Hypoglycemia in Type 2 Diabetes According to Medication Used

Metformin	2.4%
Sulfonylurea	3.3%
Insulin	11.2%

Source: United Kingdom Prospective Diabetic Study Group, 1995.

FIGURE 42-1 Monitor Sheet: Hypoglycemia

Time						
Vital signs						
B/P						
Pulse						
Respiration*						
Level of consciousness†						
Blood glucose levels						
Intake						
Parenteral						
Oral						
Output						

*D = deep, S = shallow, N = normal
†A = alert, D = drowsy, S = stuporous, C = comatose

Source: Cryer, Davis, & Shamoon, 2003.

the patient regains cognitive ability, the ICU nurse should begin to educate the patient on the prevention of future episodes of hypoglycemia. Reducing the risk means helping the patient to maintain plasma glucose levels as close to the nondiabetic range as possible. To achieve this goal, the patient should be taught to monitor glucose levels closely.

HYPERGLYCEMIC EMERGENCIES

Hyperglycemia occurs when the body has insufficient insulin to metabolize the glucose. If left untreated, elevated glucose levels can lead to a hyperglycemic crisis. DKA and HHS are two of the most serious complications seen with hyperglycemia. It is estimated that severe disabling hyperglycemia occurs on an average of once a year for patients with Type 1 diabetes (MacLeod, Hepburn, & Frier, 1993).

Diabetic Ketoacidosis

DKA is a biochemical syndrome consisting of hyperglycemia, ketosis, and acidosis (**Figure 42-2**). It is estimated that DKA occurs in anywhere from 4 to 8 persons per 1,000 patients with di-

abetes (Kitabchi et al., 2001). Approximately 5% of these patients will die (ADA, 2004). The patient with DKA will usually present with a history of omitting doses of insulin, infection, an acute illness, alcohol intoxication, or an undiagnosed case of Type 1 diabetes. Glucose levels are usually greater than 250 mg/dL but may not reflect the severity of DKA. Addressing the osmotic changes is necessary to correct the problem. The patient may also have fluid volume deficits and/or acid–base imbalances.

With DKA, the high glucose levels cause a fluid volume deficit by triggering an osmotic diuresis that ultimately results in polyuria. The patient has an increased urine production plus a loss of sodium, magnesium, calcium, and phosphorus through the urine. Dehydration can occur due to the hyperosmolarity, which puts the patient at risk for hypovolemic shock.

Acid–base imbalance occurs because cells start to break down fats and proteins in lieu of glucose. The fats break down quickly, producing more energy than can be utilized and leading to a buildup of ketone acids. Measurement of these ketone acids in the urine and pH levels of the blood can provide an estimate of the severity of ketoacidosis. As a patient's level of hydration worsens, more ketone acids accumulate, which activates the production of lactic acid, which then continues to increase the metabolic acidosis of the patient. Metabolic acidosis follows an increase in free H^+ concentration $[H^+]$, which can happen through production of ketones and lactic acid in the presence of a normal PCO_2. The high $[H^+]$ causes a reciprocal fall in the $[HCO_3^-]$. To compensate, the patient will try to reduce CO_2 through quick, shallow breaths. By lowering the CO_2, both the $[H^+]$ and the $[HCO_3^-]$ are lowered (Stavile & Sinert, 2005). A more in-depth discussion of acid–base imbalance appears in Chapter 22.

When further electrolyte imbalance occurs, shifts in potassium can be seen first as an elevation, then as a decrease once osmotic diuresis begins. Some physicians will order the calculation of an anion gap. The anion gap is normally 12 to 14

FIGURE 42-2 The Triangle of DKA

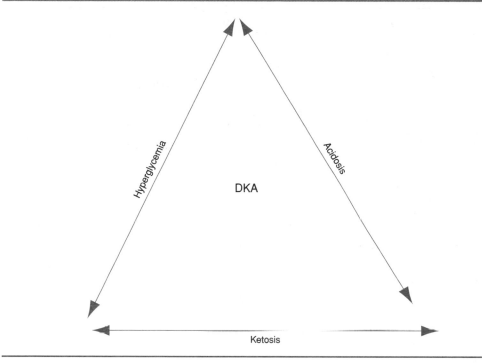

Source: Kitabchi et al., 2001.

mEq, and it is maintained at this normal level through a balance in electrolytes. When the electrolytes become unbalanced, the anion gap increases. Trending the anion gap with each set of lab results for a basic metabolic panel (i.e., electrolytes and bicarbonate) allows healthcare professionals to note an improvement or worsening of the patient's condition. To calculate an anion gap, you will need three lab values: sodium, chloride, and bicarbonate. The calculation is $Na^+ - (Cl^- + HCO_3^-)$. These calculations should be charted so that a trend can be established.

Hyperosmolar Hyperglycemic States

HHS is a life-threatening emergency that is seen most often in older adults with Type 2 diabetes. The classic signs are dehydration, hyperglycemia, high serum osmolarity, and no ketoacidosis. If ketones are present, they are very low. The lack of ketones is thought to be related to a small amount of circulating insulin in these individuals. Diagnosis of HHS is often delayed in the elderly, because these patients often present with altered mental status and dehydration. These symptoms may be incorrectly attributed to a number of other clinical conditions such as infection or factors that limit mobility and subsequently decrease fluid intake. Due to lack of population-based data, the true incidence of HHS is unknown. However, the mortality rate for this metabolic emergency is high, approximately 15% (ADA, 2005a).

Differential diagnosis of DKA and HHS can be difficult (see **Table 42-7**), because their presentations can be very similar. The difference is seen in the time of onset, the degree of dehydration, and the severity of ketosis. Restoring fluid and electrolyte balance is critical to the management of both conditions (see **Table 42-8**). The electrolyte imbalance develops due to osmotic diuresis that leads to an increase in urinary output and subsequent electrolyte loss. The results are both dehydration and sodium depletion. In addition to sodium loss, many other electrolytes and minerals are lost, so they must be replaced as well (see Table 42-8) (Kitabchi et al., 2001).

TABLE 42-7 Differential Diagnosis of DKA and HHS

	DKA			HHS
	Mild	**Moderate**	**Severe**	
Glucose (mg/dL)	> 250	> 250	> 250	> 600
Blood pH	7.25–7.3	7–7.24	< 7	> 7.3
Bicarbonate (mEq/L)	15–18	10 to < 15	< 10	> 15
Ketones (urine)	+	+	+	−/+
Ketones (serum)	+	+	+	−/+
Serum osmolarity (mOsm/kg)	Variable	Variable	Variable	> 320
Anion gap	> 10	> 12	> 12	Variable
Mention	Alert	Alert → drowsy	Stupor/coma	Stupor/coma

Source: ADA, 2004.

TABLE 42-8 Typical Deficits of Water and Electrolytes

	DKA	HHS
H_2O (mL/kg)	100	100–200
Na^+ (mEq/kg)	7–10	5–13
Cl^- (mEq/kg)	3–5	5–15
K^+ (mEq/kg)	3–5	4–6
PO_4 (mmol/kg)	5–7	3–7
Mg^{++} (mEq/kg)	1–2	1–2
Ca^{++} (mEq/kg)	1–2	1–2

Sources: ADA, 2005b; Kitabchi et al., 2001; Kitabchi & Wall, 1999.

Assessment of the patient will depend on the presence or absence of a coma. If the patient is awake, a complete history of current diabetic status is needed. All medications, complications, and symptoms should be assessed. Patients' adherence to their treatment plan should be assessed and may become a focal point for future education.

Signs and Symptoms of Hyperglycemia

Hyperglycemia should be suspected if the patient complains of an increase in thirst or hunger, increased urinary output, drowsiness, or blurred vision. Always obtain an extra blood glucose check to evaluate the patient's symptoms against the glucose level.

Diagnosis of DKA and HHS

Patients with DKA and HHS present with evidence of dehydration (dry mucous membranes, thirst, and orthostatic hypotension) as well as labored breathing (Kussmaul respiration). The breath with DKA may have a fruity odor that is caused by the presence of acetone. Laboratory assessment (see **Table 42-9**) followed by osmolarity calculation (see **Table 42-10**) are important steps to correct the identified deficits and are important nursing care measures.

TABLE 42-9 Laboratory Assessment for DKA and HHS

Plasma glucose
Electrolyte profile
Metabolic profile
Arterial blood gases
Urine ketones
Blood pH
CBC with differential
ECG

TABLE 42-10 Formulas for Osmolarity Calculation

Effective serum osmolarity:
$$2[Na^+ + K^+] + \frac{(glucose\ in\ mg/dL)}{18} + \frac{BUN}{2.8}$$

Correction of Na^+:
$$[Na^+] + 1.6 \times \frac{glucose\ in\ mg/dL - 100}{100}$$

Anion gap:
$$[Na^+] - [Cl^- + HCO_3]$$

Source: Abrahamson et al., 2004.

TREATMENT

Treatment of hyperglycemia has two major objectives. First is the restoration of both fluid volume and electrolyte homeostasis. Fluid therapy is directed at expansion of total fluid volume, both intravascular and extravascular. The rate of fluid replacement in the absence of cardiac compromise is 15 to 20 mL/kg for the first hour. In the average adult, this equates to approximately 1 to 1.5 liters. Subsequent fluid replacement depends on the level of dehydration present. The fluid of choice is 0.9% NS solution. The fluid is changed to 0.45% NS as volume and sodium levels return to normal, with conversion to 5% dextrose in water (D_5W) as plasma glucose levels fall below 250 mg/dL (**Figure 42-3**) (ADA, 2004; Gardner & Greenspan, 2001; Kitabchi & Wall, 1999).

Electrolytes must also be replaced to restore homeostasis. Sodium replacement is accomplished with the use of NS IV fluid. Potassium and bicarbonate levels must be assessed and replaced as needed. Hyperkalemia may be present with both DKA and HHS. Because of dehydration, this effect is seen even in the presence of total potassium depletion. Once dehydration has been corrected, a decrease in serum potassium levels will be noted; therefore potassium replacement is started as soon as the levels reach 5.5 mEq/L if kidney function is normal. If the patient is hypokalemic on admission, then potassium replacement is started immediately. To avoid cardiac arrhythmias and/or cardiac arrest, insulin therapy is delayed until the potassium levels reach more than 3.3 mEq/L (Gardner & Greenspan, 2001).

Bicarbonate replacement depends on blood pH. If the pH is less than 7, just the resolution of the DKA can restore the pH to normal. As yet, no randomized studies have examined the use of bicarbonate with pH levels that are less than 7.0. If they are less than 7.0, however, the current management is to add 44 mEq to 500 mL of fluid to run over six hours. This is done because adverse vascular effects may be seen in patients with a pH of less than 7.0 (see Figure 42-3) (ADA, 2005b).

FIGURE 42-3 Management of DKA/HHS Fluid and Electrolyte Balance

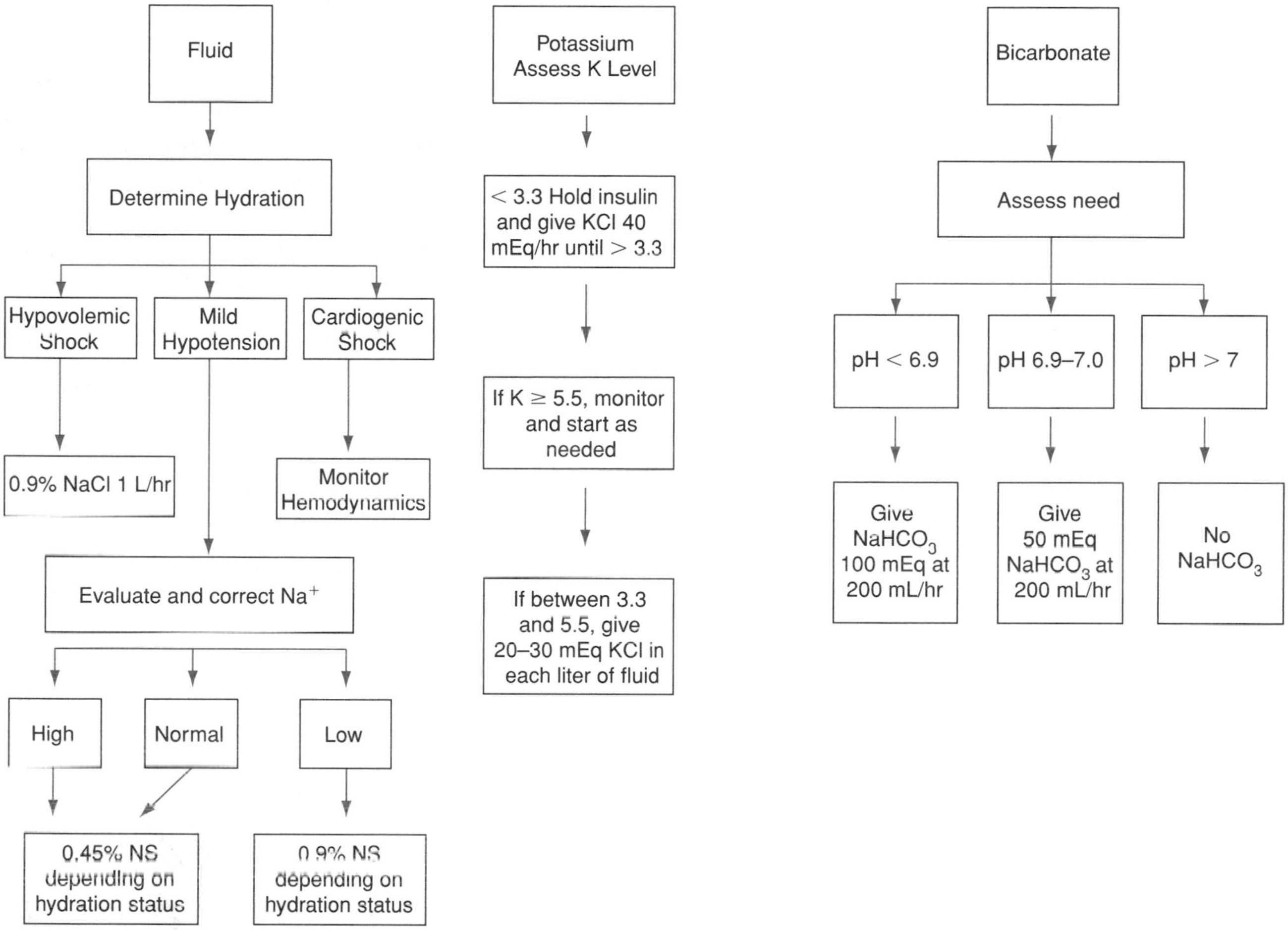

Sources: Abrahamson et al., 2004; ADA, 2004; Kitabchi et al., 2001; Kitabchi & Wall, 1999.

The second objective in treatment is to restore insulin and glucose levels. In DKA and HHS, regular insulin is administered at 10 to 20 units IV bolus and followed with a piggyback solution of 0.1 unit/kg/hr. If there is an inadequate response after two hours, the infusion rate is to be doubled. Insulin levels should be checked every hour and the rate of infusion adjusted until glucose levels are between 100 and 200 mg/dL. DKA can initially be treated with either subcutaneous (SC) or IM insulin. To start, administer 0.4 unit/kg with half the dose given IV and half given either SC or IM. The follow-up is 0.1 unit/kg/hr either SC or IM. If the glucose level does not fall to between 100 and 200 mg/dL, then administer 10 units of regular insulin hourly as an IV bolus until the glucose levels reach the desired level (see **Figure 42-4**) (ADA, 2005b). Blood sugar levels should be de-

creased by 50 to 100 mg/hr to prevent complications such as cerebral edema.

Nursing care is critical to the prevention of complications. The patient must be closely monitored and measures taken to correct the identified abnormality (Figure 42-1). Management depends on the level of dehydration, response to insulin, and electrolyte replacement. If awake, the patient may be anxious and reassurance is critical. Blood glucose levels need to be checked every hour, while electrolyte levels need to be checked every two hours. Arterial blood gases are evaluated initially every four to six hours until stable to determine the need for bicarbonate. Intake and output needs to be measured hourly, because over-replacement of fluid can also cause problems. As soon as possible, oral nutrition should be started. Start with clear liquid and progress as tolerated.

FIGURE 42-4 Insulin Administration for DKA and HHS

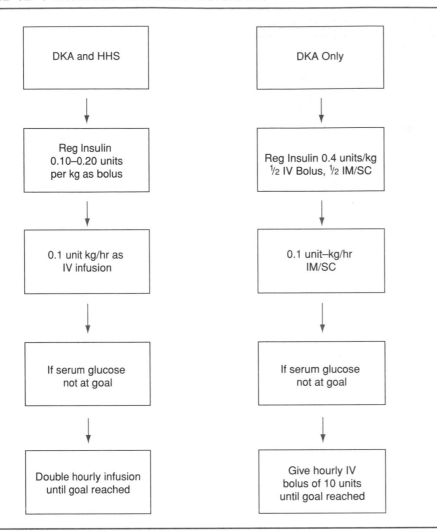

Sources: Abrahamson et al., 2004; ADA, 2004; Kitabchi et al., 2001; Kitabchi & Wall, 1999.

Level of consciousness needs to be assessed at least every hour and may require more frequent monitoring. Vital signs are recorded every hour until stable. **Figure 42-5** is an example of a flowsheet used to record the progress of both DKA and HHS (ADA, 2005b).

The most common complication of DKA and HHS is hypoglycemia. This complication can be avoided by close monitoring. Hypokalemia can occur due to both insulin and fluid administration and should be managed properly (Kitabchi et al., 2001).

PREVENTION

The best treatment for both DKA and HHS is prevention. Proper education (see **Box 42-1**), good access to health care, and effective self-monitoring can help to prevent the development of hyperglycemia. With support from the National Institute of Diabetes and the Digestive and Kidney Diseases

(NIDDKD) of the National Institutes of Health, the largest study of lifestyle changes to prevent diabetes was conducted with 3,234 people who were at high risk for developing diabetes. The Diabetes Prevention Program (DPP) enrolled adults who were overweight or obese, and who had impaired glucose tolerance (IGT). IGT is a condition in which blood sugar levels are elevated after a standardized test called the oral glucose tolerance test, but not high enough to be considered diabetic.

The DPP lifestyle program was directed at achieving long-lasting changes in the behaviors that cause weight gain and a sedentary lifestyle. Although the goals of the lifestyle intervention were not intensive, the training to change the ingrained behaviors of a lifetime was intensive.

The DPP demonstrated that diabetes can be prevented. People in the lifestyle intervention group were 58% less likely to develop diabetes over a three-year period than the people in the control group. In the United States, if these results were applied to the population at high risk to develop diabetes (such as those recruited into the DPP), which totals more than 10 million people, it would reduce the occurrence of new diabetes cases from 800,000 to fewer than 400,000 cases per year. Research into diabetes prevention has also shown that people at high risk for Type 2 diabetes can prevent or delay the onset of the disease by losing 5% to 7% of their body weight. Thirty minutes of moderate physical activity per day, coupled with a 5% to 10% reduction in body weight, produced a 58% reduction in diabetes (ADA, 2005b; Centers for Disease Control and Prevention, 2006).

As soon as the patient is receptive, education needs to begin. Patients are unique in their individual needs, and the program of education should reflect this uniqueness. If the patient is to maximize the benefits of education, ethnic origin as well as personal healthcare beliefs must be considered in the development of an education plan.

FIGURE 42-5 Flow Sheet for DKA and HHS

Vital signs						
Weight (daily)						
Mental status						
Temperature q 4 hr						
Pulse						
Respiration						
B/P						
Glucose level						
Insulin amount/route						
Complete Blood Count						
Serum ketones						
Urine ketones						
Electrolytes						
Na						
K						
Cl						
HCO$_3$						
BUN						
Effective osmolality						
Anion gap						
ABG						

(continues)

FIGURE 42-5 Flow Sheet for DKA and HHS (continued)

pH						
pO$_2$						
pCO$_2$						
O$_2$ sat						
HCO$_3$						
Fluid intake (Record type and additives)						
Output						
Urine						
Other						

Mental status: A = alert, B = drowsy, S = stuporous, C = coma
Respiratory: D = deep, S = shallow, N = normal

Sources: Abrahamson et al., 2004; ADA, 2004; Kitabchi et al., 2001; Kitabchi & Wall, 1999.

Box 42-1
Assessment of Patient Knowledge of Diabetes

Does the patient understand the disease and the interaction of food, exercise, and medication?
Does the patient know his or her unique symptoms of hypoglycemia?
Does the patient do self-monitoring of blood glucose (SMBG) on a regular basis?
Does the patient know how to treat a low glucose level found on SMBG?
Does the patient carry a high glucose source at all times?
What is the patient's meal plan, including snacks?

PATIENT OUTCOMES

Nurses can help ensure the obtainment of optimal patient outcomes such as those listed in **Box 42-2** through the use of evidence-based interventions for diabetic patients.

Box 42-2
Optimal Patient Outcomes

- Blood sugar in expected range
- Vital signs in expected range
- Patient and family knowledgeable about disease process and actions to take in the event of an emergency
- Demonstrates adequate coping of changes in lifestyle
- Fluid status in expected range
- Electrolytes in expected range

SUMMARY

Diabetic emergencies are preventable complications. Proper management of diabetes can prevent these conditions. If an emergency occurs, then a combination of proper management and education is needed to prevent recurrences. As the diabetes prevention study showed, individuals can change lifestyles to benefit their health.

CASE STUDY

J.R. is an 85-year-old male who was admitted to ICU from a nursing home in a stupor-like condition. He has a history of diabetes, hypertension, chronic heart failure (CHF), and limited mobility due to arthritis. The nursing home staff noted that he has been progressively less responsive over the last several days, and this morning they were unable to awaken him to give him his medicine.

Current Medications

Metformin 500 BID	For diabetes
Glipizide 10 mg BID	
Lasix 10 mg daily	For CHF and hypertension
Monopril 20 mg daily	
Toprol-XL 50 mg daily	
Anaprox 550 mg q 12 hours as needed for pain	

There is no other history of present illness, because the patient is unresponsive.

Physical Exam

Well-developed, slightly obese male who is responsive to deep stimulation but does not regain consciousness. Respirations are labored.

Vital Signs

Temperature 36.6°C

B/P   126/75

Heart rate 98

Respirations 15 and shallow

Skin	Dry, increased skin turgor
HEENT	Pupils round, reactive to light; mucous membranes dry
Neck	No masses
Lungs	Decreased breath sounds unilaterally; no rales or rhonchi
Heart	Regular sinus rhythm; rate 98
Abdomen	Soft
Extremities	No edema

Lab Work	Patient	Reference Range
Glucose	1950	70–110 mg/dL
Sodium	152	135–145 mEq/L
Potassium	6.2	3.6–5.0 mEq/L
Chloride	112	70–110 mEq/L
CO_2	10	21–31 mg/dL
BUN	46	6–20 mg/dL
Creatinine	3.7	0.5–1.2 mg/dL
Anion gap	14	0–15
BUN/creatinine	21:1	12:1–20:1
AST	36	10–42 IU/L
Alkaline phosphatase	160	42–120 IU/L
Serum osmolality	441	285–295 mOsm/kg

Urinalysis

Negative for ketones

> 1,000 for glucose

Large—blood

1.050 specific gravity

Chest X-Ray

Infiltrate seen in right lower lobe

Patient Diagnosis

HHS

CRITICAL THINKING QUESTIONS

1. One of the first nursing tasks is to assess the patient for dehydration. Provide a rationale for assessing the patient for dehydration.
2. What are J.R.'s signs of dehydration?
3. You start J.R. on 0.45% NS, 1 liter, to run over one hour. Discuss the management of J.R.'s IV fluids.
4. For the accurate measure of input and output, would you insert a urinary catheter? Why or why not?
5. When would you do blood work again, and what would you do?
6. There is no order for insulin even in the presence of grossly elevated blood glucose. What is the rationale for this choice?
7. As J.R. improves and becomes alert, what are some of your primary nursing responsibilities?
8. Which disciplines should be consulted to work with J.R.?
9. How would you modify your plan of care if J.R. did not speak English?
10. What types of issues may require you to act as an advocate or moral agent for this patient?
11. How will you implement your role as a facilitator of learning for this patient? Use the form to identify the top four priorities for educating this patient.

Using the Synergy Model to Facilitate Learning

	Learning Needs of the Patient	Content to Be Covered	Learning Outcome
SYNERGY MODEL			

Online Resources

Diabetes Prevention: www.ndep.nih.gov/diabetes/prev/prevention.htm

American Diabetes Association: www.diabetes.org/diabetes-prevention.jsp

National Diabetes Clearing House: diabetes.niddk.nih.gov/

American College of Endocrinology Position Statement on Inpatient Diabetes:
www.aace.com/clin/guidelines/InpatientDiabetesPositionStatement.pdf

Evidence-based Recommendations for Diabetic Hyperglycemic Crisis:
www.amda.com/caring/february2003/diabetesmanagement.htm

Solving a Hidden Problem: Low Health Literacy: www.amda.com/caring/january2003/healthliteracy.htm

Lilly Diabetes (explains how insulin works): www.lillydiabetes.com/index.jsp

REFERENCES

Abrahamson, M., Beaser, R., Carver, C., Cooppan, R., Grossman, S., Laffel, L., et al. (2004). *Guideline for management of hyperglycemic emergencies for adults.* Joslin Diabetes Center and Beth Israel Deaconess Medical Center.

American Diabetes Association. (2005a). All about diabetes. Retrieved June 18, 2005, from www.diabetes.org/about-diabetes.jsp

American Diabetes Association. (2005b). Standards of medical care in diabetes. *Diabetes Care, 28*(S1), S4–S36.

American Diabetes Association. (2004). Hyperglycemic crises in diabetes. *Diabetes Care, 27*(S1), S94–S102.

Centers for Disease Control and Prevention. (2006). Retrieved August 8, 2006, from www.cdc.gov

Cryer, P. E., Davis, S. N., & Shamoon, H. (2003). Hypoglycemia in diabetes. *Diabetic Care, 26*(6), 1902–1912.

Diabetic Control and Complications Trial Research Group. (1998). The effects of intensive treatment of diabetes on the development and progression of long-term complications in insulin dependent diabetes mellitus. *New England Journal of Medicine, 329*, 977–986.

Fletcher, B., & Lamendola, C. (2004). Insulin resistance syndrome. *Journal of Cardiovascular Nursing, 19*(5), 339–345.

Gardner, D. G., & Greenspan, F. S. (2001). Endocrine emergencies. In P. G. Greenspan & D. G. Gardner (Eds.), *Basic and clinical endocrinology* (pp. 867–892). New York: Lange Medical Books.

Kitabchi, A. E., Umpierrez, G. E., Murphy, M. B., Barrett, E. J., Kreisberg, R. A., Malone, J. I., et al. (2001). Management of hyperglycemic crisis in patients with diabetes. *Diabetes Care, 24*(1), 131–153.

Kitabchi, A. E., & Wall, B. M. (1999). Management of diabetic ketoacidosis. *American Family Physician, 60*(2), 328–341.

Laing, S. P., Swerdlow, A. J., Slater, S. D., Botha, J. L., Burden, A. C., Waugh, N. R., et al. (1999). The British Diabetic Association cohort study II: Cause-specific mortality in patients with insulin-treated diabetes mellitus. *Diabetic Medicine, 16*, 466–471.

MacLeod, K. M., Hepburn, D. A., & Frier, B. M. (1993). Frequency and morbidity of severe hypoglycemia in insulin-treated diabetic patients. *Diabetic Medicine, 10*, 238–245.

Mathur, R. (2005). Hypoglycemia. Retrieved August 8, 2006, from www.medicinnet.com/hypoglycemia/article.htm

Norman Endocrine Surgery Clinic. (2005). Type 2 Diabetes. Retrieved August 8, 2006 from www.endocrineweb.com/diabetes/2diabetes.html

Stavile, K. L., & Sinert, R. (2005). Metabolic acidosis. Retrieved August 9, 2006, from www.emedicine.com/emerg/topic312.htm

United Kingdom Prospective Diabetic Study Group. (1995). U.K. prospective diabetes study. Overview of 6 years' therapy of Type 2 diabetes: A progressive disease. *Diabetes, 44*, 1249–1258.

Renal

CHAPTER 43

Renal Anatomy, Physiology, and Assessment

Pat Ostergaard   Roberta Kaplow

LEARNING OBJECTIVES

Upon completion of this chapter, the reader will be able to:

1. Describe the anatomy and physiology of the renal system.
2. Perform a complete assessment of renal function.
3. Identify laboratory tests that may be performed to assess the renal system.
4. Explain the studies used in diagnosing renal pathologies.

To assess, plan, and implement care of the critically ill patient, the intensive care unit (ICU) nurse must have a thorough understanding of renal anatomy and physiology. Variation in any part of renal anatomy or physiology can change the condition of the patient. Renal assessments are performed based on a number of factors. These data assist the ICU nurse to plan care for the critically ill patient.

ANATOMY OF THE RENAL SYSTEM

To describe the anatomy of the renal system, it is necessary to discuss the gross and functional anatomical structures that make up this system. The renal parenchyma (medulla and cortex) and the renal sinus (renal blood vessels, pelvis, and calyces) make up the macrostructure of the kidney. **Table 43-1** describes the gross anatomical structures.

The functional units of the kidney are called nephrons. Each kidney has more than 1 million nephrons. Each nephron contains a glomerulus, Bowman's capsule, and tubule system. These components work together to maintain ion balance for optimal cell function and eliminate unnecessary material from plasma (Amerling & Levin, 2001).

Glomeruli are clumps of afferent and efferent arterioles surrounded by Bowman's capsule. The glomerulus is the filtering system of the nephron, is semipermeable and allows water and soluble waste to pass through and be eliminated as urine. Blood flows into Bowman's capsule through the afferent arteriole, is filtered through the glomerulus, and then flows out through the efferent arteriole. If the glomerulus is intact, filtrate dispensed into the Bowman's capsule should be free of red blood cells and proteins. A healthy person produces approximately 180 liters of filtrate per day, but only 1 to 1.5 liters is excreted as urine.

The tubular system emerges out of the Bowman's capsule and forms the proximal convoluted tubule, loop of Henle, distal convoluted tubule, and collecting ducts. The filtered water containing metabolic waste passes through Bowman's capsule into the proximal convoluted tubule (Amerling & Levin, 2001).

Each component of the tube system has a specific role in urine formation (Huether, 2002). The tubular system begins with the proximal convoluted tubule. (PCT) Fluid then flows into the descending and ascending limbs of the loop of Henle, to the

TABLE 43-1 Gross Anatomy of the Renal System

Anatomical Structure	Description
Renal cortex	The renal cortex is the outer portion of the kidney.
Renal medulla	The renal medulla is the innermost part of the kidney. It is made up of 8 to 18 of these conical subdivisions, called renal pyramids (Chmielewski, 2003).
Renal pyramids	Renal pyramids are cone-shaped tissues of the kidney (Chmielewski, 2003).
Renal calyces	The outer extensions of the renal pelvis into the parts of the kidneys responsible for filtering of blood (Urologyhealth.org, 2005).
Renal pelvis	The area at the center of the kidney. It is where urine collects and is funneled into the ureter (MedicineNet.com, 2005).
Ureters	The tubes that connect the kidney to the bladder (Urologyhealth.org, 2005).
Bladder	The area where urine is stored.
Urethra	The tube that connects the bladder to the outside of the body to eliminate urine (Chmielewski, 2003).

distal tubule, then to the collecting tubule, and ends up in the collecting ducts. In the tubule system, "substances are reabsorbed and secreted, and the final product of urine is excreted from the collecting ducts through the ureters into the bladder" (Henke & Eigsti, 2003, p. 129) (see **Table 43-2**).

The juxtaglomerular apparatus is composed of the macula densa and juxtaglomerular cells. It is located near the point where the afferent and efferent arterioles enter and exit each glomerulus. The macula densa consists of epithelial cells on the inner lining of the distal tubule. They have the ability to interpret signals related to pressure changes in the glomerulus. If perfusion to the kidney decreases (e.g., due to hypotension or hypovolemia), the macula densa sends a signal to the juxtaglomular cells and causes the release of renin. Renin, an enzyme that converts angiotensinogen to angiotensin I, initiates a cascade of events leading to the production of angiotensin II. Angiotensin II produces constriction of the efferent arteriole (Giuliano, 2001). **Figure 43-1** depicts the workings of the renin-angiotensin-aldosterone system (RAAS).

PHYSIOLOGY OF THE RENAL SYSTEM

The roles of the renal system include regulation of fluid volume, regulation of electrolyte balance, maintenance of acid–base balance, excretion of foreign and waste products, and regulation of systemic blood pressure and osmolarity, red blood cell production, hormone secretion, and vitamin D metabolism.

Fluid Volume Regulation and Osmolarity

Three essential processes are involved with renal function: glomerular filtration (filtering of blood into the tubule system to form urine), tubular reabsorption (reabsorption of products from the tubules that are needed by the body into the bloodstream), and tubular secretion (secretion of products from the blood to be wasted into the tubule system). The processes of filtration, reabsorption, and secretion keep the body in balance in terms of water, minerals, electrolytes, and hydrogen ion concentration and eliminate the toxic substances produced by the body (Chmielewski, 2003).

Glomerular filtration is the first step in the formation of urine. Tubular reabsorption involves water, sodium, and urea.

TABLE 43-2 Components of a Nephron and Their Roles

Glomerulus	Filtration.
Proximal tubules	100% reabsorption of vitamins, amino acids, and glucose; 65–70% reabsorption of sodium, water, potassium, bicarbonate, and urate. Hydrogen is excreted. Fluid leaves isotonic.
Loop	Sodium chloride transport. Fluid leaves hypotonic. Initiates the processes of urine concentration or dilution. The descending limb is very permeable to water (with no sodium transport). The ascending limb pumps out sodium and is impermeable to water.
Distal tubule	Sodium and bicarbonate are reabsorbed. Antidiuretic hormone (ADH) is required to reabsorb H_2O. Potassium, urate, and ammonia are excreted.
Collecting ducts	ADH required to reabsorb H_2O for final concentration. Adjustments in sodium and potassium are made due to aldosterone.

Sources: Huether, 2002; Perkins, 2005.

FIGURE 43-1 Renin-Angiotensin-Aldosterone System

Renin

↓ Cleaves

Angiotensinogen (from liver)

to form

Angiotensin I

Converted in Lung and Arteries

↓ by angiotensin-converting enzyme (ACE) into

Angiotensin II

↓ promotes the release from the adrenal cortex of:

Aldosterone (adjusts Na^+ + H_2O)

Approximately 99% of water and sodium are reabsorbed by the tubules; 50% of urea is reabsorbed. The proximal tubule is responsible for reabsorption of glucose, amino acids, sodium and other electrolytes, water, and urea. The distal tubule reabsorbs sodium (by aldosterone), chloride, and water [by antidiuretic hormone (ADH)]. The collecting ducts perform some water reabsorption (by ADH) (Henke & Eigsti, 2003).

The kidneys receive 20% to 25% of the cardiac output (the amount of blood ejected by the heart each minute). About 600 mL of this output is in the form of plasma. Twenty percent of the renal plasma flow (RPF) is filtered at the glomerulus and passes into Bowman's capsule. The glomerular filtration rate (GFR)—that is, the filtration of plasma per unit of time—is directly related to the perfusion pressure in the glomerular capillaries. The perfusion pressure moves plasma across the glomerulus, through Bowman's capsule, and into the proximal convoluted tubule. The fluid that is produced is called filtrate. Filtrate composition changes as it moves through the tubular system, as described in Table 43-2. The remaining 80% of renal blood flow (RBF) goes through the efferent arterioles to the peritubular capillaries, where only 1 to 2 mL of filtrate is reabsorbed (Huether, 2002; Rule et al., 2004).

The GFR is directly related to the RBF, which is regulated by an intrinsic autoregulatory mechanism, the nervous system, and hormones.

- The kidney has an intrinsic *autoregulatory system* to maintain a constant rate of blood flow and hence a con-

stant GFR, despite arterial pressures ranging from 80 to 180 mm Hg. This autoregulation prevents widespread fluctuations in systemic arterial pressure from being transmitted to the glomerular capillaries. The body therefore maintains a constant level of water and solute excretion, which will not be affected by arterial pressure changes.
- The *myogenic mechanism* is triggered by pressure changes. As pressure decreases, the stretch on the afferent arteriole wall decreases. Arteriole relaxation increases the RBF. Conversely, an increase in arterial pressure will cause the arterioles to constrict and decreases RBF.
- The *tubuloglomerular feedback mechanism* maintains RBF and GFR. The macula densa senses changes in flow rate and sodium chloride content, which in turn triggers compensatory changes in the efferent arteriolar resistance and thereby controls GFR.
- As part of *nervous system regulation*, the blood vessels of the kidneys are innervated by the sympathetic fibers that cause arteriole vasoconstriction. The afferent and efferent arterioles are richly supplied by nerve fibers, but the glomerular capillaries appear to have none. When blood pressure decreases, the increased renal sympathetic nerve activity is mediated through the carotid sinus and baroreceptors of the aortic arch. This activity stimulates renal arteriolar vasoconstriction, which decreases both RBF and GFR, leading to a decrease in sodium and water excretion. The end result is an increase in circulating blood volume and systemic blood pressure (Henke & Eigsti, 2003; Rule et al., 2004).

Regulation of Blood Pressure and Osmolarity

The RAAS plays a major role in control of blood pressure and RBF. As mentioned previously, renin is released by the juxtaglomerular apparatus cells. This enzyme, which is secreted by the kidney, promotes the release of angiotensin I, which is then converted into angiotensin II. Angiotensin II, a potent vasoconstrictor, stimulates secretion of aldosterone by the adrenal cortex. Aldosterone secretion, in turn, leads to an increase in sodium and water from the distal and collecting tubules into the bloodstream, which will affect blood pressure. If a patient's volume status decreases, the brain secretes more ADH into the bloodstream. This causes the kidneys to excrete less water, so that the body retains more fluid. Conversely, as fluid volume status is normalized, less ADH is secreted and urinary output increases. This control of the volume of water affects the osmolarity of the body. If the level of fluid in the body falls below normal, osmoreceptors in the hypothalamus detect an increase in osmolarity, resulting in release of ADH, which makes the person thirsty. In combination, drinking additional fluid and recovering the maximum fluid volume possible from the urine will restore fluid volume and osmolarity very rapidly, usually within minutes. If the level of fluid in the body rises above normal, this effect will also change the osmolarity of the circulating fluids. The fall in osmolarity prompts the hypothalamus to stop producing ADH. In the absence of ADH, the kidney permits fluid loss from the body. Hence, the RAAS serves to stabilize systemic blood pressure, enhance sodium reabsorption, and promote systemic vasoconstriction and sympathetic nerve stimulation (Huether, 2002).

Another group of cells, located within the right atrium, secrete atrial natriuretic peptides (ANPs). When pressure rises in the right atrium, ANP will decrease renin and inhibit the angiotensin cascade, relax vascular smooth muscle, and inhibit sodium and water absorption by the kidney tubules. This activity results in a decreased blood pressure and blood volume (Curry, 2005; Henke & Eigsti, 2003).

Electrolyte and Acid–Base Balance

Electrolyte balance is essential for normal cellular and organ function. Through the RAAS, regulation of sodium and potassium retention or excretion is established. The kidneys maintain normal acid–base status by excreting or retaining hydrogen ions and bicarbonate (Giuliano, 2001).

Elimination of Waste, Drugs, and Toxins

In addition to monitoring fluid volume status, the kidney evaluates levels of metabolic waste (i.e., blood urea nitrogen [BUN] and creatinine) as well as foreign substances and medications. As GFR varies, so does the amount of metabolic waste. If GFR is higher than normal, substances that should not be excreted appear in the urine (e.g., protein) (Giuliano, 2001).

Red Blood Cell Production

Red blood cell production occurs by the kidneys through the secretion of the hormone erythropoietin. When erythropoietin is secreted, it stimulates the bone marrow to produce more red blood cells. If the kidneys fail and the serum level of metabolic waste becomes elevated, the life span of red blood cells is shortened. This shorter life cycle partly contributes to the anemia that is seen in renal failure (Khan, Sachs, Pechet, & Snyder, 2002).

Hormone Secretion

The major known hormonal functions of the kidney influence calcium and phosphorus levels via calcitrol and parathyroid hormone and through vitamin D. Kidney hormones also influence red blood cell production, as described previously (Giuliano, 2001).

ASSESSMENT OF THE RENAL SYSTEM

If a patient develops a renal problem, the condition must be evaluated thoroughly. This evaluation should include changes in patterns of urination, the presence of incontinence, and any pain or difficulty encountered upon urination. Medications taken, including over-the-counter and herbal remedies, should be identified. The physical exam should include palpation (to assess for enlargement of the kidney) and percussion for any abnormalities.

Several methods are available to the ICU nurse to determine renal function, including patient history, laboratory tests, and a variety of procedures, depending on suspected pathology. Intake and output and daily weights should be obtained as part of the clinical picture.

Serum Laboratory Tests

Serum Creatinine

Creatinine is a substance that is produced by muscles. Serum creatinine measures the amount of creatinine in the blood and reflects how well the kidneys excrete the creatinine. Normal values range from 0.8 to 1.4 mg/dL. Abnormal results can be related to changes in muscle mass (which decreases in the elderly), liver disease (decreased muscle mass), malnutrition (decrease), large protein meat intake (increase), exercise (increase), and renal failure (increase). Medications [e.g., cimetidine (Tagamet®), trimethoprim sulfamethoxazole (Bactrim®)] can also increase serum creatinine levels (Van Biesen et al., 2006). Creatinine levels will vary with age, gender, and ethnic group as well (Manjunath, Sarnak, & Levey, 2001).

Blood Urea Nitrogen

BUN measures the amount of urea nitrogen (a product of protein metabolism) in the blood. Normal values range from 7 to 18 mg/dL. A common etiology for elevated BUN is dehydration. The ICU nurse should evaluate the BUN level with the patient's vital signs, hemodynamic status (e.g., central venous pressure, wedge pressure), intake and output, and skin turgor. An increased BUN may also be a manifestation of poor renal perfusion or renal dysfunction. BUN levels may also be elevated in patients on high-protein diets. BUN has an inverse relationship with GFR (as discussed later in this chapter). That is, as GFR levels decrease, BUN levels increase. Conversely, in patients with liver disease, BUN may be below normal levels or normal despite a decreased GFR (Churchill, Blake, Jindal, Tofflemire, & Goldstein, 1999).

Urine Laboratory Tests

Urinalysis

A urinalysis evaluates urine appearance, specific gravity, pH, presence of glucose, red blood cells, white blood cells, and protein. Specific gravity measures the kidney's ability to dilute or concentrate urine. Normal values range between 1.003 and 1.030. The appearance of normal urine is clear (versus bloody, cloudy, or turbid). Urinary pH is usually on the acidic side. If glucose is present in the urine, it may be related to increased blood sugar levels or a disorder in the tubules. Normally, no protein should be present in urine. If protein is present, it may be related to renal failure, a glomerular lesion, nephrotic syndrome, Bence-Jones syndrome, or myoglobulin. Presence of white blood cells with or without red blood cells could be indicative of a urinary tract infection. A more in-depth discussion of urinary tract infections appears in Chapter 6. The presence of red blood cells in the urine may be indicative of any of several conditions, including infection, obstruction, trauma, cancer, sickle cell disease, or menses (Khan et al., 2002).

Urine Creatinine

The urine creatinine test (spot level) determines the amount of creatinine in the urine.

Creatinine Clearance (Glomerular Filtration Rate)

Creatinine clearance is the standard by which renal function is assessed and is the test most frequently performed when renal problems are suspected. It provides an estimate of GFR and entails comparison of the levels of creatinine in urine and blood. It is usually based on measurements of a 24-hour urine sample and a blood sample drawn at the end of the 24-hour period. Creatinine clearance is inversely related to serum creatinine. That is, as the serum creatinine levels increase, creatinine clearance is decreased (Delanaye & Krzesinski, 2005; Manjunath et al., 2001). Normal GFR is 125 mL/min, but the rate depends on age, gender, and race. Among elderly patients, the nurse can expect renal function will decline with age by 1 mL/min per year on average. The most widely used clearance formula, Cockroft–Gault, which is based on serum creatinine, seems to underestimate the GFR in the elderly, whereas serum urea seems to be a better parameter (Fehrman-Ekholm & Skeppholm, 2004).

Radiology Studies

Radiographic studies of the kidney, ureters, and bladder (KUB) may help in the diagnosis of kidney disease. Abnormalities in the shape or size of the kidney may be seen. Such studies allow for the identification of renal or bladder calculi (University of Virginia Health System, 2005).

Renal Ultrasound

Ultrasound uses sound waves to create an image and is a valuable tool to diagnose kidney disease. This modality allows for visualization of the kidney, measurement of kidney size, and collection of a biopsy for an accurate diagnosis (University of Virginia Health System, 2005).

Renal Biopsy

A renal biopsy is performed to obtain a sample of kidney tissue. It is most commonly combined with ultrasound, but can also be performed with computerized tomography (CT) scan guidance. For this procedure, the patient will be required to lie in a prone position. This position can prove challenging for some ICU patients, depending on the number and types of catheters, tubes, and devices that are in place (e.g., endotracheal tube, central venous catheter). Local anesthesia is administered for this procedure. A needle is inserted into the skin and then advanced to the surface of the kidney. If able to cooperate, the patient is asked to take and hold a deep breath; the needle is then introduced into the kidney, the tissue sample is obtained, and the needle is removed. Pressure is applied to the site to stop the bleeding. The patient is requested to remain in bed for six to eight hours after the procedure. Pain medicines are prescribed. Hemorrhage should be monitored in the patient's urine upon return to the ICU (University of Virginia Health System, 2005).

Cystoscopy

Cystoscopy entails use of a tiny camera on the end of a probe, which can be used inside the urethra, vagina, or bladder to locate the ureteral openings (University of Virginia Health System, 2005).

Intravenous Pyelogram

With an intravenous pyelogram (IVP), contrast dye is given intravenously and radiographs are taken showing the dye move through the kidneys, through the ureters, and into the bladder (University of Virginia Health System, 2005). Assessment of patient allergies to iodine is critical prior to administering this diagnostic test. Those individuals who are allergic to iodine or shellfish should be evaluated for possible use of prophylactic drugs such as diphenhydramine (Benadryl®) prior to the procedure or whether the severity of the allergic reaction should preclude the test.

Renal Arteriogram

A renal arteriogram is performed to examine the blood vessels of the kidneys. Contrast material is injected into one or more arteries so they may be seen and evaluated. The site of the test is usually the groin. A local anesthetic is administered, and a needle is then inserted into the artery. A catheter is threaded up to the abdominal aorta. Next, the contrast material is injected into the renal artery and x-rays are taken. The catheter is then withdrawn. Pressure is applied to the leg at the site of insertion for 10 to 15 minutes or longer to stop the bleeding. After that time, the area is checked and a tight bandage is applied. The leg should be kept straight for an additional 12 hours after the procedure. Patients may report discomfort from the catheter insertion or feeling flushed, a burning sensation, or nausea when the contrast material is instilled. Upon return to the ICU, the nurse should observe for bleeding or clotting at the insertion site. Other complications may include internal bleeding outside the renal artery, blood clots, kidney failure, or loss of kidney function (University of Virginia Health System, 2005). Contrast material elimination is enhanced by the administration of a liter of IV fluid post procedure.

ASSESSMENT OF THE RENAL SYSTEM IN THE ICU

Assessing for kidney dysfunction should be routine with any admission to the ICU. Individuals entering the ICU are at risk for developing renal complications associated with their primary diagnosis. Numerous clinical factors place the patient at risk for developing kidney disease, including hypertension, diabetes, hypovolemia, sepsis, and shock states. Persons deemed to be at risk should be followed closely for detection of proteinuria and anuria. While receiving care in the ICU, the nurse utilizes the pattern of urinary output with regard to amount, color, clarity or sediment, and odor to analyze the patient's risk. The nurse should assess drugs ordered for the patient for the risk of nephrotoxicity. Patient complaints of frequency, urgency, hesitation, and dysuria should be reported to the physician. All diagnostic tests on the chart should be evaluated for their relationship to the renal status of the patient. Patients in the ICU often have fluid imbalance associated with their underlying condition, which requires the nurse to monitor intake with output to ensure balance. If the intake and output are not balanced, the nurse should consider notifying the physician for further orders. The most accurate reflection of the patient's fluid status is daily weights. Nurses caring for patients in the ICU need to understand the diagnostic tests for assessing renal function and have an understanding of the physiology of the kidney to ensure at least minimal clinical judgment in providing optimal patient care.

SUMMARY

A comprehensive assessment of the renal system in conjunction with application of knowledge of renal anatomy and physiology can assist the ICU nurse with developing a plan of care for the patient with actual or potential renal problems.

CRITICAL THINKING QUESTIONS

1. Describe the role of each area of the kidney in the formation of urine.
2. Describe why GFR is a more reliable indicator of renal function than serum creatinine or BUN.
3. Describe your role as a facilitator of learning in patients' renal diagnostic procedures.
4. How does the administration of furosemide (Lasix®) affect the renal system?
5. Describe the assessment data required to determine whether a patient is at risk for renal dysfunction.

Online Resources

MedicineNet.com: www.medterms.com

National Kidney Federation: www.kidney.org.uk

Nephron Information Center: www.nephron.com

RenalNet: www.renalnet.org

Urologyhealth.org. www.urologyhealth.org

REFERENCES

Amerling, R., & Levin, N. (2001). Uremia. In S. Massry & R. Glassrock (Eds.), *Textbook of nephrology* (4th ed., pp. 551–561). Philadelphia: Lippincott Williams & Wilkins.

Chmielewski, C. (2003). Renal anatomy and overview of nephron function. *Nephrology Nursing Journal, 30*(2), 185–190.

Churchill, D. N., Blake, P. G., Jindal, K. K., Tofflemire, E. B., & Goldstein, M. B. (1999). Clinical practice guidelines for initiation of dialysis. Canadian Society of Nephrology. *Journal of the American Society of Nephrology, 10*(Suppl. 13), S289–S291.

Curry, F. R. (2005). Atrial natriuretic peptide: An essential physiological regulator of transvascular fluid, protein transport, and plasma volume. *Journal of Clinical Investigation, 115*(6), 1458–1461.

Delanaye, P., & Krzesinski, J. M. (2005).The new Mayo Clinic equation for estimating glomerular filtration rate. *Annals of Internal Medicine, 142*(8), 679–680.

Fehrman-Ekholm, I., & Skeppholm, L. (2004). Renal function in the elderly (>70 years old) measured by means of iohexol clearance, serum creatinine, serum urea and estimated clearance. *Scandinavian Journal of Urology and Nephrology, 38*(1), 73–77.

Giuliano, K. (2001). Renal system. In D. Lynn-McHale & K. Carlson (Eds.), *AACN procedure manual for critical care* (4th ed., pp. 717–752). Philadelphia: Saunders.

Henke, K., & Eigsti, J. (2003). Renal physiology: Review and practical application in the critically ill patient. *Dimensions of Critical Care Nursing, 22*(3), 125–132.

Huether, S. (2002). Structure and function of the renal and urologic system. In K. McCance & S. Huether (Eds.), *Pathophysiology* (4th ed., pp. 1170–1190). St. Louis, MO: Mosby.

Khan, F., Sachs, H. J., Pechet, L., & Snyder, L. M. (2002). *Guide to diagnostic testing.* Baltimore: Lippincott Williams & Wilkins.

Manjunath, G., Sarnak, M. J., & Levey, A. S. (2001). Estimating the glomerular filtration rate. Dos and don'ts for assessing kidney function. *Postgraduate Medicine, 110*(6), 55–62.

MedicineNet.com. (2005). Retrieved October 6, 2005, from www.medterms.com

Perkins, C. (2005). Renal nursing. Utilizing physiological knowledge to care for acute renal failure. *British Journal of Nursing, 14*(14), 768–773.

Rule, A. D., Larson, T. S., Bergstralh, E. J., Slezak, J. M., Jacobsen, S. J., & Cosio, F. G. (2004). Using serum creatinine to estimate glomerular filtration rate: Accuracy in good health and in chronic kidney disease. *Annals of Internal Medicine, 141*, 929–937.

University of Virginia Health System. (2005). www.healthsystemvirginia.edu/uvahealth/peds_urology/kidneytran.cfm

Urologyhealth.org. (2005). Retrieved October 6, 2006, from www.urologyhealth.org

Van Biesen, W., Vanholder, R., Veys, N., Verbeke, F., Delanghe, J., De Bacquer, D., et al. (2006). The importance of standardization of creatinine in the implementation of guidelines and recommendations for CKD: Implications for CKD management programmes. *Nephrology Dialysis and Transplant, 21*(1), 77–83.

CHAPTER 44

Acute Renal Failure

Carol Isaac MacKusick

LEARNING OBJECTIVES

Upon completion of this chapter, the reader will be able to:

1. Describe the causes, assessment findings, and treatments unique to each type of acute renal failure.

2. Explain clinical judgment in selecting appropriate nursing interventions during the four stages of acute renal failure.

3. Use the role of facilitator of learning in delineating appropriate client and family teaching strategies related to acute renal failure.

4. Differentiate between acute renal failure, chronic kidney disease, and end-stage renal disease.

5. Recognize resources available to the nursing and healthcare community to further assist in care and education of the acute renal failure client and family.

6. List optimal outcomes that may be achieved through evidence-based management of the patient with acute renal failure.

Acute renal failure (ARF) is a commonly seen manifestation in the intensive care setting; it has been documented to affect as many as 25% of all intensive care unit (ICU) patients (Bellomo, Kellum, Mehta, Palevsky, & Ronco, 2002). Generally recognized by a sudden, rapid deterioration in renal function, ARF oftentimes occurs as part of a multisystem organ disorder such as trauma or shock. Despite new treatment strategies and surveillance methods, an increasing number of patients develop ARF annually, and mortality rates remain greater than 50% (Ronco, Kellum, Mehta, Bellomo, & Palevsky, 2002).

Three types of ARF exist, each with its own presenting signs and symptoms, nursing interventions, and treatment methods. Diagnosis is based on the point of initial renal insult: prerenal—before the kidney; intrarenal—also known as intrinsic, or within the kidney; or postrenal—injury occurring after the kidney. The most common cause of ARF is acute tubular necrosis (ATN), a form of intrarenal ARF (Richard, 2001). Each type of ARF follows its own disease course, or pattern, which includes four stages: initiation, oliguric, diuretic, and recovery. For the patient who recovers from ARF, moderate to good return of renal function should be anticipated.

RENAL FAILURE

ARF is a syndrome that is noted by a marked and oftentimes rapid decline in renal function that results in alterations in electrolyte balances, acid–base status, fluid volume status, and nitrogenous waste accumulation, as well as a decrease in the production of erythropoietin. In some cases, alteration in bone metabolism may occur, although this problem is most common in patients with longer courses of ARF. In the majority of cases, an insult to the patient results in multiple organ distress and thus affects the ability of the kidneys and renal system to function appropriately. Management of the ARF patient will vary based on the etiology and degree of renal injury. Although mortality rates remain high, for the patient who recovers from ARF, normal return of kidney function can be anticipated.

Some signs, symptoms, and treatments for ARF, chronic kidney disease (CKD), and end-stage renal disease (ESRD; see Chapter 46) are similar, because resolution of certain types of problems (e.g., fluid volume overload) requires identical treatment, though the diseases themselves are *not* identical. It is important to remember that ARF is reversible if aggressive treatment is initiated in a timely manner. Although it is possible that the patient with ARF may develop CKD or progress to ESRD, this chapter focuses on only the etiologies, assessments, and interventions appropriate for the ARF patient.

Prerenal Acute Renal Failure

At the most basic physiologic level, the etiology behind prerenal ARF is decreased blood flow to the kidneys. **Table 44-1** outlines common causes of prerenal ARF. The kidneys will attempt to compensate for decreased perfusion via autoregulation and the release of renin (Richard, 2001); if renal hypoperfusion persists and cannot be corrected by the kidney's adaptive mechanism, however, ARF develops.

Patient Assessment Findings

E.L., a 22-year-old college senior, presents to the Emergency Department after a serious motor vehicle crash. He was transported via ambulance and was unresponsive except to painful stimuli upon arrival. Vital signs on admission were blood pressure 68/palpable, pulse 143, and respirations 28 and shallow. E.L.'s temperature was not obtained, but his skin was clammy. Abdominal assessment indicated a ruptured spleen, and he was sent for immediate surgery. E.L. was also noted to have a compound fracture of the femur (which was repaired) and a hemothorax. He arrived postoperative to the ICU. He is in traction, is receiving oxygen via face mask, has a chest tube draining to wall suction, has a central venous catheter in place for fluid, and responds to verbal commands. E.L. received six

units of packed red blood cells during surgery. It was estimated that he had been at the accident scene 40 minutes prior to the arrival of the emergency medical services. He is now approximately 11 hours post accident. His mother and father sit anxiously at the bedside and appear supportive of their son.

From the preceding scenario, the nurse recognizes that E.L. is at risk for developing prerenal ARF secondary to his acute blood loss, the abdominal trauma that he sustained, and his recent surgical experience. Other history-related risk factors that should be considered when assessing for prerenal ARF include high fever (indicating infection or possible alterations in the vascular resistance of the client), recent acute myocardial infarction, anaphylactic drug or transfusion reactions, cardiac arrest with successful resuscitation, changes in dietary habits, diuretic use, and medication history (Richard, 2001). Patients at risk for development of prerenal ARF need to have strict intake and output monitoring; be frequently reassessed for fluid volume depletion; maintain strict blood pressure monitoring and records; and have frequent laboratory tests to determine the extent (if any) of renal damage (Richard). Blood pressure and oxygen saturation levels should also be frequently measured and recorded. **Table 44-2** notes common laboratory findings associated with prerenal ARF.

Two days post surgery, it is noted that E.L.'s urinary output has decreased to approximately 350 mL per 24 hours.

Nursing Interventions

Based on the assessment findings, the ICU nurse would anticipate that E.L. might have developed prerenal ARF. Treatment considerations with prerenal ARF focus on reestablishing renal perfusion. Fluid challenges for patients with prerenal ARF are common during the initial manifestation of the disease state (Richard, 2001). The ICU nurse should anticipate and prepare to deliver intravenous (IV) fluids to help increase circulatory volume. If no urinary output is present after 30 minutes, a fluid challenge may be repeated one time (Richard).

TABLE 44-1 Causes of Prerenal Acute Renal Failure

- Alterations in blood volume status: hemorrhage, burns, shock, profuse sweating, peritonitis, nephrotic syndrome, gastrointestinal losses, diuretic abuse, diabetes insipidus, malignancies
- Alterations in peripheral vascular system: sepsis, some antihypertensive medications, drug overdose, anaphylactic reactions, neurogenic shock
- Alterations in cardiac system: chronic heart failure, myocardial infarction, cardiac tamponade, cardiac arrhythmias, cardiac resuscitation
- Alterations in renal artery function: renal emboli and thrombi, renal stenosis, renal artery aneurysm, renal artery occlusion, renal trauma
- Alterations in liver/renal system: hepatorenal syndrome— cirrhosis followed by unexplained renal and liver failure

Source: Tonelli, Manns, & Feller-Kopman, 2002.

TABLE 44-2 Laboratory Findings with Prerenal ARF

- Oliguria: urinary output less than 400 mL/24 hr
- Increased urine osmolality and specific gravity
- Decreased urinary sodium and urinary urea
- Increased blood urea nitrogen (BUN), increased BUN to serum creatinine ratio
- Serum creatinine generally normal or high normal

Source: Richard, 2001.

During the fluid challenge, the ICU nurse will closely monitor E.L.'s cardiovascular and pulmonary status to ensure that no compromise in circulation or air exchange develops (Burrows-Hudson, Prowant, & Currier, 2005). The ICU nurse is also aware of the need to closely monitor E.L. during this period for urinary output, blood pressure control, change in body weight, and potential acid–base disturbances. When no actual nephron damage has occurred, recovery from prerenal ARF can be rapid (Richard, 2001). Prolonged prerenal ARF can and will lead to intrarenal ARF, which carries a much higher mortality rate.

Patient and Family Teaching

As E.L.'s status changes, both he and his family will have questions regarding the basic function of the kidneys, the relationship between the motor vehicle crash and renal health, and the role of the kidneys in the overall health of E.L. Specific teaching should initially focus on the disease state and plan of care, allowing for full expression of patient and family feelings and time for appropriate discussion regarding alternatives to treatment. The ICU nurse should encourage and respond to any patient and family member questions as accurately and succinctly as possible.

Intrarenal Acute Renal Failure

Intrarenal acute renal failure is also known as intrinsic acute renal failure or acute tubular necrosis (ATN). ATN, which accounts for the majority of ARF cases, results when renal tissue is physically damaged due to injury or insult (Dirkes & Kozlowski, 2003). The majority of the cases of ATN result in suppression of bone marrow, endocrine disturbance, coagulopathy, and cardiovascular dysfunction, because normal homeostasis can no longer be maintained. **Table 44-3** outlines causes of intrarenal acute renal failure.

TABLE 44-3 Causes of Intrarenal Acute Renal Failure

- Exposure to nephrotoxic agents: drugs, contrast agents, environmental agents, heavy metals
- Hemolysis
- Inflammatory processes
- Alteration in immune system
- Trauma: penetrating or nonpenetrating
- Intrarenal obstruction: tumors, stones, scar tissue
- Prolonged prerenal acute renal failure: prolonged hypovolemia or shock

---

Source: Richard, 2001.

Renal cellular death begins to occur when mean arterial pressure falls below 75 mm Hg (Richard, 2001). The extensiveness of the renal damage can be estimated by determining the length of time since the renal ischemia occurred. Ischemia of 25 minutes or less may cause reversible mild injury, ischemia of 40 to 60 minutes may cause damage that will take the kidneys two to three weeks to recover, and ischemia lasting longer than 1 to 1.5 hours may cause irreversible damage (Richard). As ischemia progresses, the renal tubular cells swell and become necrotic—hence the name acute tubular necrosis.

Patient Assessment Findings

As the nurse caring for E.L., you are concerned about the potential progression to ATN, and would frequently assess for the following changes:

- Oliguria
- Increased blood urea nitrogen (BUN)
- Elevated serum creatinine
- Isosthenuria (a condition in which urinary osmolality approximates plasma osmolality).

Frequent laboratory testing will be indicated, because no one physical assessment finding can differentiate ATN from prerenal ARF. ATN is characterized by the kidney's inability to conserve sodium, and it has a slower recovery process and requires more intense management than does prerenal ARF. The interventions and assessments initiated with prerenal ARF—strict intake and output, monitoring of oxygen saturation, blood pressure, and fluid status—will continue or should be initiated in any patient at risk for development of ATN or who has actually developed ATN.

Nursing Interventions

The major treatment goal in ATN is to remove the causative agent and begin the clinical recovery course. As the nurse caring for E.L., the primary goal in helping to prevent his prerenal ARF from developing into ATN would be to monitor and aid in prevention of further ischemic episodes. Additionally, some patients will demonstrate improved renal function with administration of fluids and diuretics. Calcium channel blockers and low doses of dopamine are also sometimes administered to aid in maintenance of renal perfusion (Tonelli, Manns, & Feller-Kopman, 2002). Many patients require renal replacement therapy (RRT) during the course of recovery from ATN (Dirkes & Kozlowski, 2003). RRT will be discussed in detail in Chapter 45.

Patient and Family Teaching

If RRT becomes necessary for E.L. during his recovery, the procedure—including its risks, side effects, vascular access, length of treatment, and patient positioning—should be fully explained to both the patient and the family. Explaining the clinical condition and the anticipated course of recovery will help the patient and family understand the need for invasive therapy. The nurse should answer any questions that may arise from the family and should also review the process involved in delivery of RRT (Burrows-Hudson et al., 2005).

Postrenal Acute Renal Failure

Postrenal ARF results when the flow of urine is disrupted or obstructed. **Table 44-4** lists some common causes of postrenal ARF.

When urine flow is obstructed, pressure increases in the nephron and the glomerular filtration rate (GFR) slows (Richard, 2001). Serum creatinine and BUN rise. If postrenal ARF continues for long periods of time, nephron damage can occur.

Patient Assessment Findings

The patient presenting with postrenal ARF may have a positive history for some or all of the following:

- Change in urinary volume
- Prostate enlargement or abdominal tumors
- Recent pregnancy
- Recent abdominal surgery
- Paraplegia or quadriplegia
- Bladder obstruction, urinary tract obstruction, urinary tract stones, urinary stasis

Physical assessment findings will vary based on the etiology of the postrenal ARF. Physical assessment findings will correlate with laboratory findings and historical data.

J.P. is a 78-year-old male with a past history of benign prostate hyperplasia. Recently, he has been complaining of a decrease in his urinary stream; he frequently feels the need to void, but is unable to do so. Physical assessment findings indicate a distended bladder. Laboratory findings indicate that J.P.'s

TABLE 44-4 Causes of Postrenal Acute Renal Failure

- Postrenal blockage: urethral or bladder neck obstruction, prostate enlargement, scar tissue in the retroperitoneal cavity, abdominal or pelvic tumors, bladder rupture, neurogenic bladder (a condition when the nerves that control the bladder and urination do not function properly)
- Exposure to some drugs: antihistamines, ganglionic-blocking agents
- Pregnancy

Source: Richard, 2001.

serum creatinine and BUN have risen dramatically since his last routine physical exam. Other laboratory findings that may be noted in the setting of postrenal ARF include the following:

- Change in urinary output—the patient may complain of a sudden onset of anuria, may be oliguric, or may have polyuria
- Change in urine osmolality and specific gravity, and decreases in urine urea and sodium
- Increases in serum creatinine and BUN

Nursing Interventions

After informed consent is obtained, J.P. is prepared for prostate surgery. It is explained to him that he will return with a urinary catheter in place to assist in monitoring his urinary output and to flush the surgical area as needed. The primary goal in postrenal ARF is to remove the obstruction, thereby facilitating the return of normal kidney function (Richard, 2001). Resection or removal of the prostate gland in J.P.'s case will allow for reestablishment of a normal urinary flow pattern.

Patient and Family Teaching

If surgical interventions are required to remove the postrenal obstruction, appropriate surgical teaching needs to be performed. Teaching will vary based on the type of intervention performed. In J.P.'s case, review of the procedure and the facts that urinary incontinence may be an issue post procedure, that normal sexual activity may need to be altered until healing has occurred, and that blood-tinged urine is common for several weeks post surgery are common teaching points. The patient generally is discharged to home with a urinary catheter in place. Return of normal kidney function can be anticipated in a relatively speedy manner if prompt treatment is initiated and delay had not occurred between the onset of symptoms and the time when the client sought care. The patient will need to continue to follow up for routine laboratory testing after removal of the obstruction to ensure that no reoccurrences happen and that return to kidney function baseline has resumed.

CLINICAL STAGING OF ACUTE RENAL FAILURE

The ARF patient will follow a relatively predictable course of disease state progression—initiation, oliguria, diuresis, and recovery—regardless of the type of renal failure. The total length of time from onset of renal damage to recovery can last from months to one year. Generally, patients are managed in the ICU setting until the recovery stage has begun (Ronco, Bellomo, & Kellum, 2002).

Initiation Stage

The initiation stage of ARF begins when the renal insult occurs and lasts from a few hours to a few days. Initial signs and symptoms of renal impairment are noticed, and the cause of ARF is investigated.

Initial signs and symptoms generally include a decrease in urinary output, wet lung sounds, potentially muffled cardiac sounds or development of a new-onset heart murmur, and an increase in body weight (indicating fluid volume overload). The nurse's primary responsibility for patients at risk for developing ARF is to ensure that both intake and output are recorded and accurately monitored. Failure to do so could result in a much more serious course of the disease for the patient.

Oliguric Stage

Oliguria is the decrease in urinary volume to less than 400 mL/day. Diminished urinary output may result from inadequate perfusion of the kidneys (such as with shock or dehydration), from intrarenal diseases (where the tubules can no longer appropriately collect urine), or from obstruction to renal outflow (e.g., with hydronephrosis). The oliguric stage generally lasts one to two weeks (Richard, 2001). Data suggest that the longer a patient stays in the oliguric stage, the worse the prognosis becomes, because alterations in renal endocrine functions become more severe over time (Ronco, Bellomo, et al., 2002).

Laboratory values will indicate a decrease in GFR, increases in serum creatinine and BUN, and increases in electrolytes excreted by the renal system (e.g., potassium and phosphorus). Laboratory values must be closely monitored, because a frequent cause of death during the oliguric stage is cardiac arrest secondary to hyperkalemia (Richard, 2001). Additionally, as azotemia (the buildup of nitrogenous waste products normally eliminated through urinary output) progresses, the patient is at an increased risk for infection and gastrointestinal bleeding (Dirkes & Kozlowski, 2003). Patients require intense day-to-day surveillance, because the mortality rate during the oliguric stage is greater than 50% (Ronco, Kellum, et al., 2002). Approximately half of all patients with ARF do not present with oliguria; patients with non-oliguric ARF have an increased chance of survival and faster recovery times. Renal healing begins during the diuretic phase, as the renal tubules begin to regenerate.

Nursing care and interventions for the patient in the oliguric stage of ARF include the following measures:

- Prevention of secondary infections by implementation of preventive measures; monitoring of wound drainage, vital signs, lung and heart sounds, and laboratory values; and treatment of any potential or identified infections promptly.
- Monitoring of fluid volume status through daily weights; strict monitoring of intake and output; assessment of periorbital, sacral, and extremity edema; record-

ing of color and clarity of urinary output; assessment of lung and heart sounds, pulse, blood pressure, and respiratory rate; and limiting fluid intake to 500 mL plus urinary output daily.
- Monitoring of electrolyte status to include sodium, potassium, phosphorus, and calcium, and reporting and treatment of dangerously high and low levels as appropriate; instituting and evaluating cardiac monitoring for changes in cardiac conduction related to electrolyte changes.
- Monitoring for metabolic acidosis through arterial blood gas values.
- Monitoring for gastrointestinal and cutaneous bleeding, and instituting appropriate bleeding precautions; monitoring for anemia; and administering blood products or erythropoietin products, as prescribed.
- Ensuring appropriate nutritional intake, and consulting with appropriate dietary staff to ensure that all metabolic demands are being met through a renal-regulated diet; monitoring and treating anorexia, nausea, and vomiting as appropriate.
- Reviewing medication administration and dosing to ensure that further nephrotoxicity does not occur.
- Ensuring adequate skin care to help prevent skin breakdown.
- Assisting the patient with self-concept issues that relate to the lack of privacy, change in body function, fatigue, and inability to meet personal or professional demands.
- Helping the client meet daily rest requirements.
- Preparing the client and family for RRT as indicated. Consult with the pharmacist and physician about the potential need to discontinue use of angiotensin converting enzyme (ACE) inhibitors prior to the first RRT treatment (Daugirdas, Blake, & Ing, 2001). Continuous renal replacement therapy (CRRT) or intermittent hemodialysis may be performed based on the patient's overall condition and the hospital's capabilities (Ronco, Bellomo, et al., 2002). Some facilities are now offering renal assistive devices as an alternative to CRRT (Dirkes & Kozlowski, 2003). The renal assistive device entails the use of a bio-artificial kidney to replace kidney function in the ARF patient. Phase II clinical investigations are underway to determine the applicability of this replacement cellular technology (Dirkes & Kozlowski).
- Assessing neurological status and implementing needed safety requirements.
- Assisting the patient, family, and other significant others in understanding the role of the kidneys and renal function and the relationship to testing and disease state (Burrows-Hudson et al., 2005; Richard, 2001).

Diuretic Stage

The diuretic stage begins after the oliguric stage has completed, lasts for approximately two weeks, and is evidenced by an increase in urinary output. Previously retained solutes act as osmotic agents and, as renal tubular patency is restored, diuresis begins (Richard, 2001). ARF patients who never developed oliguria tend to have shorter periods of diuresis and a faster recovery period (Ronco, Bellomo, et al., 2002). Generally, patients regain most of their initial kidney function during this stage, although this recovery is totally dependent on the initial amount of membrane damage and the length of time in the oliguric stage (Richard; Tonelli et al., 2002). As the diuresis stage nears completion, signs and symptoms of azotemia resolve.

ARF patients in the diuretic stage remain subject to a high mortality rate and are at increased risk for infection and bleeding. Care focuses on day-to-day management to ensure patient survival. Nursing care for the ARF patient in the diuretic stage includes the following measures:

- Continuation of accurate fluid assessment. Fluid volume deficit is a common problem during this stage because RRT may continue, urinary excretion is increased, and oral intake cannot compensate for the loss. Mucous membranes and skin turgor should be frequently assessed; daily weights, regular vital signs, and strict intake and output monitoring continue to be required; and monitoring for hypotension, dizziness, and hard stools should be included in the assessment.
- Coordination with a renal dietitian to ensure that an appropriate fluid and nutritional plan remain in place; oral fluids may be increased to the amount of loss plus 500 mL daily.
- Monitoring of electrolyte status as the diuretic stage continues, to include sodium, potassium, phosphorus, and calcium; monitoring for cardiac conduction changes with the potential for rapid electrolyte changes; assessment for neuromuscular irritability, constipation, or diminished reflexes.
- Monitoring and treatment of metabolic alkalosis with drugs such as acetazolamide (Diamox®).
- Continued monitoring for and treatment of infections, and implementing appropriate precautions.
- Continued monitoring for gastrointestinal and cutaneous bleeding, and instituting appropriate bleeding precautions.
- Continued routine and preventive skin care to avoid skin breakdown.
- Continued monitoring of drug dosages to help avoid further nephrotoxicity.

- Continued assisting of the patient in maintenance of daily rest patterns.
- Continued provision of appropriate disease state education for the patient and support system (Burrows-Hudson et al., 2005; Richard, 2001).

Recovery Stage

The recovery stage begins immediately after completion of diuresis and will last for several months to one year. During this time, the patient's kidney function returns to near baseline, and the renal tubules are functionally intact. Urinary output, urine solutes, and serum concentrations all return to within normal limits. Patients are generally transferred to home with follow-up instructions with both a nephrologist and other healthcare providers, and discharge instructions based on their ARF etiology (Burrows-Hudson et al., 2005; Richard, 2001).

KEY RESEARCH

Intensive care nephrology has been the target of recent quality initiatives, and the National Kidney Foundation has created a task force to implement the acute dialysis quality initiative (ADQI) (Ronco, Kellum, et al., 2002). Research into improvement and practice patterns for the ARF patient have included topics such as decision-making criteria for CRRT, appropriately defining ARF, developing consensus recommendations for best practices, establishing evidence-based guidelines when applicable, and defining future research topics (Kellum, 2002). To date, several recommendations and consensus statements have been developed and are being further explored.

PATIENT OUTCOMES

Nurses can help ensure the obtainment of optimal patient outcomes such as those listed in **Box 44-1** through the use of evidence-based interventions for acute renal failure patients.

Box 44-1
Optimal Patient Outcomes

- Acid-base balance in expected range
- Fluid and electrolyte in expected range
- Hemoglobin and hematocrit in expected range
- Cardiovascular and pulmonary status in expected range
- Knowledge of disease state and plan of care

SUMMARY

The ARF patient is generally complex, highly vulnerable, and fragile. The family and patient together may need assistance in engaging in decision-making and care processes. These patients require nurses who exhibit strong clinical judgment and caring, and are willing to collaborate with the entire healthcare team. For these reasons, application of the Synergy Model for Patient Care (AACN, 2004) is an appropriate guide to help link clinical practice to patient outcomes.

CRITICAL THINKING QUESTIONS

1. E.L. was at risk for progression to acute tubular necrosis. Why? Could anything have been done to prevent his initial acute renal failure?

2. J.P. developed a post renal obstruction resulting in postrenal ARF. What are other causes for postrenal ARF? How can they be prevented?

3. Why do you feel that the mortality rate remains almost 50% for ARF? What can be done to improve this rate?

4. Why is metabolic acidosis a concern during the oliguric stage? During the diuretic stage, alkalosis becomes a concern. What would the typical presentation of both be? Why do they occur?

5. What would be two appropriate nursing problems for all four stages of ARF? Create a care map for one of these problems.

6. Describe the pathophysiology behind ATN.

7. Why do ACE inhibitors require discontinuation prior to the first RRT treatment in some cases? What other pharmacological management would you anticipate in the client with ARF? During the diuretic stage, which type of IV fluids would you anticipate being ordered? During attempted renal reperfusion of the prerenal ARF patient, which type of IV fluids would you anticipate being ordered?

8. Develop a diet plan for the patient with ATN in the oliguric stage. How would this plan change when diuresis begins?

9. What type of electrocardiographic changes would you anticipate with alterations in electrolyte status?

CASE STUDY

P.J. is an 84-year-old female who was admitted to the ICU of your hospital after an abdominal aortic aneurysm resection. For the last seven years, P.J. has been treated for decreased cardiac output and has been noted by her cardiologist to have decreased cardiac contractility. She is a widow and has one daughter who lives out of state.

CRITICAL THINKING QUESTIONS

1. As you prepare for her care, how can you recognize that P.J. is at risk for ARF? How would you manage this concern?

2. Which signs and symptoms need to be immediately reported to the healthcare team?

3. Which nursing interventions will be unique for the patient who has ARF or who is at risk for development of ARF?

4. Which disciplines should be consulted to work with this client?

5. How will you implement your role as a facilitator of learning for this patient?

6. Given your knowledge of acute renal failure, use the form to write up a list of educational resources available for the patient and family.

7. Identify three research studies focused on acute renal failure.

Using the Synergy Model as a Facilitator of Learning

	Resource	Location of Resource
SYNERGY MODEL		

Using the Synergy Model for Clinical Inquiry

	Article	Summary
SYNERGY MODEL		

Online Resources

The following web-based resources will provide up-to-date information related to acute renal failure, and aid in professional education and development of patient teaching plans:

- **Acute Dialysis Quality Initiative:** www.ADQI.net
  The website devoted to improvement of care and research related to acute renal failure and acute dialysis topics.

- **American Association of Kidney Patients:** www.aakp.org
  A national kidney patient education organization that provides free educational materials for patients and families with or at risk for development of kidney disease.

- **American Nephrology Nurses' Association:** www.annanurse.org
  The specialty nursing organization for nurses working in or with nephrology patients, or patients at risk for developing renal problems.

- **National Kidney Foundation:** www.kidney.org
  A national advocacy organization for renal patients and healthcare professionals. Provides research and quality initiatives for renal-related issues.

- **Renal Web:** www.renalweb.com
  A news website devoted to current topics related to or about renal health issues.

- **United States Renal Data System:** www.usrds.gov
  A U.S. government tracking website that contains data and statistics related to patients with renal disease.

REFERENCES

American Association of Critical-Care Nurses. (2004). The AACN synergy model for patient care. Retrieved May 11, 2005, from AACN Certification Corporation, www.certcorp.org/certcorp/certcorp.nsf/vwdoc/SynModel?opendocument

Bellomo, R., Kellum, J., Mehta, R., Palevsky, P., & Ronco, C. (2002). The acute dialysis quality initiative II: The Vicenza conference. *Advances in Renal Replacement Therapy, 9*(4), 290–293.

Burrows-Hudson, S., Prowant, B. F., & Currier, H. (2005). *Nephrology nursing standards of practice and guidelines for care.* Pitman, NJ: American Nephrology Nurses' Association.

Daugirdas, J. T., Blake, P. G., & Ing, T. S. (2001). *Handbook of dialysis* (3rd ed.). Philadelphia: Lippincott Williams & Wilkins.

Dirkes, S. M., & Kozlowski, C. (2003). Renal assist device therapy for acute renal failure. *Nephrology Nursing Journal, 30*(6), 611–620.

Kellum, J. (2002). The acute dialysis quality initiative: Methodology. *Advances in Renal Replacement Therapy, 9*(4), 245–247.

Richard, C. (2001). Renal disorders. In L. E. Lancaster (Ed.), *Core curriculum for nephrology nursing* (4th ed., pp. 83–115). Pitman, NJ: American Nephrology Nurses' Association.

Ronco, C., Bellomo, R., & Kellum, J. (2002). Continuous renal replacement therapy: Opinions and evidence. *Advances in Renal Replacement Therapy, 9*(4), 229–244.

Ronco, C., Kellum, J., Mehta, R., Bellomo, R., & Palevsky, P. (2002). The acute dialysis quality initiative: A focused review. *Advances in Renal Replacement Therapy, 9*(4), 227–228.

Tonelli, M., Manns, B., & Feller-Kopman, D. (2002). Acute renal failure in the intensive care unit: A systematic review of the impact of dialytic modality on mortality and recovery of renal function. *American Journal of Kidney Diseases, 40*(5), 875–885.

Interventions for the Renal System

Carol Isaac MacKusick

LEARNING OBJECTIVES

Upon completion of this chapter, the reader will be able to:

1. Differentiate between hemodialysis, peritoneal dialysis, and continuous renal replacement therapies.

2. Describe appropriate patient selection for renal replacement therapy.

3. Describe evidence-based interventions for the client receiving hemodialysis, peritoneal dialysis, and continuous renal replacement therapy.

4. Delineate client and family leaching strategies related to renal replacement therapies.

5. Discuss client timing and initiation strategies for renal replacement therapies, and the differences among them based on modality selection.

6. Recognize resources available to the nursing and healthcare community to further assist in care and education of the client receiving renal replacement therapies.

7. List optimal patient outcomes that may be achieved through evidence-based management of patients with renal disease.

Since the 1960s, renal replacement therapy (RRT) has provided life-saving and life-sustaining treatment for millions of individuals affected with end-stage renal disease (ESRD) (Eknoyan & Levin, 2002). For the patient with ESRD to maintain life, dialysis therapy or transplantation must be elected. In the United States, more than 300,000 individuals are currently receiving some form of RRT (United States Renal Data System, 2002). RRT consists of hemodialysis (HD), peritoneal dialysis (PD), or continuous renal replacement therapy (CRRT). HD and PD are generally utilized for long-term maintenance of the patient with chronic kidney disease (CKD) who has progressed to stage 5 of CKD; in contrast, CRRT is generally used for the patient who has sustained renal insult related to acute renal failure or the CKD patient who is acutely ill in the intensive care unit (ICU). All three modalities and selection criteria for each are discussed throughout this chapter. Care of the patient who elects to undergo transplantation is covered in Chapter 59.

Approximately 75% of all ESRD patients suffered their first renal insult as a result of untreated or undertreated diabetes mellitus or hypertension. As the Type 2 diabetes mellitus population continues to grow, the number of individuals who are at risk for developing renal failure likewise rises. Other etiologies associated with ESRD include pyelonephritis, glomerulonephritis, congenital disorders, systemic lupus erythematosus, sickle cell disease, polycystic kidney disease, renal tubule acidosis, Fanconi syndrome, malignancies of the kidney, Wilms' tumors, renal tuberculosis, and obstructive disorders (Burrows-Hudson, Prowant, & Currier, 2005; Daugirdas, Blake, & Ing, 2001; Richard, 2001).

RENAL REPLACEMENT THERAPIES

The Need for Renal Replacement Therapy

When the glomerular filtration rate (GFR) decreases to less than 15 mL/min/1.73 m^2, an individual is statistically defined as having stage 5 CKD (National Kidney Foundation, 2002). At this level of renal functioning, the kidneys are no longer capable of maintaining their daily function and the health of the individual dramatically declines. The kidneys provide many essential life functions, including regulation of body fluid volume and osmolality; regulation of electrolyte and acid–base balance;

regulation of blood pressure; removal of metabolic waste products, toxins, and drugs; synthesis of vitamin D, prostaglandins, endothelin, and nitric oxide; performance of gluconeogenesis; and secretion of erythropoietin (Coresh, Astor, Greene, Eknoyan, & Levey, 2003). Patients with renal failure express feeling progressively worse in the months prior to entering a dialysis-dependent life, and oftentimes they are anxious to begin to "feel better" with dialysis therapy (Martin-McDonald & Biernoff, 2002).

Chronic Kidney Disease Staging

Normal kidney function is defined as a GFR between 90 and 120 mL/min/1.73 m^2 (Richard, 2001). GFR is considered to be the standard measure when defining the stages of a slowly progressive and insidious disease; it represents the volume of plasma filtered from the glomerular capillaries into the Bowman's capsule each minute and is expressed in units of mL/min/m^2. The National Kidney Foundation's Disease Outcome Quality Initiative (NKF DOQI) has developed a clinical action plan for each of the five stages of CKD.

CKD stage 1 is represented by a client clinically with a GFR greater than or equal to 90 mL/min/1.73 m^2, but who is at risk for or who has had kidney disease or comorbid conditions that indicate kidney damage over three consecutive months. During this stage, individuals should be diagnosed, and disease prevention strategies should be implemented. Steps should be taken to reduce further renal damage and to help eliminate or reduce cardiovascular damage (National Kidney Foundation, 2002). Stage 2 is represented clinically by a GFR of 60 to 89 mL/min/1.73 m^2, and further disease progression estimates should continue at this point. Clients should receive detailed education and follow-up to help slow, stop, or delay progression of the renal disease and damage (National Kidney Foundation). CKD stage 3 is represented by a GFR of 30 to 59 mL/min/1.73 m^2 (National Kidney Foundation). Complications of reduced renal function begin to manifest at this stage, and treatment for anemia, bone disease, and other metabolic disorders may be warranted at this point (McCrory et al., 2002).

As an individual progresses to CKD stage 4 (defined as a GFR of 15 to 29 mL/min/1.73 m^2), the healthcare team should begin to prepare the client for RRT (National Kidney Foundation, 2002). Metabolic signs and symptoms are clinically significant; patients complain of generalized fatigue; a "fugue" state, social isolation, and loneliness frequently develop; and depression may be manifested (Hedayati et al., 2004; McCrory et al., 2002; Molitoris, 2005; Richard, 2001).

The fifth stage of CKD is clinically represented by a GFR of less than 15 mL/min/1.73 m^2 (National Kidney Foundation, 2002). RRT (HD, PD, or scheduled transplantation) should be initiated upon evidence of uremia and will be required as a life-sustaining treatment. Treatment of the many metabolic complications becomes necessary at this point to help provide better patient outcomes upon beginning RRT (McCrory et al., 2002; Richard, 2001). Ideally, patients will begin RRT in a scheduled, non-acute care setting (Daugirdas et al., 2001). Upon initiation of RRT in stage 5 CKD, patients are also known as having ESRD and are classified as ESRD patients by the U.S. Center for Medicare Services.

Acute Renal Failure and RRT

Another patient population that frequently requires dialysis therapy comprises hospitalized, gravely ill clients with acute renal failure (Bellomo, Kellum, Mehta, Palevsky, & Ronco, 2002). These patients present with progressively deteriorating renal function, necessitating the initiation of RRT. Kidney function during initiation of therapy generally falls to 15 mL/min/ 1.73 m^2, similar to the rate seen in a chronically ill patient with stage 5 CKD. Because of the ICU patient's severely debilitated state, initiation of traditional forms of dialysis therapy is not always the best option. Instead, in many cases, CRRT is initiated.

PRINCIPLES OF DIALYSIS

The process of dialysis involves movement of molecules across a semipermeable membrane. If the blood is exposed to an artificial membrane (a dialyzer or hemodialyzer) outside the body, this process is called HD, hemofiltration, or, in some cases, CRRT (Daugirdas et al., 2001). If the exchange of molecules occurs through the peritoneal membrane, the process is called PD (Kelly, 2004). For the movement of solutes and fluids to occur during the dialysis process, the principles of diffusion, osmosis, and ultrafiltration must be applied.

Diffusion

Diffusion is the process of movement of a solute from an area of higher concentration to an area of lower concentration (Daugirdas et al., 2001). Dialysis works through diffusion, which carries the solutes and electrolytes normally removed by the kidneys from the blood through the membrane (the dialyzer or peritoneal membrane) to outside of the body for disposal. Diffusion can best be described by visualization of a tea bag in hot water. When the tea bag is placed in the water, tea (the solute) moves from inside the bag (the membrane) into the water. Tea continues moving from the area of higher concentration (inside the tea bag) to the area of lower concentration (the water in the teacup) until both sides are virtually equal. In this example, both sides would have approximately the same amount of tea.

Osmosis

Osmosis is the movement of a solvent from an area of higher concentration to an area of lower concentration (Daugirdas et al., 2001). Dialysis requires the use of osmosis to remove the fluids normally excreted by the kidneys out of the body, so the patient no longer remains in a state of fluid volume overload. Recalling the tea bag example, as diffusion occurs with the tea (the tea has leached from the bag to the warm water in the teacup), osmosis is also occurring as water leaches into the tea bag.

Ultrafiltration

Osmosis alone will not remove the necessary fluid from the client. The process of ultrafiltration is required to complete the job. Ultrafiltration is the application of force to move solvent (fluid) across a semipermeable membrane (Daugirdas et al., 2001). When preparing a cup of tea, after a proper amount of time has transpired, frequently the tea bag is removed on a spoon, with the tea bag string used to wrap around the spoon and bag, causing any remaining fluid to return to the cup. The force applied by the process of taking the tea bag string and wrapping it tightly around the spoon and bag, thereby causing the water (the solvent) to return to the cup, is ultrafiltration.

All three mechanisms are required during any type of RRT to ensure optimal solute, electrolyte, and fluid balance in the patient. Dialysis, therefore, is a process of diffusion, osmosis, and ultrafiltration by which dissolved particles move across a semipermeable membrane from one fluid compartment to another. This therapy does not cure renal disease or renal failure, but will correct the fluid overload, balance out some electrolyte disturbances, and partially restore the client to optimal acid–base balance.

HEMODIALYSIS

HD is a process where solute and fluid removal occurs as blood crosses over an artificial semipermeable membrane. This artificial semipermeable membrane is known as the hemodialyzer (or dialyzer). HD requires direct access to the vascular compartment (Daugirdas et al., 2001; Keen, Lancaster, & Binkley, 2001; Wagner, 2001). **Table 45-1** describes the differences in means of HD access.

Patients with acute or rapid-onset renal failure who require HD will need a temporary means of entry into the vascular system, generally through either femoral or subclavian venous catheters. These catheters are frequently referred to as central venous catheters (CVCs). Temporary catheters generally are used for only a short period of time, because the risk for infection with these devices is high. For chronic, maintenance HD, a permanent entryway into the vascular system is made either through a surgically created fistula (a surgical connection of a vein and artery) or through a graft (insertion of a material connecting the vein and artery). For maintenance dialysis therapy, the preferred method of vasculature access is the fistula, because it allows optimal dialysis therapy to be achieved (McGill, Healy, Marcus, Sandroni, & Brouwer, 2005).

Patient Assessment Findings

Prior to initiation of any HD treatment (whether acute or chronic in nature), several baseline physical assessment findings

---

TABLE 45-1 Types of Circulatory Access for Hemodialysis

Arteriovenous (AV) graft: A permanent access method for chronic maintenance hemodialysis. Ideal for patients whose vasculature cannot support creation of an AV fistula. The connection between the vein and artery is made surgically with a biologic, semibiologic, or synthetic material. Access is made with large-bore (15- or 16-gauge, one-inch) needles. Generally can be used for treatments approximately two weeks post insertion. Blood pressure readings and serum sampling should never be performed in the AV graft limb.

Central venous catheter (CVC): Constructed of rigid or semirigid material, generally with a double lumen design. One lumen is designated as arterial flow, and the other lumen is designated as venous return. Generally used for emergent, acute hemodialysis treatments. Most types of CVCs are not intended for use over extended periods of time. CVCs have a higher infection rate than other access types.

External AV shunt: No longer in popular use; initially developed in the 1960s. Consists of two rigid tips (generally made from Teflon) implanted into an artery and a vein. Tubing is attached to the tips and brought to the outside of the body. This tubing is connected and disconnected through a Luer lock device, allowing easy access to blood supply for hemodialysis. Blood pressure readings and serum samples should never be obtained from the limb with the AV shunt.

Native AV fistula: The preferred access method for chronic maintenance hemodialysis therapy. Requires a long time for maturation (generally 6 to 12 months). Surgical creation of an anastamosis between the artery and vein allows the fistula to develop. Hemodialysis access is made via large-bore (14- or 15-gauge, one-inch) needles for the dialysis treatment. Blood pressure readings and serum samples should never be obtained from the limb with the AV fistula.

Source: Hartigan & Breiterman-White, 2001.

should be noted. **Table 45-2** compares and contrasts assessment findings important in both the chronic maintenance HD and the acute HD patients.

HD in the hospital setting is generally performed in a designated dialysis room or clinic or, for those clients who are too acutely ill to transfer, at the bedside. HD being performed as chronic maintenance therapy for ESRD clients generally takes place at outpatient dialysis centers. In either setting, HD treatments are typically performed by specially trained registered nurses and patient care technicians.

TABLE 45-2 Predialysis Assessment

	Acute	Chronic
Baseline vital signs	Temperature, blood pressure (supine and standing, if possible), apical pulse (noting quality, rate, and rhythm), radial pulse, respiration (depth and frequency)	Temperature, blood pressure (both sitting and standing), radial and apical pulse (noting rate, rhythm, and quality)
Fluid volume status	Weight, estimated weight gain since last hemodialysis treatment (if applicable), auscultation of all lung fields, auscultation of heart sounds, neck vein distention, presence or absence of edema, pulmonary artery occlusive pressure or central venous pressure as appropriate, intake and output, skin turgor, mucous membrane assessments, presence or absence of ascites	Current body weight, weight gain since last hemodialysis treatment, respiratory status and auscultation of all lung fields, auscultation of heart sounds, assessment of neck vein distention, notation of presence or absence of edema and (if present), extent of edema as applicable
Hematological status	Latest hemoglobin/hematocrit, complaints of new-onset bruising or bleeding, bleeding from access site since last treatment	Latest hemoglobin/hematocrit, complaints of new-onset bruising or bleeding, bleeding from access site since last treatment
Review of new laboratory reports	Special note made of hematologic status, potassium, calcium, magnesium, and phosphorus levels	Serum chemistries, adequacy of dialysis studies, radiograph films, access studies
Vascular access	Status, overall condition, patency (check for thrill [buzzing sensation] and bruit [sound produced by blood flowing through a graft, fistula, or shunt), signs or symptoms of infection	Patency (check for thrill and bruit), signs or symptoms of infection, hematomas at access site, aneurysms at access site, patient complaints of pain
Neurological status	Level of consciousness, orientation, pupil response, hand strength or grip, gait	Orientation, gait
Hospitalization	Reason for current hospitalization, including general overall well-being, patient's subjective reason for hospitalization, presence of infection, presence of comorbid conditions, nutritional status	Reports of any hospitalizations since last treatment
Medications	Currently prescribed inpatient medications (intravenous or oral), presence or absence of parenteral fluids or feedings, oxygen therapy	Reports of any changes in home medications since last treatment, any updated orders for treatment medication changes
Indwelling lines or tubes	Type, reason, appropriately and securely anchored	Type, reason, appropriately and securely anchored
Patient overall status	Patient complaints or concerns, overall general feelings of health and well-being	Patient complaints or concerns, overall general feelings of health and well-being

Source: Keen, Lancaster, & Binkley, 2001.

Following any HD treatment, the nurse must perform a close physical assessment to gauge the fluid volume and solute shift. **Table 45-3** delineates post-HD treatment assessment findings that should be noted in both acute and chronic HD patients. Although most HD is performed by specially trained dialysis staff, assessment findings that are unique to the renal population should be noted during routine assessment by the critical care nurse. Upon completion of the HD treatment, appropriate transfer of care should occur between the dialysis team member and the critical care registered nurse. Assessment findings discussed in this section are of benefit to both the critical care registered nurse and the dialysis team member, and they should be noted in reports given before and after the HD treatment.

TABLE 45-3 Post-dialysis Assessment

	Acute	Chronic
Post-treatment vital signs	Temperature, blood pressure (supine and standing, if possible), comparison of blood pressure to last post-treatment blood pressure, apical pulse (noting quality, rate, and rhythm), radial pulse, respiration (depth and frequency), changes noted since initiation of treatment	Temperature, blood pressure (both sitting and standing), comparison of blood pressure to last post-treatment blood pressure, radial and apical pulses (noting rate, rhythm, and quality), changes noted since initiation of treatment
Fluid volume status	Post-treatment weight, actual weight gain or loss since initiation of treatment, auscultation of all lung fields, auscultation of heart sounds, neck vein distention, presence or absence of edema, pulmonary artery occlusive pressure or central venous pressure as appropriate, intake and output, skin turgor, mucous membrane assessments, presence or absence of ascites	Post-treatment weight, weight loss (or gain) during treatment, respiratory status and auscultation of all lung fields, auscultation of heart sounds, assessment of neck vein distention, notation of presence or absence of edema and (if present) extent of edema as applicable
Hematological status	Post-treatment bleeding time from internal access, amount of heparin received during treatment, amount of heparin placed in central venous catheter (CVC) if applicable	Post-treatment bleeding time from internal access, amount of heparin received during treatment, amount of heparin placed in CVC if applicable
Laboratory reports	Notation of any testing performed during treatment	Notation of any testing performed during treatment
Vascular access	Overall condition, patency (check for thrill and bruit), signs or symptoms of infection, hematomas at access site, aneurysms at access site, patient complaints of pain	Patency (check for thrill and bruit), signs or symptoms of infection, hematomas at access site, aneurysms at access site, patient complaints of pain
Neurological status	Level of consciousness, orientation, pupil response, hand strength or grip, gait	Orientation, gait
Discharge status	Patient stability at end of hemodialysis treatment	Patient stability at end of hemodialysis treatment
Medications	Notes of any medication changes made during treatment	Notes of any medication changes made during treatment
Indwelling lines or tubes	Notes of any changes to indwelling tubes or lines during treatment	Notes of any changes to indwelling tubes or lines during treatment
Patient overall status	Patient complaints or concerns, overall general feelings of health and well-being	Patient complaints or concerns, overall general feelings of health and well-being

Sources: Bellomo, Kellum, Mehta, Palevsky, & Ronco, 2002; Keen, Lancaster, & Binkley, 2001.

Nursing Interventions

Nursing interventions for the ICU nurse who is providing daily care for the patient receiving HD focus on comparing the physiologic changes noted in the patient before and after treatment. Additional interventions should target on maintaining vascular access patency, monitoring vital signs and hemodynamic stability, providing strategies for bowel elimination, monitoring electrolyte status, preventing infection, assessing fluid volume status, maintaining fluid intake restrictions, and maintaining optimal nutritional status while following a renal diet (Burrows-Hudson et al., 2005). Monitoring for hyperkalemia, treating anemia and renal osteodystrophy, and maintaining adequate anticoagulation are other essential interventions when providing care for these patients.

Patient and Family Teaching

Patients new to HD frequently exhibit large amounts of anxiety related to the treatment process itself. Education is key in relieving this anxiety, for both patients and family. Education should be delivered in small doses and covered in several different formats to encourage retention of the material. Patients need to be aware of appropriate diet modifications, steps to preserve access function, signs and symptoms of infection, appropriate fluid volume allowed daily, and signs to report to the nephrology healthcare team.

PERITONEAL DIALYSIS

PD is a process that uses the client's own peritoneal membrane to act as the semipermeable membrane. The process of dialysis occurs when a solution (called dialysate) is introduced through sterile technique into the peritoneal cavity. This solution is then allowed to dwell for a number of hours, permitting the processes of osmosis, diffusion, and ultrafiltration to occur before the dialysate is drained from the peritoneal cavity. In this kind of dialysis, diffusion across the peritoneal membrane is the primary mechanism for solute and fluid removal (Prowant, 2001). The three-part process of entry, dwell, and drain of the dialysate solution in the peritoneal cavity is known as an exchange. The dialysate generally consists of a dextrose-based solution that acts as an osmotic gradient; it is introduced into the peritoneal cavity through a PD catheter inserted through the subcutaneous abdominal wall and intraperitoneal cavity (Kelly, 2004). Several types of PD catheters exist, as outlined in **Table 45-4**.

Two types of PD exist: chronic ambulatory peritoneal dialysis (CAPD) and continuous cycling peritoneal dialysis (CCPD). With CAPD, PD exchanges are performed by the patient or caregiver in a clean environment under sterile conditions four to six times per day. With CCPD, patients are connected to a machine (known as a cycler) that performs exchanges throughout the night or during rest periods.

PD is contraindicated in patients with a larger body mass index, those who are hypercatabolic, and those who have many abdominal wall adhesions or scar tissue from abdominal surgeries. This therapy is an ideal choice for patients with hemodynamic instability or reduced cardiovascular capability, because it provides a gentler form of fluid removal; for patient with limited or diminished vascular access sites; for children; and for geriatric patients. PD also remains the number one choice for ESRD clients who continue to work and are unable to commit to thrice-weekly HD treatments in an outpatient clinic. Maintenance PD therapy secondary to ESRD requires a willingness to perform PD exchanges at home, a desire to undergo a strict training and education program, and the presence of a willing partner to serve as a secondary provider of care.

TABLE 45-4 Peritoneal Dialysis (PD) Catheters

Acute PD Catheters

Stylet catheter: rigid in material, inserted at bedside for immediate use, one-time use only, greater risk of organ perforation and peritonitis, easily removed

Single-cuff silicone catheters: requires surgical insertion; may be used for long-term care if necessary, most commonly used acute PD catheter

Chronic PD Catheters

Straight silicone: also known as a Tenckhoff or Schechter catheter, second most widely used PD catheter in the United States, requires six weeks healing time for use generally, double cuffed (one cuff in the abdominal muscle wall, one cuff in the subcutaneous tissue)

Curled or coiled: most widely used PD catheter in the United States, may be inserted with a trocar, lowest amount of patient-reported pain, highest survival rate

Swan-neck: straight or coiled catheter that is modified with a "U" appearance, specific for one side of the peritoneal cavity only, well suited for patients with peritoneal adhesions on one side of the body

Cruz catheter: made of polyurethane, pail-handle configuration

---

Source: Kelly, 2004.

PD that is performed in the hospital is generally performed by the nursing staff and requires training in sterile exchange technique and in the use of the cycler, should CCPD be the treatment choice. Dialysis staff generally do not perform CAPD exchanges or CCPD connection and disconnection in the hospital setting.

Patient Assessment Findings

PD is a continuous process, so the nurse responsible for care would not expect to see the rapid fluid shifts or electrolyte changes noted in a patient receiving HD treatment. Appropriate monitoring of vital signs, heart and lung sounds, and fluid volume status remains important to determine whether the PD process is functioning optimally for the patient. Notes should be made about the condition of the PD catheter and surrounding tissue. Signs of infection should be immediately reported to the nephrologist for intervention. Herniation in the peritoneal wall is not uncommon in patients receiving PD, and its presence should be carefully evaluated and brought to the attention of the nephrologist. Finally, blood glucose monitoring needs to be initiated on all acute PD clients. The most common additive in PD dialysate is dextrose, which means that hyperglycemia in PD clients is commonplace.

Nursing Interventions

Acute hyperglycemia requires an immediate response and should be treated as per hospital or physician protocol or orders. Treatment may include regular insulin therapy subcutaneously or addition of regular insulin into the dialysate itself. Weight gain from the dextrose solution is not uncommon, and appropriate dietary teaching and controls may need to be implemented. Given that PD is a continuous process, fluid and dietary restrictions are not as strict as those instituted with HD.

Peritonitis is a common problem among PD patients, and one that must be treated immediately. Signs and symptoms of infection must be immediately reported to the physician or nurse practitioner, appropriate aseptic technique utilized during exchanges, and medications administered as necessary. For suspected peritonitis, cultures of the peritoneal fluid are required prior to administration of antibiotics. Antibiotic therapy may be given orally, intravenously, or as part of the dialysate. Catheter care should be performed before every exchange. Drained dialysate should be noted for color, presence of fibrin, and clarity. Generally, drained dialysate should be light yellow, fibrin free, and clear.

Prior to any PD exchange, the PD fluid should be warmed. Microwave ovens are not recommended for warming of the dialysate because uneven warming may occur, causing burning of the peritoneal cavity (Kelly, 2004). Warming of the dialysate should be done on a specially provided dialysate warmer. These warmers can be obtained from the manufacturer of the dialysate. Failure to appropriately warm dialysate prior to infusion can cause shoulder, abdominal, and back pain in the client, alter ultrafiltration and solute removal, and crack the PD catheter (Kelly; Prowant, 2001).

As with other patients with renal disease, treatment for anemia, renal osteodystrophy, and other electrolyte imbalances may be appropriate.

Patient and Family Teaching

During hospitalization, patients and families should receive education regarding the necessity of the dialysis treatment, signs or symptoms to report during treatments, and dietary modifications and fluid restrictions currently instituted. Patients should be encouraged to play an active role in their care as appropriate to their current health status. Prior to discharge from the hospital, a newly initiated PD patient should be able to appropriately return-demonstrate PD exchanges, understand dietary modifications and fluid restrictions, recognize the importance of appropriate follow-up care, and know how and from where to order dialysis supplies.

CONTINUOUS RENAL REPLACEMENT THERAPY

CRRT is a form of dialysis therapy that lasts eight or more hours and takes place in the ICU setting. Patients who are appropriate candidates for CRRT include those who are not suited for PD and those who are hemodynamically unstable (Bellomo et al., 2002). CRRT is generally initiated by the dialysis team, with continuous monitoring being performed by the ICU nurse. Most hospitals have strict policies and procedures in place regarding who initiates, discontinues, and monitors CRRT. Strict intake and output must be recorded during the monitoring of the treatment, and appropriate safety measures must be taken to avoid potential blood loss or exsanguination.

Several types of CRRT currently exist, with the primary goal of all being to remove excess fluid volume, promote solute removal, and help balance electrolyte status. Continuous arteriovenous hemofiltration (CAVH), continuous arteriovenous hemofiltration-dialysis (CAVHD), continuous venovenous hemofiltration (CVVH), continuous venovenous hemofiltration-dialysis (CVVHD), slow continuous ultrafiltration (SCUF), continuous arteriovenous hemodiafiltration (CAVHDF), and continuous venovenous hemodiafiltration (CVVHDF) are the types of CRRT most commonly utilized in the ICU setting. As the different names imply, some types of CRRT require both arterial and venous access, whereas others require only venous access. When blood flows out of the body through an artery and back through a vein (arteriovenous), the patient's blood pressure pushes blood through the system and hemofilter. When the venovenous system is used (a vein is used to remove and return blood), a pump is required to propel blood through the system.

Some types of CRRT provide hemofiltration only (removal mostly of excess fluids, with a minimal amount of solute removal); others actively remove both solutes and fluids. With SCUF, fluid is ultrafiltrated from the patient. The main objective of SCUF is removal of fluid. With CAVH, fluid and some solutes are eliminated from the body. A percentage of the fluid that is removed each hour is replaced as intravenous fluid. CAVHD is similar to CAVH but adds a dialysate solution to the therapy. The dialysate circulates around the hemofilter and increases diffusion, which results in greater solute removal. With CVVH, there is both fluid and solute removal. CVVHD is similar to CAVHD except that a pump is required to push the blood through the system and filter.

Because each of these systems runs continuously, CRRT provides a kinder and gentler shift in fluid and electrolyte status as compared to an HD treatment, which is associated with peaks and valleys in the level of fluid and electrolytes.

Patient Assessment Findings

Patients undergoing any type of CRRT should have close monitoring and supervision at all times. Continuous vital sign measurements and assessment of hemodynamic status are necessary. A baseline electrocardiogram as well as current heart rhythm monitoring should be available prior to initiation of any CRRT treatment. Heart and lung sounds should be auscultated prior to initiation of treatment and regularly thereafter, with notes made of extra heart sounds, rubs, gallops, or murmurs. Apical and peripheral pulses should be noted, with their strength, intensity, rate, and rhythm being documented. Hemodynamic parameters should be continuously monitored throughout the treatment. Notation should be made of current oxygen saturation both prior to initiation of the CRRT treatment and regularly thereafter. Neurological status should be evaluated to include orientation, mentation changes, and cranial nerve assessment. Gastrointestinal status should be assessed fully. Skin integrity should be noted.

Accurate volume status of the client prior to initiation of the CRRT treatment is imperative. Daily or more frequent weight measurements should be obtained. Accurate intake and output should be documented. Edema, neck vein distention, types of drainage from other orifices or tubes, condition of mucous membranes, and skin turgor should all be assessed (Burrows-Hudson et al., 2005).

Nursing Interventions

Continuous monitoring of the patient undergoing CRRT is vital for a positive outcome. Care should be given to appropriately document all intake and output. Cardiac medications and infusions should be administered to help maintain hemodynamic stability. At times, use of cardiac augmentation devices may be necessary during the CRRT process (Burrows-Hudson et al., 2005). Oxygen therapy should be administered as ordered, and mechanical ventilation parameters followed as per current hospital protocol and physician orders.

Maintaining a safe environment is a key priority in the care of the patient receiving CRRT. The potential for bleeding is high, so close surveillance and monitoring of the patient are required. In cases of blood loss, care should be taken to accurately document estimated blood loss and prepare for necessary transfusions. The potential for development of an air embolism also exists. Accurate visualization of the lines whether or not the patient is connected to a CRRT machine is necessary. Alarms of the machines to detect air in the lines are necessary as well.

Nursing staff should maintain aseptic technique to limit potential infections. They should also promptly report and document any signs or symptoms of infection.

Providing psychosocial support to both the family and patient is vital during this acute phase of illness. Most patients who receive CRRT have multiple organ dysfunction syndrome, sepsis, or acute renal failure. Support systems for the family—including friends, pastoral care, or other family members—may be necessary. Pain and comfort measures will be required for the patients themselves.

Patient and Family Teaching

Teaching during this phase will initially focus on the need for CRRT and the patient's response to the treatment. Family members may be the sole receivers of educational material during this acute phase because the patient may not be receptive to learning. Updates provided to the family on a regular basis will help relieve their anxiety and fear. Further education can be provided based on the underlying cause of the renal failure and the patient's overall status.

DIALYSIS OF DRUGS

Drugs that are metabolized by the kidney will also be excreted during the dialysis process. Conversely, a client who is not scheduled to receive some form of dialysis therapy on the same day a drug is administered runs a great risk of developing drug toxicity. It is essential that nursing staff check with the pharmacy for the current schedule of dialyzability of medications prior to administering any pharmacological therapy to help avoid potential harm to the client. Medications must be timed appropriately to avoid adverse events, and to ensure safety during the dialysis process. Up-to-date lists of drugs that are removed during the dialysis process should be available from hospital pharmacists.

KEY RESEARCH

Currently, research regarding RRTs is focusing on optimal dialysis care (National Kidney Foundation, 2002). The NKF has collaborated with key thought leaders in the area of RRT to improve overall patient outcomes and survival rates. The latest data may be found through the NKF's website and the DOQI updates. Other current research is examining daily HD and nocturnal dialysis. Both areas of study have brought interesting data to the field regarding the necessary length of time needed for optimal dialysis adequacy, as well as potential cost savings and benefits with more lengthy treatments (Molitoris, 2005).

PATIENT OUTCOMES

Nurses can help ensure attainment of optimal patient outcomes such as those listed in **Box 45-1** through the use of evidence-based interventions for patients receiving RRT.

SUMMARY

Patients who are receiving any form of dialysis therapy tend to require complex care, because their illness often involves mul-

tiple organ systems. For these reasons, patients tend to be vulnerable to comorbid conditions and in fragile health upon admission. The family and patient together may need assistance in engaging in decision making and care processes. Long-term care of a chronic condition may exhaust a patient's financial resources, leading to further stressors on the family and client. Care must be tailored to meet the holistic needs of both the client and the family, and it requires nurses to exhibit strong clinical judgment, caring, and a willingness to collaborate with the entire healthcare team. Application of the Synergy Model for Patient Care (AACN, 2004) is an appropriate guide to help link clinical practice to patient outcomes.

Box 45-1
Optimal Patient Outcomes

- Weight in expected range
- Volume flow within expected range
- Dialysis access is functional and free of inflammation
- Serum electrolytes in expected range
- Coagulation status in expected range
- Demonstrates understanding about disease process
- Uses effective coping strategies
- Adjustment to changes in health status

CASE STUDY

You are a registered nurse who is working in a step-down ICU. Your assignment today is to care for three patients, all of whom have some form of renal disease requiring dialysis therapy.

E.L. is a 79-year-old male who recently suffered an acute myocardial infarction that led to acute renal failure. He is hemodynamically unstable, and the nephrologist has decided to help relieve his uremic symptoms with CRRT.

C.K. is a 45-year-old female with a 23-year history of Type 2 diabetes mellitus that is controlled by oral antidiabetic agents and insulin. She has a body mass index of 37 kg/m² and a history of hypertension and hyperlipidemia. She recently underwent a coronary artery bypass graft. She has been on HD for two years.

M.C. is a 28-year-old female who is currently employed as an accountant in a large accounting firm. She was hospitalized for a systemic lupus erythematosus flare-up. A GFR was computed by her nephrologists during this hospitalization, and it indicated renal function of 18 mL/min/1.73 m². Dialysis options are to be discussed with her today because she is experiencing uremic symptoms. M.C. appears to be interested in investigating peritoneal dialysis as a treatment choice.

CRITICAL THINKING QUESTIONS

1. Do you believe that CRRT is a wise choice for E.L.? Why or why not?

2. Could E.L. also be treated with another form of dialysis therapy?

3. How would care differ between C.K. and E.L.?

4. What important teaching strategies should be implemented with C.K. to help improve her overall health and well-being?

5. Is C.K. an ideal candidate for PD?

6. Is PD a good treatment choice for M.C.?

7. How would your assessments differ between M.C., C.K., and E.L.? What findings would you expect to see that are similar?

8. What disciplines should be consulted to work with these clients?

9. What types of issues may require you to act as an advocate or moral agent for these clients?

10. How will you implement your role as a facilitator of learning for these clients?

11. Use the form to write up data and a plan of care for a patient receiving renal replacement therapy in the clinical setting. Rate the patient as a level 1, 3, or 5 on each characteristic. Identify the level of nurse characteristics needed in the care of this patient.

12. Take one patient outcome for a patient and list evidence-based interventions found in a literature review for this patient.

Using the Synergy Model to Develop a Plan of Care

	Patient Characteristics	Level (1, 3, 5)	Subjective and Objective Data	Evidence-based Interventions	Outcomes
SYNERGY MODEL	Resiliency				
	Vulnerability				
	Stability				
	Complexity				
	Resource availability				
	Participation in care				
	Participation in decision making				
	Predictability				

Online Resources

- **American Association of Kidney Patients:** www.aakp.org
  A national kidney patient education organization that provides free educational materials for patients and families with or at risk for development of kidney disease.

- **American Diabetes Association:** www.diabetes.org
  Professional organization related to diabetes and care of the patient with diabetes. Patient education material available. Free weekly e-newsletter for health professionals.

- **American Kidney Fund:** www.akfinc.org
  An advocacy and education group for renal patients and their families.

- **American Nephrology Nurses' Association:** www.annanurse.org
  The specialty nursing organization for nurses working in or with nephrology patients or patients at risk for developing renal problems.

- **ESRD Networks Data Reports:** www.esrdnetworks.org
  Content includes a list of all data reports for all patients receiving RRT under the federal Medicare programs in the United States.

- **Kidney School:** www.kidneyschool.org
  Sponsored by the Life Options and Rehabilitation Activities Committee. The content includes patient-centered information about renal replacement therapies and compliance with treatment.

- **National Kidney Foundation:** www.kidney.org
  A national advocacy organization for renal patients and healthcare professionals. Provides research and quality initiatives for renal-related issues.

- **National Kidney Foundation Kidney Disease Outcomes Quality Initiative:** www.kdoqi.org
  This website provides the latest information on quality initiatives and evidence-based practice for renal patients. Downloadable charts, graphs, and GFR calculators are available.

- **National Kidney Foundation's Kidney Learning System:** www.kidney.org/professionals/KLS
  An educational initiative sponsored by the National Kidney Foundation for healthcare professionals and providers. Continuing education offerings available with updates provided on the latest scientific research in the nephrology community.

- **Renal Web:** www.renalweb.com
  A news website devoted to current topics related to or about renal health issues.

- **United States Renal Data System:** www.usrds.gov
  A U.S. government tracking website that contains data and statistics related to patients with renal disease.

REFERENCES

American Association of Critical-Care Nurses. (2004). The AACN Synergy Model for Patient Care. Retrieved May 11, 2005, from AACN Certification Corporation, www.certcorp.org/certcorp/certcorp.nsf/vwdoc/SynModel?opendocument

Bellomo, R., Kellum, J., Mehta, R., Palevsky, P., & Ronco, C. (2002). The acute dialysis quality initiative II: The Vicenza conference. *Advances in Renal Replacement Therapy, 9*(4), 290–293.

Burrows-Hudson, S., Prowant, B. F., & Currier, H. (2005). *Nephrology nursing standards of practice and guidelines for care.* Pitman, NJ: American Nephrology Nurses' Association.

Coresh, J., Astor, B., Greene, T., Eknoyan, G., & Levey, A. S. (2003). Prevalence of chronic kidney disease and decreased kidney function in the adult US population: Third national health and nutrition examination survey. *American Journal of Kidney Diseases, 41*(1), 1–12.

Daugirdas, J. T., Blake, P. G., & Ing, T. S. (2001). *Handbook of dialysis* (3rd ed.). Philadelphia: Lippincott Williams & Wilkins.

Eknoyan, G., & Levin, N. W. (2002). *Clinical practice guidelines for chronic kidney disease: Evaluation, classification, and stratification.* New York: National Kidney Foundation Press.

Hartigan, M. F., & Breiterman-White, R. (2001). Circulatory access for hemodialysis. In L. E. Lancaster (Ed.), *Core curriculum for nephrology nursing* (4th ed., pp. 305–330). Pitman, NJ: American Nephrology Nurses' Association.

Hedayati, S. S., Jiang, W., O'Connor, C. M., Kuchibhatia, M., Krishnan, R., Cuffe, M. S., et al. (2004). The association between depression and chronic kidney disease and mortality among patients hospitalized with congestive heart failure. *American Journal of Kidney Diseases, 44*(2), 207–215.

Keen, M. L., Lancaster, L. E., & Binkley, L. S. (2001). Hemodialysis. In L. E. Lancaster (Ed.), *Core curriculum for nephrology nursing* (4th ed., pp. 255–304). Pitman, NJ: American Nephrology Nurses' Association.

Kelly, K. T. (2004). How peritoneal dialysis works. *Nephrology Nursing Journal, 31*(5), 481–490.

Martin-McDonald, K., & Biernoff, D. (2002). Initiation into a dialysis dependent life: An examination of rites of passage. *Nephrology Nursing Journal, 29*(4), 347–353, 376.

McCrory, D., Klassen, P., Rutschmann, O., Coladonato, J., Yancy, W., Reddan, D., et al. (2002). *Evidence report: Appropriate patient preparation for renal replacement therapy*. Rockville, MD: Renal Physicians Association.

McGill, R. L., Healy, D. A., Marcus, R. J., Sandroni, S. E., & Brouwer, D. J. (2005). Nurturing "fistula culture" in a hospital environment. *Nephrology News & Issues, 19*(6), 53–55.

Molitoris, B. A. (2005). *Critical care nephrology*. Chicago: Remedica.

National Kidney Foundation. (2002). K/DOQI clinical practice guidelines for chronic kidney disease: Evaluation, classification and stratification. *American Journal of Kidney Diseases, 39*(Suppl), 19.

Prowant, B. (2001). Peritoneal dialysis. In L. E. Lancaster (Ed.), *Core curriculum for nephrology nursing* (4th ed., pp. 331–376). Pitman, NJ: American Nephrology Nurses' Association.

Richard, C. (2001). Renal disorders. In L. E. Lancaster (Ed.), *Core curriculum for nephrology nursing* (4th ed., pp. 83–115). Pitman, NJ: American Nephrology Nurses' Association.

United States Renal Data System (USRDS). (2002). *USRDS 2002 annual data report: Atlas of end-stage renal disease in the United States*. Bethesda, MD: National Institutes of Health, National Institute of Diabetes and Digestive and Kidney Diseases.

Wagner, K. D. (2001). Acute renal dysfunction. In P. S. Kidd & K. D. Wagner (Eds.), *High acuity nursing* (3rd ed., pp. 645–670). Upper Saddle River, NJ: Prentice-Hall.

CHAPTER 46

End-Stage Renal Disease and Renal Transplantation

Carol Isaac MacKusick

LEARNING OBJECTIVES

Upon completion of this chapter, the reader will be able to:

1. Describe the major etiologies of end-stage renal disease (ESRD).

2. Explain appropriate clinical judgment for the acutely ill ESRD patient.

3. Describe selection criteria and nursing interventions for the renal transplant patient.

4. Discuss criteria for living and cadaveric kidney donors.

5. Differentiate between chronic kidney disease staging and ESRD.

6. Delineate appropriate client and family teaching strategies related to the acutely ill ESRD patient and the renal transplant patient.

7. Identify resources available to the nursing and healthcare community to further assist in the care and education of ESRD patients and their families.

8. List optimal patient outcomes that may be achieved through evidence-based management of ESRD.

The number of individuals with kidney disease continues to grow annually, with the latest estimates noting that approximately one out of five Americans is at risk for developing kidney disease at some point (National Kidney Foundation, 2002). In the United States, more than 300,000 individuals are receiving some form of renal replacement therapy (RRT) (United States Renal Data System, 2002). In 2004, nearly 27,000 Americans received a solid-organ transplant, nearly an 11% increase in transplants since 2003; of this number, the majority of the transplants were in the renal and liver arena (Chartier, 2005).

Approximately three-fourths of all patients with end-stage renal disease (ESRD) suffered their first renal insult as a result of untreated or undertreated diabetes mellitus or hypertension. As the Type 2 diabetes mellitus population continues to grow, the number of individuals who are at risk for developing renal failure likewise rises. Other etiologies associated with ESRD include pyelonephritis, glomerulonephritis, congenital disorders, systemic lupus erythematosus, sickle cell disease, polycystic kidney disease, renal tubule acidosis, Fanconi syndrome, malignancies of the kidney, Wilms' tumors, renal tuberculosis, and obstructive disorders (Burrows-Hudson, Prowant, & Currier, 2005; Daugirdas, Blake, & Ing, 2001; Richard, 2001).

Chronic kidney disease (CKD) can progress to ESRD, necessitating the need for RRT to sustain life. All body systems are affected by ESRD. Unlike acute renal failure, however, ESRD is not reversible. For the patient with ESRD to maintain life, some form of RRT must be undertaken. These treatment options include either dialysis therapies or transplantation. This chapter focuses on treatment of the acutely ill ESRD patient and transplantation related to ESRD.

CHRONIC KIDNEY DISEASE STAGING

The degree of advancement of CKD is determined by a combination of evidence of kidney damage and level of kidney function as indicated by the glomerular filtration rate (GFR) (McCrory et al., 2002). The National Kidney Foundation's (NKF) Kidney Disease Outcomes Quality Initiative (KDOQI) describes the clinical progression of CKD in terms of stages. This staging progression was designed to help eliminate confusion among healthcare providers related to the progression of renal disease, and to provide evidence-based practice guidelines on care and management of the CKD patient (National Kidney Foundation, 2002).

CKD Stages 1–4

Normal kidney function is represented by a GFR between 90 and 120 mL/min/1.73 m^2. Patients who present with a clinically normal GFR but exhibit signs of kidney damage (e.g., hypertension, proteinuria, or microalbuminuria) would be classified as being in stage 1 of CKD. Clinical actions recommended for these patients would include treating the comorbid conditions to help delay or halt progression of renal disease as well as implementing a cardiovascular disease risk reduction plan (National Kidney Foundation, 2002).

Patients with a GFR between 60 and 89 mL/min/1.73 m^2 are recognized as having kidney damage with a mild decrease in GFR. This condition is also known as stage 2 of CKD. Clinicians would treat these patients by estimating renal disease progression and continuing to treat comorbid conditions (National Kidney Foundation, 2002).

Patients with a moderate decrease in GFR are noted to be in stage 3 of CKD; they have a GFR between 30 and 59 mL/min/1.73 m^2. The first signs of CKD may become manifest at this stage, and these complications should be screened for and treated (National Kidney Foundation, 2002). As CKD progresses to stages 2 and 3, erythropoietin production decreases and anemia may become clinically evident (McCrory et al., 2002).

CKD stage 4 is evidenced by a severe decrease in GFR. The patient's GFR remains between 15 and 29 mL/min/1.73 m^2 (National Kidney Foundation, 2002). At this point, a host of metabolic issues become apparent, including worsening of anemia, the onset of metabolic acidosis, alterations in bone metabolism, alterations in electrolyte balances, and fluid volume accumulation (McCrory et al., 2002). The patient may complain of symptoms associated with uremia, including burning feet, restless legs, vomiting, anorexia, disturbance in sleep patterns, fatigue, temperature intolerance, an ongoing metallic taste in the mouth, and an inability to concentrate (McCrory et al.; Molitoris, 2005; Richard, 2001). Studies have indicated that patients who reach stage 4 will likely progress to CKD stage 5 and require RRT (Hunsicker et al., 1997). Patients and healthcare providers should prepare for initiation of RRT (National Kidney Foundation).

CKD Stage 5

The fifth stage of CKD is clinically represented as a GFR less than 15 mL/min/1.73 m^2 (National Kidney Foundation, 2002). RRT (either dialysis or scheduled transplantation) should be initiated upon evidence of uremia and will be required as a

life-sustaining treatment. Treatment of the many metabolic complications is necessary at this point to help provide better patient outcomes upon beginning RRT (McCrory et al., 2002; Richard, 2001). Ideally, patients can begin RRT in a scheduled, non-acute care setting (Daugirdas et al., 2001). Upon initiation of RRT in stage 5, patients are also considered to have ESRD and are classified as ESRD patients by the U.S. Center for Medicare and Medicaid Services.

THE ACUTELY ILL ESRD PATIENT

Table 46-1 identifies the many systemic effects that renal failure has on a patient. Although many of these problems will continue to be addressed during the acute care hospital admission, most are handled in the chronic, outpatient setting (Burrows-Hudson et al., 2005; Lancaster, 2001; McGill, Healy, Marcus, Sandroni, & Brouwer, 2005; Molitoris, 2005). More serious problems include pulmonary issues, issues related to infection, and cardiovascular issues. In fact, the leading cause of death for all patients with ESRD is cardiovascular disease (Lancaster; National Kidney Foundation, 2003). It is also the second leading reason for long-term hospitalizations for ESRD patients (National Kidney Foundation), following closely behind hospitalizations secondary to systemic infections (Klevens, Tokars, & Andrus, 2005). Because of the multisystem organ involvement, ESRD patients are frequently admitted to the intensive care unit (ICU) for treatment and stabilization of these problems.

Patient Assessment Findings

B.W., a 57-year-old African American male, was admitted to the renal ICU from the emergency department (ED) with a diagnosis of chronic heart failure (CHF) on Sunday, two days after his normally scheduled chronic hemodialysis treatment. He has been receiving maintenance hemodialysis for approximately four months. Upon admission to the ICU, B.W.'s vital signs were blood pressure 210/118 mm Hg (sitting at side of bed), pulse 108, respiration 32 and deep, and temperature 99.2 °F. He is unable to lie supine. You note use of accessory muscles during respiration, and his neck veins are engorged. B.W. states, "I feel like I am suffocating." His weight is 73.2 kg, and he is anuric. A serum electrolyte panel was drawn in the ED; results are pending. On telemetry, you note a slight loss of the P wave and a slight widening of the QRS complex. B.W. states that his legs feel "like they are asleep," and his hand grips are weak bilaterally. You note bilateral crackles throughout the lung fields, with a questionable pleural rub in the left cavity. You note S$_1$, S$_2$, and S$_3$ heart sounds. The patient's primary nephrologist was notified by the ED and further orders are pending.

TABLE 46-1 Comorbid Conditions Associated with End-Stage Renal Disease

- Acid–base disorders: metabolic acidosis
- Bone metabolism disorders: changes noted in calcium and phosphate levels, vitamin D absorption, renal osteodystrophy, hyperparathyroidism, aluminum toxicity
- Cardiovascular disorders: hyperlipidemia, coronary artery disease, atherosclerosis, arterial hypertension, left ventricular hypertrophy, cardiomyopathy, pericarditis, cardiac tamponade, pericardial effusion
- Electrolyte disorders: alterations in sodium, potassium, calcium, phosphate, magnesium, hydrogen, bicarbonate, and aluminum
- Elimination disorders: problems with constipation and bowel elimination
- Endocrine disorders: decreased availability of growth hormone, decreased reproductive function, male impotence
- Fluid volume disorders: fluid volume overload, as evidenced by pulmonary edema, chronic heart failure, hypertension, pitting or nonpitting edema, ascites
- Gastrointestinal disorders: gum and mouth ulcerations, fetor uremicus, anorexia, nausea, vomiting, gastrointestinal bleeding
- Infection: vascular access infections, bacteremia, sepsis, antibiotic resistance infection, immune suppression
- Hematological disorders: anemia, iron deficiency, decreased platelet aggregation, decreased white blood cell function
- Neuromuscular disorders: peripheral neuropathy, uremic encephalopathy
- Nutritional imbalances: alterations in carbohydrate metabolism, alterations in glycemic control
- Pulmonary disorders: depressed cough reflex, pleural effusion, pulmonary edema, pleuritic pain
- Sexuality disorders: male impotence, altered body image issues, lack of desire, decreased reproductive ability
- Skin disorders: bruising, discoloration, dryness, pallor, pruritis, uremic frost
- Sleep disorders: nighttime wakefulness, daytime drowsiness, insomnia, snoring, sleep apnea, restless legs syndrome
- Vascular access issues: hemodialysis access stenosis or clotting, hemodialysis access infection, peritoneal dialysis catheter infection, peritoneal dialysis membrane infection

Sources: Burrows-Hudson, Prowant, & Currier, 2005; Lancaster, 2001; McGill, Healy, Marcus, Sandroni, & Brouwer, 2005; Molitoris, 2005.

B.W. is exhibiting classic symptoms of CHF. Upon retrieval of the chronic hemodialysis records, you note that his last recorded weight (after his last dialysis treatment) was 68.8 kg. Other findings that would indicate fluid volume overload would be pitting edema of feet, ankles, hands, and fingers; periorbital edema; sacral edema; cough; liver enlargement; and ascites. An elevated blood pressure and respirations that are increased in both depth and frequency are common findings as well (Lancaster, 2001). A serum albumin level should be evaluated, because it is often decreased in severe cases of fluid volume overload (Legg, 2005).

B.W. is also exhibiting signs of hyperkalemia (Molitoris, 2005). Muscle weakness generally does not occur until the potassium level exceeds 8.0 mEq/L. B.W.'s muscle weakness combined with the loss of the P wave would indicate an approximate potassium level between 8 and 9 mEq/L. Patients with potassium readings between 6 and 7 mEq/L will exhibit tall, tented T waves and prolonged PR intervals (Lancaster, 2001; Ludlow, 2003).

Nursing Interventions

When you become aware of the findings noted in this case, you immediately notify the nephrologist and the dialysis nurse on call. Although both peritoneal dialysis and hemodialysis work to remove potassium, hemodialysis is the treatment of choice with dangerously high levels of potassium, because rapid solute removal can occur. You follow up with the laboratory to determine serum electrolyte levels, and you prepare to administer insulin and glucose, calcium, or a cation-exchange resin enema per orders. Sodium bicarbonate also may be utilized for correcting acidosis and driving potassium into cells, but would not be utilized in B.W.'s case, because it may further increase total vascular volume. Serial serum potassium measurements must be drawn and monitored, and continuous cardiac monitoring used to evaluate decreases in potassium levels (Burrows-Hudson et al., 2005; Lancaster, 2001).

You also recognize that B.W. is at risk for infection and inflammation due to his hospitalization, decreased immune system function (white blood cell function is altered in renal failure), and frequent vascular access cannulations (Klevens et al., 2005). You immediately institute appropriate precautions to keep B.W. infection free throughout his hospitalization. Additionally, you contact the hospital dietitian to ensure that his renal diet is being followed and is not contributing further to his issues related to fluid volume overload, electrolyte imbalances, or inflammation (Wells, 2003).

Patient and Family Teaching

Emergent hemodialysis is initiated for B.W. Pharmacologic interventions do not become necessary, because his serum potassium level was noted to decrease to 4.8 mEq/L post hemodialysis. Additionally, 3.5 kg of fluid is removed during the hemodialysis session, and B.W. reports being able to breathe "better" and is able to lie supine. His neck vein engorgement has diminished, and his breath sounds are clear.

Several educational needs were presented during this short, but serious, ICU stay. Prior to discharging B.W. to the medical floor for further observation, you begin a teaching plan that would include the following issues:

- Management of fluid volume status: the role the kidneys played in fluid removal; the substitution of the fluid removal act by the dialysis machine; the need for B.W. to take daily weights and report unusual increases; accurate assessment of his oral intake; monitoring his blood pressure for signs of increase; managing thirst and oral care; the role of sodium, thirst, and fluid volume; and signs and symptoms of fluid volume overload.
- Review of the renal diet. You request a consult with the renal dietitian for follow-up with B.W. in his regular hospital room, but also encourage B.W. to limit his intake of high-potassium foods and use of salt substitutes, and provide him with a list of high-potassium foods. You remind him that for patients on hemodialysis, 40 to 70 mEq of potassium daily is the maximum that the body can tolerate, and you educate him regarding the role of potassium in electrical activity of the heart (Green & Hoffart, 2001).
- How to take his blood pressure at home, and when to notify his healthcare provider.

RENAL TRANSPLANTATION

Since the 1950s, renal transplantation has been a viable option for the ESRD patient. By the 1970s, the use of cadaver organs became accepted practice, and more organs became available for transplantation (Bartucci & Schanbacher, 2001). As improvements in immunosuppressive coverage have emerged, patients receiving kidney transplants have enjoyed longer, more successful graft function. Unfortunately, despite the increases in the number of families donating cadaver organs and the number of successful transplants, the number of people on transplant waiting lists continues to grow, and a critical shortage of available organs exists (Molzahn, Starzomski, & McCormick, 2003). In response to this alarming trend, the organ donation breakthrough collaborative was initiated, with best practices being determined and reported to the U.S. Department of Health and Human Services (U.S. Health and Human Services, 2003).

Currently, there are three available methods for receiving a kidney donation. Living donation can be related or nonrelated. Individuals who are willing to donate to a family member, to a friend, or as an anonymous donation must meet strict evaluation and assessment criteria (Bartucci & Schanbacher, 2001; Mitzel & Snyders, 2002), as outlined in **Table 46-2**. Cadaver donation—by far the most common solid-organ donation process—also has strict qualification standards, which are outlined in **Table 46-3** (Bartucci & Schanbacher).

TABLE 46-2 Evaluation Criteria for Living Kidney Donation

Psychosocial evaluation of donor with assessment of willingness to donate

Medical assessment of donor:

- Compatibility testing
- Health history and physical examination
- Diagnostic testing: chest radiograph, electrocardiogram (ECG), serum chemistry analysis, urinalysis, renal studies by computerized tomography or magnetic resonance imaging and renal arteriogram

Review of expectations of donation process
Financial considerations of the donation process

Sources: Bartucci & Schanbacher, 2001; Mitzel & Snyders, 2002.

Prior to receiving an organ from a cadaver or living donor, recipient candidates must be thoroughly assessed. Considerations are given for overall general health and ability to maintain organ viability after transplantation (Bartucci & Schanbacher, 2001; Ehlers, 2002). Other general assessment criteria are outlined in **Table 46-4**.

Pre-transplant Nursing Interventions

Several months later, B.W. returns to your ICU as a direct admission. The local organ procurement agency has matched him with a cadaver organ, and you are assigned to provide his care preoperatively. Nursing care for the patient preparing for renal organ transplantation includes the following measures:

- Collaborating with the organ procurement agency, the organ transplant coordinator, and the surgical team, to ensure a timely and successful graft placement
- Assisting in dialysis, which may be performed before surgery, depending on electrolyte and fluid status

---

TABLE 46-3 Qualifications for Cadaver Kidney Donation

Must meet criteria for brain death or have irreversible brain injury with life support

Must meet medical criteria:

- Absence of carcinomas or other malignancies
- Absence of active systemic infections
- Absence of significant renal disease
- Absence of uncontrolled hypertension

Must have appropriate medical power of attorney consent for donation

Source: Bartucci & Schanbacher, 2001.

TABLE 46-4 Assessment for Renal Transplantation

Prior to being accepted as a transplant candidate, the following body systems and comorbid conditions are evaluated to help ensure transplantation success:

1. Cardiovascular system health
2. Dental and oral health
3. Endocrine system
   - Diabetes should be well managed
   - Consideration should be given to dual renal–pancreas transplantation
4. Gastrointestinal system health
5. Gynecological health for female patients
   - Includes recent Pap testing and mammogram
6. Immune system
   - Patients should be infection free
   - Screening for viral, fungal, and bacterial infections
   - Free of neoplastic disease
7. Physiologic age
8. Psychosocial exam
9. Pulmonary system health
10. Primary renal disease cause and current state of control
11. Urinary tract capabilities

Sources: Bartucci & Schanbacher, 2001; Ehlers, 2002.

- Maintaining the patient as nothing by mouth (NPO) to help minimize nausea and vomiting immediately postoperatively and prevent intraoperative aspiration
- Performing a thorough nursing assessment
  - Baseline vital signs and weight should be documented for later comparison
  - Extremity pulses should be assessed and documented for later comparison
- Reviewing current medical history and implementing the following medical orders
  - Delivering appropriate medication administration (some facility protocols dictate immunosuppressive coverage and antibiotic coverage preoperatively)
  - Obtaining blood work to make sure that the patient has electrolytes within normal limits, is infection free, and is the appropriate cross match for the organ donation
  - Initiating telemetry and obtaining an electrocardiogram (ECG)
  - Obtaining a chest radiograph and forwarding the results to the surgical team
  - Obtaining vascular access
  - Skin preparation, which may include clipping hair in the surgical area (Bartucci & Schanbacher, 2001; Burrows-Hudson et al., 2005)

Post-transplant Nursing Interventions

B.W. returns from surgery several hours later. In report, you learn that the surgical procedure went well and that the cadaver kidney was placed extraperitoneally in the anterior iliac fossa. B.W. had immediate urinary output during the surgical procedure. If he had not, or if urinary output is scant or electrolytes are not maintained at normal levels, you would recognize that a need may exist for him to have one or more post-transplant dialysis treatments.

Maintaining optimal graft function is the immediate goal postoperatively and requires the following interventions:

- Ambulation as soon as possible, with assistance
- Frequent assessment for complications such as graft rupture, acute rejection, acute tubular necrosis, or urologic complications
- Assessment of circulatory function and comparison with preoperative baselines
- Bowel elimination
- Daily weights and assessment of fluid volume status
- Diuretic administration as ordered
- Immunosuppressive coverage as ordered
- Laboratory testing daily
- Pain and comfort management
- Prevention of infection
- Pulmonary toilet and maintenance of adequate respiratory function
- Strict intake and output recording, with details on color and clarity of urine noted
- Wound care

PATIENT AND FAMILY TEACHING

B.W. inquires as to why he has a dressing on his abdomen. He tells you that he thought that his "new kidney would be where my old one was." You explain to him that surgical placement in the extraperitoneal space will allow for easier assessment and needle biopsies in the future, eliminate the need to remove his "old" kidney, and made it easy to connect the vasculature and ureters to the newly transplanted organ (Bartucci & Schanbacher, 2001).

Families and transplant recipients also may have psychosocial adjustment issues post transplantation. Referral to a social worker, psychotherapist, or psychiatrist is not uncommon, and may help aid in the transition to wellness. Patients may have difficulties adjusting to wellness, have difficulties in coping with the new medication regimen, may have sexuality issues, or may even feel a sense of guilt after receiving an organ from someone who is deceased (Bartucci & Schanbacher, 2001; Burrows-Hudson et al., 2005). Allowing the patient and family to openly express these concerns during the postoperative period in a nonjudgmental manner is key to facilitating caring practices.

Discharge planning must begin immediately to help ensure a successful transition for the patient (Bartucci & Schanbacher, 2001). The teaching plan for a post-renal transplant patient will include the following issues:

- Activities of daily living: importance of regular exercise, type of activity restrictions, when to return to work or school
- Alcohol consumption: moderate consumption at most, unless otherwise contraindicated
- Consultation with the dietitian: drug–food interactions, ability to increase fluids, the components of a well-balanced diet
- Dental care: need for regular dental exams and good oral care
- Financial concerns: referral to social services as needed to help plan for expenses associated with medication coverage, referral with vocational rehabilitation as applicable
- Follow-up care: the importance of attending all regularly scheduled healthcare provider and lab appointments
- Infection: signs and symptom of perioperative site infection, signs and symptoms of generalized infection, practices to prevent infections, annual physical exams, continuing with appropriate immunizations
- Medications: administration, interactions, herbal remedies and over-the-counter interactions, importance of follow-up lab visits for medication trough levels
- Rejection: signs and symptoms of rejection, causes of rejection, how and when to contact the transplant team
- Sexuality: safe sex practices, need to resume contraception practices as applicable, emotional changes, need for wellness exams (breast self exam, Pap Smear, testicular self exam, prostate exam)
- Smoking cessation (Bartucci & Schanbacher, 2001; Burrows-Hudson et al., 2005)

Graft and patient survival issues may also be a concern expressed by B.W. and his family. Patient survival is generally greater than 95% at one year. Cadaveric graft survival is approximately 85% at the first year, and living donor graft survival is approximately 90% at the end of year 1 (Bartucci & Schanbacher, 2001).

KEY RESEARCH

Research into the improvement of quality of care and evidence-based practices for the ESRD patient is being pursued aggressively by the NKF through KDOQI. Improvements in infection issues related to ESRD patients are actively being pursued by the Centers for Disease Control and Prevention (CDC). Evidence-based practice guidelines are also being investigated and outlined for all organ transplant recipients through the organ donation breakthrough collaborative. Links to updated information regarding these and other ESRD issues may be found in the Online Resources section of this chapter.

PATIENT OUTCOMES

Nurses can help ensure attainment of optimal patient outcomes such as those listed in **Box 46-1** through the use of evidence-based interventions for patients with end-stage renal disease.

SUMMARY

Both the renal transplant patient and the acutely ill ESRD patient require care to be tailored to their individual needs and circumstances. These patients tend to be initially unstable, with multiple disease states and highly complex issues, which leave patients quite vulnerable. Resource availability for long-term and chronic care management may be an issue. The care delivered to these patients requires the nurse to act as a facilitator of learning, provide strong clinical judgment and coordination of care, and act as a patient advocate.

Box 46-1

Optimal Patient Outcomes

- Demonstrates understanding of disease process
- Uses effective coping strategies
- Adjustment to changes in health status
- Hemoglobin/hematocrit in expected range
- Serum electrolytes in expected range
- Physical comfort in expected range
- Absence of signs and symptoms of infection

CRITICAL THINKING QUESTIONS

1. B.W. initially presents with hyperkalemia and CHF. What other problems might a patient who is relatively new to dialysis experience?
2. If you had received orders for medications to help with B.W.'s hyperkalemia, what would they have been, and in what doses? What type of routine medications would you expect a hemodialysis patient to be on? Why?
3. As ESRD progresses, which comorbid conditions would you expect to see?
4. What are the primary electrolyte levels that should be reviewed on a regular basis for the ESRD patient? Why? What would normative values be, and what would alert values be? What type of disease progression would you expect to see when values remain abnormal?
5. Review the pharmacology for a renal transplant patient. What type of immunosuppressive coverage would you expect B.W. to be on initially? Assuming he does not experience acute or chronic rejection, which changes would you expect to see in his medications six months post transplant? What are some long-term side effects of immunosuppressive coverage?
6. Develop a list of potential nursing diagnoses for the ESRD patient admitted to the ICU with hyperkalemia and CHF.
7. Develop a list of potential problems for the renal transplant patient.
8. Renal failure rates continue to rise in the United States. What steps could be taken to help curb this epidemic?
9. Develop a diet plan for the ESRD patient.
10. Describe the pathophysiology of decreased GFR in the diabetic patient. How does this differ for the patient with a decreased GFR who has renal hypertension?
11. Use the form to plan care for this patient. Rate the patient as a level 1, 3, or 5 on each characteristic.

Using the Synergy Model to Develop a Plan of Care

	Patient Characteristics	Level (1, 3, 5)	Subjective and Objective Data	Evidence-based Interventions	Outcomes
SYNERGY MODEL	Resiliency				
	Vulnerability				
	Stability				
	Complexity				
	Resource availability				
	Participation in care				
	Participation in decision making				
	Predictability				

CASE STUDY

S.W. is 38 years old and has been on maintenance hemodialysis for the last three years. She is admitted to the ICU setting with a diagnosis of sepsis. She is to be treated with an aminoglycoside.

CRITICAL THINKING QUESTIONS

1. As you perform S.W.'s initial assessment, what type of changes would you expect to see related to her cardiac status, skin, bone health, peripheral vascular system, hematology, and metabolism?

2. Which drug would you expect to see ordered for S.W., and at what rate? How would this differ if S.W. were in stage 3 of CKD?

3. What would you expect to see during her assessment that indicates S.W.'s sepsis?

4. If S.W. does not respond to the aminoglycoside, what type of agents might also be prescribed?

5. During her hospitalization, S.W. expresses interest in receiving a transplant. What steps need to be taken before S.W. can be transplanted? What assessments will be performed to determine whether she is a suitable candidate?

6. As you prepare for her care, how can you recognize that S.W. is at risk for acute renal failure?

7. How would you manage acute renal failure?

8. What signs and symptoms need to be immediately reported to the healthcare team?

9. What nursing interventions will be unique for the patient with ESRD?

10. Which disciplines should be consulted to work with this client?

11. How will you implement your role as a facilitator of learning for this patient?

12. Take one patient outcome for this patient and list evidence-based interventions found in a literature review.

Online Resources

The following Web-based resources will provide up-to-date information related to acute renal failure and aid in professional education and development of patient teaching plans:

- **American Diabetes Association:** www.diabetes.org
  Professional organization related to diabetes and care of the patient with diabetes. Patient education material available. Free weekly e-newsletter for health professionals.
- **American Kidney Fund:** www.akfinc.org
  An advocacy and education group for renal patients and their families.
- **American Nephrology Nurses' Association:** www.annanurse.org
  The specialty nursing organization for nurses working in or with nephrology patients or patients at risk for developing renal problems.
- **Centers for Disease Control and Prevention—prevention of dialysis-related infections and tracking site:**
  www.cdc.gov/ncidod/hip/dialysis/dsn.htm
  A CDC-developed website to help monitor and track infections in dialysis patients. Provides provider education and statistics.
- **ESRD Networks Data Reports:** www.esrdnetworks.org
  Content includes a list of all data reports for all patients receiving RRT under the U.S. federal Medicare programs.

- **Kidney School:** www.kidneyschool.org

  Sponsored by the Life Options and Rehabilitation Activities Committee. Content includes patient-centered information about renal replacement therapies and compliance with treatment.
- **National Kidney Foundation:** www.kidney.org

  A national advocacy organization for renal patients and healthcare professionals. Provides research and quality initiatives for renal-related issues.
- **National Kidney Foundation Kidney Disease Outcomes Quality Initiative:** www.kdoqi.org

  This website provides the latest information on quality initiatives and evidence-based practice for renal patients. Handheld downloadable charts, graphs, and GFR calculators are available.
- **National Kidney Disease Education Program:** www.nkdep.nih.gov

  A government-affiliated resource and statistic site related to care of the renal patient.
- **Renal Web:** www.renalweb.com

  A news website devoted to current topics related to or about renal health issues.
- **United States Renal Data System:** www.usrds.gov

  A U.S. government tracking website that contains data and statistics related to patients with renal disease.
- **United Network for Organ Sharing (UNOS):** www.patients.unos.org

  Transplant statistics, information about approaching potential donor families, and information for patients awaiting organ donation. Subdivided into organ category. Professional and patient information provided.

REFERENCES

Bartucci, M. R., & Schanbacher, B. (2001). Renal transplantation. In L. E. Lancaster (Ed.), *Core curriculum for nephrology nursing* (4th ed., pp. 501–522). Pitman, NJ: American Nephrology Nurses' Association.

Burrows-Hudson, S., Prowant, B. F., & Currier, H. (2005). *Nephrology nursing standards of practice and guidelines for care.* Pitman, NJ: American Nephrology Nurses' Association.

Chartier, K. (2005). Organ transplants hit record high in 2004. *Nephrology News and Issues, 19*(6), 31.

Daugirdas, J. T., Blake, P. G., & Ing, T. S. (2001). *Handbook of dialysis* (3rd ed.). Philadelphia: Lippincott Williams & Wilkins.

Ehlers, S. E. (2002). Financial aspects of organ transplantation. *Nephrology Nursing Journal, 29*(3), 285–291.

Green, J. H., & Hoffart, N. (2001). Nutrition in renal failure, dialysis, and transplantation. In L. E. Lancaster (Ed.), *Core curriculum for nephrology nursing* (4th ed., pp. 203–220). Pitman, NJ: American Nephrology Nurses' Association.

Hunsicker, L. G., Adler, S., Caggiula, A., England, B. K., Greene, T., Kusek, J., et al. (1997). Modification of diet in renal disease study group: Predictors of the progression of renal disease in the modification of diet in renal disease study. *Kidney International, 51*(6), 1908–1919.

Klevens, R. M., Tokars, J. I., & Andrus, M. (2005). Electronic reporting of infections associated with hemodialysis. *Nephrology News and Issues, 19*(7), 37–43.

Lancaster, L. (2001). Systemic manifestations of renal failure. In L. E. Lancaster (Ed.), *Core curriculum for nephrology nursing* (4th ed., pp. 119–158). Pitman, NJ: American Nephrology Nurses' Association.

Legg, V. (2005). Complications of chronic kidney disease: Renal osteodystrophy, nutritional disturbances, and inflammation. *American Journal of Nursing, 105*(6), 40–50.

Ludlow, M. (2003). Renal handling of potassium. *Nephrology Nursing Journal, 30*(5), 493–498.

McCrory, D., Klassen, P., Rutschmann, O., Coladonato, J., Yancy, W., Reddan, D., et al. (2002). *Evidence report: Appropriate patient preparation for renal replacement therapy.* Rockville, MD: Renal Physicians Association.

McGill, R. L., Healy, D. A., Marcus, R. J., Sandroni, S. E., & Brouwer, D. J. (2005). Nurturing "fistula culture" in a hospital environment. *Nephrology News & Issues, 19*(6), 53–55.

Mitzel, H., & Snyders, M. (2002). Anonymous donation: A transplant center's experience. *Nephrology Nursing Journal, 29*(3), 275–277.

Molitoris, B. A. (2005). *Critical care nephrology.* Chicago: Remedica.

Molzahn, A., Starzomski, R., & McCormick, J. (2003). The supply of organs for transplantation: Issues and challenges. *Nephrology Nursing Journal, 30*(1), 17–28.

National Kidney Foundation. (2002). K/DOQI clinical practice guidelines for chronic kidney disease: Evaluation, classification and stratification. *American Journal of Kidney Diseases, 39*(Suppl. 19).

National Kidney Foundation. (2003). K/DOQI clinical practice guidelines for managing dyslipidemias in chronic kidney disease. *American Journal of Kidney Disease, 41*(4 Suppl. 3).

Richard, C. (2001). Renal disorders. In L. E. Lancaster (Ed.), *Core curriculum for nephrology nursing* (4th ed., pp. 83–115). Pitman, NJ: American Nephrology Nurses' Association.

United States Department of Health and Human Services. (2003). *The Organ Donation Breakthrough Collaborative: Best Practices Final Report.* Washington, DC: Health Resources and Services Administration, U.S. Department of Health and Human Services. www.organdonor.gov/bestpractice.htm

United States Renal Data System. (2002). *Annual Data Report: Atlas of End-Stage Renal Disease in the United States.* Bethesda, MD: National Institutes of Health, National Institute of Diabetes and Digestive and Kidney Diseases.

Wells, C. (2003). Optimizing nutrition in patients with chronic kidney disease. *Nephrology Nursing Journal, 30*(6), 637–648.

Hematology

Oncologic Emergencies

Jennifer S. Webster

LEARNING OBJECTIVES

Upon completion of this chapter, the reader will be able to:

1. Describe the pathophysiology and symptoms of six oncologic emergencies that may be encountered: cardiac tamponade, hypercalcemia, spinal cord compression, superior vena cava syndrome, syndrome of inappropriate antidiuretic hormone secretion, and tumor lysis syndrome.

2. Review the medical and nursing interventions to provide care for patients experiencing these selected oncologic emergencies.

3. Delineate appropriate patient and family teaching strategies in cases involving acutely ill oncology patients.

4. Recognize resources available to the nursing and healthcare community to further assist in care and education of the oncology patient and the family.

5. List optimal patient outcomes that may be achieved through evidence-based management of oncologic emergencies.

An oncologic emergency is defined as a critical or life-threatening complication resulting from malignant disease or the treatment of that disease. The emergency may be the presenting symptom of the cancer in previously undiagnosed patients but is usually a sign of progressive disease (Johnston & Spence, 2002; Otto, 2004). As our population ages, a concomitant increase in cancer diagnoses is expected. Therefore, increasing numbers of these emergencies can be anticipated in the intensive care unit (ICU).

CARDIAC TAMPONADE

Definition and Etiology

Cardiac tamponade is an acute low cardiac output syndrome caused by an excessive accumulation of fluid in the pericardial space or constriction of the pericardium by fibrous tissue, which results in restriction of the heart's ability to pump. Ventricular filling time is impaired, which in turn decreases cardiac output (the amount of blood ejected by the heart each minute) and systemic perfusion (Flounders, 2003a; Shelton, 2004a).

Cancer and its treatment are the most common causes of pericardial effusion and subsequent cardiac tamponade. Tumors of the breast and lung may spread into the pericardium, lymphomas frequently involve the mediastinum and pericardium, and leukemias may infiltrate the myocardium. Radiation therapy in large cumulative doses to the chest may cause pericarditis. Certain chemotherapies—namely, the anthracyclines—can cause cardiomyopathy and pericardial effusion (Flounders, 2003a; Kaplow, 2005; Keefe, 2000; Shelton, 2004a).

Diagnosis

The most sensitive diagnostic method is the echocardiogram, although an electrocardiogram (ECG) and a chest radiograph may be used for initial evaluation. The latter will reveal a "water bottle heart," an enlarged heart and a widened mediastinum. ECG findings include sinus tachycardia, dysrhythmias, elevated ST segments, T-wave changes, and a QRS with low voltage (Gullatte, Kaplow, & Heidrich, 2005; Kaplow, 2005).

Clinical Findings

Development of signs and symptoms depends on the rate and volume of the pericardial effusion. When accumulation of fluid is slow, large volumes can be accommodated without obvious symptoms due to the stretchiness of the pericardial fibers. Rapid accumulation of fluid does not allow for the pericardium to compensate, and symptoms quickly appear (Dulak, 2005; Flounders, 2003a).

Early symptoms of tamponade include the following (Flounders, 2003a; Goldman, 2004; Otto, 2004; Shelton, 2004a):

- Dyspnea (usually the most common presenting symptom).
- Cough, hiccups, dysphagia, or hoarseness as the nerves of the esophagus and trachea are compressed.
- Retrosternal chest pain related to compression of the heart. The pain is relieved by leaning forward and intensified by lying supine.
- Agitation, dizziness, or other signs of hypoxia.
- Weakness and fatigue as cardiac output decreases.
- Muffled or decreased heart sounds, or a pericardial friction rub.
- Weak apical pulse.

Late symptoms appear when the pericardium is no longer able to compensate and there is a sudden rise in intrapericardial pressure (Flounders, 2003a; Goldman, 2004; Kaplow, 2005; Otto, 2004):

- Progressive dyspnea, tachypnea, and orthopnea
- Tachycardia greater than 100 beats per minute, palpitations
- Hepatomegaly, abdominal pain
- Progressive retrosternal chest pain causing patients to remain in a forward-leaning position
- Neck vein distention
- Decreased systolic blood pressure and increased diastolic blood pressure, resulting in a narrowing pulse pressure, pulsus paradoxus greater than 10 mm Hg
- Jugular vein distention
- Edema
- Decreased stroke volume (the amount of blood ejected by the heart with each beat)
- Elevated central venous pressure, hypotension
- Electrical alternans (pulse waves varying between greater and lesser amplitude with successive beats)
- Skin cool and clammy to touch, pallor or cyanosis
- Oliguria progressing to anuria
- Change in level of consciousness
- Circulatory collapse or cardiac arrest

Medical Management and Nursing Care

Treatment of mild tamponade may include diuretics and corticosteroids, oxygen therapy, anxiolytics, analgesics, blood product administration, and fluid support. Vasoactive drugs [e.g., dopamine (Intropin®)] may be added (Dulak, 2005; Flounders, 2003a; Goldman, 2004; Kaplow, 2005; Otto, 2004; Shelton, 2004a).

A patient in acute distress requires emergency pericardiocentesis with ECG, echocardiogram, or fluoroscopic guidance. After initial removal of the pericardial fluid by needle and syringe, a small catheter may be left in place to continue drainage of the fluid. Reaccumulation of fluid may require sclerosing the pericardium with agents such as bleomycin sulfate (Blenoxane®), thiotepa (Thioplex®), or nitrogen mustard (Mustargen®). Sclerosing creates an inflammatory reaction that causes the two layers of the pericardium to fibrose, thereby eliminating the space (Dulak, 2005; Flounders, 2003a; Goldman, 2004; Kaplow, 2005; Otto, 2004; Shelton, 2004a).

Chronic effusions may require a pericardial window, defined as a partial removal of the pericardium, which allows drainage into the mediastinal or peritoneal compartment. Treating the underlying malignancy with appropriate chemotherapy or radiation therapy may prevent recurrence of the effusion. Radiation-induced constrictive pericarditis may require a total pericardiectomy; the heart does not need the pericardial sac to maintain adequate function.

Nursing care of the patient requires accurate and ongoing assessment of cardiopulmonary and hemodynamic status. Early recognition of signs and symptoms of pericardial effusion is important and requires strict monitoring of vital signs, pulse pressure, pulsus paradoxus (arterial blood pressure is different by more than 10 mm Hg between exhalation and inhalation), respiratory status, level of consciousness, fluid balance, and ECG tracings. Administration of volume expanders such as normal saline, red blood cells, and/or fresh frozen plasma will improve cardiac filling pressures. Elevating the head of the bed and maintaining a calm environment may improve patient oxygenation and comfort (Dulak, 2005; Flounders, 2003a; Goldman, 2004; Kaplow, 2005; Otto, 2004; Shelton, 2004a). The nurse must also prepare and educate the patient and family about any impending procedures such as periocardiocentesis (Flounders).

HYPERCALCEMIA

Definition and Etiology

Hypercalcemia entails greater than normal amounts of calcium in the blood, commonly defined as a serum calcium of more than 11.0 mg/dL (Keenan & Wickham, 2005).

Hypercalcemia is estimated to occur in up to 20% of patients with cancer (Olsen & Finley, 2004a; Richerson, 2004). Common etiologies include metastatic bone disease in patients with breast, lung, renal cell, multiple myeloma, lymphoma, or prostate cancer; hyperparathyroidism; prolonged immobility; dehydration; and poor nutrition with low serum albumin (Keenan & Wickham, 2005; Olsen & Finley). Some cancer therapies (e.g., estrogen, antiestrogen agents) may increase hypercalcemia as well (Kaplow & Reid, 2006).

Pathophysiology

Hypercalcemia is a complex metabolic disorder that results when increased bone resorption (destruction) exceeds both bone formation and the ability of the kidney to excrete extracellular calcium. Bone remodeling is an ongoing process that balances the resorption of old or damaged bone by osteoclasts with the building of new bone by osteoblasts. (*Hint:* CC and BB = osteoclasts chew up old bone; osteoblasts build new bone). The parathyroid gland, kidneys, and thyroid gland all assist in the regulation of calcium levels. When serum calcium falls below normal levels, the parathyroid gland releases parathyroid hormone protein (PTH), which stimulates the osteoclasts to increase resorption. PTH also stimulates the kidneys to reabsorb calcium in the tubules. When serum calcium increases above normal levels, the thyroid gland releases calcitonin, a PTH antagonist, which suppresses osteoclast activity and increases renal excretion of calcium (Otto, 2004; Richerson, 2004).

Tumors may cause hypercalcemia by direct bone destruction, such as in cancers with bony metastases. The malignant cells may also secrete PTH-like substances or other osteoclast-activating factors that increase osteoclast-activity so significantly that the kidneys and osteoblasts are unable to maintain the normal calcium balance (Keenan & Wickham, 2005; Olsen & Finley, 2004a).

Clinical Findings

The clinical signs and symptoms of hypercalcemia depend on the degree of alteration in the serum calcium and the rapidity of the change (Flombaum, 2000). Age, performance status, renal function, and general health of the patient also affect the clinical findings. For example, elderly patients are less able to tolerate small changes in calcium level and, therefore, will exhibit more severe symptoms earlier in the course of the disorder (Olsen & Finley, 2004a). Bone pain is the most common symptom of hypercalcemia in metastatic disease and frequently is the reason patients seek medical attention (Otto, 2004).

Mild, moderate, and severe hypercalcemia are difficult to define precisely due to the variation in symptom severity. The serum levels listed below are suggested by Stewart (2005).

Signs and Symptoms of Mild Hypercalcemia (serum calcium < 12.0 mg/dL)

- Polydypsia and polyuria, with nocturia (These are the earliest signs of hypercalcemia, but are commonly overlooked or ignored by patients if their onset is gradual.)
- Anorexia, nausea, constipation
- Affect changes, lethargy, restlessness, difficulty concentrating
- Weakness, fatigue
- Mild hypertension with orthostasis

Signs and Symptoms of Moderate Hypercalcemia (serum calcium of 12.0–13.9 mg/dL)

- Vomiting, increased abdominal pain and cramping, abdominal bloating
- Confusion, drowsiness, mental status changes
- Generalized muscle weakness
- ECG changes, cardiac arrhythmias (tachycardia, if early; bundle branch block, ventricular dysrhythmias), increasing hypertension
- Increasing polydypsia, dehydration

Signs and Symptoms of Severe Hypercalcemia (serum calcium >13.9 mg/dL)

- Paralytic ileus
- Stupor, seizures, coma
- Diminished deep tendon reflexes, ataxia, skeletal fractures
- Bradycardia, heart block, cardiac arrest
- Renal insufficiency, renal failure

Diagnostic Tests

The primary diagnostic test is serum calcium greater than 11 mg/dL (normal = 8.5–10.5), although patients may be asymptomatic with levels up to 14 to 16 mg/dL. The physical status of the patient, the rapidity of the increase in calcium, and other variables will affect the timing of the onset of visible symptoms. Low albumin levels will mask the severity of hypercalcemia and require a correction in the calculation of serum calcium to accurately measure the serum levels. *Corrected serum calcium* is calculated by determining that if the albumin is low (less than 4.0 Gm/dL), the serum Ca^{++} must be increased by 0.8 mg/dL for every 1 Gm/dL of albumin below normal. The level of ionized calcium (the amount of calcium available for use; normal = 1.13–1.32 mmol/L) may also be measured independently of the total serum calcium, because it is unaffected by serum albumin (Richerson, 2004; Stewart, 2005).

Other diagnostic tests include elevated urinary calcium and a prolonged PR interval and shortened QT interval on ECG (Olsen & Finley, 2004a).

Medical Management and Nursing Care

Long-term management of hypercalcemia can be achieved only by treating the underlying cancer with appropriate chemotherapy or radiation therapy. Immediate medical management focuses on addressing the acute emergency. Normal saline is administered to reverse dehydration, increase renal flow, and promote excretion of the excess calcium. As much as 3 to 8 L of fluid may be required to reverse the dehydration associated with hypercalcemia (Kaplow & Reid, 2006). Furosemide (Lasix®) may be ordered to block calcium reabsorption in the kidneys and promote renal excretion; however, furosemide is administered only after the dehydration has been corrected (Keenan & Wickham, 2005; Olsen & Finley, 2004b).

Administration of antiresorptive therapy, which inhibits osteoclast activity, is highly effective in restoring calcium balance. Currently, two antiresorptive therapies are used in the United States: pamidronate (Aredia®) and zoledronate acid (Zometa®). Both are administered intravenously and have an onset of action of 24 to 48 hours (Keenan & Wickham, 2005; Olsen & Finley, 2004b).

In extremely urgent situations, calcitonin (Miacalcin®) may be administered. This agent has the most rapid onset of action (4 to 6 hours) but a shorter duration of action (less than 72 hours); it is considered less effective than other antiresorptive therapies. Calcitonin inhibits osteoclast activity and promotes urinary excretion of calcium. Dialysis may be required if the patient is experiencing severe hypercalcemia with renal insufficiency (Flombaum, 2000).

Nursing care focuses on keeping the patient safe, managing the symptoms of hypercalcemia, monitoring for side effects of the administered therapies, and minimizing the risk of recurrence. Monitor vital signs, fluid status, cardiovascular status, mental status, and neurological status. Place the patient on seizure and safety precautions, and protect the patient from falls and injury due to the high risk of fractures. Increase the patient's physical activity and mobility with attention to safety. Pain management may be a priority if the patient suffers pain from bony metastases or fractures. The ICU nurse may also need to administer stool softeners and antiemetics to manage the constipation and nausea associated with hypercalcemia. Due to the likelihood of recurrence with hypercalcemia, an essential nursing intervention is to educate the patient and family on this disorder's common signs and symptoms to report to the healthcare team (Keenan & Wickham, 2005; Otto, 2004).

SUPERIOR VENA CAVA SYNDROME
Definition and Etiology

Superior vena cava syndrome (SVCS) is an internal or external obstruction of the superior vena cava causing reduced blood return to the heart. The resulting congestion impairs cardiac output and can result in life-threatening pulmonary and cerebral compromise. Although SVCS is not a common oncologic emergency, it is often the presenting sign of malignancy. Approximately 85% to 97% of SVCS cases are due to cancer, especially lung cancer (approximately 75%), lymphoma (15%), and breast cancer (10%). As the use of central venous catheters, pacemaker wires, and ports has increased, the rate of SVCS associated with internal thrombus appears to be increasing (Johnston & Spence, 2002; Moore, 2005; Shelton, 2004c).

Pathophysiology

Obstruction of the superior vena cava may be either by external pressure, such as that caused by a tumor or enlarged lymph nodes, or by internal pressure, such as that caused by a thrombus (Otto, 2004; Shelton, 2004c). The superior vena cava returns blood from the head, neck, upper extremities, and upper thorax to the heart (Moore, 2005); when compressed, it causes a backflow of blood in these same areas (Flounders, 2003b; Shelton, 2004c). Upper body edema and venous engorgement are the hallmark signs of SVCS.

Clinical Findings

Symptoms of SVCS vary in their frequency and severity based on how rapidly the obstruction develops (Aurora, Milite, & Vander Els, 2000; Flounders, 2003b; Johnston & Spence, 2002; Kaplow & Reid, 2006). The ICU nurse will need to assess for the following conditions:

- Dyspnea (the most common symptom)
- Cough, hoarseness
- Tachypnea, stridor, increasing respiratory distress
- Upper extremity, trunk, and facial edema (including tongue swelling and papilledema)
- Neck and chest vein distention
- Hypotension
- Cyanosis of the upper torso
- Headache
- Changes in mental status including stupor, seizures, and coma
- Stridor (in severe cases)
- Reddish face or cheeks
- Tightness of the neck (Stokes' sign)

Diagnostic Tests

Diagnostic tests for SVCS include a chest radiograph (to confirm a mass) and computerized tomography (CT) or magnetic resonance imaging (MRI) scans (to precisely show the location and size of the tumor or enlarged lymph nodes). A biopsy may be performed or a cytology specimen collected if a tumor has not been previously diagnosed. If no tumor or enlarged lymph nodes are detected, a venogram will be ordered to confirm the presence of thrombosis. MRI or ultrasound may also assist in locating a thrombus (Gucalp & Dutcher, 2001).

Medical Management and Nursing Care

Medical management depends on the etiology of the SVCS. If the emergency is the result of malignant disease, it is treated with radiation therapy or chemotherapy, depending on the tumor type and the patient's response to therapy. On the rare occasion when SVCS related to malignant disease is rapidly progressing with life-threatening symptoms, immediate treatment without tissue diagnosis of the tumor may be warranted. The treatment of choice without tissue diagnosis is irradiation (Flounders, 2003b; Moore, 2005). Corticosteroids and diuretics may also be used to decrease inflammation and edema, although controversy about their effectiveness exists (Flounders; Moore; Rowell & Gleeson, 2001). Patients with chronic or recurrent SVCS may benefit from vascular stenting of the vena cava, which is a surgical procedure (Flounders; Greillier et al., 2004). Diuretics may be administered to decrease the amount of volume returning to the heart, thereby lessening the pressure on the superior vena cava. If diuretics are used, the patient must be observed for signs of dehydration (Gullatte et al., 2005).

SVCS related to catheter thrombosis is treated with thrombolytic therapy—tissue plasminogen activator, streptokinase (Streptase®), or urokinase (Abbokinase®)—to lyse the clots in the catheter. Anticoagulant therapy may be used to prevent further thrombus formation although its use remains controversial. The once-common practice of administering low-dose warfarin (Coumadin®) or low-molecular-weight heparin as prophylaxis for catheter-associated thrombosis in cancer patients is no longer recommended (Couban et al., 2005; Levine & Kakkar, 2005). Catheter removal may be warranted. Insertion of a stent to reopen the superior vena cava has been suggested and has been reported effective more than 90% of the time (Gucalp & Dutcher, 2001).

ICU nurses are uniquely situated to notice subtle changes in patient status, and their assessment for changes in cardiopulmonary status should be ongoing. Nursing interventions include measures to reduce dyspnea, maintain adequate cardiopulmonary function, and improve comfort. The ICU nurse should promote measures to maintain a patent airway and prevent airway compromise or tracheal obstruction (Gullatte et al., 2005). The nurse should closely monitor fluid intake and output, vital signs, and mental status and watch for the side effects of steroids or anticoagulants as warranted. The head of the bed should be elevated 45° and supplemental oxygen administered. Remove rings, watches, and clothing that may restrict blood flow in the upper extremities. Avoid invasive or constrictive procedures—for example, venipunctures, intravenous (IV) fluid administration, and blood pressure measurements—in the upper extremities. A central venous catheter may be necessary to ensure the upper extremities are avoided. Maintain a calm, quiet environment and provide explanations and instructions to patients and families regarding the management of SVCS (Flounders, 2003b; Moore, 2005; Otto, 2004; Shelton, 2004c).

SYNDROME OF INAPPROPRIATE ANTIDIURETIC HORMONE SECRETION

Definition and Etiology

Syndrome of inappropriate antidiuretic hormone (SIADH) secretion is a condition characterized by the excessive production and release of antidiuretic hormone (ADH) that changes the body's fluid and electrolyte balance by increasing water retention, resulting in hyponatremia (Flounders, 2003c). Lung cancer is the most common cause of SIADH; it is responsible for approximately 80% of all cases. Several chemotherapeutic agents are responsible for the development of SIADH (Kaplow & Reid, 2006).

Pathophysiology

Body fluid balance is tightly controlled by a series of complex mechanisms. One of the most importance substances in this balance is ADH, a hormone secreted by the pituitary gland. In response to decreased intake of fluids or other reductions in the body's fluid volume, ADH acts on the kidneys to increase water reabsorption, resulting in water retention and dilution of the blood. In SIADH, ADH is produced in uncontrolled amounts by tumor cells directly or by those cells stimulating the pituitary gland. The overproduction leads to excessive water retention and a dilution of sodium ions in the plasma. At the same time, water is conserved in the kidney, leading to production of concentrated urine with a high sodium content (Keenan, 2005; Olsen & Finley, 2004b; Richerson, 2004).

Normal serum sodium levels are 135 to 145 mEq/L. As the concentration of the sodium decreases, water moves out of the blood vessels and into the cells. Severe SIADH can result in cerebral edema and death.

Clinical Findings

Symptoms of SIADH are related to the severity of the hyponatremia and the movement of fluid out of the circulatory system into the cells (Richerson, 2004). As the sodium level decreases, an associated increase in symptoms will occur. Serum sodium of 125 to 134 mEq/L is considered a mild hyponatremia. Other early signs and symptoms include the following (Flombaum, 2000; Flounders, 2003c; Langfeldt & Cooley, 2003):

- Thirst
- Headache, irritability, lethargy, behavioral changes
- Decreasing urine output, weight gain
- Peripheral edema
- Muscle cramps
- Anorexia

Serum sodium levels of 115 to 125 mEq/L indicate moderate hyponatremia, and levels below 115 mEq/L are severe. Moderate to severe signs and symptoms include the following:

- Confusion, irritability, weakness, tremors
- Combativeness, agitation, hallucinations, areflexia (decreased tendon reflex)
- Seizures, coma
- Oliguria
- Respiratory failure, inability to maintain a patent airway or mobilize secretions
- Death

Diagnostic Tests

Several laboratory values are assessed when diagnosing SIADH. The primary findings are decreased serum sodium of less than 130 mEq/L, a decreased serum osmolality of less than 280 mOsm/kg, with concurrent increases in urine sodium of greater than 20 mEq/L and urine osmolality of greater than 300 mOsm/L. Hypokalemia, hypomagnesemia, and hypocalcemia will also be evident due to the dilution of the plasma (Flombaum, 2000; Flounders, 2003c; Langfeldt & Cooley, 2003).

Medical Management and Nursing Care

Long-term control of SIADH requires that the underlying cause—usually a cancer—be treated. Therefore the initial interventions are aimed at immediate management until the cause can be identified and a treatment plan developed. Mild to moderate SIADH may be managed with a fluid restriction of 500 to 1,000 mL/day only (Flombaum, 2000; Flounders, 2003c; Richerson, 2004).

Severe SIADH may require an infusion of a 3% hypertonic saline solution to increase water movement from cells to plasma. The infusion is administered over several hours to gradually increase serum sodium. A correction in sodium that

is too rapid may lead to seizures and possibly even death (Olsen & Finley, 2004b; Richerson, 2004). If the patient has hyponatremia for more than 48 hours, correction should not exceed 0.5 to 1 mEq/hr (Gucalp & Dutcher, 2001). Furosemide may be administered concurrently to assist with diuresis and prevent fluid overload.

The antibiotic demeclocycline hydrochloride (Declomycin®) may be used as an agent in the management of SIADH. Demeclocycline interferes with the action of ADH but requires several days to take effect. It may cause gastrointestinal distress, photosensitivity, and hematologic changes. Other agents that are effective in treating SIADH include lithium and urea, but both have side effects that make their use uncommon.

Nursing care is directed toward management of fluids and the side effects of hyponatremia and its treatment. Patients must maintain a fluid restriction of 500 to 1,000 mL/day, so management includes strict monitoring of intake and output, overseeing the variety of infusions ordered to ensure the minimum fluid volume, and supporting the patient in complying with the restrictions. Further assessments and interventions include daily weights; monitoring of blood and urine chemistry levels; frequent review of the cardiopulmonary, neuromuscular, and renal systems; and placing the patient on seizure precautions. The nurse must also teach the patient and family which signs of hyponatremia to report and how to respond to seizures (Held-Warmkessel, 2005; Olsen & Finley, 2004b).

TUMOR LYSIS SYNDROME
Definition and Etiology

Tumor lysis syndrome (TLS) is a metabolic imbalance resulting from the rapid release of large amounts of intracellular components during cell death. It can occur between one and five days after initiation of chemotherapy in patients who have a bulky tumor that is responsive to chemotherapy. The lysing of tumor cells releases large amounts of potassium, phosphorus, and uric acid into the blood, which leads to a reciprocal decrease in serum calcium (Kaplow, 2002; Otto, 2004; Richerson, 2004). TLS is commonly associated with hematologic tumors that grow rapidly and have a large number of cells, such as leukemia and non-Hodgkin's lymphoma, although it may occur in solid tumors as well (Doane, 2002; Flombaum, 2000).

Pathophysiology

Potassium, phosphorus, and nucleic acids are intracellular ions that are present in higher amounts in cancer cells than in normal cells (Kaplow, 2002). Destruction of these cancer cells in large numbers precipitates a rapid release of these intracellular components into the circulation, overwhelming the kidney's ability to excrete them. The resulting metabolic abnormalities include hyperkalemia, hyperphosphatemia, a reciprocal decrease in serum calcium as it binds to the phosphorus, and hyperuricemia from the conversion of the nucleic acids into uric acid by the liver. Renal failure may occur due to increased formation of uric acid crystals and calcium phosphate salts that obstruct renal flow. Fatal cardiac arrhythmias may result from the hyperkalemia (Flombaum, 2000; Kaplow; Lydon, 2005).

Clinical Findings

Laboratory results indicating TLS include hyperkalemia, hyperphosphatemia, and increased uric acid. Serum calcium and, concurrently, magnesium, will be decreased. Physical findings are related to the effects of the metabolic changes on the organ systems:

- Renal—flank pain, decreased urine output, hematuria, weight gain, edema
- Gastrointestinal—nausea, vomiting, anorexia, diarrhea, abdominal cramping, and/or pain
- Cardiac—dysrhythmias, which are usually atrial
- Neuromuscular—muscle cramps, tetany, weakness, confusion, seizures

Medical Management and Nursing Care

Early recognition and timely management of TLS will greatly minimize the severity of its effects. If patients at risk for TLS can be identified, preventive measures can be put in place before and during treatment. Preventive measures include aggressive hydration to dilute the electrolytes and enhance excretion. A sodium bicarbonate ($NaHCO_3$) solution may be used to alkalinize the urine, thereby increasing uric acid solubility and minimizing precipitation. Diuretics may be added to promote urine excretion. Administration of allopurinol in an oral (Zyloprim®) or IV (Aloprim®) formulation is used to prevent uric acid formation. Finally, monitoring serum electrolytes every 6 to 12 hours to detect increases in potassium or decreases in calcium quickly will assist in prompt recognition of the TLS (Cantril & Haylock, 2004; Flombaum, 2000; Richerson, 2004; Tan, 2002).

Once TLS has been identified, medical management will depend on the severity of the syndrome. Common interventions include the administration of aluminum hydroxide, to bind with phosphate, and the administration of exchange resins, such as sodium polystyrene sulfonate (Kayexalate®), to promote potassium elimination through the feces. Rasburicase (Elitek®) may also be administered to promote uric acid metabolization and excretion in the urine once hyperuricemia

exists. If electrolyte abnormalities persist or when renal failure is evident, hemodialysis may be initiated (Ambrosio, 2004; Cantril & Haylock, 2004).

Nursing management focuses on the maintenance of fluid and electrolyte balance and monitoring the patient for side effects of the TLS or its treatment (Richerson, 2004). Patients will need education about the "paradox of treatment": While TLS can be a critical outcome of cancer treatment, it also suggests that the tumor is responsive to treatment and may be viewed as a positive sign. Management includes close monitoring of intake and output, serial weights, and frequent assessment for signs of fluid overload such as peripheral edema, distended neck veins, and shortness of breath. The nurse must also regularly monitor laboratory values including blood urea nitrogen (BUN)/creatinine and serum electrolytes. Prompt recognition of the signs of hyperkalemia, hyperphosphatemia, hypocalcemia, and hyperuricemia is essential. In addition, the nurse must educate the patient and family about TLS and the signs that should be reported to the healthcare provider (Gobel, 2002; Lydon, 2005; Richerson).

SPINAL CORD COMPRESSION

Definition and Etiology

Spinal cord compression (SCC) is a neurological emergency resulting from pressure on the spinal cord. This pressure may be due to direct tumor invasion of the spinal cord or tumor invasion of the vertebrae, causing destruction and collapse onto the spinal cord (Flounders & Ott, 2003; Otto, 2004). SCC is usually seen in patients with metastatic breast, lung, prostate, kidney, lymphoma, and multiple myeloma malignancies and develops in 2% to 5% of all patients with systemic cancer (Prasad & Schiff, 2005).

Pathophysiology

The spinal cord is a long mass of nervous tissue that contains the motor, sensory, and autonomic functions of the body. The effects of its compression relate to the position and extent of the malignant invasion or vertebral collapse and range from temporary numbness to devastating paralysis (Flounders & Ott, 2003; Held-Warmkessel, 2005; Otto, 2004).

Clinical Findings

The presenting symptoms of SCC vary with the location and severity of the cord compression. Neck or back pain is the most common symptom; this pain may be constant or initiated with movement, and it usually worsens with strains on the neck and back such as during coughing or sitting up. The pain progresses over time and is the primary reason patients seek medical attention (Flaherty, 2005; Flounders & Ott, 2003). Tingling and sensory loss are also early symptoms of compression and may occur before the onset of pain. Weakness or paralysis will occur below the level of the cord that is being compressed (Gullatte et al., 2005). As the compression increases, the severity of the symptoms increases, progressing from the sensory to the motor to the autonomic nervous system. Therefore, symptoms may include muscle weakness, loss of deep tendon reflexes, paralysis, loss of bowel and/or bladder function, and sexual dysfunction or impotence (Wilkes, 2004).

Diagnosis

The diagnosis of SCC is based on findings on physical exam and patient history. CT scan or MRI of the spine is used to confirm the diagnosis (Kaplow & Reid, 2006).

Medical Management and Nursing Care

The goal of medical management is to quickly halt or reverse the compression; therefore the treatment of choice for SCC is radiation to the tumor. Surgical decompression can be used if the tumor does not respond to radiation or if the area has already been treated with radiation. Corticosteroids may be administered concurrently to reduce edema around the area of compression, and pain management is a priority. Chemotherapy agents may be used for tumors sensitive to these agents and if radiation or surgery is contraindicated (Kaplow & Reid, 2006).

Early recognition and prompt management are essential to prevent paralysis. Nursing management focuses on safety, symptom relief, and supportive care. The ICU nurse should provide a safe environment of care, especially when moving the patient, and implement a comprehensive program for pain management. Frequent (every 1 to 2 hours) assessment of neuromuscular status and monitoring for changes in bowel and bladder function are also essential. The patient will require immobility to prevent further damage; this will include bedrest and logrolling for turning. Strategies to prevent complications of immobility should be implemented (e.g., deep vein thrombosis and pressure ulcer prevention) (Kaplow & Reid, 2006). If the patient has a cervical compression, respiratory assessments and intubation to ensure airway patency will be required (Kaplow & Reid).

Pain management for SCC is equally essential. Medications may include steroids, nonsteroidal anti-inflammatory drugs, opioids, antidepressants, or anticonvulsants (Kaplow & Reid, 2006).

The nurse should teach the patient and family signs of SCC to report and may need to consult with rehabilitative services to implement a strengthening and mobility program and obtain assistive devices (Flaherty, 2005; Shelton, 2004b; Wilkes, 2004). Measures to help meet the patient's psychosocial needs must be considered. This can be facilitated by collaborating with the multidisciplinary team.

PATIENT OUTCOMES

Nurses can help ensure attainment of optimal patient outcomes such as those listed in **Box 47-1** through the use of evidence-based interventions for patients with oncologic emergencies.

SUMMARY

As our population ages, ICU nurses will encounter increasing numbers of patients with a diagnosis of cancer. Along with the diagnosis comes the risk of developing an oncologic emergency. Nurses who are familiar with the most common oncologic emergencies provide an essential service to their patients by recognizing and providing nursing management of these emergencies, and by contributing to the education and support of patients and families.

Box 47-1

Optimal Patient Outcomes

- Vital signs in expected range
- Oxygen saturation in expected range
- Serum electrolytes within normal limits
- 24-hour intake and output balanced
- Demonstrates understanding of the disease process and complications
- Reports satisfaction with symptom control

CASE STUDY 1

M.B. is a 76-year-old male with a diagnosis of prostate cancer that has recently metastasized to his pelvis. Over the past few days, he has become weak, irritable, and confused. He refuses to eat because he feels nauseated and has no appetite, and he complains constantly of being thirsty. M.B. has not had a bowel movement in several days. When he is admitted to the hospital, he is restless and agitated, complaining continuously about his care, the lack of attention from his wife, and the ride in the ambulance. His wife describes him as usually a mild, very kind man and states that she has "never seen him like this before." Laboratory values include a serum calcium level of 11.4 mg/dL.

CRITICAL THINKING QUESTIONS

1. Is a serum calcium level an accurate correlate of the severity of symptoms?
2. Which other factors may be contributing to M.B.'s severity of symptoms?
3. Which other laboratory value would assist you in determining the true nature of M.B.'s hypercalcemia?
4. List the nursing management priorities for this patient.
5. What types of issues may require you to act as an advocate or moral agent for this patient?
6. How will you implement your role as a facilitator of learning for this patient?
7. Which disciplines should be consulted to work with a client who is experiencing an oncologic emergency?

CASE STUDY 2

A 28-year-old female is newly diagnosed with advanced non-Hodgkin's lymphoma. Her physician describes seeing a "large mediastinal mass" on the chest radiograph and admits her to the hospital for close monitoring during her initial chemotherapy treatment to observe her for potential onset of tumor lysis syndrome.

CRITICAL THINKING QUESTIONS

1. Why is this patient at risk for TLS?
2. Which laboratory values can the nurse be expected to closely monitor and why?
3. List the nursing management priorities for this patient.
4. Which interventions will the ICU nurse plan to prevent TLS?
5. What signs and symptoms will the ICU nurse look for to detect the onset of TLS?
6. Use the form to write up data and a plan of care for a patient with TLS.

Using the Synergy Model to Develop a Plan of Care

	Patient Characteristics	Level (1, 3, 5)	Subjective and Objective Data	Evidence-based Interventions	Outcomes
SYNERGY MODEL	Resiliency				
	Vulnerability				
	Stability				
	Complexity				
	Resource availability				
	Participation in care				
	Participation in decision making				
	Predictability				

Online Resources

American Cancer Society—Oncologic Emergencies: www.ncbi.nlm.nih.gov/books/bv.fcgi?rid=cmed.chapter.41500

Cancernetwork.com—Oncologic Emergencies: www.cancernetwork.com/textbook/morev42.htm

Oncology Nursing Society—Oncologic Emergencies: www.ons.org/publications/journals/ONF/Volume30/Issue2/3002224.asp

REFERENCES

Ambrosio, K. L. (2004). Tumor lysis syndrome. In B. K. Shelton, C. R. Ziegfeld, & M. M. Olsen (Eds.), *Manual of cancer nursing* (2nd ed., pp. 578–588). Philadelphia: Lippincott Williams & Wilkins.

Aurora, R., Milite, F., & Vander Els, N. J. (2000). Respiratory emergencies. *Seminars in Oncology, 27*(3), 256–269.

Cantril, C. A., & Haylock, P. J. (2004). Emergency: Tumor lysis syndrome. *American Journal of Nursing, 104*(4), 49–52.

Couban, S., Goodyear, M., Burnell, M., Dolan, S., Wasi, P., Barnes, D., et al. (2005). Randomized placebo-controlled study of low-dose warfarin for the prevention of central venous catheter-associated thrombosis in patients with cancer. *Journal of Clinical Oncology, 23*(18), 4063–4069.

Doane, L. (2002). Overview of tumor lysis syndrome. *Seminars in Oncology Nursing, 18*(Suppl. 3), 2–5.

Dulak, S. B. (2005). Hands-on help: Cardiac tamponade. *RN, 68*(4), 32.

Flaherty, A. M. (2005). Spinal cord compression. In C. H. Yarbro, M. H. Frogge, & M. Goodman (Eds.), *Cancer nursing: Principles and practice* (6th ed., pp. 910–924). Boston: Jones and Bartlett.

Flombaum, C. D. (2000). Metabolic emergencies in the cancer patient. *Seminars in Oncology, 27*(3), 322–334.

Flounders, J. A. (2003a). Cardiovascular emergencies: Pericardial effusion and cardiac tamponade. *Oncology Nursing Forum Online Exclusive, 30*(2), E48–E55.

Flounders, J. A. (2003b). Superior vena cava syndrome. *Oncology Nursing Forum Online Exclusive, 30*(4), E84–E90.

Flounders, J. A. (2003c). Syndrome of inappropriate antidiuretic hormone. *Oncology Nursing Forum Online Exclusive, 30*(3), E63–E70.

Flounders, J. A., & Ott, B. B. (2003). Oncology emergency modules: Spinal cord compression. *Oncology Nursing Forum Online Exclusive, 30*(1), E17–E23.

Gobel, B. H. (2002). Management of tumor lysis syndrome: Prevention and treatment. *Seminars in Oncology Nursing, 18*(Suppl. 3), 12–16.

Goldman, D. (2004). Effusions. In C. H. Yarbro, M. H. Frogge, & M. Goodman (Eds.), *Cancer Symptom Management* (3rd ed., pp. 420–436). Boston: Jones and Bartlett.

Greillier, L., Barlesi, F., Doddoli, C., Durieux, O., Torre, J. P., Gimenez, C., et al. (2004). Vascular stenting for palliation of superior vena cava obstruction in non-small cell lung cancer patients: A future "standard" procedure? *Respiration, 71*(2), 178–183.

Gucalp, R., & Dutcher, J. (2001). Oncologic emergencies. In E. Braunwald, A. S. Fauci, D. L. Kasper, S. L. Hause, D. L. Longo, & J. L. Jameson (Eds.), *Harrison's principles of internal medicine* (15th ed., pp. 642–650). New York: McGraw-Hill.

Gullatte, M., Kaplow, R., & Heidrich, D. (2005). Oncology. In K. K. Kuebler, M. P. Davis, & C. D. Moore (Eds.), *Palliative practices: An interdisciplinary approach* (pp. 197–245). St. Louis, MO: Elsevier.

Held-Warmkessel, J. (2005). Managing three critical cancer complications. *Nursing 2005, 35*(1), 58–63.

Johnston, P. G., & Spence, R. A. (2002). Cardiovascular emergencies. In J. Gea-Banocloche, S. Chanock, & T. Walsh (Eds.), *Oncologic emergencies* (pp. 20–24). New York: Oxford University Press.

Kaplow, R. (2002). Pathophysiology, signs, and symptoms of acute tumor lysis syndrome. *Seminars in Oncology Nursing, 18*(Suppl. 3), 6–11.

Kaplow, R. (2005). Cardiac tamponade. In C. H. Yarbro, M. H. Frogge, & M. Goodman (Eds.), *Cancer nursing: Principles and practice* (6th ed., pp. 873–886). Boston: Jones and Bartlett.

Kaplow, R., & Reid, M. (2006). Oncologic emergencies. In H. M. Schell & K. A. Puntillo (Eds.), *Critical care nursing secrets.* Philadelphia: Hanley & Delfus.

Keefe, D. L. (2000). Cardiovascular emergencies in the cancer patient. *Seminars in Oncology, 27*(3), 244–255.

Keenan, A. K. (2005). Syndrome of inappropriate antidiuretic hormone. In C. H. Yarbro, M. H. Frogge, & M. Goodman (Eds.), *Cancer nursing: Principles and practice* (6th ed., pp. 940–945). Boston: Jones and Bartlett.

Keenan, A. K., & Wickham, R. S. (2005). Hypercalcemia. In C. H. Yarbro, M. H. Frogge, & M. Goodman (Eds.), *Cancer nursing: Principles and practice* (6th ed., pp. 791–807). Boston: Jones and Bartlett.

Langfeldt, L. A., & Cooley, M. E. (2003). Syndrome of inappropriate antidiuretic hormone secretion in malignancy: Review and implications for nursing management. *Clinical Journal of Oncology Nursing, 7*(4), 425–430.

Levine, M., & Kakkar, A. K. (2005). Catheter-associated thrombosis: Thromboprophylaxis or not? *Journal of Clinical Oncology, 23*(18), 4006–4008.

Lydon, J. (2005). Tumor lysis syndrome. In C. H. Yarbro, M. H. Frogge, & M. Goodman (Eds.), *Cancer nursing: Principles and practice* (6th ed., pp. 946–958). Boston: Jones and Bartlett.

Moore, S. (2005). Superior vena cava syndrome. In C. H. Yarbro, M. H. Frogge, & M. Goodman (Eds.), *Cancer nursing: Principles and practice* (6th ed., pp. 925–939). Boston: Jones and Bartlett.

Olsen, M., & Finley, J. P. (2004a). Hypercalcemia. In B. K. Shelton, C. R. Ziegfeld, & M. M. Olsen (Eds.), *Manual of cancer nursing* (2nd ed., pp. 510–519). Philadelphia: Lippincott Williams & Wilkins.

Olsen, M., & Finley, J. P. (2004b). Syndrome of inappropriate antidiuretic hormone (SIADH). In B. K. Shelton, C. R. Ziegfeld, & M. M. Olsen (Eds.), *Manual of cancer nursing* (2nd ed., pp. 571–577). Philadelphia: Lippincott Williams & Wilkins.

Otto, S. E. (2004). *Oncology nursing clinical reference.* St. Louis, MO: Mosby.

Prasad, D., & Schiff, D. (2005). Malignant spinal-cord compression. *Lancet Oncology 2005, 6,* 15–24.

Richerson, M. T. (2004). Electrolyte imbalances. In C. H. Yarbro, M. H. Frogge, & M. Goodman (Eds.), *Cancer symptom management* (3rd ed., pp. 440–453). Boston: Jones and Bartlett.

Rowell, N. P., & Gleeson, F. V. (2001). Steroids, radiotherapy, chemotherapy and stents for superior vena caval obstruction in carcinoma of the bronchus. *Cochrane Database of Systematic Reviews, 4*(CD001316).

Shelton, B. K. (2004a). Neoplastic cardiac tamponade. In B. K. Shelton, C. R. Ziegfeld, & M. M. Olsen (Eds.), *Manual of cancer nursing* (2nd ed., pp. 520–535). Philadelphia: Lippincott Williams & Wilkins.

Shelton, B. K. (2004b). Spinal cord compression. In B. K. Shelton, C. R. Ziegfeld, & M. M. Olsen (Eds.), *Manual of cancer nursing* (2nd ed., pp. 548–559). Philadelphia: Lippincott Williams & Wilkins.

Shelton, B. K. (2004c). Superior vena cava syndrome. In B. K. Shelton, C. R. Ziegfeld, & M. M. Olsen (Eds.), *Manual of cancer nursing* (2nd ed., pp. 560–570). Philadelphia: Lippincott Williams & Wilkins.

Stewart, A. F. (2005). Hypercalcemia associated with cancer. *New England Journal of Medicine, 352*(4), 373–379.

Tan, S. J. (2002). Recognition and treatment of oncologic emergencies. *Journal of Infusion Nursing, 25*(3), 182–188.

Wilkes, G. M. (2004). Spinal cord compression. In C. H. Yarbro, M. H. Frogge, & M. Goodman (Eds.), *Cancer symptom management* (3rd ed., pp. 359–371). Boston: Jones and Bartlett.

CHAPTER 48

Human Immunodeficiency Virus and Acquired Immune Deficiency Syndrome

Dianne Weyer

LEARNING OBJECTIVES

Upon completion of this chapter, the reader will be able to:

1. Discuss the epidemiology of HIV/AIDS.

2. Explain the routes of transmission of HIV.

3. Review tests used to diagnose and monitor HIV/AIDS.

4. Describe current management strategies of HIV/AIDS.

5. List rationales for patients with HIV/AIDS to be admitted to the ICU.

6. List optimal patient outcomes that may be achieved through evidence-based management of patients with HIV and AIDS.

Acquired immune deficiency syndrome (AIDS) marched into the medical community in 1981. At the beginning of the AIDS epidemic in the United States, much confusion reigned regarding the etiology of this devastating disease. It led to high mortality among young, otherwise healthy individuals. The origination date of the AIDS epidemic is considered June 1981, when the Centers for Disease Control and Prevention (CDC) reported unusual clusters of *Pneumocystis carinii* pneumonia (PCP) seen in homosexual men in Los Angeles. Over the next 18 months, other parts of the country began seeing unusually high rates of another opportunistic infection, Kaposi's sarcoma (Farthing, Brown, & Staughton, 1988).

Many names have been used over the course of the epidemic to label those individuals who had what appeared to be a sexually transmitted disease as well as a blood borne pathogen infecting homosexual men, hemophiliacs, and heterosexual intravenous drug users (IVDUs). After a number of names for this phenomenon were put forth, in 1986 the International medical community agreed on human immunodeficiency virus (HIV) (American Foundation for AIDS Research, 2005).

TRANSMISSION

HIV is a blood-borne pathogen. As such, it is transmitted through body fluids containing high concentrations of blood cells, particularly those body fluids with high concentrations of infected white blood cells (CDC, 1998). Transmission routes of HIV include the exchange of sexual body fluids among individuals, including semen and vaginal secretions; blood transfusions; sharing of blood-contaminated drug-use equipment; mother-to-child transmission during pregnancy and delivery; breastfeeding; and occupational exposures to infected body fluids. Each mode of transmission bears a wide-ranging level of risk. For this reason, the epidemic may differ in different parts of the world, with varying levels of infection rates being noted in particular regions. The main route of transmission in the United States remains men who have sex with men, heterosexual transmission from males to females, and injecting drug users who share their drug-using equipment. Transmission rates continue to climb, with the greatest numbers found to come from the heterosexual male-to-female route. There continues to be a strong correlation between sexually transmitted infections (STIs) and HIV transmission (CDC, 2005).

One of the major success stories in the United States regarding HIV infection has been the enormous drop in perinatal transmission over the last few years. This trend is believed to result from the clinical trials conducted in the 1990s, which demonstrated that if HIV-infected pregnant women used zidovudine (AZT, Retrovir®) while they were pregnant, and received intravenous AZT intrapartum, transmission of the virus to the infant was much less likely. In addition to using antiretroviral therapy for the mother, the newborn is given AZT upon delivery, and this therapy is continued for eight weeks. The success of this regimen has resulted in an agreed-upon philosophy that all pregnant women in the United States should be offered HIV testing and, if found to be positive, antiretroviral medications should be offered to the expectant mother. Presently, reducing the possible risk of perinatal transmission to as low as 2% seems to be an attainable goal in the United States (American Foundation for AIDS Research, 2005).

HIV/AIDS AND THE IMMUNE SYSTEM

Pathogenesis

HIV is a retrovirus family member of the genus Lentivirus. Retroviruses tend to have longer latency periods, more potent virulence, and easier transmission. Two types of HIV infect humans: HIV-I and HIV-II. While the predominant virus in the United States and most other parts of the world is HIV-I, individuals in West Africa are infected primarily with HIV-II (Sande & Volberging, 1999). The life cycle of the HIV infection is described in **Table 48-1**.

The opportunity for HIV infection depends on two factors: the number of infective HIV virions in the body fluid that comes into contact with a host and the number of CD4 receptor cells available at the site of contact. Because HIV uses the CD4 cells to replicate, eventually these cells will succumb while the virus continues to thrive on newly found CD4 cells. This pattern will lead to the HIV-infected individual's loss of CD4 cells while replication of HIV continues apace. The person is said to be "immunocompromised" or "immunodeficient." Once a person becomes immunodeficient, the body is more likely to develop symptoms of HIV progression or opportunistic infections. When the population of CD4 cells drops below a total of 200 or the individual develops one of 26 opportunistic infections associated with HIV, the term AIDS is used to describe the disease. The term really does not indicate the status of HIV, but rather means that the individual has met the AIDS criteria in the course of the HIV disease (Sande & Volberding, 1999).

Acute HIV Infection

Usually, HIV antibodies develop within six weeks to three months after the initial infection. Individuals are rarely aware of their new HIV infection even though acute HIV symptoms are common among the newly infected. Because the symptoms of acute HIV infection resemble more common conditions such as influenza, mononucleosis, drug reaction, and secondary syphilis, individuals may or may not seek medical care. Even if medical care is sought, medical care providers often overlook the symptoms.

The main tool used to sort out HIV infection from common impersonators is a complete and focused risk assessment. Symptoms of acute HIV infection are usually transient and last only a few weeks, adding to the challenge of reaching an accurate diagnosis. Acute HIV infection results in a high rate of viral replication with unopposed HIV antibody. Thus the individual is highly infectious during this period. Some experts also argue that this short period offers treatment possibilities, which might result in a better prognosis (Bartlett & Gallant, 2004).

TABLE 48-1 Life-Cycle Steps of HIV Infection and Dissemination

Attachment and Entry	RNA to DNA Replication	Integration	Assembly	Budding of New Virus
HIV attaches itself to protein receptors on the outside of CD4 cells. After binding with the CD4 cell, the virus enters the cell.	Using an enzyme called reverse transcriptase, HIV merges its RNA with the cell's genetic material (DNA). This allows the DNA in the CD4 cell to make copies of HIV (replication).	HIV DNA enters the nucleus, the command center of the cell. Once inside the nucleus, HIV uses another enzyme, integrase, to reprogram the cell, integrating the virus with the cell's DNA.	Another enzyme called protease helps the formation of the HIV proteins line up to produce an effective virus.	The new viruses break out of the CD4 cell, almost like a flower budding off a stem. These new "buds" have the capacity to infect more cells, leading to HIV dissemination and CD4 destruction.

Source: U.S. Department of Health and Human Services, 2005a.

Clinical Manifestations

HIV disease may first present within a few weeks of infection with a seroconversion illness as described in the previous section. Symptoms such as fatigue and night sweats and relatively minor medical problems such as shingles and oral thrush usually precede the development of major opportunistic infections or tumors. At this point in the course of the disease, the individual does not yet meet the case-defining criteria for AIDS. The actual syndrome of AIDS may not occur for many years after infection.

"Minor" manifestations of HIV disease include fatigue, lymphadenopathy, night sweats, diarrhea, oral cavity disease, skin disease, and thrombocytopenia. Although they are seldom life-threatening and rarely require hospitalization, their presence is very important in both diagnosis and management of HIV disease. The most common opportunistic infections include the following conditions (Farthing et al.,1988):

- PCP
- Primary or secondary central nervous disease
- Esophageal candidiasis
- Tuberculosis
- Cervical cancer
- Non-Hodgkin's lymphoma
- Cryptococcal meningitis

LABORATORY TESTS

HIV Testing

A standard enzyme immunoassay (EIA) is used to screen for HIV infection and, if it is positive, a diagnostic Western Blot is necessary. Western Blot testing can have one of three results: negative, positive, or indeterminate. An indeterminate test must be repeated, and only a confirmatory Western Blot can definitively diagnose HIV infection (Bartlett & Gallant, 2004).

CD4 Count

The CD4 or T-cell count reflects the competence of the immune system. As more copies of the virus are replicated and more CD4 cells are destroyed, the individual's immune system begins to deteriorate. The CD4 count is believed to be the most reliable indicator of prognosis. Because the CD4 count can be affected by many variables, including current illnesses, it is important to look at CD4 progressions rather than single random values (Bartlett & Gallant, 2004).

Some key CD4 values are known to be important in the management of HIV disease. If the absolute CD4 count drops below 200 cells/mm^3 in the HIV-infected individual, then an AIDS diagnosis has been reached. In addition, the patient with a CD4 count of less than 200 cells/mm^3 should be placed on PCP prophylaxis. When a CD4 count of less than 100 cells/mm^3 is obtained, prophylaxis for toxoplasmosis is initiated. A CD4 count of less than 50 cells/mm^3 requires additional prophylaxis protection from *Mycobacterium avium* complex (MAC).

CD4 measurements also guide antiretroviral management. A CD4 count of less than 350 cells/mm^3 would indicate the patient should be considered for antiretroviral therapy, according to most experts. As patients continue on their highly active antiretroviral therapy (HAART) regimens, CD4 counts are intermittently measured as a way to determine the efficacy of treatment and the need to modify failing regimens (Mountain Plains AIDS Education and Training Center, 2005).

Quantitative Plasma HIV RNA (Viral Load)

Quantitative plasma HIV RNA, a common HIV laboratory test, is useful in supporting the diagnosis of acute HIV infection, determining the probability of transmission of virus to another individual, predicting the progression of HIV in the chronically infected, and monitoring the efficacy of antiretroviral therapy. While CD4 counts reflect the competence of the immune system, viral load monitoring reflects the viral replication pattern. The viral load count is believed to measure only 2% of the total viral replication and viral load in the body. Factors affecting the viral load count include ongoing illnesses, antiretroviral treatment failure, and possibly immunization interaction, although the latter is usually a transient effect persisting for only two to four weeks. Newer viral load testing assays allow the virus to be measured at levels of less than 50 copies per milliliter. This value is also termed undetectable (Bartlett & Gallant, 2004).

Mutations

Given the distinctive replication pattern of retroviruses, errors in copying are not uncommon, resulting in what is called a mutated virus. These mutations are unpredictable and lead to resistance, which in turn results in treatment failure and disease progression. Resistance testing allows the virus to be evaluated by looking at both genetic mutations (genotypic testing) and the level of medication required to suppress the virus (phenotypic testing). If the virus does not appear to be responding to a drug or combination of drugs, the viral genome is examined for mutations. Genotypic assays look for the key mutations associated with resistance to a particular drug. Unlike genotypic testing, phenotypic assays do not examine the actual genes or RNA of the virus but instead measure the ability of the virus to reproduce in a test tube when a particular drug is present and determine how much of the drug is needed in that test tube to suppress replication. Both laboratory tests can add value in differentiating disease progression (Bartlett & Gallant, 2004).

TREATMENT

When considering HIV suppression, one thinks only of medication. In some individuals, however, the virus does not progress as expected. Other patients experience a very slow progression, so medications are not immediately indicated.

For the individual in which viral replication is greater than 100,000 copies/mL or whose CD4 count drops below 350 cells/mm^3, antiretroviral medication is usually indicated. There is growing concern about the long-term side effects of some antiretroviral agents, and some experts would argue for a delay in initiation of therapy until the CD4 count is closer to 200 cells/mm^3. Treatment must be individualized to enhance efficacy (U.S. Department of Health and Human Services, 2005b).

Antiretroviral Medications

The first class of antiretrovirals developed consisted of the nucleoside/nucleotide reverse transcriptase inhibitors (NRTIs). These medications alter the ability of the virus to reverse the RNA to DNA, thereby limiting copying of HIV at this step of replication. Examples of NRTI agents include didanosine (ddI, Videx®), lamivudine (3TC, Epivir®), and stavudine (d4T, Zerit®).

In the mid- to late 1990s, HIV mortality changed significantly when the protease inhibitors (PIs) were released for wide use. These medications block the effectiveness of the viral enzyme protease. PIs bind to the enzyme's active site and block its activity; as a consequence, the budding viral particles are not infectious. Examples of PIs include amprenavir (Agenerase®) and nelfinavir (Viracept®).

The third and newest class of antiretrovirals was approved in 2003 and is known as entry/fusion inhibitors. Presently, only one drug has been approved in this class, enfuvirtide (T20, Fuzeon™). Enfuvirtide interferes with the virus's entry by binding to gp41 and preventing the virus from fusing to the CD4 cell. The only route of administration for this drug is subcutaneous injection (American Foundation for AIDS Research, 2005).

Side Effects of Drugs

All HIV medications have the potential to cause gastrointestinal, skin, and nervous system side effects. Certain drugs have greater capacity for these general side effects than others. Long-term metabolic side effects seen with the use of antiretrovirals include those listed in **Box 48-1**.

The number of hospital beds required for patients with HIV disease has declined over the last 10 years with the widespread use of HAART. However, due to increasing resistance

---

Box 48-1

Long-Term Metabolic Side Effects of Antiretroviral Therapy

Diabetes mellitus and insulin resistance—usually with PIs (Mehta, Moore, Thomas, Chaisson, & Sulkowski, 2003)

Lipodystrophy—greatest with NRTIs and especially Zerit (Andersen et al., 2003)

Hyperlipidemia—seen with both PIs and NRTIs (Dube et al., 2003)

Lactic acidosis—usually with NRTIs (Carr, 2003)

---

and virulent virus mutations, demand for these hospital beds could potentially begin to rise again.

Patients with HIV/AIDS may be admitted to the intensive care unit (ICU) for a number of reasons, including sepsis or septic shock from toxoplasmosis, cytomegalovirus (CMV), resistant tuberculosis, or cryptococcal meningitis; respiratory failure from PCP; and hemorrhage from hemorrhoids, colonic lesions, or CMV-induced colitis. Central nervous system dysfunction is not uncommon in patients with AIDS, and may be related to toxoplasmosis, lymphoma, or other causes. Other reported reasons for admission to the ICU include PCP-related pneumothorax, bacterial infection, tuberculosis-associated pneumothorax, cerebral toxoplasmosis, and severe dilated cardiomyopathy (Broch & Kaiser, 2005; Fingerhood, 2001; Holzman, Schirmer, & Nasraway, 2005).

Patients with HIV/AIDS are also admitted to the ICU for treatment-related toxicities. In one study, admissions to the ICU related to sepsis increased from 16.3% to 22.6% from pre-HAART to post-HAART treatment use. In the same study, AIDS-related admissions significantly decreased. No difference in mortality rates in the two groups of patients was observed (Casalino et al., 2004). In a similar study, the researchers compared pre-HAART and HAART patients. The patients in the latter group required significantly more ICU stays, but ICU survival did not differ in the two groups (Vincent et al., 2004). A case report of a patient with late HIV disease who received HAART revealed esophageal varices and non-cirrhosis cholestasis. The patient was admitted to the ICU for worsening acidosis, which was attributed to HAART (Shahmanesh, Cartledge, & Miller, 2002).

When patients are admitted to the ICU and placed on mechanical ventilation, oftentimes oral medications are held if an intravenous preparation of the medication is not available. Many antiretroviral therapies are not available in intravenous form. Withholding antiretroviral treatment may result in increased resistance and increased immunosuppression due to viral load rebound. Some medications, when given enterally, may be inadequately absorbed. This, too, may lead to drug resistance. ICU nurses must also observe for serious toxicities of these drugs, such as pancreatitis and lactic acidosis (Soni & Pozniak, 2001).

As with other disease processes, HIV care is complicated and labor-intensive. One of the major issues in management is not a medical challenge but rather a psychosocial one. Mental health patients or those individuals with a dual or triple diagnosis require care that may tax even the most resource-rich sites. Adherence to HIV drug regimens is critical for viral suppression but difficult to assess and even harder to provide solutions to the nonadhering individual.

PATIENT OUTCOMES

Nurses can help ensure attainment of optimal patient outcomes such as those listed in **Box 48-2** through the use of evidence-based interventions for patients with HIV or AIDS.

Box 48-2
Optimal Patient Outcomes

- Immune function in expected range
- Oxygen saturation in expected range
- Demonstrates understanding of disease process and mechanism of transmission
- Nutritional status in expected range
- Perceived importance of following expected health practices
- Effective coping patterns present
- Adherence to treatment plan
- Physical comfort in expected range

SUMMARY

Nursing staff are constantly challenged with not only the nursing care needed for HIV/AIDS but also the support needed by patients and their families. HIV patient education is critical for the nursing care plan and will advance a timely recovery.

CASE STUDY

D.M. is a 42-year-old who presents to the emergency department (ED) for evaluation of fever and respiratory symptoms. He was diagnosed with HIV infection eight years ago and has intermittently received care for his HIV disease. His last CD4 count was 135 cells/mm³ and his HIV RNA was measured at 53,000 copies/mL. Trimethoprim-sulfamethoxazole (Bactrim®, Septra®), one tablet a day, was prescribed for prophylaxis at that time, and D.M. was scheduled to follow up one week later to discuss starting antiretroviral therapy. He did not return for the follow-up appointment and now presents with a one- to two-week history of fever, fatigue, nonproductive cough, and dyspnea on exertion. He admits that he did not take any of the trimethoprim-sulfamethoxazole. His examination shows a respiratory rate of 26. Room air resting O_2 saturation was 91%, and arterial blood gas shows pH 7.48, CO_2 29 mm Hg, and pO_2 68 mm Hg. The chest radiograph shows bilateral opacities with an increase in interstitial markings. D.M. has no known drug allergies.

D.M. was admitted to the ICU as his shortness of breath worsened. Ultimately, he was intubated because of progressive and refractory hypoxemia and hypercarbia (pH 7.28, pO_2 52, pCO_2 55, SaO_2 84%). Once intubated, D.M. underwent a bronchoscopy with bronchoalveolar lavage, and his *Pneumocystis carinii* pneumonia was confirmed. He was started on intravenous trimethoprim-sulfamethoxazole and a 21-day course of prednisone.

D.M. responded to his PCP treatment, was extubated after three days, and remained in the hospital for an additional week before being discharged home to continue his 21-day course of therapy. His intravenous therapy was switched to an oral regimen, and he continued both his PCP treatment and the antiretroviral regimen begun during his hospitalization.

Emphasis was placed on his continuing the PCP therapy, the antiretroviral regimen, and a prophylaxis regimen for PCP once his 21 days of therapy were complete.

CRITICAL THINKING QUESTIONS

1. What information in this case study suggests that D.M. has *Pneumocystis carinii* pneumonia?
2. What is the recommended treatment for PCP?
3. What are the indications for use of steroid therapy with this patient?
4. Which disciplines should be consulted to work with this client?
5. What types of issues may require you to act as an advocate or moral agent for this patient?
6. How will you implement your role as a facilitator of learning for this patient?
7. Using the website www.clinicaltrials.gov, list the current trials that are in progress for patients with HIV or AIDS.
8. Use the form to write up data and a plan of care for a patient with HIV in the ICU. Rate the patient as a level 1, 3, or 5 on each characteristic. Identify the level of nurse characteristics needed in the care of this patient.
9. Take one patient outcome for an HIV patient and list evidence-based interventions found in a literature review for this patient.

Using the Synergy Model to Develop a Plan of Care

	Patient Characteristics	Level (1, 3, 5)	Subjective and Objective Data	Evidence-based Interventions	Outcomes
SYNERGY MODEL	Resiliency				
	Vulnerability				
	Stability				
	Complexity				
	Resource availability				
	Participation in care				
	Participation in decision making				
	Predictability				

Online Resources

AIDS information: www.aidsinfo.nih.gov

AIDS Fact Sheet: www.aids.org

UNAIDS (the Joint United Nations Program): www.unaids.org

CDC, Division of HIV/AIDS Prevention: www.cdc.gov/hiv/dhap.htm

AIDS Education Global Information System (AEGIS): aegis.com

HIV Knowledge Base: www.hivinsite.ucsf.edu/Insite

FDA HIV/AIDS Program: www.fda.gov/oashi/aids/hiv.html

HIV/AIDS Bureau: www.hab.hras.gov

REFERENCES

American Foundation for AIDS Research. (2005). Retrieved October 7, 2005, from www.amfar.org

Andersen, O., Haugaard, S. B., Andersen, U. B., Friis-Moller, N., Storgaard, H., Volund, A., et al. (2003). Lipodystrophy in human immunodeficiency virus patients impairs insulin action and induces defects in beta-cell function. *Metabolism, 52*(10), 1343–1353.

Bartlett, J. G., & Gallant, J. E. (2004). *Medical management of HIV infection.* Baltimore, MD: Johns Hopkins Medicine Health Publishing Business Group.

Broch, K. C., & Kaiser, A. B. (2005). Central nervous system infections. In M. P. Fink, E. Abraham, J. Vincent, & P. M. Kochanek (Eds.), *Textbook of critical care* (5th ed., pp. 1295–1308). Philadelphia: Saunders.

Carr, A. (2003). Lactic acidemia in infection with human immunodeficiency virus. *Clinical Infectious Disease, 36,* S96–S100.

Casalino, E., Wolff, M., Ravaud, P., Choquet, C., Bruneel, F., & Regnier, B. (2004). Impact of HAART advent on admission patterns and survival in HIV-infected patients admitted to an intensive care unit. *AIDS, 18*(10), 1429–1433.

Centers for Disease Control and Prevention (CDC). (1998). Guidelines for treatment of sexually transmitted diseases. *Morbidity and Mortality Weekly Report, 47*(RR-1).

Centers for Disease Control and Prevention (CDC). (2005). Retrieved September 5, 2005, from www.cdc.gov/hiv/stats/htm

Dube, M. P., Stein, J. H., Aberg, J. A., Fichtenbaum, C. J., Gerber, J. G., Tashima, K. T., et al., Adult AIDS Clinical Trials Group Cardiovascular Subcommittee, HIV Medical Association of the Infectious Disease Society of America. (2003). Guidelines for the evaluation and management of dyslipidemia in human immunodeficiency virus (HIV)-infected adults receiving antiretroviral therapy: Recommendations of the HIV Medical Association of the Infectious Disease Society of America and the Adult AIDS Clinical Trials Group. *Clinical Infectious Disease, 37*(5), 613–627.

Farthing, C. F., Brown, S. E., & Staughton, R. C. (1988). *Color atlas of AIDS and HIV disease* (2nd ed., pp. 6–7). London: Wolfe Medical Publications.

Fingerhood, M. (2001). Full recovery from severe dilated cardiomyopathy in an HIV-infected patient. *AIDS Read, 11*(6), 333–335.

Holzman, N. L., Schirmer, C. M., & Nasraway, S. A. (2005). Gastrointestinal hemorrhage. In M. P. Fink, E. Abraham, J. Vincent, & P. M. Kochanek (Eds.), *Textbook of critical care* (5th ed., pp. 973–982). Philadelphia: Saunders.

Mehta, S. H., Moore, R. D., Thomas, D. L., Chaisson, R. E., & Sulkowski, M. S. (2003). The effect of HAART and HCV infection on the development of hyperglycemia among HIV-infected persons. *Journal of Acquired Immune Deficiency Syndrome, 33*(5), 577–584.

Mountain Plains AIDS Education and Training Center. (2005). *HIV: 2005 Sourcebook for the primary care provider* (pp. 2–5). www.mpaetc.org

Sande, M. A., & Volberging, P. A. (1999). *The medical management of AIDS* (4th ed., p. 24). Philadelphia: Saunders.

Shahmanesh, M., Cartledge, J., & Miller, R. (2002). Lactic acidosis and abnormal liver function in advanced HIV disease. *Sexually Transmitted Infections, 78*(2), 139–142.

Soni, N., & Pozniak, A. (2001). Continuing HIV therapy in the ICU. *Critical Care, 5*(5), 247–248.

U.S. Department of Health and Human Services. (2005a). Guidelines for the use of antiretroviral agents in HIV-infected adults and adolescents. www.aidsinfo.nih.gov/guidelines/default_db2.asp?id=50

U.S. Department of Health and Human Services. (2005b). HIV life cycle. Retrieved March 26, 2006, from http://aidsinfo.nih.gov/other/hivlifecycle.html

Vincent, B., Timsit, J., Auburtin, M., Schortgen, F., Bouadma, L., Wolff, M., et al. (2004). Characteristics and outcomes of HIV-infected patients in the ICU: Impact of the highly active antiretroviral treatment era. *Intensive Care Medicine, 30,* 859–866.

CHAPTER 49

Thrombocytopenia

Hildy Schell

LEARNING OBJECTIVES

Upon completion of this chapter, the reader will be able to:

1. Identify four potential causes of thrombocytopenia.

2. List the clinical manifestations of thrombocytopenia.

3. Discuss potential treatment interventions for thrombocytopenia.

4. Conduct a nursing assessment and select appropriate interventions for patients with thrombocytopenia.

5. List optimal patient outcomes that may be achieved through evidence-based management of thrombocytopenia.

Thrombocytopenia is defined as an abnormally low number of platelets in circulating blood. A platelet count of less than $100,000/mm^3$ is considered thrombocytopenia. Thrombocytopenia is one of the more common coagulation disorders observed in critically ill patients. This chapter reviews normal platelet function, causes of thrombocytopenia and platelet dysfunction, and the essential nursing monitoring and management for patients with thrombocytopenia.

PLATELETS AND NORMAL HEMOSTASIS

Platelets are essential for normal hemostasis (arresting of bleeding). These small disc-shaped cells are manufactured in the bone marrow and released into the bloodstream. Megakaryocytes, the precursor cells for platelets, are found in the bone marrow.

Platelets have a lifespan of 7 to 10 days. If they are not used to form a clot, they are destroyed by the liver or spleen.

Platelets are activated at the site of vascular injury or by inflammatory mediators. The essential platelet reactions needed to maintain normal hemostasis are adhesion, aggregation, and granule secretion. Adhesion is the deposition of platelets on the subendothelial matrix layer of a blood vessel. The interaction of platelets with collagen fibrils of the matrix layer results in activation of other platelets. These cells contain signaling proteins and membrane surface receptors, which enable them to activate other platelets in an effort to create a vascular plug. The platelet-activating substances, thromboxane-A_2 and adenosine diphosphate (ADP), are secreted into circulation. After adhesion, platelets begin to aggregate (clump together) to form a platelet plug. Proteins or granules that help platelets aggregate at the site are secreted from the platelets. When glycoproteins (GPIIb/IIIa)—receptors for fibrinogen that are located on the platelet membrane surface—are activated, platelets bind to fibrinogen proteins circulating in the bloodstream, resulting in more aggregation.

PLATELET DISORDERS

Two types of platelet disorders are distinguished: qualitative and quantitative. In a qualitative disorder, the platelets present do not function normally. In a quantitative disorder, the person has an abnormally low or high number of platelets.

Qualitative Platelet Disorders

When the platelets have a structural or functional defect, the person is considered to have a qualitative platelet disorder. The platelet count may be normal, but the platelets' adhesion, aggregation, and/or secretion response is abnormal. Some qualitative platelet disorders are related to inherited disorders resulting in GP defects or von Willebrand's disease, uremia, and medications [e.g., aspirin, clopidogrel bisulfate (Plavix®), dextran, dipyridamole (Persantine®), and GPIIb/IIIa inhibitors—abciximab (Reopro®), eptifibatide (Integrilin®), and tirofiban hydrochloride (Aggrastat®)]. Patients with qualitative platelet disorders require prophylactic treatment prior to invasive procedures (e.g., surgery, central venous catheter placement, biopsy). Treatments include stopping the medication causing platelet dysfunction, providing renal replacement therapy when uremia is present, administering desmopressin (DDAVP®), administering Factor VIII concentrate, and/or transfusing platelets. Desmopressin increases plasma Factor VIII and von Willebrand factor, both of which enhance the adhesion of platelets to blood vessels. These same treatments are implemented when active bleeding is present.

Quantitative Platelet Disorders

A normal platelet count is in the range of 150,000 to 450,000/mm³. A count less than 100,000/mm³ is considered thrombocytopenia. Patients are at risk for spontaneous bleeding—usually gastrointestinal or intracranial bleeding—when the platelet count is less than 20,000/mm³. The risk of a life-threatening bleed is highest when the count is less than 5,000/mm³ (Hardin, 2005).

The mechanisms that cause thrombocytopenia are related to five issues: (1) impaired platelet production; (2) accelerated destruction of platelets; (3) dilution from massive transfusion; (4) abnormally high distribution to the spleen; and (5) excessive consumption of platelets. It is important to recognize that a low platelet count may be a spurious laboratory value and not true thrombocytopenia. This situation is referred to as "pseudothrombocytopenia." Such a laboratory artifact may be related to the anticoagulant, ethylene diamine tetraacetic acid (EDTA®), used in lab tubes. EDTA can cause platelets to adhere to the white blood cells in the test tube sample (Hardin, 2005). To eliminate this problem, blood samples can be redrawn in tubes with other anticoagulant substances, such as sodium and lithium heparin (green top) or sodium citrate (blue top).

Pseudothrombocytopenia may also be due to overfilling of the vacuum tubes, which results in inadequate anticoagulation of the sample and platelet clumping within the sample (Baldwin, 2003). **Table 49-1** summarizes the etiologies of thrombocytopenia.

CLINICAL PRESENTATION OF THROMBOCYTOPENIA

Patients with thrombocytopenia may present with either subtle or overt signs and symptoms. Thrombocytopenia is typically asymptomatic until the platelet count drops below 20,000/mm³. **Table 49-2** describes key areas of nursing assessment for the patient with thrombocytopenia.

Heparin-Induced Thrombocytopenia

Heparin-induced thrombocytopenia (HIT) is considered an adverse reaction to heparin therapy. HIT is thought to be caused by formation of an immunoglobulin G (IgG)–heparin immune complex (Franchini, 2005). Patients should be suspected of having HIT if their platelet counts are less than 100,000/mm³ or are reduced by 50% from their baseline measurements. Thrombocytopenia usually begins between 3 and 15 days after heparin therapy is started, but it has been reported within hours of the beginning of heparin therapy in patients who were previously exposed to the drug. The platelet count usually returns to the patient's baseline level within 4 days after heparin is stopped. HIT is estimated to develop in as many as 3% of patients exposed to heparin (Chong & Chong, 2004) and is associated with a reported mortality rate of 30% and amputation rate of 20% (Picker & Gathof, 2004). Some of the more severe complications associated with HIT include arterial or venous thromboembolism, limb gangrene, and skin necrosis (Menajovsky, 2005). The fact that the thrombocytopenia seen in HIT usually resolves within 3 to 7 days of heparin withdrawal is a useful aid in diagnosing HIT. The thrombotic tendency associated with HIT can last for as long as 30 days and can develop well after heparin discontinuation and platelet count recovery. Management of HIT involves the elimination of heparin and use of newer anticoagulants such as lepirudin (Refludan®), agratroban (Argatroban®), and danaparoid sodium (Orgaran®). Monitoring the platelet levels of patients receiving heparin will aid in early diagnosis of HIT.

Heparin-induced hemorrhage is controlled with protamine sulfate. This heparin antagonist neutralizes heparin within 5 minutes after intravenous (IV) administration. Repeated doses may be required given the drug's short duration of 2 hours. Protamine sulfate should be administered as a slow IV push; 1 mg can neutralize 90 to 115 units of heparin. Give no more than 50 mg over a 10-minute period. Protamine sulfate may cause bleeding if the amount given exceeds the amount of heparin that it is trying to neutralize.

Idiopathic Thrombocytopenic Purpura

Idiopathic thrombocytopenic purpura (ITP) is an autoimmune blood disorder in which an IgG autoantibody forms and binds

TABLE 49-1 Thrombocytopenia: Mechanisms and Associated Clinical Conditions

Mechanisms of Thrombocytopenia	Associated Clinical Conditions
Decreased bone marrow production	• Bone marrow abnormalities: dysplasia, aplasia, fibrosis, infiltration with malignant cells (leukemia, myeloma) • Malnutrition: iron, folic acid, or vitamin B_{12} deficiency • Chronic liver disease • Congenital disorders • Cytotoxic medications: cyclophosphamide, azathioprine, chemotherapeutic agents
Accelerated destruction	• Idiopathic thrombotic purpura • Thrombocytopenic thrombotic purpura • Hemolytic uremic syndrome • Antiphospholipid syndrome • Heparin-induced thrombocytopenia • Vasculitis • Medications
Dilutional	• Massive transfusion with non-platelet-containing blood products (RBCs, WBC, FFP, cryoprecipitate), crystalloid, or colloid over short period of time
Distributional	• Splenomegaly • Portal hypertension • Chronic liver disease (cirrhosis) • Myeloproliferative or lymphoproliferative disorders with splenic involvement
Consumptive	• Disseminated intravascular coagulation • Heparin-induced thrombocytopenia
Medications and other	• Medications: antifungal agents, furosemide, phenytoin, digoxin, acetaminophen, rifampin, penicillin, heparin • High fever • Pre-eclampsia • HELLP syndrome (hemolysis, elevated liver function test results, low platelets)

Sources: George, 2006; Horell & Rothman, 2001; Matthai, 2005.

to platelets (Kaplow, 2006). Patients with platelet counts greater than 50,000/mm^3 often have no signs of bleeding. However, when the platelet count drops below this level, signs of bleeding may be observed. Diagnosis of ITP is based on clinical history and presentation, along with exclusion of other causes of thrombocytopenia. Peripheral blood cell morphology may reveal platelets that are slightly enlarged (megathrombocytes).

Treatment is required in patients with severe thrombocytopenia (less than 30,000/mm^3) with prednisone (Deltasone®), 1 to 2 mg/kg/day. Prednisone decreases the binding of the antibody to the platelet surface. An alternative steroid regimen is high-dose dexamethasone (Decadron®), 40 mg/day for 4 days. High-dose immunoglobulin (1 Gm/kg for 1 to 2 days) is highly effective in increasing platelet counts for 1 to 2 weeks, but this therapy is reserved for bleeding emergencies or to prepare severely thrombocytopenic patients for a splenectomy. A splenectomy is indicated in patients who do not respond to prednisone initially or when unacceptably high doses are required. Bleeding usually decreases within a day after beginning treatment with prednisone. Platelet counts usually increase within 1 week. Responses are typically seen within 3 weeks (Kaplow, 2006).

Thrombotic Thrombocytopenic Purpura

Thrombotic thrombocytopenic purpura (TTP) is a rare disorder of platelet aggregation that is often precipitated by estrogen use, pregnancy, medications, or infections in patients who are 20 to 50 years of age. Even though 80% to 90% of patients recover when treated, 20% of patients with TTP may have a relapse. Symptoms include anemia, bleeding, and neurologic abnormalities (e.g., headache, confusion, aphasia, and changes in level of consciousness ranging from lethargy to coma). The key laboratory finding is seen on a peripheral blood smear in the form of fragmented red blood cells. Other laboratory findings include anemia, thrombocytopenia (platelet count less than 20,000/mm^3), and marked reticulocytosis. Treatment includes daily large-volume plasmapheresis, prednisone (Deltasone®), antiplatelet agents (e.g., acetylsalicylic acid, 325 mg once daily), and dipyridamole (Persantine® 75 mg three times a day [TID]). Nurses should monitor for signs of bleeding (i.e., petechiae or unusual bruising) (Kaplow, 2006).

EVALUATION AND DIAGNOSIS

Identifying the etiology of thrombocytopenia is essential to choose the best treatment option. Evaluation of a patient with

TABLE 49-2 Systematic Assessment of a Patient with Thrombocytopenia and Potential Findings

Assessment Criteria	Potential Findings
Patient history	• Hematologic disorders (e.g., aplastic anemia, myelodysplasia, myeloma, leukemia) • Non-hematologic disorders that are associated with thrombocytopenia (e.g., sepsis, eclampsia, liver disease, HIV, SLE) • Recent or past platelet transfusion • Malnourished state • Prolonged bleeding or ease of bruising history
Medication review	• Medications that can cause thrombocytopenia or that increase risk of bleeding: aspirin, nonsteroidal anti-inflammatory agents, herbs (ginger, gingko, kelp), heparin, enoxaparin, activated protein C
General observation	• Evidence of bleeding from mouth, nose, or exposed skin
Neurologic	• Altered mental status, confusion, pupil changes, coma potentially related to intracranial bleeding
Skin	• Petechiae (tiny red/purple spots), purpura (small areas of hemorrhage into skin/mucosa), ecchymosis (bruises) • Bleeding from IV sites, incisions, wounds
Gastrointestinal/genitourinary	• Abdominal distention related to splenomegaly or hepatomegaly • Occult-blood-positive stool, bloody stool, or melena • Hemetemesis or heme-positive NG drainage • Hematuria or heme-positive urine • Heavy-flow menses
Respiratory	• Hemoptysis • Bloody chest tube drainage
Laboratory values	• Platelet count (low) • Hematocrit and hemoglobin (may be low) • Abnormal coagulation studies (PT/INR, PTT, fibrinogen, fibrin degradation products) • Abnormal platelet aggregation studies (confirm HIT) • Abnormal autoimmune disorder tests (e.g., antinuclear antibodies) • Abnormal peripheral smear results

Source: Menajovsky, 2005.

SLE = Systemic Lupus Erythematosus   PTT = Partial Thromboplastin Time
HIV = Human Immunodeficiency Virus   PT = Prothrombin Time
NG = Nasogastric   INR = International Normalized Ratio

clumping and the cell counts and shapes. Giant platelets are associated with ITP, whereas schistocytes (fragments) are seen in TTP and disseminated intravascular coagulation (DIC). The bone marrow is examined for cell types and shapes as well as for presence of megakaryocytes.

If the patient has an enlarged spleen and normal bone marrow, the thrombocytopenia is usually related to abnormal distribution or sequestration. This problem may be caused by congestive splenomegaly, liver disease, or tumor infiltration of the spleen. When splenomegaly and abnormal bone marrow are present, the patient likely has a hematologic disorder such as leukemia, lymphoma, or myeloma. Thrombocytopenia with a normal spleen and normal bone marrow is caused by excessive destruction or use of platelets to form clots. The immune- or non-immune-related causes of platelet destruction need to be considered and worked up (e.g., by sending serum for autoantibodies). Impaired production of platelets is the cause of thrombocytopenia when the spleen is normal and the bone marrow is abnormal.

TREATMENT AND MANAGEMENT

Treatment will depend on the severity of thrombocytopenia and the presence of active bleeding. The initial aim is identification and treatment of the underlying cause of thrombocytopenia. If the patient with thrombocytopenia is actively bleeding or has a life-threatening bleed, platelet transfusion is indicated. If a medication is suspected as the etiology, it should be discontinued when possible. When fever or an infection is causing thrombocytopenia, the source of infection should be identified and treated appropriately with antibiotics and source control measures (e.g., removal of the

a low platelet count usually starts with a review of the patient's medical history, current condition, and all medications. The spleen is assessed by palpation, ultrasonography, and/or computerized tomography (CT) scan. A peripheral blood film/smear and bone marrow biopsy or aspirate may be indicated to diagnose the cause of thrombocytopenia. The blood smear is examined under the microscope to assess the presence of platelet

infected device or tissue). Close monitoring of platelet counts, hematocrit levels, and signs of bleeding is essential during treatment. It is also important to evaluate whether the discontinuation of a medication or administration of a platelet transfusion improved the clinical condition. Corticosteroids or IgG may be administered to block the reticuloendothelial system's phagocytic clearance of antibody-coated platelets. A splenectomy may be indicated for refractory thrombocytopenia related to ITP and other immunologic etiologies (e.g., collagen vascular or lymphoproliferative disorders).

Platelet transfusions are indicated for active bleeding with concomitant thrombocytopenia or as prophylaxis with severe thrombocytopenia (less than 5,000/mm^3). The evidence supports the safety of performing major surgical or invasive procedures with a platelet count in the range of 40,000 to 50,000/mm^3 (Schiffer et al., 2001). Caution should be taken when transfusing platelets in patients with TTP or HIT, however, because this intervention may increase the severity of these thrombotic disorders (Symonette & Hoffman, 2005). Platelets for transfusion are either pooled from multiple donors or apheresed from a single donor. Pooled platelet packs come from 6 to 10 donors. The risk of adverse reactions and sensitization to platelet antigens is lower when single-donor platelets are used. Platelets arrive from the blood bank in either a bag or syringe and are transfused over 10 to 20 minutes. Patients should be closely monitored during and after the transfusion for signs of a reaction: itching, rash, fever, and shivering/chills. A post-transfusion platelet count should be obtained to evaluate the efficacy of the transfusion, when possible.

Some patients become refractory to platelet transfusions—that is, their platelet count does not increase after platelets are transfused. Although dependent on patient size, the usual increase in platelet levels after transfusion is 2,000 to 10,000/mm^3 in an average-sized adult (Schiffer et al., 2001). Refractoriness may be the result of either non-immune causes

(high fever, enlarged spleen, medications) or immune causes (antibodies recognize donated platelets as non-self and destroy them). The donor platelets can be HLA-A and HLA-B matched and/or cross matched to prevent further sensitization by the recipient's antibodies.

PATIENT OUTCOMES

Nurses can help ensure attainment of optimal patient outcomes such as those listed in **Box 49-1** through the use of evidence-based interventions for patients with thrombocytopenia.

SUMMARY

Thrombocytopenia is a potentially life-threatening condition. The underlying cause or condition associated with the low platelet count must be identified and treated. Astute nursing assessments and implementation of appropriate nursing interventions can aid in the evaluation of the condition, prevent serious complications, and contribute to the treatment of the disorder causing thrombocytopenia. The nurse who integrates assessment findings with clinical knowledge about the disorder, causes, and risks can positively influence patient outcomes by identifying and implementing the appropriate actions necessary to meet the needs of the patients and families.

Box 49-1
Optimal Patient Outcomes

- Absence of overt signs of bleeding
- Platelet count in expected range
- Neurologic status in expected range
- Distal pulses palpable
- Verbalizes strategies to prevent bleeding

CASE STUDY

A 55-year-old male patient with chronic obstructive pulmonary disease and hypertension, status post thyroidectomy for cancer, is admitted to the ICU with respiratory distress. He is afebrile, tachypneic, and diaphoretic, and has an oxygen saturation of 91% on 50% oxygen via face mask. He complains of right leg pain, and the leg is edematous. Serum laboratory tests reveal a platelet count of 30,000/mm^3. An ultrasound of the patient's leg reveals a DVT.

The patient's son asks if he could shave his dad's beard per his father's request. The nurse reinforced the risks of bleeding and suggested use of an electric razor.

The nurse received an order to remove the CVC, which had two clotted lumens, after the scheduled peripherally inserted central catheter (PICC) was inserted. The nurse contacted the PICC team nurse and reviewed the patient's history, labs, and precautions; clarified the order for CVC removal with the physician; and reported the latest platelet count of 28,000/mm^3. The physician came to the bedside and assisted with the procedure. Pressure was held on the CVC exit site for 15 minutes until the bleeding stopped. The nurse monitored that site closely for signs of bleeding and/or hematoma formation over the shift. The need for close monitoring of that site was communicated to the oncoming nurse.

CRITICAL THINKING QUESTIONS

1. What are important assessment criteria related to the thrombocytopenia for the admitting ICU nurse?

2. What are the potential causes of this thrombocytopenia?

3. What are essential nursing interventions, related to thrombocytopenia for this patient?

4. Take one patient outcome for this patient and list evidence-based interventions found in the literature.

5. Write an education plan for this patient based on his request to shave.

6. Use the form to write up a plan of care based upon patient characteristics. Identify specific interventions and outcomes.

Synergy Model to Develop a Plan of Care

	Patient Characteristics	Subjective and Objective Data	Evidence-based Interventions	Outcomes
SYNERGY MODEL	Resiliency			
	Vulnerability			
	Stability			
	Complexity			
	Resource availability			
	Participation in care			
	Participation in decision making			
	Predictability			

Online Resources

Thrombotic Thrombocytopenic Purpura: www.netdoctor.co.uk/diseases/facts/ttp.htm

American Society of Clinical Oncology Clinical Practice Guidelines:
www.asco.org/ac/1,1003,_12-002032-00_18-0011068-00_19-0011069-00_20-001,00.asp

Platelet Disorder Support Association: www.itppeople.com/

REFERENCES

Baldwin, P. D. (2003). Thrombocytopenia. *Clinical Journal of Oncology Nursing, 7*(3), 349–352.

Chong, B. H., & Chong, J. H. (2004). Heparin-induced thrombocytopenia. *Expert Review of Cardiovascular Therapy, 2*(4), 547–559.

Franchini, M. (2005). Heparin-induced thrombocytopenia: An update. *Thrombosis Journal, 3*, 14.

George, J. N. (2006). Evaluation and management of thrombocytopenia by primary care physicians. Retrieved February 11, 2006, from http://patients.uptodate.com/topic.asp?file=prim_hem/5430#1

Hardin, R. I. (2005). Disorders of the platelet and vessel wall. In Kasper, D. L., Braunwald, E., Fauci, A., Hauser, S., Longo, D., & Jameson, J. L., *Harrison's principles of internal medicine* (16th ed., pp. 673–679). New York: McGraw-Hill.

Horell, C. J., & Rothman, J. (2001). The etiology of thrombocytopenia. *Dimensions of Critical Care Nursing, 20*(4), 10–16.

Kaplow, R. (2006). Thrombocytopenia: HIT, ITP, and TTP. In H. Schell and K. A. Puntillo (Eds.), *Critical care nursing secrets.* Philadelphia: Hanley & Belfus.

Matthai, W. H. (2005). Thrombocytopenia in cardiovascular patients: Diagnosis and management. *Chest, 127*(Suppl. 2), 46S–52S.

Menajovsky, L. B. (2005). Heparin-induced thrombocytopenia: Clinical manifestations and management strategies. *American Journal of Medicine, 118*(Suppl. 8A), 21S–30S.

Picker, S. M., & Gathof, B. S. (2004). Pathophysiology, epidemiology, diagnosis and treatment of heparin-induced thrombocytopenia (HIT). *European Journal of Medical Research, 9*(4), 180–185.

Schiffer, C. A., Anderson, K. C., Bennett, C. L., Bernstein, S., Elting, L. S., Goldsmith, M., et al. (2001). Platelet transfusion for patients with cancer: Clinical practice guidelines of the American Society of Clinical Oncology. *Journal of Clinical Oncology, 19*(5), 1519–1538.

Symonette, D., & Hoffman, E. (2005). Thrombotic purpura. Retrieved July 22, 2005, from www.emedicine.com/EMERG/topic579.htm

CHAPTER 50

Disseminated Intravascular Coagulation

Jan Teal

LEARNING OBJECTIVES

Upon completion of this chapter, the reader will be able to:

1. Identify diseases associated with disseminated intravascular coagulation (DIC).

2. Explain laboratory tests that may be performed to diagnose DIC.

3. Recognize how DIC affects each body system as a secondary syndrome.

4. Discuss potential treatment for DIC.

5. List optimal patient outcomes that may be achieved through evidence-based management of DIC.

Disseminated intravascular coagulation (DIC) is a complex syndrome that is characterized by intravascular overstimulation of the clotting cascade and results in thrombosis and hemorrhage (Krimmel, 2003). The DIC Subcommittee of the International Society on Thrombosis and Hemostasis has suggested the following definition for DIC: "An acquired syndrome characterized by the intravascular activation of coagulation with loss of localization arising from different causes. It can originate from and cause damage to the microvasculature, which if sufficiently severe, can produce organ dysfunction" (Furlong & Furlong, 2005). The process may occur slowly or rapidly, as a localized or a systemic coagulopathy. DIC may be either chronic or acute. The primary presentation of DIC in the critically ill patient is acute. Importantly, DIC is secondary to another primary illness.

DIC has a long history in the literature. It has been called a variety of names in the past: consumption coagulopathy, defibrination syndrome, diffuse intravascular thrombosis, and consumption thrombohemorrhagic disorder. While possibly described earlier, beginning in the 1950s patient descriptions of illness met today's definition of DIC (Ratnoff, Pritchard, & Colopy, 1955). Until recently, very little evidence-based research related to treatment of DIC had been undertaken, which may be explained by the lack of clarity until now in the definition (Levi, 2004).

ETIOLOGIC FACTORS

Systemic activation of coagulation may occur with a variety of disorders. Two major pathways may lead to DIC: (1) a systemic inflammatory response, leading to an activation of cytokines and a subsequent activation of coagulation (sepsis or major trauma); or (2) release of a procoagulant (clotting factor) material in the bloodstream (e.g., in cancer or pregnancy). Systemic infections with other microorganisms such as viruses or parasites may also produce DIC (Levi, 2004). **Table 50-1** lists conditions known to be associated with DIC.

ACUTE VERSUS CHRONIC DIC

DIC is distinguished as acute or chronic, based on the rapidity of the initiating event in showing signs and symptoms or changes in lab values. Sepsis and massive trauma

TABLE 50-1 Conditions That May Be Associated with DIC

Acid-base disturbances	Gram-positive or -negative bacteria
	Sepsis
Trauma	Pancreatitis
Burns	Malignancies (e.g., acute promyelocytic leukemia)
Hepatitis	Cirrhosis
Crush injuries	
Retained placenta	Acute respiratory distress syndrome
Abruptio placenta	Vascular abnormalities (aneurysm)
	Multiple transfusions
Septic abortion	Toxins (snake bite, aspirin poisoning)
	Tissue necrosis
Embolism (fat, amniotic, or pulmonary)	Transplant rejection
	Septicemia
Transfusion reaction	Viremia

Sources: Aysola & Lopez-Plaza, 1999; Krimmel, 2003; Levi, 2004; Toh & Dennis, 2003.

may lead to acute DIC, whereas chronic DIC may be caused by a retained dead fetus, cancer, or a large abdominal aneurysm (Labelle & Kitchens, 2005). Chronic DIC may be characterized by minimally heightened coagulation. Laboratory values may reflect mildly reduced platelets or slightly increased D-dimer levels (Geitner, 2003). Patients with chronic DIC may exhibit little bleeding or even no symptoms at all. Acute DIC is manifested as generalized bleeding, which ranges from petechiae to exsanguinating hemorrhage, as well as microcirculatory and macrocirculatory thrombosis. The end result is hypoperfusion, infarction, and organ damage.

To understand the pathophysiology of DIC, it is essential to review the normal clotting cascade.

COAGULATION

Platelets

In response to vascular injury, the first line of defense is platelets. Following a break in the endothelial lining, platelets are exposed to subendothelial tissue. Platelets rush to the site of the injury and adhere to the exposed collagen of a damaged blood vessel. These cells also release a number of substances that assist in controlling bleeding: serotonin (a vasoconstrictor), adenosine diphosphate (ADP) (an aggregating agent), and platelet factor 3, which stimulates the clotting cascade (see **Figure 50-1**). Platelets aggregate at the site of injury and form a plug. This kind of platelet aggregation may be explained as the attachment of platelets to other platelets that are

bound to the endothelial wall. Circulating von Willebrand factor causes platelets to attach themselves to the exposed collagen of the injured endothelium. Thus coagulation is initiated by platelet adhesion and activation of the clotting cascade (Morgan, 2005). Activated platelets also stimulate the production of prostaglandin thromboxane A_2 (TXA_2) and ADP, and TXA_2 in turn stimulates platelet adhesion and aggregation (Morgan). Platelet aggregation opens up the platelet so that it can fit into binding sites on the platelet surface known as glycoproteins IIb and IIIa, further enhancing aggregation and a platelet plug. Additionally, activation of the clotting cascade initiates thrombin, which initiates the conversion of fibrinogen to fibrin.

Coagulation Pathways

Intrinsic and Extrinsic Pathway Activation

Coagulation may be initiated by either the intrinsic pathway (may also be known as the Contact Activation pathway) or extrinsic pathway (may also be known as the Tissue Factor pathway). The intrinsic pathway is so named because all of the factors in it are intrinsic to the blood. The extrinsic pathway is named because the stimulus that initiates clotting from this pathway is tissue-based (extrinsic to blood). Tissue factor, a protein that extends from the surfaces of cells (also known as thromboplastin and formerly known as factor III) is released when there is tissue injury. The extrinsic pathway is the primary mechanism for clot development. Both the intrinsic and extrinsic pathways lead to the common pathway. The intrinsic pathway constantly generates small amounts of thrombin, resulting in slow amounts of turnover of fibrinogen (Labelle & Kitchens, 2005).

Clotting Cascade

Normal endothelium will inhibit coagulation by producing nitric oxide and prostacyclin, which respectively promote vasodilation and platelet inhibition (Morgan, 2005). An injured endothelium loses its natural anticoagulant property at the site of the injury and stops producing nitric oxide and prosta-

FIGURE 50-1 Coagulation Cascade

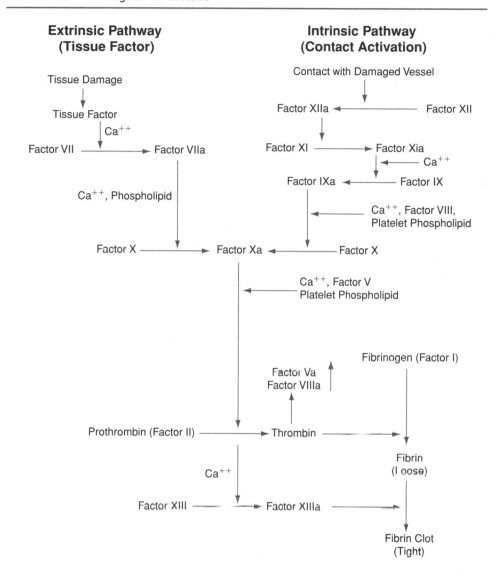

cyclin. An injured endothelium initiates platelet adhesion by producing adhesion molecules and von Willebrand factor.

The coagulation cascade (Fig. 50-1) consists of a series of enzymatic reactions that result in the formation of a clot. This series primarily begins because tissue factor is expressed when a vessel is injured. It can be viewed as a chain reaction that ultimately leads to the generation of thrombin at an injury site. The activation of one specific factor of the cascade leads to the activation of another factor. The initiation of the coagulation pathway is believed to occur as a result of the activation of the intrinsic or extrinsic pathway.

The intrinsic pathway is activated when a vascular injury exposes blood and collagen to subendothelial tissue. When another clotting factor, factor XII, comes in contact with the ex-

posed subendothelial tissue, the coagulation cascade is set into motion (Geitner, 2003). When factor XII gets activated, it activates factor XI; factor XIa activates factor IX. Together factor IXa and factor VIIIa form a complex, which activates factor X (Liebman & Weitz, 2005).

The extrinsic pathway is activated by exposure of blood to tissue factor bearing cells as a result of tissue disruption. Damage causes endothelial cells to release a chemical known as tissue thromboplastin (tissue factor). When tissue thromboplastin comes in contact with factor VII, factor VII becomes activated and it forms a complex (TF-FVIIa) the extrinsic pathway is activated. TF-FVII activates factors IX and X. Factor Xa, together with factor V form a complex, which activates prothrombin and converts it to thrombin. Thrombin is needed to convert fibrinogen to fibrin, which will form a fibrin clot (Goodsell, 2006).

Both of these pathways converge to become one common pathway when factor Xa and Va are combined. Factor Xa/Va is responsible for the conversion of prothrombin to thrombin.

Anticoagulation

The coagulation cascade is subject to control by a checks-and-balances system, the fibrinolytic system. Without the fibrinolytic system, blood would exist as a gel. Once the clotting cascade is activated, circulating antithrombin binds to thrombin, causing an inactivation of thrombin activity (Morgan, 2005). Antithrombin inactivates Factors Xa, IXa, XIa, and XIIa. The body's endogenous heparin accelerates antithrombin–thrombin binding, thereby enhancing thrombin inhibition. Thrombin generates the conversion of protein C to activated protein C, which is a potent anticoagulant. Thrombin inhibition prolongs activated partial thromboplastin time.

Fibrinolysis

Fibrinolysis begins with tissue plasminogen activator (tPA), which is released in response to fibrin generation (Morgan, 2005). tPA converts plasminogen to plasmin; plasmin then causes fibrinolysis (i.e., the dissolution of a formed clot). Clot dissolution results in the circulation of fibrin degradation products (FDPs), which serve as functional anticoagulants in four ways:

- They coat platelets and diminish their adhesiveness.
- They inhibit thrombin action.
- They attach to fibrinogen (inhibit polymerization).
- They produce a defective fibrin clot.

PATHOPHYSIOLOGY

DIC is a complex systemic disorder involving the generation of intravascular fibrin and the consumption of coagulation factors and platelets. It results from an excessive activation of coagulation. The pathophysiology involves initiation of coagulation via endothelial injury or tissue injury with the subsequent release of procoagulant materials in the form of cytokines and tissue factor. Interleukin (IL-6) and tumor necrosis factor (TNF) may be the most influential cytokines involved in coagulation activation. In DIC, clots are formed in the absence of injury. Thrombin production is both uncontrolled and excessive, leading to fibrin deposition throughout the microcirculation (especially in the kidneys and skin). Nevertheless, a stable clot cannot form at an injury site. Instead, circulating red blood cells (RBCs) are sheared by the mechanical stress of the fibrin strands, leading to a microangiopathic hemolytic anemia.

Excessive fibrin deposition leads to platelet aggregation and consumption of coagulation factors. Additionally, excessive plasmin that is produced in response to widespread intravascular thrombi acts to degrade fibrinogen, fibrin, and other coagulation factors, and fibrinolysis in turn enhances hemorrhage.

Several factors are associated with the development of DIC; all have in common the generation of thrombin. These triggering mechanisms include the following:

- Endothelial cell damage → activation of the intrinsic system
- Tissue injury → activation of the extrinsic system
- RBC or platelet injury → release of phospholipids

Some conditions associated with the development of DIC are listed in Table 50-1.

As DIC develops, thrombin and plasmin become activated and circulate systemically. The balance of plasmin and thrombin determines whether there will be a bleeding or clotting tendency. Additionally, plasmin and thrombin initiate platelet abnormalities. Thrombin cleaves to fibrinogen to form fibrin monomers and potentiates the coagulation cascade, leading to small- and large-vessel clots. The end result is organ ischemia and multiple organ dysfunction syndrome (MODS).

Inhibitors of coagulation are overwhelmed by the continuous activation of coagulation. Once these inhibitors are exhausted, plasmin and thrombin are free to circulate unbound and mediate the clinical syndrome of DIC.

DIAGNOSIS

The diagnosis of DIC is made in the context of the patient's history, clinical presentation, and lab values. Clinical manifestations include bleeding and thrombosis with possible ensuing organ dysfunction. Bleeding is typically acute and occurs from multiple sites. Intravenous (IV) lines, old injuries, or surgical sites may begin (inexplicably) to ooze blood. Nose (epistaxis) and gum bleeding are common, as are petechiae and purpura. Blood or hemoglobin (or both) may appear in the urine. Hemodynamic instability and shock may be present in acute DIC.

No single, definitive test for DIC exists. However, laboratory results (various tests or a DIC panel) confirm suspicions of DIC. These tests include platelet count, prothrombin time (PT), activated partial thromboplastin time (a-PTT), thrombin time (TT), FDP assay, D-dimer assay, and peripheral blood smear (Labelle & Kitchens, 2005). (See **Table 50-2**.) The use of DIC tests or a DIC panel may vary according to the healthcare facility.

Platelet Count

A platelet count is the first test that may show something is amiss. Abnormalities in the platelet count may be picked up on a routine complete blood count (CBC). If DIC is present, the platelet count will be decreased to less than $150,000/mm^3$. Thirty percent of platelets are kept in the spleen, from which they are released into circulation as needed by the body to maintain homeostasis. A drop of the platelet level to $50,000/mm^3$ or less or a drop of 50% from the patient's baseline may lead to suspicion of massive clot formation and the possibility of DIC (Geitner, 2003).

Fibrin Degradation Products

FDP, also termed fibrin split products, are measured in an effort to determine fibrinolytic (clot breakdown) activity. When plasmin dissolves fibrin blood clots, FDPs are formed. FDPs are

TABLE 50-2 Tests for DIC

Lab Test	Normal Range	Comments
Platelet count	150,000–400,000/mm^3	Critical value < 50,000/mm^3 Falling count DIC
Fibrin degradation products (FDPs)	<10 mcg/mL	Critical value > 40 mcg/mL Rising values DIC
D-dimer	Negative (none present)	Levels increased when thrombin clots are lysed
Fibrinogen	200–400 mg/dL	Critical value < 100 mg/dL Falling value DIC
Prothrombin time (PT)	11–12.5 seconds*	Critical value > 20 seconds Increasing clotting time in DIC
Partial thromboplastin time (PTT)	60–70 seconds*	Critical value >100 seconds Increasing clotting time in DIC
Activated partial thromboplastin time (aPTT)	30–40 seconds*	Critical value > 70 seconds Increasing clotting time in DIC
Thrombin time	11.3–18.5 seconds*	Prolonged due to the inhibition of thrombin Prolonged with DIC
Blood smear	Normal numbers of WBCs, RBCs, and platelets; normal size, shape, and color of RBCs	Abnormal numbers, size, shape or color may be seen May see schistocytes if the RBC has been sheared by fibrin
Antithrombin III	Plasma: > 50% of control Serum: 15%–34% lower than plasma	Values vary along with laboratory method Decreased levels in DIC

*Normal range may vary based on institutional equipment used in measurement.
Source: Pagana & Pagana, 2001.

also formed by the breakdown of circulating fibrinogen or free fibrin that has not yet been incorporated into a clot. During acute DIC, rapid clot formation and clot dissolution directly lead to a much higher level of FDPs. FDPs, when circulating, have an anticoagulant effect.

D-Dimer

A D-dimer is a specific FDP that is formed only by plasmin degradation of fibrin. The presence of D-dimers indicates that fibrin has been formed and broken down or degraded. Low levels of D-dimers are normal, because the body is always forming and dissolving clots. The higher the D-dimer level, the more rapid the clot dissolution. Cancer patients often have positive tests for D-dimers and FDPs, which may indicate a chronic level of DIC. D-dimer tests can be positive with DIC or a thrombosis such as deep vein thrombosis, pulmonary embolus, or myocardial infarction. Anticoagulant therapy with an agent such as heparin would also cause an increase in FDP or D-dimer levels.

Fibrinogen

Fibrinogen normally remains at a steady state within the body. In DIC, clots form rapidly, and consequently the body's production of fibrinogen cannot meet the rate of consumption. The body will attempt to increase production, such that near-normal levels may be found in mild or chronic DIC. Fibrinopeptide A is a breakdown product of fibrinogen and indicates thrombin activity. Fibrinogen levels are abnormal in 88% of patients with DIC (Furlong & Furlong, 2005). Of note, patients with cancer or sepsis may have elevated fibrinogen levels. Hence, fibrinogen levels in these patients should not be used as a diagnostic criterion for DIC.

Prothrombin Time

The PT measures the clotting time from the activation of Factor VII through the formation of a fibrin clot. It is calculated as the time in seconds it takes for a fibrin clot to form after the initiation of the extrinsic pathway. Additionally, the PT test measures the integrity of the extrinsic and common pathways of coagulation. The prolongation of clotting times may reflect the consumption and depletion of coagulation factors (II, V, VII, or X). This test is also used to measure the effects of warfarin (Coumadin®). Each lab converts a normal PT to an international normalized ratio (INR) of 1 (Morgan, 2005).

Activated Partial Thromboplastin Time

aPTT measures the clotting time from the activation of Factor XII through the formation of a fibrin clot. This test analyzes the integrity of the intrinsic pathway and common pathway from Factor X to fibrin. In DIC, the aPTT is prolonged as clotting factors (VIII, IX, XI, or XII) are depleted. aPTT may also be prolonged if the patient is on an anticoagulant such as heparin or any of the direct thrombin inhibitors.

Thrombin Time

The TT is the time that is required for the blood to clot following the administration of thrombin. This test assesses the lower half of the common pathway, and the TT will be prolonged if the fibrinogen level is low.

Blood Smear

A blood smear may demonstrate fragmented red blood cells (schistocytes) in half of all cases of DIC (Labelle & Kitchens, 2005). Schistocytes are generated when hemolyzed red blood cells become severed by flowing through fibrin strands. The blood smear can also confirm thrombocytopenia.

Factor VII

Factor VII is beginning to gain favor as a lab test to monitor DIC. Most clotting is initiated when tissue factor combines with Factor VII. If tissue factor is increased, Factor VII will be low or depleted.

Antithrombin III

Antithrombin III (AT III) is a glycoprotein produced in the liver. This protease inhibitor irreversibly inhibits several enzymes involved in hemostasis and serves a prominent role in controlling coagulation by limiting the extent of thrombus formation. AT III binds to the catalytic site of thrombin (Factor IIa) and Factors IXa, Xa, XIa, and XIIa.

TREATMENT

Removal of the Trigger

DIC is a syndrome secondary to another disease process, so treatment should focus on removing the causing factor (if possible). Removal of the trigger or causative factor enhances the patient's chance of recovery. Antibiotics may assist in control of DIC in the patient who has sepsis. Additionally, debridement of devitalized tissue in a burn patient may accomplish control of DIC (Labelle & Kitchens, 2005). If the causative factor cannot be removed, therapy may be simply supportive and the prognosis may be poor. There is no consensus on the optimal treatment of DIC, given that there are so many potential causes for this disorder (Labelle & Kitchens).

Therapies to Consider

The key to therapy is balancing clot formation, clot dissolution, and clot inhibition (Geitner, 2003). Replacement of consumed factors is sometimes all that can be done. MODS is frequently present in DIC patients; it may develop related to a lack of perfusion from the presence of emboli or bleeding.

Platelet Transfusions

Caution should be used with platelet transfusions, because administration of platelets may lead to the development of antiplatelet antibodies, which in themselves can initiate DIC (Geitner, 2003). Platelet transfusion is indicated for individuals with active bleeding and whose platelet counts have fallen to less than 40,000/mm^3. Petechiae, ecchymosis, and spontaneous bleeding may occur when the platelet count dips below 20,000/mm^3 (Pagana & Pagana, 2001). Platelet transfusion may be needed for patients following surgery or another procedure whose platelet counts exceed 40,000/mm^3 if bleeding is prolonged (Pagana & Pagana). The dose of platelets is 1 unit/10 kg (Lewis, 2005). Platelets must be administered immediately when they are received on the unit. Platelet tubing with a filter is used for administration. The rate of infusion is 4 to 8 mL/kg/hour. As with any other blood product administration, informed consent is required.

Packed Red Blood Cells and Fresh Frozen Plasma

Packed RBCs should be given as needed to maintain adequate oxygen delivery. Replacement may be necessary due to prolonged bleeding or the destruction of RBCs. Packed RBCs must be administered through a filter and not left hanging more than four hours. Note that RBCs that have been stored in the blood bank are usually deficient in Factors V and VIII.

Infusion of fresh frozen plasma (FFP) may assist the control of hemostasis and replace depleted clotting factors. Prolonged PT/INR levels can be lowered by administering FFP. One unit of FFP is commonly given for every four to six units of packed RBCs administered. However, there is no evidence of a ratio of FFP to PRBC administration (Hirshberg et al.,

2003). The adult dose of FFP is 15 to 20 mL/kg IV (Furlong & Furlong, 2005).

Cryoprecipitate

Cryoprecipitate replaces fibrinogen and is typically given to patients with fibrinogen levels less than 50 to 60 mg/dL (Labelle & Kitchens, 2005). Each bag contains 80 to 100 units of Factor VIII. As many as 10 units of cryoprecipitate may be needed to restore the fibrinogen level to 100 mg/dL. Administration of cryoprecipitate does not require compatibility testing (Morgan, 2005).

Controversy continues to surround the decision to administer platelets, FFP, or cryoprecipitate to a patient with DIC. The primary concern is that administration may be "adding fuel to the fire" by providing factors that can be used for additional clot formation.

Heparin

Heparin administration remains controversial in the treatment of DIC. In theory, giving heparin or other anticoagulants to reduce thrombin generation would seem effective, because it interrupts the cycle with the hope of slowing down production of thrombin. Little clinical evidence or research supports the benefit of heparin in acute, severe DIC, however (Gobel-Holmes, 2002; Lewis, 2005). Heparin may be beneficial in obstetrical events such as retained placenta or incomplete abortion, in cases of severe arterial occlusion, or in individuals with significant thrombosis (Geitner, 2003). Heparin is contraindicated for a DIC patient with an acute head injury. Some clinicians still consider heparin to be the mainstay of DIC treatment. Future research related to DIC and heparin use may better elucidate heparin's role. The adult dose of heparin is 80 to 100 units/kg subcutaneously every 4 to 6 hours or 20,000 to 30,000 units/day per continuous IV infusion (Furlong & Furlong, 2005).

Other Treatments

Antithrombin III Therapy

AT III therapy is used with a therapeutic goal of achieving supernormal levels of AT III (more than 125% to 150%). Experimental treatment trials have indicated that this therapy has a beneficial effect in individuals who experience DIC while in septic shock (Lewis, 2005). Many treatments are currently in clinical trials, but as yet their benefits are unknown. Dosing of AT III (ATnativ®, Thrombate III®) is calculated as 0.6 times the body weight in kilograms, with greater than 125% AT III; it may also be given as a loading dose of 100 units/kg IV over 3 hours, followed by a continuous infusion of 100 units/day (Furlong & Furlong, 2005).

Other Therapies

Tissue factor pathway inhibitor (TFPI) is currently being studied as a treatment for DIC, and initial results are promising (Lewis, 2005). TFPI complexes with tissue factor, Factor VIIa, and Factor Xa to inhibit the conversion of prothrombin to thrombin. Tissue factor inhibition may produce anti-inflammatory effects.

Antifibrinolytic therapy is rarely indicated in DIC, because fibrinolysis is needed to clear thrombi from the microcirculation. Indeed, use of an antifibrinolytic agent can lead to a fatal disseminated thrombosis (Lewis, 2005). Antifibrinolytic therapy may be used in cases involving bleeding that has not responded to other therapies, laboratory evidence of overwhelming fibrinolysis, and evidence that intravascular coagulation has ended. Antifibrinolytics may also prove helpful in cases of DIC secondary to hyperfibrinolysis associated with some forms of cancer (Furlong & Furlong, 2005).

SYSTEMIC ASSESSMENT AND SUPPORT

Skin

Bleeding, which may begin suddenly and become severe quickly, is the most obvious sign of DIC. Bleeding may come from drainage tubes, old surgical sites, the nose, or either recent or older venipuncture sites. If bleeding continues, the patient may go into shock.

Thrombosis may be evident and may be seen as microclots enter the capillaries. Evidence of thrombosis may be seen in the patient as perhaps toes, fingers, nose, ears, or other parts of the body become cyanotic. Cyanosis may progress to sloughing of skin and gangrene. Petechiae, ecchymoses, or hematomas may be present (Owen & Webster, 1998).

Care of the patient with DIC should include avoiding venipunctures, intramuscular injections, or invasive treatments unless absolutely necessary. Patient care activities such as mouth care, suctioning, backrubs, vital signs, turning, or use of nonpaper adhesive tapes should be performed gently related to risk of bleeding or injury (Owen & Webster, 1998). Manual and automatic blood pressure cuffs should be avoided, if possible, to prevent bruising. It is hoped that an arterial line is already in place for blood pressure monitoring.

Perform mouth care gently with alcohol-free swabs to decrease the risk of injury. Avoid rectal temperatures and shave the patient, if necessary, with an electric razor. If a venipuncture is necessary, provide pressure for 3 to 5 minutes or longer if the patient has not stopped bleeding. If an arterial puncture was required, pressure will be required for 10 to 15 minutes or longer (Dennison, 2000).

It is imperative that areas of cyanosis be kept free from pressure. Watch pressure points such as the sacrum, elbows, ears, heels, shoulders, and hips carefully. A therapeutic, pressure-reducing bed may be helpful in preventing ulceration.

Do not disrupt dressings with old blood, because their dislodgement may lead to further bleeding. If you are worried that the family may be upset by dressings with dried blood, perform patient and family teaching to increase their understanding of the need not to disrupt the clot.

Pain

The patient's pain level should be assessed frequently and aggressively, because thrombosis, bleeding into joints and tissues, and tissue ischemia may create a level of moderate to severe pain. Pain medication is best given by the IV route. Suppositories, intramuscular injections, and subcutaneous injections should be avoided, given their potential for causing bleeding. Although medicating for pain is important, medications that are ordered for pain should not have side effects that disrupt clotting (Owen & Webster, 1998).

Respiratory Care

Maintain the patient's airway (i.e., monitor the ABCs). Administer oxygen to maintain a PaO_2 of 80 mm Hg and an SpO_2 of 95% unless contraindicated (Dennison, 2000). Oxygen should be humidified—breathing passages bleed easily if dry gas is used. If hypoxia is present, the patient may experience dyspnea or tachypnea. Assist with intubation and initiation of mechanical ventilation as necessary. Nursing interventions that decrease oxygen demand and consumption are essential. Decreasing oxygen demands may be accomplished by sedating the patient, keeping the temperature under control, and giving the patient adequate rest periods (Urden, Stacy, & Lough, 2002). The respiratory system should be aggressively supported to prevent hypoxia and acidosis. However, suctioning should be done gently in an effort to minimize trauma to the airway tissues. Blood products may be given to improve the patient's oxygen-carrying capacity. Hemoptysis, pulmonary embolus, and acute respiratory distress syndrome are all potential consequences of DIC.

Cardiac Care

Perform frequent cardiovascular assessment to include auscultation, vital signs, and palpation of pulses. If you are unable to palpate a pulse, use a Doppler device to determine the presence of the pulse. Prepare to administer volume replacement with IV fluids and blood products to restore the intravascular volume. Some patients may develop a fluid volume deficit related to bleeding and third spacing of bodily fluids. An infusion of a vasopressor, such as dopamine (Intropin®), may be needed to maintain cardiac output. The patient may be experiencing tachycardia as the body attempts to increase oxygenation to the tissues. Cardiac arrhythmias may be present if the patient develops hypoxia or a shift in electrolytes. In addition, the patient may experience chest pain or a myocardial infarction if there is inadequate oxygenation or a shortage of RBCs to carry the oxygen. If the patient becomes acidotic, a shift of potassium will occur. When blood pH falls, potassium levels rise. This potassium shift may lead to more cardiac arrhythmias.

Neurological Care

Patients with DIC may experience changes in their level of consciousness (LOC) related to the lack of oxygen. Headache, change in LOC, or pupillary changes may indicate that a cerebral hemorrhage has taken place, whereas visual changes may indicate that a retinal hemorrhage has occurred. Additionally, altered LOC, lethargy, restlessness, confusion, seizures, or coma may signify a thrombotic event within the brain. The patient should have frequent neurological assessments, perhaps as often as hourly, to determine whether any neurological changes have taken place. The Glasgow Coma Scale is a standard assessment tool to evaluate neurological changes.

Gastrointestinal Care

The gastrointestinal system may be affected by DIC, and symptoms of hemorrhage such as hematemesis or melena may be present. The patient may complain of gastric pain or discomfort. Bowel sounds may be absent or decreased. However, if clotting/thrombosis is the cause, the patient may develop bowel ischemia or infarction, which if left unchecked will lead to dead bowel. High-pitched, tinkling bowel sounds may be heard above the infarction. Abdominal distention or rebound tenderness may indicate a retroperitoneal hemorrhage. All stool samples should be guaiaced to test for occult blood.

Nutritional support should be initiated, as hypermetabolism may be present. The goal of nutritional support is to preserve organ structure and function. Enteral feeding is preferred (if possible) and is given distal to the pylorus to prevent pulmonary aspiration (Urden et al., 2002). During a major stressor such as critical illness, the body is in a "fight or flight" mode (sympathetic nervous system response), and consequently blood is diverted from the gut. Without the rich blood supply to the gut, the epithelial layer may weaken and allow gut bacteria to migrate upward. Enteral feeding may limit this translocation of bacteria from the gut (Urden et al.).

Genitourinary Care

The genitourinary (GU) system may be affected by DIC-related hemorrhage or thrombosis. Signs of hemorrhage may include vaginal bleeding or hematuria. A minimum of 0.5 mL/kg/hr of urine should be present. Possible consequences of DIC for the GU system may be acute tubular necrosis, proteinuria, or anuria. There may also be further electrolyte imbalances.

Patient/Family Support/Education

The diagnosis of DIC is often terrifying for the patient, family, or significant others. Patients and families will inevitably require education. Preparation regarding what to expect and interventions to be avoided until DIC has resolved are essential aspects to be reinforced. High anxiety and the sense of crisis, however, will likely decrease the ability to comprehend or remember what has been taught. The patient, family, or significant others may have some difficult decisions ahead of them regarding treatment options. Emotional support may be the biggest gift that the nurse can give the patient and loved ones.

DETECTION OF DIC

It is essential that DIC is detected early and the primary cause found. Early detection may minimize morbidity and mortality. Because DIC is a secondary complication associated with a primary problem, mortality is estimated at 50% despite aggressive treatment (Owen & Webster, 1998). Medical management must include treatment of the underlying disorder. Nurses must identify patients who are at high risk for developing DIC. Frequent and thorough assessment of all body systems and testing of all body secretions for occult blood should be done for these high-risk patients. Although the onset of DIC cannot be prevented, early recognition may improve the outcome.

PATIENT OUTCOMES

Nurses can help ensure attainment of optimal patient outcomes such as those listed in **Box 50-1** through the use of evidence-based interventions for patients with DIC.

SUMMARY

DIC is a secondary syndrome (disorder) featuring uncontrolled activation of coagulation and secondary fibrinolysis. It can occur in both acute and chronic forms and can be systemic or localized. Many conditions—such as trauma, sepsis, cancer, obstetric complications, and liver disease—can trigger DIC. Once DIC is triggered, thrombin is activated. Thrombin causes the conversion of fibrinogen into fibrin, promotes platelet aggregation, and eventually leads to the formation of thrombi in the microvasculature. Plasmin generation increases with thrombin activation, such that fibrinolysis develops. The combination of fibrinolysis and thrombocytopenia then leads to a bleeding diathesis. The end result of DIC may be multiple-organ failure and death. The hallmark of DIC therapy is treatment of the underlying disorder, supportive treatment, and replacement of coagulation factors (Aysola & Lopez-Plaza, 1999).

Box 50-1
Optimal Patient Outcomes

- Oxygen saturation in expected range
- Heart rate in expected range
- Coagulation profile—no deviation from expected range
- Demonstrates knowledge of DIC process
- Physical comfort in expected range
- Strong distal pulses

CASE STUDY

D.J., a 75-year-old male, was admitted to the ICU yesterday with a diagnosis of pneumonia. Initial blood culture results were positive for a gram-negative organism. Broad-spectrum antibiotics were begun yesterday. Over the past several hours, D.J.'s condition has progressively worsened. He was intubated earlier today and is now on a ventilator receiving FiO_2 of 60%. Vital signs were HR 140, BP 140/80, and RR 22. D.J.'s temperature has been steadily rising over the last several hours (temperature 104.8°F). You have placed the patient on a hypothermia blanket and administered acetaminophen via a rectal suppository. Dopamine (Intropin®) 5 mcg/kg/min is infusing, and you have just initiated a fluid challenge of 250 mL of NS.

D.J. seems to respond to therapy as his HR decreases to 120 bpm, temperature to 101 °F, and BP to 105/60. As you are performing his routine assessment, you notice fresh blood on the bed. As you investigate, you notice blood oozing from D.J.'s IV site, antecubital vein, and urinary catheter. You also observe that the tips of his fingers and toes are blue-tinged. You obtain an order for a DIC lab panel.

CRITICAL THINKING QUESTIONS

1. Which lab tests might be ordered?
2. What do you think would be an appropriate treatment plan for D.J.'s DIC?
3. Would you consider giving heparin? Why or why not?
4. Which blood products might you consider administering to this patient?
5. Why is heparin a controversial treatment for DIC?
6. Which disciplines should be consulted to work with this client?
7. How would you modify your plan of care for patients of diverse backgrounds?
8. What types of issues may require you to act as an advocate or moral agent for this patient?
9. How will you implement your role as a facilitator of learning for this patient?

D.J. begins to show signs of renal failure. His output is less than 0.25 mL/kg/hr (despite fluid resuscitation). Serum BUN = 40 mg/dL and creatinine = 10 mg/dl.

The laboratory has called in the results for this patient: platelets 35,000/mm^3, hemoglobin 8 Gm/dL, hematocrit 28%, D-dimers elevated, FDPs increased, and fibrinogen decreased. Four units of packed red blood cells and two units of fresh frozen plasma are administered. Twenty units of platelets have been ordered.

The following day D.J.'s pneumonia begins improving and his vital signs, labs, and clinical status seem to be improving.

CRITICAL THINKING QUESTIONS

10. Use the form to write up data and a plan of care for a patient with DIC in the clinical setting. Rate the patient as a level 1, 3, or 5 on each characteristic. Identify the level of nurse characteristics needed in the care of this patient.
11. Take one patient outcome for a patient and list evidence-based interventions found in a literature review for this patient.

Using the Synergy Model to Develop a Plan of Care

	Patient Characteristics	Level (1, 3, 5)	Subjective and Objective Data	Evidence-based Interventions	Outcomes
SYNERGY MODEL	Resiliency				
	Vulnerability				
	Stability				
	Complexity				
	Resource availability				
	Participation in care				
	Participation in decision making				
	Predictability				

Online Resources

Global Statistics for DIC: www.nationmaster.com/graph-t/mor_dis_int_coa_def_syn

Topic Overview of DIC: http://my.webmd.com/hw/blood_disorders/tp22265.asp

Dr. Coop: www.drcoop.com/ency/93/000573.html

REFERENCES

Aysola, A., & Lopez-Plaza, I. (1999). Disseminated intravascular coagulation. *Transfusion Medicine Update*. Retrieved July 15, 2005, from www.itxm.org/TMU1998/tmu3 99.htm

Dennison, R. D. (2000). *Pass CCRN!* St. Louis, MO: Mosby.

Furlong, M. A., & Furlong, B. R. (2005). Disseminated intravascular coagulation. Retrieved May 28, 2005, from www.emedicine.com/med/topic577.htm

Geitner, H. (2003). Disseminated intravascular clotting. *Dimensions of Critical Care Nursing, 22*(3), 108–114.

Gobel-Holmes, B. (2002). Disseminated intravascular coagulation in cancer: Providing quality care. *Topics in Advanced Practice Nursing eJournal, 2*(4). www.medscape.com/viewarticle/442737_print

Goodsell, D. S. (2006). The molecular perspective: Tissue factor. *The Oncologist, 11*(7), 849–850.

Hirsberg, A., Dugas, M., Banez, E. I., Scott, B. G., Wall, M. J., & Maddox, K. L. (2003). Minimizing dilutional coagulopathy in exsanguinating hemorrhage: A computer simulation. *Journal of Trauma, 54*(3), 454–463.

Krimmel, T. (2003). Disseminated intravascular coagulation. *Clinical Journal of Oncology Nursing, 7*(4), 479–481.

Labelle, C., & Kitchens, C. S. (2005). Disseminated intravascular coagulation: Treat the cause, not the lab values. *Cleveland Clinic Journal of Medicine, 72*(5), 377–397.

Levi, M. (2004). Current understanding of disseminated intravascular coagulation. *British Journal of Haematology, 124*, 567–576.

Lewis, K. (2005). Disseminated intravascular clotting. *Society of Critical Care Medicine*. Retrieved July 2005, from www.sccm.org

Liebman, H. A., & Weitz, I. C. (2005). Disseminated intravascular coagulation. In R. Hoffman, E. J. Benz, S. J. Shattil, B. Furie, H. J. Cohen, L. E. Silberstein, et al. *Hematology basic principles and practice* (4th ed., pp. 2169–2182). Philadelphia: Elsevier.

Morgan, B. (2005). Inflammation and coagulation overview. *Critical Care Concepts*, 1–8.

Owen, D. C., & Webster, J. S. (1998). Hematology disorders. In M. Kinney, S. B. Dunbar, J. Brooks–Brunn, N. Molter, & J. M. Vitello-Cicciu (Eds.), *AACN's clinical reference for critical care nursing* (4th ed., pp. 908–913). St. Louis, MO: Mosby.

Pagana, K. D., & Pagana, T. J. (2001). *Mosby's diagnostic and laboratory test reference* (5th ed.). St. Louis, MO: Mosby.

Ratnoff, O. D., Pritchard, J. A., & Colopy, J. E. (1955). Hemorrhagic states during pregnancy. *New England Journal of Medicine, 253*, 63–69.

Toh, C., & Dennis, M. (2003). Disseminated intravascular clotting: Old disease, new hope. *British Medical Journal, 327*(7421), 974–977.

Urden, L. D., Stacy, K. M., & Lough, M. E. (2002). Systemic inflammatory response syndrome and multiple organ dysfunction syndrome. In L. D. Urden, K. M. Stacy, & M. E. Lough (Eds.), *Thelan's critical care nursing* (4th ed., pp. 956–959). St. Louis, MO: Mosby.

Systems
Thinking

PART V

CHAPTER 51

Systemic Inflammatory Response Syndrome and Sepsis

Mary Fran Tracy

Upon completion of this chapter, the reader will be able to:

1. Describe the pathophysiology of systemic inflammatory response syndrome (SIRS) and sepsis.

2. Describe the clinical manifestations of SIRS and sepsis.

3. Discuss current management strategies for sepsis.

4. List optimal patient outcomes that may be achieved through evidence-based management of SIRS.

It is estimated that more than 750,000 cases of sepsis or septic shock occur in the United States each year, with mortality rates at approximately 30% (Angus et al., 2001). The incidence of sepsis is increasing due to several factors. While diagnosis of sepsis can be difficult, greater awareness has led to better recognition and diagnosis of this condition. The population considered to be at high risk for sepsis, which includes immunocompromised individuals and the elderly, is also growing. More extensive utilization of short-term and long-term invasive devices (such as vascular access devices) increases the risk for sepsis as well. Finally, there is an ever-present risk of encountering organisms in our daily lives that are resistant to the current antibiotic regimens.

Critically ill patients are at particularly high risk for sepsis with resulting high mortality and morbidity. Nurses play a vital role in the recognition and early treatment of sepsis.

DEFINITIONS

The human response to infection ranges along a severity continuum from systemic inflammatory response syndrome (SIRS) to multiple organ dysfunction syndrome (MODS). Traditionally, a multitude of definitions have been used in describing and communicating about sepsis, resulting in a lack of clarity about the diagnosis. In 1991, the American College of Chest Physicians and the Society of Critical Care Medicine convened a Consensus Conference to standardize the use of terms and criteria in defining sepsis (Bone et al., 1992). **Figure 51-1** outlines the definitions and criteria agreed upon for the different stages of sepsis. In 2001, 11 international organizations again met to review, confirm, and refine these definitions and criteria as well as to update and expand the compilation of signs and symptoms based on current evidence in an effort to improve awareness and recognition of sepsis. These additional criteria include the following signs and symptoms:

- Hypotension
- Decreased urine output
- Edema
- Skin mottling

FIGURE 51-1 Systemic Inflammatory Response Syndrome

Presence of more than one of the following signs:
- Temperature > 38°C or < 36°C
- Heart rate > 90 beats/minute
- Tachypnea with respiratory rate > 20 breaths/minute or $PaCO_2$ < 32 mm Hg
- White blood cell count > 12,000 cells/mm^3 or < 4,000 cells/mm^3 or > 10% immature neutrophils

↓

Sepsis
SIRS resulting from a bacterial, viral, parasitic, or fungal infection

↓

Severe Sepsis
Sepsis that involves at least one organ dysfunction, hypoperfusion, or hypotension

↓

Septic Shock
Sepsis-related hypotension after adequate fluid resuscitation

↓

Multiple Organ Dysfunction Syndrome
Two or more organ dysfunctions to the point that maintaining homeostasis requires active interventions

Source: Bone et al., 1992.

- Elevated glucose
- Unexplained mental status changes (Levy et al., 2003).

It is imperative that SIRS and sepsis be identified early and treated aggressively to minimize as much as possible the risk of complications and mortality. Progression from SIRS to severe sepsis and possibly death is difficult to predict at this stage given our current knowledge base. It is important that nurses be aware of populations who are at particular risk for developing sepsis so that they can achieve early recognition. These patients include those who meet the following criteria:

- Ages less than 1 year and greater than 85 years
- Immunocompromised
- Severe community-acquired pneumonia
- Intra-abdominal surgery
- Meningitis
- Chronic diseases such as cardiovascular disease, renal disease, and diabetes
- Cellulitis
- Urinary tract infection (Eli Lilly and Company, 2005)

PATHOPHYSIOLOGY

The pathophysiology of sepsis is complex and not yet fully understood. Although an in-depth analysis of the pathophysiology is beyond the scope of this chapter, understanding the basics of sepsis will assist in comprehending the assessment measures and interventions undertaken by nurses.

The human body attempts to maintain a fine physiologic balance between compensatory inflammatory and anti-inflammatory responses to immune system activation. The complications of sepsis become manifest when this balance becomes misaligned. Three main processes occur simultaneously in severe sepsis: inflammation, coagulation, and impaired fibrinolysis. In addition, the role of endothelium activation is important to understanding the ensuing complications.

Endothelial cells make up the majority of the cells lining the vasculature and, therefore, are in close and frequent contact with blood. Previously, it was believed that the endothelium acted only as a simple layer between the two. It is now known that the endothelium has many functions, including preventing coagulation, regulating movement of blood cells from the vasculature into the tissue, participating in the regulation of vascular arteriole tone (and thereby influencing blood pressure), and altering vascular permeability (Hack & Zeerleder, 2001; Vallet & Wiel, 2001).

Inflammation

During the inflammatory process, white blood cells (WBCs) release cytokines (substances that carry out biologic activity) that are proinflammatory, such as tumor necrosis factor-α (TNF-α) and interleukin-1 (IL-1). This activity attracts more neutrophils to the site to assist in fighting infection. Myocardial depressant factor, another proinflammatory mediator, causes a decrease in ejection fraction (the amount of blood ejected by the heart with each beat in relation to the amount of blood remaining in the left ventricle at the end of filling), a decrease in response to fluid resuscitation, and a decreased response to catecholamines (which may be used to enhance blood pressure). In an attempt to achieve balance, anti-inflammatory cytokines are released as well. This process activates the endothelium, resulting in a change of its function to become procoagulant (in an attempt to isolate the infection), increase production of TNF–α and IL-1, and produce more vasoactive components such as nitric oxide and prostacyclin, which act as vasodilators (Hack & Zeerleder, 2001). It is believed that excessive inflammation and coagulation can damage the endothelium, resulting in dysfunction and capillary leak. This process can lead to a shift of fluid and cells into tissue, promoting further inflammation and edema. In such a scenario, there is difficulty in maintaining homeostasis, and organ dysfunction can occur (Kleinpell, 2003).

Coagulation

In the coagulation component of sepsis, inflammation initiates the coagulation cascade related to endothelial injury and cytokine release, ultimately promoting thrombin production. Making this situation perpetuate itself, thrombin, which is needed for coagulation, causes further inflammation, which in turn causes yet more endothelial injury. Compounding the activated coagulation through the cascade are decreased levels of protein C and antithrombin III, both of which are vital to anticoagulation. This decline contributes to the procoagulant state and unregulated functioning of thrombin. Thrombin transforms the previously soluble fibrinogen into fibrin, which combines with circulating platelets to form clots. These clots can become microemboli that may block the microvasculature in the body (Tazbir, 2004), which negatively impacts cell and organ function. [Refer to Chapter 50 on disseminated intravascular clotting (DIC).]

Fibrinolysis

In a healthy individual, a compensatory mechanism removes fibrin through fibrinolysis (breakdown of fibrin), which prevents excessive deposition of fibrin. In contrast, in severe sepsis, endothelial injury causes production of substances that impairs fibrinolysis. When fibrinolysis is delayed, the delicate balance between normal clot development and clot removal becomes disrupted.

In severe sepsis, what is normally a local response to an infection becomes overwhelming and excessive and eventually leads to a systemic imbalance of the compensatory mechanisms. Over time, these alterations and unmitigated function of the coagulation cascade may lead to full-blown DIC (Osborn, 2005).

Many organ systems can be affected in sepsis depending on the underlying diagnosis and the progression of the syndrome. Assessment of the patient is the first step in early recognition. **Box 51-1** lists the common symptoms of sepsis and septic shock according to the system affected.

NURSING ASSESSMENTS

Cardiovascular Assessment

Cardiovascular dysfunction is frequently seen with sepsis. Release of mediators causes endothelium vasoregulation abnormalities that in turn produce persistent hypotension.

Hypotension in severe sepsis is defined as a systolic blood pressure less than 90 mm Hg or a 40 mm Hg decrease in systolic blood pressure from baseline with no other known causes. As sepsis progresses to septic shock, hypotension may become unresponsive to aggressive fluid administration. Tachycardia may be present with or without ectopic beats.

Some patients may initially present with an elevated cardiac output (CO; the amount of blood ejected by the heart each minute) and low systemic vascular resistance (SVR) (the amount of work the heart has to do to eject blood). As sepsis progresses, however, mediator release causes myocardial depression leading to diminished CO, elevated central venous pressure (CVP) and pulmonary artery (PA) pressures, cooler skin temperature, sluggish capillary refill, and pale skin color (Robson, 2005).

Pulmonary Assessment

Lung dysfunction is common in sepsis and frequently prompts the use of mechanical ventilation. Signs of impending respiratory failure include tachypnea with a respiratory rate greater than 20 breaths per minute and respiratory alkalosis with a $PaCO_2$ less than 32 mm Hg due to hyperventilation. Monitoring oxygen saturation (SpO_2) through pulse oximetry can help in assessing oxygen delivery and, therefore, appropriate tissue perfusion. Auscultation of lung sounds will assist in identifying crackles and wheezes from pulmonary edema or constriction. In addition, respiratory status can be tracked over time by following the PaO_2 to FiO_2 ratio (P/F ratio). Performing this simple calculation by using the PaO_2 value from an arterial blood gas and the FiO_2 value from the supplemental oxygen can assist in ensuring early recognition of acute lung injury (P/F ratio $\leq$ 300) or the more severe acute respiratory distress syndrome (ARDS) (P/F ratio $\leq$ 200).

If mechanical ventilation is required, pulmonary status can be tracked by monitoring the patient's response to ventilator settings such as increasing FiO_2 and changes in positive end-expiratory pressure (PEEP) and tidal volume. Changes in SpO_2 and inspiratory pressures can be early indicators of changes in the compliance or elasticity of the lungs themselves (Osborn, 2005).

Renal Assessment

The kidneys depend on adequate perfusion through CO to ensure that they maintain good function. Assessment of kidney function entails monitoring urine output every one to two hours, assessing for peripheral edema, and monitoring creatinine and blood urea nitrogen levels. As kidney function declines, oliguria and azotemia will worsen. Assessing urine characteristics is also important, because cloudy and foul-smelling urine are signs that need to be explored as a potential underlying cause for the sepsis, particularly in elderly patients (Robson, 2005).

Box 51-1

Signs and Symptoms of Sepsis and Septic Shock by System

System	Sepsis	Septic Shock
General	Fever; chills; fatigue; malaise; rigors; warm, pink periphery	
CNS	Confusion, anxiety, disorientation, apprehension, agitation, obtunded, comatose	
Cardiovascular	Tachycardia, increased pulse pressure, hypotension	Refractory hypotension, tachycardia, decreased CO, myocardial depression, decreased SVR
Pulmonary	Hyperventilation, respiratory alkalosis, shortness of breath, tachypnea, acute lung injury	Tachypnea, hypoxemia, respiratory failure, acute lung injury
GI/GU	Nausea, vomiting, decreased albumin, jaundice, oliguria	Decreased motility, ileus, liver function test abnormalities, nausea, vomiting, diarrhea
Hematologic	Increased or decreased WBCs, increased INR, increased aPTT, DIC, thrombocytopenia	Coagulopathies, increased D-dimers, decreased protein C, DIC, leukocytosis or leukopenia
Metabolic/endocrine		Changes in carbohydrate, fat, and glucose metabolism; increased glucose production; insulin resistance; lactic acidosis; electrolyte abnormalities

CO = cardiac output   INR = international normalized ratio
SVR = systemic vascular resistance   aPTT = activated partial thromboplastin time
WBC = white blood cell   DIC = disseminated intravascular coagulation
Source: Balk, Ely, & Goyette, 2001.

Hematologic Assessment

Due to the activation of the coagulation cascade that takes place in severe sepsis, a decrease in platelets may be observed as these cells quickly become depleted as a result of systemic microclot formation. This can increase the patient's risk for bleeding. Monitoring for bleeding will include assessing bruising, petechiae, nasogastric returns, urine, stool, and hemoglobin levels (Robson, 2005).

Gastrointestinal Assessment

Gastrointestinal (GI) function is interrupted during evolving sepsis. Decreased perfusion affects the ability of the liver, stomach, and intestines to function normally. Gastroparesis (damage in the stomach that causes slow digestion and emptying) can be a result of impaired motility. Bilirubin, glucose, and liver function tests can be elevated from liver dysfunction.

Nutrition is already a priority in critically ill patients to support their full recovery, but GI dysfunction makes achieving adequate nutrition even more of a challenge. Gastroparesis can result in nausea and vomiting as well as high enteral feeding residuals. Diminished liver function can pose a challenge to the use of parenteral nutrition (Robson, 2005).

Close assessment of GI function provides additional information for the overall assessment of organ function and patient status. The intensive care unit (ICU) nurse should routinely assess for nausea, vomiting, diarrhea, jaundice, high enteral feeding residuals, diminished or absent bowel sounds, and increased abdominal girth from distention.

Neurological Assessment

Critically ill patients frequently experience changes in their neurological status, and sepsis can exacerbate those changes. Patients may exhibit confusion and delirium along with periods of agitation. These changes can be attributed to many potential issues—hypoxemia, circulating toxins, infection, organ dysfunction, use of multiple medications, the ICU environment itself, and disruption of sleep-wake cycles (Robson, 2005).

Patients may receive sedation to optimize their oxygen consumption and relieve any anxiety and agitation. Neurological status should be routinely assessed to enable the nurse to quickly recognize a decline. As sepsis progresses, patients may become increasingly lethargic and eventually obtunded or comatose. The Glasgow Coma Scale is an effective way to track changes in neurological status over time.

Integumentary Assessment

Ongoing and frequent skin assessment is key when working with critically ill septic patients. Pressure ulcers may develop quickly, even when pressure relief is a priority and the nurse performs meticulous skin care. Hypoperfusion, hypoxemia, decreased mobility, altered nutrition, and the clotting-bleeding cycle of DIC can all contribute to skin breakdown. Assessing the skin from head to toe on a routine basis is key to early intervention. Signs to watch for include purulent drainage, redness, and inflammation (all signs of infection) as well as skin mottling or blanching, microemboli showers, and breakdown from incontinence or pressure areas. Even with meticulous skin care regimens, skin breakdown may be inevitable in case of sepsis (Robson, 2005).

Lab Values

Nurses will be drawing frequent laboratory specimens to track patient status and response to interventions. Some of the laboratory values found to be abnormal with sepsis have already been mentioned. **Table 51-1** identifies additional lab values that should be monitored closely.

INTERVENTIONS

Interventions to treat sepsis can be categorized by the aggressive treatment of the source of the infection, if known, and optimizing organ function. In 2003, 11 international organizations developed the *Surviving Sepsis Guidelines* based on current evidence related to the early and aggressive treatment of sepsis (Dellinger et al., 2004). **Table 51-2** highlights key evidence-based recommendations from these guidelines.

In general, identifying the source of infection as soon as possible is essential. It not only helps to assess the extent of the infection, but also assists in tailoring treatment to the individual patient. Obtaining blood cultures prior to administration of antibiotics offers the best chance to identify causative organisms. Ideally, the nurse will draw two sets of cultures from two different sites. Obtaining cultures from at least one

TABLE 51-1 Selected Altered Laboratory Values in Sepsis

Lab Test	Potential Causes
Increased or decreased electrolytes (e.g., sodium, potassium, magnesium)	• Renal dysfunction • Fluid imbalances
Elevated glucose	• Liver dysfunction • Insulin resistance • Increased glucose production
Elevated bilirubin Elevated liver function tests (e.g., AST, ALT, LDH)	• Liver dysfunction
Decreased platelets	• Hematologic
Elevated INR and aPTT Elevated D-dimer	• Coagulopathy • Liver dysfunction
Elevated WBC or decreased WBC	• Infection • Immunocompromise
Elevated serum lactate	• Anaerobic metabolism
Decreased pH	• Hypoperfusion-induced acidemia
Decreased PaO_2	• Respiratory failure
Decreased $PaCO_2$ or elevated $PaCO_2$	• Hyperventilation • Respiratory failure

AST = aspartate aminotransferase
ALT = alanine aminotransferase
LDH = lactate dehydrogenase
INR = international normalized ratio
aPTT = activated partial thromboplastin time
WBC = white blood cell
PaO_2 = partial pressure of arterial oxygen
$PaCO_2$ = partial pressure of arterial carbon dioxide
Source: Balk, Ely, & Goyette, 2001.

venipuncture site is recommended due to the potential for contamination of cultures taken from central or peripheral access lines. Antibiotics should be initiated within one hour of the onset of signs of severe sepsis. Antibiotic selection will be based on the extent of knowledge of the causative organism, mode of acquisition of the infection (either nosocomial or community acquired), and institutional variables.

Cardiovascular Interventions

The goals of supporting the cardiovascular system include reversing hypotension and maintaining adequate CO and vascular tone. These goals may be achieved through fluid resuscitation using crystalloids, colloids, or, in some cases, blood products. Aggressive fluid resuscitation involves fluid challenges of as much as one liter of crystalloids or 500 mL of colloids

TABLE 51-2 Selected Evidence-based Interventions for the Treatment of Sepsis

Initial resuscitation	Goals: • Central venous pressure 8–12 mm Hg • Mean arterial pressure ≥ 65 mm Hg • Urine output ≥ 0.5 mL/kg/hr • SvO_2 ≥ 70% (venous oxygen saturation)
Diagnosis	• Two blood cultures, with at least one from venipuncture
Source control	• Evaluation for source control intervention such as drainage of infection, debridement, or prompt removal of an infected device
Anti-infective therapy	• Initiate antimicrobials within one hour of severe sepsis recognition • Initiate empiric anti-infective agents with reassessment after 48–72 hours based on diagnostic and culture results • Stop antimicrobial therapy immediately if syndrome discovered to be due to noninfectious cause
Fluid therapy	• May use colloids or crystalloids • Administer fluid challenge
Vasopressor therapy	• May initiate after fluid resuscitation • First-line vasopressors should be norepinephrine or dopamine • Vasopressin may be used for refractory shock • Place arterial catheter with use of vasopressors
Inotropic therapy	• Dobutamine may be used for decreased cardiac output despite fluid resuscitation
Mechanical ventilation	• Goal is tidal volume of 6 mL/kg • Goal is to maintain end-inspiratory plateau pressures < 30 cm H_2O • Use minimum amount of positive end-expiratory pressure • Maintain head of bed at 45° to prevent ventilator-associated pneumonia • Utilize ventilator weaning protocol
Glucose control	• Maintain tight glucose control • Preference for use of enteral route for nutrition
Deep venous thrombosis prophylaxis	• Prophylaxis with heparin, sequential compression devices, and/or antiembolism stockings is recommended
Stress ulcer prophylaxis	• Recommended for all patients with severe sepsis
Consideration for limitation of support	• Promote communication with patient and family regarding likely outcomes and treatment plan • Limitation of support may be appropriate for consideration

Source: Dellinger et al., 2004.

are used to optimize CVP and PA filling pressures.

If a patient with septic shock has been adequately fluid resuscitated but still requires vasopressor medications to achieve adequate blood pressure, anticipate the use of corticosteroids as a method to reverse the shock and reduce mortality. While corticosteroids may be effective in patients exhibiting adrenal insufficiency, there is no known benefit from administering them in the absence of adrenal insufficiency unless the patient's endocrine history warrants continuation of maintenance steroid therapy. A corticostimulation test may be used to determine adrenal function status (Dellinger et al., 2004).

Pulmonary Interventions

Interventions to support the pulmonary system are aimed at optimizing oxygen exchange, delivery, and consumption. It is key to intervene quickly when the patient develops hypoxemia. An estimated 85% of patients with severe sepsis will require mechanical ventilation, and 40% will progress to develop ARDS (Kleinpell, 2003). Oxygen should be titrated to the lowest level needed to maintain SpO_2 greater than 90%. Barotrauma can be an additional insult to the lungs; for this reason, use of PEEP and higher tidal volumes needs to be closely monitored so as to not exacerbate already compromised pulmonary function.

over 30 minutes and may need to be repeated (Dellinger et al., 2004). If fluid resuscitation is not adequate to reverse the hypotension, vasoactive medications such as dopamine (Intropin®), norepinephrine bitartrate (Levophed®), or vasopressin (Pitressin®) may be administered. An inotropic medication such as dobutamine (Dobutrex®) may be indicated to counteract myocardial depression and improve contractility. All of these medications

Good pulmonary care includes suctioning for secretions as needed, administration of nebulized medications, and positioning to promote optimal oxygen exchange. Oral care is also indicated to prevent oral bacterial colonization from being aspirated and potentially leading to another infection (i.e., ventilator-associated pneumonia). Oral care should be performed in intubated patients at least every two to four hours. It should entail removing plaque buildup, removing secretions that have pooled in the glottic region, and keeping oral mucosa moist to prevent cracking, thereby avoiding another potential portal for infection.

Renal Interventions

Judicious use of both fluids and diuretics may be required to maintain optimal fluid balance. Successful fluid resuscitation should improve renal perfusion. Restoring adequate circulation and addressing the infection so as to reduce circulating toxins are the best support measures for the kidneys. The goal of therapy is to maintain urine output of at least 0.5 mL/kg/hr. If the patient progresses to renal failure, hemodialysis or continuous renal replacement therapy may be initiated to manage fluid balance and electrolytes and to normalize creatinine.

Hematologic Interventions

Blood product utilization is not automatic treatment for the septic patient. Typically packed red blood cells are transfused only if the hemoglobin is 7.0 Gm/dL or less. Giving blood may be warranted if the hemoglobin is greater than 7.0 Gm/dL if the patient is actively bleeding or is exhibiting myocardial ischemia. Fresh frozen plasma is usually reserved for patients who are bleeding with a coagulopathy.

Patients with septic shock have decreased amounts of circulating protein C. Furthermore, protein C is less likely to become activated in patients with sepsis due to endothelial damage. Infusions of activated protein C (drotrecogin alfa, Xigris®) may prove beneficial for patients with severe sepsis who are at high risk for death. This substance targets all three of the main processes occurring in sepsis: It reduces inflammation, prevents coagulation by inactivating part of the clotting cascade, and increases fibrinolysis. Since there is a risk of bleeding with administration of activated protein C, its use should be avoided in patients who have active bleeding or who have experienced recent hemorrhagic incidents (Baillie & Murray, 2006).

The risk of developing deep vein thrombosis (DVT) is always present in critically ill patients. DVT prophylaxis should be considered and initiated if appropriate, including use of heparin, sequential compression devices, and/or antiembolism stockings.

Gastrointestinal Interventions

To avoid complications of enteral nutrition, feeding residuals should be checked routinely and the elevation of the head of bed maintained at least 30 degrees. If the residual is twice the rate of enteral feed infusion, the feedings should be stopped for an hour and the residual then rechecked. These interventions will assist in preventing aspiration of gastric contents into the lungs. Medications intended to promote GI motility or to reduce gastric reflux may be ordered. Interventions to avoid diarrhea will help maintain normal bowel function.

Neurological Interventions

Patients may require sedation to relieve anxiety and agitation, to promote respiratory synchrony with mechanical ventilation, and to optimize oxygen consumption. In addition, pain medication should be administered to provide adequate comfort for what can be a painful ICU stay due to the frequent procedures and interventions, hypoperfusion, invasive lines, and immobility. Uncontrolled pain can impair healing.

It is all too easy to oversedate patients in the process of attempting to keep them comfortable. Ideally, patients will be sedated appropriately so as to maintain comfort while remaining arousable so that the nurse can assess neurological status, pain control, and changes in condition. This is not an easy balance to achieve. Consider complementary therapies to promote comfort and relaxation. Reorient the patient frequently, and promote a conducive, healing environment through lighting, massage, music, and other therapies. Promote adequate sleep to prevent the onset of delirium and worsened confusion. (Other consequences of sleep disturbances are discussed in Chapter 5.)

Integumentary Interventions

Attention to skin care is essential to prevent skin breakdown in the patient with sepsis. Maintain fecal and urinary continence to avoid perineal and perianal excoriation. Use available skin products and barriers to protect the skin. Not only is breakdown a painful condition, but it creates another potential site of infection. Pay particular attention to positioning of the patient, and take advantage of specialty mattresses when appropriate to maximize pressure relief. Repositioning the patient at least every two hours, unless clinically contraindicated, is ideal.

Other areas that can frequently break down but may be missed include the heels, face, and head. Keeping heels elevated off the bed, rotating the position of the endotracheal tube, and alleviating pressure areas from endotracheal security devices are interventions that prevent breakdown of these areas.

Additional Laboratory Value Interventions

In addition to the laboratory values already mentioned, the nurse must anticipate that frequent interventions to correct abnormal lab values will be necessary. Achieving balance with electrolytes such as potassium and magnesium can be a challenge when dealing with patients who exhibit renal failure and fluid imbalances. Elevated glucose levels negatively impact the patient in many ways, not the least of which is the impairment of WBC functioning leading to slow healing. Tight glucose control (80 to 110 mg/dL) through continuous insulin infusion should be initiated. This intervention will require frequent assessments of blood glucose—at a minimum, every hour on initiation of the infusion and every two hours when the glucose is stable.

PREVENTION OF INFECTION

While this chapter has focused on the early recognition and treatment of sepsis, prevention of infection cannot be overemphasized. Nurses play a key role in preventing nosocomial infections. Good handwashing is the most important intervention to prevent the spread and occurrence of infections. Follow standard precautions when working with body secretions, wear gowns and gloves when indicated, and strictly adhere to isolation precautions.

Likewise, providing oral and skin care reduces the risk of infection. In addition, particular attention to the care of invasive lines helps maintain skin integrity and prevent infection. Ensure that dressings remain intact, perform routine entry-site care, and discontinue invasive lines—including vascular access lines, urinary drainage catheters, and drains—as soon as possible.

PATIENT AND FAMILY EDUCATION AND COMMUNICATION

Good communication with and effective education of the patient and family are essential during the critical phase of a sepsis episode. Many organs can be failing at the same time and multiple acute interventions may need to occur rapidly. This can be overwhelming and stressful for the patient and family. Educate them as appropriate and reinforce information frequently. Depending on the source of the infection and the patient's underlying medical history, the sepsis may be reversed with little long-term sequelae, it may evolve into a long-term recovery with significant deficits, or it may progress into an end-of-life situation. Provide the family with honest, compassionate information with realistic estimated outcomes of the treatment. As the care decisions are made, consider the need for discussions regarding the patient's quality of life wishes and the potential for limitation or withdrawal of support consistent with anticipated outcomes and patient wishes.

PATIENT OUTCOMES

Nurses can help ensure attainments of optimal patient outcomes such as those listed in **Box 51-2** through the use of evidence-based interventions for patients with SIRS or sepsis.

SUMMARY

Nurses play a vital role in the prevention, early recognition, and treatment of sepsis. Identification of subtle changes and analysis of the comprehensive medical condition of the patient, including risk factors for sepsis, is the first step in rapid intervention to avoid the downward spiral from SIRS to MODS.

Box 51-2
Optimal Patient Outcomes

- Vital signs in expected range
- Coagulation profile in expected range
- Absence of signs and symptoms of bleeding
- Peripheral pulses strong
- Patient/family uses effective coping strategies
- Skin intact
- Glucose levels are maintained in expected range
- Oxygen delivery and consumption levels are optimized

CASE STUDY

A 50-year-old female is admitted to the medical ICU with severe right upper quadrant pain rated as a 10 on a scale of 1 to 10. Her past medical history is significant for end-stage liver disease due to history of alcohol abuse and infection with hepatitis C virus, diabetes, and asthma. The patient is slightly confused. Her abdomen is firm and distended. The patient's husband is present with her. Assessments and labs on admission are as follows:

Sodium 136 mEq/L
Potassium 3.1 mEq/L
Chloride 109 mEq/L
BUN 10 mg/dL
Creatinine 0.68 mg/dL
Glucose 169 mg/dL

ALT 48 IU/L
AST 95 IU/L
Albumin 1.9 Gm/dL
Total bilirubin 9.4 mg/dL

WBC 6,400/mm^3
INR 1.80
Platelets 176,000/mm^3

Oxygen saturation is 91% on FiO$_2$ 1.00 via non-invasive positive pressure ventilation. The patient's right lung sounds clear, but expiratory wheezes are heard in the left lower lobe. She is jaundiced, has positive bowel sounds, but has no edema, nausea, or vomiting. She has guarding with palpation of her abdomen.

Temperature 96.8°F
Respiratory rate 32 breaths/min
Pulse 94 beats/min
Blood pressure 86/44 mm Hg

CRITICAL THINKING QUESTIONS

1. Discuss the patient's hemodynamic and lab assessments.
2. Where does the patient fall on the continuum from SIRS to MODS?
3. Which interventions should you anticipate?

The patient is intubated and started on dopamine. Cultures are drawn, and broad-spectrum antibiotics are initiated. The patient remains in stable condition. Twenty-four hours later, she has an acute deterioration in her status. Sputum, blood, and urine cultures are all negative. An abdominal CT is negative for an abscess. An endoscopic retrograde cholangiopancreatography is done for removal of a gallstone, but no abscess is noted. A pulmonary artery catheter is placed. Now her labs and assessments are as follows:

Sodium 135 mEq/L	Total bilirubin 9.4 mg/dL	WBC 20,700/mm^3
Potassium 2.8 mEq/L	Serum lactate 6.7 mmo/L	Hemoglobin 13.0 Gm/dL
BUN 18 mg/dL	D-dimer 3.2 ng/mL	Platelets 100,000/mm^3
Creatinine 1.2 mg/dL	Fibrinogen 472 mg/dL	PTT 37 sec
Glucose 208 mg/dL	Cortisol 199.8 mcg/dL	INR 2.16
Magnesium 1.3 mg/dL		

ABGs: pH 7.24 PaCO$_2$ 51 PaO$_2$ 78 HCO$_3$ 21 on FiO$_2$ .80
Pulmonary artery occlusive pressure 20 mm Hg   Systemic vascular resistance 367 dynes/sec/cm^{-5}
Cardiac Output 10 L/min   Central venous pressure 6 mm Hg

The patient has low urine output despite the use of furosemide (Lasix®) and fluid challenges. A clear source of infection has not yet been found. The patient now has 2+ peripheral edema. Her chest radiograph confirms a new right pneumonia and pulmonary edema. She is obtunded, yet requires a small amount of sedation for intermittent agitation.

CRITICAL THINKING QUESTIONS

4. Identify and support with evidence the organ systems that are not functioning in this patient.
5. Discuss the nursing interventions that should be initiated or maintained.
6. Discuss the anticipated medical interventions.
7. Which disciplines should be consulted to work with this client?
8. How would you modify your plan of care for patients of diverse backgrounds?
9. What types of issues may require you to act as an advocate or moral agent for this patient?
10. How will you implement your role as a facilitator of learning for this patient?
11. Write a case example for a patient with SIRS or sepsis from the clinical setting. Rate the patient as a level 1, 3, or 5 on each characteristic. Identify the level of nurse characteristics needed in the care of this patient.
12. Use the form to write up a plan of care for one client with SIRS or sepsis in the clinical setting. Take one patient outcome and list evidence-based interventions for this patient.

Using the Synergy Model to Develop a Plan of Care

	Patient Characteristics	Subjective and Objective Data	Evidence-based Interventions	Outcomes
SYNERGY MODEL	Resiliency			
	Vulnerability			
	Stability			
	Complexity			
	Resource Availability			
	Participation in Care			
	Participation in Decision Making			
	Predictability			

Online Resources

Eli Lilly and Company: www.sepsis.com

Surviving Sepsis Campaign Guidelines: www.sccm.org

Institute for Healthcare Improvement: www.ihi.org

VHA Research Series 2004—Improving Sepsis Care in the Intensive Care Unit: An Evidence-based Approach: www.vha.com

***Promoting a Better Understanding of Sepsis* booklet:** www.sepsisforum.org

National Initiative in Sepsis Education: www.nise.cc

REFERENCES

Angus, D. C., Linde-Zwirble, W. T., Lidicker, J., Clermont, G., Carcillo, J., & Pinsky, M. R. (2001). Epidemiology of severe sepsis in the United States: Analysis of incidence, outcomes, and associated costs of care. *Critical Care Medicine, 29*(7), 1303–1310.

Baillie, J. K., & Murray, G. (2006). Drotrecogin alfa (activated) in severe sepsis. *New England Journal of Medicine, 34*(1), 94–96.

Balk, R. A., Ely, E. W., & Goyette, R. E. (2001). *Sepsis handbook.* Vanderbilt University Medical Center: National Initiative in Sepsis Education.

Bone, R. C., Balk, R. A., Cerra, F. B., Dellinger, R. P., Fein, A. M., Knaus, W. A., et al. (1992). ACCP/SCCM Consensus Conference: Definitions for sepsis and organ failure and guidelines for the use of innovative therapies for sepsis. *Chest, 101,* 1644–1655.

Dellinger, R. P., Carlet, J. M., Masur, H., Gerlach, H., Calandra, T., Cohen, J., et al. (2004). Surviving sepsis campaign guidelines for management of severe sepsis and septic shock. *Critical Care Medicine, 32*(3), 858–873.

Eli Lilly and Company. (2005). www.sepsis.com

Hack, C. E., & Zeerleder, S. (2001). The endothelium in sepsis: Source of and target for inflammation. *Critical Care Medicine, 29*(7), S21–S27.

Kleinpell, R. (2003). Advances in treating patients with severe sepsis: Role of drotecogin alfa (activated). *Critical Care Nurse, 23*(3), 16–29.

Levy, M. M., Fink, M. P., Marshall, J. C., Abraham, E., Angus, D., Cook, D., et al. (2003). 2001 SCCM/ESICM/ACCP/ATS/SIS International Sepsis Definitions Conference. *Critical Care Medicine, 31*(4), 1250–1256.

Osborn, T. M. (2005). Emergency medicine and the surviving sepsis campaign: An international approach to managing severe sepsis and septic shock. *Annals of Emergency Medicine, 46*(3), 228–231.

Robson, W. (2005). Assessing treating and managing patients with sepsis. *Nursing Standard, 19*(50), 56–64, 66, 68.

Tazbir, J. (2004). Sepsis and the role of activated protein C. *Critical Care Nurse, 24*(6), 40–45.

Vallet, B., & Wiel, E. (2001). Endothelial cell dysfunction and coagulation. *Critical Care Medicine, 29*(7), S36–S41.

Burns

Frank Costello

Upon completion of this chapter, the reader will be able to:

1. Differentiate burn injuries with respect to their depth, extent, and severity.

2. Discuss the assessment and management principles involved in the emergent phase of a burn injury.

3. Identify the special considerations involved in the assessment and management of inhalation injuries ("chemical tracheobronchitis") and circumferential, electrical, and chemical burns.

4. Discuss the primary characteristics of the acute and rehabilitative phases of a burn injury and the general management principles inherent within each phase.

5. List optimal patient outcomes that may be achieved through evidence-based management of a patient with a burn injury.

In the United States, more than 1 million people sustain burn injuries each year. Although the overall death rate from burns declined approximately 50% between 1978 to 1998, morbidity and mortality from major burns still account for more than 4,500 deaths, 45,000 hospitalizations, and 700,000 annual emergency room visits (Alson, 2005; American Burn Association, 2004). Burns pose significant challenges and disruptions to one's physical, psychological, and social functioning. The multisystem nature of burn injuries demands not only a nursing competence capable of interpreting a vast array of physiological parameters but also the development of an intuitive, ethical, and emotional expertise. This chapter provides an overview and promotes an understanding of the multisystem assessment and management principles inherent in the three phases (emergent, acute, and rehabilitative) of a burn injury.

BURN ASSESSMENT

Type and Depth

The most common etiologies of burn injuries are thermal, chemical, and electrical. The depth of tissue damage depends on the temperature and duration of exposure and is diagnosed clinically by assessing and inspecting the anatomical layers of the skin involved. First-degree burns are superficial and involve an avascular epidermis composed of stratified epithelial cells, keratinocytes (new cells), and melanocytes (pigmentation). It can be characterized as a zone of hyperemia because it receives the least amount of cell damage and generally appears red from blood vessel dilatation.

Second-degree burns (superficial and/or deep partial thickness) involve the epidermis and part of the dermis. The dermis forms the structure, nutrition, and vascular support of the skin and is composed of connective tissue (lymphocytes, nerve endings, sebaceous and sweat glands, hair follicles, blood vessels, and subcutaneous tissue) and fibroblast cells for collagen formation. It can be characterized as a zone of stasis, where circulation is sluggish and variable but some degree of perfusion remains. Burns in this zone can convert from superficial to deep partial thickness to full thickness if blood flow becomes impaired or if perfusion is not maintained during fluid resuscitation.

Third-degree burns (full thickness) involve the entire epidermal and dermal layers. The affected area can be characterized as a zone of coagulation, where the prolonged source of heat results in tissue damage, injury, and necrosis. Subdermal burns extend below the dermis into subcutaneous tissue, fat, muscle, or bone, usually as the result of an electrical injury or massive tissue destruction of a body part. They appear as charred, devitalized, and/or mummified (see **Table 52-1**).

Burn Extent

The extent (size) of the body surface area (BSA) burned is important in determining the severity and appropriate management of the injury and deciding whether the victim meets the criteria for transfer to a specialized burn facility as outlined by the American Burn Association. (See **Table 52-2**.)

TABLE 52-1 Depth and Characteristics of Burn Wounds

Depth (Degree)	Characteristics
First degree (superficial)	• Pink to red • Hypersensitive and painful to touch • Weepy and edematous • Complete healing expected because basic skin functions are not impaired
Second degree (superficial or deep partial thickness)	• Red to pale ivory • Moist, bullous, and edematous • Pain can be severe since nerve endings are generally only partially damaged • Exudate forms a crust-like surface and epithelialization (epithelium growth) occurs beneath the crust and may take 14 to 21 days to heal as the crust falls off, leaving a healed surface beneath
Third degree (full thickness)	• White, cherry red, black, charred-like appearance • Thrombosed vessels • Marked edema and inelasticity of dermis • Dry, hard, leathery appearance • Generally painless to touch • Requires grafting

Sources: American Burn Association, 2001; Danks, 2003.

TABLE 52-2 Burn Referral Criteria

Burn Injuries That Should Be Referred and/or Transferred to a Burn Unit/Center
Second- and third-degree burns of more than 10% for ages < 10 years and > 50 years and more than 20% for all other ages
Third-degree burns of more than 5%
Burns of face, hands, eyes, ears, feet, or perineum
All inhalation injuries, electrical and chemical burns
Circumferential burns of extremities and/or chest
All burns complicated by fractures and trauma
All burns in poor-risk children, including all children younger than age 2
All burns with preexisting medical conditions

Sources: American Burn Association, 2001; Carrougher, 1998.

Several methods can be used to determine the extent of the burn wound. One method popular in the prehospital setting is the Rule of Nines, which divides the total BSA into anatomical areas worth 9% each. For children, this formula is adjusted to better approximate their BSA, with the legs receiving 14% instead of 18% each and the head 18% instead of 9%. Another quick method of determining the burn extent is the palmar method, wherein an individual's palm surface is estimated to be 1% of a person's BSA. The most accurate and acceptable method, which is especially useful in pediatric patients, is the Lund and Browder chart, which divides the total BSA into anatomical areas worth a certain percentage according to age-based growth and development standards (see **Figure 52-1**).

BURN MANAGEMENT

The management and treatment of burn injuries can be divided into three phases: emergent, acute, and rehabilitative. Each phase has its own characteristics and management modalities.

Emergent (Shock) Phase

The emergent phase extends from the time of injury to the time of diuresis (fluid mobilization). It is distinguished by increased capillary permeability and massive fluid shifts (third space edema). Attention to the basic ABC principles of trauma resuscitation and intervention need to be applied. Application of the primary (ABCDEFG) and secondary surveys (head-to-toe physical exam, additional history, lab and chemistry values) is an organized approach to assess and manage a burn injury

FIGURE 52-1 Rule of Nines and Lund and Browder Chart

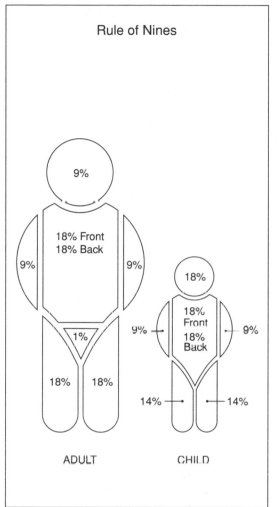

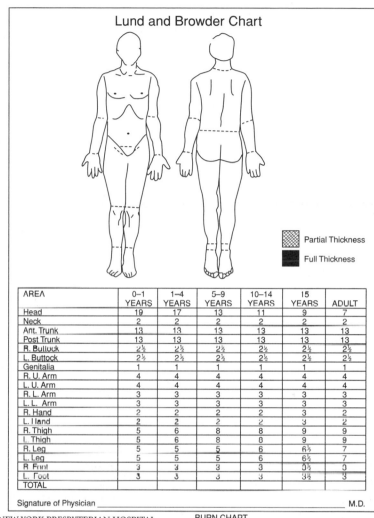

Lund and Browder Chart

AREA	0–1 YEARS	1–4 YEARS	5–9 YEARS	10–14 YEARS	15 YEARS	ADULT
Head	19	17	13	11	9	7
Neck	2	2	2	2	2	2
Ant. Trunk	13	13	13	13	13	13
Post Trunk	13	13	13	13	13	13
R. Buttock	2½	2½	2½	2½	2½	2½
L. Buttock	2½	2½	2½	2½	2½	2½
Genitalia	1	1	1	1	1	1
R. U. Arm	4	4	4	4	4	4
L. U. Arm	4	4	4	4	4	4
R. L. Arm	3	3	3	3	3	3
L. L. Arm	3	3	3	3	3	3
R. Hand	2	2	2	2	3	2
L. Hand	2	2	2	2	3	2
R. Thigh	5	6	8	8	9	9
L. Thigh	5	6	8	8	9	9
R. Leg	5	5	5	6	6½	7
L. Leg	5	5	5	6	6½	7
R. Foot	3	3	3	3	3½	3
L. Foot	3	3	3	3	3½	3
TOTAL						

Partial Thickness

Full Thickness

Signature of Physician _____ M.D.

NEW YORK PRESBYTERIAN HOSPITAL   BURN CHART

Source: Illustrated by James R. Perron; Adapted from NY Presbyterian Hospital.

(American Burn Association, 2001; American College of Surgeons Committee on Trauma, 1999; Jacobs & Hoyt, 2000).

Airway/Breathing (Ventilation/Oxygenation)

The patient's airway and breathing need to be assessed immediately because inhalation injuries are present in as many as half of major burns and account for more than 50% of all burn injury deaths (American Burn Association, 2001). Three types of inhalation injuries are distinguished: carbon monoxide poisoning, upper airway obstruction/edema, and lower airway injury. The diagnosis is made from the circumstances of the fire (history of being in a closed versus open space), physical exam (neck and facial burns, singed nasal hairs, soot-coated tongue,

hoarseness, inflamed and edematous nasal and oral mucosa, carbonaceous sputum) and laboratory tests (arterial blood gases (ABGs), carboxyhemoglobin levels, fiber-optic bronchoscopy).

Ventilation and oxygenation compromise can also occur when deep second- and-third degree circumferential chest burns restrict chest excursion, causing increased work of breathing, decreased lung compliance, and impaired gas exchange. This restrictive process usually involves intubation, mechanical ventilation, and chest escharotomies (surgical incision within constricting eschar of a circumferentially burned chest or limb to allow expansion through eschar—dead tissue—separation) to avoid further pulmonary compromise and deterioration (Bird, 1999; Fitzpatrick & Cioffi, 1997).

Carbon Monoxide Poisoning

Carbon monoxide (CO), a by-product of oxygen combustion, binds to hemoglobin with a much greater affinity than oxygen does. It results in tissue hypoxia and eventual asphyxiation (see **Table 52-3**). Treatment for CO poisoning is administration of 100% oxygen, which reduces the concentration of carboxyhemoglobin by half for every 30 minutes of high-flow oxygen administration. Depending on the clinical situation, a high FiO$_2$ can be administered either through a rebreather mask or an endotracheal tube. This therapy is continued until the CO levels are less than 10%. If available and as long as there is pulmonary and hemodynamic stability, hyperbaric therapy (HBO) can be useful. HBO delivers 100% oxygen systemically at levels two to three times greater than atmospheric pressure (sea level). This elevated pressure results in a 10- to 15-fold increase in plasma oxygen concentration, producing a four-fold increase in the diffusion of oxygen from the capillaries to the tissue cells (Bird, 1999; Demling & DeSanti, 2005; Walker & Neubauer, 1998).

Upper Airway Obstruction/Edema (Inhalation Injury above Glottis)

Direct inhalation of superheated air can not only cause external facial/neck burns but also damage the airway mucosa, leading to laryngeal erythema and edema and potential airway obstruction. Upper and lower airway injuries can be exacerbated by fluid resuscitation because increased capillary permeability promotes intravascular fluid shifts into the interstitial and alveoli. Based on the patient's history, physical evidence, and results of ABGs and fiber-optic bronchoscopy, it must be decided whether the airway can be maintained with or without intubation. A rule of thumb is this: When in doubt, intubate—airway edema is a progressive and continuous process that can

last up to 24 hours (American Burn Association, 2001; Bird, 1999; Costello & Dungca, 1988).

Lower Airway Injury below the Glottis (Chemical Tracheobronchitis)

The amount and type of noxious substances and products of incomplete combustion inhaled may cause varying lower airway tissue injuries. The tissue response to the injury is often delayed in its onset and presentation (two to three days post injury) and becomes clinically unpredictable. An acute respiratory distress syndrome (ARDS)-like pattern develops with increased work of breathing and impaired gas exchange, so it may become necessary to promote ventilatory support through intubation and to employ lung-protective mechanical ventilation strategies to improve functional residual capacity [positive end-expiratory pressure (PEEP)]. When airway injury is accompanied by significant cutaneous burns, hemodynamic monitoring may be necessary to monitor fluid resuscitation and avoid exacerbation (Bird, 1999; Herndon, 2001; Tasaki et al., 1997).

C-Spine/Circulation/Circumferential Burns

Concomitant trauma frequently accompanies burn injuries. Potential or suspected C-spine injuries need to be stabilized immediately. Internal and external hemorrhage must be controlled and absolute emergencies (e.g., cardiac arrest, tension pneumothorax/hemothorax, cardiac tamponade, myocardial contusion/infarction, and shock) quickly recognized and treated. Treatment and resuscitation of burn shock will be discussed shortly.

In addition to the restrictive chest burns as mentioned earlier, circumferential extremity burns (arms and legs) need to be monitored promptly because they may act like a tourniquet and compromise and/or impair perfusion, thereby creating a potential site for ischemia and necrosis. Circulatory compromise as assessed through color, capillary refill, sensation, pain, and monitoring of peripheral pulses by Doppler ultrasound is best treated with escharotomies to release the pressure and allow expansion through separated eschar (American Burn Association, 2001; American College of Surgeons Committee on Trauma, 1999; Jacobs & Hoyt, 2000).

Determination of Disability and Exposure/Examination of the Injury

Determination of level of consciousness and orientation can best be assessed by use of the AVPU method (Alert, Verbal stimuli response, Painful stimuli response, Unresponsive) and the Glasgow Coma scale (eye opening, best verbal and motor response). If any neurological deficits are present, associated

---

TABLE 52-3 Carbon Monoxide Poisoning

Level of Poisoning	Characteristics
< 20% HbCO	Headache, confusion, decreased function
20–40% HbCO	Nausea, irritability, impaired function, disorientation
40–60% HbCO	Confusion, obtundation, ataxia, hallucinations, visual changes
> 60% HbCO	Combativeness, shock, coma

Key—HbCO = carboxyhemoglobin
Sources: Bird, 1999; Demling & DeSanti, 2005; Tasaki et al., 1997.

circumstances need to be considered (e.g., chemical abuse, hypoxia, preexisting medical conditions). However, control of agitation, emotional support, and pain management with narcotics, sedatives, and analgesics should be provided intravenously in sufficient amounts to control pain and relieve anxiety without masking hypoxemia or compromising hemodynamic stability.

Exposure and examination of the burn injury involves stopping the burning process, and removing all clothing and restrictive apparel that could obstruct circulation due to edema. The loss of intact skin causes loss of temperature regulation and protection against infection and necessitates appropriate temperature warming measurements, universal precautions, and tetanus wound prophylaxis if not current (American Burn Association, 2001; American College of Surgeons Committee on Trauma, 1999; Jacobs & Hoyt, 2000).

Fluid Resuscitation/Foley Catheter/Gastric Tube

A burn injury is characterized by extensive fluid and electrolyte losses that cause massive third space fluid shifts and a concomitant low-flow perfusion state. This hypovolemic phase (burn shock) begins at the onset of the burn injury and lasts until diuresis begins (mobilization of fluids). The first 24 to 48 hours is characterized by capillary permeability (third space edema), protein losses (hypoproteinemia), hemoconcentrated hematocrit and hemoglobin, oliguria from the low-flow state, hyponatremia from the fluid sequestration and losses, hyperkalemia from damaged cells, and metabolic acidosis from inadequate oxygen delivery (cardiac output) and tissue perfusion (American Burn Association, 2001; Hilton, 2001).

While intravenous (IV) access is necessary in all burn injuries, burns over 15% to 20% of the BSA generally require guided fluid resuscitation to prevent further shock and tissue damage. This therapy is initiated through large-bore IV lines with isotonic crystalloid fluids (lactated Ringer's or 0.9% normal saline). To accurately monitor urine output and the adequacy of fluid resuscitation, an indwelling urinary catheter should be in place. A gastric ileus that could lead to a stress ulcer (Curling's ulcer) is common after a major burn/trauma due to decreased perfusion to the gastrointestinal (GI) tract. To counter this possibility, a nasogastric tube is initially inserted to decompress the stomach, protect against aspiration, and monitor changes in gastric mucosa and occult bleeding through pH testing and guaiac of stomach contents. A soft feeding tube should subsequently replace the nasogastric tube, and enteral feedings should be started as soon as possible.

In the presence of massive burns, inhalation injuries, concomitant trauma, or preexisting medical conditions, invasive hemodynamic monitoring may be considered. Placement of an arterial line for continuous blood pressure measurement and blood drawing, central venous catheter for multiple access and CVP monitoring, and pulmonary artery catheters for core temperatures, filling pressures, cardiac output/index, vascular resistance, and oxygen delivery/consumption may be necessary to better ascertain tissue oxygen requirements (American Burn Association, 2001; Carrougher, 1998; Hilton, 1998).

Although there are many resuscitation formulas, the consensus formula advocated by the American Burn Association is 2 to 4 mL of lactated Ringer's $\times$ (weight in kilograms) $\times$ (percentage BSA burned). One-half of the total amount is given in the first eight hours from the time of injury; the second half is given over the remaining 16 hours. A maintenance formula is usually added to the amount given by this calculation for pediatric patients, because their greater BSA per pound of body weight leads to greater evaporative losses and increased fluid needs (Carvajal & Parks, 1998; Herndon, 2001).

After the initial 24 hours and for the next three to seven days, capillary permeability begins to subside as the edematous fluid shifts back into vessels, increasing vascular volume and in turn causing an increase in renal blood flow and diuresis. The amount and composition of the resuscitative fluids change during this period. In particular, more hypotonic dextrose and saline with electrolyte replacement as needed are used to replenish evaporative losses. In large burns and optionally in smaller burns, colloid therapy may be initiated in an attempt to replenish protein stores, move third space fluids back into the vasculature, and enhance diuresis (American Burn Association, 2001; Demling, 2001).

It is during this period that many complications can occur. In those patients with preexisting cardiopulmonary conditions, fluid mobilization with the onset of oliguria can lead to heart failure (cardiogenic shock) and pulmonary edema and may require hemodynamic monitoring (e.g., arterial lines, central venous and pulmonary pressures, cardiac output/index). Inhalation injuries with or without burns can begin to exhibit an ARDS-like syndrome (e.g., infiltrates, atelectasis, hypoxia despite increasing FiO_2), necessitating increased lung-protective ventilation and oxygenation strategies. Following resuscitation of large burns and lasting for days to weeks, one may observe a hyperdynamic phase (vasodilation, hypermetabolism, and increased cardiac output/index) as a result of a systemic inflammatory response syndrome (SIRS) response and the release of systemic inflammatory mediators (cytokines). This leads to periods of perfusion deficits, maldistribution of circulating volume, and inability of tissues to adequately extract and use oxygen (Carrougher, 1998; Demling, 2001; Holm, Melcer, Horbrand, von Donnersmarck, & Muhlbauer, 2000).

The overall goal of the emergent period is to maintain organ perfusion and avoid either excessive resuscitation with its concomitant fluid overload and edema or insufficient resuscitation that leads to a worsening hypovolemic shock, renal failure, and eventually multiple organ dysfunction syndrome (MODS). Appropriate clinical responses and signs of adequate resuscitation include clear sensorium, appropriate ventilation and oxygenation, blood pH between 7.35 and 7.45, temperature greater than 37°C, pulse less than 120 bpm, systolic blood pressure (SBP) greater than 90 mm Hg and/or mean arterial pressure (MAP) greater than 60 mm Hg, and adequate urine output (0.5 to 1.0 mL/kg/hr) (American Burn Association, 2001; Barret & Herndon, 2004; Wald, 1998; Wiebelhaus & Hansen, 1999).

Secondary Survey

An ongoing secondary survey is obtained and completed throughout the entire emergent phase, which includes a head-to-toe assessment of associated injuries, additional history, and laboratory studies (see **Table 52-4**).

Special Considerations (Electrical/Chemical Burns)

Electrical burns occur as energy is converted to heat, causing thermal injury; direct damage to tissue, muscle, and bone; and interference with the body's electrical conduction system. All body tissues, to varying degrees, are conductive to current flow, making these injuries difficult to clinically evaluate. The severity of the burn depends on the voltage, strength, and path of the current; the resistance; and the type and duration of contact. Low-voltage injuries (less than 1,000 volts) are characteristic of household current, whereas high-voltage (more than 1,000 volts) injuries can cause extensive and progressive damage to all body organ systems.

In addition to attention to the immediate ABCs, IV access, insertion of a urinary catheter, and fluid resuscitation should begin as soon as possible. Because of the likelihood of unseen deep and extensive tissue and muscle damage (iceberg effect), resuscitation formulas can underestimate fluid requirements. Therefore, a minimum urine output of 0.5 to 1.0 mL/kg/hr should be maintained. In the presence of hemoglobinuria/myoglobinuria (reddish to brown), urine output of more than 1 mL/kg/hr should be maintained along with sodium bicarbonate in the IV fluids to alkalinize and raise the pH of the urine. IV mannitol (Osmitrol®) should be used to clear the renal tubules of pigment and potential obstruction to flow. The immediate principles of care also include early debridement and/or amputation of necrotic tissue with immediate closure, topical therapy for cutaneous burns, monitoring of the peripheral circulation for the presence of compartment syndrome (increased pressure and decreased perfusion within a confined space causing tissue ischemia), and continuous electrocardiogram (ECG) monitoring with cardiac enzymes and electrolytes for at least 24 hours (Herndon, 2001; Koumbourlis, 2002; Wolf & Herndon, 1999).

Chemical burns are classified into those caused by acids, alkali, and organic compounds (e.g., gasoline, phenols, tar). The agent used, its concentration, its volume, and the duration of contact determine the severity of the injury. Regardless of the chemical agent, treatment consists of removing all clothing, brushing off any solid chemicals, and flushing with copious amounts of water. Healthcare personnel should wear

---

TABLE 52-4 Secondary Survey

Head-to-Toe Physical Assessment
Head (depressions, lacerations, fractures)
Eye (PERL)
Mouth (foreign bodies, blood, vomitus)
Neck (tenderness, deviations)
Chest (expansion, breath and heart sounds, open wounds)
Abdomen (open wounds, pain, tenderness, distention, rigidity)
Pelvis (stability)
Back (deviations, fractures)
Extremities (fractures, open wounds, pulses)

Additional History
Circumstances of injury (closed versus open space, chemicals, related trauma)
Previous morbidity (illness, medication, allergies, tetanus immunization)
AMPLE (Allergies, Medications, Previous illness/history, Last meal, Events preceding injury)

Laboratory Studies
ABGs, carboxyhemoglobin
CBC, type and crossmatch
Electrolytes, BUN/creatinine, metabolic profile
Urinalysis
X-rays

Sources: American Burn Association, 2001; American College of Surgeons Committee on Trauma, 1999.

protective clothing so as not to be injured by contact with the offending agent. It should be assumed that the depth of the wound will be deeper than initial presentation, and standard fluid resuscitation guidelines should be initiated.

Certain chemical burns need more specific care and closer monitoring. Ocular burns are best treated with topical eye anesthetics and copious irrigation through a Morgan lens. An ophthalmology consult should be obtained to assess and manage further injury. Contact with gasoline, fuel, and phenol can not only lead to a deeper burn but also result in the absorption of hydrocarbons, which can cause pulmonary dysfunction, central nervous system (CNS) disturbance, and renal and hepatic failure. The fluoride ion in hydrofluoric acid burns penetrates and destroys tissue and is extremely painful. Aside from irrigation, the neutralization of fluoride and pain relief is best achieved through topical calcium gels, subcutaneous calcium gluconate injection, or IV infusions of magnesium. These measures assist in increasing the local blood supply and the body's endogenous calcium and magnesium stores. The debridement of tar burns can be painful. The use of petroleum-based products can often assist in softening the tar for easier removal (American Burn Association, 2001; Herndon, 2001; Roth & Hughes, 2004; Wolf & Herndon, 1999).

Acute Phase

The acute phase extends from the time of diuresis (fluid mobilization) to wound healing and/or closure. Wound care, surgical wound management, and infection control through metabolic and nutritional support are the primary concerns of care during this period.

Wound Care

The goal of wound care is to cleanse and debride the wound daily of dead tissue (eschar) to prepare it for healing or grafting, prevent infection, and minimize scarring and contractures. Topical antimicrobials, especially silver, are the primary nonsurgical method used to control burn wound microbial growth (see **Table 52-5**). The value of the silver ion lies in its relative nontoxicity, anti-inflammatory ability to block microbial cellular growth, and capacity to stimulate re-epithelialization. Recent clinical evidence has demonstrated that a continuous silver release system such as Acticoat™ provides even more rapid antimicrobial activity and accelerated re-epithelialization of the wound bed (Demling, DeSanti, & Orgill, 2005; Yurt, 1999).

Another evidence-based method of nonsurgical treatment of burn wounds has been the use of negative-pressure wound therapy, known as vacuum-assisted closure (VAC). Through the use of a piece of foam sized to the wound shape, controlled negative pressure (suction) is applied, which removes excessive wound fluids (debridement), thereby allowing endogenous

TABLE 52-5 Commonly Used Topical Antimicrobials

Topical	Characteristics
Silver sulfadiazine (Silvadene®)	• Bacteriocidal for gram-negative and -positive organisms, yeast • Allergies to silver/sulfur • Can cause leukopenia, rash
0.5% silver nitrate ($AgNO_3$)	• Effective for gram-positive organisms and *Pseudomonas* • Allergy to silver • Electrolyte leeching (especially potassium and sodium) • Increased evaporative water and heat loss • Used to avoid Silvadene's side effects (leukopenia and/or rash) • Skin discoloration
Sulfamylon (Mafenide®)	• Bacteriostatic for gram-negative and -positive organisms, especially *Pseudomonas* • Diffuses through devascularized tissue • Absorbed systemically; allergy to sulfur • Carbonic anhydrase inhibitor (metabolic acidosis with a compensatory respiratory alkalosis) • Painful
Diluted Dakin's solution	• Bacteriostatic • Used to avoid Silvadene's side effects (leukopenia and/or rash) • Can reduce septic/hypermetabolic wound response • Painful
Petroleum-based ointments (e.g., bacitracin,® Bactroban,® gentamicin)	• Clear on application; painless; allows for easy wound observation • Commonly used for treatment of facial burns, graft sites, healing donor sites, and small partial-thickness burns • Bactroban effective against methicillin-resistant *Staphylococcus aureus* (MRSA)

Sources: Costello & Dungca, 1988; Warden, 1998; Yurt, 1999.

re-epithelialization to take place until the wound is closed or can be covered with skin graft. The vacuum pressure can also stabilize a grafted wound bed by preventing the pooling of tissue fluids that might otherwise destabilize the graft (Barret & Herndon, 2004; Bishop, 2004; Johnson & Richard, 2003; Warden, 1998; Yurt, 1999).

With full-thickness burns or burns that do not heal spontaneously, surgical intervention is necessary. Excision and closure of the burn wound not only reduces the extent of the injury but also minimizes the potential for infection and complications. If sufficient donor sites are available, autograft (tissue taken from one area and grafted to another area on the same person) is the preferable means of wound closure. The skin taken from unburned areas of the body (donor sites) can be either split thickness (consisting of the epidermis and a portion of dermis) or full thickness (consisting of the epidermis and the full depth of the dermis). Grafts, in turn, can be either meshed, so as to cover a greater area, or sheet-like (unmeshed), applied to the more visible parts of the body such as face, neck, and hands to keep scarring at a minimum and achieve better cosmetic reconstruction or functionality. Donor sites, which themselves are partial-thickness wounds, must be properly cared for to prevent infection and encourage re-epithelialization because the site could be used again (recropped) for future grafting (Herndon, 2001; Warden, 1998; Yurt, 1999).

In large burns where donor sites are limited, wound closure may need to be accomplished with organic or biosynthetic biological dressings and/or skin substitutes until permanent closure can be accomplished or donor sites become available. Biological dressings are temporary coverings meant to keep the wound from drying, reduce the loss of body heat and fluids, weaken bacterial proliferation, reduce pain and discomfort, and ultimately prepare the wound for a permanent graft.

Unlike biologic dressings, skin substitutes become incorporated as either a temporary or permanent part of the wound closure. The advent of skin substitutes has allowed for more rapid and greater wound covering, improved functional and cosmetic outcomes, and greatly increased survival from major burn injuries (see **Table 52-6**). Skin substitutes are bilayer structures possessing the epidermal and dermal material necessary for skin regeneration. The outer epidermal layer acts as a protective barrier, allowing healing to

take place in the dermal layer beneath. The dermal layer possesses factors that activate and stimulate re-epithelialization and wound healing. These dermal elements may be either temporary or permanent. Temporary dermal elements provide the framework for healing but are eventually removed and replaced with a permanent autograft. Permanent dermal layers act as a template on which the body can create and organize its own permanent dermal regeneration, with the epidermis eventually being replaced by a very thin autograft (Demling et al., 2005; Herndon, 2001; Yurt, 1999).

Metabolic and Nutritional Support

The initial emergent response to a burn injury is a low-flow state (ebb phase) marked by low cardiac output, decreased metabolism, vasconstriction, and capillary leakage. It is not uncommon, however, to witness a hyperdynamic and hypermetabolic response (flow phase) following the resuscitation of large burns. This hyperdynamic response, which can last from days to weeks, is characterized by vasodilation, increased cardiac output/index, and increased energy expenditure as a result of a SIRS response to the burn injury. Normally, the body's inflammatory response to injury remains localized and maintains a homeostatic balance between inflammation, coagulation, and fibrinolysis. This SIRS response can become grossly distorted and amplified when the synergistic release of inflammatory mediators (cytokines) causes excessive inflammation and coagulopathy, impaired fibrinolysis, decreased tissue oxygen extraction and utilization, and susceptibility to infection (sepsis) and MODS (Jacobs & Hoyt, 2000).

The hypermetabolic response produces a catabolic state marked by accelerated protein catabolism (gluconeogenesis); increases in caloric expenditure, oxygen consumption, and carbon dioxide production (hypercatabolism); and activation

TABLE 52-6 Biological Dressings and Skin Substitutes

Skin Substitute	Types
Temporary organic biological dressings	• Allograft or homograft (skin from an individual of the same species) • Xenograft (pig skin)
Temporary biosynthetic skin substitutes	• Biobrane • Transcyte
Permanent biosynthetic skin substitutes	• Integra • Alloderm (donated human dermal tissue) • Cultured epidermal autograft (autologous skin graft cultured and grown from the patient's own cells)

Sources: Demling, DeSanti, & Orgill, 2005; Yurt, 1999.

of a neural and endocrine response (stress response) mediated by increases in catecholamines, cortisol, and glucagon. Energy requirements may increase as much as 50% to support both this immune, inflammatory, and hormonal response and the ongoing wound and tissue repair (Bessey, 2002; Herndon, 2001; Yurt, 1999).

Management of this hyperdynamic/hypermetabolic response is multisystemic in nature and aimed at preventing the progression of injury and secondary sequelae through adequate resuscitation of the microcirculation, ventilatory support as needed, optimization of oxygen delivery and consumption, early removal of necrotic tissue followed by wound closure, antimicrobial therapy guided by culture-specific surveillance, and metabolic and nutritional support (Barret & Herndon, 2004; Yurt, 1999).

Such a maladaptive inflammatory and hormonal environment can be greatly attenuated through early and appropriate nutritional support. Research findings now advocate feeding the gut within 72 hours of traumatic injury to allay the effects of the hyperdynamic and hypermetabolic states that ensue following a traumatic injury. Oral and/or enteral nutrition is the preferred delivery route of nutrients because it promotes immunocompetence of the GI tract, improves GI blood flow, maintains the mucosal integrity of the endothelium, and makes colonic bacterial translocation less likely. Parenteral nutrition should be reserved as a supplemental nutritional route if the complete nutritional needs of the body cannot be met orally or enterally.

The preferred feeding route is post pyloric (duodenum, jejunum). Nutritional absorption begins in the small intestine, so feedings given by this route can be safer and better tolerated. Although gastric (stomach) feeding can be used, it may not be as beneficial since gastric atony and paralytic ileus are often post-traumatic sequelae.

Nutritional goals are to have carbohydrates provide 55% to 60% and fat and proteins 20% to 25% of total calories along with micronutrients (vitamins and trace minerals). The assessment of energy needs is based on the basal metabolic rate (BMR), total daily requirements (growth and activity), and a stress component, which factors in the hypermetabolism that accompanies severe trauma or injury. The calculation of nutritional needs can be accomplished through the use of several empiric formulas, with the most familiar one being the Harris–Benedict equation (Bessey, 2002; Herndon, 2001).

Rehabilitative and Reentry Phase

The rehabilitative phase extends from the time of injury to the time of societal reentry. A major burn injury is one of the most disastrous events that can happen to the patient, family, friends, and significant others. Restoration of physical, emotional, psy-

chological, and social function through multidisciplinary supportive services must be aggressively and progressively provided and maintained from admission to discharge and beyond.

Physical/Occupational Function and Therapy

The intent of physical and occupational therapy is early and complete restoration of function. To prevent complications of prolonged bedrest, especially during the critical period of injury, positioning and passive range of motion exercises are immediately implemented. As healing and recovery take place, activities of daily living and ambulation become part of the daily rehabilitation program to encourage normal movement and provide a feeling of accomplishment. When burned skin heals, it has a tendency to tighten. Left untreated, this effect could cause deformities (contractures). Involved joints are positioned to maintain function with specially measured molded splints. Daily exercise programs are individually designed to maintain strength, coordination, and active exercise. To prevent scarring, which frequently happens after a deep burn heals, custom-designed pressure garments are employed to control scar tissue formation (hypertrophy) (Carrougher, 1998; Herndon, 2001; Roth & Hughes, 2004).

Emotional/Psychological/Social Function and Therapy

While rendering emotional and psychological support begins on admission, it becomes most necessary during the rehabilitation and reentry phase. In the emergent or shock phase, a major concern is the fear of death. As survival and recovery become more likely, this fear is replaced by feelings of grief, depression, and anxiety; worries of deformity and disfigurement; anger at the circumstances that caused this event; and perhaps feelings of guilt that the patient or significant others may have contributed to this injury. Compounding this cascade of emotions is the immense pain and suffering incurred from the daily care and surgical procedures, disruption of lifestyle, loss of control and independence, apprehension of a prolonged hospitalization and convalescence, and dread of lifelong debt and expense.

The focus of therapy is to provide appropriate counseling, pharmacotherapy (e.g., pain management, anxiety) and support services not only to the patient, but also to family members and significant others. The primary interventions are to assist patients to work through feelings of anger or guilt, accept the present circumstances despite losses, invest in their own physical and vocational rehabilitation, and reflect on the changes that recovery presents in terms of their self-identity and changes in lifestyle. The physical and emotional trauma of the injury must be balanced against the functional, vocational, and cosmetic needs of the patient through an individualized, staged, and multidisciplinary plan of rehabilitation, retraining, and reconstruction. The ultimate goal is to achieve the physical and psychosocial reentry and reintegration of the patient into society, a process that may extend for several years after discharge (Herndon, 2001; Ptacek, Patterson, & Heimbach, 2002; Sheffield et al., 1988).

PATIENT OUTCOMES

Nurses can help ensure attainment of optimal patient outcomes such as those listed in **Box 52-1** through the use of evidence-based interventions for patients with a burn injury.

SUMMARY

It has been this chapter's intent to increase the nurse's understanding of the multisystem management and multidisciplinary competence and concern involved in the care of a burn patient from time of injury through recovery, rehabilitation, and societal reentry. Since burns are often viewed as adhering to the trauma model, primary and secondary surveys were emphasized as the initial systematic means of managing the burn shock of the emergent phase. An overview of the clinical advances of wound care, surgical wound management, and meta-

bolic and nutritional support was underscored as the hallmark of the acute phase of care. The chapter concluded with a discussion of how best to meet the complex physical, psychological, and social needs of the burn patient in the stage of recovery. Over the past 25 years, advances in resuscitation, wound management, and critical care have not only increased survival from a burn injury but also emphasized and provided a true quality of life after injury.

Box 52-1
Optimal Patient Outcomes

- 24-hour intake and output balanced
- Uses effective coping strategies
- Physical comfort within expected range
- Serum electrolytes in expected range
- Airway remains patent
- SpO_2 in expected range
- Breathing pattern within normal limits
- Adjusts to alterations in body image

CASE STUDY

A 30-year-old male who is the father of two young children and who worked in a steel plant experienced a hot sheet of steel fall on his entire anterior body. The steel sheet fell on top of him, causing him to fall onto his back. He sustained third-degree burns to 50% of his body. Injuries included loss of ear cartilage, eyelids, and nose cartilage.

Upon admission to the ED, he was intubated and placed on mechanical ventilation. Intravenous fluids were started with lactated Ringer's with infusion rates guided by the American Burn Association recommendations. An arterial line and central venous catheter were inserted for hemodynamic monitoring. The patient was 6 feet tall and weighed 185 pounds.

Upon admission to the burn ICU, he was placed in a whirlpool bath, and his wounds were cleaned and subsequently dressed. After one week, the ICU nurse noted that the patient had a "black fuzzy growth" on his dressing and on the bed linen. He was diagnosed with aspergillosis and was started on amphotericin B. As a complication, he developed acute renal failure, requiring hemodialysis.

CRITICAL THINKING QUESTIONS

1. Calculate the fluid requirement for this patient for the first 24 hours.
2. Which disciplines should be consulted to work with this client?
3. What types of issues may require you to act as an advocate or moral agent for this patient?
4. How will you implement your role as a facilitator of learning for this patient and his family?
5. Use this case example to rate the patient as a level 1, 3, or 5 on each characteristic. Identify the level of nurse characteristics needed in the care of this patient.
6. Take one patient outcome for the patient and list evidence-based interventions for this patient.

Using the Synergy Model to Develop a Plan of Care

	Patient Characteristics	Level (1, 3, 5)	Subjective and Objective Data	Evidence-based Interventions	Outcomes
SYNERGY MODEL	Resiliency				
	Vulnerability				
	Stability				
	Complexity				
	Resource availability				
	Participation in care				
	Participation in decision making				
	Predictability				

Online Resources

National Institutes of Health (interactive tutorial): www.nlm.nih.gov/medlineplus/tutorials/burns/htm/index.htm

Merck Manual of Medical Information (includes photos and treatment of burns): www.merck.com/mmhe/sec24/ch289/ch289a.html

American Burn Association: www.ameriburn.org

National Institutes of Health: www.clinicaltrials.gov

National Institute of General Medical Sciences: www.nigms.nih.gov/news/facts/traumaburnfactsfigures.html

REFERENCES

Alson, R. (2005). Burns, thermal. Retrieved on May 29, 2005, from http://www.emedicine.com/emerg/topic72.htm

American Burn Association. (2004). Burn incidence and treatment in the U.S. Retrieved May 29, 2005, from www.ameriburn.org/pub/BurnIncidence FactSheet.htm

American Burn Association. (2001). *Advanced burn life support provider manual.* Chicago: American Burn Association.

American College of Surgeons Committee on Trauma. (1999). *Resources for the optimal care of the injured patient.* Chicago: American College of Surgeons Committee on Trauma.

Barret, J., & Herndon, D. (2004). *Principles and practice of burn surgery.* Monticello, NY: Marcel Dekker.

Bessey, P. (2002). Metabolic response to critical illness and nutritional support. In D. Wilmore (Ed.), *ACS surgery: Principles and practice* (pp. 1495–1549) New York: WebMD Professional Publishing.

Bird, D. (1999). Inhalation injuries. *Emergency Nurse, 7*(7), 19–23.

Bishop J. F. (2004). Burn wound assessment and surgical management. *Critical Care Nursing Clinics of North America, 16*(1), 145–177.

Carrougher, G. J. (1998). *Burn care and therapy: Quick reference for burn care and therapy.* St. Louis, MO: Mosby.

Carvajal, H. F., & Parks, D. H. (1998). *Burns in children: Pediatric burn management.* Chicago: Year Book Medical.

Costello, F., & Dungca, C. (1988). Burns. In B. Johanson (Ed.), *Standards for critical care* (3rd ed., pp. 561–570). St. Louis, MO: Mosby.

Danks, R. R. (2003). Burn management: A comprehensive review of the epidemiology and treatment of burn victims. *Journal of Emergency Medical Services, 28*(5), 118–139, quiz 140–141.

Demling, R. (2001). Burn care in the early post resuscitation period and burn care after first post burn week. In D. W. Wilmore (Ed.), *ACS surgery: Principles and practice* (pp. 479–505). New York: WebMD Professional Publishing.

Demling, R., & DeSanti, L. (2005). Carbon monoxide toxicity. Retrieved May 28, 2005, from http://www.burnsurgery.org/

Demling, R., DeSanti, L., & Orgill, D. (2005). The use of skin substitutes and beneficial effects of silver. Retrieved May 13, 2005, from www.burnsurgery.org/

Fitzpatrick, J. C., & Cioffi, W. G. (1997). Ventilatory support following burns and smoke-inhalation injury. *Respiratory Care Clinics of North America, 3*(1), 21–49.

Herndon, D. N. (2001). *Total burn care* (2nd ed.). Philadelphia: Saunders.

Hilton, G. (2001). Emergency thermal burns. *American Journal of Nursing, 101*(11), 32–34.

Holm, C., Melcer, B., Horbrand, F., von Donnersmarck, G. H., & Muhlbauer, W. (2000). The relationship between oxygen delivery and oxygen consumption during fluid resuscitation of burn-related shock. *Journal of Burn Care Rehabilitation, 21*(2), 147–154.

Jacobs, B., & Hoyt, K. (Eds.). (2000). *Trauma nursing core course* (5th ed.). Bedford Park, IL: Emergency Nurses Association.

Johnson, R. M., & Richard, R. (2003). Partial-thickness burns: Identification and management. *Advances in Skin and Wound Care, 16*(4), 178–187; quiz 188–189.

Koumbourlis, A. C. (2002). Electrical injuries. *Critical Care Medicine, 30*(11 Suppl.), S424–S430.

Ptacek, J. T., Patterson, D. R., & Heimbach, D. M. (2002). Inpatient depression in persons with burns. *Journal of Burn Care Rehabilitation, 23,* 1–9.

Roth, J., & Hughes, W. (2004). *Essential burn unit handbook.* St. Louis, MO: Quality Medical Publishing.

Sheffield, C. G., Irons, G. B., Muehal, P., Malie, J. F., Ilstrup, D. M., & Stonnington, H. H. (1988). Physical and psychological outcome after burn. *Journal of Burn Care & Rehabilitation, 9,* 172–177.

Tasaki, O., Goodwin, C. W., Saitoh, D., Mozingo, D. W., Ishihara, S., Brinkley, W. W., et al. (1997). Effects of burns on inhalation injury. *Journal of Trauma, 43*(4), 603–607.

Wald, D. A. (1998). Burn management: Systematic patient evaluation, fluid resuscitation and wound management. *Emergency Medicine Reports, 19,* 45–52.

Walker, M., & Neubauer, R. (1998). Using HBOT to treat burns. In R. A. Neubauer & M. Walker (Eds.), *Hyperbaric oxygen therapy* (pp. 75–80). New York: Penguin Group (USA).

Warden, G. D. (1998). Burns and wound care and wound healing. In S. I. Schwartz (Ed.), *Principles of surgery* (7th ed., pp. 223–296). New York: McGraw-Hill.

Wiebelhaus, P., & Hansen, S. (1999). Burns. Handle with care. *RN, 62*(11), 52–58.

Wolf, S., & Herndon, D. (1999). *Burn care.* Georgetown, TX: Landes Bioscience.

Yurt, R. (1999). Burns. In J. Norton, P. Barie, R. Bollinger, A. Chang, S. Lowry, S. Mulvihill, et al. (Eds.), *Surgery: Basic science and clinical evidence* (pp. 327–341). New York: Springer Verlag.

CHAPTER 53

Managing the Transition from the Hospital

Evelyn Koenig

LEARNING OBJECTIVES

Upon completion of this chapter, the reader will be able to:

1. Describe the importance of planning transitional care.

2. Explain the significance of a collaborative approach to transitional planning.

3. Analyze the domains for assessment in transitional planning.

4. Discuss the nursing role in assessment and planning for the next level of care.

5. Utilize clinical judgment in designing nursing priorities in the transition of care.

6. List optimal patient outcomes that may be achieved through evidence-based management of the patient transitioning from the hospital.

Changes in healthcare financing from fee-for-service to largely fixed payment systems have driven changes in the organization of health care. The financial survival of any healthcare organization is supported by ensuring that patients receive the right care in the right setting, and by using appropriate resources within an optimal length of stay. Recognizing the importance of carefully planning for patients as they move through the healthcare system is essential to ensuring optimal patient outcomes. Given accrediting and regulatory bodies' mandates for an assessment and planning process, nurses must demonstrate competence in transfer and discharge of clients to prevent inconsistent delivery of care. For example, the Joint Commission requires that hospitals have a process that addresses the need for continuing care, treatment, and services after discharge or transfer; that any transfer or discharge must be based on a patient's assessed need; that planning for transfer or discharge includes the patient and all staff involved in the patient's care; and that appropriate information related to care, treatment, and services be exchanged with those accepting care at the time of transfer or discharge (Joint Commission, 2005).

The Centers for Medicare and Medicaid Services (CMS) requires hospitals participating in the Medicare program to establish a discharge planning process for all patients. That process must include a discharge planning evaluation, early identification of the need for post-discharge services, preparation of patient and family for post-discharge care, and appropriate communication of care needs to any facilities or agencies providing posthospital care (CMS, 2004).

The emphasis of both The Joint Commission and CMS is not just excellence during an episode of care but the need for continuity of care between settings. To reflect this change in focus, the term *discharge planning*, which reflects an ending of care, is being supplanted by *transitional planning*, which reflects the beginning of a new phase of care (Cesta & Tahan, 2003). Transitional planning identifies and organizes the services necessary to address deficits in a patient's health and functional status. Comprehensive transitional planning requires thorough and ongoing assessment of the healthcare needs of the patient and family during a course of illness; identification of the settings and services necessary to meet predicted care needs; timely confirmation of patient eligibility for and the availability of desired services; and ultimate coordination of services at the time of transition from acute care.

TRANSITIONAL PLANNING AS COLLABORATIVE PRACTICE

Because of the complexity of payment and care systems, the multiplicity of community facilities and agencies providing varying levels of care (see **Box 53-1**), and the complexity of patient needs, transitional planning has become a specialty within hospital systems. Professionals variously labeled social workers, case managers, or discharge planners assume the responsibility for ensuring that assessment and planning lead to continuity between settings and to an uninterrupted course of care. However, by its nature, transitional planning is a collaborative process in which each healthcare team member works as a subunit of the whole, thereby allowing the team to achieve results that individual providers could not accomplish in isolation. Patient and family are primary contributors in the process, and information is required from every member of the healthcare team.

The more complex a patient's need, the more disciplines will be required to complete an adequate assessment and transitional plan. Information from disciplines such as physical, respiratory, occupational, and speech therapies; social work; pharmacy; and clinical nutrition may be critical to the development of this plan.

The nurse is integral to the transitional planning process. The American Nurses Association (ANA), in its *Code of Ethics for Nurses*, states that nursing care is directed toward meeting the comprehensive needs of patients and their families across the continuum of care and that the nurse must promote multidisciplinary planning that ensures the availability and accessibility of quality health services (ANA, 2001). Nurses, by virtue of their role, have the most consistent contact with the patient and, therefore, have the most consistent opportunity to collect information, make observations, identify care needs, and understand patient/family concerns. This unique opportunity makes the nurse's contribution to transitional planning invaluable.

ASPECTS OF TRANSITIONAL PLANNING AND THE NURSING ROLE

Comprehensive transitional planning requires in-depth assessment in four functional domains: physical, psychological, social, and economic.

Physical

Physical function is the ability to perform self-care, self-maintenance, and physical activities. It is divided between activities of daily living (ADLs) and instrumental activities of daily living (IADLs). ADLs include bathing, dressing, toileting, transferring, continence, and feeding. These activities can represent a natural progression in both the loss of function and the return of ability on recovery or rehabilitation. IADLs include meal preparation, shopping, transportation, laundry, housekeeping, and medication administration.

Significance

Physical function is one of the most significant determinants of posthospital needs and the level of care, services, and settings available to the patient. Given this fact, it becomes imperative that hospital care prevents unnecessary loss of function and promotes independence wherever possible. Assessment of physical function gives a picture of the patient's assets and/or deficits and creates a baseline that allows monitoring for changes so that decline can be prevented, function enhanced, and transitional planning needs identified.

Nursing Role

"Nurses in the acute care setting are in a pivotal position to assess function and target interventions to prevent loss of function and maintain an individual's self-care ability" (Kresevic & Mezey, 1997, p. 220). By obtaining information from the patient and family, the nurse should assess the patient's prehospital ability to perform ADLs and should, through observation and patient/family feedback, regularly reassess the ability to perform ADLs during the course of care. The nursing care plan should include interventions necessary to maintain independence and promote self-care. Attention to appropriate skin care, nutrition, and adequate rest and mobility can prevent complications that might hinder function. As the patient's condi-

---

Box 53-1
Post-Acute Care Alternatives

- Home health: Intermittent skilled services to a homebound patient
- Assisted living: Provision of supervision or assistance with ADLs and IADLs
- Nursing home: Provision of 24-hour care, custodial or skilled, including personal care and health services
- Subacute care: Intensive nursing, rehabilitation, and restorative care for patients of higher acuity
- Rehabilitation: Active rehabilitation services at minimum of three hours daily
- Long-term acute care: Intensive specialty hospital services to complex patients over an extended period of time
- Hospice: Care when prognosis for survival is six months or less and no life-prolonging care is desired

tion allows, referral to physical and occupational therapy to assist in preventing deconditioning or in regaining self-care capabilities may be appropriate. Given that a sudden decline in function could signal underlying complications, any observed decline in functional abilities should be immediately communicated to the healthcare team.

Psychological

Psychological function includes thinking and perception, cognition (alertness, orientation, memory, insight, judgment), and affect (emotional expression). One recent study has shown that individual attitudes, prior experiences, the intensive care unit (ICU) experience, and the support of family and friends all influence physical and psychological recovery following discharge to the community from an ICU (Maddox, Dunn, & Pretty, 2001).

Significance

A person's thinking, emotion, and behavior have significant impact on the ability to provide for the individual's essential needs, either directly or by allowing others to meet those needs. Depression, delirium, and anxiety are of particular concern in hospitalized patients. Delirium is a disturbance in consciousness that develops over a short period, tends to fluctuate over the course of a day, and is manifested by reduced clarity of awareness; impaired ability to focus, sustain, or shift attention; recent memory disturbance; perceptual disturbance such as misinterpretations, illusions, or hallucinations; and disorientation to time and place. Depression is characterized by a persistently depressed mood, tearfulness, hopelessness, and a diminished interest in activities. Anxiety is the apprehensive anticipation of future danger or misfortune and is accompanied by dysphoria and increased arousal with difficulty falling or staying asleep, irritability, difficulty concentrating, and hypervigilance (American Psychiatric Association, 1994).

Problems such as delirium, depression, and anxiety may be indicative of underlying factors that should be promptly corrected (e.g., infection or medication reaction). Left untreated, they may interfere with the patient's ability to cooperate with and thereby benefit from care and treatment, learn about an illness and provide appropriate self-care, and exercise appropriate judgment and make appropriate decisions. Problems with thinking, affect, and behavior often result in extended hospitalizations, physical functional decline, and the need for increased care and services as a part of any transitional plan.

Nursing Role

The nurse should continuously assess and reassess the patient's cognitive and emotional status. Observation of the patients, their reactions and interactions, and more formal testing of orientation and memory will allow appropriate and timely intervention. If delirium is present, the nurse should immediately notify the physician so that any underlying causes can be identified and treated. The nurse should act to ensure patient safety, because there is a potential for harm from poor judgment or agitation. With the depressed or anxious patient, listening to concerns, educating the patient and family about the occurrence of depression and anxiety in acute illness, and reassuring the patient and family that interventions are forthcoming is helpful. If further assessment or intervention is required, initiating referrals to social work, psychiatry, or chaplaincy would be appropriate.

Social

Assessment of *social function* helps determine the amount of physical and social support available to patients and their level of satisfaction with that support. Elements of social function include the living situation (alone, spouse, children, communal), social contacts (frequency of contact with family, friends, and others), social activities, social resources and environment (accessibility of services, safety, transportation), social support (who helps with emergency and daily needs), caregivers/caregiver burden (stress on health, finances, and emotional resources from provision of care), and quality of life (level of satisfaction with life).

Significance

The level of social function in relationship to physical care needs assists in determining patients' ability to return to their preadmission living circumstances, the need for additional resources, or the need for an alternative level of care. Caregiver stress has particular impact on the success of a transitional plan, and caregivers require a clear idea of what responsibilities care provision will entail.

Nursing Role

The initial nursing assessment should always include an understanding of patients' prehospital living situation. During the course of treatment, the nurse should be cognizant of the patients' physical function in relation to their living situation and communicate concerns to the transitional planning team. The nurse is instrumental in helping the patient and family make appropriate decisions about transitional plans. Many families want to take even very complex patients home but have no clear understanding of what 24-hour care entails. The nurse should provide education about the disease, disease process, and caregiving activities. If caregivers seem particularly unrealistic in their determination to provide care, the nurse should have them provide daily care, under supervision, to gain an understanding of its complexity, demand, and burden, thus better informing their decisions.

Economic

The *economic domain* includes income and insurance. Income could be in the form of a monthly Social Security check, pension, or dividends from investments. Many individuals will have long-term care insurance that may provide extensive resources for alternative care modalities outside of the hospital.

Significance

The assessment of a patient's economic situation defines the number and kinds of resources available for transitional planning. Collaboration with social work, families, and significant others can provide important information in defining the economic resources available to the patient.

Nursing Role

The nurse does not assume responsibility for assessment of the patient's financial and insurance situation. However, when resources are limited, the nurse may be able to assist the team with suggestions that will make a transitional plan more economically feasible. For example, suggestions about changing from intravenous to oral drug therapy or changing to a less expensive but equally efficacious medication, adapting a patient's bed rather than renting a hospital bed, or consolidating follow-up appointments to limit the expense of transportation would reduce the cost of care.

SCREENING

The ICU nurse should identify patients who are at risk for encountering problems on or after discharge. To facilitate this step, the use of a risk-screening instrument can improve postdischarge problems. The Blaylock Risk Assessment Screening Score (BRASS; see **Figure 53-1**) has been shown to be effective in those patients who are at risk for a prolonged hospital stay and in need of discharge planning resources. The nurse scores

---

FIGURE 53-1 Blaylock Discharge Planning Risk Assessment Screen

Circle all that apply and total. Refer to the Risk Factor Index.

Age

0 = 55 years or less
1 = 56 to 64 years
2 = 65 to 79 years
3 = 80 + years

Living Situation/Social Support

0 = Lives only with spouse
1 = Lives with family
2 = Lives alone with family support
3 = Lives alone with friends' support
4 = Lives alone with no support
5 = Nursing home/residential care

Functional Status

0 = Independent in activities of daily living and instrumental activities of daily living

Dependent in:
1 = Eating/feeding
1 = Bathing/grooming
1 = Toileting
1 = Transferring
1 = Incontinent of bowel function
1 = Incontinent of bladder function
1 = Meal preparation
1 = Responsible for own medications
1 = Handling own finances
1 = Grocery shopping
1 = Transportation

FIGURE 53-1 Blaylock Discharge Planning Risk Assessment Screen (continued)

Cognition

0 = Oriented
1 = Disoriented to some spheres* some of the time
2 = Disoriented to some spheres all of the time
3 = Disoriented to all spheres some of the time
4 = Disoriented to all spheres all of the time
5 = Comatose

Behavior Pattern

0 = Appropriate
1 = Wandering
1 = Agitated
1 = Confused
1 = Other

Mobility

0 = Ambulatory
1 = Ambulatory with mechanical assistance
2 = Ambulatory with human assistance
3 – Nonambulatory

Sensory Deficits

0 = None
1 = Visual or hearing deficits
2 = Visual and hearing deficits

Number of Previous Admissions/Emergency Room Visits

0 = None in the last 3 months
1 = One in the last 3 months
2 – Two in the last 3 months
3 = More than two in the last 3 months

Number of Active Medical Problems

0 = Three medical problems
1 = Three to five medical problems
2 = More than five medical problems

Number of Drugs

0 = Fewer than three drugs
1 = Three to five drugs
2 = More than five drugs

Total Score: _____

Risk Factor Index: Score ≤ 10 = at risk for home care resources; score of 11–20 = at risk for extended discharge planning; score greater than 20 = at risk for placement other than home. If the patient's score is 10 or greater, refer the patient to the discharge planning coordinator or discharge planning team.

*Spheres = person, place, time, and self.

Source: Copyright 1991 Ann Blaylock. Reprinted with permission from Blaylock, A., & Cason, C. L. (1992). Discharge planning predicting patients' needs. *Journal of Gerontological Nursing, 18*(7), 5–10.

the patient on 10 items: age, living situation/emotional support, functional status, cognition, behavior pattern, mobility, sensory deficits, previous admissions/emergency room visits, active medical problems, and drugs. The total score can range from 0 to 40. The index categorizes patients into three groups: A score of 10 or less suggests a low risk for having post-discharge problems; a score ranging from 11 to 20 suggests that the patient's problems are more complicated and require extensive discharge planning; and a score of greater than 20 suggests that the patient is at risk for a discharge destination other than home. All patients with a score greater than 10 should be referred to the discharge planning team (Mistiaen, Duijnhouwer, Prins-Hoekstra, Ros, & Blaylock, 1999).

PATIENT OUTCOMES

Nurses can help ensure attainment of optimal patient outcomes such as those listed in **Box 53-2** through the use of evidence-based interventions for patients transitioning from the hospital.

SUMMARY

Comprehensive transitional planning is a critical component of acute care. It is based on comprehensive assessment and support of a patient's physical, psychological, social, and economic function. The nurse supports transitional planning through assessment, intervention to prevent loss of function, patient/family education, and timely communication with the healthcare team. One study reported that the ICU nurse faced at least three obstacles in hospital discharge planning: patient acuity, time constraints, and limited experience with the discharge process (Chaboyer, Foster, Kendall, & James, 2002). While ICU nurses are aptly placed to manage discharge planning, they cannot be expected to undertake this important role without a systematic approach to its implementation through the use of tools such as care maps, pathways, and clinical decision trees.

Box 53-2
Optimal Patient Outcomes

- Patient and family participate in planning and providing care
- Performs prescribed health behaviors
- No demonstration of transfer anxiety
- Social support present at transfer
- Satisfied with health status
- Economic and other resources available to the patient

CASE STUDY

L.M. is a 57-year-old man who was recently in a motor vehicle crash, which resulted in long-term ventilation and tracheostomy. During his time in the ICU, he had an acute exacerbation of chronic obstructive pulmonary disease. He has a history of being a three-pack-per-day tobacco smoker. This is his second admission to the hospital this year. Six months prior, L.M. had pneumonia that required a two-night stay on the telemetry unit. The patient is on day 32 in the ICU; he is hemodynamically stable but cannot be weaned. He is off antibiotic therapy for a previously diagnosed pneumonia. A decision is made to transfer him to a portable ventilator so as to prepare him for home.

L.M. has a wife who is from Korea and does not speak English, and her frail elderly mother lives with the couple in a two-story home. There is a master bedroom on the main floor. L.M. is able to feed himself, but requires a one-person assist to stand and pivot to the chair and assistance with activities of daily living.

L.M. is alert and oriented ×3 and is optimistic about returning home. He states, "I want to get off the ventilator in the next month." "I think that if I get some rest I will be able to come off the ventilator." He is currently receiving nebulizer treatments twice a day, which will continue in the home. His medication list includes bronchodilators, antihypertensive agents, antidepressants, and daily ASA.

CRITICAL THINKING QUESTIONS

1. Utilizing the BRASS, score the patient in this case study and determine his needs prior to discharge.
2. Which disciplines should be consulted to collaborate with this client? Identify their roles.
3. What types of issues may require you to act as an advocate or moral agent for this patient?
4. How will you implement your role as a facilitator of learning for this patient?
5. Use the form to write up data and a plan of care for a patient with discharge planning needs. Rate the patient as a level 1, 3, or 5 on each characteristic.

Using the Synergy Model to Develop a Plan of Care

	Patient Characteristics	Subjective and Objective Data	Evidence-based Interventions	Outcomes
SYNERGY MODEL	Resiliency			
	Vulnerability			
	Stability			
	Complexity			
	Resource availability			
	Participation in care			
	Participation in decision making			
	Predictability			

Online Resources

Case Management Resource Guide: www.cmrg.com

Guide for Interfacility Patient Transfer: www.nhtsa.dot.gov/people/injury/ems/interfacility/images/interfacility.pdf

REFERENCES

American Nurses Association. (2001). *Code of ethics for nurses with interpretative statements.* Washington, DC: American Nurses Publishing.

American Psychiatric Association. (1994). *Diagnostic and statistical manual of mental disorders* (4th ed.). Washington, DC: American Psychiatric Association.

Centers for Medicare and Medicaid Services. (2004). Conditions of participation: Discharge planning. In *Conditions of Participation* (Chapter IV, 482.43). Washington, DC: Department of Health and Human Services.

Cesta, T., & Tahan, H. (2003). Transitional planning and case management. In *The case manager's survival guide* (pp. 113–133). St. Louis, MO: Mosby.

Chaboyer, W., Foster, M., Kendall, E., & James, H. (2002). ICU nurses' perceptions of discharge planning: A preliminary study. *Intensive Critical Care Nursing, 18*(2), 90–95.

Joint Commission on Accreditation of Healthcare Organizations. (2005). Provision of care, treatment and services. In *Comprehensive accreditation manual for hospitals: The official handbook* (PC-46). Oakbrook, IL: Joint Commission Resources.

Kresevic, D., & Mezey, M. (1997). Nurses are in a position in all care settings to assess elders' functional status. *Geriatric Nursing, 18,* 216–222.

Maddox, M., Dunn, S. V., & Pretty, L. E. (2001). Psychosocial recovery following ICU: Experiences and influences upon discharge to the community. *Intensive Critical Care Nursing,17*(1), 6–15.

Mistiaen, P., Duijnhouwer, E., Prins-Hoekstra, A., Ros, W., & Blaylock, A. (1999). Predictive validity of the BRASS index in screening patients with post-discharge problems. Blaylock Risk Assessment Screening Score. *Journal of Advanced Nursing, 30*(5), 1050–1056.

Collaboration

PART VI

Recovery of the Postanesthesia Patient

Teresa Dozier

LEARNING OBJECTIVES

Upon completion of this chapter, the reader will be able to:

1. Compare the various anesthetic agents.

2. Compare the two major categories of neuromuscular blocking agents.

3. Discuss the nursing management of the postanesthesia patient.

4. Describe common postanesthesia complications.

5. List optimal patient outcomes that may be achieved through evidence-based management of postanesthesia patients.

The specialties of surgery and anesthesia have greatly evolved over the years. Not until the 1940s, however, did the benefits of a specialized unit to care for these patients become apparent. During this time, the Anesthesia Study Commission of the Philadelphia Medical Study published the results of a study that looked at mortality rates after general anesthesia. The study determined that 47% of the deaths could have been prevented. To decrease the mortality rates, the Commission recommended the development "and maintenance of post anesthesia rooms . . . staffed by specially trained nurses" (Litwack & Ledbetter, 1995, p. 4).

The initial area to which patients were sent to recover from anesthesia was envisioned a combination of postanesthesia recovery and surgical intensive care units (SICUs). In actuality, intensive care units (ICUs) evolved from recovery areas as the trend changed to separate postanesthesia care units (PACUs) from the SICU (Barone, Pablo, & Barone, 2003).

Based on the decisions of the surgeon and/or anesthesiologist, surgical patients may bypass the PACU and be transferred directly to the ICU. For this reason, ICU nurses must possess the basic knowledge and skills required to care for a patient recovering from anesthesia.

OVERVIEW OF ANESTHETIC AGENTS AND ADJUNCTS

Inhalation Agents

Inhalation anesthetics produce a rapid loss of consciousness and are eliminated primarily through the lungs. They contain no analgesic properties, except for nitrous oxide. The amount of an inhalation agent that moves from the alveoli to the arterial blood depends on the patient's cardiac output. The blood transports the anesthetic agent to the tissues (Drain, 2003). Therefore, the more blood-rich the tissue is (e.g., brain, heart, kidneys), the more saturated it becomes with the anesthetic agent. Once the gas is discontinued, the reverse is also true.

Some of the inhalation agents are also fat soluble, so they are absorbed in the adipose tissue. Since adipose tissue is not very vascular, it has a prolonged recovery from the inhalation agent. Hence, overweight patients will take longer to recover following administration of these drugs.

The most commonly used inhalation anesthetics are enflurane (Ethrane®), halothane (Fluothane®), isoflurane (Forane®), sevoflurane (Ultane®), desflurane (Suprane®), and nitrous oxide.

Enflurane is very popular among anesthesia providers because it is rapid acting. It causes muscle relaxation and enhances the effect of nondepolarizing skeletal muscle relaxants (Drain, 2003). Effects of enflurane include cerebral vasodilation; decreased arterial blood pressure, stroke volume, and systemic vascular resistance; increased heart rate; and sensitization of the heart to the effects of catecholamines. Enflurane may cause mild hepatic dysfunction (Drain). The patient usually regains consciousness quickly and experiences little to no postoperative nausea and vomiting (PONV).

Halothane has bronchodilator properties, so it is useful in patients with preexisting pulmonary diseases. This agent also decreases the mucociliary function of the airway for as long as six hours postoperatively, which places patients at an increased risk for atelectasis and pneumonia (Litwack & Ledbetter, 1995). Like enflurane, halothane is associated with a low incidence of PONV. It does sensitize the heart to the effects of catecholamines. Halothane also causes myocardial depression and peripheral vasodilation (Drain, 2003).

Isoflurane is another very popular inhalation agent. Unlike other members of this drug class, it does not sensitize the heart to catecholamines. Other advantages of isoflurane are that it stabilizes the cardiovascular system, has no hepatotoxicity, causes the least increase in cerebral blood flow, and increases heart rate without compromising cardiac output (Drain, 2003).

Sevoflurane is a very rapid-acting agent. It does not sensitize the heart to the effects of catecholamines and is nonirritating to the respiratory tract. Sevoflurane may cause hypotension by decreasing the systemic vascular resistance. No evidence of hepatotoxicity has been observed with sevoflurane. This agent decreases cerebrovascular resistance and can increase intracranial pressure depending on the dosage (Drain, 2003).

Like sevoflurance, desflurane is extremely rapid acting and does not sensitize the heart to catecholamines. This drug decreases both blood pressure and cardiac output. The bitterness of desflurane makes it a respiratory tract irritant—it causes coughing, breath holding, and laryngospasm (Drain, 2003).

Nitrous oxide is considered the "patriarch of the family." A high incidence of PONV is associated with its use. Nitrous oxide is the only inhalation agent to have some analgesic properties. It can be used alone or in combination with other inhalation agents. This drug has minimal cardiovascular effects and does not sensitize the heart to catecholamines. Nitrous oxide will expand closed gas-filled spaces, so its use should be avoided in intestinal, thoracic, or middle ear surgeries (Drain, 2003).

Nursing implications to be considered for a patient recovering from inhalation anesthesia include oxygen administration, because these agents are eliminated primarily through the lungs; deep breathing and coughing, to facilitate gas exchange; monitoring of respirations and pulse oximetry, because all inhalation agents are respiratory depressants; monitoring vital signs, because of cardiovascular effects; treatment of PONV; and prompt pain management, because none of the inhalation anesthetics except nitrous oxide have analgesic properties.

Muscle Relaxants

Neuromuscular blocking agents (NMBAs) are used as adjuncts to general anesthesia. These drugs are used to facilitate endotracheal intubation and to optimize surgical working conditions. They work by providing relaxation of skeletal muscles (Litwack & Ledbetter, 1995). NMBAs are also used on patients requiring mechanical ventilation to decrease the work of breathing, eliminate "fighting the ventilator," and treat laryngospasms. Two types of NMBAs are distinguished: depolarizing and nondepolarizing. The nondepolarizing agents are further classified as long acting, intermediate acting, and short acting.

NMBAs produce their effect at the neuromuscular junction by interacting with acetylcholine either by depolarizing the motor end plate (depolarizing NMBAs) or by competing with acetylcholine for binding sites on the motor end plates (nondepolarizing NMBAs). This interaction prevents motor transmission, which then prevents patient movement (Levins, 2002). **Table 54-1** compares common NMBAs on physiologic variables.

After administration of the NMBAs, paralysis begins at the smaller muscle groups and progresses to the larger muscle groups until complete paralysis is obtained. The recovery process then occurs in the reverse order, from large to small muscle groups. It is also imperative that nurses remember that NMBAs do not provide amnesia, analgesia, or loss of consciousness, so appropriate medications need to be provided to the patient for those purposes (e.g., benzodiazepines, propofol, and/or opioids).

The effects of nondepolarizing NMBAs are reversed by administration of anticholinesterase drugs, such as neostigmine (Prostigmin®). These drugs restore neuromuscular function by binding to the enzyme acetylcholinesterase (AChe) and inactivating it. Acetylcholine shifts the nondepolarizing muscle relaxant, allowing for restoration of normal neuromuscular transmission (Litwack & Ledbetter, 1995).

The anticholinesterase drugs also stimulate muscarinic receptors located in the central nervous system, heart, and sali-

TABLE 54-1 Common Neuromuscular Blocking Agents

	Atracurium Besylate (Tracrium®)	Pancuronium (Pavulon®)	Vecuronium (Norcuron®)	Mivacurium Chloride (Mivacron®)	d-Tubocurarine	Succinylcholine (Anectine®)
Nondepolarizing	Yes	Yes	Yes	Yes	Yes	No
Depolarizing	No	No	No	No	No	Yes
Reversible	Yes	Yes	Yes	Yes	Yes	No
Cumulative effects	No	Yes	Slight	Slight	Yes	No
Fasciculations and muscle soreness	No	No	No	No	No	Yes
Risk of histamine release	Minimal	Slight to none	No	Yes	Significant	Possible
Cardiovascular effects	Few	Slight ↑ in pulse and ↑ BP	None	Minimal	Hypotension	Slight ↓ in pulse

Sources: Arbour, 2000; Drain, 2003; McManus, 2001.

vary glands. Effects commonly experienced include bradycardia, hypotension, bronchoconstriction, and excessive salivation. Therefore, in addition to the reversal agent, the patient is also given an anticholinergic drug (e.g., atropine or glycopyrrolate [Robinul®]) to prevent these undesired symptoms.

Depolarizing NMBAs [e.g., succinylcholine (Anectine®)] are metabolized by the enzyme pseudocholinesterase, so their effects cannot be reversed pharmacologically. The disadvantages of using succinylcholine include bradycardia, hyperkalemia, increased intraocular pressure, increased intracranial pressure, muscle fasciculation, and it is a known trigger for malignant hyperthermia (MH), which will be discussed later in this chapter. However, due to its rapid onset and short duration of muscle relaxation, succinylcholine is an excellent NMBA when used appropriately.

Intravenous Anesthetics

Intravenous anesthetics may be used to induce or maintain anesthesia, promote sedation, and administer monitored anesthesia care (MAC) (Litwack & Ledbetter, 1995). These anesthetics can be classified as barbiturates [e.g., thiopental sodium (Pentothal®), brevital sodium (Methohexital®)], nonbarbiturates [etomidate (Amidate®), propofol (Diprivan®)], tranquilizers-benzodiazepines [midazolam (Versed®), lorazepam (Ativan®)], and dissociative agents [ketamine (Ketalar®)]. Since these anesthetics are injected directly into the bloodstream, their onset of action is very rapid. As with inhalation agents, the more blood-rich tissue groups are exposed to the medication more quickly. This group of drugs is metabolized primarily by the liver.

In general, barbiturates are used to induce rapid, pleasant sleep prior to the administration of other slower, less pleasant anesthetic agents. These central nervous system depressants cause rapid loss of consciousness after administration. They also suppress cardiac function, with a resulting decrease in cardiac output, blood pressure, and peripheral vascular resistance. Barbiturates are respiratory depressants and, at higher dosages, can cause a loss of laryngeal reflexes, making the patient prone to aspiration (Litwack & Ledbetter, 1995).

The nonbarbiturates include etomidate and propofol. Etomidate is an excellent intravenous (IV) anesthetic choice for patients with preexisting cardiovascular disease because it causes less hypotension than barbiturates and has minimal effect on the cardiac output. Adverse effects after administration include PONV, hiccoughs, involuntary tremors, and suppressed adrenal function (Litwack & Ledbetter, 1995).

Propofol, a sedative-hypnotic, is very rapid acting. Patients generally awaken more responsive after its use than with the other agents. This is one primary reason why propofol is also a very popular choice for sedating ventilated patients. This drug is associated with little to no PONV. Propofol is a respiratory depressant and causes hypotension when given too rapidly. This agent contains lecithin so its use should be avoided in patients with known allergies to eggs. Because of its milky white appearance, propofol is fondly referred to as "milk of anesthesia" (Leffler, 2004).

The benzodiazepines, midazolam and lorazepam, are generally used as a premedication before the patient is brought to surgery. These drugs are useful for providing sedation during MAC procedures such as synchronized cardioversion and during regional anesthetic techniques. These drugs produce amnesia, respiratory depression, and a reduction in anxiety. In cases of profound respiratory depression, the effects of benzodiazepines can be reversed with the antagonist flumazenil (Romazicon®).

Ketamine causes a loss of consciousness described as dissociative anesthesia. The patient appears cataleptic (i.e., has loss of voluntary muscle control and a rigid body and limbs) and experiences amnesia and profound analgesia that persists into the postoperative period (Litwack & Ledbetter, 1995). Ketamine is a derivative of the street drug PCP, so vivid hallucinations are possible postoperatively. Patients who receive this drug should be placed in an area that is dark and very quiet and should receive minimal stimulation. Ketamine is also a cardiac stimulant, so an increase in blood pressure may occur shortly after its administration.

Local Anesthetics

Local anesthetics inhibit excitation of nerve endings or block conduction in peripheral nerves (Revis & Seagel, 2005). These drugs can be used topically, by infiltration, and for regional anesthesia. Local anesthetics are categorized as amides, which are metabolized in the liver, or as esters, which are broken down by plasma pseudocholinesterase. Epinephrine, a vasoconstrictor, may be added to some local anesthetic agents to prolong the agent's activity (Drain, 2003). The esters include cocaine, procaine (Novocain®), chloroprocaine (Nesacaine®), and tetracaine (Pontocaine®). The amides include lidocaine (Xylocaine®), mepivacaine (Carbocaine®), bupivacaine (Marcaine®), ropivacaine hydrochloride (Naropin®), and dibucaine (Nupercaine®).

The complications that a nurse should be aware of after a patient has received a local anesthetic include contact dermatitis, anaphylaxis, and systemic toxicity. Systemic toxicity is caused by an accidental injection of the local agent intravenously or by administration of an excessive amount of the drug. Signs and symptoms can range from mild to severe and may include lightheadedness, dizziness, tinnitus, muscular irritability, seizures, disorientation, unconsciousness, increased PR interval, increased QRS duration, decreased cardiac output, decreased blood pressure, bradycardia, AV blocks, asystole, or respiratory arrest. If these signs and symptoms occur, support of the ABCs (airway, breathing, circulation) is very important, and the anesthesiologist should be notified immediately.

Regional Anesthesia

Regional anesthesia techniques use local anesthetic agents to block nerve conduction in an extremity or a region of the body (Drain, 2003). Advantages of regional anesthesia include the avoidance of general anesthesia, better postoperative pain management, faster recovery time, decreased incidence of PONV, and decreased cardiac and respiratory risk. The primary disadvantage of regional anesthesia is the increased anxiety in patients because they remain awake during the procedure.

Local infiltration is designed to achieve a sensory blockade and to block a nerve stimulus at its origin without blocking a specific nerve. Lidocaine is usually the drug of choice for this purpose. Common uses of local infiltration include IV starts, placement of invasive lines, and numbing at the location of a spinal, epidural, or peripheral nerve block (Litwack & Ledbetter, 1995).

Peripheral nerve blockade is accomplished by injecting a local anesthetic into or around a specific nerve or group of nerves (Litwack & Ledbetter, 1995). The most common of these procedures is the axillary or brachial plexus block. The axillary block is appropriate for surgical procedures involving the upper extremity below the elbow. The brachial plexus (interscalene) block is used for procedures performed on the upper arm and the shoulder. Immediate postoperative nursing care of these patients should include proper positioning of the affected extremity to prevent undue pressure. Patients should be instructed that, until the block recedes, they will not have full motor function and should not attempt to move their arm so as to prevent injury. A known complication with the interscalene approach is a pneumothorax. The nurse should monitor respiratory effort and pulse oximetry, and should report any complaint of chest pain or difficulty breathing by the patient.

If the supraclavicular approach is chosen for the brachial plexus block, Horner's syndrome may result. This problem occurs when the anesthetic agent spreads and involves the stellate ganglion (Drain, 2003). Signs and symptoms of Horner's syndrome include facial flushing, pupil constriction, drooping eyelid, and stuffy nose. These symptoms occur on the same side that the block was done and disappear as the block recedes. Other complications with the supraclavicular approach include phrenic nerve block, in which patients complain of chest heaviness, or recurrent laryngeal nerve block, which produces hoarseness and feeling like the patient has a lump in the throat. These patients should not be allowed to eat or drink (NPO) until the block recedes to prevent aspiration.

Epidural anesthesia involves injection of a local anesthetic into the epidural space through either a thoracic or a lumbar approach. Local anesthetics act by binding to the nerve roots entering and exiting the spinal cord. With use of a low concentration of local anesthetic, sensory pathways are blocked and motor fibers remain intact (Litwack & Ledbetter, 1995).

The local anesthetic can be combined with a narcotic (e.g., fentanyl or morphine) to provide ongoing postoperative pain relief. This technique is commonly used for nonemergent cesarean section. Contraindications for epidural anesthesia include hypovolemia; infection, either systemically or at the injection site; and use of anticoagulants.

During the administration of the epidural anesthetic, a catheter can be threaded over the epidural needle into the space for later use to manage postoperative pain. Side effects seen with epidural anesthesia include respiratory depression (with epidural narcotics), pruritus, nausea and vomiting, urinary retention, and hypotension. Complications include accidental subarachnoid puncture and inadvertent intravascular injection of the anesthetic. Immediate postoperative nursing care of the patient who had epidural anesthesia entails assessment for and management of any side effects. Adverse effects of epidural anesthesia are rare, however. Those reported are in the form of case studies and include spinal epidural hematoma (Litz, Gottschlich, & Stehr, 2004), foot drop (Uzunlar, Duman, Eroglu, Topcu, & Erciyes, 2004), angina and electrocardiogram (ECG) changes (Easley, Rosen, & Lindeman, 2003), spinal subdural hematoma (Constantoyannis, Shahidi, & Kourtopoulos, 2003), cardiac and respiratory arrest (Lee & Kim, 2000), pressure sores (Shah, 2000), and postural hypotension (Roffey, Thangathura, Mogos, Black, & Mikhail, 2001).

Spinal anesthesia involves the injection of a local anesthetic into the lumbar intrathecal space. This technique requires a smaller amount of local anesthetic than epidural anesthesia because the local anesthetic comes in direct contact with the spinal cord and nerve roots (Litwack & Ledbetter, 1995).

Three types of blockade occur after the injection of the agent. The smallest nerves— the autonomic nerves—are the most sensitive to the anesthetic, resulting in a sympathetic block first. Patients may become hypotensive as a reaction to the sympathetic block and venous pooling, especially if they are hypovolemic.

Sensory nerves are medium in size and, therefore, the second to block. Assessment of this block is done by analyzing der-matome levels in the operating room (OR) as well as during the patient's recovery. **Figure 54-1** depicts the dermatomes.

Motor nerves are the largest nerves and are the third block to occur. Motor blockade is assessed by having the patient attempt general movement of the lower extremities as well as more controlled movement, such as a straight leg raise.

Advantages of spinal anesthesia include good postoperative pain management and use as an alternative for patients unable to tolerate general anesthesia. Contraindications include hypovolemia, uncooperative patients, infection at the injection site or systemically, increased intracranial pressure, patients who are on anticoagulants or who have a history of a bleeding disorder, previous back surgery, or spinal disorders such as multiple sclerosis or paralysis (Litwack & Ledbetter, 1995).

Complications related to spinal anesthesia include hypotension, bradycardia, nausea and vomiting, spinal headache,

FIGURE 54-1 Dermatomes

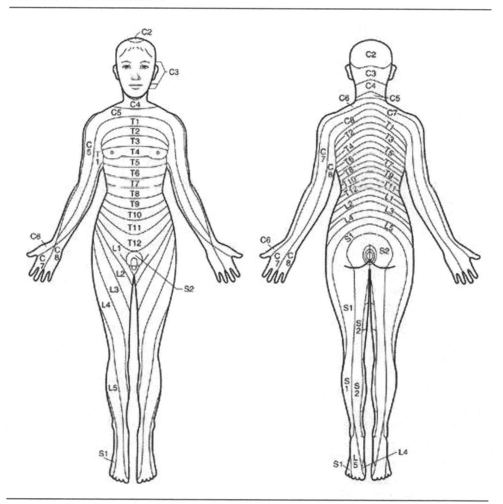

Source: Reproduced with permission from The Wister Institute: Keegan, J. J. & Garrett, F. D. (1948). Sensory dermatomes. *Anatomical Record,* 102, 409–437.

urinary retention, palsies and paralysis, and a high spinal block. Hypotension is treated with IV fluid bolus and/or vasopressors. Bradycardia may be treated with IV fluids or atropine. Nausea and vomiting usually occurs secondary to the hypotension and should be treated with IV fluids and notifying anesthesia. A spinal headache may result from a cerebrospinal fluid (CSF) leak through the puncture in the dura mater. Treatment includes bedrest, analgesics, hydration, and caffeine. In some cases, the headache may be severe enough to require an epidural blood patch. Any palsies or paralysis should be reported immediately. Urinary retention may cause hypertension, restlessness, or bladder distention. The nurse should assess the bladder and, if the patient is unable to void, an order should be obtained for catheterization. Symptoms of a high spinal block include apprehension, agitation, nausea and vomiting, hypotension, respiratory insufficiency, apnea, and unconsciousness (Litwack & Ledbetter, 1995). These symptoms will resolve when the block recedes. Nursing care consists of oxygenation, assisting ventilation, and blood pressure support. The nurse also needs to explain to patients what is occurring when they are conscious and provide reassurance as necessary.

Patients who are receiving systemic anticoagulation and have an epidural catheter in place or being removed are at risk for development of spinal hematoma (Keegan & Horlocker, 1999). The decision to perform spinal or epidural anesthesia and the timing of catheter insertion and removal in a patient who is receiving anticoagulation should be made on an individual basis (American Society of Regional Anesthesia and Pain Medicine, 2005). Recommendations from the American Society of Regional Anesthesia and Pain Medication appear in **Table 54-2.**

MODERATE SEDATION/MAC

Moderate sedation/MAC is useful for several procedures that may be conducted in the ICU, such as synchronized cardiover-

TABLE 54-2 Anticoagulation and Epidural Catheters

	Epidural Catheter Insertion	Catheter Removal
Unfractionated heparin	Heparin administration should be delayed for 1 hour after needle placement.	Catheters should be removed 2–4 hours after the last heparin dose and the patient's coagulation status should be evaluated with labs. Heparin reinitiation should occur 1 hour after catheter removal.
Low-molecular-weight heparin (LMWH)	Patients receiving LMWH preoperatively should have needle placement occur at least 10–12 hours after the LMWH dose. Patients on higher doses of LMWH require delays of at least 24 hours.	Epidural catheters should be removed prior to initiation of postoperative LMWH. For patients on twice-daily dosing, the first dose of LMWH can be administered after at least 2 hours of catheter removal. In patients receiving single-daily dosing of LMWH, the epidural catheter should be removed a minimum of 10–12 hours after the last dose of LMWH. Subsequent dosages should occur at a minimum of 2 hours after catheter removal.
Oral anticoagulation	Anticoagulant therapy must be stopped, ideally 4–5 days prior to a planned procedure. Caution should be used when inserting an epidural catheter in a patient who recently had chronic oral anticoagulant therapy discontinued.	The catheter can be removed when the INR < 1.5.
Antiplatelet medications	Timing of use of an epidural catheter is dependent on the medication used, ranging from 7 to 14 days (until platelet function has been restored).	Antiplatelet medications are contraindicated within 4 weeks of surgery. If administered in the postoperative period (following having an epidural catheter), the patient should be carefully monitored neurologically for 8 hours.

Source: American Society of Regional Anesthesia and Pain Medicine, 2005.

sion, endoscopic procedures, or other diagnostic or minimally invasive procedures. Moderate sedation is achieved by administering an amnestic, analgesic, and sedative intravenously. With this approach, patients have a depressed level of consciousness but are able to maintain a patent airway and respond to verbal and physical stimuli (Litwack, 1999; U.S. Dept. of Veterans Affairs, 2006). Nursing care should be aimed at monitoring the patient's respiratory status, since all of the drugs given are respiratory depressants. Pain assessment and management should be included.

INITIAL POSTOPERATIVE CARE

If the patient is admitted directly to the ICU from the OR, standards of postoperative monitoring must be upheld. Basic life-sustaining needs are of the highest priority and constant vigilance is required during the immediate postoperative period because the needs of the patient are neither minimal nor episodic (American Society of PeriAnesthesia Nurses, 2004a).

Assessment

When patients arrive from the OR, they are immediately attached to the appropriate monitors: pulse oximetry, automatic blood pressure, cardiac monitor, and any invasive hemodynamic monitoring equipment. Patient reports must include, but are not limited to, the patient's preoperative status and pertinent history; anesthesia technique and agents; length of surgery/anesthesia; medications administered, including reversal agents; type of procedure; estimated blood loss during the surgery; IV fluid and blood replacement given; urine output during the procedure; position of the patient on the operating table; types and locations of dressings, drains, and packing; and any complications, including treatment and response.

Once the patient is attached to the monitoring equipment, the next focus is on the ABCs. The patient's airway should be assessed for patency and for the presence of an artificial airway, such as a jaw-thrust maneuver, nasal or oral airway, or endotracheal tube. The respiratory status, method of oxygen delivery, breath sounds, oxygen saturation, and patient's color should also be noted. Circulation assessment includes cardiac rhythm, blood pressure, heart rate, palpable peripheral pulses, and any invasive monitoring results. The initial assessment should also include the patient's level of consciousness, temperature, and presence of any pain or PONV. Vital signs should be monitored and documented every 5 minutes for 20 minutes and then every 15 minutes and as needed until the patient is stable.

Once the nurse has ascertained that the patient's ABCs are stable, the rest of the assessment may be completed. This phase of assessment is patient surgery specific, based on the report received upon admission. It entails assessment of IV sites; loca-

tion and condition of any dressings or drainage devices; pertinent neurovascular checks; skin condition, as related to the patient's position in surgery; any swelling, redness, or drainage related to the surgical site; dermatome levels on spinals; and ventilator settings and details about the endotracheal tube (i.e., size, location). This list is not all-inclusive and will vary according to the specific patient. This assessment and appropriate documentation should be completed on admission and then every 15 minutes and as needed until the patient is stable, regardless of the setting in which the patient is recovering.

Extubation Criteria

If the patient arrives in the ICU intubated, the nurse must maintain this airway and provide appropriate oxygenation. Some patients are not ready for extubation in the OR, or this step may not be clinically indicated given the critical nature of the patient's condition. Once clinically indicated, in collaboration with the intensivist or anesthesiologist, the ICU nurse must monitor the patient for signs of meeting extubation criteria. Criteria for extubation include strong spontaneous ventilation, adequate respiratory rate, a patient who is awake and following directions, sustained head lift of greater than five seconds, strong hand grips, and a strong cough. If in doubt about the patient's readiness, notify the anesthesiologist and do not extubate.

The patient's mouth is suctioned prior to extubation, and the tape securing the tube is removed. The cuff on the endotracheal tube is deflated with a syringe. Presence of an air leak must be ascertained prior to extubation. Such an air leak can be either heard or felt. The patient is then asked to take a deep breath and cough. The tube is removed toward the end of the cough. Supplemental humidified oxygen is then applied (Litwack & Ledbetter, 1995).

Oxygen Therapy

Patients who have received general anesthesia must receive supplemental oxygen until they are awake enough to maintain their own oxygen saturation equal to or greater than 93%. Oxygen may be supplied through a nasal cannula or face mask. If the patient is unable to maintain oxygen saturation equal to 95% while using the nasal cannula, humidified oxygen is given by face mask. It is very important to prevent hypoxia in the immediately postoperative patient.

Stir-up Regime

All patients who received an inhalation anesthetic require the "stir-up regime" in the immediate postoperative period. All inhalation agents are respiratory depressants and are eliminated through pulmonary ventilation. Gases travel from areas of higher to lower concentration (Litwack & Ledbetter, 1995).

Patients need to be "stirred up" by elevating the head of the bed, unless contraindicated, and then having them deep breathe and cough at regular intervals. This technique facilitates the gas exchange by moving the inhalation agent from the area of higher concentration (the patient's lungs) to the area of lower concentration (room air). Further, oxygen is in higher concentration in the room (through the nasal cannula or face mask) and in lower concentrations in the patient's lungs.

Temperature Regulation

Temperature regulation is very important in all postoperative patients because every patient who undergoes surgery is at a risk for hypothermia. Hypothermia can cause many detrimental effects and is defined as a core temperature of less than 36°C (96.8°F) (American Society of PeriAnesthesia Nurses, 2004b). The patient's temperature should be measured on admission and at the end of the postanesthesia period. Temperature should also be monitored every 15 to 30 minutes during active rewarming. Methods used to rewarm the hypothermic patient include warm blankets, heat lamps, warmed IV fluids, hyperthermia blankets, covering the top of the patient's head, and/or increasing the ambient room temperature.

Discharge Criteria

A patient in the immediate postoperative period must meet the criteria for discharge from anesthesia's care. Discharge criteria may vary among hospitals but generally include those listed in **Table 54-3**.

TABLE 54-3 Anesthesia Discharge Criteria

1. Patent airway, adequate respiratory function, and oxygen saturation
2. Vital signs are stable
3. Temperature greater than or equal to 96.8 °F
4. Level of consciousness and muscular strength stable
5. Adequate pain control
6. Mobility stable or at preoperative status (Patients who received regional anesthesia will need special criteria based on the method utilized.)
7. Adequate patient comfort and anxiety levels
8. Patent tubes, catheters, drains, and IV lines
9. Skin color or condition stable or at preoperative status
10. Satisfactory condition of dressing and/or surgical site
11. Adequate intake and output
12. Postanesthesia Recovery Score (PARS or Aldrete) (see **Table 54-4**) adequate or a return to preoperative status

---

Source: American Society of PeriAnesthesia Nurses, 2004c.

TABLE 54-4 Postanesthesia Recovery Score (PARS)

Activity
Score = 2	Moves all extremities
Score = 1	Moves two extremities
Score = 0	Unable to move

Respiration
Score = 2	Able to deep breathe/cough independently
Score = 1	Respiratory effort limited/airway management required
Score = 0	Mechanical assistance

Circulation
Score = 2	BP ± 20 points of preanesthetic level
Score = 1	BP ± 20 to 50 points of preanesthetic level
Score = 0	BP ± 50 points of preanesthetic level

Consciousness
Score = 2	Oriented to time, place, and person
Score = 1	Responds to verbal stimuli
Score = 0	No response

Color
Score = 2	Normal color
Score = 1	Pale, dusky, flushed
Score = 0	Cyanotic

Some PARS may have a fifth criteria for pain level with 2 = no pain, 1 = minimal pain, and 0 = moderate to severe pain.
Source: Reproduced with permission from DeKalb Medical Center, Decatur, GA.

Miscellaneous

Documentation is a vital part of patient care. The written report should be accurate and complete and maintained throughout the patient's stay in ICU. Assessments, vital signs, medications, IV fluids, and intake and output should be documented according to hospital policy. Any complication, treatments, and response to treatments should also be documented in the patient's medical record.

While a patient is recovering in the ICU, it is vital for the nurse to communicate with the patient's family and significant others at regular intervals. The surgical experience is stressful enough, as is the process of waiting and wondering how their significant other is doing after surgery. One phone call to the family can ease their anxiety and make the surgical experience less unpleasant. Open and honest communication is the key to excellent customer service. Another way to interact with the family is by allowing them to visit the patient during recovery. A complete discussion of family-focused care appears in Chapter 2.

MANAGEMENT OF POSTOPERATIVE COMPLICATIONS

Hypoventilation/Hypoxemia

Hypoventilation is one of the most common complications seen in the immediate postoperative period due to the anesthetics and medications given to the patient; it may also be related to certain surgical procedures. Hypoventilation may be accompanied by shallow respirations. Institutional policy varies regarding the use of naloxone (Narcan®) for patients with shallow respirations or slow respiratory rates.

Hypoxemia, another potential complication, is defined as an oxygen saturation of less than 90%. Other signs of hypoxemia include cyanosis, agitation, somnolence, tachycardia, bradycardia, hypertension, and hypotension. Hypoxemia can have numerous undesirable effects, such as cardiac dysrhythmias, myocardial ischemia, and postoperative wound complications.

Prompt assessment of the patient with hypoventilation or hypoxemia is required by the ICU nurse. Oxygen should be applied and the "stir-up regime" should be initiated. If the respiratory rate remains insufficient, oxygen delivery via a bag-valve-mask may be necessary, especially if other symptoms are occurring.

If the hypoventilation or hypoxemia is not corrected with these simple interventions, the anesthesiologist should be summoned to the bedside immediately. Note whether the patient also has nasal flaring, use of accessory muscles, stridor, wheezing or crackles on auscultation, unequal chest movement, or frothy sputum. These assessment findings, along with a chest radiograph or arterial blood gases, will assist the anesthesiologist in diagnosing the patient. Depending on the cause of the hypoventilation or hypoxemia, the treatment will vary. Application of supplemental oxygen may be all that is required. If the hypoventilation is related to narcotics, naloxone (Narcan®) may be given in a dose sufficient to reverse the respiratory depression but not the analgesia effects. However, depending on the severity of the symptoms or the presence of prolonged hypoxemia, more aggressive interventions may be required, such as reintubation and mechanical ventilation. Prompt identification of the problem by the ICU nurse is essential. Pulse oximetry monitoring and assessment of the patient's respiratory status at regular intervals is the key to preventing this complication.

Laryngospasm

Laryngospasm (bronchospasm) can occur at any time in the ICU and can be a life-threatening situation. Patients can experience a partial or complete obstruction of the airway due to this spasm. Common causes include aspiration, endotracheal intubation (from the tube passing through the vocal cords), tracheal or pharyngeal suctioning, histamine release secondary to medications, or an allergic response (Litwack & Ledbetter, 1995). Signs of a laryngospasm include "rocking" respirations, wheezing, stridor, dyspnea, use of accessory muscles, or tachypnea. The ICU nurse should summon the anesthesiologist immediately while retrieving the bag-valve-mask. The patient should be encouraged to cough, because this measure may be enough to relieve a partial obstruction. The treatment for a complete or partial laryngospasm is positive-pressure ventilation with a bag-valve-mask. If a laryngospasm does not respond to positive pressure-ventilation within one minute, the patient is usually treated with the administration of succinylcholine and reintubation (Drain, 2003).

It is important to remember that the patient is awake throughout this experience and is very anxious. Reassurance and explanation of the treatments should be provided. After the laryngospasm is reversed, the patient requires ongoing monitoring and assessment. The anesthesiologist may order aerosolized bronchodilator treatments or a follow-up chest radiograph.

Noncardiogenic Pulmonary Edema

Noncardiogenic pulmonary edema may follow an episode of acute upper airway obstruction or the relief of chronic upper airway obstruction (Van Kooy & Gargiulo, 2000). Protein and fluid accumulate in the alveoli, but this buildup is not associated with elevated pulmonary artery occlusive pressure (Colucci, 2005). The symptoms of this type of edema, which can occur relatively quickly, include agitation, tachypnea, tachycardia, decreased pulse oximetry readings, and/or frothy, pink sputum. The patient will have crackles present when auscultating the lungs.

In such a case, the ICU nurse should maintain supplemental oxygen and notify the anesthesiologist. The nurse should also provide reassurance to the patient. A chest radiograph is usually obtained and may show findings of pulmonary edema. Treatment of noncardiogenic pulmonary edema includes supplemental oxygen, respiratory support, and diuretics.

Hypotension

Hypotension is a common postoperative complication in the perianesthesia setting and is associated with increased morbidity and mortality rates (Cowling & Haas, 2002). The primary cause of hypotension in the immediate postoperative setting is hypovolemia, usually due to the patient's NPO status, unreplaced fluid loss, or blood loss during surgery. The patient is treated with an IV fluid bolus of 500 mL of isotonic fluid (e.g., lactated Ringer's or 0.9% normal saline). If the blood pressure responds to the fluid bolus, then hypovolemia can be assumed. Subsequent IV fluid boluses may be required. Other potential causes of hypotension include position of the patient, positive end-expiratory pressure (PEEP), cardiac dysfunction, low systemic vascular resistance, anaphylaxis, sepsis, dysrhythmias, hypoventilation, and hypoxemia. Treatment is directed toward relieving the underlying cause. The ICU nurse should always provide supplemental oxygen and notify the anesthesiologist.

Depending on the surgical procedure and resulting blood loss, a hematocrit may be ordered and use of blood replacement products may be warranted. If the hypotension occurred after the head of the bed was elevated (especially in patients with spinal anesthesia), the head of the bed should be lowered, if not contraindicated. Also, the patient's legs may be raised with the head of the bed flat (modified Trendelenburg position). Other treatments of hypotension include vasoconstrictors [e.g., neosynephrine (Phenylephrine®), ephedrine (Pseudoephrine®)], inotropes [dopamine (Intropin®)], or afterload reduction [high-dose nitroglycerin or nitroprusside (Nipride®)]. Anaphylaxis is treated with antihistamines [diphenhydramine (Benadryl®)] and epinephrine (Adrenaline®). Ongoing assessment by the ICU nurse is warranted.

Hypertension

Hypertension is another common complication seen in the postoperative patient. Postoperative hypertension is defined as a significant elevation in arterial blood pressure during the immediate postoperative period (Haas & LeBlanc, 2004). It may be attributed to elevated levels of two catecholamines, epinephrine and norepinephrine, secondary to sympathetic stimulation from stress and pain. Peripheral vascular resistance (PVR) is also increased because of hypothermia and vasoconstriction. This increase in PVR and elevation of catecholamines may combine to produce hypertension (Nunnelee & Spaner, 2000).

The ICU nurse should look at the patient's preoperative and intraoperative blood pressure readings to determine whether a blood pressure reading is actually elevated for that particular patient. The anesthesiologist should be notified of persistent elevated blood pressure readings and supplemental oxygen should be provided. Medications used to treat hypertension include labetalol (Normadyne®), nicardipine (Cardene®), esmolol (Brevibloc®), clonidine (Catapres®), angiotensin converting enzyme (ACE) inhibitors, nitroglycerin, sodium nitroprusside, and analgesics. Sodium nitroprusside is less likely to be used in this scenario due to the need for invasive hemodynamic monitoring. Postoperative hypertension usually lasts for less than six hours. Prior to administration of antihypertensive agents, possibly reversible causes—such as pain, anxiety, hypothermia, and hypoxemia—should be considered (Haas & LeBlanc, 2004).

Cardiac Dysrhythmias

The postoperative patient is at risk for developing cardiac dysrhythmias—most commonly, bradycardias, tachycardias, and premature ventricular contractions. Other dysrhythmias that may be seen include ventricular tachycardia or ventricular fibrillation in hypokalemia and conduction blocks associated with hypoxemia or hypothermia (Drain, 2003). Treatment is aimed at relieving the underlying cause. If the dysrhythmia is life-threatening, treatment should be guided by the recommendations published by the American Heart Association.

Hypothermia

Hypothermia can cause many detrimental effects, especially if left untreated. Factors that predispose a patient to hypothermia relate to age, health status, surgical procedure, exposed body areas, body surface area, duration of anesthesia or surgery, ambient room temperature, prepping and irrigation solutions, administration of cool IV fluids, burns, peripheral vascular disease, and neuromuscular disease. Effects of hypothermia can include decreased level of consciousness due to decreased cerebrovascular blood flow; vasoconstriction with increased blood pressure, increased afterload, increased oxygen demand, increased thrombus formation, angina, or myocardial infarction; decreased platelet function; decreased activation of the clotting cascade; and decreased myocardial contractility leading to decreased cardiac output, decreased heart rate, or dysrhythmias. Shivering increases oxygen demand; increases blood viscosity, which leads to delayed drug metabolism and increased risk for metabolic acidosis; causes hyperventilation, hypoventilation, hypoxia, and lactic acidosis; increases bleeding times; and suppresses the immune system. Active rewarming is required in all patients with a temperature of less than 96.8 °F. Hypothermia can also cause decreased patient satisfaction (Abelha, Castro, Neves, Landeiro, & Santos, 2005).

Malignant Hyperthermia

MH is a genetic condition. In MH triggering agents (e.g., anesthetic agents) interfere with the reentry of calcium into the sarcoplasmic reticulum. With each neuronal stimulus, more calcium is released, forcing the cell into a state of hypermetabolism (Litwack & Ledbetter, 1995). Triggering agents include certain inhalation agents (e.g., halothane, enflurane, isoflurane, desflurane) and the muscle relaxant succinylcholine. Patients who are at higher risk for the development of MH include those with a family history of MH; a patient history of muscular disorders, such as Duchenne muscular dystrophy; a central nervous system disorder; and other myopias. The only definitive diagnostic test for MH is a muscle biopsy.

Many signs and symptoms are associated with MH. The most sensitive method to diagnose MH in the OR is the unanticipated doubling or tripling of end-tidal carbon dioxide levels (ETCO2)(Litwack & Ledbetter, 1995). Other signs include muscle rigidity, especially of the jaw (masseter rigidity); unexplained tachycardia; tachypnea; cyanosis; respiratory and metabolic acidosis; myoglobinuria; hyperkalemia, elevated creatine kinase (CK) and high fever. Contrary to what its name would suggest, a high fever in MH is a late sign and spells trouble for the patient. Most cases of MH occur in the OR, but this complication can develop as long as 24 hours postoperatively (Litman & Rosenberg, 2005).

MH progresses rapidly. It is essential that all locations where MH-triggering agents are administered have a fully stocked MH cart, and that the entire staff be familiar with the cart contents (Redmond, 2003). Once MH is suspected, the potential triggering agent should be immediately discontinued. The ICU nurse should call the anesthesiologist and have someone obtain the MH cart. The patient should be hyperventilated with 100% oxygen both while waiting for the cart and after its arrival. All interventions should occur simultaneously, because this situation can be life-threatening.

The drug used to treat MH, dantrolene sodium (Dantrium®), is given as an initial dose of 2.5 mg/kg IV up to a maximum of 10 mg/kg. Dantrolene inhibits the release of calcium. It is packaged as a powder in 20 mg vials and needs to be reconstituted with 60 mL of preservative-free sterile water. Dantrolene is difficult to reconstitute due to the volume involved, and one person should be assigned this task. Once the initial dose is administered, dantrolene is continued at a dose of 1 mg/kg every 4 hours for at least 48 hours.

Other treatments for MH include administration of sodium bicarbonate, initiation of active cooling, monitoring of urine output, and treatment of associated symptoms such as hypertension or dysrhythmias. Lab tests that may be ordered include arterial blood gases, serum electrolytes, liver enzymes, renal function studies, blood counts, and a coagulation profile. Any suspected case of MH should be reported to the Malignant Hyperthermia Association of the United States (MHAUS).

Box 54-1 lists recommended contents of a malignant hyperthermia cart, which should be available in the PACU, the OR, and any other area where general anesthesia is administered (Redmond, 2005).

Pseudocholinesterase Deficiency

Pseudocholinesterase deficiency is another hereditary condition in which the body has a deficiency in this enzyme or a variation of the enzyme (Dell & Kehoe, 1996). Acquired deficiencies are also seen in patients with liver disease, severe anemia, malnutrition, and recent dialysis. Pseudocholinesterase is necessary for the metabolism of succinylcholine. A patient who presents with this condition will, therefore, have a delayed recovery from the effects of succinylcholine (prolonged paralysis). These patients will present as intubated and requiring mechanical ventilation until the effects of succinylcholine have worn off. No medication can be given to the patient to relieve this condition; time is the only factor involved at this point. The ICU nurse must remember that the patient is awake and probably very anxious and should provide reassurance and administer medications such as amnestics (midazolam) and analgesics [fentanyl (Sublimaze®) or morphine]. When the patient meets the criteria for extubation, the anesthesiologist should be notified. In this situation, it is best to have the anesthesiologist perform the extubation. The patient and family should be instructed to notify any future surgeons and anesthesiologists that the patient had a prolonged recovery from succinylcholine.

Problems Related to OR Positioning

Every surgery requires the patient to be placed in a particular position, usually after induction of anesthesia, which can put each patient at risk for injury (Litwack & Ledbetter, 1995). The circulating nurse should take care to pad all bony prominences, and extremities should be positioned so as to prevent nerve compression. Any time a person remains in the same position for an extended period of time, pressure is exerted on the tissue, especially over bony prominences. The skin should be examined in the ICU for redness, blanching, induration or edema, or skin breakdown in areas related to the patient's position in the OR. Also, when the patient is moved off of the OR table, shearing of the skin may occur, especially in the elderly patient. If any rolls or pillows were used during surgery, the skin in contact with them should also be assessed for signs of pressure damage.

It is possible for the patient to sustain nerve injuries secondary to direct stretching of a nerve through improper positioning or compression against bone or equipment (Litwack & Ledbetter, 1995). The patient should be assessed for neurovascular status of affected extremities, and any abnormalities should be reported to the anesthesiologist. If any skin breakdown or nerve damage is assessed, the circulating nurse should also be notified to ensure proper follow-up.

Box 54-1

Recommended Malignant Hyperthermia Cart Contents

Medications

- Dantrolene sodium (36 vials) and sterile water for injection (without a bacteriostatic agent) to reconstitute dantrolene sodium—1,000 mL
- Sodium bicarbonate 8.4%—50 mL
- Mannitol 20%—500 mL
- Furosemide 160 mg
- $D_{50}W$—100 mL
- Regular insulin 100 units/mL
- Standard antidysrhythmic drugs (excluding calcium channel blockers)

General Equipment

- Syringes to dilute dantrolene sodium
- IV transfer sets to reconstitute dantrolene sodium
- IV insertion equipment (multiple sizes for intravenous access and arterial line)
- Nasogastric tubes with a nasogastric tube irrigation tray with piston syringe
- Disposable cold packs

Monitoring Equipment

- Esophageal temperature probes
- Central venous pressure kits

IV Supplies

- D_5W 250 mL, IV tubing

Nursing Supplies

- Large sterile Steri-Drape (for rapid drape of wound)/personal protective equipment
- Three-way irrigating Foley catheters (sizes appropriate for patient population)
- Urine meter
- Rectal tubes—sizes 14F, 16F, 32F, 34F

Laboratory Testing Supplies

- Arterial blood gas kits
- Blood specimen tubes for creatine kinase, myoglobin, SMA-19 (lactate dehydrogenase, electrolytes, thyroid studies) PT/PTT, fibrinogen, fibrin split products; complete blood count, platelets; lactic acid level
- Urine specimen tubes × 2 (myoglobin level)
- Urine dipstick (hemoglobin)

Source: Redmond, 2005.

Pain Management

Pain assessment is sometimes referred to as the "5th vital sign." Pain assessment and management should begin upon the patient's admission. This section focuses on pain management through patient-controlled analgesia (PCA) and epidural analgesia. The majority of the patients receive IV narcotics for pain, an issue that is discussed further in Chapter 4.

PCA allows the patient some control over pain management and allows for earlier ambulation and compliance with care regime. The PCA tubing is connected to the existing IV at the nearest port to the insertion site. The ordered parameters are entered into the machine and are verified by a second registered nurse. Proper documentation should be initiated and should reflect the starting amount of the medication in the syringe; ordered parameters including the basal rate (the continuous infusion rate that is administered to the patient without the patient pushing the button), if appropriate; time at which the infusion was initiated; the lockout interval (the minimum amount of time between the delivery of two doses of medication); the patient's status, including level of consciousness, respiratory rate, and pain level; and the signatures of the two registered nurses. The nurse should also document the patient's response to the treatment, patient education on the use of the PCA pump, and any changes in status or infusion rate.

Depending on the surgery, a patient may have orders for a continuous epidural infusion postoperatively for pain management. After verifying the orders and obtaining the medication, the appropriate equipment is obtained (epidural pump, epidural tubing, labels, and documentation forms). The nurse should assess the epidural catheter site for dislodgement of the catheter, kinks in the catheter, breakage of the catheter, and appearance of the insertion site prior to the initiation of the epidural pump. The catheter is usually secured in place with a large transparent occlusive dressing and taped securely to the patient's back. A microfilter should be present to prevent air from entering during the infusion. The medication bag (usually fentanyl and bupivacaine) is attached to the special epidural tubing. This tubing is thicker in diameter and contains no injection ports. Some epidural tubing is also a different color than regular IV tubing, allowing for its ready identification. Once the tubing is primed, the epidural pump is programmed with the ordered parameters. A bolus dose of the medication is usually ordered at the initiation of the infusion. The epidural tubing and pump should be labeled to designate that they are both for epidural use only. The patient's response to the treatment should be documented.

A common complication associated with continuous epidural analgesia is hypotension. In this case, the patient's epidural infusion should be placed on hold and the anesthesiologist should be notified. Also, if the head of the bed is elevated, it should be lowered, if not contraindicated, and an IV fluid bolus may be appropriate. The anesthesiologist may order a reduction in the infusion rate. Documentation required with a continuous epidural infusion includes the medication, rate of infusion, any boluses administered, time the infusion was initiated, patient's response, complications, patient's level of consciousness, respiratory rate, and pain level. Continuous epidural analgesia is an excellent method for treatment of post-operative pain and patients will have better compliance with their care regime, as with the PCA pump (D'Arcy, 2004).

Postoperative Nausea and Vomiting

Postoperative nausea and vomiting is a common occurrence in the immediate postoperative period due to the medications administered and certain surgical procedures. If a patient has been identified preoperatively to be prone to motion sickness or has a history of PONV, preventive treatment should have been initiated prior to surgery [e.g., scopolamine (Hyoscine hydrobromide®), premedication with an antiemetic]. Certain types of surgery may also predispose the patient to PONV, such as gynecological procedures, abdominal surgeries, and middle ear operation. Other risk factors for the development of PONV include the patient's gender (females are more prone to PONV), age, health status, and failure to maintain an NPO status before surgery. The ideal situation is these patients should receive antiemetics intraoperatively; however, that is not always the case. PONV can occur at any time in the postoperative period. The nurse should ascertain whether the PONV is related to risk factors, the surgical procedure, hypotension, or a reaction to medication. If hypotension is the cause of the nausea and vomiting, IV fluid boluses are the treatment of choice. If the PONV is related to anything else, antiemetic therapy is warranted. Medications used to treat PONV include ondansetron (Zofran®), promethazine (Phenergan®), and prochlorperazine (Compazine®). Any PONV not relieved with two doses of antiemetics should be reported to the physician. Patients who are actively vomiting should be positioned to prevent aspiration of gastric contents, and splinting of the surgical site may be needed.

PATIENT OUTCOMES

Nurses can help ensure attainment of optimal patient outcomes such as those listed in **Box 54-2** through the use of evidence-based interventions for postanesthesia patients.

Box 54-2
Optimal Patient Outcomes

- Vital signs in expected range
- Oxygen saturation in expected range
- Physical comfort in expected range
- Expressed satisfaction with pain control
- Absence of adverse effects of anesthesia
- Breathing pattern within normal limits

SUMMARY

Postanesthesia nursing has evolved over time into a specialty care unit. The ICU nurse who is caring for the postoperative patient should possess a basic knowledge of anesthetics and surgical procedures and receive intensive training in the care of immediately postoperative patients. Patients may be scared or anxious and usually require aggressive pain management. The interaction with the patient and all of the treatments provided can make the surgical experience a pleasant one for the patient and the family.

CASE STUDY

I.S. is a 63-year-old patient in the ICU with an acute exacerbation of chronic obstructive pulmonary disease (COPD). He has been a two-pack-per-day tobacco user for 45 years and continues to use tobacco between hospital admissions. This is his third episode warranting hospitalization. His previous two admissions were significant for intubation and prolonged mechanical ventilation. In an effort to avoid intubation, he is on bilevel positive airway pressure (BiPAP). His medical and surgical histories are otherwise unremarkable.

I.S. reported acute onset of right upper quadrant abdominal pain that radiated to his back. The pain began 30 minutes earlier. He was taken to the OR for exploratory surgery and possible cholecystectomy, which was ultimately done for gallstones.

I.S. received fentanyl, halothane, and succinylcholine intraoperatively. The OR course was uncomplicated. Upon arrival back to the ICU, I.S. was intubated and was being ventilated by the anesthesia provider with a bag-valve-device. He was connected to a ventilator and back to the monitoring equipment. The ICU nurse noted that the patient's blood pressure was elevated and he was tachycardic with a rate of 147. His temperature was 104.2°F (40.2°C). I.S. was also tachypneic with a spontaneous respiratory rate of 35. The ICU nurse noted muscle rigidity upon assessment. An arterial blood gas was obtained: pH 7.06, $PaCO_2$ 60, PaO_2 98, HCO_3 12.

The ICU nurse summoned anesthesia back to the bedside and began hyperventilating the patient with a bag-valve-device. The MH cart was obtained and dantrelene sodium was administered. Patient cooling was implemented with a hypothermia blanket and by covering I.S.'s head with cool towels. His vital signs eventually normalized, and I.S. was successfully extubated 72 hours later.

CRITICAL THINKING QUESTIONS

1. What caused this patient's condition to occur?
2. Which symptoms did the ICU nurse recognize that were clues that the patient had MH?
3. Why is hyperventilation with a bag-valve-device essential as the initial intervention for a patient with MH?
4. How will you implement your role as a facilitator of learning for this patient?
5. What other complications should the ICU nurse observe for in this patient?
6. Use the form to write up a plan of care for one patient in the immediate postoperative period. Rate the patient as a level 1, 3, or 5 on each characteristic. Identify the level of nurse characteristics needed in the care of this patient.
7. Take one outcome for the patient and list evidence-based interventions for this patient.

Using the Synergy Model to Develop a Plan of Care

	Patient Characteristics	Level (1, 3, 5)	Subjective and Objective Data	Evidence-based Interventions	Outcomes
SYNERGY MODEL	Resiliency				
	Vulnerability				
	Stability				
	Complexity				
	Resource availability				
	Participation in care				
	Participation in decision making				
	Predictability				

Online Resources

American Society of PeriAnesthesia Nurses: www.aspan.org

Association of PeriOperative Registered Nurses: www.aorn.org

Malignant Hyperthermia Association of the United States: www.mhaus.org

PACU Standards: www.asahg.org/publicationsAndServices/standards/36.pdf

REFERENCES

Abelha, F. J., Castro, M. A., Neves, A. M., Landeiro, N. M., & Santos, C. C. (2005). Hypothermia in a surgical intensive care unit. *BMC Anesthesiology, 5*(1), 7.

American Society of PeriAnesthesia Nurses. (2004a). Resource 6: American Society of Anesthesiologists (ASA) standards. In *2004 standards of perianesthesia nursing* (pp. 36–37). Cherry Hill, NJ: American Society of PeriAnesthesia Nurses.

American Society of PeriAnesthesia Nurses. (2004b). Resource 12: American Society of PeriAnesthesia Nurses clinical guideline for the prevention of unplanned perioperative hypothermia. In *2004 standards of perianesthesia nursing* (pp. 50–59). Cherry Hill, NJ: American Society of PeriAnesthesia Nurses.

American Society of PeriAnesthesia Nurses. (2004c). Resource 4: Criteria for initial, ongoing, and discharge assessment and management. Discharge assessment: Phase I. In *2004 standards of perianesthesia nursing* (p. 29). Cherry Hill, NJ: American Society of PeriAnesthesia Nurses.

American Society of Regional Anesthesia and Pain Medicine. (2005). Retrieved December 10, 2005, from www.asra.com/Consensus_Conferences/Consensus_Statements.shtml

Arbour, R. (2000). Mastering neuromuscular blockade. *Dimensions of Critical Care Nursing, 19*(5), 4–18.

Barone, C. P., Pablo, C. S., & Barone, G. W. (2003). A history of the PACU. *Journal of PeriAnesthesia Nursing, 18*(4), 237–241.

Colucci, W. S. (2005). Noncardiogenic pulmonary edema. Retrieved November 23, 2005, from http://patients.uptodate.com/topic.asp?file=hrt_fail/12162

Constantoyannis, C., Shahidi, S., & Kourtopoulos, H. (2003). Spinal subdural haematoma after epidural anaesthesia: A diagnosis not to be missed. *Hospital Medicine (London), 64*(11), 682–683.

Cowling, G. E., & Haas, R. E. (2002). Hypotension in the PACU: An algorithmic approach. *Journal of PeriAnesthesia Nursing, 17*(3), 159–163.

D'Arcy, Y. (2004). Using thoracic epidural catheters for pain management. *Nursing, 34*(9), 18.

Dell, D. D., & Kehoe, C. (1996). Plasma cholinesterase deficiency. *Journal of PeriAnesthesia Nursing, 11*(5), 304–308.

Drain, C. B. (2003). *Perianesthesia nursing: A critical care approach* (4th ed.). St. Louis, MO: Saunders.

Easley, R. B., Rosen, R. E., & Lindeman, K. S. (2003). Coronary artery spasm during initiation of epidural anesthesia. *Anesthesiology, 99*(4), 1015–1017.

Haas, C. E., & LeBlanc, J. M. (2004). Acute postoperative hypertension: a review of therapeutic options. *American Journal of Health-System Pharmacy, 61*(16), 1661–1673.

Keegan, M. T., & Horlocker, T. T. (1999). Epidural catheter removal before unanticipated anticoagulation: The pharmacy fail-safe. *Anesthesiology, 91*(1), 328.

Lee, P. K., & Kim, J. (2000). Lumbar epidural blocks: A case report of a life threatening complication. *Archives of Physical Medicine and Rehabilitation, 81*(12), 1587–1590.

Leffler, T. M. (2004). Propofol for sedation in the endoscopy setting: Nursing considerations for patient care. *Gastroenterology Nursing, 27*(4), 176–180.

Levins, T. T. (2002). NMBAs: Manage with caution. *Nursing Management, 33*(8), 38–40.

Litman, R. S., & Rosenberg, H. (2005). Malignant hyperthermia. *Journal of the American Medical Association, 293*, 2918–2924.

Litwack, K. (1999). *Core curriculum for perianesthesia nursing practice* (4th ed.). Philadelphia: W.B. Saunders.

Litwack, K., & Ledbetter, M. S. (Eds.). (1995). *Post anesthesia care nursing* (2nd ed.). St. Louis, MO: Mosby-Year Book.

Litz, R. J., Gottsschlich, B., & Stehr, S. N. (2004). Spinal epidural hematoma after spinal anesthesia in a patient treated with clopidogrel and enoxaparin. *Anesthesiology, 101*(6), 1467–1470.

McManus, M. C. (2001). Neuromuscular blockers in surgery and intensive care, part 2. *American Journal of Health-System Pharmacy, 58*(24), 2381–2399.

Nunnelee, J. D., & Spaner, S. D. (2000). Assessment and nursing management of hypertension in the perioperative period. *Journal of PeriAnesthesia Nursing, 15*(3), 163–168.

Redmond, M. C. (2003). Perianesthesia care of the patient with gastroesophageal reflux disease. *Journal of PeriAnesthesia Nursing, 18*(5), 335–344.

Redmond, M. C. (2005). Malignant hyperthermia: Perianesthesia recognition, treatment, and care. Retrieved December 10, 2005, from www.aspan.org/EdCeMalHyper.htm

Revis, D. R., & Seagel, M. B. (2005). Local anesthetics. Retrieved November 23, 2005, from www.emedicine.com/ent/topic20.htm

Roffey, P., Thangathura, D., Mogos, M., Black, D., & Mikhail M. (2001). Postural hypotension blamed on epidural. *Journal of Pain and Symptom Management, 22*(2), 634–635.

Shah, L. (2000). Postoperative pressure sores after epidural anaesthesia. *British Medical Journal, 321*(7266), 941–942.

U.S. Department of Veterans Affairs. (2006). JCAHO 2001 Standards pain management sedation. Retrieved September 4, 2006, from www.anesthesia.med.va.gov/anesthesia/page.cfm?pg=7

Uzunlar, H. I., Duman, E. N., Eroglu, A., Topcu, B., & Erciyes, N. (2004). A case of "foot drop" following combined spinal epidural anesthesia. *Internet Journal of Anesthesiology, 8*(1), 8p.

Van Kooy, M. A., & Gargiulo, R. F. (2000). Postobstructive pulmonary edema. *American Family Physician, 62*(2), 401–404.

CHAPTER 55

Trauma

Andy Betz   Sally Betz   Kelly Nadeau

LEARNING OBJECTIVES

Upon completion of this chapter, the reader will be able to:

1. Discuss the continuum of trauma care delivery.

2. Correlate findings from the primary and secondary assessments with initial resuscitation of the trauma patient.

3. Explain specific system injuries.

4. Describe considerations in the critical care of the injured patient.

5. List optimal patient outcomes that may be achieved through evidence-based management of trauma patients.

The term *trauma* describes a variety of injuries and poses a major challenge for prehospital care, emergency care, critical care, surgical care, and rehabilitation. In the United States, trauma is the leading cause of death for people of ages 1 to 44 years. In this country, there are approximately 2.9 million injuries, and nearly 150,000 people die as a result of traumatic injuries every year (National Highway Traffic Administration, 2003). The lifetime economic cost to society for each fatality exceeds $977,000, more than 80% of which is directly related to lost workplace and household productivity (Blincoe et al., 2002). Hundreds of thousands of people experience non-fatal injuries, many resulting in significant lifelong disabilities (Centers for Disease Control and Prevention, 2004). Motor vehicle crashes (MVCs) in the United States in the year 2000 cost $230.6 billion, the equivalent of 2.3% of the U.S. gross domestic product (Blincoe et al., 2002). The future is often challenging and uncertain for those who survive a serious injury because a lifelong disability takes a toll on not just the victims and their families, but also society.

Findings from the National Trauma Data Bank (NTDB) show that the majority of trauma patients are male. The age range that one is most likely to experience trauma is 16 through 24 years (American College of Surgeons, 2002).

Trauma has been a part of the human experience since the beginning of time and the care of the injured has always been of interest, especially in times of war. In 1966, *Accidental Death and Disability: The Neglected Disease of Modern Society* was published by the National Academy of Sciences. It marked the beginning of a "systems approach" to trauma care. Cook County Hospital in Chicago and the University of Maryland were both pioneers in the development of regional systems that extended from prehospital care through rehabilitation. Educational courses—for example, the Advanced Trauma Life Support Course—were developed to teach healthcare professionals a standardized approach to trauma care.

TRAUMA SYSTEMS

Optimal trauma care depends on an organized approach to care that includes prehospital, acute care, and rehabilitation (Moore, Feliciano, & Mattox, 2004). An organized system gets the right patient to the right place in the right amount of time and by the right mode of transport. Literature supports the principle that the care and treatments delivered within that first hour of severe injury are likely to mean the difference between temporary and permanent disabilities as well as between life and death.

There are four recognized levels of trauma centers as defined by the American College of Surgeons Committee on Trauma in *Resources for Optimal Care of the Injured Patient*. A Level I trauma center provides the highest level of care and is a regional resource center for other trauma centers and non-trauma hospitals. Level I centers are also required to conduct trauma research. Level II trauma centers have similar clinical resources as Level I centers and are capable of providing optimal care to trauma patients; however, they do not meet the research requirements of the Level I centers. Level III centers are community hospitals that commit to providing care to trauma patients but have varying levels of capabilities for specialty care. Level IV trauma centers stabilize trauma patients but will generally transfer them to a higher level of care if they require operative intervention or specialty care (Emergency Nurses Association [ENA], 2000; McQuillan, Von Rueden, Hartsock, Flynn, & Whalen, 2002).

PHASES OF TRAUMA CARE

Trauma deaths occur at three different phases following the initial injury. The level of care provided in each phase can dramatically affect the patient's chance of survival. Early deaths usually occur at the scene and happen in the first minutes after the trauma. These deaths are usually the result of large-vessel disruption and exsanguination, or catastrophic neurological injuries. The second death peak occurs within the first two hours of the injury. With appropriate assessment and interventions, a significant number of these patients can be saved. The third peak occurs days to weeks after the traumatic event and is usually the result of multiple organ dysfunction syndrome and infection. Initial resuscitative care can greatly influence these death rates by reducing the risk of infection and preventing the consequences of hypoxia and hypovolemia (ENA, 2000).

Multiple phases of care for the trauma patient are distinguished. The first phase of care starts in the field with field stabilization. The "golden hour" of trauma refers to that initial time when interventions are most effective in decreasing disabilities and saving lives. Prehospital care is provided by emergency medical technicians at basic, intermediate, and advanced (paramedic) levels as they assess, triage, stabilize, and transport the trauma patient. A patient may require specialized techniques of extrication from the scene of the event or particular stabilizing interventions prior to transportation.

As the patient arrives in the Emergency Department (ED), prehospital providers transfer resuscitative care to the ED trauma team. The patient is further evaluated and stabilized, and the decision is made to admit, discharge, or transfer the patient depending on the hospital capabilities and the severity of the patient's injuries. The admitted patient will go to the operating room (OR), intensive care unit (ICU), or general floor, depending on the extent of the injuries. Upon discharge from the hospital, many trauma patients require further care in a post-acute facility such as a rehabilitation center or skilled nursing facility. Outpatient speech, physical, and occupational therapy may also be required. To provide optimal care to the trauma patient, all elements of the system—from prehospital care through rehabilitation—must work synergistically.

TRAUMA AND MECHANISM OF INJURY

Trauma is injury to human tissue. Three broad categories of trauma are defined: blunt, penetrating, and burns. Blunt trauma is a result of blunt forces such as MVCs, motorcycle crashes, assault, and falls. Penetrating trauma occurs from an object piercing or penetrating the body and causing injury, such as gunshot wounds or stab wounds from a sharp object (Moore et al., 2004). Burn trauma is tissue injury as a result of thermal energy, electrical energy, chemical injury, or radiating source (ENA, 2000).

The mechanism of injury (MOI) looks at the forces and energy transfer involved in the event, and its identification is an important part of the patient assessment. The MOI raises the index of suspicion for injuries and predicts injury patterns. The kinetic energy equation, which describes the amount of energy absorbed to the body, is important because it considers mass and velocity (ENA, 2000; Moore et al., 2004). The speed surrounding an MVC, the height of a fall, and whether penetrating trauma is high velocity or low velocity are all critical considerations. For example, aortic rupture is the most common cause of death following an MVC or a fall from height (Mechem, 2005).

MVCs remain the overall number one cause of injury in the United States. Note that crashes are no longer called motor vehicle "accidents" because the majority of traumatic injuries are preventable. A primary goal of any trauma system is to identify preventable causes of injury so that prevention programs can be designed and implemented.

PHYSIOLOGY OF TRAUMA AND INJURY

When a significant traumatic injury occurs, the consequences begin at the cellular level. An acute injury can result in inadequate gas exchange or fluid volume deficit. The care and treatment of traumatic injuries seeks to maintain normal ventilation and circulation so as to avoid the consequences created by hypoxia at the cellular level. Patients with significant trauma will encounter an oxygen supply demand mismatch at the cellular level that may result in shock. The most common cause for shock in an injured patient is hypovolemia from blood loss. Patient survival depends on controlling bleeding and replacing lost volume, thereby maintaining adequate perfusion throughout the body.

A burn victim can develop nonhemorrhagic hypovolemic shock from fluid leaking from the intravascular spaces due to increased capillary permeability. These patients need massive fluid replacement to optimize organ perfusion.

Obstructive shock in the trauma patient may occur from tension pneumothorax or cardiac tamponade. Patient survival depends on accurate assessment and immediate intervention of these conditions.

Cardiogenic shock in trauma may be the result of blunt cardiac injury or a pre-event myocardial infarction in at-risk patients.

Distributive shock states occur with neurogenic shock initially and later from a septic focus. These patients typically have enough circulating volume, but they may require vasopressors to restore adequate circulation.

TRAUMA ASSESSMENT

Trauma assessment is conducted in a systematic, organized manner. The primary survey comes first, along with any appropriate life-saving interventions; it is followed by a secondary survey. The same approach should be used for reassessment throughout the patient's care regardless of the patient's location.

The primary assessment (or survey) is a rapid evaluation of airway, breathing, and circulation (ABCs) and disability (D) of the trauma patient. Life-threatening injuries found during the primary survey are treated immediately.

The airway is the first priority in the primary assessment. It is visually inspected for foreign bodies. Any foreign materials should be suctioned and removed from the mouth and pharyngeal area. In a patient with a decreased level of consciousness (LOC), the tongue may create an obstruction. To lift the tongue from blocking the airway, a modified jaw-thrust maneuver can be used. The use of airway adjuncts to keep the tongue from falling back to the posterior pharynx may be necessary. Intubation may be required in four circumstances: (1) the patient is unable to maintain a patent airway; (2) oxygenation or ventilation is inadequate; (3) the patient's LOC is decreased (Glasgow Coma Scale [GCS] score < 8); or (4) or there is a risk

of loss of a patent airway or airway control is desired (Galler, Skinner, & Ng, 2005). Simultaneously with the airway evaluation, the healthcare provider will manually provide in-line stabilization of the cervical spine.

The patient is observed for spontaneous breathing and the rate, depth, and effort of the respirations are noted. The patient is also assessed for presence of grunting, wheezing, and use of accessory muscles (Galler et al., 2005). The chest is inspected and palpated for symmetry of expansion and obvious injuries. If a patient is significantly compromised and unstable, the neck should be inspected for signs of tension pneumothorax such as a deviated trachea, jugular venous distention, tachycardia, and hypotension (Galler et al.). Auscultate for the presence of breath sounds, symmetry, and adventitious sounds. Percussion may be useful if breath sounds are compromised, looking for areas of dullness that may be indicative of a hemothorax or hyperresonance with a tension pneumothorax. All trauma patients should be given the maximum amount of oxygen possible. In the spontaneously ventilating patient, a non rebreather mask is initiated. In a case of respiratory compromise, the patient may be endotracheally intubated and provided manual volume ventilation. Chest tube placement may be necessary at this point to relieve a pneumothorax or hemothorax.

Evaluation of circulation begins with checking the patient's pulse for presence, rate, regularity, and quality. Time is not taken on initial arrival to obtain a full set of vital signs. If a patient is compromised, a weak, rapid, thready pulse will manifest in an attempt to compensate for blood loss. It is estimated that a patient with a radial pulse has a systolic blood pressure of at least 80 to 90 mm Hg. A palpable femoral pulse indicates a systolic pressure of at least 70 to 80 mm Hg. If only a palpable carotid pulse is evident, the systolic blood pressure is estimated at 60 to 70 mm Hg. Skin color, temperature, and diaphoresis are assessed as well. A rapid inspection is made for any areas of uncontrolled bleeding. Place pressure on bleeding areas to gain control of them. Fluid volume resuscitation is initiated via two large-bore intravenous catheters, and warmed crystalloid fluid boluses are given. Remember to draw blood for typing as lines are started. Lactated Ringer's (LR) is the primary fluid of choice for resuscitation, although a line with normal saline (NS) is necessary to administer blood. Injured patients frequently present tachycardic and cool to touch. Once the patient has been warmed and a fluid bolus of 2 to 3 liters has been given, transfusion of packed red blood cells may be necessary if the patient has not responded to crystalloids. If blood is required, the first choice is to administer typed and cross-matched blood. If time does not permit, then type-

TABLE 55-1 Primary Assessment of the Trauma Patient

Airway with c-spine stabilization	The airway is evaluated for patency The airway may be opened with jaw-thrust maneuver Debris or foreign material is suctioned or removed from airway Airway adjuncts (e.g., nasal or oral airway) may be utilized to open the airway Manual c-spine immobilization maintained in a neutral position
Breathing	Adequacy of ventilation evaluated • Skin color • Respiratory rate, depth, symmetry, and effort • Breath sounds If respiration is adequate, start O_2 per non-rebreather mask If inadequate respirations, provide bag-valve-mask assist Intubate the patient with no spontaneous respirations
Circulation	Adequacy of circulation evaluated • Pulse presence, rate, quality • Skin color, moisture, temperature • Breath sounds Observe for areas of uncontrolled bleeding Initiate cardiac compressions if no spontaneous pulse Initiate two large-bore IVs and initiate fluid bolus of warm NS or LR Control any uncontrolled bleeding
Disability	Rapid neurological evaluation (AVPU) Glasgow Coma Scale • Pupil check

Source: ENA, 2000.

specific blood is the next choice; O-negative blood is the next choice for the trauma patient.

The disability (D) check entails a quick assessment of the patient's neurological status. It includes the pupils' response to light, LOC, and identification of any posturing (i.e., decerebrate or decorticate) (Galler et al., 2005). The AVPU (Alert, responds to Verbal commands, responds to Pain, and Unresponsive) scale provides a quick determination of responsiveness or the GCS score may be calculated. **Table 55-1** describes the primary assessment of a trauma patient.

Once the primary assessment is completed and the appropriate interventions for life-threatening conditions have been completed, the secondary survey should be conducted. This next phase of the initial resuscitation consists of exposing (E) the patient by removing clothing and beginning external warming. The room should be warmed and kept free of drafts, warming lights placed on the patient, and the intravenous (IV) fluids warmed. Later in the patient's care, warmth remains a major focus. Critically injured trauma patients who are hypothermic have a higher rate of complications and mortality (Tsuei & Kearney, 2004; Wang, Callaway, Peitzman, &

Tisherman, 2005), so warmth is more than a comfort measure.

The next step in the secondary survey includes getting a full set of vital signs (F). A full set of vital signs is not taken until this point. Many assessment signs, such as pulse presence and quality, skin color, and temperature, are excellent indicators of stability that will serve as initial indicators until a full set of vital signs may be obtained.

The patient is placed on a cardiac monitor and pulse oximeter, and labs are drawn. A gastric tube is considered and usually placed nasally unless there is any concern that the patient has facial or basilar skull fractures. In the latter case, the tube is placed orally. A urinary catheter is inserted if there are no contraindications such as blood at the urinary meatus indicating the possibility of urethral disruption (usually associated with pelvis fracture).

Family involvement and presence are also essential. Visitation should be included as early and frequently as possible.

Giving comfort (G) measures is part of the secondary survey. This step may include explanation of procedures, reassurance of care, and pain medication administration.

A history (H)—including the mechanism of injury, safety devices (e.g., seat belts, helmets), medication history, previous illness/injuries, and allergies—should be obtained from the patient directly or the family. The history also reminds the nurse to complete a head-to-toe assessment. This check is certainly important upon initial patient presentation to begin to identify injuries, but it is even more critical throughout the patient's hospitalization to assess for changes. Many injuries— especially contusions—evolve over time and require vigilance. The goal of the head-to-toe assessment is to visualize and palpate (inspect [I]) every inch of the patient's body:

1. *Head and face.* Assess and palpate for abrasions, contusions, lacerations, and bony deformities, paying particular attention to the maxilla and mandible because of the potential for airway obstruction. Check for

drainage of cerebrospinal fluid (CSF) or blood from the nose and ears. Look for the development of raccoon eyes and Battle's sign, which are indicative of a basilar skull fracture.

2. *Neck.* If the cervical spine is still immobilized in a hard collar, assistance must be obtained to hold manual in-line stabilization while the neck is examined. The trachea position should be midline and the neck veins should not be distended. Assess and palpate the rest of the neck, including the cervical areas, noting areas of pain, deformities, and crepitus.

3. *Chest.* Assess and palpate the chest for symmetrical movement, color, rate and depth of respirations, open wounds, and use of accessory muscles. Percussion determines dullness or hyperresonance. Auscultation of lung fields and heart tones is essential.

4. *Abdomen.* The abdomen is first observed for distention, open wounds, abrasions, and contusions. Bowel sounds are then auscultated. Palpate the abdomen for distention, rigidity, guarding, and pain. If the patient complains of abdominal discomfort, that area should be palpated last.

5. *Pelvis and perineum.* The pelvis and perineal area are assessed for open wounds, contusions, and blood at the urinary meatus and vaginal area. The pelvis is checked initially for stability by placing the hands on the iliac crests and compressing downward and inward. Pelvic instability must be immobilized to minimize bleeding.

6. *Extremities.* All four extremities are assessed and palpated for abrasions, contusions, lacerations, and deformities. Palpate the pulses and assess for capillary refill.

After the anterior head-to-toe assessment, the patient's posterior surface is inspected (I). If the spine has not yet been cleared, the patient should be carefully log-rolled with assistance. The entire posterior surface should be inspected for lacerations, abrasions, contusions, and open wounds. Palpate the entire spine for pain and deformities.

In review, the primary and secondary assessment alphabet is

A   Airway

B   Breathing

C   Circulation

D   Disability

E   Exposure

F   Full set of vitals, five interventions, and family

G   Give comfort

H   History and head-to-toe assessment

I   Inspect the posterior surface (ENA, 2000)

This primary and secondary assessment may be started or completed at the prehospital scene or in the ED. Sometimes the assessment may not have been completed prior to ICU admission. This systematic approach should be followed on an ongoing basis throughout the patient's ICU admission. **Table 55-2** identifies the monitoring equipment and diagnostic studies that can be used to help with this assessment.

TABLE 55-2 Monitoring Equipment and Diagnostic Studies

Monitoring Equipment/ Diagnostic Study	Purpose
Cardiac monitor	Ongoing evaluation and trending of heart rate and dysrhythmias
Noninvasive BP	Ongoing evaluation and trending of BP
Pulse oximetry	Ongoing evaluation of oxygenation
End-tidal CO_2	Trending indicating adequacy of ventilation
Nasal/oral gastric tube	Decompress the stomach
Foley catheter	Ongoing monitoring of volume status
Chest x-ray	Evaluate for life-threatening thoracic injuries
Pelvis x-ray	Evaluate for pelvic trauma cause of hemodynamic instability
Focused abdominal sonogram for trauma (FAST)	Evaluate intra-abdominal blood cause of hemodynamic instability
Computed axial tomography	Evaluate head, neck, thoracic, abdomen for injuries
Angiography	Evaluate vascular disruption with intervention to control bleeding

Source: ENA, 2000.

HEAD INJURY

Traumatic brain injury (TBI) is the leading cause of death in trauma. An estimated 180 to 220 cases per 100,000 population occur annually. In the United States, approximately 600,000 new TBIs occur each year. Approximately 90% of these patients survive (Shepard, 2004).

Head injury may occur from blunt or penetrating trauma resulting in areas of hemorrhage, contusion, swelling, and/or diffuse axonal injuries. Any injury can result in changes in the balance of blood, CSF, and brain tissue. The primary injury is a direct result of the trauma, but bleeding and swelling within the rigid skull can cause secondary trauma. The goal of treatment for head injury is to minimize secondary injury.

Skull fractures may be classified as either linear or comminuted fractures. Linear fractures have no displacement. In a comminuted fracture, the skull is in distinct pieces, which may be depressed and pressed against brain tissue. A depressed skull fracture may have to be surgically lifted and repaired. Open fractures increase the chances of infection.

Significant blunt force may result in a fracture to the base of the skull, such that the patient may have physical findings of periorbital ecchymosis (raccoon eyes) or bruising behind the ear at the mastoid area (Battle's sign). With a disruption in the base of the skull, CSF may leak out through the nose (rhinorrhea) or ears (otorrhea) (ENA, 2000).

A concussion is a brain injury with no structural injury. The patient may experience a brief loss of consciousness, possibly memory loss, headache, confusion, dizziness, and nausea and vomiting. An associated post-concussive syndrome may be manifested as headache, memory loss, and problems with concentration that may last as long as a year after the initial injury (ENA, 2000).

Epidural hematomas (EDHs) are usually arterial bleeds between the inner table of the skull and the dura. The patient may exhibit a decreased LOC immediately post injury, followed by a lucid interval with a return to the decreased LOC. An EDH is usually the result of an arterial bleed and tends to expand rapidly. A linear skull fracture in the temporal area is a common location. The fracture disrupts the middle meningeal artery, allowing the resulting hematoma to expand rapidly. Immediate surgical intervention is required, and there is an excellent prognosis with early intervention (ENA, 2000).

An acute subdural hematoma (SDH) is a collection of blood between the dura and the brain. SDHs are more common than epidurals and usually entail venous bleeding from the tearing of the bridging veins. The subdural may be acute (within 48 hours) or chronic (as long as two weeks after an event) in nature. Acute SDHs are usually the result of a high-velocity impact; because of the underlying brain injury, more than 50% of these patients will not survive (O'Carroll, 2000). The high mortality rate can be lowered by rapid identification of the injury, aggressive medical management, and emergent surgical intervention.

A chronic SDH may be seen in elderly patients (as the brain atrophies, the bridging vessels get stretched), chronic alcoholics, and individuals on anticoagulants (from their tendency to bleed). Such a patient may show a steady decline in LOC. A patient with a chronic SDH may have it surgically evacuated. If the area of bleeding is small and of no consequence, however, it may not require surgical evacuation (ENA, 2000).

Intracerebral hematomas are hemorrhages within the brain parenchyma that result from blunt or penetrating injury with a contusion. These hematomas include intraparenchymal hematomas and subarachnoid hemorrhages. The significance and management of these injuries depend on where they are located and how large they are. They may be managed medically or surgically.

Diffuse axonal injury (DAI) is a result of shearing and disrupting of brain tissue. It is usually a result of blunt acceleration–deceleration forces and is associated with prolonged coma that is not the result of an identifiable lesion. In the clinical setting, it may be difficult to determine if the coma is due to hypoxic injury versus DAI; indeed, a combination of those factors may be involved (ENA, 2000).

Management of Traumatic Brain Injury

Regardless of the origin of the brain injury, initial management efforts focus on stabilizing the ABCs so as to maintain cerebral perfusion. Treatment may include the interventions listed in **Table 55-3**.

Key measures include diligent ongoing serial neurological assessments of LOC, pupillary size/reactivity, motor exam, and vital signs. The GCS will provide a quantitative evaluation of the patient's best response to eye opening, verbal response, and extremity movement.

SPINE TRAUMA

Approximately 11,000 spinal cord injuries (SCIs) occur each year in North America (Spinal Cord Injury Information Network, 2005). Most of these injuries (55%) involve the cervical region, with another 15% noted in the thoracic region, 15% in the thoracolumbar junction, and 15% in the lumbosacral area (American College of Surgeons, 2004). The consequences of SCI with neurological deficit have catastrophic implications for the patient and the family.

TABLE 55-3 Treatment of Traumatic Brain Injury

- Airway management: Rapid sequence intubation to maintain ventilation. Hyperventilation is reserved for herniation or significant rapid deterioration.

- Maintain cerebral perfusion pressure (CPP) > 60 mm Hg in adults. Cerebral blood flow is optimal with a CPP between 50 and 150 mm Hg.

- Maintain ICP as close as possible to normal value of 0 to 15 mm Hg; ICP > 20 mm Hg requires treatment.

- Elevate the head: This helps manage swelling and increased ICP but remains controversial—while head elevation lowers ICP, there is concern that it may decrease CPP and compromise cerebral blood flow.

- Osmotic diuretic: Mannitol 1 Gm/kg may be administered to decrease cerebral edema in normotensive or hypertensive patients.

- Mechanical decompression: Consider craniectomy will allow room for swelling; ventriculostomy to drain CSF to accommodate swelling.

Source: ENA, 2000.

The majority of injuries occur from MVCs, followed by falls, assault, and sporting injuries (O'Carroll, 2000). Injuries to the spine may also result from penetrating trauma. Physical findings relate to the area of injury, with varying levels of motor, sensation, and proprioception being observed. Dermatome measurements designate the level of injury, indicating at what level loss of sensation has occurred. (Refer to Figure 54-1.) Correlating myotome readings indicate levels of muscle movement.

Any patient with significant blunt trauma is assumed to have a spine injury until proven otherwise. Part of the initial stabilization of the injured patient includes stabilizing and supporting the spine in alignment. This effort continues until the patient can be assessed and cleared of any injury to the spine.

Injury to the spine may be associated with spinal shock, which occurs after complete or incomplete severing of the spinal cord. Motor, sensory, autonomic, and reflex functions below the level of the lesion are lost. The patient may experience flaccid paralysis and loss of reflex activity in the same areas. This effect may last days to several months.

Neurogenic shock may occur with sudden transection of the cord at T6 or above. This condition causes an impairment of the sympathetic pathways, with a loss of all vasomotor activity below the level of the lesion. The disruption in the pathway leads to vasodilation, decreased venous return, and cardiac

deceleration that will be demonstrated by bradycardia, hypotension, and temperature abnormalities.

Bony injuries of the spine include facet dislocation and subluxations. Bone fractures of the spine are classified as simple, compression, wedge, burst, or comminuted fractures. These injuries may or may not be associated with injury to the spinal cord. Fractures are also classified as stable or unstable. Stable fractures do not have movement that would encroach on the cord. Unstable injuries have a disruption of ligaments or bony elements that allow for abnormal movement of the spine.

SCIs are classified as complete when they involve a loss of motor and sensory function below the level of the lesion. The patient will have flaccid paralysis, paraparesis, loss of autonomic function, hypotension, bradycardia, loss of voluntary bowel/bladder control, and loss of reflexes. An incomplete SCI spares some motor or sensory function below the level of the lesion. Incomplete SCIs are described in terms of the area of the cord involved (ENA, 2000):

- Central cord: loss of motor and sensory function below lesion; arms > legs
- Anterior cord: loss of pain and temperature and motor function below the lesion; proprioception, touch, pressure, and vibration preserved
- Brown-Sequard Syndrome: loss of motor function, position sense, and vibration on the same side as the injury; pain and temperature loss on the opposite side

Diagnosis of SCI starts with a physical exam. It includes assessing for complaints of neck/back pain, palpating for deformities and point tenderness, and assessing for motor and sensory function, reflexes, and rectal sphincter tone (absent in complete SCI). Immediate interventions include immobilizing the vertebral column, maintaining spinal alignment, and logrolling the patient. All patients will continue to be maintained in spinal alignment until the possibility of spine injury has been fully evaluated and ruled out.

Further evaluation is done through multiple studies including anterior, posterior, and lateral radiographs (cervical spine lateral films must include the top of T1 to be adequate); thoracic and lumbar spine films as indicated; computerized tomography (CT) scan; and magnetic resonance imaging (MRI).

Management of Spinal Cord Injury

Patients with acute SCI with neurological deficit may be treated with high-dose steroids initially. Methylprednisolone (Solu-Medrol®) may be administered within 8 hours of injury at a dose of bolus 30 mg/kg followed by an infusion at 5.4 mg/kg/hr for 23 hours (ENA, 2000). Although somewhat controversial, the actions of methyprednisolone that are believed to be of benefit in SCI include improved blood flow, decreased lactic acid, promotion of extracellular calcium recovery, reduction of lipids and free radicals, and stabilization of cell membranes.

Surgical stabilization may be required to restore alignment, stabilize the spine, decompress the neural tissue, and allow for earlier mobilization. Open reduction and internal fixation of acute spine injuries may be delayed in unstable patients.

Conservative or nonoperative management may be used if alignment is achieved through traction or positioning. External orthopedic devices such as a halo device for cervical fractures may provide the necessary stability and alignment if there is no need for operative reduction or removal of fragments. It is critical to do whatever it takes to get patients mobile once stable.

Patients with cervical SCI and resultant paralysis are at significant risk for a myriad of problems associated with immobility. Potential complications include pulmonary problems and hypoxia because of decreased vital capacity, ineffective cough, poor secretion clearance, risk of aspiration, and pneumonia. Deep venous thrombosis and pulmonary embolus require preventive measures [e.g., anticoagulant therapy, pneumatic sequential devices, range of motion (ROM), and physical therapy]. Immobility also predisposes the patient to pressure ulcers. Appropriate positioning and ROM exercises are important to decrease contractures and deformities.

The psychosocial implications for SCI patients are also very significant. Anger and depression can be severe. There are ongoing issues with self-esteem, sexuality, loss of independence, and financial challenges. It is critical to employ a team approach to care that includes not only the healthcare team but also friends and family.

ABDOMINAL TRAUMA

The evaluation of the injured abdomen looks for hemorrhage or spillage of bowel contents. Patients with blunt or penetrating abdominal trauma with continuing unanticipated blood loss should be further evaluated for overlooked intra-abdominal injury (Mechem, 2005).

Abdominal evaluation for trauma presents special problems. The unconscious, intoxicated, or spinal cord injured patient's exam provides virtually no clues, because the patient cannot adequately participate in an exam. Even in alert patients, the level of pain and the reaction to palpation are of little help in differentiating severe from trivial injury during the critical early period following injury. Significant peritoneal signs may not develop until hours after an injury. The abdomen contains a multitude of organs whose functions remain largely invisible. When the patient presents with pain, the location and quality of that pain help very little in identifying the injured organ. Instead, more imaging or surgical intervention is necessary for diagnosis.

Any penetrating injury from the nipples to groin should be considered as a potential abdominal injury. Patients with clinical signs of peritonitis or with evisceration of the bowel should be taken immediately to the operating room after satisfactory stabilization.

The goals of assessment for blunt or penetrating abdominal trauma are to identify any injuries requiring surgical repair and to avoid unnecessary surgery along with its associated morbidity. A large number of penetrating traumas present with superficial tenderness around the wound site, but no signs of peritoneal inflammation. Likewise, many blunt abdominal traumas present with few or no visible signs of trauma to the abdomen. For these hemodynamically normal trauma patients, several options may be pursued for the evaluation of abdominal trauma; see **Table 55-4**.

Serial Physical Examination

Serial physical examinations remain one of the best screening methods for delayed identification of intra-abdominal injury (Nast-Kolb, Bail, & Taeger, 2005). **Table 55-5** lists the pertinent points to be included in an abdominal physical examination.

Imaging Modalities
FAST

The role of focused assessment with sonography for trauma (FAST) in abdominal trauma continues to be evaluated. A negative FAST does not exclude significant abdominal injury (Nast-Kolb et al., 2005). Therefore, it should be considered only as a part of the assessment of penetrating and blunt injury. Ultrasound cannot detect small amounts of fluid that may be associated with a hollow viscous injury. A positive FAST indicates fluid in the abdomen presumably from peritoneal disruption, but is a poor choice for discriminating which injuries require intervention.

CT Scan

As the technology has improved, CT is finding a greater role in the evaluation of blunt and penetrating abdominal injury. Most studies recommend a multi-detector (multi-slice) scanner with triple-contrast protocol (IV, oral, and rectal), although more recent research may demonstrate that the administration of polonium (PO) contrast in the initial trauma

TABLE 55-4 Evaluation of the Hemodynamically Stable Patient with Abdominal Trauma

Chest radiograph	An erect chest radiograph may identify subdiaphragmatic air. This must be interpreted with some caution in the absence of peritonitis, because air may be entrained into the peritoneal cavity with a bowel rupture from a stab, gunshot wound, or blunt injury. The presence of subdiaphragmatic air signals peritoneal disruption.
Nasogastric tube	Blood drained from the stomach will identify a gastric injury.
Urinary catheter	Gross hematuria indicates a renal or bladder injury. Microscopic injury suggests, but is not characteristic of, a ureter injury.
Rectal examination	Rectal blood indicates rectal or sigmoid penetration. Proctoscopy, sigmoidoscopy, or CT with rectal contrast should be performed.
Abdominal x-ray	An AP and lateral radiograph with the use of radiopaque markers placed near entrance and exit wounds can help identify the potential track of a penetrating object. In the absence of an entrance and exit wound, the surgeon may identify the location and depth of any retained foreign bodies.
Options for continued evaluation	The hemodynamically stable patient with blunt or penetrating trauma to the abdomen who requires further evaluation using one or more of the following diagnostic modalities: • Serial physical examination • Local wound exploration • Diagnostic peritoneal lavage • Ultrasound (FAST) • CT scan • Laparoscopy • Laparotomy

Source: ENA, 2000.

setting yields little information due to the emergent nature of administration. Of all the diagnostic modalities listed, CT gives the best assessment of retroperitoneal structures (ENA, 2000).

Computed abdominal tomography with a helical scanner, with and without IV contrast media, is currently the gold standard of imaging techniques to identify traumatic abdominal injuries. It has a sensitivity of 97.2% and a specificity of 94.7%. False-negative findings must be expected with hollow-organ injuries (Nast-Kolb et al., 2005).

Management of Abdominal Trauma

Nursing management of the patient with abdominal trauma includes frequent monitoring of vital signs, hemodynamic monitoring, maintaining adequate IV access, preparation of the patient for serial abdominal examinations (including administration of oral and IV contrast per hospital protocols), and traveling with patients to imaging studies.

THORACIC TRAUMA

The thoracic cavity contains a number of life-sustaining organs—the heart, lungs, aorta, vena cava, trachea, esophagus, and spinal cord. Overall, the mortality following thoracic trauma is approximately 10%. Thoracic trauma can result in hypoxia, hypercarbia, acidosis, hypovolemia, ventilation/perfusion deficits, and shock (ENA, 2000).

MOI is important because blunt and penetrating injuries have different pathophysiologics and clinical courses. Most blunt injuries are managed nonoperatively, with interventions such as intubation, mechanical ventilation, and chest tube insertion. Pulmonary contusion is the most common lung injury of blunt chest trauma (Mechem, 2005). Diagnosis of blunt injuries may be more difficult and require additional investigative measures such as CT scanning. In contrast, penetrating thoracic injuries are less likely to need additional imaging studies but are more likely to require operative interventions. Patients with penetrating trauma may deteriorate rapidly, but recover much faster than patients with blunt injury.

In the primary assessment, examine the chest immediately after the airway is controlled. Inspect for open wounds, tenderness, crepitus, and unequal respiratory motion. Listen to breath sounds. Life-threatening injuries must be treated before proceeding with the assessment.

Following any intervention, it is imperative that the chest be reexamined to determine treatment efficacy. In almost all trauma patients, a chest radiograph will be obtained, because severe internal injuries may be present without external tenderness. Repeat chest films should follow any invasive intervention to determine accurate placement of lines and tubes.

TABLE 55-5 Abdominal Physical Exam

Inspect	• Is there bleeding present?
	• Is the incision approximated, oozing, red?
	• Is the abdomen distended?
Auscultate	• Are bowel sounds present in all four quadrants?
Palpate	• Is the abdomen firm?
	• Does the patient have rebound tenderness, focal tenderness, or other peritoneal signs of irritation?
Percuss	• What sound is present with percussion?
	• Is there pain with percussion?
Assess pelvic stability	• Manual horizontal compression of the iliac crests may elicit abnormal movement suggesting pelvic fracture
History	• Last meal
	• Last bowel movement
	• Frequency of bowel movements prior to admission
	• Diet at home

Source: ENA, 2000.

TABLE 55-6 Primary and Secondary Survey

Primary Survey

Life-threatening conditions requiring immediate treatment	• Tension pneumothorax
	• Massive hemothorax
	• Open pneumothorax
	• Cardiac tamponade
	• Flail chest
Monitoring adjuncts	• Oxygen saturation
	• End-tidal CO_2 (if intubated)
	• Diagnostic adjuncts
	• Chest radiograph
	• FAST ultrasound
	• Arterial blood gas
	• Interventions
	• Chest tube drainage
	• Thoracotomy

Secondary Survey

The secondary survey is a more detailed and complete examination, aimed at identifying all injuries and planning further investigation and treatment	• Rib fractures and flail chest
	• Pulmonary contusion
	• Simple pneumothorax
	• Simple hemothorax
	• Blunt aortic injury
	• Blunt myocardial injury

Source: ENA, 2000.

The presence of respiratory distress is ominous. Hypoxia and hypoventilation are the primary killers of acute trauma patients. Assessment of ventilation is therefore assigned a high priority in the primary survey. It may be obvious that the patient has a ventilatory problem during assessment of the airway. Similarly, the identification or actual severity of certain conditions may be determined only after assessment of the circulation or use of monitoring or diagnostic adjuncts.

Some injuries may develop over time and become life-threatening during the course of resuscitation. Reassessment and ongoing evaluation are therefore extremely important, especially if the patient's condition deteriorates. **Table 55-6** reviews those injuries that should be first identified in the primary and secondary surveys.

Physical Examination

Physical examination is the primary tool for diagnosis of acute thoracic trauma. While the initial primary survey may identify some conditions, an initial normal examination does not exclude any of them; serial examinations and use of diagnostic adjuncts are important. **Table 55-7** describes pertinent physical examination findings.

The size of the injury and position of the patient will affect the clinical findings. For example, a small hemothorax may have no clinical signs. A moderate hemothorax will be dull to percussion with absent breath sounds at the bases in the erect patient, whereas signs will be posterior in the supine patient. This difference is also reflected in chest radiograph findings. **Table 55-8** compares findings for selected thoracic injuries.

Monitoring Adjuncts

Oxygen Saturation

Pulse oximetry allows for continuous, noninvasive assessment of arterial hemoglobin oxygen saturation. Continuous oxygen saturation monitoring should be used during the resuscitation and ongoing management of all trauma patients. Pulse oximetry is discussed in more detail in Chapter 21.

TABLE 55-7 Physical Examination of the Patient with Thoracic Trauma

Inspect	• Determine the respiratory rate and depth
	• Look for chest wall asymmetry, paradoxical chest wall motion
	• Look for bruising, seat belt or steering wheel marks, penetrating wounds
Palpate	• Feel for the trachea for deviation
	• Assess whether there is adequate and equal chest wall movement
	• Feel for chest wall tenderness or rib "crunching" indicating rib fractures
	• Feel for subcutaneous emphysema
Auscultate	• Listen for normal, equal breath sounds on both sides
	• Listen especially in the apices and axillae and at the back of the chest (or as far as you can get while supine)
Percuss	• Percuss both sides of the chest looking for dullness or resonance

Source: ENA, 2000.

End-Tidal Carbon Dioxide Monitoring

End-tidal carbon dioxide monitoring ($ETCO_2$) should be used in all intubated trauma patients. $ETCO_2$ is a key method of confirming placement of a tracheal tube by sensing the presence of carbon dioxide during exhalation. It is also used to monitor trends in carbon dioxide levels while intubated. $ETCO_2$ monitoring is discussed in more detail in Chapter 21.

Diagnostic Adjuncts for Blunt and Penetrating Trauma

Chest Radiograph

The plain anterior/posterior chest radiograph remains the standard initial diagnostic study for the evaluation of chest trauma. The indications and techniques are slightly different for blunt and penetrating trauma.

All blunt trauma patients should have a portable chest radiograph performed in the trauma resuscitation room. The discussion of the physical examination highlighted the inaccuracy of clinical signs in the trauma patient. The chest radiograph is a rapid screening examination that will identify significant thoracic problems requiring intervention. Chest radiographs in blunt trauma patients are taken in the supine position. Unstable spinal fractures have not been ruled out at this stage, eliminating the option of sitting the patient upright for the film.

Patients with a stab wound that may have violated the thoracic cavity or mediastinum should have a chest radiograph. In practice, this means all patients with stab wounds between the neck and the umbilicus in either the front or the back require a film study. For gunshot wounds, all patients with wounds between the neck and the pelvis/buttock area should have a chest film. This is especially true if the bullet track is unclear, there is a missing bullet, or the patient has an odd number of entry/exit wounds. The chest radiograph in penetrating trauma should be taken with the patient sitting upright if possible, but only if spine injury is ruled out. This strategy will increase the sensitivity for detecting a small hemothorax, pneumothorax, or diaphragm injury.

FAST Examination

FAST is a rapid ultrasound examination that is performed in the trauma resuscitation room looking specifically for blood in the peritoneum or pericardium or for a hemothorax.

TABLE 55-8 Physical Exam Findings of the Thoracic Trauma Patient

	Trachea	Expansion	Breath Sounds	Percussion
Tension pneumothorax	Deviated away from affected side	Decreased; chest may be fixed in hyperexpansion	Diminished or absent	Hyperresonant
Simple pneumothorax	Midline	Decreased	May be diminished	May be hyperresonant; usually normal
Hemothorax	Midline	Decreased	Diminished if large; normal if small	Dull, especially posteriorly
Pulmonary contusion	Midline	Normal	Normal; may have crackles	Normal
Lung collapse	Deviated toward affected side	Decreased	May be reduced	Normal

Sources: Dincer & Lipchik, 2005; ENA, 2000; Herzig & Biffl, 2005; Keough & Pudelek, 2001; McRoberts, McKenchnie, & Leigh-Smith, 2005; Neale, 2006.

Arterial Blood Gas Analysis

An arterial blood gas (ABG) sample should be drawn from all intubated and ventilated trauma patients and from any patient with significant chest trauma or evidence of respiratory or hemodynamic instability. ABG analysis is discussed in more detail in Chapter 21.

Further Investigation/Definitive Care

The results of the preceding examinations and findings in other body regions are used to determine the subsequent disposition of the trauma patient. Further investigations may include CT scan, angiography, esophagoscopy/esophagram, or bronchoscopy. Definitive care may include chest drain, thoracotomy, and transfer to the ICU for ventilatory and hemodynamic monitoring or observation.

ORTHOPEDIC TRAUMA

Orthopedic injuries run the gamut from noncritical to life-threatening. Although the majority of musculoskeletal injuries are minor, they do contribute to significant short- and long-term disabilities. These injuries are most often associated with blunt mechanisms of injury, such as MVCs and falls, but can result from penetrating trauma. Musculoskeletal injuries account for approximately 8,000 deaths per year, and an estimated 85% of patients who sustain blunt trauma will have musculoskeletal injuries (ENA, 2000).

While minor injuries such as strain and sprains may affect ambulation, fractures can be significant injuries. The most common fractures are located in the femur, tibia, ankle, hip, pelvis, acetabulum, and distal radius. Eight fracture types are distinguished: open, closed, complete, incomplete, comminuted, greenstick, impacted, and displaced.

A femur fracture is usually a result of major trauma. A closed femur fracture can result in a loss of 1,500 to 3,000 mL of blood. Signs and symptoms include shortened appearance, deformity, rotation, and evidence of shock. Treatment includes immobilization, possible application of traction devices, and definitive stabilization in the OR with intramedullary nailing, open reduction, and internal fixation (ENA, 2000).

Pelvic fractures may be stable or unstable. Approximately two-thirds of all cases involve unstable injuries. Unstable pelvic fractures can be life-threatening and are often accompanied by large blood loss and injury to the genitourinary system. The pelvis is a ring, so it may break in more than one place. Signs and symptoms include pain or bony instability on palpation, shortening or abnormal leg rotation, and evidence of hypovolemic shock. Rapid evaluation and intervention to stabilize the pelvis to stop the ongoing blood loss must occur simultaneously with other life-saving interventions. The pelvis may be stabilized with external compressive devices such as a sheet tied around the pelvis, commercially available pelvic stabilizers that are applied externally, or application of an external skeletal fixation device. Ongoing management is directed at restoring circulating volume and stopping the bleeding process (ENA, 2000).

Significant patient considerations with orthopedic trauma beyond fracture stabilization include assessment of the patient for and early identification of complications. Many complications are of concern in the orthopedic trauma patient.

Compartment syndrome occurs in the muscle sheath due to swelling from bleeding and edema. This compression can disrupt both the circulation and nerve impulses. Signs and symptoms include pain out of proportion to the injury, pain with muscle stretching or passive movement, tense swollen area, elevated muscle compartment pressure, sensory deficits, and loss of pulse. Ongoing assessment focuses on the five P's: pain, pallor, pulselessness, paresthesia, and paralysis. If compartment syndrome occurs, immediate release of pressure is required through an incision into the fascial compartment (a fasciotomy). It is important to remember that a cast can lead to compartment syndrome by external pressure because of swelling of the casted extremity. Ongoing assessment is essential.

Deep vein thrombosis (DVT) is a complication frequently noted in orthopedic trauma patients. Signs and symptoms may include calf tenderness, redness, swelling, fever, and positive Homan's sign. Efforts to prevent DVT include early ambulation, anticoagulant therapy, and pneumatic compression devices.

The threat of a pulmonary embolism (PE) exists with any immobilized patient but is of particular concern in orthopedic patients. PE is discussed in more detail in Chapter 22.

The release of fat emboli from long bone fractures has been documented to occur. It is not well understood why some patients experience this phenomenon whereas others do not. A fat embolus will usually manifest itself 24 to 48 hours after injury and may prove difficult to differentiate from PE. The signs and symptoms are similar to those noted in PE, with additional symptoms of altered mental status and a petechiae rash—that is, flat, tiny, round red spots under the skin surface caused by bleeding into the skin that do not blanch when pressed upon.

ICU CONSIDERATIONS

Following stabilization in the ED or operative intervention, the trauma patient may be transferred to the ICU for ongoing monitoring and resuscitation. Acidosis, coagulopathies, and hypothermia are three complications that can be corrected (Mechem, 2005). The patient should immediately be assessed for ABCs (Richards & Mayberry, 2004). Breath sounds should be auscultated, and the position of the endotracheal tube should be determined as indicated. The patient's cardiovascular and neurological status should similarly be assessed. The patient should be completely but briefly exposed to evaluate external injuries. The primary and secondary assessments should be completed.

Meticulous monitoring for potential missed diagnosis of injuries is essential (ENA, 2003). For example, intra-abdominal pressure monitoring should be initiated in patients with abdominal trauma (Mechem, 2005). Signs and symptoms of pulmonary contusion may not become manifest for several hours following an injury and may be present despite the absence of any apparent chest wall injury. ICU nurses may suspect pulmonary contusion in patients who manifest dyspnea, hemoptysis, tachypnea, crackles, wheezing, hypoxemia, and hypercarbia (Mechem). Management of pulmonary contusion is supportive. If the patient does not have signs of shock, judicious use of fluids is recommended to prevent increasing edema in the contused lung. Aggressive pulmonary toileting and administration of analgesics can minimize complications and the need for intubation. Intercostal nerve blocks and epidural opioids are recommended to decrease the incidence of respiratory depression (Mechem). In one study, missed injuries and complications included meningitis, retroperitoneal abscess, bowel infarction, bleeding gastric ulcer, pneumonia, PE/infarction, thoracic spine fracture with epidural hemorrhage, ruptured esophageal varices, central venous catheter erosion, myocardial infarction, lacerated tricuspid papillary muscle, hemoperitoneum greater than 500 mL, pancreatitis/fat necrosis, subarachnoid hemorrhage, liver and/or spleen laceration, gastric ulcer, duodenal ulcer, and small lung abscess (Ong et al., 2002).

Patients with a significant crush injury or multiple trauma are at risk for the development of rhabdomyolysis. Rhabdomyolysis—the breakdown of muscle with the release of muscle fiber contents into the systemic circulation—can lead to the development of renal failure. Its symptoms include muscle pain, edema, weakness, and dark urine. Not all patients have all of these symptoms, however (Mechem, 2005). Management includes fluid resuscitation and maintaining a high urine output (100 to 300 mL/hr) (Mechem). Use of bicarbonate and mannitol has been shown to decrease myoglobin toxicity to the renal tubules (Mechem), but this treatment is now considered questionable (Brown et al., 2004).

In addition to monitoring for delayed and missed injuries, ICU care may include management of complications of initial management or evaluation. It includes assessment of complications from transfusions, administration of contrast media, venous thromboembolism, and upper GI bleeding.

Complications of transfusions may include hypothermia, coagulopathies, hypocalcemia, acute lung injury, and non-cardiogenic pulmonary edema (Lapointe & Von Rueden, 2002; Mechem, 2005). Administration of contrast media can cause nephrotoxicity. Assessment of renal function is essential (Mechem).

Patients with traumatic injuries are at risk of developing DVT or PE due to such factors as prolonged immobilization, injuries to the pelvis or leg, or direct vascular injuries (Stannard et al., 2006). Because they are at risk for gastric stress ulcers, trauma patients admitted to the ICU should receive prophylactic measures (Mechem, 2005).

Patients who are intubated and receiving mechanical ventilation are at risk for the development of ventilator-associated pneumonia (VAP). Preventive measures for VAP are discussed in Chapter 6. Use of empiric antibiotic therapy is essential to minimize this risk. Critically ill trauma patients who do not receive adequate antibiotic therapy have increased morbidity and mortality rates (Mueller et al., 2005).

While the primary damage of a TBI can often be reversed, measures to decrease the incidence of secondary brain damage can also be implemented. If the patient had been intubated prior to ICU admission, steps to decrease the FiO_2 from 100% will usually begin once the patient is in the ICU. The goal is to keep the PaO_2 at 70 mm Hg or greater (Marik, Varon, & Trask, 2002). Hypoventilation to a $PaCO_2$ of 25 mm Hg was formerly recommended to prevent increased intracranial pressure (ICP). Most recent data suggest maintaining $PaCO_2$ levels in the 35–40 mm Hg range (Brain Trauma Foundation, American Association of Neurological Surgeons, Joint Section on Neurotrauma and Critical Care, 2000; Marik et al.).

Attaining and maintaining normal circulating volume is also indicated for the patient with severe TBI. A mean arterial pressure of 90 mm Hg or greater is the recommended target to maintain cerebral perfusion pressure at more than 70 mm Hg (Brain Trauma Foundation, American Association of Neurological Surgeons, Joint Section on Neurotrauma and Critical Care, 2000). Administration of LR or NS is recommended (Rafie et al., 2004). Use of vasoactive agents to maintain blood pressure is controversial (Marik et al., 2002). ICP monitoring is recommended if the patient has a GCS score of less than 8 (Marik et al.). ICP monitoring is described in Chapter 27.

Patients in the ICU with TBI need pain medication and sedation even if they are comatose. These measures are indicated to help minimize increases in blood pressure and ICP. Morphine or fentanyl (Sublimaze®) is considered first-line therapy for pain management. Propofol (Diprivan®) is also a popular choice because it can be easily titrated and reversed quickly when the infusion is stopped. Propofol can also decrease the cerebral metabolic rate (Kaisti et al., 2003). If ICP remains greater than 20 mm Hg even with traditional measures, CSF drainage or mannitol administration can be initiated. Administration of hypertonic saline can be considered as an alternative to mannitol to decrease ICP and increase cerebral perfusion pressure (Khanna et al., 2000; Marik et al., 2002).

Patients with TBI in the ICU also require monitoring of their electrolyte status. These individuals are at risk for hyponatremia and hypomagnesemia. The etiology of hyponatremia may be syndrome of inappropriate secretion of antidiuretic hormone, described in Chapter 47, and cerebral salt wasting (Marik et al., 2002).

TBI puts the patient in a hypermetabolic and catabolic state. Early initiation of enteral feedings is encouraged to help minimize complications. Parenteral nutrition should be avoided because of its associated complications and increased mortality (Marik et al., 2002).

Hypotension in critically ill trauma patients is associated with an increased mortality rate. The results of one study indicated that patients who experienced even a brief (less than 10 minutes) episode of hypotension during the first 24 hours in the ICU had increased mortality rates. The longer the hypotensive episode lasted, the higher the mortality rate (Zenati, Billiar, Townsend, Peitzman, & Harbrecht, 2002).

Geriatric patients who sustain trauma have unique issues that can prove challenging to nurses in the ICU. These patients may have preexisting health conditions that can complicate their care. For example, alterations in cardiac and respiratory systems reduce physiologic reserve, which is needed to respond to hypoxia and shock (Pudelek, 2002).

While stabilizing and managing the trauma patient in the ICU are essential, communication with the family on an ongoing basis is equally important. Including family members on daily critical care rounds has been reported to be successful in the literature and warrants consideration (Schiller & Anderson, 2003). Leske (2003) reported that family members of a patient with a gunshot wound have more stress and demonstrate less effective coping than families of patients from an MVC. It is suggested that ICU nurses develop and implement interventions to assist the family to form or initiate coping strategies and help them address their stress.

PATIENT OUTCOMES

Nurses can help ensure attainment of optimal patient outcomes such as those listed in **Box 55-1** through the use of evidence-based interventions for patients sustaining trauma.

SUMMARY

Our greatest success would be to prevent the trauma injury from ever occurring. Many initiatives have been directed at public education, especially in the highest-risk age groups. These programs attempt to modify risky behavior by providing education about the consequences of actions that can have a catastrophic result.

After primary prevention, we turn to secondary prevention of the consequences that follow significant trauma. Trauma is a national health problem that would be best dealt with by the development of a coordinated system ensuring prompt access to optimal care. Despite the amount of care and extended ICU admission, a coordinated multidisciplinary approach can result in most trauma patients ultimately being discharged and being functional and independent. These patients, however, may not be at their pre-injury level (Miller, Patton, Graham, & Hollins, 2000).

Box 55-1
Optimal Patient Outcomes

- Vital signs in expected range
- Airway patent
- No overt signs of bleeding
- Cognitively intact
- Physical comfort in expected range
- Musculoskeletal injuries stabilized
- Heart & breath sounds normal
- Fluid status in expected range
- Tissue perfusion in expected range

CASE STUDY

You are doing a clinical in a busy ED of a level I trauma center. Your preceptor informs you that you are assigned to the first trauma team. You have just been notified that a patient is being brought in by helicopter from the scene of a single-car MVC. A report from the EMS indicates the patient was the restrained driver in a pickup truck that struck a tree. The patient was hauling 300-pound hydraulic cylinders that were in the bed of the truck and became projectiles, causing significant damage to the driver's passenger compartment.

The patient had a GCS score of 8 at the scene. He was intubated to protect his airway and is now being ventilated. Currently, he has a heart rate of 120 and a blood pressure of 80 systolic. He is receiving an NS bolus through two large-bore IVs. EMS indicates that he continues to have bleeding from an open perineal wound where he experienced blunt trauma from the hydraulic cylinder. The patient is in complete c-spine immobilization.

Multiple other members of the trauma team are ready and waiting when the patient arrives. The flight crew gives details of the mechanism of injury, findings at the scene, rescue issues, initial patient presentation, interventions, and response to interventions. The controlled chaos begins with rapid reassessment of the patient.

Airway: # 7.5 oral endotracheal tube, taped at 23 cm at the lip.

Breathing: No spontaneous respirations currently due to sedation and paralytics. He assists easily with bag-valve-device with clear bilateral breath sounds.

Circulation: Femoral pulse present but no radial pulse; patient is pale, cool, and diaphoretic. There is blood coming from under the patient's pelvic area. Two 16-gauge IVs are in the right hand and antecubital area, and the IV fluids are switched over to the rapid infuser for rapid flow and warming of the fluids to body temperature.

Disability: The patient is currently unresponsive due to paralytic and sedative medications but his pupils are both sluggishly reacting. His GCS score before medications was 8.

The patient looks young (late teens), and healthy, although he is very pale, cool, and diaphoretic. The patient is exposed, and a large bleeding perineal wound is noted and packed in an attempt to stop the bleeding. Simultaneously, the patient is placed on a cardiac monitor, noninvasive blood pressure monitoring, pulse oximetry, and EtCO$_2$ monitoring. A FAST is performed and is negative for intra-abdominal bleeding. The chest radiograph shows bilateral pulmonary contusions, and the pelvis film shows an open pelvic fracture. The patient also has fractures of the left humerus, radius, and femur. Those injuries are splinted, and the pelvis fracture is treated with compression via sheet stabilization.

The patient remained very unstable throughout his emergency resuscitation phase and was given multiple transfusions of O-negative blood. A rapid secondary exam reveals facial fractures but no additional injuries.

You are instructed to prepare to transport the patient to the OR for placement of an external fixator to stabilize his pelvic fracture. He remains unstable throughout the operative procedure to stabilize his pelvis and intramedullary rod placement for his femur fracture.

The ICU nurse receives the patient postoperatively and assesses the patient. He is still sedated, chemically paralyzed, intubated, ventilated, and continuing to receive blood products and crystalloid fluid resuscitation. He continues to bleed from the open perineal wound. The patient is transported to interventional radiology, where coils and Gelfoam® are used and successfully tamponade the bleeding of the branch of the iliac vessel that had continued to cause his blood loss. He returns to the ICU.

The patient remained critical for many days and experiences many complications associated with hemorrhagic shock with hypoperfusion at the tissue cellular level, including acute respiratory distress syndrome requiring ventilator support and positive end-expiratory pressure (PEEP); acute renal failure requiring dialysis; blood pressure support with fluids, blood products, and vasopressor drug therapy, pulmonary embolus treated with anticoagulants and a filter placement to catch the clots; and infection with septic shock treated with antibiotic, fluids, and vasopressor drug therapy. He underwent a diverting loop colostomy to prevent contamination to the perineal wound. He underwent five operative procedures aimed at stabilizing fractures, providing abdominal treatment, and cleaning out wounds. Through the first 48 hours of his hospitalization, he received more than 100 blood products.

After a month in the ICU with intense multidisciplinary care, the patient was transferred for a short stay on the stepdown unit. His acute hospital stay was followed by a month of rehabilitation for cognitive, occupational, and physical therapy. Today, this patient is married with a healthy baby boy, has graduated from college, and is a high school math/science teacher and an assistant football coach. The challenge of caring for critically injured patients requires attention to detail, sequential physical exams, cutting-edge technology, and astute caring healthcare providers working as a team toward a common goal.

CRITICAL THINKING QUESTIONS

1. Which disciplines should be consulted to work with this client?
2. What types of issues may require you to act as an advocate or moral agent for this patient?
3. How will you implement your role as a facilitator of learning for this patient?
4. Use the form to write up a plan of care for one client in the clinical setting who is a trauma patient. Rate the patient as a level 1, 3, or 5 on each characteristic. Identify the level of nurse characteristics needed in the care of this patient.
5. Take one outcome for a patient and list evidence-based interventions for this patient.

Using the Synergy Model to Develop a Plan of Care

	Patient Characteristics	Level (1, 3, 5)	Subjective and Objective Data	Evidence-based Interventions	Outcomes
SYNERGY MODEL	Resiliency				
	Vulnerability				
	Stability				
	Complexity				
	Resource availability				
	Participation in care				
	Participation in decision making				
	Predictability				

Online Resources

Coalition for American Trauma Care Washington Reports: http://204.3.196.9/CATC/coalition.html

Society of Trauma Nurses: www.traumanursesoc.org

Trauma.org: www.trauma.org

Trauma Practice Guidelines: www.east.org/tpg.html

World Health Organization, *Guidelines to Essential Trauma Care:*
http://whqlibdoc.who.int/publications/2004/9241546409.pdf

REFERENCES

American College of Surgeons. (2002). *National Trauma Data Bank Report.* Chicago: American College of Surgeons.

American College of Surgeons. (2004). Spine and spinal cord trauma. In *Advanced trauma life support for doctors. Student course manual* (pp. 178–203). Chicago: American College of Surgeons Committee on Trauma.

Blincoe, L. J., Seay, A., Zaloshnja, E., Miller, T. R., Romano, E. O., Lychter, S., & Spicer, R. S. (2002). *The Economic Impact of Motor Vehicle Crashes.* COT HS 809 446, Washington, DC: National Highway Traffic Safety Administration.

Brain Trauma Foundation, American Association of Neurological Surgeons, Joint Section on Neurotrauma and Critical Care. (2000). Hyperventilation. *Journal of Neurotrauma, 17,* 513–520.

Brown, C. V., Rhee, P., Chan, L., Evans, K., Demetriades, D., & Velmahos, G. C. (2004). Preventing renal failure in patients with rhabdomyolysis: Do bicarbonate and mannitol make a difference? *Journal of Trauma, 56,* 1191–1196.

Centers for Disease Control and Prevention. (2004). Traumatic Occupational Injuries. Available at www.cdc.gov/niosh/injury/traumamv.html

Dincer, H. W., & Lipchik, R. J. (2005). The intricacies of pneumothorax. Management depends on accurate classification. *Postgraduate Medicine Online.* Retrieved February 14, 2006, from www.postgradmed.com/issues/2005/12_05/dincer.htm

Emergency Nurses Association. (2000). *Trauma nursing core course provider manual* (5th ed.). Des Plaines, IL: Emergency Nurses Association.

Emergency Nurses Association. (2003). *Course in advanced trauma nursing II: A conceptual approach to injury and illness* (2nd ed.). Des Plaines, IL: Emergency Nurses Association.

Galler, D., Skinner, A., & Ng, A. (2005). Critical care considerations in trauma. Retrieved January 25, 2006, from www.emedicine.com/med/topic3218.htm#section~neurotrauma

Herzig, D., & Biffl, W. Z. (2005). Thoracic trauma. In M. P. Fink, E. Abraham, JL. Vincent, & P. M. Kochanek (Eds.), *Textbook of critical care* (5th ed., pp. 2077–2087). Philadelphia: Saunders.

Kaisti, K. K., Langsjo, J. W., Aalto, S., Oikonen, V., Sipila, H., Teres, M., et al. (2003). Effects of sevoflurane, propofol, and adjunct nitrous oxide on regional cerebral blood flow, oxygen consumption, and blood volume in humans. *Anesthesiology, 99*(3), 603–613.

Keough, V., & Pudelek, B. (2001). Blunt chest trauma: Review of selected pulmonary injuries focusing on pulmonary contusion. *AACN Clinical Issues, 12*(2), 270–281.

Khanna, S., Davis, D., Peterson, B., Fisher, B., Tung, H., O'Quigley, J., et al. (2000). Use of hypertonic saline in the treatment of severe refractory posttraumatic intracranial hypertension in pediatric traumatic brain injury. *Critical Care Medicine, 28,* 1144–1151.

Lapointe, L. A., & Von Rueden, K. T. (2002). Coagulopathies in trauma patients. *AACN Clinical Issues, 13*(2), 192–203.

Leske, J. S. (2003). Comparison of family stresses, strengths, and outcomes after trauma and surgery. *AACN Clinical Issues, 14*(1), 33–41.

Marik, P. E., Varon, J., & Trask, T. (2002). Management of head trauma. *Chest, 122*(2), 699–711.

McQuillan, K., Von Rueden, K., Hartsock, R., Flynn, M., & Whalen, E. (2002). *Trauma nursing: From resuscitation to rehabilitation* (3rd ed.). Philadelphia: Saunders.

McRoberts, R., McKenchnie, M., & Leigh-Smith, S. (2005). Tension pneumothorax and the forbidden CXR. *Emergency Medical Journal, 22,* 597–598.

Mechem, C. C. (2005). Intensive care unit management of the trauma patient. Retrieved January 25, 2006, from www.uptodate.com

Miller, R. S., Patton, M., Graham, R. M., & Hollins, D. (2000). Outcomes of trauma patients who survive prolonged lengths of stay in the intensive care unit. *Journal of Trauma: Injury, Infection, and Critical Care, 48*(2), 229–234.

Moore, E. E., Feliciano, D. V., & Mattox, K. L. (Eds.). (2004). *Trauma* (5th ed.). New York: McGraw-Hill.

Mueller, E. W., Hanes, S. D., Croce, M. A., Wood, G. C., Boucher, B. A., & Fabian, T. C. (2005). Effect from multiple episodes of inadequate empiric antibiotic therapy for ventilator-associated pneumonia on morbidity and mortality among critically ill trauma patients. *Journal of Trauma: Injury, Infection, and Critical Care, 58*(1), 94–101.

Nast-Kolb, D., Bail, H. J., & Taeger, G. (2005). Moderne diagnostik des bauchtraumas. *Der Chirurg, 76,*10, 919–926.

National Highway Traffic Administration Facts 2003. (2003). A compilation of motor vehicle crash data from the fatality analysis reporting system and the general estimates system. Retrieved February 14, 2006, from www.nhtsa.dot.gov

Neale, D. A. (2006). Blunt thoracic trauma. Retrieved February 14, 2006, from www.trauma.org/bluntthoracic.html

O'Carroll, B. M. (2000). *Principles of basic trauma nursing.* Brockton, MA: Western Schools.

Ong, A., Cohn, S., Cohn, K., Jaramillo, D., Parbhu, R., McKenney, M., et al. (2002). Unexpected findings in trauma patients dying in the intensive care unit: Results of 153 consecutive autopsies. *Journal of American College of Surgeons, 94*(8), 401–406.

Pudelek, B. (2002). Geriatric trauma: Special needs for a special population. *AACN Clinical Issues, 13*(1), 61–72.

Rafie, A. D., Rath, P. A., Michell, M. W., Kirschner, R. A., Deyo, D. J., Prough, D. S., et al. (2004). Hypotensive resuscitation of multiple hemorrhages using crystalloid and colloids. *Shock, 22*(3), 262–269.

Richards, C. F., & Mayberry, J. C. (2004). Initial management of the trauma patient. *Critical Care Ethics, 20*(1), 1–11.

Schiller, W. R., & Anderson, B. F. (2003). Family as a member of the trauma rounds: A strategy for maximized communication. *Journal of Trauma Nursing, 10*(4), 93–101.

Shepard, S. (2004). Head trauma. Retrieved August 29, 2006, from www.emedicine.com/med/topic2820.htm

Spinal Cord Injury Information Network. (2005). Spinal cord injury facts and figures at a glance June 2005. Retrieved February 13, 2006, from www.spinalcord.uab.edu/show.asp?durki=21446

Stannard, J. P., Lopez-Ben, R. R., Volgas, D. A., Anderson, E. R., Busbee, M., Karr, D. K., et al. (2006). Prophylaxis against deep-vein thrombosis following trauma: A prospective, randomized comparison of mechanical and pharmacologic prophylaxis. *Journal of Bone and Joint Surgery, 88*(2), 261–266.

Tsuei, B. J., & Kearney, P. A. (2004). Hypothermia in the trauma patient. *Injury, 35,* 7–15.

Wang, H. E., Callaway, C. W., Peitzman, A. B., & Tisherman, S. A. (2005) Admission hypothermia and outcome after major trauma. *Critical Care Medicine, 33,* 1296–1301.

Zenati, M. S., Billiar, T. R. Townsend, R. N., Peitzman, A. B., & Harbrecht, B. G. (2002). A brief episode of hypotension increases mortality in critically ill trauma patients . . . including discussion. *Journal of Trauma: Injury, Infection, and Critical Care, 53*(2), 232–237.

CHAPTER 56

Drug Overdose and Poisonings

Michael Neville   Roberta Kaplow

LEARNING OBJECTIVES

Upon completion of this chapter, the reader will be able to:

1. Describe the manifestations of selected overdoses or poisonings.

2. Describe the management of selected overdoses or poisonings.

3. List optimal patient outcomes that may be achieved through evidence-based management of patients experiencing a drug overdose or poisoning.

In 2002, poison control centers in the United States received 2.1 million calls related to accidental poisonings. The total number of cases of poisoning or overdose was 2,386,292 in that year (Anonymous, 2005a). This number does not account for all deaths that could possibly be attributed to poisoning or overdose. This chapter describes the management of selected poisonings or overdose.

ACETAMINOPHEN

Background

Acetaminophen (Tylenol®) is the most widely used analgesic worldwide. It is also a leading cause of overdose. More than 100,000 calls occur each year to poison control centers in the United States, and more hospitalizations are related to acetaminophen exposure than from any other widespread medication (Bizovi & Smilkstein, 2002). Acetaminophen toxicity is a burden on the healthcare system and contributes significantly to admission to the intensive care unit (ICU) and cost of hospitalization (Gyamlani & Parikh, 2002). When taken in amounts greater than are recommended, acetaminophen can be toxic to the liver and damage a person's DNA (Bender, Lindsey, Burden, & Osheroff, 2004). Hepatic failure from acetaminophen poisoning is the most common indication of liver transplantation in the United States and Europe (Pajoumand, Jalali, Abdollahi, & Shadnia, 2003).

Acetaminophen ingestion of 7.5 Gm or 150 mg/kg is considered the lowest amount capable of causing toxicity. This ingestion must take place within a four-hour period (Bizovi & Smilkstein, 2002). Approximately 5% to 15% of acetaminophen is oxidized and forms a toxic metabolite, N-acetyl-p-benzoquinone imine (NAPQI). When acetaminophen is taken in excess amounts, an increased amount is metabolized to this toxic metabolite. The toxicity of acetaminophen overdose is attributed to the excess production of NAPQI (Bender et al., 2004; Bizovi & Smilkstein). Acetaminophen can cause hepatic necrosis within 2 to 5 days of ingestion and renal tubular necrosis and failure within 14 days of ingestion (Amirzadeh & McCotter, 2002).

Clinical Manifestations

Manifestations of acetaminophen toxicity are described in phases. In phase I, which occurs 0.5 to 24 hours after ingestion, the patient usually reports anorexia, nausea, vomiting, and diaphoresis, and has pallor. In phase II (24 to 72 hours post ingestion), patients develop renal insufficiency, right upper quadrant pain, and elevated liver enzymes, international normalized ratio (INR), and bilirubin due to hepatic damage. Approximately 72 to 96 hours post ingestion, patients develop hepatic encephalopathy, coagulation defects, jaundice, renal failure, nausea, and vomiting. Hepatic encephalopathy progressing to coma is a main symptom of significant liver damage from acetaminophen overdose (Ala, Schiano, Burroughs, & Keshav, 2004). Hepatic failure is the main cause of death. Death can also occur from complications of multiple organ dysfunction syndrome (e.g., hemorrhage, acute respiratory distress syndrome, sepsis, and cerebral edema) (Bender et al., 2004). Renal dysfunction may occur in the absence of hepatic failure (von Mach et al., 2005). Other symptoms, including pancytopenia, metabolic acidosis, shock, hypothermia, hyperglycemia, and rhabdomyolysis, have been reported in a case study of a patient who ingested an unknown quantity of acetaminophen (Yang, Deng, & Lin, 2001).

Management

Following an overdose of acetaminophen, the greater part of absorption takes place after two hours. Levels usually peak within four hours (Bizovi & Smilkstein, 2002). The antidote for acetaminophen toxicity is oral N-acetylcysteine (NAC, Mucomyst®). One way NAC prevents liver damage is by stopping toxic metabolites from binding with protein molecules in liver cells (Hoffman & Gibel, 2005). Rapid administration of NAC is essential. The incidence of hepatotoxicity is low if NAC is administered within eight hours of ingestion, but thereafter increases incrementally for each hour that treatment is delayed (Amirzadeh & McCotter, 2002). The loading dose of NAC is 140 mg/kg; maintenance doses are 70 mg/kg every four hours for a total of 17 doses. The total amount of time the patient receives NAC is 72 hours (Kociancic & Reed, 2003). The doses are diluted to a 1:4 ratio with water, a carbonated beverage, or juice to make the medicine more palatable. The dose is repeated if the patient vomits within one hour of taking a dose. Antiemetics may be prescribed or a nasogastric tube inserted if vomiting persists (Bizovi & Smilkstein).

Shorter-duration therapy (e.g., 24 or 36 hours) has been suggested, but requires further evaluation (Kociancic & Reed, 2003). Researchers who conducted one study suggested that 72 hours of NAC may be too much in many cases of acetaminophen poisoning. They suggest that hepatic toxicity is preventable when intravenous (IV) administration of NAC is initiated within 8 to 10 hours after ingestion and continued for 20 hours (Yip & Dart, 2003). Intravenous NAC, however, has not been approved by the Food and Drug Administration (FDA). Therapy is considered complete when serum acetaminophen concentrations fall to less than 10 mcg/mL.

If the patient is in fulminate hepatic failure, if ingestion occurred more than eight hours earlier, or if the patient cannot tolerate oral dosing after a trial with antiemetics, intravenous NAC is preferred. However, only oral NAC has proven efficacy. Patients with severe hepatic toxicity or hepatic encephalopathy are admitted to the ICU for frequent neurological checks, monitoring of vital signs, and assessment of laboratory data. Consultation with a gastroenterologist and notification to the poison control center are completed. Patients should also undergo psychiatric evaluation to determine if they are eligible for transplant (Bizovi & Smilkstein, 2002).

AMPHETAMINE AND METHAMPHETAMINE

Background

Ma Huang (ephedrine), one of the earliest identified sympathomimetics (agents that "mimic" the sympathetic nervous system), has been used in folk medicines for thousands of years but was not formally identified until 1885 (Aaron, 1990). Amphetamine and methamphetamine, which are both synthetic sympathomimetics, were discovered in 1887 and 1914, respectively. Amphetamines continued to gain popularity and were prescribed for narcolepsy, exhaustion, weight loss, and fatigue during the early and mid-1900s.

In 2006, a wide variety of legal sympathomimetics [e.g., dextroamphetamine (Dexedrine®), methylphenidate (Ritalin®)] continue to be widely prescribed for the same indications. Conversely, methamphetamine ("speed," "crank," "ice," or "lemon drops") is considered an illicit substance and is responsible for the presentation of many who report to emergency departments (EDs) (Turnipseed, Richards, Kirk, Diercks, & Amsterdam, 2003). Although one study found that federal regulations had few effects on reducing the number of methamphetamine-related admissions, by July 2005 more than 40 states had placed restrictions on the sale of over-the-counter pseudoephedrine (Sudafed®), a medication that can be used to produce methamphetamine, in an effort to decrease its illegal production and consumption (Anderson, 2005).

Clinical Manifestations

When patients consume amphetamine and methamphetamine, they may experience a wide variety of pharmacologic effects. When exposed to sympathomimetics, the body increases the release of the endogenous sympathetic neurotransmitters, norepinephrine and epinephrine. Dopamine and serotonin are also released, but to a lesser extent (Rothman et al., 2001). These hormones have receptor targets located on numerous target organs and tissues, including the heart, blood vessels, lungs, and brain.

Central nervous system (CNS) and cardiovascular toxicities are commonly seen in those who present for care. Apprehension, confusion, agitation, hyperthermia, seizures, and coma exemplify CNS effects, whereas hypertension, tachydysrhythmias, and sinus tachycardia that result in chest pain, encephalopathy, and even myocardial ischemia characterize cardiovascular effects (Olson, 2004). Gastrointestinal toxicity that manifests as diarrhea, cramping, constipation, or mesenteric ischemia may also occur. Unfortunately, the pulmonary and renal systems may be affected as well. Pulmonary hypertension or infarcts and renal failure may occur (van Wolferen, Vonk, Boonstra, & Postmus, 2005).

Management

Adequate airway, breathing, and circulation (ABCs) must be established in patients who overdose on sympathetomimetics. IV lines are placed for rehydration and medication administration. A 12-lead electrocardiogram (ECG) is advised to detect rhythm disturbances—normal readings lower the likelihood of acute coronary syndrome. Sedation and cooling are also recommended (White, 2002). Serum chemistries are useful to detect electrolyte disturbances and the presence of rhabdomyolysis. Serum and urine toxicology screening reveals the presence of other drugs (Pittman, 2005).

Gastric lavage with activated charcoal (1 to 2 Gm/kg up to 90 Gm) given with sorbitol through a large-bore orogastric tube may be considered in patients who present within one to two hours of sympathomimetic consumption (Gussow, 2003a). Syrup of ipecac should be avoided, because sympathomimetic-induced emesis may precipitate seizures. Neither hemodialysis (not effective) nor urine acidification (may worsen rhabdomyolysis) is recommended to increase elimination of sympathomimetics (Olson, 2004).

Benzodiazepines [e.g., lorazepam (Ativan®) 2 to 6 mg IV] and neuroleptics [e.g., haloperidol (Haldol®) 5 mg IV] have been used to manage agitation (Gussow, 2003a). However, the use of neuroleptics for agitation management may exacerbate hyperthermia, another problem frequently seen in these patients (Gelander & Kleber, 2004). Hypertension can be managed with IV labetalol (Normadyne®; 10 to 20 mg every 10 minutes up to a maximum of 150 mg) until blood pressure is controlled (Pittman, 2005). Rhabdomyolysis (breakdown and release of

muscle fibers into the circulation, which can lead to renal failure) is managed with administration of fluids to maintain a urine output of 1 to 2 mL/min (Gussow).

Finally, a search of body cavities should be considered if there is a suspicion of "body stuffing" (ingesting or concealing substances to avoid police detection) of these agents (Norfolk, 2006).

BARBITURATES

Background

When malonylurea was discovered in 1863, it was named "barbituric acid" for Saint Barbara by its discoverer, Johan Adolf (Cozanitis, 2004). In the early 1900s, two scientists, Fischer and von Mering, were instrumental in having this chemical produced in mass quantities. Over the last century, multiple barbiturates have been produced and used for their hypnotic effects, anesthetic qualities, "truth serum effects," and anticonvulsant qualities.

A wide variety of barbiturates remain on the market today. They vary widely in their pharmacokinetic profiles as well as their FDA indications. Examples include thiopental sodium (Pentothal®), amobarbital (Amytal®), pentobarbital (Nembutal®), secobarbital (Seconal®), butalbital (Fiorinal/Fioricet®), butabarbital (Butisol®), and phenobarbital (Luminal®) (Anonymous, 2005b).

Clinical Manifestations

Patients in acute barbiturate overdose situations present with symptoms such as hypothermia, drowsiness, confusion, decreased or lost reflexes, shortness of breath, bradycardia, unusual movements of the eyes, and slurred speech (Anonymous, 2005c). Over time, these symptoms may progress to a shock syndrome (respiratory arrest, apnea, circulatory collapse, and death).

Healthcare providers may be confounded by the fact that extreme barbiturate overdoses can be associated with a "flat line" electroencephalogram (EEG) (no electrical brain activity), but this finding should not be interpreted as clinical brain death unless severe hypoxia occurs simultaneously (Anonymous, 2005c).

As with overdoses involving many substances discussed in this chapter, the unusual presentations of poisoning patients in EDs or ICUs may reflect the fact that multiple substances are involved. Because barbiturates and ethanol are both CNS depressants, their combination can increase the mortality risk (Lisanti, 1998).

Management

As with many overdose situations, supportive care is a cornerstone of treatment of barbiturate poisoning. Many patients will require standard procedures (ABCs, IV access, oxygen). Cardiac monitoring, administration of normal saline through a large-gauge needle, insertion of a urinary catheter to monitor output, nasogastric tube placement to sample gastric contents and administer medications, and obtaining toxicology screens are all important steps (Lisanti, 1998).

Absorption of barbiturates may be decreased by administration of syrup of ipecac if the patient is conscious and has an intact gag reflex. Activated charcoal (30 to 60 Gm given with sorbitol) is also effective in these patients. Gastric lavage and endotracheal intubation followed by a dose of activated charcoal may be considered in an unconscious patient after being placed in a face-down position. Saline laxative administration should be considered following this therapy (Anonymous, 2005c).

Forced diuresis and alkalinization of the urine are both measures that can be used to enhance elimination of these agents. Although hemodialysis and hemoperfusion are not recommended, they may be considered in patients with severe poisonings who develop anuria or who progress to shock (Anonymous, 2005c).

BENZODIAZEPINES

Background

Sedative hypnotics (also known as anxiolytics or tranquilizers) are used to produce a calming effect and minimize excitability. They may also be administered to stimulate drowsiness and sleep. Benzodiazepines are the most frequently prescribed of these sedatives. While anxiolysis and sedation are the two most common reasons that benzodiazepines are prescribed, temazepam (Restoril®) and triazolam (Halcion®) are prescribed for sleep. Death from benzodiazepine ingestion is rare unless these drugs are taken in combination with other agents (Lee, 2002). Alprazolam (Xanax®), however, is reportedly more toxic than other benzodiazepines when overdosed (Ibister, O'Regan, Sibbritt, & White, 2004).

All sedatives cause CNS depression. They generate this effect by enhancing function of the γ-aminobutyric acid (GABA) system. GABA inhibits neurotransmitter conduction in the CNS. Sedative hypnotic toxicity is related to these agents' effects on GABA receptors (Lee, 2002).

Clinical Manifestations

Patients who have experienced benzodiazepine overdose usually exhibit slurred speech, ataxia, and uncoordinated movements. Patients with moderate to severe overdose may be stuporous or comatose. Those with the most serious toxicity may lose all neurological response. The greater the CNS depression, the greater the chance for respiratory depression.

Respiratory depression is manifested as a decrease in tidal volume (the amount of gas exchange in each breath) and minute ventilation (the amount of gas exchange in one minute). Patients then develop a respiratory acidosis from hypoventilation. Respiratory compromise can lead to cardiovascular depression (Lee, 2002).

Management

Flumazenil (Romazicon®) is a benzodiazepine antagonist and an inhibitor of the GABA receptor. It therefore counteracts the effects of benzodiazepine overdose (Melo, Nogue, Trullas, Aguilo, & Maciel, 2004). The dose of flumazenil used for this purpose is 0.1 mg/min to a maximum of 1 mg. The duration of effect of flumazenil is shorter than the effect of most benzodiazepines, so repeat dosing may be required. Resedation may occur in 20 to 120 minutes (Howland, 2002). When a patient's other medical conditions may extend the half-life of a benzodiazepine, use of a continuous infusion of flumazenil may be indicated to prevent resedation and respiratory insufficiency (Maxa, Ogu, Adeeko, & Swaner, 2003).

Flumazenil administration may cause seizures or other withdrawal symptoms in patients who are tolerant to benzodiazepines. It does not reverse respiratory depression that might occur but will counteract CNS depression. Note that flumazenil may increase intracranial pressure if it is administered to patients who have previously received midazolam (Versed®) for severe head injury (Howland, 2002).

If the patient ingested a significant amount of sedatives, administration of activated charcoal is indicated. Patients will require admission to the ICU for 8 to 12 hours, maintenance of a patent airway, and adequate ventilation. Oxygen therapy should be provided, and implementation of measures to prevent aspiration is essential. The main cause of death from sedative hypnotic overdose, in general, is respiratory failure (Lee, 2002).

Hemodynamic instability usually ensues from respiratory compromise. Hypotension should be treated with volume resuscitation. Vasopressors may be required if volume repletion alone is inadequate to sustain blood pressure or if the patient develops signs of fluid overload (e.g., pulmonary edema). Most patients see improvement in their level of consciousness within 12 to 36 hours after a benzodiazepine overdose. Supportive care is the basis of treatment (Lee, 2002).

CARBON MONOXIDE

Background

Carbon monoxide (CO), a colorless, odorless, tasteless gas, is a leading cause of morbidity and mortality from poisoning in the United States. Approximately 10,000 people seek medical attention or lose time from work, and 5,600 people die from CO poisoning each year (Jaslow, Ufberg, Ukasik, & Sananman, 2001). Young children and elderly persons are among those victims killed most often in the United States by sitting in an idling automobile with an obstructed exhaust pipe. Others at risk for exposure include (1) individuals who live or work around gasoline engines or defective furnaces; (2) persons in the fire fighting, coal mining, and mechanic professions; and (3) those who smoke cigarettes, pipes, and cigars (McCance, 2005).

CO is dangerous because its affinity for hemoglobin is 300 times greater than that of oxygen (McCance, 2005). Deleterious consequences result from an impaired oxygen carrying capacity and decreased oxygen delivery to the tissues. Many victims develop increased lactic acid levels, increased myoglobin concentrations, and sharp rises in carboxyhemoglobin (COHb, hemoglobin bound to CO) as a sign of this exposure (Gussow, 2003b).

Clinical Manifestations

Patients who present with CO poisoning often have a myriad of symptoms that affect the cardiovascular (chest pain, dysrhythmias, palpitations), ophthalmologic (blurred vision, retinal hemorrhage), respiratory (tachypnea, dyspnea, respiratory alkalosis), central nervous (dizziness, confusion, headache, ataxia), gastrointestinal (nausea, vomiting), and metabolic (lactic acidosis, rhabdomyolysis) systems (Gussow, 2003b).

Management

ABCs, placement of an IV line, and administration of 100% oxygen (through a mask or endotracheal tube) are all crucial measures in case of CO poisoning (Gussow, 2003b). Continuous monitoring of COHb levels until they fall below 5% to 10%—rather than pulse oximetry measurements—is suggested. Pulse oximetry may read COHb as oxyhemoglobin (oxyHb) and lull the healthcare provider into a false sense of security related to the patient's oxygenation status (Gussow). Oxygen administration is even more critical in the pregnant patient because fetal COHb is 10% to 15% greater than maternal levels; clinicians should be even more aggressive with oxygen treatment in this population.

The rate of conversion of COHb to oxyHb depends on the concentration of oxygen and the atmospheric pressure. The half-life of COHb is about 270 minutes on room air, 90 minutes with 100% normobaric oxygen, and 20 minutes with hyperbaric oxygen (Gussow, 2003b; Mak, Kam, Lai, & Tang, 2000). Indications for hyperbaric oxygen in one London hospital were reported in the literature as follows: (1) loss of consciousness, cognitive, or neurological abnormalities; (2) ECG

evidence of ischemia in the cardiac tissues; (3) COHb >20%; or (4) pregnancy (Mak et al.).

Although some animal data suggest that hyperbaric oxygen therapy can reduce CO-associated mortality and prevent cognitive dysfunction, data are inconclusive as to whether oxygen (even hyperbaric) can prevent the delayed neurological injuries noted with this type of poisoning (Gilmer, Kilkenny, Tomaszewski, & Watts, 2002).

COCAINE

Background

Use of recreational drugs continues to increase (Broderick, 2003). Cocaine is one of the most widely available drugs of abuse. Several million people are believed to be occasional or regular users of cocaine. This widespread use has made toxicity more prevalent (Finnell & Harris, 2000). Cocaine can be sniffed, inhaled (smoked), or intravenously injected. It may also be combined with heroin and injected. Crack is a freebase form of cocaine that is produced by combining it with sodium bicarbonate to create an alkaline aqueous solution, which is then dried (Olson, 2004). The onset of action for cocaine ranges from 3 seconds to 5 minutes, depending on the route of administration. The effects of cocaine last 5 to 90 minutes (Mouhaffel, Madu, Satmary, & Fraker, 1995).

Cocaine acts as a CNS stimulant and inhibits the reuptake of catecholamines (e.g., norepinephrine and dopamine), which results in sympathetic stimulation. The toxic dose of cocaine depends on tolerance of the user, route of administration, and concomitant use of other drugs. Intake of more than 1 Gm of cocaine is probably fatal (Finnell & Harris, 2000).

Clinical Manifestations

Several body systems are affected by the intake of cocaine. CNS toxicity may become manifest within minutes of smoking or IV intake, or the effect may be delayed for up to one hour. Users experience an initial sense of euphoria or "high." This effect is especially prevalent in users who smoke cocaine, as this method allows large doses to reach the brain quickly. The euphoria from snorting cocaine may last 15 to 30 minutes, but only 5 to 10 minutes if the drug is smoked (National Institute on Drug Abuse, 2006). The euphoria may precede anxiety, agitation, delirium, psychosis, tremors, muscle rigidity, hyperactivity, or seizures. The seizures are usually short and stop without intervention (Middleton, 2004).

Numerous cardiac effects are likely following cocaine intake, with these effects being mediated by overactivity of the sympathetic nervous system. Chest pain is the most common complaint in the ED, with a reported 6% of these patients experiencing a myocardial infarction (MI) (Weber et al., 2000).

Cocaine overdose will cause a discernible increase in blood pressure, heart rate, and, therefore, myocardial oxygen demand. Coronary vessels constrict, and the resulting hypertension can lead to hemorrhagic stroke or aortic dissection. The increased demand for oxygen by the heart in the face of decreased supply leads to myocardial ischemia, which in turn can cause MI, dysrhythmias, and acute pulmonary edema. Lethal cardiac arrhythmias include tachyarrhythmias, ventricular tachycardia, ventricular fibrillation, or heart block. Coronary artery spasm and/or thrombosis may lead to MI. Shock may be caused by myocardial, intestinal, or brain infarction; hyperthermia; or hypovolemia. The user may also develop chest pain, which may suggest MI but is more likely related to rhabdomyolysis (Finnell & Harris, 2000). In addition, users of cocaine may develop infective endocarditis, myocarditis, or cardiomyopathy (Finnell & Harris).

High doses of cocaine may cause hyperventilation or respiratory arrest. Renal failure may be a consequence of shock or renal artery spasm (Gitman & Singhal, 2004).

Management

Seizures and death are the more significant toxic consequences related to cocaine overdose (Macedo et al., 2004). The most essential initial intervention for a patient with cocaine overdose is maintaining patency of the airway and, if necessary, assisting with ventilation. No specific antidote for cocaine is available. Emergent treatment may include administration of activated charcoal if cocaine was ingested. Inducing vomiting is not recommended due to the possibility of seizure activity.

Treatment should also be directed at decreasing the sympathomimetic effects of cocaine. This goal may be accomplished with the administration of diazepam (Valium®) 5 mg IV every 5 minutes to a maximum dose of 20 mg, which should lower sympathomimetic effects. Lorazepam (Ativan®) 2 mg IV per minute to a maximum dose of 8 to 10 mg may be considered as an alternative (Finnell & Harris, 2000).

Propranolol (Inderal®) was recommended as a cocaine antidote in the past. However, because this drug may exacerbate cocaine-associated hypertension, its use is no longer recommended. If the possibility exists that the patient has coronary artery spasms, admission to the ICU is advised for continuous monitoring of vital signs, dysrhythmias, and electrocardiographic changes. Nitrates or calcium channel blockers may be used to treat chest pain. Tachyarrhythmias may be treated with propranol (Inderal®) 0.01 to 0.03 mg/kg IV or esmolol (Brevibloc®) 25 to 100 mcg/kg/min IV. For supraventricular tachycardia, sedation with administration of benzodiazepine and oxygen is usually adequate. If this measure is not successful, rapid IV administration of 6 mg adenosine (Adenocard®) is advised, followed by 12 mg and then another 12 mg if necessary. Labetalol (Trandate®) 2 mg/min or 20 mg can be administered intravenously initially, followed by 20 to 80 mg every 10 to 15 minutes to a maximum dose of 300 mg. Ventricular fibrillation or pulseless ventricular tachycardia should be treated with defibrillation, cardiopulmonary resuscitation, and antiarrhythmic therapy. Lidocaine must be used with caution because of the potential for increased cocaine toxicity when these two substances are used together. Sedation may be effective in cases of stable ventricular tachycardia. Labetalol given according to the previously described regimen may also be tried. Heart block may be treated with either atropine sulfate or pacemaker. Seizures may be controlled with any of the benzodiazepines, phenobarbital (Luminal®), or phenytoin (Dilantin®) (Finnell & Harris, 2000).

Patients with chest pain should receive oxygen, aspirin, and a benzodiazepine. If chest pain persists, sublingual nitroglycerin (0.4 mg) or nitropaste (Nitro-Bid® ointment) (1 inch) may be used, followed by an infusion that is titrated until the pain resolves. Morphine sulfate may be needed to alleviate the chest discomfort. In patients with suspected cocaine-induced chest pain, a 12-hour observation period is reasonable (Finnell & Harris, 2000), because these patients may still develop dysrhythmias or MI (National Institute on Drug Abuse, 2006).

Initial management of hypertension should consist of sedation and oxygen. If the patient shows limited or no response, an infusion of nitroprusside (Nipride®) at a rate of 0.5 to 10 mcg/kg/min or phentolamine (Regitine®) 5 mg IV is recommended (Finnell & Harris, 2000).

CYANIDE

Background

Before the eighteenth century, cyanide had not been specifically identified but was nevertheless extracted from bitter almonds and used by the Greeks and Romans to poison their enemies (Brueske, 1997). Since that time, cyanide has gained much notoriety as a poison and has been used to kill both individuals and entire populations (Cummings, 2004; Gracia & Shepherd, 2004). One of the most infamous incidents of mass suicide with this agent occurred in the 1980s, when more than 900 individuals in Jonestown, Guyana, were killed after drinking beverages that contained the poison (Brueske).

Accidental cyanide poisoning occurs most commonly in Western countries when victims are exposed during residential house fires and industrial accidents when burning plastics release cyanide compounds into the air (Megarbane, Delahaye, Goldgran-Toledano, & Baud, 2003). Victim exposure may also occur during suicide attempts, terrorist attacks, rodent extermination, occupational injuries (nylon manufacturing, Plexiglass, and electroplating), or dietary consumption (bitter almonds, cherry laurel, cassava) (Cummings, 2004).

Cyanide causes injury by binding to and disabling an important cellular enzyme, cytochrome oxidase, which is crucial for normal cellular respiration. Although the body can metabolize cyanide to a certain extent, necessary metabolic substrates (e.g., sulfur donors) eventually become depleted and cellular hypoxia results (Cummings, 2004; Gracia & Shepherd, 2004).

Clinical Manifestations

Although exposure to high levels of cyanide may cause death within minutes, clinicians may be baffled by the initial symptoms, which may masquerade as anxiety (Gracia & Shepherd, 2004). Early stages of cyanide toxicity are often exemplified by restlessness, confusion, shortness of breath, tachypnea, tachycardia, and nausea. With continued cellular hypoxia, mydriasis, seizures, dysrhythmias, apnea, cardiac arrest, and death may occur (Brueske, 1997).

Elevated serum lactate levels are one of the most common laboratory signs in these patients. As cellular hypoxia shifts from aerobic to anaerobic metabolism, the accumulation of lactic acid results in an anion gap metabolic acidosis (Gracia & Shepherd, 2004). Cellular mitochondria lose their ability to use arterial oxygen, and supranormal concentrations of oxygen in venous blood occur. Their presence indicates that the tissues are not taking up (extracting) oxygen effectively. What may baffle clinicians is the fact that pulse oximetry measurements will show higher than normal oxygenation in the patient. Oxygen saturation of the blood is not the issue, but rather the use of oxygen by the tissues. During the physical examination, the clinician may see clear evidence of this during funduscopic examination—the arterioles and venules will have the same red color (Gracia & Shepherd).

Management

History of exposure to cyanide is often unavailable to healthcare workers, and serum cyanide levels may not become available for hours or even days (Gracia & Shepherd, 2004). This lack of information is alarming because the detrimental effects of cyanide occur rapidly.

Healthcare workers should exercise great caution when caring for these patients. Cyanide-soaked clothing, skin, or emesis from the victim may be absorbed by the care provider either through direct contact or through aerosolization of cyanide from these sources. To minimize exposure, caregivers should wear personal protective equipment, including gloves, gown, and a face mask, and work in a well-ventilated area (Brueske, 1997).

Based on the evidence, oxygen administration may seem counterintuitive in case of cyanide poisoning. In fact, oxygen administration may serve two useful purposes: It may decrease cyanide's harmful metabolic effects and it may potentiate the beneficial effects of antidotes (Brueske, 1997).

Cyanide absorption from the gastrointestinal tract is often rapid and complete. Gastric decontamination through orogastric lavage and administration of activated charcoal are reasonable steps if the treatment begins within one hour of cyanide exposure (Gracia & Shepherd, 2004). They have limited value if their administration is delayed, however. There is international disagreement about which antidotes are most appropriate to manage cyanide toxicity (Cummings, 2004). Mild poisonings may be effectively managed with rest, oxygen, and inhaled amyl nitrite (Donoghue, 2003). Amyl nitrite pearls can be crushed, placed in a cloth (or inside the rim of a bag-valve-mask device), and waved in front of the patient's mouth for 15 to 30 seconds every 3 minutes in those with no IV access.

More severe cases require IV administration of sodium nitrite 3% 300 mg given in 10 mL of sterile water over 4 to 10 minutes (2.5 mL/min). Nitrites may increase methemoglobin levels (methemoglobinemias) and reduce the oxygen and CO_2 carrying capacity of red blood cells. Methylene blue may be administered parenterally if methemoglobin levels reach critical levels. Sodium thiosulfate, which aids in renal administration of cyanide metabolites, is also administered (12.5 Gm in 50 mL of sterile water over 10 minutes) immediately following nitrites and may be repeated in 2 hours if the patient has not improved (Brueske, 1997). A cyanide antidote kit that contains all of the necessary medications (amyl and sodium nitrite and sodium thiosulfate) is available.

METHANOL

Background

Methanol (wood alcohol) is a common component of many compounds, including windshield washer fluid and paint remover. It is occasionally ingested as a substitute for ethanol by people with alcoholism. Methanol is metabolized to formaldehyde and then to formic acid (formate). A fatal dose is approximately 30 to 240 mL (20 to 150 Gm). Blood levels greater than 20 mg/dL are considered toxic, and levels exceeding 40 mg/dL are very serious (Olson, 2004).

Clinical Manifestations

In the first few hours following ingestion of methanol, patients appear inebriated and report gastritis. Systemic acidosis would not be present at this time because metabolism has not yet occurred. Patients may also develop acute renal insufficiency in the early stages of methanol poisoning. The metabolic effects of methanol can lead to development of a metabolic acidosis, visual disturbances or blindness, coma, and death approximately 30 hours following ingestion (Verhelst et al., 2004). Other symptoms include headache, tachycardia, hypotension, CNS depression, seizures, dizziness, hypothermia, abdominal pain, anorexia, gastritis, nausea, vomiting, pancreatitis, blurred vision, mydriasis, respiratory depression, and hyperventilation (Olson, 2004).

Management

The most essential initial intervention for a patient with methanol overdose is maintaining patency of the airway and, if necessary, assisting with ventilation. Emergency management includes gastric lavage. Activated charcoal does not absorb methanol and, therefore, is not recommended. Vomiting should not be induced. Administration of fomepizole (4-MP, Antizol®) blocks methanol metabolism, thereby preventing the formation of toxic metabolites. Ethanol infusions have been used for the same effect. Folic acid 50 mg IV every four hours may promote the conversion of formate to carbon dioxide and water. If a metabolic acidosis exists, it should be treated with sodium bicarbonate. Hemodialysis, which removes methanol and formate, may be considered in patients with a severe metabolic acidosis or a methanol level greater than 40 mg/dL (Olson, 2004).

OPIATES

Background

Opioids are widely used analgesics. If taken appropriately, they are safe and effective. An overdose, however, can cause coma and life-threatening respiratory depression (Williams & Erikson, 2000). Opioids have several clinical effects. Although the primary effect is analgesia, the secondary effect of euphoria is likely to lead to abuse. Euphoria is mediated by release of dopamine. Whereas some opioids cause euphoria (e.g., heroin), others do not (e.g., morphine sulfate) (Nelson, 2002). Extreme dosages of opioids, regardless of the intent, can lead to significant morbidity and mortality.

Clinical Manifestations

Large doses of opioids can produce serious toxicity. Respiratory depression is an expected effect. Other problems may include a decreased level of consciousness, hypoventilation, miosis, and decreased bowel motility (Olson, 2004).

Respiratory depression may be manifested as a decrease in respiratory rate or tidal volume. This outcome is the result of either a decreased sensitivity to high levels of carbon dioxide or a decreased ventilatory response to hypoxia. If there is no stimulus to breathe, the patient will become apneic.

Several minutes to hours after they awake from an opioid coma or following administration of an opioid antagonist, patients may develop signs of pulmonary edema (hypoxia, crackles, and pink frothy sputum). Pulmonary edema is likely to occur following a heroin overdose (Mabry, Greller, & Nelson, 2003).

Opioids cause arteriolar and venous dilation, which may in turn lead to hypotension. Orthostatic changes in heart rate and blood pressure may occur. The decrease in heart rate may be attributed to decreased CNS stimulation; hypotension is due to release of histamine. Opioids have different ability to release histamine—for example, meperidine (Demerol®) causes the greatest release of histamine, and fentanyl (Sublimaze®) causes the least (Nelson, 2002). Propoxyphene (Darvon®) can instigate wide-complex dysrhythmias and a decrease in contractility (Nelson).

Miosis is due to stimulation of the parasympathetic neurons, which will cause constriction of pupils. Morphine sulfate also increases pupil response to light. In contrast, meperidine and propoxyphene usually do not affect pupil size (Nelson, 2002).

In acute opioid overdose, the patient may develop seizures, most likely as a result of hypoxia. Other subtle but common symptoms of opioid toxicity include hypoglycemia, hypoxia, and hypothermia (Nelson, 2002; Williams & Erikson, 2000).

Management

The most concerning effects of opioid overdose are CNS and respiratory depression. The patient's oxygenation and ventilatory status require support. In particular, an opioid antagonist, naloxone (Narcan®), should be administered. Naloxone works by preventing the binding of opioid agonists to the opioid receptors, thereby promoting spontaneous breathing. The lowest possible dose of this agent should be given so that opioid withdrawal can be avoided. Most patients improve with 0.05 mg IV, with the usual initial dose ranging from 0.4 to 2 mg. The dose can be repeated every two to three minutes up to a total of 10 mg (Anonymous, 2005d; Nelson, 2002). Given that the half-life of naloxone is shorter than that of many of the opioids whose effects it reverses, a rebound effect is likely and further dosing will be required. Patients who overdosed on long-acting opioids [e.g., methadone (Dolophine®)] may require a continuous infusion of naloxone to ensure that they continue to breathe. The infusion rate may either be 0.4 mg/hr or two-thirds of the initial dose that reversed the respiratory depression (Anonymous; Nelson). All patients with opioid overdose require frequent assessment of their respiratory status. If the respiratory depression is not reversed by the management measures described here, intubation is required (Nelson).

Adverse effects of naloxone administration have been reported. In one study of patients who overdosed on heroin, for example, the most common adverse effects were related to opioid withdrawal (e.g., gastrointestinal disorders, aggressiveness, tachycardia, shivering, sweating and tremors). Confusion and restlessness were observed and were attributed to opioid withdrawal or to the effect of the heroin in combination with other drugs. Headache and seizures were attributed to hypoxia. Most events in this study were not serious (Buajordet, Naess, Jacobsen, & Brors, 2004).

Data suggest that naloxone may also potentiate normeperidine-induced seizures (Nelson, 2002). Normeperidine is a toxic hepatic metabolite of chronic meperidine (Demerol®).

Patients who developed extreme hypoventilation or hypoxia following opioid overdose are at risk of developing acute lung injury or post-hypoxic encephalopathy. These patients require observation for more than 24 hours (Nelson, 2002). Psychosocial intervention is required for all patients with intentional opioid overdose (Nelson).

SALICYLATES

Background

Aspirin (acetylsalicylic acid) is widely available without a prescription. Although self-poisoning is rare, if it is extreme, salicylate overdose is potentially life-threatening (Wood, Dargan, & Jones, 2005; Wrathall, Sinclari, Moore, & Pogson, 2001). Acetylsalicylate is the active ingredient in aspirin. The effects of salicylic acid and acetylsalicylate on cardiac mitochondrial function may contribute to the toxicity associated with salicylate overdose (Nulton-Persson, Szweda, & Sadek, 2004).

In case of a salicylate overdose, serum levels may not be reached for four to six hours. Salicylates have a longer half-life when they are at toxic levels: When salicylate levels increase,

40% of the elimination pathways become saturated and elimination patterns change. Levels in excess of 30 mg/dL usually accompany signs and symptoms of toxicity (Flomenbaum, 2002).

Clinical Manifestations

Salicylates stimulate the respiratory center in the brainstem, which in turn promotes hyperventilation and a respiratory alkalosis. **Table 56-1** lists manifestations of salicylate overdose. Impaired renal function may develop due to the accumulation of acid. The combination of a metabolic acidosis and respiratory alkalosis is not due to any compensatory mechanisms, however, but rather to a mixed acid–base disturbance. This mixed picture is usually seen with salicylate levels exceeding 40 mg/dL. Salicylates also interfere with the Krebs cycle, which will limit the production of adenosine triphosphate (ATP). The result of this disruption is accumulation of lactic acid and generation of excessive amounts of heat (Flomenbaum, 2002).

The first signs of salicylate overdose are nausea and vomiting, diaphoresis, and tinnitus. As salicylate levels continue to increase, decreased auditory acuity replaces tinnitus. Other early symptoms may include vertigo, hallucinations, hyperventilation, hyperactivity, seizures, lethargy, and stupor (Flomenbaum, 2002).

TABLE 56-1 Clinical Manifestations of Salicylate Overdose

System	Associated Symptoms
Acid–base imbalance/metabolic	Metabolic acidosis, respiratory alkalosis, hypernatremia or hyponatremia, hypokalemia, hyperthermia. Presence of a respiratory acidosis indicates a poor patient prognosis.
CNS	Tinnitus, hallucinations, vertigo, agitation, hyperactivity, delirium, stupor, coma, lethargy, seizures, cerebral edema, syndrome of inappropriate secretion of antidiuretic hormone, decreased glucose levels in cerebrospinal fluid.
Pulmonary	Deep or rapid breathing, acute lung injury, pulmonary edema.
Renal	Tubular damage, proteinuria, sodium and water retention, hyperuricemia or hypouricemia, impaired renal function.
Hepatic/gastrointestinal	Decreased liver enzymes, altered glucose metabolism, nausea, vomiting, hemorrhagic gastritis, decreased GI motility.
Coagulation	Decreased prothrombin levels; inhibition of coagulation factors V, VII, and X; platelet dysfunction.
Cardiovascular	Hypotension, tachycardia, heart failure.
Other	Diaphoresis, extreme fatigue.

Source: Flomenbaum, 2002, p. 511.

Hypokalemia is a frequent consequence of salicylate poisoning. It results from movement of potassium into the cell in exchange for hydrogen ions generated by alkalosis, potassium loss in the urine, and vomiting (Flomenbaum, 2002).

Management

Initial management of salicylate overdose is administration of activated charcoal. Multiple dosing has been suggested but remains controversial (Flomenbaum, 2002). Volume repletion will be required due to the fluid losses from tachypnea, vomiting, hyperthermia, and diaphoresis. In addition, the kidneys respond to salicylate overdose by eliminating bicarbonate, sodium, and potassium (Flomenbaum).

Since salicylates are weak acids, alkalinization of blood and urine will increase their excretion and prevent salicylates from reaching the brain. Alkalinization is accomplished with the administration of sodium bicarbonate 1 to 2 mEq/kg IV bolus, followed by addition of 132 mEq to each liter of intravenous fluid. These fluids should infuse at 1.5 to 2 times the maintenance fluid range, with fluid replacement being initiated when salicylate levels exceed 35 mg/dL. Urinary pH should be maintained in the range of 7.5 to 8 (Flomenbaum, 2002).

Hemodialysis may be considered if the patient cannot tolerate sodium bicarbonate administration; if renal failure, acute lung injury, hepatic compromise with coagulation defects, extreme acid–base or electrolyte imbalance, or heart failure is present; if there is progressive decline in vital signs; or if salicylate levels are greater than 100 mg/dL (Flomenbaum, 2002). Use of continuous renal replacement therapies—specifically, continuous venovenous hemodiafiltration—may be effective as well (Wrathall et al., 2001). All patients who ingested significant amounts of salicylates require frequent monitoring of arterial blood gas (ABG) results; a discussion of ABG interpretation appears in Chapter 21. Arterial pH should be maintained at less than 7.55 to avoid the consequences of an alkalosis (i.e., hemoglobin having a higher affinity for oxygen) (Flomenbaum).

TRICYCLIC ANTIDEPRESSANTS

Background

Tricyclic antidepressants (TCAs) were originally developed for the sedative properties and were used to manage patients with agitation and psychosis (Liebelt & Francis, 2002). By the 1960s and into the late 1980s, TCAs were recognized as the primary medication class to treat depressive disorders. Their beneficial therapeutic effects on depressive illness were offset by their toxicity, however. The toxic profile of TCAs motivated the development of newer agents (e.g., tetracyclics and dibenzoxap-

ines) with wider therapeutic indices (Liebelt & Francis). Although TCAs have been replaced by even newer, less toxic antidepressants [e.g., selective serotonin reuptake inhibitors, such as fluoxetine (Prozac®)], they continue to be widely prescribed for other illnesses, including chronic pain conditions, attention deficit hyperactivity disorder, and obsessive-compulsive disorder (Liebelt & Francis).

In the 1980s, TCAs consistently ranked high among agents involved in fatal overdose situations (Cantilena, 2001). One study reported 5.52 deaths per 100,000 prescriptions of TCAs (Reith, Fountain, Tilyard, & McDowell, 2003). What makes these agents so toxic? The myriad of pharmacologic properties—alpha$_1$-antiadrenergic action, adrenergic reuptake inhibition, fast sodium channel blockade, and anticholinergic action—that all characterize TCAs is most likely responsible (Thanacoody & Thomas, 2005; Vieweg & Wood, 2004).

Clinical Manifestations

Clinical presentations of patients with TCA toxicity may vary substantially and pose great challenges for healthcare providers. A majority of those individuals who present will exhibit sedation or other anticholinergic side effects [e.g., mydriasis (pupil dilation)] and will recover with supportive care (Bailey, Buckley, & Amre, 2004). Pharmacodynamic (e.g., receptor binding and channel-mediated) differences between agents, coupled with the pharmacokinetic variations (e.g., metabolism and clearance) of patients who consume them, may complicate matters further (Bailey et al.).

Cardiovascular complications are commonplace in cases of TCA poisoning. Mild ECG changes occur in as many as 20% of patients who are taking therapeutic doses (Singh & Singh, 2002). Ventricular dysrhythmias, which occur most often in patients with wide QRS complexes, are often fatal. Coexistent acidosis, hypoxia, hyperthermia, and concurrent beta-agonist therapy further amplify this probability (Liebelt & Francis, 2002). Hypotension frequently makes the cardiovascular picture even more complex and may prove refractory to conventional treatments.

Generalized seizures, which typically transpire in the first two hours after overdose, occur in approximately 4% of overdose situations and in approximately 13% of fatal cases of TCA overdose (Liebelt & Francis, 2002). Early nervous system manifestations, such as hallucinations, psychosis, delirium, and disorientation, may eventually give way to lethargy, obtundation, and, coma (Liebelt & Francis). In an attempt to predict which patients might develop seizures in TCA overdose situations, Bailey and colleagues (2004) examined 18 clinical trials and noted that elevated TCA concentrations and ECG changes were highly correlated.

Management

Supportive care and treatment with sodium bicarbonate are considered first-line treatment options in patients with TCA overdoses. Cardiac monitoring and ECG evaluation are critical and should be coupled with ABG and laboratory assessments of glucose and electrolytes in all individuals with an altered mental status (Liebelt & Francis, 2002).

Wide QRS complexes call for alkalinization with sodium bicarbonate. Repeat boluses of one ampule and maintenance infusions have been used when necessary.

INITIAL NURSING MANAGEMENT

As described in this chapter, the clinical manifestations of drug overdose and poisonings vary widely and are based on the agents ingested and the individual's response to them. In addition to neutralizing and promoting elimination of the ingested agent, ongoing patient assessment is a required part of caregiving in such cases. Initial assessment entails focus on the ABCs, neurological status, and safety status (Poor, 2000).

Airway assessment and management includes insertion of a nasal airway. Oral airway insertion is not recommended due to the high risk of vomiting. If the patient is semiconscious or unconscious, positioning on the left side in reverse Trendelenburg position to help prevent aspiration is suggested. If the patient vomits, this position will allow the vomitus to drain rather than to be aspirated (Poor, 2000).

Insertion of an endotracheal tube and initiation of mechanical ventilation may be required in some patients—namely, those who have an inadequate respiratory effort, are comatose, have a decreased or absent gag reflex, are in status epilepticus, or have ingested a substance that causes rapid deterioration. Post-intubation nursing assessment includes verification of tube placement with a colorometric device, auscultation to check for equal and bilateral breath sounds, monitoring of oxygen saturation by pulse oximetry and carbon dioxide level with end-tidal CO_2 monitoring, ensuring that a chest radiograph is obtained to verify tube placement, and ABG analysis (Poor, 2000).

Circulation assessment entails observing for cardiac dysrhythmias, hypotension, or hypertension. Poisoning/overdose agents have variable hemodynamic effects that require ongoing monitoring (Poor, 2000).

Patients who have overdosed or ingested a toxic substance require monitoring of their neurological status. Initial management of a patient with a decreased level of consciousness includes administration of naloxone (to reverse opioids) and thiamine (vitamin B_1, if the patient is in an alcohol-induced coma). Determination of the patient's blood sugar can be made with a bedside glucometer. If the patient experiences seizure activity, it can be managed with diazepam (Valium®), phenytoin (Dilantin®), or phenobarbital (Luminal®) (Poor, 2000).

Another essential component of the ongoing nursing assessment focuses on patient safety. Patients may require frequent orientation, especially if they are hallucinating or are agitated. Administration of haloperidol (Haldol®) or a benzodiazepine is suggested for patients who are deemed at risk for self-injury. Propofol (Diprivan®) is recommended if the patient is intubated. Once patients have regained consciousness, they must be assessed for suicidal ideation. Until the patient has been cleared by a member of the psychiatric department as not being at risk, the nurse is responsible for maintaining suicide precautions and close monitoring to ensure that the environment is safe for the patient. As a consequence, the nurse may need to remove any potentially harmful equipment, devices, or items that could be utilized for self-suffocation (e.g., pillow cases). All patient personal items will need to be examined and documented as returned to the family if family is present. No medications should be left at the patient's bedside. IV pumps should be locked to prevent patients from changing the rate and placed at a distance to prevent the utilization of the IV tubing for self-strangulation. Patients should be placed within viewing of the nurse's station to facilitate frequent observation. These suicide precautions should be maintained according to institutional policy, and in collaboration with members of the psychiatry department to determine whether the patient is a risk to self is essential (Poor, 2000).

PATIENT OUTCOMES

Nurses can help ensure attainment of optimal patient outcomes such as those listed in **Box 56-1** through the use of evidence-based interventions for patients experiencing poisoning or drug overdose.

Box 56-1
Optimal Patient Outcomes

- Oxygen saturation in expected range
- Vital signs in expected range
- Modified lifestyle present
- Physical comfort in expected range
- Sleep patterns in expected range
- Perception that health is a high priority in making lifestyle changes
- Uses effective coping strategies
- Cognitive status in expected range

SUMMARY

Overdose, regardless of the substance, can cause serious or life-threatening effects that can result in admission to the ICU. Correct identification of the substance followed by emergent management is essential to optimize patient outcomes. Considerable morbidity and mortality may result if patients are not managed effectively. **Table 56-2** lists emergency measures to counteract some of the more common overdoses.

TABLE 56-2 Select Poisonings and Emergency Management

Agent	Activated Charcoal (AC)?	Induced Vomiting?	Antidote?	Gastric Emptying?	Enhanced Elimination?
Acetaminophen	Yes, if less than 3–4 hours since ingestion unless delayed absorption is suspected		N-acetylcysteine	Not necessary if AC is given promptly	Hemoperfusion, but usually not necessary since antidote is effective
Amantadine	Yes	No	None	Not necessary if AC is given promptly	
Ammonia	No	No	None	Gastric lavage	No role
Amphetamines	Yes	No	None	Not necessary if AC is given promptly	Not effective
Anesthetics, local	Yes	No	None	Gastric lavage if recent ingestion	May be effective if massive overdose
Antiarrhythmics	Yes		Type Ia or Ic, prolonged QRS, bradyarrhythmias, or hypotension: $NaHCO_3$ 1–2 mEq/kg IV	Gastric lavage if large ingestion	Not effective
Antibiotics: Trimethoprim (Bactrim®)	Yes	No	Leukovorin (folinic acid)	Not necessary if AC is given promptly	Maintain adequate urine flow
Anticholinergics	Yes		Physostigmine (Antilirium®) 0.5–1 mg IV if severe toxicity	Not necessary if AC is given promptly	Not effective
Antidepressants (noncyclic)	Yes		If suspect serotonin syndrome, methysergide (Sansert®) 2 mg q 6 hr × 3 doses		Not effective
Antidiabetic agents: Sulfonylurea	Yes		$D_{50}W$ 1–2 mL/kg Octreotide (Sandostatin®)	Not necessary if AC is given promptly	Alkalinization of urine to pH ≥ 8
Metformin HCl (Glucaphage®)	Yes				Hemodialysis
Antihistamines	Yes		None Possibly physostigmine for severe delirium or tachycardia	Gastric lavage for massive ingestion	Not effective

TABLE 56-2 Select Poisonings and Emergency Management (continued)

Agent	Activated Charcoal (AC)?	Induced Vomiting?	Antidote?	Gastric Emptying?	Enhanced Elimination?
			NaHCO$_3$ 1–2 mEq/kg IV may be useful for myocardial depression and prolonged QRS after massive diphenhydramine (Benadryl®) overdose		
Arsenic	Yes		Dimercaprol (BAL) 3–5 mg/kg IM q 4–6 hr	Consider in large ingestions	Hemodialysis if patient has renal failure
Barbiturates	Yes		No	Consider in large ingestions	Alkalinization of urine for phenobarbital only. Hemodialysis or hemoperfusion may be necessary for severely intoxicated patients who do not respond to supportive care
Benzodiazepines	Yes		Flumazenil (Romazicon®) 0.1–0.2 mg/dose up to 3 mg	Not necessary if AC is given promptly	No
Beta blockers	Yes		Glucagon (Glucagen®) 5–10 mg IV bolus, followed by 1–5 mg/hour infusion. Epinephrine 1–4 mcg/min titrated to effect. NaHCO$_3$ if wide complex conduction defects. Magnesium sulfate, isoproterenol (Isuprel®), or overdrive pacing for QT prolongation	Consider gastric lavage for large ingestions	May be useful if medication has a small volume of distribution
Beta stimulants	Yes		Propranolol (Inderal®) 0.01–0.02 mg/kg or Esmolol (Brevibloc®) 25–50 mcg/kg/min IV	Not necessary if AC is given promptly	No role

continues

TABLE 56-2 Select Poisonings and Emergency Management (continued)

Agent	Activated Charcoal (AC)?	Induced Vomiting?	Antidote?	Gastric Emptying?	Enhanced Elimination?
Calcium channel blockers	Yes		Calcium chloride 10% 10 mL (0.1–0.2 mL/kg) or calcium gluconate 10 mL 20% (0.3–0.4 mL/kg IV); repeat q 5–10 min Glucagon and epinephrine may also increase heart rate Amrinone (Inocor®) 0.75 mg/kg followed by infusion of 5–10 mcg/kg/min for refractory hypotension		Not effective
Carbon monoxide	No		Oxygen 100%	No	Hyperbaric oxygen
Cardiac glycosides	Yes	Yes, if used at the scene	Digoxin-specific antibodies (Digibind®)	Not necessary if AC is given promptly	Not effective
Clonidine (Catapres®) and related drugs	Yes	No	Naloxone	Not necessary if AC is given promptly	Not effective
Cocaine	Yes		None	Not necessary if AC is given promptly	Not effective
Cyanide	Yes	No, unless patient is > 20 minutes from a medical facility and AC is not available	Amyl nitrite pearl broken and placed under nose and sodium nitrite 300 mg IV Sodium thiosulfate 12.5 Gm IV	Insert gastric tube and then perform gastric lavage	Not effective
Ethylene glycol and other glycols	No	No	Fomepizole (4-methylpyrazole) or alcohol	Gastric lavage as quickly as possible	Yes
Isopropyl alcohol	Yes		None	Gastric lavage for very large ingestions	When levels are extremely high
Methanol	No	No	Fomepizole or alcohol Folic acid 50 mg IV q 4 hr	Gastric lavage	Yes, if significant metabolic acidosis
Monoamine oxidase inhibitors	Yes	Yes	Alpha-adrenergic blockers (phentolamine, Regitine®) or combined alpha- and beta-adrenergic blockers (labetalol, Trandate®)	Gastric lavage if large overdose suspected	Not effective

TABLE 56-2 Select Poisonings and Emergency Management (continued)

Agent	Activated Charcoal (AC)?	Induced Vomiting?	Antidote?	Gastric Emptying?	Enhanced Elimination?
Nonsteroidal anti-inflammatory drugs	Yes	Yes	None	Not necessary if AC is given promptly	Not effective
Opiates and opioids	Yes	No	Naloxone 0.4–2 mg IV Nalmefene (Revex®) 0.1–0.2 mg IV up to 10–20 mg NaHCO₃ for QRS prolongation from propoxyphene (Darvon®) poisoning	Not necessary if AC is given promptly	Not effective
Phencyclidine (PCP)	Yes	No	None	Not necessary if AC is given promptly	Not effective
Phenothiazines and other antipsychotic drugs	Yes	No	No specific antidote Dystonic reactions: diphenhydramine (Benadryl®) 0.5–1 mg/kg IM or IV NaHCO₃ 1–2 mEq/kg IV for prolonged QRS	Not necessary if AC is given promptly	Not effective
Phenytoin (Dilantin®)	Yes	Yes	None	Not necessary if AC is given promptly	Not effective
Salicylates	Yes	Yes	NaHCO₃ 100 mEq/L D₅W to prevent acidemia and promote elimination	Not necessary for small ingestions (< 300 mg/kg) if AC is given promptly	Hemodialysis and hemoperfusion are very effective Urinary alkalinization enhances elimination
Sedative hypnotics	Yes	No	Flumazenil (Romazicon®)	Not necessary if AC is given promptly. Gastric lavage may be considered for massive ingestions	Not effective
Strychnine	Yes	No	None	Not necessary if AC is given promptly or for small ingestion	Not needed
Tricyclic antidepressants	Yes	No	NaHCO₃ 1–2 mEq for prolonged QRS	Gastric lavage for large ingestion only	Not effective

Source: Olson, 2004.

CASE STUDY

N.H., a 16-year-old female, was brought to the ED by her mother after ingesting twenty 500-mg tablets of acetaminophen (Tylenol Extra Strength®) in an attempted suicide. N.H.'s boyfriend of three months had broken up with her earlier that day. N.H.'s mother denies that her daughter uses recreational drugs or drinks alcohol. She has a history of GI bleeding related to a peptic ulcer. She is allergic to ibuprofen (Motrin®).

Upon admission, N.H. complained of nausea and had two bouts of vomiting. She was diaphoretic and pale. Her vital signs are as follows: BP 90/60; HR 78; RR 22; temperature 98°F; SpO$_2$ 95%.

N.H. was placed on a cardiac monitor, oxygen via nasal cannula at 5 L/min, as well as a pulse oximeter, a peripheral IV was inserted, and blood specimens were taken for several tests, including a comprehensive metabolic profile, complete blood count, coagulation profile, toxicology screen, liver function tests, and acetaminophen level. An infusion of isotonic saline (0.9%) was started. A nasogastric tube was inserted, and N.H. received 140 mg/kg of NAC. The patient was also transferred to the ICU for further monitoring. She did not receive activated charcoal, because the ingestion likely occurred more than four hours earlier.

N.H. had no bouts of hypoglycemia or other manifestations of hepatic failure. She received a consult from the psychiatry department and was deemed not to pose a further threat to herself. She completed NAC treatment with no adverse effects and was discharged home under her mother's care.

CRITICAL THINKING QUESTIONS

1. If N.H. complained about a headache, how would you intervene?
2. Which disciplines should be consulted to work with this patient?
3. What types of issues may require you to act as an advocate or moral agent for this patient?
4. How would you implement your role as a facilitator of learning for this patient?
5. List three caring practices that can be utilized to promote a compassionate, supportive, and therapeutic environment for N.H.
6. Using the evidence-based literature (e.g., on the Internet), describe the incidence of teenage suicide and compare the literature to N.H.'s case.
7. Which strategies can be implemented to prevent N.H. from future toxic ingestions?
8. Use the form to write up data and a plan of care for a patient who sustained an overdose or poisoning in the clinical setting. Rate the patient as a level 1, 3, or 5 on each characteristic. Identify the level of nurse characteristics needed in the care of this patient.
9. Take one outcome and list evidence-based interventions for this patient.

Using the Synergy Model to Develop a Plan of Care

	Patient Characteristics	Level (1, 3, 5)	Subjective and Objective Data	Evidence-based Interventions	Outcomes
SYNERGY MODEL	Resiliency				
	Vulnerability				
	Stability				
	Complexity				
	Resource availability				
	Participation in care				
	Participation in decision making				
	Predictability				

Online Resources

American Association of Poison Control Centers: www.aapc.org

American Association of Poison Control Centers—Toxic Exposure Surveillance System: www.aapc.org/poison.htm

American Association of Poison Control Centers Poison Prevention and Education: www.aapc.org/education.htm

Rocky Mountain Poison & Drug Center: www.rmpdc.org

REFERENCES

Aaron, C. K. (1990). Sympathomimetics. In W. L. Augenstein (Ed.), *Emergency medicine clinics of north america* (pp. 513–523). Philadelphia: Saunders.

Ala, A., Schiano, T., Burroughs, A., & Keshav, S. (2004). Recognition of nonhepatic coma in the setting of acetaminophen overdose. *Digestive Diseases & Sciences, 49*(11–12), 1977–1980.

Amirzadeh, A., & McCotter, C. (2002). The intravenous use of oral acetyl-cysteine (Mucomyst) for the treatment of acetaminophen overdose. *Archives of Internal Medicine, 162*(1), 96–97.

Anderson, V. (2005). Anti-meth law roils drugstores. Retrieved November 13, 2005, from www.ajc.com/metro/content/metro/0705/01meth.html

Anonymous. (2005a). American Association of Poison Control Centers. Retrieved October 28, 2005, from www.aapcc.org/

Anonymous. (2005b). Barbiturates. Retrieved November 13, 2005, from www.streetdrugs.org/barbiturates.htm

Anonymous. (2005c). Barbiturates (systemic). In T. Micromedex (Ed.), *USP DI drug information for the health care professional* (25th ed.). Greenwood Village: Thomson Micromedex.

Anonymous. (2005d). Rx.com. Retrieved October 29, 2005, from www.rx.com

Bailey, B., Buckley, N. A., & Amre, D. K. (2004). A meta-analysis of prognostic indicators to predict seizures, arrhythmias or death after tricyclic antidepressant overdose. *Journal of Toxicology Clinical Toxicology, 42*(6), 877–888.

Bender, R. P., Lindsey, R. H., Burden, D. A., & Osheroff, N. (2004). N-acetyl-p-benzoquinoneimine, the toxic metabolite of acetaminophen, is a topoisomerase II poison. *Biochemistry, 43*(12), 3731–3739.

Bizovi, K. E., & Smilkstein, M. J. (2002). *Acetaminophen* (7th ed.). New York: McGraw-Hill.

Broderick, M. (2003). Spotting drug use. *RN, 66*(9), 48–53.

Brueske, P. (1997). ED management of cyanide poisoning. *Journal of Emergency Nursing, 23*(6), 569–573.

Buajordet, I., Naess, A. C., Jacobsen, D., & Brors, O. (2004). Adverse events after naloxone treatment of episodes of suspected acute opioid overdose. *European Journal of Emergency Medicine, 11*(1), 19–23.

Cantilena, L. (2001). *Casarett and Doull's toxicology: The basic science of poisons* (6th ed.). New York: McGraw-Hill.

Cozanitis, D. A. (2004). One hundred years of barbiturates and their saint. *Journal of the Royal Society of Medicine, 97*, 594–598.

Cummings, T. F. (2004). The treatment of cyanide poisoning. *Occupational Medicine, 54*(2), 82–85.

Donoghue, A. M. (2003). Alternative methods of administering amyl nitrite to victims of cyanide poisoning. *Occupational and Environmental Medicine, 60*(2), 147.

Finnell, J. T., & Harris, C. R. (2000). Cardiovascular toxicity of selected drug overdoses. *Topics in Emergency Medicine, 22*(1), 29–41.

Flomenbaum, N. E. (2002). *Salicylates* (7th ed.). New York: McGraw-Hill.

Gelander, M., & Kleber, H. D. (2004). Treatment of acute intoxication and withdrawal from drugs of abuse. Adapted or excerpted from *Textbook of substance abuse treatment*. Retrieved February 11, 2006, from www.chce. researchmed.va.gov/chce/pdfs/Doaacutetreatment.pdf

Gilmer, B., Kilkenny, J., Tomaszewski, C., & Watts, J. A. (2002). Hyperbaric oxygen does not prevent neurologic sequelae after carbon monoxide poisoning. *Academic Emergency Medicine, 9*(1), 1–8.

Gitman, M. D., & Singhal, D. C. (2004). Cocaine-induced renal disease. *Expert Opinion on Drug Safety, 3*(5), 441–448.

Gracia, R., & Shepherd, G. (2004). Cyanide poisoning and its treatment. *Pharmacotherapy, 24*(10), 1358–1365.

Gussow, L. (2003a). Amphetamine poisoning. In J. Schaider, S. R. Hayden, R. Wolfe, R. M. Barkin, & P. Rosen (Eds.), *Rosen and Barkin's 5-minute emergency medicine consult* (2nd ed., pp. 24–25). Philadelphia: Lippincott Williams & Wilkins.

Gussow, L. (2003b). Carbon monoxide poisoning. In J. Schaider, S. R. Hayden, R. Wolfe, R. M. Barkin, & P. Rosen (Eds.), *Rosen and Barkin's 5-minute emergency medicine consult* (2nd ed., pp. 178–179). Philadelphia: Lippincott Williams & Wilkins.

Gyamlani, G. G., & Parikh, C. R. (2002). Acetaminophen toxicity: Suicidal vs. accidental. *Critical Care (London), 6*(2), 155–159.

Hoffman, C., & Gibel, L. (2005). Acetaminophen overdose. *Nursing, 35*(1), 88.

Howland, M. A. (2002). *Sedative hypnotics*. New York: McGraw-Hill.

Ibister, G. K., O'Regan, L., Sibbritt, D., & White, I. M. (2004). Alprazolam is relatively more toxic than other benzodiazepines in overdose. *British Journal of Clinical Pharmacology, 58*(1), 88–95.

Jaslow, D., Ufberg, J., Ukasik, J., & Sananman, P. (2001). Routine carbon monoxide screening by emergency medical technicians. *Academic Emergency Medicine, 8*(3), 288–291.

Kociancic, T., & Reed, M. D. (2003). Acetaminophen intoxication and length of treatment: How long is enough? *Pharmacotherapy, 23*(8), 1052–1059.

Lee, D. C. (2002). *Sedative hypnotics*. New York: McGraw-Hill.

Liebelt, E. L., & Francis, P. D. (2002). *Cyclic antidepressants*. New York: McGraw-Hill.

Lisanti, P. (1998). Barbiturate overdose. *American Journal of Nursing, 98*(10), 38.

Mabry, B., Greller, H. A., & Nelson, L. S. (2003). Patterns of heroin overdose-induced pulmonary edema. *American Journal of Emergency Medicine, 21*(1), 32–34.

Macedo, D. S., Vaconscelos, S. M., Belchior, L. D., Santos, R. S., Viana, G. S., & Sousa, F. C. (2004). Alterations in monoamine levels after cocaine-induced status epilepticus and death in striatum and prefrontal cortex of mice. *Neuroscience Letters, 362*(3), 185–188.

Mak, T. W., Kam, C. W., Lai, J. P., & Tang, C. M. (2000). Management of carbon monoxide poisoning using oxygen therapy. *Hong Kong Medical Journal, 6*(1), 113–115.

Maxa, J. L., Ogu, C. C., Adeeko, M. A., & Swaner, T. G. (2003). Continuous-infusion flumazenil in the management of chlordiazepoxide toxicity. *Pharmacotherapy, 23*(11), 1513–1516.

McCance, K. L. (2005). Altered cellular and tissue biology. In K. L. McCance & S. E. Heuther (Eds.), *Pathophysiology: The biologic basis for disease in adults and children* (5th ed.). St. Louis, MO: Mosby.

Megarbane, B., Delahaye, A., Goldgran-Toledano, D., & Baud, F. (2003). Antidotal treatment of cyanide poisoning. *Journal of Chinese Medical Association, 66*(4), 193–203.

Melo, O. L., Nogue, S., Trullas, J. C., Aguilo, S., & Maciel, A. (2004). Seizures after flumazenil administration in a case of combined benzodiazepine and tricyclic antidepressant overdose. *Revista de Toxicologia, 21*(1), 38–40.

Middleton, P. M. (2004). Cerebrovascular effects of cocaine. *Internet Journal of Emergency Medicine, 2*(1). Retrieved February 11, 2006, from www.ispub.com/ostia/index.php?xmlFilePath=journals/ijem/vol2n1/cocaine.xml

Mouhaffel, A. H., Madu, E. C., Satmary, W. A., & Fraker, T. D. (1995). Cardiovascular complications of cocaine. *Chest, 107*(5), 1426–1434.

National Institute on Drug Abuse. (2006). NIDA InfoFacts: Crack and cocaine. Retrieved February 11, 2006, from www.nida.nih.gov/Infofacts/cocaine.html

Nelson, L. S. (2002). *Opioids*. New York: McGraw-Hill.

Norfolk, G. A. (2006). The fatal case of a cocaine body-stuffer and a literature review—towards evidence based management. *Clinical Journal of Forensic Medicine, 24*. Retrieved February 11, 2006, from www.ncbi.nlm.nih.gov.libproxy.lib.unc.edu/entrez/query.fcgi?cmd=Retrieve&db=pubmed&dopt=Abstract&list_uids=16442337&query_hl=18&itool=pubmed_DocSum

Nulton-Persson, A. C., Szweda, L. I., & Sadek, H. A. (2004). Inhibition of cardiac mitochondrial respiration by salicylic acid and acetylcysteine. *Journal of Cardiovascular Pharmacology, 44*(5), 591–595.

Olson, K. R. (2004). *Poisonings and drug overdose* (4th ed.). New York: McGraw-Hill.

Pajoumand, A., Jalali, N., Abdollahi, M., & Shadnia, S. (2003). Successful treatment of acetaminophen overdose associated with hepatic failure. *Human & Experimental Toxicology, 22*(8), 453–458.

Pittman, H. J. (2005). Methamphetamine overdose. *Nursing 2005, 35*(4), 88.

Poor, K. (2000). Drug overdose. Retrieved November 23, 2005, from www.tchpeducation.com/homestudies/generalinterest/drug_overdose/drugbook_web.pdf

Reith, D., Fountain, J., Tilyard, M., & McDowell, R. (2003). Antidepressant poisoning deaths in New Zealand for 2001. *Journal of the New Zealand Medical Association, 116*(1184). Retrieved February 11, 2006, from www.nzma.org.nz/journal/116-1184/646/

Rothman, R. B., Baumann, M. H., Dersch, C. M., Romero, D. V., Rice, K. C., Carroll, F. I., et al. (2001). Amphetamine-type central nervous system stimulants release norepinephrine more potently than they release dopamine and serotonin. *Synapse, 39*(1), 32–41.

Singh, N., & Singh, H. K. (2002). Serial electrocardiographic changes as a predictor of cardiovascular toxicity in acute tricyclic antidepressant overdose. *American Journal of Therapeutics, 9*(1), 75–79.

Thanacoody, H. K., & Thomas, S. H. (2005). Tricyclic antidepressant poisoning: Cardiovascular toxicity. *Toxicological Reviews, 24*(3), 205–214.

Turnipseed, S. D., Richards, J. R., Kirk, J. D., Diercks, D. B., & Amsterdam, E. A. (2003). Frequency of acute coronary syndrome in patients presenting to the emergency department with chest pain after methamphetamine use. *Journal of Emergency Medicine, 24*(4), 369–373.

Van Wolferen, S. A., Vonk, N. A., Boonstra, S., & Postmus, P. E. (2005). Pulmonary arterial hypertension due to the use of amphetamines as drugs or doping. *Nederlands Tijdschrift voor Geneekunde, 149*(23), 1283–1288.

Verhelst, D., Moulin, P., Haufroid, V., Wittebole, X., Jadoul, M., & Hantson, P. (2004). Acute renal injury following methanol poisoning: Analysis of case series. *International Journal of Toxicology, 23*(4), 267–273.

Vieweg, W. V., & Wood, M. A. (2004). Tricyclic antidepressants, QT interval prolongation, and torsade de pointes. *Psychosomatics, 45*(5), 371–377.

Von Mach, M. A., Hermanns-Clausen, M., Koch, I., Hengstler, J. G., Lauterbach, M., Kaes, J., et al. (2005). Experiences of a poison control center network with renal insufficiency in acetaminophen overdose: An analysis of 17 cases. *Clinical Toxicology, 43*(1), 31–37.

Weber, J. E., Chudnofsky, C. R., Boxzar, M., Boyer, E. W., Wilkerson, M. D., & Hollander, J. E. (2000). Cocaine-associated chest pain: How common is myocardial infarction? *Academic Emergency Medicine, 7*(8), 873–877.

White, S. R. (2002). Amphetamine toxicity. *Seminars in Respiratory and Critical Care Medicine, 23*(1), 27–36.

Williams, R. H., & Erikson, T. (2000). CE update—drugs of abuse I. Emergency diagnosis of opioid intoxication. *Laboratory Medicine, 31*(6), 334–342.

Wood, D. M., Dargan, P. I., & Jones, A. L. (2005). Measuring plasma salicylate concentrations in all patients with drug overdose or altered consciousness: Is it necessary? *Emergency Medicine Journal, 22*(6), 401–403.

Wrathall, G., Sinclari, R., Moore, A., & Pogson, D. (2001). Three case reports of the use of haemodiafiltration in the treatment of salicylate overdose. *Human & Experimental Toxicology, 20*(9), 491–495.

Yang, C. C., Deng, J. F., & Lin, T. J. (2001). Pancytopenia, hyperglycemia, shock, coma, rhabdomyolysis, and pancreatitis, associated with acetaminophen poisoning. *Veterinary & Human Toxicology, 43*(6), 344–348.

Yip, L., & Dart, R. C. (2003). A 20-hour treatment for acute acetaminophen overdose. *New England Journal of Medicine, 348*(24), 2471–2472.

Management of the Critically Ill Bariatric Patient

Catherine Head

LEARNING OBJECTIVES

Upon completion of this chapter, the reader will be able to:

1. Discuss the three major types of bariatric surgery: Roux-en-Y gastric bypass (RYGB), laparoscopic adjustable banding, and duodenal switch.

2. Describe the criteria utilized for identifying candidates for bariatric surgery.

3. Describe the preoperative teaching for the bariatric surgery patient.

4. Relate the nursing care for postoperative bariatric surgery patients to the Synergy Model.

5. Discuss the potential complications of bariatric surgery and evidence-based interventions.

6. Discuss the nursing assessment and interventions for the postoperative bariatric patient.

7. List optimal patient outcomes that may be achieved through evidence-based interventions for the bariatric patient.

Obesity is a chronic disease and the second most common cause of death in the United States (Stocker, 2003). According to the latest data from the National Center for Health Statistics, more than 60 million people in the United States are obese. Current data indicate that the prevalence of obesity is increasing and that costs related to obesity and its associated comorbidities exceed $117 billion per year (Centers for Disease Control and Prevention, 2006).

Given the prevalence and complications of obesity, significant efforts have been directed toward developing effective treatment for it. Conservative treatments for obesity, such as diet intervention, exercise, behavior modification, and lifestyle intervention, have shown limited success with the morbidly obese. The National Institutes of Health (NIH) Technology Assessment Conference concluded that many morbidly obese individuals—defined as a body mass index (BMI) greater than 40 kg/m^2 or a BMI between 35 and 40 with one comorbidity—had not successfully achieved long-term weight loss with conservative methods, and gastric bypass surgery was recommended as the best treatment option for these patients (NIH Consensus Conference Statement, 1991).

This chapter reviews the various types of bariatric (or weight reduction) surgery and associated complications. Sometimes, patients who have undergone bariatric surgery are admitted to the intensive care unit (ICU). Management of these patients will be described.

INDICATIONS FOR BARIATRIC SURGERY

The NIH developed indications for bariatric surgery in 1991. These indications, which remain consistent with generally accepted guidelines, appear in **Table 57-1**. Prior to undergoing any bariatric surgery, prospective patients are assessed by a multidisciplinary team with medical, surgical, psychological, and nutrition expertise.

TYPES OF BARIATRIC SURGERY

A variety of operations have been performed for the purpose of weight loss. All of these procedures employ one or both of two primary mechanisms to promote weight loss: gastric restriction and intestinal malabsorption. Examples of the former include vertical banded gastroplasty (VBG) and laparoscopic adjustable gastric banding (LAGB). A

TABLE 57-1 Surgical Candidate for Bariatric Surgery

1. Patient must be obese:
   a. BMI $\geq$ 35 kg/m^2 with at least one obesity-related comorbidity, or
   b. BMI $\geq$ 40 kg/m^2
2. Patient must have failed nonoperative approaches (e.g., diet, exercise).
3. Patient must be psychologically stable through methods of evaluation.
4. Patient must be medically stable preoperatively.
5. Patient must be willing to adapt to and participate in the required life changes, including changes in dietary patterns.
6. Patient must be willing to embrace a modified lifestyle.

Source: National Institutes of Health, 1991.

duodenal switch, biliopancreatic diversion with duodenal switch, and Roux-en-Y gastric bypass (RYGB) are types of malabsorptive and restrictive procedures.

Restrictive Surgery

VBG and LAGB procedures result in weight loss by decreasing the reservoir capacity of the stomach. Following such surgery, absorption occurs in the small intestine. The weight loss associated with restrictive procedures is more gradual than that associated with other types of procedures (Sanchez, Schneider, & Mun, 2006a).

VBG, also known as stomach stapling, partitions the stomach with staples. Food is directed into a small pouch, thereby limiting food intake. The outlet from the pouch to the remainder of the stomach is restricted by a band. The band slows food emptying from the stomach, which maintains a "full" feeling (U.S. National Library of Medicine, 2004). VBG procedures are performed less frequently now than in the past.

LAGB involves partitioning the upper stomach with a band. The band comprises a ring that is connected to an infusion port, which itself is placed in the subcutaneous tissue. Saline may be instilled into the port with a needle and syringe. This results in a decrease in the diameter of the band, thereby increasing the degree of restriction (O'Brien et al., 1999) (see **Figure 57-1**).

Advantages of LAGB include the following: It has the lowest mortality rate of all bariatric procedures; it lacks staple lines that might otherwise erode and lead to weight gain; the band is adjustable in the event increased caloric or fluid intake is required (e.g., in pregnancy); the procedure does not entail division of the stomach or intestinal resection; and it offers reported improvement in obesity-associated comorbidities (e.g., diabetes, obstruc-

FIGURE 57-1 Laparoscopic Banding

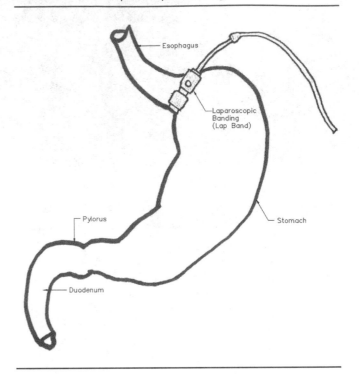

Source: Illustrated by James R. Perron.

tive sleep apnea, hypertension) (Dixon, Dixon, & O'Brien, 2001; Dixon & O'Brien, 2002; Food and Drug Administration, 2005; O'Brien & Dixon, 2003). LAGB is also associated with a shorter hospital stay, reduced risk of early complications (especially a leak), and avoidance of vitamin and mineral supplements. The band does require four to six band adjustments in the first year and, there is the possibility of infection erosion or slippage, which can cause peritonitis. Although the procedure is reversible, it is not recommended due to a potential for weight gain. Weight loss is an average of 41% at one year post band placement, and attained at a progressively slower rate as compared with the RYGB (Ren, Horgan, & Ponce, 2002).

Malabsorptive and Restrictive Surgery

The duodenal switch procedure (also called the biliopancreatic diversion or biliopancreatic duodenal switch) involves dividing the stomach vertically (removing the remaining 85% versus creating a pouch with the RYGB), preserving the pylorus, and diverting the majority of the small intestine from the ingested food. The duodenum is divided at the connection near the lower stomach in an effort to divert pancreatic juice and bile. Food travels along one section of the intestine, and digestive juices travel along another section of the intestine. This anatomical change reduces the amount of fat emulsification and calorie absorption (see **Figure 57-2**).

FIGURE 57-2 Duodenal Switch

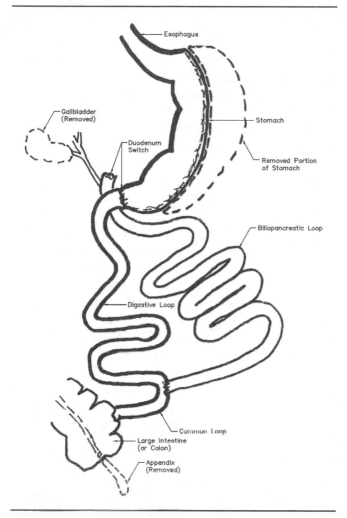

Source: Illustrated by James R. Perron.

Malabsorptive procedures decrease nutrient absorption by decreasing the length of functional small intestine. Although the patient experiences a significant weight loss, this benefit may be counteracted by protein calorie malnutrition and micronutrient deficiencies associated with this type of procedure.

The RYGB is an example of a bariatric procedure with both restrictive and malabsorptive elements. It is the gold standard and most successful bariatric surgical procedure performed in the United States (Nguyen, 2004). The RYGB involves creating a small pouch by transecting the proximal stomach (restrictive) and then connecting this pouch to a portion of the small intestine, after bypassing the distal stomach and a portion of the small intestine (malabsorptive) (see **Figure 57-3**). The combination of restriction of stomach contents with the inability to absorb as much food in the intestine results in suc-

cessful weight loss. RYGB may be associated with the development of dumping syndrome with nausea, diarrhea, abdominal pain, and lightheadedness when the patient consumes a meal high in sugar (Kellum et al., 1990).

COMPLICATIONS OF BARIATRIC SURGERY

Despite its benefits, bariatric surgery does carry the risk of potential complications. Obesity adds another dimension to the needs and challenges of caring for the critically ill patient. According to the International Bariatric Society Registry, the primary cause of death after bariatric surgery is pulmonary embolism (PE). Patients at greatest risk for PE include those with a BMI of 60 kg/m² or greater, chronic edema of the legs, obstructive sleep apnea, or history of PE (Sapala, Wood, Schuhknecht, & Sapala, 2003; Savel, Gropper, Macura, & Lazzaro, 2006). Signs of PE include unexplained shortness of breath, chest pain that worsens with a deep breath or coughing, coughing up blood, anxiety or feelings of dread, lightheadedness, increased respiratory rate, tachycardia, decreased oxygen saturation, and diaphoresis.

Patients who have undergone bariatric surgery are also at risk for death from anastomotic leak or respiratory failure. Signs and symptoms of anastomotic leak include sustained

FIGURE 57-3 Roux-en-Y Gastric Bypass

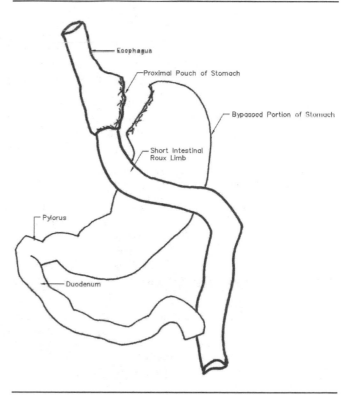

Source: Illustrated by James R. Perron.

tachycardia, severe abdominal pain, fever, rigors, and hypotension (Savel et al., 2006).

A variety of other complications are also associated with each of the bariatric procedures (see **Table 57-2**). Overall mortality for all procedures ranges from 0.1% to 4.6%. The higher mortality rates reflect procedures performed in older patients and procedures done by surgeons who performed fewer cases (Buchwald et al., 2005; Flum et al., 2005; Maggard et al., 2005; Santry, Gillen, & Lauderdale, 2005).

MANAGEMENT OF THE BARIATRIC SURGERY PATIENT IN THE ICU

Patients may be admitted to the ICU following bariatric surgery for management of complications following surgery or from obesity-related comorbidities. The ICU nurse must be knowledgeable of and observe for signs and symptoms of these complications. As many as 20% of patients who undergo bariatric surgery may require admission to the ICU or have an increased length of stay. Caring for critically ill obese patients can present a potential challenge for the ICU staff from both a medical and psychological perspective. The technical aspects of intubation and extubation, placement of central venous catheters, medication dosing, routine skin care, nutrition, and patient positioning all require special attention in this population.

Patients who are morbidly obese may feel they are a burden to healthcare providers. Regardless of the challenges, it is essential that these patients are treated with care, dignity, and respect at all times (Savel et al., 2006). Each member of the ICU multidisciplinary team must manage any prejudice and avoid all unbefitting or immoral comments, because these are very destructive to the patient–healthcare provider relationship (Drake, McAuliffe, Edge, & Lopez, 2006). A review of patients' experiences revealed that patients continue to feel misunderstood and mistreated by medical personnel. This prejudice is likely due to a lack of understanding of morbid obesity, its underlying causes, the consequences if left untreated, and the benefits of weight loss procedures (Kaminsky & Gadaleta, 2002).

The majority of bariatric patients present with an average of 6.8 comorbidities, the most common of which are hypertension, diabetes, gastroesophageal reflux disease (GERD), hypercholesterolemia, obstructive sleep apnea, degenerative joint disease, coronary heart disease, urinary stress incontinence, asthma, and pulmonary hypertension (Stocker, 2003). Because of the severity and multitude of their comorbidities, these patients have less tolerance for complications. An increased incidence of complications is noted in male patients with a BMI of more than 60 kg/m^2, age greater than 50, and associated cardiac and pulmonary comorbidities (Pieracci, Barie, & Pomp, 2006).

Obesity Pathophysiology

The typical respiratory pattern of the obese patient is hypoventilation from restrictive ventilation secondary to decreased lung expansion. This pattern results in a decrease in oxygenation due to ventilation/perfusion mismatch, an increase in carbon dioxide due to hypoventilation, pulmonary hypertension, and ultimately right-sided heart failure (Wilson & Clark, 2003). The consequences of restrictive breathing pattern include decreased residual capacity, inspiratory capacity, and expiratory reserve volume (Ray, Sue, Bray, Hansen, & Wasserman, 1983). Obstructive sleep apnea is characterized by partial obstruction of the upper airway causing oxygen desatura-

TABLE 57-2 Complications of Bariatric Procedures

Procedure	Associated Complications
Vertical banded gastroplasty	Staple line disruption, band erosion, gastroesophageal reflux disease (GERD), nausea, vomiting, ulcers, stomal stenosis, weight gain
Laparoscopic adjustable gastric banding	Infection, esophagitis, stomal obstruction, band erosion, stomach wall prolapse, gastric obstruction, band slippage, port or tubing malfunction, esophageal dilation
Duodenal switch and biliopancreatic diversion	Protein calorie malnutrition, fat-soluble vitamin deficiency, vitamin B_{12} deficiency, anemia
Roux-en-Y gastric bypass	Pulmonary embolism, deep vein thrombosis, anastomotic leak, infection, ulcer, small bowel obstruction, hernia, stomal stenosis, bleeding, gastric remnant distention (leading to peritonitis), cholelithiasis, metabolic and nutritional derangements

Sources: Angrisani et al., 2003; Balsiger, Murr, Poggio, & Sarr, 2000; Cadiere et al., 2002; Champion & Williams, 2003; Christou, Jarand, Sylvestre, & McLean, 2004; DeMaria, 2003; DeMaria et al., 2001; Guedea et al., 2004; Mason, 2003; Mun, Blackburn, & Matthews, 2001; Papasavas et al., 2002; Podnos, Jiminez, Wilson, Stevens, & Nguyen, 2004; Poole et al., 2004; Ren, Horgan, & Ponce, 2002; Rubenstein, 2002; Sanchez, Schneider, & Mun, 2006b; Sapala, Wood, Sapala, & Flake, 1998; Sapala, Wood, Schuhknecht, & Sapala, 2003; Shiffman, Sugerman, Kellum, Brewer, & Moore, 1991; Spaulding, 1997.

tion, thereby leading to nocturnal dysrhythmias, polycythemia, and systemic and pulmonary hypertension (Gibson, 2004).

Preexisting pulmonary disease can lead to postoperative pulmonary complications. Most patients present with short necks and associated excessive adipose tissue. Intubations are difficult, and patients desaturate quickly due to poor residual lung capacity. The laryngeal mask airway allows for easier ventilation and intubation. Postoperative respiratory insufficiency requires early intervention with arterial blood gas (ABG) evaluation. The head of the bed should be elevated to prevent aspiration. If a nasogastric tube is placed, its insertion should be done with caution to avoid rupturing the gastrojejunostomy anastomosis (pouch).

Continuous positive airway pressure (CPAP) may be initiated if the patient's CO_2 level is stable and acceptable. Although CPAP may cause gastric distention at increased pressures, its use has not been associated with anastamotic leak failure. In a series of 1,067 patients, Livingston and colleagues (2002) noted similar leak rates of 1.3% in both patients wearing CPAP and those not wearing CPAP. If the patient is retaining CO_2 or it is not possible to maintain the adequate oxygenation, mechanical ventilation may be required.

Patients who are morbidly obese have a decrease in functional residual capacity and expiratory reserve volume, especially when they are placed in the supine position. They may manifest increased work of breathing due to a decrease in chest wall compliance (Ladosky, Botelho, & Albuquerque, 2001). These physiologic changes predispose the patient to atelectasis with resultant severe hypoxemia secondary to intrapulmonary shunting (Savel et al., 2006).

If mechanical ventilation is required, the tidal volume should be set for 8 mL/kg ideal body weight (IBW) versus the actual body weight (ABW) to avoid extreme airway pressures and alveolar distention (Pieracci et al., 2006). Changes in ventilator settings are subsequently based on ABG results and peak airway pressures. Plateau pressures should be maintained below 35 cm H_2O. A positive end-expiratory pressure of 5 to 10 cm H_2O will help improve atelectasis and reserve volume (Champion, 2006).

Respiratory distress, especially within the first 24 hours post bariatric surgery, may be reflective of respiratory compensation secondary to lactic acidosis. Lactic acidosis, which is induced by poor tissue perfusion and hypovolemia, could be an early sign of an impending abdominal complication (Davidson & Callery, 2001).

The increased body mass in the obese patient results in an increase in circulatory volume, causing a corresponding increase in preload and afterload. The heart responds with elevated levels of aldosterone, renin, mineralocorticoids, and catecholamines to increase the afterload, which in turn leads to diastolic dysfunction, myocardial hypertrophy, decreased cardiac compliance, and ventricular failure (Messerli, 1982). This chronic hyperdynamic state decreases oxygen delivery to the tissues, because oxygenation to the cells of the body depends on adequate ventilation, diffusion, and perfusion into the tissues.

Most patients do not require central venous access for hemodynamic monitoring. If it is necessary, catheter placement may be difficult due to obscured landmarks. Noninvasive hemodynamic monitoring requires appropriate-sized blood pressure cuffs to obtain accurate pressures. A cuff that is too small can overestimate the systolic pressure by as much as 10 to 50 mm Hg. The length of the cuff bladder should be 75% to 80% of the upper arm length, and the width should be 40% of the circumference of the upper arm (Beevers, Lip, & O'Brien, 2001).

Obesity affects both immune and metabolic reserves. The extra adipose tissue in the obese individual is related to increased levels of tumor necrosis factor and interleukin-6, which result in an increased inflammatory response (Kern, Ranganathan, Li, Wood, & Ranganathan, 2001). The neutrophils in the obese patient have impaired chemotaxis and activation correlating with a reduced immune response (Dixon & O'Brien, 2006). Higher concentrations of fibrinogen and plasminogen activator inhibitor 1 and lower concentrations of antithrombin III and fibrinolysis are associated with the obese population, leading to an increased risk for deep vein thrombosis (DVT) and pulmonary emboli (Sapala et al., 2003). Vascular insufficiency, venous stasis, and pulmonary hypertension also contribute to the hypercoagulability noted in these patients.

Routine thromboprophylaxis is the standard of care in the preoperative and postoperative periods, although no universal regimen has been identified. Most bariatric protocols include early ambulation, pneumatic compression stockings, unfractionated heparin, and low-molecular-weight heparin (LMWH) (Wu & Barba, 2000). Prophylactic dosing of unfractionated heparin with 5,000 to 8,000 units every 8 to 12 hours or LMWH [e.g., enoxaparin (Lovenox®)] 40 mg every 12 hours initiated 1 to 2 hours preoperatively and continued throughout the hospital stay, pending laboratory results. Currently, no data support weight-based dosing of LMWH using the criterion of 1 mg per unit BMI (Champion, 2006). Patients with a history of venous thromboembolism or pulmonary embolism may have an inferior vena cava filter placed at the time of surgery or prior to the weight loss procedure.

Pharmacology

The increased ratio of adipose tissue to lean body mass and volume distribution in obese patients alters the distribution of lipophilic drugs in these individuals. Lipophilic drugs, which are distributed in the adipose tissue, may necessitate a larger bolus to achieve a desired effect and produce a longer half-life (Savel et al., 2006). The effects of hydrophilic drugs, which have poor penetration into the adipose tissue, relate better to the amount of lean body mass. When administering drugs, it is important to remember the increase in circulating volume and connective tissue found in obese patients. Serum concentrations of these drugs should be monitored when possible. Dosing of lipophilic drugs is best based on *actual* body weight, whereas dosing of hydrophilic drugs, which have an affinity for water, is based on *ideal* body weight. The critical care pharmacist should be consulted regarding appropriate dosing (Erstad, 2004). **Table 57-3** shows the dosing calculations for drugs commonly administered to the bariatric surgical patient.

Sedation and Extubation

If patients need to be adequately sedated, fentanyl (Sublimaze®) appears to have the fewest hemodynamic side effects (Gehlbach & Kress, 2002; Kress et al., 2003). The level of sedation should be assessed to avoid oversedation. Because of poor alveolar ventilation in the obese patient, excessive opiate administration can potentiate respiratory failure. Extubation may require immediate positive-pressure ventilation and ABG monitoring (den Herder, Schmeck, Appelboom, & de Vries, 2004). If respiratory depression manifests, a patient may require prolonged mechanical ventilation and a tracheostomy may be considered. An elongated tracheostomy tube may be required due to the anatomy of the neck and trachea (El-Solh, 2004).

Nutrition

As mentioned earlier, RYGB involves both a restrictive component (small stomach pouch) and a malabsorptive component (portion of small bowel bypassed), which leads to decreased absorption of vitamins, electrolytes, minerals, and salts.

TABLE 57-3 Dosing Guidelines for Bariatric Patients

Drug	Dosing Weight
Propofol	ABW
Benzodiazepine	Single dose: ABW Continuous infusion: IBW
Vancomycin	ABW
Aminoglycosides	IBW + (0.40 × [ABW − IBW])
Fluoroquinolones	IBW + (0.40 × [ABW − IBW])

ABW = actual body weight; IBW = ideal body weight.
Source: Pieracci, Barie, & Pomp, 2006.

Patients may require total parental nutrition or a Rally pack if in the hospital for a lengthy stay. A Rally pack contains intravenous fluids (e.g., D_5W or 0.9% NS) supplemented with vitamins and minerals.

It is hypothesized that humoral effects brought on by the bypassed stomach, duodenum, and jejunum correlate with diabetes or insulin resistance improvement in bariatric surgery patients, prior to any appreciable weight loss (Wickremesekera, Miller, Naotunne, Knowles, & Stubbs, 2005). Tight glucose control should be an important consideration, especially with the insulin-dependent patient, to achieve glucose homeostasis and decrease potential wound infection (Elamin, 2005; Savel et al., 2006).

All post-gastric bypass patients who present to the ICU should be considered for a FAST-HUG: feeding (total parenteral nutrition), analgesia, sedation, thromboembolic prophylaxis, head of bed elevated, ulcer prophylaxis, and glucose control (Vincent, 2005).

Hemodynamic Instability

RYGB is often performed laproscopically with carbon dioxide pneumoperitoneum (CO_2-filled abdomen under pressure) and associated physiologic effects include systemic absorption of CO_2 and physiologic alteration from the increased intra-abdominal pressure (Nguyen & Wolfe, 2005). The most likely cause of acute hypotension is hypovolemia from bleeding or use of sedatives. Initial management of hypotension is a fluid challenge with 500 to 1,000 mL of isotonic crystalloid and possible ABG monitoring, cardiac enzymes, and electrocardiogram if the hypotension is accompanied by respiratory and cardiac distress. If fluid resuscitation results in improved blood pressure, tachycardia, and urine output, hypovolemia was the likely cause of hypotension. If there is no improvement in hypotension with fluid resuscitation, acute hemorrhage and anastomotic leak are possible causes. Both are surgical emergencies (Savel et al., 2006).

Patients who are obese usually have an increased cardiac output and total blood volume, and are considered to be in a hyperdynamic state. Over time, the hyperdynamic state can lead to a decrease in cardiac performance, left ventricular contractility, and cardiac compliance, as well as diastolic ventricular dysfunction and left ventricular hypertrophy. These cardiac changes may decrease the patient's ability to tolerate fluid boluses (Savel et al., 2006).

Anastomotic Leak

Although the incidence of anastomotic leak is rare—ranging from 0.1% to 5% with an average of 2% to 3%—it is the second most common cause of mortality post gastric bypass (Papasavas et al., 2002). Initially, the patient may present with tachycardia (heart rate greater than 120 beats/min for 4 hours) and progressive tachypnea. Other signs include leukocytosis, decreased urinary output, abdominal pain (sometimes radiating to the shoulder), abdominal distention, and fever. Patients often have the feeling of impending doom. A leak is usually confirmed with computerized tomography (CT) of the abdomen, although this imaging study may not be feasible due to the weight limitations of most tables. In addition to emergent surgery, other treatment may include a drain, G-tube insertion, broad-spectrum bacterial and *Candida* coverage, DVT prophylaxis, and nutrition support (Champion, 2006).

Venous Thromboembolism/Pulmonary Embolism

The obese patient is at a higher risk for a DVT and PE due to the hypercoagulable state, decreased mobility, venous stasis, and pulmonary hypertension (Sapala et al., 2003). Symptoms of PE may include chest pain that gets worse with a deep breath, unexplained shortness of breath, tachycardia, tachypnea, coughing up blood, anxiety or feelings of dread, diaphoresis, lightheadedness, and hypoxemia. The D-dimer level is an unreliable diagnostic test in this scenario because it is elevated postoperatively and in the obese patient (Champion, 2006). A contrast-enhanced spiral CT is the best diagnostic test to rule out a PE, although some scanners have weight limitations (Fedullo & Tapson, 2003). Treatment may consist of unfractionated heparin or LMWH, compression hose, and a vena cava filter (Geerts et al., 2004; Savel et al., 2006; Wu & Barba, 2000).

Gastrointestinal Bleeding

Postoperative bleeding can occur either early—from any of the anastomotic sites—or late—occurring from an ulcer in the gastric remnant (leftover stomach) or duodenum (Ukleja & Stone, 2004). Early symptoms (within 24 hours) include hematemesis, bright red hematachezia, hemodynamic instability, and abdominal distention and tenderness. A later (after 24 hours) symptom of a gastrointestinal (GI) bleed is melena stools. Patients may require fluid resuscitation, blood transfusions, or upper endoscopy. Most GI bleeding episodes stop spontaneously. Hemodynamic changes, oliguria, and pallor (especially within six hours of surgery), may be signs of progressive bleeding and necessitate surgical intervention.

Aspiration

Patients who have undergone bariatric surgery are at risk for aspiration. Positioning in reverse Trendelenburg at 45 degrees is recommended to avoid this complication (Savel et al., 2006).

Pressure-Induced Rhabdomyolysis

Although rhabdomyolysis is most commonly caused by a crush injury, pressure-induced rhabdomyolysis has been documented in bariatric patients. This condition, although rare, is due to unrelieved pressure to the muscles (Bostanjian, Anthone, Hamoui, & Crookes, 2003). In a retrospective study of 100 bariatric patients with a median BMI of 67 kg/m^2, 6 patients developed gluteal necrosis with a creatine kinase (CK) between 26,000 and 29,000 IU/L (Bostanjian et al.). Presenting symptoms include numbness and muscular pain. The patient may also have an elevated CPK that peaks on the second to fifth day from intracellular myoglobin secondary to muscle breakdown. Treatment is initiated with aggressive hydration, diuresis with mannitol, and alkalization of urine with sodium bicarbonate (Pieracci et al., 2006).

Infection and Sepsis

Sepsis is the most common cause of death in the ICU setting, with a 40% mortality rate (Champion, 2006). The pathophysiology of sepsis comprises an infectious, inflammatory response complicated by increased coagulation and decreased fibrinolysis, leading to microvascular thrombosis, endothelial dysfunction, hypoperfusion, and ultimately organ dysfunction (Bone et al., 1992). The bariatric surgery patient is at a greater risk of developing infection and sepsis due to poor ventilation, diffusion, and perfusion of oxygen to the tissues; impaired wound healing; presence of diabetes and hyperglycemia; and elevated baseline inflammatory state (Savel et al., 2006; Wilson & Clark, 2003). Most obese patients are in a hypercoagulable, inflammatory state with an underlying diabetic comorbidity that further potentiates the possibility of sepsis.

Hemodynamic support for management of sepsis involves aggressive volume resuscitation to maintain the mean arterial pressure (MAP) greater than 65, urine output greater than 0.5 mL/kg/hr, oxygen saturation greater than 92%, and central venous pressure between 6 and 12 mm Hg (Savel et al., 2006). Norepinephrine (Levophed®) is usually a first choice if vasopressor therapy is required; vasopressin is considered second-line therapy (Dellinger, 2003). Sepsis is discussed in more detail in Chapter 51.

Anastomotic Strictures

RYGB purposely leaves a small opening at the gastrojejunostomy anastomosis (pouch) to minimize how much food passes through. As this opening heals (4–6 weeks), scar tissue can form making the opening between the stomach (pouch) and bowel too small to allow food to pass through. Patients should be educated on the usual presentation of a stricture as a gradual onset of dyspagia, over 7–10 days, with associated nausea and vomiting with the average postoperative time frame of 4–6 weeks. An endoscopy is diagnostic, in addition to determining possible ulcer formation, and a dilatation is performed if indicated. Anastomotic strictures have a low occurrence of approximately 5% (Carrodeguas, Szomstein, Zundel, Lo Menzo, & Rosenthal, 2006).

PATIENT OUTCOMES

Nurses can help ensure obtainment of optimal patient outcomes such as those listed in **Box 57-1** through the use of evidence-based interventions for the bariatric surgery patients.

SUMMARY

Morbid obesity has reached epidemic proportions. It is predicted that obesity, over the course of the next 20 years, will be the number one health problem throughout the world (SAGES, 2006). An increasing number of patients are undergoing bariatric surgery each year. A meta-analysis of 22,094 bariatric patients, between 1990 and 2003, revealed an operative mortality of 0.5% with an average excess weight loss of 61% at one year (Christou, Jarand, Sylvestre, & McLean, 2004). These procedures also lead to significant resolution of diabetes (77%), hyperlipidemia (70%), hypertension (62%), and osteoarthritis (86%) (Buchwald et al., 2005). With the increasing obesity population and more successful outcomes and resolution of comorbidities, even more patients are likely to undergo bariatric procedures in the future. Caring for the postoperative

bariatric patient requires special equipment, professional psychological interaction, specific nutritional therapy, and an understanding of the physiological needs and demands of the body systems. An important component of any multidimensional program is an enhanced understanding of the complications that may occur with bariatric surgery and ultimately result in an ICU admission. The interactions of the healthcare team are integral in promoting a successful outcome for the bariatric surgery population.

Box 57-1
Optimal Patient Outcomes

- Knowledge of basic anatomy post surgery
- Absence of postoperative complications
- Presence of psychological coping
- Adequate nutritional status
- Electrolytes within expected range
- Compliance with vitamin supplement therapy
- Understanding of postoperative diet
- Understanding of postoperative complications

CASE STUDY

A 52-year-old female with a history of hypertension, diabetes, gastroesophageal reflux disease, hypercholesterolemia, obstructive sleep apnea, degenerative joint disease, coronary heart disease, urinary stress incontinence, and pulmonary hypertension is admitted following 2 weeks post RYGB. She smokes two packs of cigarettes per day, and has a BMI of 52 kg/m^2. She is admitted with vague abdominal pain, tachycardic, vomiting, and nausea.

CRITICAL THINKING QUESTIONS

1. How should the potential risk for a postoperative infection be addressed?
2. Which postoperative complications should the nurse be alert for, and what are the best management techniques if a complication occurs?
3. Would a consult to the nutritionist be required for this case and, if so, why?
4. Use the form to write a plan of care for a bariatric surgery patient in the clinical setting. Rate the patient as a level 1, 3, or 5 on each characteristic.
5. Take one patient outcome for a patient and list evidence-based interventions found in a literature review for this patient.

6. Develop a list of potential postoperative complications that are associated with four of the Synergy Model patient characteristics in the table below.

Patient Characteristics	Potential Postoperative Complications
Vulnerability	
Resource Availability	
Participation in Care	
Participation in Decision Making	

7. Identify one nurse characteristic that would be crucial in providing care to the bariatric surgery patient, and provide a rationale for choosing the characteristics as it relates to this patient population.

Using the Synergy Model to Develop a Plan of Care

	Patient Characteristics	Level (1, 3, 5)	Subjective and Objective Data	Evidence-based Interventions	Outcomes
SYNERGY MODEL	Resiliency				
	Vulnerability				
	Stability				
	Complexity				
	Resource availability				
	Participation in care				
	Participation in decision making				
	Predictability				

Online Resources

Psychological Assessment for Bariatric Surgery: www.asbs.org/html/pdf/PsychPreSurgicalAssessment.pdf

2004 ABS Consensus Statement: www.asbs.org/html/pdf/2004_ASBS_Consensus_Conference_Statement.pdf

NIH Consensus Statement: http://consensus.nih.gov/1991/1991GISurgeryObesity084html.htm

Medicare Criteria: www.cms.hhs.gov/MLNMattersArticles/downloads/MM5013.pdf

REFERENCES

Angrisani, L., Furbetta, F., Doldi, S. B., Basso, N., Lucchese, M., Giacomelli, F., et al. (2003). Lap band adjustable gastric banding system: The Italian experience with 1863 patients operated on 6 years. *Surgical Endoscopy, 17*(3), 409–412.

Balsiger, B. M., Murr, M. M., Poggio, J. L., & Sarr, M. G. (2000). Bariatric surgery: Surgery for weight control in patients with morbid obesity. *Medical Clinics of North America, 84,* 477–489.

Beevers, G., Lip, G. Y., & O'Brien, E. (2001). ABC of hypertension. Blood pressure measurement. Part I. Sphygmomanometry: Factors common in all techniques. *British Medical Journal, 322*(7292), 981–985.

Bone, R. C., Balk, R. A., Cerra, F. B., Dellinger, R. P., Fein, A. M., Knaus, W. A., et al. (1992). Definitions for sepsis and organ failure and guidelines for the use of innovative therapies in sepsis. The ACCP/SCCM Consensus Conference Committee. American College of Chest Physicians/Society of Critical Care Medicine. *Chest, 101*(6), 1644–1655.

Bostanjian, D., Anthone, G. J., Hamoui, N., & Crookes, P. F. (2003). Rhabdomyolysis of gluteal muscles leading to renal failure: A potentially fatal complication of surgery in the morbidly obese. *Obesity Surgery, 13*(2), 302–305.

Buchwald, H., Avidor, Y., Braunwald, E., Jensen, M. D., Pories, W., Fahrbach, K., et al. (2005). Bariatric surgery: A systematic review and meta-analysis. *Journal of the American Medical Association, 292,* 1724–1737.

Cadiere, G. B., Himpens, J., Hainaux, B., Gaudissart, G., Favretti, S., & Segato, G. (2002). Laparoscopic adjustable gastric banding. *Seminars in Laparoscopic Surgery, 9*(2), 105–114.

Carrodeguas, L., Szomstein, S., Zundel, N., Lo Menzo, E., & Rosenthal, R. (2006). Gastrojejunal anastomotic strictures following laparoscopic Roux-en-Y gastric bypass surgery: Analysis of 1291 patients. *Surgery for Obesity and Other Related Diseases, 2*(2), 92–97.

Centers for Disease Control and Prevention. (2006). Retrieved June 13, 2006, from www.cdc.gov/nccdphp/dnpa/obesity/

Champion, J. K. (2006). Obesity hypoventilation, respiratory failure and DVT prophylaxis in the bariatric surgical patient. Presentation at American Society of Bariatric Surgery, San Francisco. June 26–July 1, 2006.

Champion, J. K., & Williams, M. (2003). Small bowel obstruction and internal hernias after laparoscopic Roux-en-Y gastric bypass. *Obesity Surgery, 13*(4), 596–600.

Christou, N. V., Jarand, J., Sylvestre, J. L., & McLean, A. P. (2004). Analysis of the incidence and risk factors for wound infections in open bariatric surgery. *Obesity Surgery, 14,* 16–22.

Davidson, J. E., & Callery, C. (2001). Care of the obesity surgery patient requiring immediate-level care or intensive care. *Obesity Surgery, 11*(1), 93–97.

Dellinger, R. P. (2003). Cardiovascular management of septic shock. *Critical Care Medicine, 31*(3), 946–955.

DeMaria, E. J. (2003). Laparoscopic adjustable silicone gastric banding: Complications. *Journal of Laparoendoscopic and Advanced Surgical Techniques, Part A, 13*(4), 271–277.

DeMaria, E. J., Sugerman, H. J., Meador, J. G., Doty, J. M., Kellum, J. M., Wolfe, L., et al. (2001). High failure rate after laparoscopic adjustable silicone gastric banding for treatment of morbid obesity. *Annals of Surgery, 233*(6), 809–818.

Den Herder, C., Schmeck, J., Appelboom, D. J., & de Vries, N. (2004). Risks of general anaesthesia in people with obstructive sleep apnoea. *British Medical Journal, 329*(7472), 955–959.

Dixon, J. B., Dixon, M. E., & O'Brien, P. E. (2001). Quality of life after lap-band placement: Influence of time, weight loss, and comorbidities. *Obesity Research, 9,* 173–721.

Dixon, J. B., & O'Brien, P. E. (2002). Changes in comorbidities and improvements in quality of life after lap-band placement. *American Journal of Surgery, 184*(6B), 51S–54S.

Dixon, J. B., & O'Brien, P. E. (2006). Obesity and the white blood cell count: Changes with sustained weight loss. *Obesity Surgery, 16*(3), 251–257.

Drake, K. J., McAuliffe, M. S., Edge, M. J., & Lopez, C. C. (2006). Postoperative nursing care of patients after bariatric surgery. *Perspectives, 6*(4), 1, 5–7.

Elamin, E. M. (2005). Nutritional care of the obese intensive care unit patient. *Current Opinion in Critical Care, 11*(4), 300–303.

El-Solh, A. A. (2004). Clinical approach to the critically ill, morbidly obese patient. *American Journal of Respiratory Critical Care Medicine, 169*(5), 557–561.

Erstad, B. L. (2004). Dosing of medications in morbidly obese patients in the intensive care unit setting. *Intensive Care Medicine, 30*(1), 18–32.

Fedullo, P. F., & Tapson, V. F. (2003). Clinical practice. The evaluation of suspected pulmonary embolism. *New England Journal of Medicine, 349*(13), 1247–1256.

Flum, D. R., Salem, L., Elrod, J. A., Dellinger, E. P., Cheadle, A., & Chan, L. (2005). Early mortality among Medicare beneficiaries undergoing bariatric surgical procedures. *Journal of the American Medical Association, 294*(15), 1903–1908.

Food and Drug Administration. (2005). FDA trial summary of safety and effectiveness data: The lap-band adjustable gastric banding system (P000008). Retrieved July 20, 2006, from www.fda.gov

Geerts, W. H., Pineo, G. F., Heit, J. A., Bergqvist, D., Lassen, M. R., Colwell, C. W., et al. (2004). Prevention of venous thromboembolism: The Seventh ACCP Conference on Antithrombotic and Thrombolytic Therapy. *Chest, 126*(Suppl.), S338–S400.

Gehlbach, B. K., & Kress, J. P. (2002). Sedation in the intensive care unit. *Current Opinion in Critical Care, 8*(4), 290–298.

Gibson, G. (2004). Obstructive sleep apnea syndrome: Underestimated and undertreated. *British Medical Bulletin, 72*(1), 49–64.

Guedea, M. E., Arribas del Amo, D., Solanas, J. A., Marco, C. A., Bernado, A. J., Rodrico, M. A., et al. (2004). Results of biliopancreatic diversion after five years. *Obesity Surgery, 14*(6), 766–772.

Kaminsky, J., & Gadaleta, D. (2002). A study of discrimination within the medical community as viewed by obese patients. *Obesity Surgery, 12*(1), 14–18.

Kellum, J. M., Kuemmerle, J. F., O'Dorisio, T. M., Rayford, P., Martin, D., Engle, K., et al. (1990). Gastrointestinal hormone responses to meals before and after gastric bypass and vertical banded gastroplasty. *Annals of Surgery, 211*(6), 763–770.

Kern, P. A., Ranganathan, S., Li, C., Wood, L., & Ranganathan, G. (2001). Adipose tissue tumor necrosis factor and interleukin-6 expression in human obesity and insulin resistance. *American Journal of Physiology and Endocrinology Metabolism, 280*(5), E745–E751.

Kress, J. P., Gehlbach, B., Lacy, M., Pliskin, N., Pholman, A. S., & Hall, J. B. (2003). The long-term psychological effects of daily sedative interruption on critically ill patients. *American Journal of Respiratory Critical Care Medicine, 168*(12), 1457–1461.

Ladosky, W., Botelho, M. A., & Albuquerque, J. P. (2001). Chest mechanics in morbidly obese non-hypoventilated patients. *Respiratory Medicine, 95*(4), 281–286.

Livingston, E. H., Huerta, S., Arthur, D., Lee, S., DeShields, S., & Heber D. (2002). Male gender is a predictor for morbidity and age a predictor of mortality for patients undergoing bypass surgery. *Annals of Surgery, 236,* 576–582.

Maggard, M. A., Sugerman, L. R., Suttorp, M., Maglione, M., Sugerman, H. J., Livingston, E. H., et al. (2005). Meta-analysis: Surgical treatment of obesity. *Annals of Internal Medicine, 142*(7), 547–559.

Mason, E. E. (2003). Voluntary or obligatory? *IBSR Newsletter,* 18. Retrieved July 21, 2006, from www.surgery.uiowa.edu/ibsr/wsummer03.htm

Messerli, F. (1982). Cardiovascular effects of obesity. *Lancet, 1,* 1165–1168.

Mun, E. C., Blackburn, G. L., & Matthews, J. B. (2001). Current status of medical and surgical therapy for obesity. *Gastroenterology, 120*(3), 669–681.

National Institutes of Health. (1991). Available at http://consensus.nih.gov/1991/1991GISurgeryObesity084html.htm

NIH Consensus Conference Statement. (1991). Retrieved July 17, 2006, from http://consensus.nih.gov/cons/084/084_statement.htm

Nguyen, N. (2004). Open versus laparoscopic procedures in bariatric surgery. *Journal of Gastrointestinal Surgery, 86*(4), 393–395.

Nguyen, N., & Wolfe, B. (2005). The physiologic effects of pneumoperitoneum in the morbidly obese. *Annals of Surgery, 241*(2), 219–226.

O'Brien, P. E., Brown, W. A., Smith, A., McMurrick, P. J., & Stephens, M. (1999). Prospective study of a laparoscopically placed adjustable gastric band in the treatment of morbid obesity. *British Journal of Surgery, 86*(1), 113–118.

O'Brien, P. E., & Dixon, J. B. (2003). Lap-band: Outcomes and results. *Journal of Laparoendoscopic and Advanced Surgical Techniques, Part A, 13*(4), 265–270.

Papasavas, P. K., Hayetian, F. D., Caushaj, P. F., Landreneau, R. J., Maurer, J., Keenan, R. J., et al. (2002). Outcome analysis of laparoscopic Roux-en-Y gastric bypass for morbid obesity. The first 116 cases. *Surgical Endoscopy, 16*(12), 1653–1657.

Pieracci, F., Barie, P., & Pomp, A. (2006). Critical care of the bariatric patient. *Critical Care Medicine, 34*(6), 1796–1804.

Podnos, Y. D., Jimenez, J. C., Wilson, S. E., Stevens, C. M., & Nguyen, N. T. (2004). Complications after laparoscopic gastric bypass: A review of 3464 cases. *Archives of Surgery, 138*, 957–961.

Poole, N., Al Atar, A., Bidlake, L., Fienness, A., McCluskey, S., Nussey, S., et al. (2004). Pouch dilatation following laparoscopic adjustable gastric banding: psychobehavioral factors (can psychiatrists predict pouch dilatation?). *Obesity Surgery, 14*(6), 798–801.

Ray, C., Sue, D., Bray, G., Hansen, J. E., & Wasserman, K. (1983). Effects of obesity on respiratory function. *American Review of Respiratory Disease, 128*(3), 501–506.

Ren, C. J., Horgan, S., & Ponce, J. (2002). US experience with the Lap-band system. *American Journal of Surgery, 184*(6B), 46S–50S.

Rubenstein, R. B. (2002). Laparoscopic adjustable gastric banding at a U.S. center with up to 3-year follow-up. *Obesity Surgery, 12*(3), 380–384.

SAGES Guidelines to Bariatric Surgery. (2006). Retrieved on July 24, 2006, from www.lapsurgery.com/BARIATRIC%20SURGERY/SAGES.htm

Sanchez, V. M., Schneider, B. E., & Mun, E. C. (2006a). Surgical management of severe obesity. Retrieved July 14, 2006, from www.utdol.com/utd/content/topic.do?topicKey=gi_dis/32649&type=A&selectedTitle=3~14

Sanchez, V. M., Schneider, B. E., & Mun, E. C. (2006b). Complications of bariatric surgery. Retrieved July 14, 2006, from www.utdol.com/utd/content/topic.do?topicKey=gi_dis/33257&type=A&selectedTitle=1~14

Santry, H. P., Gillen, D. L., & Lauderdale, D. S. (2005). Trends in bariatric surgical procedures. *Journal of the American Medical Association, 294*(15), 1909–1917.

Sapala, J. A., Wood, M. H., Sapala, M. A., & Flake, T. M. (1998). Marginal ulcer after gastric bypass: A prospective 3-year study of 173 patients. *Obesity Surgery, 8*, 505–516.

Sapala, J. A., Wood, M. H., Schuhknecht, M. P., & Sapala, M. A. (2003). Fatal pulmonary embolism after bariatric operations for morbid obesity: A 24-year retrospective analysis. *Obesity Surgery, 13*, 819–825.

Savel, R. H., Gropper, M. A., Macura, J. M., & Lazzaro, R. S. (2006). Management of the critically ill bariatric patient. Retrieved June 14, 2006, from www.utdol.com/utd/content/topic.do?topicKey=cc_medi/30895&type=A&selectedTitle=5~14

Shiffman, M. L., Sugerman, H. J., Kellum, J. M., Brewer, W. H., & Moore, E. W. (1991). Gallstone formation after rapid weight loss: A prospective study in patients undergoing gastric bypass surgery for treatment of morbid obesity. *American Journal of Gastroenterology, 86*(8), 1000–1005.

Spaulding, L. (1997). The impact of small bowel resection on the incidence of stomal stenosis and marginal ulcer after gastric bypass. *Obesity Surgery, 7*, 485–487.

Stocker, D. (2003). Management of the bariatric patient. *Endocrinology and Metabolism Clinics, 32*(2), 1–16.

Ukleja, A., & Stone, R. L. (2004). Medical and gastroenterologic management of the post-bariatric surgery patient. *Journal of Clinical Gastroenterology, 38*(4), 312–321.

U.S. National Library of Medicine. (2004). Vertical banded gastroplasty. Retrieved July 21, 2006, from www.nlm.nih.gov/medlineplus/ency/imagepages/19498.htm

Vincent, J. (2005). Give your patient a fast hug (at least) once a day. *Critical Care Medicine, 33*(5), 1225–1230.

Wickremesekera, K., Miller, G., Naotunne, T. D., Knowles, G., & Stubbs, R. S. (2005). Loss of insulin resistance after Roux-en-Y gastric bypass surgery: A time course study. *Obesity Surgery, 15*(4), 474–481.

Wilson, J. A., & Clark, J. J. (2003). Obesity: Impediment to wound healing. *Critical Care Nursing Quarterly, 26*(2), 119–132.

Wu, E. C., & Barba, C. A. (2000). Current practices in the prophylaxis of venous thromboembolism in bariatric surgery. *Obesity Surgery, 10*(1), 7–13.

Advocacy and Moral Agency

PART VII

CHAPTER 58

Bioethical Issues Concerning Death in the ICU

Shirlien Metersky

LEARNING OBJECTIVES

Upon completion of this chapter, the reader will be able to:

1. Identify state and federal laws regarding advance directives and community-based do-not-resuscitate orders.

2. Apply ethical principles in the analysis of complex end-of-life care issues, recognizing the influence of morals, professional codes, and patient preferences.

3. Recognize professional misconceptions related to management of end-of-life care.

4. Describe strategies utilized by the ICU nurse in advocating for the patient and family during an ethical dilemma.

Bioethics revolves around making choices about life and death based on moral principles of what is perceived as right or wrong. Advances in science and medical technology have enabled the prolongation of life, resulting in society moving from a perception of dying as a natural event to a drive to find a cure to all illnesses and diseases. Consequences of the prolongation of life at any cost include provision of futile care, an increased economic burden, and poor quality of life. Despite advances in technology, one in five Americans dies using critical care services, with many of these deaths due to the withholding or withdrawal of life support. Many barriers exist in the decision-making process for transitioning from curative treatment to comfort care and the withholding or withdrawal of life-sustaining treatment. This chapter discusses the challenges in the promotion of optimal end-of-life care (EOLC) that allows patients to die with dignity by examining advance directives (ADs), ethical dilemmas faced in complex EOLC dilemmas, and misconceptions related to provision of EOLC.

ADVANCE DIRECTIVES

Definition and Purpose

Advance directive is a general term for legal documents that communicate the healthcare wishes of individuals should they become incapacitated and unable to participate in their medical care (Maxfield, Pohl, & Colling, 2003). Documentation of individuals' healthcare wishes through ADs assists in individuals' right to die with dignity by making their wishes known in advance. By giving individuals control over how they will die, important decisions regarding EOLC will not be left to physicians, family members, or others who are unaware of individuals' personal values, beliefs, or preferences (Robb-Nicholson, 2004). The burden is removed from family members in making important and personal EOLC choices for their loved ones.

ADs do not become effective until the individual is unable to participate in making medical decisions at a time when such a decision is necessary. Some of the terms found in ADs require clarification because they can be ambiguous and open to interpretation, such as *terminal*, *extraordinary means*, and *incurable*. It is important to note that individuals' informed decision will take precedence over any written predetermined directive as long as individuals have the capacity to make their own decisions (Klein, 2005). Of course, the definition of *capacity* is open to interpretation and vague, implying that the individuals have the ability to understand health-related information, can reason and deliberate about healthcare choices, and apply the information to their condition. If and when the individual's health improves, the patient's verbal preferences supercede the AD.

If individuals do not have an AD, their personal wishes concerning treatment and EOLC can be respected. For example, if an individual has verbalized care wishes to healthcare providers, family, or friends, and these wishes have been documented, appropriate EOLC decisions can be addressed. Several persons may be the individual's representative, in the following order (although laws may vary from state to state):

- Legal guardian
- Spouse
- Adult children (18 or older)—the majority of the adults who are available within a reasonable length of time
- Parents
- Adult siblings (18 or older)—the majority of the adults who are available within a reasonable length of time
- Aunts, uncles, or any other known blood relatives who can be located within a reasonable length of time

When there is disagreement between co-equals (adult children, parents, adult siblings), the healthcare team should try to reach an agreement among decision-making family members. A harmonious decision is not always attainable, however, further emphasizing the need for individuals to have completed ADs for their EOLC wishes to be honored.

Types of Advance Directives

Two primary categories of ADs exist: instructive and proxy. Instructive ADs include living wills. Proxy ADs assign a durable power of attorney for health care. Two witnesses must sign the AD as well as the individual to whom it applies. Certain criteria must be met to be a witness to an AD. The witnesses cannot be the primary care or attending physician, the administrator of a nursing home if the individual resides in a nursing home, the designated healthcare proxy agent, or anyone related by blood, marriage, or adoption such as a spouse or adult children. In some states, living wills may be signed by a Notary Public instead of two witnesses (some states require signatures from two witnesses and the signature of a Notary Public). It is important to know the specific requirements for your state. Once the AD has been appropriately signed, copies should be kept by the individual's attorney, primary care physician, family members, and healthcare proxy. ADs should be kept in an accessible place ready to be easily produced whenever the in-

dividual becomes a patient in a healthcare facility and should be placed in the patient's medical record (Maxfield et al., 2003).

A community- or state-based Do-Not-Resuscitate (DNR) order is not an AD but does delineate resuscitative instructions. For example, in the state of North Carolina, only a valid North Carolina DNR order will be honored by emergency medical services (EMS) in the out-of-hospital setting. This DNR order is written by the physician on a special goldenrod-colored form with a bright red stop sign. It is recognized throughout North Carolina as a state-based DNR order and instructs healthcare providers to withhold cardiopulmonary resuscitation (CPR) and other heroic measures. Other states may use different methods to ensure that an individual's wishes are carried out by EMS. Specific state laws may be accessed by obtaining state statutes.

Living Wills

Living wills, instructive ADs, direct or guide physicians regarding withholding or withdrawing of life-sustaining treatment (LST) when an individual is in a terminal condition or a permanently unconscious state. A terminal condition is defined as an irreversible, incurable, or untreatable condition from which there can be no recovery and because of which death is likely to occur within a relatively short period of time if LST is not provided. The diagnosis of a permanently unconscious state must be based on several components and confirmed by the second opinion of a physician who specializes in such conditions. Permanently unconscious patients are irreversibly unaware of self and the environment and have a total loss of cerebral functioning so that they cannot experience pain or suffering. Living wills help determine how aggressive medical treatment should be while honoring patients' wishes and preventing prolonged painful and futile care against their wishes.

Living wills do not address all EOLC decisions. Indeed, EOLC decisions are rarely simple. Terms such as *quality of life* and *terminal condition* are open to interpretation by the physician, patient, and family members. In many instances, a patient's medical condition requires making decisions regarding LST, yet the patient is not in a terminal or permanent unconscious state. Even though an individual has a living will, it is imperative that frank communication take place between the physician and the patient so choices are made in the individual's best interest. Living wills do, however, address important medical issues such as withholding and withdrawing LST, including CPR, defibrillation, mechanical ventilation, artificial nutrition (tube feedings), and hydration.

All 50 states recognize the concept of living wills; however, living wills are not standardized from state to state. For example, some states directly address dialysis and use of vasopressors to support blood pressure. State-specific living wills can be found on the Internet (see the Online References section at the end of this chapter).

Durable Health Care Power of Attorney

The durable health care power of attorney (DHCPA), a proxy AD, designates another person to make healthcare decisions for the individual in the event that the individual loses capacity to do so. The individual's representative is the person or persons named by the individual on the DHCPA form. Examples of conditions in which a DHCPA takes effect are when a patient suffers from confusion, hallucinations, chronic sedation, or coma. The DHCPA representative has the legal and moral duty to make decisions that are consistent with the individual's previously stated wishes. If the individual's wishes are unknown, the DHCPA is supposed to decide what is best for the patient, based on knowing the type of person the patient is. A DHCPA is not allowed to change any restrictions established by the individual. If there is a conflict between what the living will designates and what the DHCPA says, the living will takes precedence.

Choosing a DHCPA as a health agent proxy is an important decision. Legally, some people are unable to serve as healthcare proxies, and restrictions may vary from state to state. Primary care or attending physicians are prohibited from serving as healthcare proxies, and the healthcare proxy must be at least 18 years of age. Most DHCPAs are family members, although they need not be. When an individual is estranged from the family, a close personal friend may be a better choice. Considerations when choosing a DHCPA include the following issues (Robb-Nicholson, 2004):

- Does the person know the individual well enough to make important healthcare decisions?
- Can the person make important decisions without becoming too emotionally involved?
- Is the person comfortable in going along with the individual's wishes?
- Will the person be persistent by advocating the individual's desired wishes?
- Will the person be readily available to serve as the individual's DHCPA?

Community- or State-Based Do-Not-Resuscitate Orders

DNR orders vary greatly within the community or state. These orders are not ADs, but rather assist with the level of LST and resuscitative efforts that may be initiated or withheld. For example, if an individual's AD indicated that he or she does not want LST if he or she has a terminal illness or is in a perma-

nently unconscious state, then the individual's primary or attending physician would complete a DNR order when that patient is admitted to a healthcare facility and/or has met the criteria designated by the AD. In other words, ADs help guide the initiation of DNR orders.

DNR orders also have implications for the *code status* assigned to the patient: Is the patient a *full code*, meaning that all levels of LST and resuscitative efforts are employed, or is the patient's care tailored by varying degrees of DNR? Each healthcare facility may develop its own distinct classification system for code status, which can cause confusion within the healthcare facility, community, and state. Does DNR mean just not performing CPR and defibrillation, or can emergency medications and intubation take place? Does DNR mean to continue administering LST until the patient has a cardiopulmonary arrest? Does it mean to withdraw all LST? Or should each patient and legal representative be allowed to tailor a list of which treatments to employ with different circumstances? It is imperative that every nurse fully understand how DNR orders are implemented within the respective healthcare facility, community, and state.

For example, two levels of DNR orders are state-approved forms in the state of Ohio. State law indicates that the DNR orders are recognized and are transferable from facility to facility or from a facility to an individual's home. A facility is defined as any hospital, nursing home, assisted living apartment, home care agency, hospice, or emergency medical service. The two levels of DNR orders recognized in Ohio are DNR Comfort Care (DNRCC) and DNR Comfort Care—Arrest (DNRCC-Arrest). A DNRCC order means that individuals want comfort care only from the time the order is written until the time they die, which would include the withdrawal of LST such as mechanical ventilation and vasopressors. DNRCC-Arrest means that any resuscitative efforts *may* be instituted until the heart or lungs stop. Although these two levels of care do not entirely eliminate any misinterpretation or ambiguous areas, their creation does help provide consistency between healthcare facilities within the state.

Legal Application for Healthcare Facilities

In 1991, the Patient Self-Determination Act became federal law. This legislation requires any healthcare facility that receives Medicare or Medicaid reimbursement to determine upon admission whether a patient has or wishes to make an AD (Dobbins, 2005). If a patient does not have an AD, then written information regarding the legal rights as designated by state law must be provided along with assistance in completing one if the patient wishes. Documentation of whether the patient has an AD must be evident in the patient's medical record (Maxfield et al., 2003). Furthermore, patients and their legal representatives need to be informed to bring in a copy of the AD to be placed in the medical record for reference.

ETHICAL DILEMMAS

Definitions

Some of the major ethical dilemmas for intensive care unit (ICU) nurses center on DNR orders and EOLC issues. To provide optimal patient care, nurses need to acquire knowledge of patient rights and ethical principles and have opportunities to explore and resolve clinical ethical dilemmas in realistic situations (Kish, 2001). Even though codes of ethics provide direction in the provision of humane patient care, they do not provide a clear-cut decision tree for handling complex clinical issues or relieve the ensuing moral distress that is encountered in such situations (Kyba, 2002).

Before discussing common ethical dilemmas encountered with EOLC issues, it is essential to have an understanding of the definition of ethics and ethical principles. *Ethics* is a branch of philosophy that deals with morality and moral reasoning—principles that guide an individual's sense of what is right or wrong. *Bioethics* centers on what is right or wrong in relation to life and life-and-death decisions. *Ethical dilemmas* are problems that arise in clinical situations where decisions must be made between alternatives that are equally undesirable (Gray, Anderson, & Kish, 2001). Such a decision is guided by morally defensible principles; however, neither choice is ideal because people are guided by their values, which place different weights on the competing moral principles under evaluation. There is no choice that soundly preserves both sides of the competing values and morals. Ethical dilemmas are resolvable but not solvable (Kish, 2001).

Ethical decisions are based on the ethical principles of autonomy, beneficence, nonmaleficence, justice, respect, fidelity, and veracity. Autonomy, beneficence, nonmaleficence, and justice are the primary principles that guide our moral justification for our professional decisions with EOLC issues (Kyba, 2002). Respect, *fidelity* (the duty to be faithful to commitments and to maintain privacy and confidentiality), and *veracity* (the duty to tell the truth) are ethical principles that guide our everyday practice.

Autonomy is the individuals' freedom to choose and make decisions for themselves. Autonomy is applied when individuals are given the ability to make their own decisions regarding EOLC issues after being informed.

The ethical principles of beneficence and nonmaleficence are closely related. *Beneficence* implies making sure that the good outweighs the harm. *Nonmaleficence* is the obligation to avoid causing harm, intentionally or unintentionally. With all patient care, it is expected that patients will be protected from harm (nonmaleficence). The administration of LST applies the principle of beneficence when evaluating the benefits versus the risks of instituting and maintaining such treatment.

Justice or fair treatment implies that treatment decisions, including allocation of resources, will not be based on factors such as age, gender, sexual orientation, religion, ethnic group, or socioeconomic status. Allocation of resources is especially pertinent when patients are utilizing costly LST against their consent or as delineated in their ADs (Kyba, 2002).

Ethical Dilemma Case Study

M.J., a 58-year-old male, is admitted to the ICU after developing severe hypotension that progressed to cardiopulmonary arrest during his hemodialysis therapy at an extended care facility. His past medical and surgical history include end-stage renal disease, diabetes, hypertension, and left above-the-knee amputation. Upon admission to the ICU, M.J. is intubated, unresponsive, and hypotensive requiring vasopressors. He does not have any ADs. On hospital day 2, M.J. remains ventilator dependent and responds only to painful stimuli with purposeful movements without sedation. Hemodialysis is not tolerated related to his hypotension. Continuous renal replacement therapy (CRRT), a gentler around-the-clock dialysis therapy, is offered as a treatment option to M.J.'s wife as the legal next-of-kin. Even though the attending and consulting physicians have documented a poor prognosis, no discussion or family conference has been held to communicate M.J.'s chance of recovery.

The preceding scenario is a common one in the ICU setting. The majority of adults do not have ADs, placing the burden of EOLC decision making on healthcare providers and family members. The first step that needs to take place is a family conference. It is imperative that the appropriate individuals participate in this meeting. The attending physician, primary nurse, pastoral care, and family members who are the legal next-of-kin or healthcare proxies who are authorized to make decisions are key members. Prior to the family conference, physicians need to reach a consensus regarding the prognosis of the patient along with the consequences of continuation of treatment. A common problem is family members *hearing* different opinions from various physicians.

During the family conference, the physician needs to apply the ethical principle of *veracity* (the duty to tell the truth) by communicating to the family M.J.'s clinical status, prognosis, treatment options including rationale for withholding or withdrawing LST, and likely quality of life. Even though M.J.'s physician had applied *justice* (fair treatment to all) by suggesting

CRRT as a treatment option, he did not employ the ethical principle of *beneficence* (do the benefits or good outweigh the risks?). Since M.J. does not have any ADs that would have taken effect now that his condition is terminal, he no longer can exercise his *autonomy* (freedom to make decisions for himself). In this situation, the family conference should center on what M.J.'s wishes for EOLC would be. The conference should be patient-centered, exploring any past discussions concerning EOLC if the present situation did occur. If M.J. has never communicated his wishes, then questions pertaining to what his views are on quality of life should be asked. An ethical dilemma will occur if M.J.'s legal representation is uncertain of what EOLC decisions should be made if the patient never communicated his wishes. The healthcare providers can maintain M.J.'s clinical status with LST (one choice) versus withdrawal of LST (another choice).

Table 58-1 provides strategies that nurses can use in dealing with ethical dilemmas in the ICU.

PROFESSIONAL MISCONCEPTIONS IN MANAGEMENT OF EOLC

Pain and Symptom Management

Many physicians and nurses are uncomfortable with administration of high doses of pain medication and sedatives to relieve pain and discomfort, because such measures may be viewed as hastening the individual's death. The doctrine of *double effect* provides moral justification for the healthcare provider's good intention of pain and symptom management (Kyba, 2002). For example, if the use of analgesics to control pain unintentionally shortens the individual's life, the doctrine of double effect states that the good intention (pain control) balances the less good effect (hastened death).

The dose of analgesics and sedatives should not be based solely on *recommended* maximal doses. The starting doses may be irrelevant because most patients will have already received these medications and developed some tolerance to their

TABLE 58-1 Strategies for Challenging Issues in the ICU

Issue	Strategies
Patient considers a hastened death	The nurse needs to examine the patient's mental health, symptom management, advance directives, and decision making.
	The nurse needs to respect the patient's autonomy.
	An ethics consultation or a consultation with pastoral or chaplain services may help staff with religious or moral objections to discuss this issue and their professional obligations in a therapeutic environment.
	Questions should be nonjudgmental and open ended (e.g., Why hasten death now?).
Advocacy	Provide pain relief and discussion options with the patient and family.
	Provide interventions to treat symptoms.
	Support the patient's AD in the face of family disagreement with the patient's decision.
Communication	Provide frequent communication.
	Discuss end-of-life preferences with documentation of clear mental status.
	Discuss hospice care with any dying patients.
	Provide support and coaching to help patients communicate their wishes, concerns, and needs to their physicians and loved ones.
	Ensure that the physician talks plainly with the families about the nearness of death and the option of hospice, and families know what to expect in the dying process.
Decision making	Show respect for patient autonomy.
	Provide direction for advance planning.
Education	Provide education, accurate facts, and options for end-of-life care and other treatment.
	Nurses can offer to be present, by encouraging advance directives or by documenting the patient's concerns and wishes.
Family support	Provide reassurance to families that everything possible was done and that death was beyond their control.
	Provide coaching to family members to help them ask the physician for information about the trajectory of the patient's illness.
	Support family EOLC decision even when not consistent with own preference/opinions.

Source: Valente, 2004.

effects. Instead, analgesics and sedatives should be titrated to effect (Trugg et al., 2001).

Withdrawal of Life Support

No set guidelines exist for the withdrawal of life support, only recommendations. Withdrawal of cardiac support by discontinuing vasopressors is often enough to satisfy these criteria. When withdrawal of cardiac support proves insufficient, withdrawal of ventilator support follows. There are both advantages and disadvantages to performing either a terminal wean or a terminal extubation. Regardless of which ventilator withdrawal method is chosen, the consensus is that paralyzing agents be discontinued and allowed to wear off prior to the withdrawal of ventilator support (Trugg et al., 2001).

A *terminal wean* occurs when the ventilator rate and oxygen level are gradually titrated down along with administration of analgesics and sedatives to prevent any symptoms of acute air hunger. This method is especially useful when the patient is conscious or semiconscious and likely to experience distress. A terminal wean is also viewed as a less active procedure, minimizing the burden on the family.

A *terminal extubation* takes place when the artificial airway is removed. This method does not prolong the dying process and allows the patient to be free from an unnatural airway. Terminal extubation is recommended for patients who are unlikely to experience distress, such as unconscious patients. Regardless of the method chosen for withdrawal of ventilator support, appropriate analgesia and sedation need to be administered prior to withdrawal to minimize discomfort (Trugg et al., 2001).

SUMMARY

Bioethical issues in the intensive care setting produce ethical dilemmas in which decisions must be guided by ethical principles of what is right or wrong. These uncomfortable situations need to be addressed to respect the individuals' wishes and to allow them to die with dignity. Knowledge of ADs is essential to educate patients and their families on the available options. Courageous conversations about EOLC—an unpleasant topic for most—must then occur. Unfortunately, when a patient is admitted to the ICU, it is often not the patient but rather the family or legal representative who is approached about EOLC choices. ADs are an integral component of EOLC decisions because they guide the withholding and withdrawal of LST.

CRITICAL THINKING QUESTIONS

1. Which disciplines should be consulted when an ethical dilemma occurs in the ICU?
2. Identify one ethical dilemma that could occur with a patient of a diverse background.
3. Which strategies would you use if a patient refuses further treatment and the family members request that all interventions be undertaken to maintain life? How would you advocate for the patient?
4. How will you implement your role as a facilitator of learning for a patient requesting information on advance directives?
5. Use the form to write up a plan of care for one client in the clinical setting who is having therapies withheld or withdrawn.
6. Write a case example from the clinical setting. Rate the patient as a level 1, 3, or 5 on each characteristic. Identify the level of nurse characteristics needed in the care of this patient.
7. Interview a healthcare provider about an example of a challenging ethical dilemma and its resolution. Identify the ethical principles underlying the strategies of resolution in this case.
8. Summarize the laws related to advance directives in any of the U.S. territories: Puerto Rico, U.S. Virgin Islands, Guam, and Samoa.

Online Resources

Individual state living wills: www.uslegalforms.com

Free copies of living wills: www.partnershipforcaring.org

Information on living wills and healthcare proxies: www.health.harvard.edu/LW

Information on advance directives: www.abanet.org/publiced/practical/patient_self_determination_act.html

Federal Patient Self-Determination Act Final Regulations: www.dgcenter.org/acp/pdf/psda.pdf

Peaceful Death: Recommended Competencies and Curriculum Guidelines for End-of-Life Nursing Care: www.aacn.nche.edu/Publications/deathfin.htm

REFERENCES

Dobbins, E. H. (2005). Helping your patient to a "good death." *Nursing 2005, 35*(2), 43–45.

Gray, P., Anderson, M., & Kish, C. (2001). Foundations for an ethical practice. In D. Robinson & C. Kish (Eds.), *Core concepts in advanced practice nursing* (pp. 205–223). Philadelphia: Mosby.

Kish, C. P. (2001). Case studies for ethical analysis. In D. Robinson & C. Kish (Eds.), *Core concepts in advanced practice nursing* (pp. 237–246). Philadelphia: Mosby.

Klein, C. A. (2005). The importance of advance directives. *Nurse Practitioner, 30*(4), 11.

Kyba, F. C. (2002). Legal and ethical issues in end-of-life care. *Critical Care Nursing Clinics of North America, 14*(2), 141–155.

Maxfield, C. L., Pohl, J. M., & Colling, K. (2003). Advance directives: A guide for patient discussions. *Nurse Practitioner, 28*(5), 38–47.

Robb-Nicholson, C. (January 2004). Living wills and health care proxies. *Harvard Women's Health Watch,* 6–7. Retrieved June 6, 2005, from www.health.harvard.edu

Trugg, R. D., Cist, A. F., Brackett, S. E., Burns, J. P., Curley, M. A., Danis, M., et al. (2001). Recommendations for end-of-life care in the intensive care unit: The Ethics Committee of the Society of Critical Care Medicine. *Critical Care Medicine, 29*(12), 2332–2347.

Valente, S. M. (2004). End-of-life challenges: Honoring autonomy. *Cancer Nursing, 27*(4), 314–319.

Organ Donation

Jesse Scruggs   Kenneth Wood   Alista "Cozzie" Watkins

LEARNING OBJECTIVES

Upon completion of this chapter, the reader will be able to:

1. Define brain death.
2. List patients who meet the inclusion criteria for organ donation.
3. Describe management of potential donors.
4. Describe the physiology of brain death.
5. List optimal patient outcomes that may be achieved through evidence-based management of patients agreeing to organ donation.

Organ transplantation is an important treatment modality for patients with end-stage organ disease refractory to medical treatment. Currently, more than 89,000 patients in the United States are on lists awaiting transplantation. On average, 17 people die each day because of a shortage of available organs. There were 14,155 organ donations in 2004: 7,151 from deceased donors and 7,004 from living donors. Over the last 10 years, organ donations from deceased donors have increased by 33%, while donations from living donors have increased by 101% (Organ Procurement and Transplantation Network, 2005). According to federal mandates, hospitals are required to notify a local organ procurement agency regarding a death or imminent death. When it is suitable, the agency will send a representative to the institution to ascertain that the family is approached to discuss the option of organ donation. Another method of increasing the supply of potentially transplantable organs from brain dead donors is to optimize the care of the potential donor. This chapter reviews the optimal care of the brain dead organ donor as well as the organ recipient.

CONTRAINDICATIONS FOR DONORSHIP

Few absolute exclusions to organ donation exist. No patient should be excluded as a potential donor until the situation is discussed with the local organ procurement organization. Generally accepted infective exclusions include a person with the human immunodeficiency virus or septic shock (Tuttle-Newhall, Collins, Kuo, & Schoeder, 2003). Uncomplicated bacteremia, fungemia, and localized infections are not absolute exclusions (Angelis, Cooper, & Freeman, 2003). Donors infected with hepatitis B and C may donate organs to recipients with the same disease (Lopez-Navidad & Caballero, 2003). Those infected with cytomegalovirus may donate to any recipient because post-transplant cytomegalovirus-induced morbidity has been reduced by routine prophylaxis (Wood, Becker, McCartney, D'Alessandro, & Coursin, 2004). Malignancy is generally an absolute contraindication, except in donors with certain intracranial primary brain malignancies and nonmelanoma skin cancers. Donors with diabetes mellitus and hypertension may often donate kidneys. Smokers with less than a 30-pack year history may donate their lungs if the chest radiograph is normal (Tuttle-Newhall et al.).

According to federal rule, any hospital that receives Medicare or Medicaid reimbursement must attempt to obtain consent for organ or tissue donation from the family of the deceased patient. The Health Care Financing Administration further mandates that the consent be attempted by a specially trained individual (Federal Register Final Rule, 2000).

Consent remains the largest obstacle to successful donation, but several psychosocial factors have been shown to increase consent rates. Prior to any discussion of organ donation, it is crucial for families to understand that brain death means their family member is dead. (Further discussion of brain death appears in Chapter 28.) Decoupling, or separating the notification of death from the request for organ donation, has been reported to enhance consent rates. Many hospitals and organ procurement agencies have added family support coordinators to their staffs in an effort to assist the families of potential organ donors.

Families in crisis typically do not understand the hospital process (e.g., visiting times and restrictions). During such situations, the family support coordinator evaluates the needs of the family and becomes a part of a liaison structure of the communication system. Families often do not understand and process the meaning of neurological death. For this reason, the request for consent should be made by experienced personnel involving the coordinator of the local organ procurement organization and be undertaken in a private setting (Williams et al., 2003). The family must be reassured that the procurement procedure will not disfigure the body or prevent viewing at the funeral.

The federal conditions of participation in the Medicare program require timely notification of local organ procurement organization in cases of impending death. In many hospitals, clinical criteria are used to help make the appropriate referral of potential organ donors. The hospital will agree on certain triggers to evaluate the potential donor, and a referral will then be made. Such a process would be initiated, for example, in a case of a patient with a Glasgow Coma Scale score of 5 or less, head trauma, and anoxia, this patient would be referred as a potential organ donor and family support would be consulted.

BRAIN DEATH PHYSIOLOGY

Recognizing and understanding the physiology and process of brain death is crucial for several reasons: It facilitates the recognition of the patient with incipient herniation, stabilization is enhanced when the physiology is understood, and declaration occurs in a more timely manner when brain death is appropriately recognized.

Brain death (neurological death) is an irreversible ischemic process that will inevitably result in cardiac death within 24 to 48 hours in the absence of medical stabilization. The term *coning* refers to the rostral-caudal progression of ischemia due to brain swelling, which leads to increased intracranial pressure and ultimately results in herniation and brain death. Initial cerebral ischemia manifests as increased vagal tone with resultant bradycardia. Pontine ischemia results in increased sympathetic tone and increased blood pressure. Cushing's response is characterized by hypertension, tachycardia, and irregular respirations. As intracranial pressure rises, systemic pressure must rise to preserve brain perfusion. Thus Cushing's response is an adaptive mechanism to preserve cerebral perfusion pressure. Caudal progression of ischemia to the medullary area precipitates a massive catecholamine surge, which is a final attempt to maintain cerebral perfusion pressure. With herniation, the spinal cord becomes ischemic and the sympathetic system is deactivated, leading to vasodilation and hypotension.

Brain death disrupts the hypothalamic-pituitary axis, resulting in thermoregulatory dysfunction, diabetes insipidus, and several consequences of thyroid and cortisol depletion. Low levels of circulating thyroid hormone, for example, cause impaired mitochondrial function and bring about a transition from aerobic to anaerobic metabolism. Low levels of cortisol result in hypotension and electrolyte abnormalities.

MEDICAL MANAGEMENT

Early referral of potential organ donors is crucial to successful medical management in such cases. Hemodynamic instability is common in donors and can contribute to impaired organ function and cardiac arrest, resulting in failed procurement. Management goals are to maintain normovolemia, systolic blood pressure greater than 100 mm Hg, and urinary output greater than 1 mL/kg/hr. Failure to achieve these goals or instability in a previously stable donor should prompt consideration for right heart catheterization with a pulmonary artery catheter. This measure allows for the monitoring of the central venous pressure, cardiac output, pulmonary artery occlusive pressure, cardiac index, and systemic vascular resistance. Incorporating diagnostic assessments and therapeutic interventions with the use of the pulmonary artery catheter into donor management protocols has been reported to increase organ procurement rates (Wood et al., 2004). **Figures 59-1** and **59-2** are critical pathways that can guide the nurse in organ donation and after cardiac death that have been published by United Network for Organ Sharing (UNOS).

Hypovolemia is common in potential donors. It can result from the initial injury, inadequate resuscitation, or treatment of elevated intracranial pressures with fluid restriction, mannitol, or other diuretics. Other causes include hyperglycemia-induced osmotic diuresis, diabetes insipidus, and hypothermic diuresis.

FIGURE 59-1 Critical Pathway for Donation after Cardiac Death

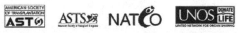

Collaborative Practice	Phase I Identification & Referral	Phase II Preliminary Evaluation	Phase III Family Discussion & Consent	Phase IV Comprehensive Evaluation & Donor Management	Phase V Withdrawal of Support /Pronouncement of Death/Organ Recovery
The following health care professionals may be involved in the Donation After Cardiac Death (DCD) donation process: Check all that apply: ○ Physician (MD) ○ Critical Care RN ○ Nurse Supervisor ○ Medical Examiner / Coroner ○ Respiratory Therapy (RT) ○ Laboratory ○ Pharmacy ○ Radiology ○ Anesthesiology ○ OR/Surgery Staff ○ Clergy ○ Social Worker ○ Organ Procurement Coordinator (OPC) ○ Organ Procurement Organization (OPO)	Prior to withdrawing life support, contact local OPO for any patient who fulfills the following criteria: ○ Devastating neurologic injury and/or other organ failure requiring mechanical ventilatory or circulatory support ○ Family and/or care giving team initiate conversation about withdrawal of support Following referral, additional evaluation is done collaboratively to determine if death is likely to occur within one hour (or within a specified timeframe as determined by caregiving team and OPO) following withdrawal of support Patient conditions might include the following: ○ **Ventilator dependent for respiratory insufficiency:** apneic or severe hypopneic; tachypnea ≥ 30 breaths /min after DC ventilator ○ **Dependent on mechanical circulatory support** (LVAD, RVAD, V-A ECMO; Pacemaker with unassisted rhythm < 30 beats per minute. ○ **Severe disruption in oxygenation:** PEEP≥ 10 and SaO2 ≤ 92%; FiO2 ≥ .50 and SaO2 ≤ 92%; V-V ECMO requirement ○ **Dependent upon pharmacologic circulatory assist:** Norephinephrine, epinephrine, or phenylephrine ≥ 0.2 ug/kg/min; Dopamine ≥ 15 ug/kg/min ○ **IABP and inotropic support:** IABP 1:1 and dobutamine or dopamine ≥10 ug/kg /min and CI ≤ 2.2 L/min/M2; IABP 1:1 & CI ≤ 1.5 L/min/M2	Physician ○ Supportive of withdrawal of care and has communicated grave prognosis to family ○ Review DCD procedure with OPC ○ Will be involved in withdrawal/ pronouncement ○ Will designate a person to be involved with withdrawal and/or pronouncement Family ○ Has received grave prognosis ○ Understands prognosis ○ In conjunction with care giving team, decide to withdraw support Patient ○ Age _____ ○ Weight _____ ○ Height _____ ○ ABO _____ ○ Medical Hx _____ ○ Surgical Hx _____ ○ Social Hx ○ Death likely < 1 hour following withdrawal (determined collaboratively by evaluating: injury, level of support, respiratory drive assessment)	○ Support services offered to family ○ OPC/Hospital Staff approach family about donation options ○ Legal next-of-kin (NOK) fully informed of donation options and recovery procedures ○ Legal NOK grants consent for DCD following withdrawal of support ○ Family offered opportunity to be present during withdrawal of support ○ OPC obtains ____ Witnessed consent from legal NOK for DCD ____ Signed consent Time _____ Date _____ ____ Detailed med/soc history Notification of donation ○ Hospital supervisor ○ ME/Coroner notified ____ ME/Coroner releases for donation ____ ME/Coroner has restrictions *Stop Pathway if—* ○ *Family, ME/Coroner denies consent* ○ *Patient determined to be unsuitable candidate for DCD* ○ *Patient progresses to brain death during evaluation – refer to brain dead pathway*	○ MD, in collaboration with OPO, implements management guidelines. ○ Establish location and time of withdrawal of support ○ Review plan for withdrawal to include: - Pronouncing MD (should be in attendance for duration of withdrawal of support, determination of death, and may not be a member of the transplant team) - Comfort Care - Extubation and discontinuation of ventilator support - Establish plan for continued supportive care if pt survives > one hour or predetermined time interval after withdrawal of support ○ Notify OR/Anesthesia ____ Review patient's clinical course, withdrawal plan and potential organ recovery procedures ____ Schedule OR Time ○ Notify recovery teams ○ Prepare patient for transport to pre-arranged area for withdrawal of support ○ Patient transported to prearranged area ○ Note: Should the clinical situation require premortum femoral cannulation, the following should be reviewed: - family consent or understanding - MD inserting cannula - Time and location of cannula insertion - If death does not occur, determine if cannula should be removed	○ Withdrawal occurs in ____ OR ____ ICU ____ Other ____ ○ Family present for withdrawal of support ____ yes ____ no ○ OR/Room prepared and equipment set up ○ Transplant team in the OR (not in attendance during withdrawal) ○ Care giving team present ○ Administration of pre-approved medication (e.g. Heparin/Regitine) ○ **Withdrawal of support according to hospital/MD practice guidelines** Time _____ Date _____ ○ **Vital signs are monitored and recorded every minute (See attached sheet)** ○ **Pt pronounced dead and appropriate documentation completed** Time _____ Date _____ MD _____ ○ **Transplant Team initiates surgical recovery at prescribed time following pronouncement of death** ○ Allocation of organs per OPTN/UNOS policy ○ *If cardiac death not established within 1 hour or predetermined time interval after withdrawal of support – Stop Pathway. Patient moved to predetermined area for continuation of supportive care.* ○ *Post mortem care administered*
Labs / Diagnostics		○ ABO ○ Electrolytes ○ LFTs ○ PT/PTT ○ CBC with Diff ○ Beta HCG (female pts) ○ ABG		Repeat full panel of labs additionally: ○ Serology Testing infectious disease profile ○ Blood cultures X 2 ○ UA & Urine culture ○ Sputum Culture ○ Tissue typing	

continues

FIGURE 59-1 Critical Pathway for Donation after Cardiac Death (continued)

Respiratory	○ Maintain ventilator support ○ Pulmonary toilet PRN	○ Respiratory drive assessment RR _____ VT _____ VE _____ NIF _____	○ ABGs as requested ○ Notify RT of location and time of withdrawal of support	○ Transport with mechanical ventilation using lowest FiO$_2$ possible while maintaining the SaO$_2$ >90%	
		Minutes off ventilator _____ ○ Hemodynamics while off ventilator HR _____ BP _____ SaO$_2$ _____			
Treatments / Ongoing Care	Maintain standard nursing care to include: ○ Vital signs q 1 hour ○ I & O q 1 hour				○ Post mortem care at conclusion of case
Medications				○ Provide medications as directed by MD in consult with OPC	○ Heparin and other medications prior to withdrawal of support
Optimal Outcomes	The potential DCD donor is identified & a referral is made to the OPO.	The donor is evaluated & found to be a suitable candidate for donation.	The family is offered the option of donation & their decision is supported.	Optimal organ function is maintained, withdrawal of support plan is established, and personnel prepared for potential organ recovery.	Death occurs within one hour of withdrawal of support and all suitable organs and tissues are recovered for transplant.

This work supported by HRSA contract 231-00-0115.

Source: Reprinted with permission from NATCO.

FIGURE 59-2 Critical Pathway for the Organ Donor

Patient name: _____

ID number: _____

Collaborative Practice	Phase I Referral	Phase II Declaration of Brain Death and Consent	Phase III Donor Evaluation	Phase IV Donor Management	Phase V Recovery Phase
The following professionals may be involved to enhance the donation process. *Check all that apply.* ○ Physician ○ Critical care RN ○ Organ Procurement Organization (OPO) ○ OPO coordinator (OPC) ○ MedicalExaminer (ME)/ Coroner ○ Respiratory ○ Laboratory ○ Pharmacy ○ Radiology ○ Anesthesiology ○ OR/Surgery staff ○ Clergy ○ Social worker	○ Notify physician regarding OPO referral ○ Contact OPO ref: Potential donor with severe brain insult ○ OPC on site and begins evaluation Time _____ Date _____ ○ Ht_____ Wt_____ as documented ○ ABO as documented _____ ○ Notify house supervisor/ charge nurse of presence of OPC on unit	○ Brain death documented Time _____ Date _____ ○ Pt accepted as potential donor ○ MD notifies family of death ○ Plan family approach with OPC ○ Offer support services to family (clergy, etc) ○ OPC/Hospital staff talks to family about donation ○ Family accepts donation ○ OPC obtains signed consent & medical/social history Time _____ Date _____ ○ ME/Coroner notified ○ ME/Coroner releases body for donation ○ *Family/ME/Coroner denies donation—stop pathway— initiate post-mortem protocol—support family.*	○ Obtain pre/post transfusion blood for serology testing (HIV, hepatitis, VDRL, CMV) ○ Obtain lymph nodes and/or blood for tissue typing ○ Notify OR & anesthesiology of pending donation ○ Notify house supervisor of pending donation ○ Chest & abdominal circumference ○ Lung measurements per CXR by OPC ○ *Cardiology consult as requested by OPC (see reverse side)* ○ *Donor organs unsuitable for transplant—stop pathway—initiate post-mortem protocol—support family.*	○ OPC writes new orders ○ Organ placement ○ OPC sets tentative OR time ○ Insert arterial line/ 2 large-bore IVs ○ Possibly insert CVP/Pulmonary Artery Catheter ○ **See reverse side**	○ Checklist for OR ○ Supplies given to OR ○ Prepare patient for transport to OR ○ IVs ○ Pumps ○ O$_2$ ○ Ambu ○ Peep valve ○ Transport to OR Date _____ Time _____ ○ OR nurse ○ reviews consent form ○ reviews brain death documentation ○ checks patient's ID band

FIGURE 59-2 Critical Pathway for the Organ Donor (continued)

Labs/Diagnostics		○ Review previous lab results ○ Review previous hemody-namics	○ Blood chemistry ○ CBC + diff ○ UA ○ C & S ○ PT, PTT ○ ABO ○ A Subtype ○ Liver function tests ○ Blood culture X 2 / 15 minutes to 1 hour apart ○ Sputum Gram stain & C & S ○ Type & Cross Match ____ # units PRBCs ○ CXR ○ ABGs ○ EKG ○ Echo ○ Consider cardiac cath ○ Consider bronchoscopy	○ Determine need for additional lab testing ○ CXR after line placement (if done) ○ Serum electrolytes ○ H & H after PRBC Rx ○ PT, PTT ○ BUN, serum creatinine after correcting fluid deficit ○ Notify OPC for ___ PT >14 ___ PTT > 28 ___ Urine output ___ < 1 mL/Kg/hr ___ > 3 mL/Kg/hr ___ Hct < 30 / Hgb <10 ___ Na >150 mEq/L.	○ Labs drawn in OR as per surgeon or OPC request ○ Communicate with pathology: Bx liver and/or kidneys as indicated
Respiratory	○ Pt on ventilator ○ Suction q 2 hr ○ Reposition q 2 hr	○ Prep for apnea testing: set FiO₂ @ 100% and antici-pate need to decrease rate if PCO₂ < 45 mm Hg	○ Maximize ventilator settings to achieve SaO₂ 98 - 99% ○ PEEP = 5cm O₂ challenge for lung placement FiO₂ @ 100%, PEEP @ 5 X 10 min ○ ABGs as ordered ○ VS q 1°	○ Notify OPC for ___ BP < 90 systolic ___ HR < 70 or > 120 ___ CVP < 4 or > 11 ___ PaO₂ < 90 or ___ SaO₂ < 95%	○ Portable O₂ @ 100% FiO₂ for transport to OR ○ Ambu bag and PEEP valve ○ Move to OR
Treatments/ Ongoing Care		○ Use warming/cooling blanket to maintain temperature at 36.5° C - 37.5 °C ○ NG to low intermittent suction	○ Check NG placement & output ○ Obtain actual Ht ____ & Wt ____ if not previ-ously obtained		○ Set OR temp as directed by OPC ○ Post-mortem care at conclusion of case
Medications			○ Medication as requested by OPC	○ Fluid resuscitation—con-sider crystolloids, colloids, blood products ○ DC meds except pressors & antibiotics ○ Broad-spectrum antibiotic if not previously ordered ○ Vasopressor support to maintain BP > 90 mm Hg systolic ○ Electrolyte imbalance: consider K, Ca, PO₄, Mg replacement ○ Hyperglycemia: consider insulin drip ○ Oliguria: consider diuretics ○ Diabetes insipidus: con-sider antidiuretics ○ Paralytic as indicated for spinal reflexes	○ DC antidiuretics ○ Diuretics as needed ○ 350 U heparin/kg or as directed by surgeon
Optimal Outcomes	The potential donor is iden-tified & a referral is made to the OPO.	The family is offered the option of donation & their decision is supported.	The donor is evaluated & found to be a suitable candi-date for donation.	Optimal organ function is maintained.	All potentially suitable, con-sented organs are recovered for transplant.

Shaded areas indicate Organ Procurement Coordinator (OPC) Activities.

This Critical Pathway was developed under contract with the U.S. Department of Health and Human Services, Health Resources and Services Administration, Division of Transplantation.

Source: Reprinted with permission from NATCO.

Specific goals for volume status are a pulmonary artery occlusive pressure of 8 to 12 mm Hg and a central venous pressure of 6 to 8 mm Hg. Intravenous fluids or diuretics are the initial treatment used in attaining these goals. Lactated Ringer's solution should be administered to prevent hypernatremia. Sodium bicarbonate, 50 mEq/L, or D_5W can be given when acidemia is present. Packed red blood cells should be transfused to reach a target hemoglobin of 10 Gm/dL. Blood glucose should be monitored and insulin infusions given to maintain blood glucose between 80 and 150 mg/dL. Before their administration to the patient, all fluids should be warmed to 37 °C.

Cardiac dysfunction is another important cause of hemodynamic instability. Mechanisms of initial injury to the heart include myocardial contusion, pericardial tamponade, and myocardial ischemia or infarct. The process of brain death can cause cardiac dysfunction through either catecholamine damage or ischemia-reperfusion injury. Metabolic depression can occur from acidosis, hypothermia, hypophosphatemia, hypocalcemia, hypoxia, or endocrine dysfunction associated with brain death. Volume overload can result in heart failure, and arrhythmias can be caused by catecholamines, ischemia, hypokalemia, and hypomagnesemia.

Specific goals for cardiac function are a cardiac index greater than 2.4 L/min/m^2, a left ventricular stroke work index greater than 15 Gm/m^2/beat, and urine output greater than 1 mL/kg/hr. Inotropic agents such as dopamine (Intropin®), dobutamine (Dobutrex®), and epinephrine (Adrenaline®) are the initial treatments. Vasoactive medications should be given in the doses required to attain these goals. High vasoactive requirement is not a contraindication to donation, because minimal association has been demonstrated between vasoactive drug requirements and recipient graft outcome (Schnuelle, Berger, de Boer, Persijn, & van der Woude, 2001; Wood et al., 2004). Dopamine is commonly the first-line agent. When dose requirements exceed 10 mcg/kg/min, additional agents are indicated. No specific vasopressor combination has been shown to be superior. Agents that work primarily through alpha-adrenergic mechanisms should be avoided in high doses. Arginine vasopressin (Pitressin®) is another acceptable second-line agent.

Arrhythmias are common in potential organ donors and often prove refractory to treatment. Lidocaine (Xylocaine®) and amiodarone (Cordarone®) are appropriate therapies for ventricular arrhythmias, and amiodarone is recommended for supraventricular arrhythmias. Bradyarrhythmias that result from vagal disruption will not respond to atropine but rather will require isoproterenol (Isuprel®) or epinephrine. Standard advanced cardiac life support algorithms should be used in case of cardiac arrest.

Vasodilation is usually coincident with cardiac dysfunction and may be caused by spinal shock, catecholamine depletion, and loss of vasomotor control with herniation, spinal cord ischemia, and acquired sepsis. Specific goals are a mean arterial pressure greater than 60 mm Hg, and systemic vascular resistance between 800 and 1200 dynes/sec/cm^{-5}. Vasopressors such as norepinepherine (Levophed®) and epinephrine should be the initial treatment. In contrast, primarily alpha-adrenergic agents should be avoided. Failure to achieve the preceding goals with conventional pulmonary artery catheter-guided therapy necessitates the use of hormonal resuscitation. **Table 59-1** delineates the hemodynamic management of the potential donor.

A growing body of literature supports the use of hormone replacement therapy in hemodynamically unstable donors. In the absence of randomized controlled trials and formal consensus, hormone replacement therapy should commence in donors requiring dopamine at doses greater than 10 mcg/kg/min and those with a left ventricular ejection fraction of less than 45%. Thyroid replacement with triiodothyronine (T3) should be given in a bolus dose of 4 mcg and an infusion of 3 mcg/hr, or with thyroxine (T4) in a bolus dose of 20 mcg and an infusion of 10 mcg/hr. Glucocorticoid support with methylprednisolone should be initiated with a bolus dose of 15 mg/kg and may be repeated in 24 hours. Vasopressin requires a bolus dose of 1 U, followed by an infusion of 0.5 to 4 U/hr. An insulin bolus of 10 U should be given along with 50% dextrose, followed by an insulin infusion beginning at 1 U/hr with a goal blood glucose level between 80 and 150 mg/dL (Wood et al., 2004).

Traditional criteria for the ideal lung donor include age less than 55 years, clear chest radiograph, partial pressure of oxygen (PaO_2) greater than 300 mm Hg on FiO_2 of 1.0 and positive end-expiratory pressure (PEEP) of 5 cm H_2O, less than 20-pack-year tobacco history, no chest trauma, absence of aspiration or sepsis, and absence of bacteria, fungus, or WBCs on sputum examination. Given the shortage of lung donors and deaths on

TABLE 59-1 Hemodynamic Management of the Potential Organ Donor

Tissue perfusion	• Pulmonary artery pressure monitoring • Vasoactive agents • Volume repletion with 500 mL over 15 min to keep the mean arterial pressure > 60 mm Hg
Tissue oxygenation	• Mechanical ventilation
Milieu presentation	• Fluid and electrolyte balance and acid–base balance • Hormonal stability • Prevent and treat infection

Source: Smith, 2003.

the lung transplant recipient waiting list, many marginal lungs may be transplanted successfully (Pierre, Sekine, Hutcheon, Waddell, & Keshavjee, 2002).

Optimizing the donor's respiratory status may maximize the chances for successful procurement of organs. The goals for mechanical ventilation include fraction of inspired oxygen less than or equal to 40%, PaO_2 greater than 100 mm Hg, partial pressure of carbon dioxide ($PaCO_2$) between 35 and 40 mm Hg, arterial pH between 7.35 and 7.45, tidal volume of 8 to 10 mL/kg ideal body weight, PEEP less than 5 cm of H_2O, and static airway pressure less than 30 cm of H_2O. Patients with intracranial hypertension will often be treated with high minute ventilation and correspondingly low $PaCO_2$. After brain death, pH and $PaCO_2$ should be normalized. Hypoxemia often results from atelectasis. Early bronchoscopy and chest radiography should be used liberally. Bronchoscopy allows for anatomical evaluation, assessment, removal of foreign bodies, and location and suctioning of secretions and infection. Selection of appropriate antibiotic therapy, when indicated, can be based on Gram staining of suctioned secretions (Wood et al., 2004).

The optimal fluid status of donated organs varies. Lung transplantation is more successful when central venous pressure is kept between 6 and 8 mm Hg. Education of the respiratory therapy department is essential to communicate needs of the medical and nursing staff managing the potential organ donor. Most organ procurement agencies have developed routine orders for management of potential organ donors.

Diabetes insipidus can result from ischemia or infarction of the posterior pituitary. The excessive loss of free water can result in hypernatremia, hypokalemia, hypomagnesemia, hypophosphatemia, hypocalcemia, hyperosmolarity, and hemodynamic instability. When urine output is less than 200 mL/hr, it should be matched volume-for-volume with 5% dextrose in water. Urine output greater than 200 mL/hr is an indication for administration of either arginine vasopressin or 1-desamino-8-D-arginine vasopressin. Serum electrolytes should be measured every 2 to 4 hours. Insulin infusions should be used to maintain plasma glucose in the range of 80 to 150 mg/dL (Davidson et al., 2003).

Coagulation abnormalities can also complicate brain death. Cytomegalovirus-negative, leukocyte-filtered packed red blood cells should be transfused to maintain hemoglobin at a level greater than 10 Gm/dL. In addition, platelets should be transfused to maintain their availability at greater than 80,000 cm^3. The international normalized ratio (INR) should be corrected to less than 2.

Hypothermia should be avoided. Methods to maintain a core body temperature of 35 °C (95 °F) include warming blankets, warming of all intravenous infusions, and heating and humidification of ventilator gases (Wood et al., 2004).

CARE OF THE ORGAN RECIPIENT

Following solid-organ transplantation, the nurse is responsible for monitoring for complications. Some complications are general for any organ transplanted; others pertain to transplant of specific organs.

A number of complications related to solid-organ transplant have been reported in the literature. They are listed in **Table 59-2**.

The signs and symptoms of rejection will vary depending on the organ that was transplanted. In all cases, organ dysfunction is the primary symptom. For example, renal transplant patients may develop a decrease in urinary output. Patients may also report generalized discomfort. Patients may develop rejection immediately following transplantation, a situation termed hyperacute graft rejection.

Immunosuppressive agents are used to repress immune system function so as to prevent graft rejection following transplantation. The five categories of immunosuppressive therapy are described in **Table 59-3**.

The literature also describes complications related to transplantation of specific organs. These potential problems are listed in **Table 59-4**.

TABLE 59-2 Complications Reported Following Solid Organ Transplant

Complication	Reference
Graft rejection	Pizzolitto, Boscutti, Falconieri, & Montanaro, 2004
Delayed graft function	McKenna, Takemoto, & Terasaki, 2000
Bleeding	Lee, Kumar, & Lai, 1991
Lymphoproliferative disorders (e.g., lymphoma) and other malignancies	Jain et al., 2005; Taylor, Marcus, & Bradley, 2005; Trofe et al, 2004
New-onset diabetes	Mora, 2004; Obayashi, 2004; Pavlakis, 2005; Salifu, Tedla, Murty, Aytug, & McFarlane, 2005; Wilkinson et al., 2005
Infection	Chiu, Domagala, & Park, 2004; Mayo, Galan, Moreno, Llacer, & Moreno, 2005
Nontuberculous *Mycobacterium*	Doucette & Fishman, 2004
Invasive aspergillosis	Singh, 2005
Hypertension	Park & Luan, 2005
Psychiatric problems	Dew et al., 2001
Neurotoxic effects	Wijdicks, 2000

TABLE 59-3 Immunosuppressive Therapies

Category	Mechanism of Action	Example(s)
Corticosteroids	Blocks T-cell expression	Prednisone (Deltasone®)
Calcineurine inhibitors	Inhibits calcineurin, which inhibits IL-2 secretion	Cyclosporine (Sandimmune®), Tacrolimus (Prograf®)
Monoclonal antibodies	Blocks T-cell activation	Muromonab-CD3 (Orthoclone OKT3®), interleukin-2 receptor antagonist (Basiliximab, Simulect®), daclizumab (Zenapax®)
Polyclonal antibodies	Depletes T-cell concentration by binding lymphocytes with specific cell antigens	Antithymocyte globulin—equine (Atgam®), antithymocyte globulin—rabbit (RATG, Thymoglobulin®)
Antiproliferative agents	Blocks the proliferative phase of acute cellular rejection	Mycophenolate mofetil (Cellcept®), azathioprine (Imuran®)

Source: Immunosuppressive Drug, 2005.

The incidence of hepatitis C associated with cardiac transplantation is linked to donors who have the virus (File, Mehra, Nair, Dumas-Hicks, & Perrillo, 2003). It has been suggested that the incidence of complications of heart transplantation such as infection, osteoporosis, renal insufficiency, and malignancy may be decreased by minimizing immunosuppression. Once these complications develop, routine pharmacological management can be implemented to treat them (Mathier & McNamara, 2004). Development of dyslipidemia following heart transplant is believed to be related to diet, inactivity, and immunosuppressive therapy (Wenke, 2004).

Results from one study identified three predictors of a poor outcome after liver transplantation: lack of immediate production of bile in the operating room, platelet transfusion, and urinary output less than 2 mL/kg/hr. The researchers suggest that early retransplantation should be considered if these parameters have been identified (Markmann et al., 2003). Risk factors for infection following liver transplantation include hepatitis C virus cirrhosis, history of diabetes mellitus, respiratory distress syndrome, acute

renal insufficiency, neurological alterations, postoperative bleeding, reperfusion syndrome, and graft dysfunction (Mayo, Galan, Moreno, Llacer, & Moreno, 2005). Respiratory complications following liver transplantation include pleural effusion, pneumonia, respiratory insufficiency, pulmonary hypertension, pulmonary edema, pneumothorax, and atelectasis (Zheng

TABLE 59-4 Complications Associated with Transplantation of Specific Organs

Organ	Complications	Reference
Heart	Hepatitis C	File, Mehra, Nair, Dumas-Hicks, & Perrillo, 2003
	Infection	Chen et al., 2004; Mathier & McNamara, 2004
	Hypertension	Mathier & McNamara, 2004
	Diabetes	Mathier & McNamara, 2004
	Dyslipidemia	Mathier & McNamara, 2004; Wenke, 2004
	Osteoporosis	Mathier & McNamara, 2004
	Graft coronary disease	Mathier & McNamara, 2004
	Renal insufficiency	Mathier & McNamara, 2004
	Malignancy	Mathier & McNamara, 2004
	Medical noncompliance	Dew et al., 2004
	Mental health limitations	Dew et al., 2004
	Quality of life limitations	Dew et al., 2004
Liver	Suboptimal graft function	Markmann et al., 2003
	Infection	Mayo, Galan, Moreno, Llacer, & Moreno, 2005
	Hepatitis B	Poordad, 2004
	Respiratory complications	Zheng et al., 2004
	Anemia	Maheshwari, Mishra, & Thuluvath, 2004
	Central nervous system (CNS) complications	Wijdicks, 2000
Kidney	Cardiovascular disease	Montanaro et al., 2004
	Rejection	Pizzolitto, Boscutti, Falconieri, & Montanaro, 2004
	Delayed graft function	Perico, Cattaneo, Sayegh, & Remuzzi, 2004
	Anemia	Vanrenterghem, 2004
Pancreas	Anastomotic leak	Nath et al., 2005

et al., 2004). Meticulous nursing care in the ICU may lead to early recognition or avert development of some of these complications. Development of anemia is common following liver transplantation. In most cases, its cause is unknown (Maheshwari, Mishra, & Thuluvath, 2004).

Cardiovascular disease is frequently observed following kidney transplantation. Its emergence may be attributed to the presence of risk factors before and after transplant (e.g., hypertension, diabetes, hyperlipidemia) and immunosuppressive therapy. Modification of risk factors may eliminate this complication (Montanaro et al., 2004). Delayed graft function, which is a type of acute renal failure, may be related to ischemia and reinstitution of blood flow to damaged kidneys (Perico, Cattaneo, Sayegh, & Remuzzi, 2004).

PATIENT OUTCOMES

Nurses can help ensure attainment of optimal patient outcomes such as those listed in **Box 59-1** through the use of evidence-based interventions for patients undergoing organ transplantation.

SUMMARY

The management of the potential organ donor fundamentally involves the simultaneous care of the seven potential recipients. After brain death has been declared, it is crucial to continue optimal medical management so that the donor somatically survives to the point of procurement and the organs are maintained in the best possible condition. The most immediate and practical solution to the organ donor shortage is the maximal utilization and optimal management of the existing donor pool. Care of the organ recipient is essential for prevention and early recognition of possible complications.

Box 59-1
Optimal Patient Outcomes

- Free of transplant rejection
- Free of graft-vs-host response
- Physical comfort in expected range
- Free of transplantation complications
- Absence of complications from immunosuppressive therapy
- Adheres to prescribed regimen
- Demonstrates knowledge of signs and symptoms of rejection and complication
- Satisfaction with health status

CASE STUDY 1

B.R. is a 58-year-old male who was admitted to the hospital with a diagnosis of sepsis. He had prolonged periods of hypotension requiring aggressive fluid resuscitation and vasopressor therapy. He was on broad-spectrum antibiotic coverage, including aminoglycoside therapy to treat his infection. As a result of these therapies, B.R. developed acute renal failure. He was treated with hemodialysis as a patient in the ICU and subsequently as an outpatient once discharged from the hospital. His renal failure persisted, however, and B.R. was later diagnosed with chronic kidney disease. He was placed on the list to receive a kidney transplant and continued his hemodialysis therapy. During his wait for a transplant, his serum creatinine remained in excess of 2.3 mg/dL. B.R. also had several bouts of hyperkalemia and fluid overload.

B.R. was fortunate enough to receive a kidney transplant. Post transplant, he was started on tacrolimus (Prograf®) to prevent rejection. Several weeks following his transplant, B.R. was readmitted to the ICU from the ED with mental status changes associated with hyperglycemia (his blood sugar was 356 mg/dL). He had no history of diabetes mellitus. B.R.'s condition was stabilized and he was discharged from the hospital three days later.

CRITICAL THINKING QUESTIONS

1. Which conditions led to the development of renal failure in B.R.?
2. What was a possible cause of hyperglycemia in B.R.?

3. Which disciplines should be consulted to work with B.R.?

4. What types of issues may require you to act as an advocate or moral agent for B.R.?

5. How will you implement your role as a facilitator of learning for B.R.?

6. What complications is B.R. at risk for with a diagnosis of diabetes mellitus?

7. Use the form to write up data and plan of care for a patient who is an organ donor or recipient in the clinical setting. Rate the patient as a level 1, 3, or 5 on each characteristic. Identify the level of nurse characteristics needed in the care of this patient.

8. Take one outcome for a patient and list evidence-based interventions found in a literature review for this patient.

Using the Synergy Model to Develop a Plan of Care

	Patient Characteristics	Level (1, 3, 5)	Subjective and Objective Data	Evidence-based Interventions	Outcomes
SYNERGY MODEL	Resiliency				
	Vulnerability				
	Stability				
	Complexity				
	Resource availability				
	Participation in care				
	Participation in decision making				
	Predictability				

CASE STUDY 2

An unidentified patient was found in a car in an abandoned parking deck. The patient was emergently airlifted to a nearby trauma hospital in a metropolitan city, with attempted homicide being suspected.

Chief Complaint

A 28-year-old female with a gunshot wound to the head presented to the emergency department with the following vital signs: BP 126/62, HR 128, RR 24 and shallow, temperature 90°F. Seizure activity was noted to last approximately 45 seconds. An oral gastric tube was inserted and connected to low intermittent suction. The patient was orally intubated. A subclavian intravenous catheter was inserted. Phenytoin (Dilantin®) 1 Gm was given as an intravenous slow push. A computed tomography (CT) scan without contrast was ordered immediately on the patient's arrival. The CT scan results showed a single transcranial gunshot wound with fragmentation; they suggested a low-caliber projectile lodged in the superior temporal gyrus. Scan results further showed blood in the 3rd and 4th ventricles, with a notable brain midline shift to the left. The patient's hemoglobin was 6 Gm/dL, with a hematocrit of 22%. The trauma attending ordered the patient to be typed and crossed for 4 units of packed red blood cells. Three units of fresh frozen plasma were given.

Physical Exam Two Hours After Admission

Glasgow Coma Scale score = 3. The patient was not responding to deep pain stimuli. Pupils were dilated 3 mm and showed no response to light. A paradoxical respiratory pattern was noted with spontaneous respirations of 26 breaths per minute. Blood pressure was 180/112 mm Hg. A sudden drop in blood pressure to 80/40 mm Hg occurred, and no spontaneous respirations were noted for 15 minutes. Urinary output was greater than 350 mL/hr. Vasopressin (Pitressin®) was ordered to control diabetes insipidus and prevent hypernatremia. The patient responded with a reduction in urinary output to 90 to 100 mL/hr.

Family Support

The family support coordinator (FSC) and chaplain were with the family from the time of family's arrival to the hospital. The FSC prepared the family by sharing information that the nursing and medical staff had made available. The FSC and the chaplain collaborated with the doctors, nurses, staff, and the organ recovery specialist about the patient's condition and neurological testing. The FSC identified the next of kin and gauged the family's readiness to hear the results of tests to determine neurological death.

Test Results and Outcome

The physicians found no spontaneous respirations after withdrawal of ventilatory support for 5 to 10 minutes and an increase of $PaCO_2$ to more than 55 from a normal baseline. No pupillary response or response to noxious stimuli was noted on clinical exam. The patient was pronounced neurologically dead, and the family was given time to acclimate the information before being approached about organ and tissue donation.

CRITICAL THINKING QUESTIONS

1. What criteria did this patient exhibit to meet the brain death definition?
2. Describe how and when to call the transplant team.
3. Vasopressin (Pitressin®) was ordered to control diabetes insipidus and prevent hypernatremia for this patient. How is this drug titrated?
4. How do you determine if the patient has exclusion criteria for organ donation?
5. Describe how you would approach the family regarding organ donation.
6. The family is approached about organ donation and they are not sure of their daughter's wishes. The mother asks you what she should do. How would you reply?
7. What level of urine output should be maintained with the organ donor?
8. What are the goals for mechanical ventilation for this patient?

Online Resources

ClinicalTrials.gov: www.clinicaltrials.gov

Donate Life: www.organdonor.gov

TransWeb.org—all about transplantation and donation: www.transweb.org

U.S. Department of Health and Human Services: www.4woman.gov/faq/organ_donation.htm

REFERENCES

Angelis, M., Cooper, J. T., & Freeman, R. B. (2003). Impact of donor infections on outcome of orthotopic liver transplantation. *Liver Transplantation, 9,* 451–462.

Chen, Z. Q., Chen, H., Hai, H., Wang, C. S., Zhao, Q., Hong, T., et al. (2004). Infection after cardiac transplantation: Prevention and management. *Chinese Medical Journal, 117*(3), 342–346.

Chiu, L. M., Domagala, D. M., & Park, J. M. (2004). Management of opportunistic infections in solid-organ transplantation. *Progress in Transplantation, 14*(2), 114–129.

Davidson, J., Wilkinson, A., Dantal, J., Dotta, F., Haller, H., Hernandez, D., et al. (2003). New-onset diabetes after transplantation: 2003 international consensus guidelines. *Transplantation, 75*(10 Suppl.), SS3–SS24.

Dew, M. A., Goycoolea, J. M., Harris, R. C., Lee, A., Zomak, R., Dunbar-Jacob, J., et al. (2004). An Internet-based intervention to improve psychosocial outcomes in heart transplant recipients and family caregivers: Development and evaluation. *Journal of Heart and Lung Transplantation, 23*(6), 745–758.

Dew, M. A., Kormos, R. L., DiMartini, A. F., Switzer, G. E., Schulberg, H. C., Roth, L. H., et al. (2001). Prevalence and risk of depression and anxiety-related disorders during the first three years after heart transplantation. *Psychosomatics, 42*, 300–313.

Doucette, K., & Fishman, J. A. (2004). Nontuberculous mycobacterial infection in hematopoietic stem cell and solid organ transplant recipients. *Clinical Infectious Diseases, 38*(10), 1428–1439.

Federal Register Final Rule. (2000). Hospital conditions for participation for organ donation (42 CFR Part 482). Retrieved August 29, 2005, from www.scha.org/documents/medicareCoPforHospitals_1.pdf

File, E., Mehra, M., Nair, S., Dumas-Hicks, D., & Perrillo, R. (2003). Allograft transmission of hepatitis C virus infection from infected donors in cardiac transplantation. *Transplantation, 76*(7), 1096–1100.

Immunosuppressive Drug. (2005). Retrieved October 23, 2005, from http://enwikipedia.org/wiki/immunosuppressive_drug

Jain, M., Badwal, S., Pandey, R., Srivastava, A., Sharma, R. K., & Gupta, R. K. (2005). Post-transplant lymphoproliferative disorders after live donor renal transplantation. *Clinical Transplantation, 19*(5), 668–673.

Lee, T. L., Kumar, A., & Lai, F. O. (1991). Extraoperative management of the liver transplant patient. *American Academy of Medicine Singapore, 20*(4), 543–548.

Lopez-Navidad, A., & Caballero, F. (2003). Extended criteria for organ acceptance: Strategies for achieving organ safety and increasing organ pool. *Clinical Transplant, 17*, 308–324.

Maheshwari, A., Mishra, R., & Thuluvath, P. J. (2004). Post-liver transplant anemia: Etiology and management. *Liver Transplantation, 10*(2), 165–173.

Markmann, J. F., Markmann, J. W., Desai, N. M., Baquerizo, A., Singer, J., Yersiz, H., et al. (2003). Operative parameters that predict the outcomes of hepatic transplantation. *Journal of the American College of Surgeons, 196*(4), 566–572.

Mathier, M. A., & McNamara, D. M. (2004). Management of the patient after heart transplant. *Current Treatment Options in Cardiovascular Medicine, 6*(6), 459–469.

Mayo, M. M., Galan, T. J., Moreno, G. A., Llacer, B. E., & Moreno, P. I. (2005). Prevalence and risk factors for early postoperative infection after liver transplantation. *Revista Espanola di Anestsiologia y Reanimacion, 52*(4), 200–207.

McKenna, R. M., Takemoto, S., & Terasaki, P. (2000). Anti-HLA antibodies after solid organ transplantation. *Transplantation, 69*(3), 319–326.

Montanaro, D., Gropuzzo, M., Tulisso, P., Boscutti, G., Risaliti, A., Baccarani, U., et al. (2004). Cardiovascular disease after renal transplantation. *Transplantation Proceedings, 37*(2), 991–993.

Mora, P. F. (2005). Post-transplantation diabetes mellitus. *American Journal of the Medical Sciences, 329*(2), 86–94.

Nath, D. S., Gruessner, A., Kandaswamy, R., Gruessner, R. W., Sutherland, D. E., & Humar, A. (2005). Late anastomotic leaks in pancreas transplant recipients—clinical characteristics and predisposing factors. *Clinical Transplantation, 19*(2), 220–224.

Obayashi, P. A. (2004). Posttransplant diabetes mellitus: Cause, impact, and treatment options. *Nutrition in Clinical Practice, 19*(2), 165–171.

Organ Procurement and Transplantation Network. (2005). Retrieved August 29, 2005, from www.optn.org

Park, J. M., & Luan, F. L. (2005). Management of hypertension in solid-organ transplantation. *Progress in Transplantation, 15*(1), 17–22.

Pavlakis, M. (2005). New-onset diabetes after transplantation. *Current Diabetes Reports, 5*(4), 300–304.

Perico, N., Cattaneo, D., Sayegh, M. H., & Remuzzi, G. (2004). Delayed graft function in kidney transplantation. *Lancet, 364*(9447), 1814–1827.

Pierre, A. F., Sekine, Y., Hutcheon, M. A., Waddell, T. K., & Keshavjee, S. H. (2002). Marginal donor lungs: A reassessment. *Journal of Thoracic and Cardiovascular Surgery, 123*(3), 421–427.

Pizzolitto, S., Boscutti, G., Falconieri, G., & Montanaro, D. (2004). Clinicopathologic correlations in acute renal graft rejection. *Giornale Italiano de Nefrologia, 21*(Suppl. 26), S19–S27.

Poordad, F. F. (2004). Liver transplant and recurrent disease. *Clinics in Liver Disease, 8*(2), 461–473.

Salifu, M. O., Tedla, F., Murty, P. V., Aytug, S., & McFarlane, S. I. (2005). Challenges in the diagnosis and management of new-onset diabetes after transplantation. *Current Diabetes Reports, 5*(3), 194–199.

Schnuelle, P., Berger, S., de Boer, J., Persijn, G., & van der Woude, F. J. (2001). Effects of catecholamine application to brain dead donors on graft survival in solid organ transplantation. *Transplantation, 72*(3), 455–463.

Singh, N. (2005). Invasive aspergillosis in organ transplant recipients: New issues in epidemiologic characteristics, diagnosis, and management. *Medical Mycology, 43*(Suppl. 1), S267–S270.

Smith, S. L. (2003). Organ and tissue donation and recovery. *Organ Transplant.* Retrieved March 25, 2005, from www.medscape.com/viewarticle/451208

Taylor, A. L., Marcus, R., & Bradley, J. A. (2005). Post-transplant lymphoproliferative disorders (PTLD) after solid organ transplantation. *Critical Reviews in Oncology-Hematology, 56*(1), 155–167.

Trofe, J., Beebe, T. M., Buell, J. F., Hanaway, M. J., Alloway, R. R., Gross, T. G., et al. (2004). Posttransplant malignancy. *Progress in Transplantation, 14*(3), 193–200.

Tuttle-Newhall, J. E., Collins, B. H., Kuo, P. C., & Schoeder, R. (2003). Organ donation and treatment of the multi-organ donor. *Current Problems in Surgery, 40*(5), 266–310.

Vanrenterghem, Y. (2004). Anaemia after renal transplantation. *Nephrology Dialysis Transplantation, 19*(Suppl. 5), V54–V58.

Wenke, K. (2004). Management of hyperlipidaemia associated with heart transplantation. *Drugs, 64*(10), 1053–1068.

Wijdicks, E. F. (2000). Coma in the critically ill, part 2: The transplant patient; management overview: Recognizing pharmacologic, ischemic, metabolic, and infectious causes. *Journal of Critical Illness, 15*(12), 646–655.

Wilkinson, A., Davidson, J., Dotta, F., Home, P. D., Keown, P., Kiberd, B., et al. (2005). Guidelines for the treatment and management of new-onset diabetes after transplantation. *Clinical Transplantation, 19*(3), 291–298.

Williams, M. A., Lipsett, P. A., Rushton, C. H., Grochowski, E. C., Berkowitz, I. D., Mann, S. L., et al. (2003). The physician's role in discussing organ donation with families. *Critical Care Medicine, 31*(5), 1568–1573.

Wood, K. E., Becker, B. N., McCartney, J. G., D'Alessandro, A. M., & Coursin, D. B. (2004). Care of the potential organ donor. *New England Journal of Medicine, 351*(26), 2730–2739.

Zheng, S. S., Lu, A. W., Liang, T. B., Wang, W. L., Shen, Y., & Shang, M. (2004). Causes and management of respiratory complication after liver transplantation. *Journal of Zhejiang University: Medical Sciences, 33*(2), 170–173.

CHAPTER 60

Palliative Care and End-of-Life Care in the ICU

Donna Arena   Roberta Kaplow

LEARNING OBJECTIVES

Upon completion of this chapter, the reader will be able to:

1. Define palliative care according to the World Health Organization's criteria.

2. Describe the goals of palliative care in the ICU.

3. Describe common symptoms that patients in the ICU encounter that require palliation.

4. Use the AACN Synergy Model for patient care to identify nurse characteristics needed to provide optimal palliative care.

5. List optimal patient outcomes that may be achieved through evidence-based management of patients requiring palliative care in the ICU.

The World Health Organization (WHO; 2005) defines palliative care (PC) as an approach that improves the quality of life of patients and their families when facing life-threatening illness through the prevention, assessment, and treatment of pain and other physical, psychosocial, and spiritual problems. The WHO further illuminates PC by specifying that it

Is applicable early in the course of illness

Affirms and enhances quality of life
- Positively influences the course of illness
- Neither hastens nor postpones death
- Regards dying as a normal process

Uses a team approach to address the needs of patients and families

Provides relief from pain and other distressing symptoms

Integrates the physical, psychological, and spiritual aspects of patient care throughout the illness trajectory

Is often rendered in conjunction with other therapies

Promotes participation in clinical trials that advance understanding and management of complications

Offers support systems to help
- the patient live as actively as possible until death
- the family throughout their loved one's illness and during their bereavement period (WHO, 2005)

GOALS OF PALLIATIVE CARE

"Palliative nursing care in the new millennium is unique because it strives to intervene at the time of diagnosis, is driven by individual and family needs, and remains consistent through initial curative attempts, beginning palliative medicine, comfort care, terminal care, and bereavement" (Super, 2001, p. 27). Upon diagnosis of a potentially life-threatening illness, PC should be initiated and continued whether or not treatment is directed at the disease process. Its intent is to provide comfort and maintain the highest possible quality of life for as long as life remains. The focus is not on death, but rather on compassionate specialized care for the living and control of any physical or emotional symptoms that may cause distress (Growthhouse, Inc., 2005). The goals of PC should be consistent with the patient's wishes. PC does not equate with, but may include, end-of-life (EOL) care.

Meyer and Sieger (2005) list five goals of PC, as delineated by the Center to Advance Palliative Care:

- Relieve of pain and distressing symptoms
- Help with difficult decision making
- Help patients complete prescribed treatments
- Enhance patient and family satisfaction
- Increase ease of referral to other appropriate care settings (e.g., hospice)

They further report that patients with critical illness want the same benefits that PC provides: aggressive treatment of pain and symptoms; relief from worry, anxiety, and depression; communication about their care over time; coordinated care throughout the course of illness; support for family caregivers; and a sense of safety in the healthcare system.

THE ICU ENVIRONMENT

Patients in the United States are living longer and with chronic illnesses such as heart disease, obstructive lung disease, cancer, and diabetes. Complications of these and other illnesses are frequently managed in the intensive care unit (ICU) and, despite the high-tech environment and complex interventions of the ICU, account for the majority of deaths (Hurst & Whitmer, 2003). In one study of patients with chronic illness who died in the hospital, almost 50% were in the ICU within three days of their death and 33% spent at least ten days in the ICU during their last hospitalization (SUPPORT Principal Investigators, 1995). In 1995, approximately 20% of patients who died in the United States were in an ICU at the time (Rocker & Curtis, 2003). In fact, hundreds of thousands of patients die in ICUs each year, but few of these patients receive PC (Seery, 2004).

The disparity that has existed between "critical illness" and "terminal illness" has resulted in patients in the ICU not receiving palliation of symptoms until death was forthcoming. PC is appropriate for all critically ill patients, regardless of where they are on a disease or treatment trajectory. This integrated model of care seems appropriate for optimizing patient outcomes. Nevertheless, data are limited on how to implement this model of care (Nelson & Danis, 2001), and a need exists to devise exemplary models.

Compounding the need for an integrated model of care are reported data that delineate the physical and psychological

suffering incurred while receiving treatment in the ICU (Nelson et al., 2001; Somogyi-Zalud et al., 2000) and data that suggest the physiologic effects of symptom distress are maladaptive. Effective symptom management may enhance healing. Today's health professionals are making strides in initiating clinical interventions focused on palliation. Comfort care should begin before all curative therapies are attempted or have been proven unsuccessful in curtailing the disease process.

END-OF-LIFE CARE

A disparity exists between the actual and desired state of EOL care in the United States. Awareness of this inadequacy is being recognized, and change is slowly occurring (Orlando Regional Healthcare, Education, and Training, 2002). In some cases, EOL care now starts only when the patient is actively dying, generally during the last days of the person's life.

An example of an unfolding scenario related to EOL care often evolves in a situation where a patient is hospitalized with a malignant terminal illness; the prognosis is guarded. The patient is admitted to a general unit, where he stays for approximately 7 to 10 days. During this time, it becomes apparent to the health team that the patient has a minimal chance of surviving due to the severity and progressive nature of the disease. A discussion of code status with the patient and family has not occurred, nor has a Do-Not-Resuscitate (DNR) order been obtained. The idea that recovery is improbable is negated either consciously or unconsciously, and the focus remains on cure. The patient and family are often uninformed and unaware that death may be imminent.

What are the subsequent events? The patient stops breathing, an emergency code is called, cardiopulmonary resuscitation is initiated, and the patient is transferred to ICU. No discussion about EOL wishes among the physicians, nurses, patient, and/or surrogates has occurred prior to this emergency. Instead, the discussion begins simultaneously as heroic medical interventions are initiated. En route to the ICU, as tensions mount, the family is confronted with the decision: "What do they want done?" The family is forced to decide in a crisis moment if they wish everything to be attempted to prolong the patient's life. Generally, the family who has not discussed EOL wishes will respond, "Yes, we want everything available; do everything." During emergencies, families are forced to struggle with a myriad of medical choices, which often cause them to unwillingly and unknowingly make decisions that may prolong and complicate their loved ones' dying process.

The luxury of time for the health team to discuss with the family what "everything" entails in terms of medical interventions and outcomes is forfeited in this situation. Heroic measures begin. Yet, in all probability, such life-saving interventions will not alter the patient's prognosis.

Technology used in the ICU is perceived by the professional team as standard. Interventions used on a patient in the ICU may include intubation, placement on mechanical ventilation, and possibly application of restraints to prevent self-extubation and removal of lines and catheters. Routinely, the patient is placed on a cardiac monitor. The patient may have an arterial line, central venous catheter, and several intravenous (IV) lines for fluid maintenance, medication administration, and/or hemodynamic monitoring. A urinary catheter may be inserted for hourly assessment of output. If the patient experiences renal failure, renal replacement therapy may be indicated. Based on the medical diagnosis, a nasogastric tube or small bore tube may be inserted either to decompress the stomach or to administer tube feeding respectively. These standard ICU interventions will be applicable for a patient based on acuity, diagnosis, and medical stability on admission to the unit as well as the goals of care for the patient. A discussion between health professionals, patients, and families early in the disease trajectory prior to an emergent situation may have diverted this event before it occurred.

ADVANCE DIRECTIVES

One way proposed to influence a patient's quality of life at the EOL is through the completion of an advance directive (AD). ADs include a living will (LW) and a durable power of attorney (DPA) for health care. These instruments are discussed further in Chapter 58. People who have remained in control throughout their entire life are usually unwilling to relinquish this control when confronted with the dying process. Therefore, discussing completed ADs with the family gives an individual some measure of control over the last phase of life.

Decisions regarding EOL issues rarely fit into neat, mutually exclusive categories; instead, they are complex and often fall into a nondelineated "gray zone." This gray zone relates to particular medical interventions not specifically addressed in an LW. The ICU nurse should ensure that a copy of the AD, if available, is placed in the patient's medical record. A nurse often refers to the AD if discrepancies are perceived between the patient wishes and the medical interventions being implemented.

SYMPTOMS AND MANAGEMENT AT THE END OF LIFE

Often pain and other symptoms are inadequately controlled at the EOL (Paice, Muir, & Shott, 2004). The symptoms a patient manifests at this stage may vary based on medical diagnosis, comorbidities, and condition upon admission to the ICU.

Respirations may become shallow and rapid, and the nail beds may become cyanotic or dusky in color. The patient's hands and feet become cold when the blood shunts to the vital organs. The patient's legs may also be mottled in color. The patient's eyes may elicit a blank stare or may roll back.

A Cheyne-Stokes respiratory pattern often occurs simultaneously with the noisy respirations from secretions, known as a "death rattle." This pattern alternates between a series of rapid, shallow breaths interspersed with periods of apnea. The interval between rapid breaths and no breaths lengthens over time. The Cheyne-Stokes pattern is a very disturbing symptom for the family to watch; the patient seems to be struggling for every breath.

Pain

Over the past three decades, tremendous advances have been made in the care of acute and critically ill patients. Care in a high-tech environment, while being curative in nature, also has the potential to cause unintentional pain and suffering (Hurst & Whitmer, 2003). ICU patients from one study reported substantial pain related to use of standard ICU equipment (e.g., endotracheal tubes, urinary catheters, central and peripheral vascular lines, nasogastric tubes) and procedures (e.g., endotracheal suctioning, turning, transferring into a chair, mechanical ventilation) (Nelson et al., 2001). Many patients die with treatable pain, even in the ICU. The reason underlying this finding is that ICU care has traditionally focused on disease versus symptom management (SUPPORT Principal Investigators, 1995). PC, in contrast, encourages symptom management in conjunction with curative measures. Patients reportedly are most fearful of EOL pain, and it is the symptom with the highest incidence. Data suggest that patients with a chronic illness such as heart failure, chronic obstructive pulmonary disease (COPD), or end-stage renal disease experience the same degree of pain as patients with cancer (Paice & Fine, 2001). Pain management is a major concern in PC (SUPPORT Principal Investigators; Truog et al., 2001). A more complete discussion of pain assessment in the critically ill appears in Chapter 4.

The assessment of pain requires alternative assessment strategies in patients who are dying. In these circumstances, evaluation can be complicated by a patient's level of consciousness, breathing patterns, and hemodynamic status. Assessment of breathing patterns can be challenging in patients who are dying. Irregular breathing patterns are common at this time, yet may not be a source of discomfort for the patient. The term "agonal breathing" is not synonymous with "agony." Likewise, the death rattle may not be a source of distress or discomfort for the patient, even though it is interpreted as such by a clinician or the family (Truog et al., 2001).

A patient may experience varying degrees of pain based on the diagnosis and the extent of the disease process. Both non-opioid and opioid medications are useful in management depending on the degree of pain (Fine, 2005). Opioids have long been a basis for the treatment of pain in dying patients. Morphine sulfate is used most often in the ICU; hydromorphone (Dilaudid®) or fentanyl (Sublimaze®) are other options. The IV route is used most often in the ICU, because most patients have this form of access. However, other routes of administration are possible if IV access is not available (e.g., oral, sublingual, subcutaneous, rectal, transdermal) (Truog et al., 2001).

The WHO has created a three-step ladder for managing pain. Although it was initially developed for patients with cancer pain, this ladder is useful in PC situations for other patients (Fine, 2005). Medications are often used in combination with nonpharmacological treatments, such as massage, acupuncture, transcutaneous electrical nerve stimulation, physical therapy, and music therapy (Fine). The degree and type of pain a patient is experiencing require frequent evaluation. Depending on the cause and nature of the pain, a combination of pharmacological medications may equate to better management. In any event, the ICU nurse should manage pain effectively (see Chapter 4).

Shortness of Breath/Dyspnea

Shortness of breath (SOB) is an unpleasant sensation for the patient. In one study, 33% of patients in the ICU reported feelings of dyspnea (Nelson et al., 2001). Dyspnea has been reported to be experienced by patients in the ICU who were receiving mechanical ventilation and in the weaning process as well as those shortly before death (Somogyi-Zalud et al., 2000).

In addition to worsening respiratory failure, dyspnea has several possible etiologies in patients who may or may not be dying—namely, heart failure, anxiety, and infection. Attempts to identify possible treatable causes should accompany symptom management (Truog et al., 2001).

Opiate medications are the mainstay of pharmacological therapy for dyspnea. Morphine is effective in reducing the sensation of struggling to breathe; it also has the capacity to diminish the respiratory center in the brain and may relieve pulmonary congestion due to its vasodilator effects (Truog et al., 2001). Treatment with oxygen given by nasal cannula at 4 to 6 L/min is helpful when nonventilated patients are gasping for breath. It appears the dying patient feels claustrophobic because of frequent attempts to remove the oxygen, although a nasal cannula may be better tolerated than a mask. Data on the effectiveness of oxygen therapy in relieving dyspnea have shown inconsistent results from this approach. Some patients obtain relief from air from a fan blowing gently on their face (Truog et al.). Patients also may benefit from the judicious use of bronchodilators and diuretics to relieve small airway obstruction and pulmonary vascular congestion (Truog et al.).

As death draws near, the patient becomes unable to clear fluid in the lungs due to a loss of the swallowing reflex. The accumulation of fluid in the lungs precipitates the death rattle. The ICU nurse should not attempt to suction these secretions, because suctioning can cause more discomfort. Treatment with drugs such as antitussives helps with cough; anticholinergics [e.g., scopolamine (Trans-Derm®)] help reduce secretions. Scopolamine and atropine can decrease oral secretions associated with the death rattle. Anxiolytics [e.g., lorazepam (Ativan®)] can reduce the anxiety component of dyspnea (Weissman, 2000).

Hydration and Nutrition

Hydration and nutrition are issues that need to be discussed with great sensitivity because they often elicit concerns among the medical team and the family (Weissman, 2000). In light of recent litigation and extensive coverage by the media, some believe that the dying should always receive nutrition and hydration and that feeding tube insertion is indicated if the patient is no longer able to be administered these substances orally. PC practices, by contrast, recognize that loss of hunger and thirst are part of the dying process and that administration of hydration and nutrition does not enhance patient comfort (Truog et al., 2001). Further, the metabolic imbalances that may occur tend to contribute to sedation and diminished consciousness. Decisions surrounding hydration and nutrition must be consistent with the patient's wishes. The consensus is that hydration and nutrition should be provided if desired by the patient and contribute to the patient's comfort; otherwise, they may be forgone (Truog et al.).

Nausea and Vomiting

Nausea and vomiting are two symptoms often experienced at the end of life. Potentially treatable etiologies should be investigated. Nausea and vomiting can be managed with antiemetic agents. Nasogastric drainage may relieve symptoms associated with an ileus or small bowel obstruction. However, it has been suggested that the discomfort associated with presence of the tube itself may be more uncomfortable than intermittent emesis (Truog et al., 2001).

Fever

Fever is a symptom that commonly develops in critically ill and dying patients. Methods to alleviate the discomfort associated with fever, such as administration of antipyretics and treatment of the underlying cause (e.g., infection), are suggested. The use of hypothermia blankets or ice packs, however, may cause more discomfort than the fever itself (Truog et al., 2001).

Delirium

Delirium is a state of acute confusion (Truog et al., 2001). Approximately, 80% of all patients in the ICU develop delirium at some point during their ICU admission. Risk factors include increased severity of illness, advanced age, comorbidities, preexisting cognitive impairment, sleep deprivation, and medications (Dubois, Bergeron, Dumont, Dial, & Skrobik, 2001). Delirium can also occur at the EOL. The use of physical restraints should be avoided, if possible. Pharmacological management should be geared toward enhancement of the patient's comfort, rather than resolution of delirium. Administration of neuroleptics may be helpful in patients with delirium. Haloperidol (Haldol®) is effective in the management of delirium (Truog et al.). Haloperidol may not be indicated for use in elderly patients, however. Delirium recognition is complicated because it is often confused with anxiety, and its level may vary on a given day (Truog et al.).

BARRIERS TO IMPLEMENTING PALLIATIVE CARE IN THE ICU

Critical care clinicians have long recognized that PC of critically ill patients is inadequate, especially for those who are dying in the ICU (Truog et al., 2001). Several impediments to implementing PC in the ICU have been identified, including the underlying culture of the ICU (i.e., the drive to save lives), cost, time constraints, fear of causing addiction, restrictions on use of opioids in the clinical setting, and the severity of the critically ill patient's condition. A patient in multiple organ dysfunction syndrome (MODS), for example, may not be seen as physiologically able to tolerate PC measures because of fear of worsening the clinical status with use of pharmacological interventions. All of these factors may impair the ICU nurse's ability to alleviate patient distress from symptoms (Truog et al.). Finally, healthcare providers who work in an ICU have to accept that many ICU patients have terminal illness and deserve compassionate care, including symptom management (Levy & Carle, 2001; Truog et al.).

THE SHIFT FROM CURATIVE TO COMFORT CARE

Health providers must acknowledge that patients and families need information about which medical interventions have the highest probability of success in relation to risk. The team should thoroughly explain—in a language the patient and family understand—the risks versus the potential benefits of every intervention. This discussion allows the patient and family to make an informed decision about whether to consent to the treatment. As the patient's condition changes and deteriorates, discussions about the withholding and withdrawal of life-sustaining interventions should be readdressed. The health team needs to remind the family that the focus of care may change daily.

If the potential to significantly improve or enhance the patient's overall prognosis and quality of life is minimal, the focus should shift from curative to comfort care. This transition should be somewhat gradual, with frequent explanations related to the rationale for changes in the plan of care being given. If the physician considers particular medical therapies to be futile, these interventions should not be presented as an option.

If the ultimate focus of care becomes comfort, then daily laboratory values, radiograph studies, arterial blood gas monitoring, antibiotics, and any unnecessary tests or procedures causing discomfort should be discontinued. At this time, all interventions should revolve solely around comfort options, avoiding heroic measures that prolong the patient's life, especially those causing discomfort. A family decision to decelerate aggressive treatments and allow a natural death must be supported by the health team.

If clinically indicated, the patient can be transferred from the ICU to a general unit after the deceleration is initiated or the focus of care shifts from curative to comfort care. Patients may benefit from a transfer out of the ICU to another unit or environment that may be more optimal for PC. Some patients, however, may be too unstable to transfer (Truog et al., 2001). The transfer between clinical units often evokes feelings of anxiety and concerns among family. These feelings may originate from the fact that the patient and family have developed a comfortable working relationship with the ICU nurses. The family may also believe the patient will not receive the same caliber, intense monitoring, or quality of nursing care on the clinical units as was received from the ICU nurses. Families may vacillate about their decision to decelerate care since the perception becomes their loved one is no longer a high priority for intensive observation. Some individuals have an impression that "deceleration of care" equates to "do not treat." These fallacies must be negated and factual information provided.

The Bedside Vigil

Flexible ICU visiting hours remain a significant amenity for families who are experiencing the death of a loved one. As a result of their feelings of helplessness during this seemingly endless "vigil," family members may become overly concerned watching the cardiac monitor visible above the patient's bedside. As the patient advances toward death, changes in values shown on the monitor will normally occur. As the vital signs decrease, the family's anxiety often increases. Family education includes information about what to expect regarding changes in vital signs during the dying process and activities that can be comforting to the patient.

Communication

Communicating with the patient and family is as important as effectively managing the physical symptoms the patient develops. The best strategies are those that keep the patient's wishes and needs in the forefront. This tactic may minimize potential conflicts among family members.

Information about EOL choices should be shared with significant others. The patient and family have the right to receive truthful information. Effective communication about prognosis requires clear, specific explanations.

Although communication with the healthcare team is an important need of critically ill patients and families, this need is rarely met today. Further, EOL topics pose additional communication challenges for the healthcare team (Truog et al., 2001). Nurses, both novice and experienced, are often uncomfortable openly talking with the patient and family about death. Novice nurses are uncomfortable because they are unfamiliar with the topic, medical interventions, and sequence of events that occur with dying. Experienced nurses are more comfortable with symptom management and subsequent events. According to Schulman-Green and colleagues (2005), if a nurse sees a physician hesitate in telling a patient and family the prognosis, the nurse may also be reluctant to lead a discussion with the patient and family. Thus nurses avoid EOL discussions, often leaving families with unanswered questions and unrealistic expectations about the death process. Physicians' hesitancy may also keep nurses from speaking to patients about prognosis and referral to hospice care (Schulman-Green, McCorkle, Cherlin, Johnson-Hurzeler, & Bradley, 2005). When families are unaware of unfolding events, stress increases, feelings of being "out of control" escalate, demands multiply, and the goal of providing a comfortable memory for families becomes practically impossible to attain.

Role confusion is not the only reason why nurses avoid discussing EOL issues. Communicating with the dying is a skill. Nurses may be at a loss for the words to use to communicate with these patients and their families. When communicating with the dying, nurses fear diminishing a patient's hope, feeling out of control, feeling helpless, and overstepping professional boundaries (Schulman-Green et al., 2005). It takes courage and skill to have a dialogue with those experiencing death. As nurses become increasingly skilled, they realize they will never have all the answers. Active listening and the willingness to "be present" with the dying are more meaningful than words.

Family-Focused Care

An in-depth discussion of family-focused care appears in Chapter 2. A family-focused approach to care is essential at the EOL (Truog et al., 2001). In the case of a dying patient, family members and significant others should be encouraged to remain at the patient's bedside as much as they desire (Truog et al.). In fact, pets have been allowed to visit in some hospitals (Campbell, 1998).

Patients' cultural beliefs should be respected, as feasible (Truog et al., 2001). Collaboration with the chaplaincy service and speaking with the family with regard to special rituals' specifications should take place. Discussion of some preferences appears in Chapter 8.

PATIENT OUTCOMES

Nurses can help to ensure optimal patient outcomes such as those listed in **Box 60-1** through the use of evidence-based interventions for patients receiving palliative care and end-of-life care in the ICU.

SUMMARY

Patients may live several years after receiving a diagnosis or developing an acute exacerbation of an illness. They reportedly appreciate efforts that address their vast symptom distress and caregiver burden over the course of their treatment (Meyer & Sieger, 2005). All critically ill patients deserve aggressive care, whether cure or comfort is the goal (Hurst & Whitmer, 2003). The philosophy of the ICU to include palliative care in addition to therapeutic interventions has been slowly changing. Palliative care in the ICU is certainly of benefit to patients, families, and healthcare providers. The ICU nurse has an obligation to continue moving this agenda forward so as to enhance optimal patient outcomes. Championing high-

---

Box 60-1
Optimal Patient Outcomes

- Physical comfort in expected range
- Cognitive status in expected range
- Remains calm and tranquil
- Reported satisfaction with symptom control
- Expresses readiness for death
- Arranges finances and makes preparation for death
- Reports satisfaction with physiological and psychological well-being
- Uses effective coping patterns
- Uses social support

quality PC should be a goal for all ICU nurses and critical care units (Nelson-Marten, Braaten, & English, 2001). Healthcare providers need several skills to provide effective PC. For example, education in symptom identification and management as well as training in breaking bad news under difficult conditions are two essential skills (Meyer & Sieger, 2005). In addition to palliation of symptoms, nurses in the ICU are challenged to address family issues, deal with the emotional and spiritual needs of the patient and family, and improve communication among the patient, family, and healthcare team (Hurst & Whitmer, 2003).

Treatment of critical illness and palliation of symptom distress are not mutually exclusive goals. To the contrary, PC may enhance patient outcomes, whereas failure to provide symptom management can adversely affect morbidity and mortality in the ICU. Symptom distress may increase oxygen consumption, increase coagulation, promote the inflammation associated with systemic inflammatory response syndrome, increase nitrogen wasting, increase physiologic stress, decrease immunocompetence, increase the work of breathing, and lead to muscle weakness. Pain may also cause spiritual distress and decrease a patient's emotional well-being. Further, patients with symptom distress are less likely to be able to participate in care activities that promote healing (Fine, 2005; Truog et al. 2001).

CASE STUDY

B.I. is a 68-year-old male who was admitted to the ICU following a decreased level of consciousness—and a grand mal seizure at home. In the ED, he was intubated for airway protection and placed on mechanical ventilation. On admission to the ICU, he had decerebrate posturing when he was touched, had a Glasgow Coma Scale score of 6, was not breathing spontaneously, and had conjugate eye movements. A CT scan revealed basilar artery occlusion.

The patient's wife reported that he experienced a sense of vertigo just prior to having the seizure. B.I.'s cardiopulmonary status remained stable, and he was treated with thrombolytic therapy. His mean arterial pressure was maintained greater than 100 mm Hg. Neither of these measures improved his neurological status. B.I. continued to receive antiseizure therapy with benzodiazepines. Comfort measures were provided, as per ICU protocol.

After two days in the ICU, the patient's pupils were midline, dilated, and nonreactive to light. The multidisciplinary team met with the wife and explained B.I.'s condition. They discussed his prognosis and the long-term plan. Although the intensivist painted a grim picture, the wife asked when she would be able to take her husband home.

Two days later, another family meeting was held with the multidisciplinary team. A discharge planner attends this meeting. Options presented to the wife included planning to discharge B.I. home with a ventilator and 24-hour home care, transfer to a chronic care facility that accepts patients on a ventilator, transfer to a medical-surgical floor extubated to die, or keeping him in the ICU with ongoing comfort measures and symptom management, as needed. After considering all of these options, she decided on the last one. She was invited to be at B.I.'s bedside whenever she wished and was provided ongoing updates and communication from the multidisciplinary team. B.I. died a peaceful death in the ICU three days later.

CRITICAL THINKING QUESTIONS

1. What types of issues may require you to act as an advocate or moral agent for the wife of this patient?
2. How will you implement your role as a facilitator of learning for this patient's wife?
3. Which comfort measures would you ensure took place?
4. Which symptoms would you anticipate seeing as B.I. was approaching death?
5. Would you anticipate Cheyne-Stokes respirations? Why or why not?
6. Write a case example of a patient receiving palliative care strategies in the clinical setting. Rate the patient as a level 1, 3, or 5 on each characteristic. Identify the level of nurse characteristics needed in the care of this patient.
7. Use the form to write up a plan of care for one client in the clinical setting. Take one patient outcome and list evidence-based interventions found in a literature review for this patient.

Using the Synergy Model to Develop a Plan of Care

	Patient Characteristics	Level (1, 3, 5)	Subjective and Objective Data	Evidence-based Interventions	Outcomes
SYNERGY MODEL	Resiliency				
	Vulnerability				
	Stability				
	Complexity				
	Resource availability				
	Participation in care				
	Participation in decision making				
	Predictability				

Online Resources

- **Center to Advance Palliative Care (CAPC):** www.capcmssm.org
  Provides technical assistance needed to establish palliative care programs as well as opportunities to network with colleagues in the palliative care community; features CAPC publications, education calendar, and information about advocacy activities.

- **National Hospice and Palliative Care Organization:** www.nhpco.org
  This organization is the industry's largest association and leading resource for professionals and volunteers committed to and providing service to patients and their families during the end of life.

- **Growth House, Guide to Death, Dying, Grief, Bereavement and End-of-Life Resources:** www.growthhouse.org
  Search engine offers access to the Internet's most comprehensive collection of reviewed resources for end-of-life care.

- **Hospice and Palliative Nurses Association (HPNA):** www.hpna.org/abouthpna.asp
  This organization promotes understanding of the specialties of hospice and palliative nursing, and studies and promotes hospice and palliative nursing research.

- **Oncology Nursing Society Evidence-Based Practice Resource Area:** www.onsopcontent.ons.org/toolkits/evidence
  Contains a topic review on palliative care. It includes evidence and extensive literature reviews within the past five years relevant to palliative care.

- **Promoting Excellence in End-of-Life Care:** www.promotingexcellence.org
  Manages 22 grant-funded projects designed to demonstrate excellence in EOL care in diverse institutional settings. The project is a National Program Office of the Robert Wood Johnson Foundation, headquartered in Montana.

- **End-of-Life Nursing Education Consortium (ELNEC):** www.aacn.nche.edu/elnec/
  A comprehensive, national education program to improve EOL care by nurses, ELNEC is funded by a major grant from the Robert Wood Johnson Foundation. Its primary goals are to develop a core of expert nursing educators and coordinate national nursing education efforts in EOL care.

- **Americans for Better Care of the Dying (ABCD):** www.abcd-caring.org/
  ABCD attempts to change what people face as they come to the end of life. Every dying person needs to be able to count on excellent care. ABCD aims to improve EOL care by learning which social and political changes will lead to enduring, efficient, and effective programs.

- **Oncology Nurses Association:** www.ons.org
  ONS Online is an information service for oncology nurses, other healthcare providers, people with cancer, and their families and friends.

- **Griefnet:** www.Griefnet.org
  An Internet community of persons dealing with grief, death, and major loss. It includes 47 e-mail support groups and 2 websites. The integrated approach to online grief support provides help to people working through loss and grief issues of many kinds. The companion site, KIDSAID, provides a safe environment for kids and their parents to find information and ask questions.

- **Hospice and Palliative Nurses Association:** www.hpna.org
  The purpose of the HPNA is to exchange information, experiences, and ideas; to promote understanding of the specialties of hospice and palliative nursing; and to study and promote hospice and palliative nursing research

- **Center for Hospice and Palliative Care:** www.palliativecare.org
  A continuum of health and mental health services for persons experiencing the impact of serious illness and loss.

- **Pain scales with evaluations:** www.chcr.brown.edu/pcoc/Physical.html

- **Pain scales in several languages:** www.britishsociety.org/pain_scales.html

- **Information on complementary therapies:** http://nccam.nih.gov

- **Palliative Care Formulary Online:** www.palliativedrugs.com

REFERENCES

Campbell, M. L. (1998). *Foregoing life-sustaining therapy.* Aliso Viejo, CA: American Association of Critical-Care Nurses.

Dubois, M. J., Bergeron, N., Dumont, M., Dial, S., & Skrobik, Y. (2001). Delirium in an intensive care unit: A study of risk factors. *Intensive Care Medicine, 27,* 1297–1304.

Fine, P. G. (2005). The last chance for comfort: An update on pain management at the end of life. Available at www.medscape.com/viewprogram/4550_pnt

Growthhouse, Inc. Retrieved October 9, 2005, from www.growthhouse.org/palliat.html

Hurst, S., & Whitmer, M. (2003). Palliative care services. *Dimensions of Critical Care Nursing, 22*(1), 35–38.

Levy, M. M., & Carle, J. (2001). Compassionate end-of-life care in the intensive care unit. *Critical Care Medicine, 29*(2, Suppl.), N1–N61.

Meyer, D., & Sieger, C. (2005). Case for hospital-based palliative care. Retrieved October 8, 2005, from www.capc.org

Nelson, J. E., & Danis, M. (2001). End-of-life care in the intensive care unit: Where are we now? *Critical Care Medicine, 29*(2 Suppl.), N2–N9.

Nelson, J. E., Meier, D. E., Oei, E. J., Nierman, D. L., Senzel, R. S., Manfredi, P. L., et al. (2001). Self-reported symptom experience of critically ill cancer patients receiving intensive care. *Critical Care Medicine, 29*(2), 277–282.

Nelson-Marten, P., Braaten, J., & English, N. K. (2001). Critical caring: Promoting good end-of-life care in the intensive care unit. *Critical Care Nursing Clinics of North America, 13*(4), 577–585.

Orlando Regional Healthcare, Education, and Training. (2002). *MP14. Improve End-of-Life Care.* Orlando, FL.

Paice, J. A., & Fine, P. G. (2001). Pain at the end of life. In B. R. Ferrell & N. Coyle (Eds.), *Textbook of palliative nursing* (2nd ed., pp. 76–90). New York. Oxford University Press.

Paice, J. A., Muir, J. C., & Shott, S. (2004). Palliative care at the end of life: Comparing quality in diverse settings. *American Journal of Hospice and Palliative Care, 21*(1), 19–27, 80.

Rocker, G. M., & Curtis, J. R. (2003). Caring for the dying in the intensive care unit: In search of clarity. *Journal of the American Medical Association, 290*(6), 820–822.

Schulman-Green, D., McCorkle, R., Cherlin, E., Johnson-Hurzeler, R., & Bradley, E. H. (2005). Nurses' communication of prognosis and implications for hospice referral: A study of nurses caring for terminally ill hospitalized patients. *American Journal of Critical Care, 14*(1), 64–70.

Seery, D. (2004). Shifting gears: From cure to comfort. *RN, 67*(11), 52–58.

Somogyi-Zalud, E., Zhong, Z., Lynn, J., Dawson, N. V., Hamel, M. B., Desbiens, N. A., et al. (2000). Dying with acute respiratory failure or multiple organ system failure with sepsis. *Journal of the American Geriatric Society, 48*(5 Suppl.), S140–S145.

Super, A. (2001). The context of palliative care in progressive illness. In B. R. Ferrell & N. Coyle (Eds.), *Textbook of palliative nursing* (pp. 27–36). New York: Oxford University Press.

Support Principal Investigators. (1995). A controlled trial to improve care for seriously ill hospitalized patients. The study to understand prognosis and preference for outcomes and risks of treatment (SUPPORT). *Journal of the American Medical Association, 274*(20), 1634–1636.

Truog, R. D., Cist, A. F., Brackett, S. E., Burns, J. P., Curley, M. A., Danis, M., et al. (2001). Recommendations for end-of-life care in the intensive care unit:

The Ethics Committee of the Society of Critical Care Medicine. *Critical Care Medicine, 29*(12), 2332–2348.

Weissman, D. E. (2000). Fast fact and concept #027: Dyspnea at end-of-life. American Academy of Hospice and Pallative Medicine. Retrieved September 4, 2005, from www.aahpm.org/cgi-bin/wkcgi/view?status=A%20&search=154&ID=157&offset=O&limit=25

World Health Organization. Retrieved October 9, 2005, from www.who.int/hiv/topics/palliative/care/en/

Index

Page numbers followed by f denote figures; those followed by t denote tables.

AAA. *See* Abdominal aortic aneurysm
AACN Certification Corporation, 3, 5, 8
Abbokinase® (urokinase), 581
ABC. *See* Airway, breathing, and circulation evaluation
Abciximab (Reopro®), 598
Abdomen
  abdominal paracentesis, 419
  assessment of, 417
  four quadrants of, 417f
  imaging of, 477
  muscles of, 273
  radiograph of, 445
  trauma of, 671, 674–675, 675t, 676t, 679
Abdominal aortic aneurysm (AAA), 261–263
ABG. *See* Arterial blood gas
Abiomed AB 5000, 214
Abiomed BVS 5000, 213–214, 213f, 217
Abiomed's AbioCor Replacement Heart, 215, 216f
Acculate® (zafirlukast), 329
ACE inhibitors. *See* Angiotensive converting enzyme inhibitors
Acetaminophen, 46t, 460, 685–686, 696t
Acetazolamide (Diamox®), 548
Acetylsalicylate, 693
Acid-base balance, 286, 538
Acidosis, 286, 678
Acquired immune deficiency syndrome. *See* AIDS and HIV
Acromegaly, 513
ACS. *See* Acute coronary syndrome
ACTH. *See* Adrenocorticotropic hormone
Action potential, 350–351, 351f
Activated partial thromboplastin time, 610
Acuity systems, 8

Acute coronary syndrome (ACS), 181–194
  case study, 193
  complications, 187–188
  diagnostic tests, 183–187
  ECG changes with, 184–185t
  imaging studies, 186–187
  interventions of critical care patient, 191–192
  myocardial infarction, 181–182, 182f
  NSTEMI *vs.* STEMI, 183f
  online resources, 194
  patient assessment, 182–183
  pharmacological treatment, 189–190
  revascularization procedures, 190–191
  treatment of, 188–191
  unstable angina, 181
Acute decompensated heart failure, 199–200, 203
Acute hepatic failure, 453–454, 454t
Acute hepatitis. *See* Hepatitis
Acute lung injury, 337
Acute pain. *See* Pain
Acute pancreatitis. *See* Pancreatitis
Acute renal failure. *See* Renal failure
Acute respiratory distress syndrome (ARDS), 311, 337–344, 632
  care-related problems with, 342t
  case study, 343
  clinical manifestations, 339
  complications/nursing interventions, 341–343, 342t
  definition/etiology, 337–338
  investigational therapies, 341
  medical management, 339–341
  online resources, 345
  pathophysiology, 338–339

Acute respiratory distress syndrome (ARDS)—*continued*
  patient outcomes, 343
  phases, 338t
  positive end expiratory pressure (PEEP), 340
  predisposing factors for, 338t
  shock and, 253
Acute ventilatory failure, 308
Acyclovir (Zovirax®), 382
Addison's disease, 492t, 505
Adenoma, 513
Adenosine (Adenocard®), 187, 690
Adefovir (Hepsera®), 468
ADH. *See* Antidiuretic hormone
Adrenal disorders, 491, 503–509
  adrenal insufficiency, 505–506
  case study, 508
  Cushing's syndrome, 506–507
  online resources, 509
  patient outcomes, 508
  pheochromocytoma, 504
  primary hyperaldosteronism, 504–504
Adrenal venous sampling, 505
Adrenaline® (epinephrine), 43, 503, 654, 732
Adrenocorticotropic hormone (ACTH), 512, 513
Advance directives, 719–722, 741
  cultural approaches to, 102
  do-not-resuscitate orders, 721
  durable health care power of attorney, 721
  living wills, 720–721
Advocacy/moral agency, 4, 6
Advocates, family. *See* Family-focused care
AeroBid® (flunisolide), 329
Afferent division, 353–354
Afferent neuron, 349
African Americans
  with advanced heart failure, 202
  cancer risk of, 101
  drug therapy and, 101
  organ donations, 102
Afterload, 141–142, 234, 245
Agenerase® (amprenavir), 592
Aggrastat® (tirofiban hydrochloride), 598
Aging. *See also* Gerontological issues
  coronary artery disease and, 162
  drug dosages and, 81
  "failure to thrive," 83t
  gastrointestinal tract, 82–83
  healthcare-associated infections and, 67
  heart failure and, 197
  hormonal function, 83–84
  immune system, 84
  neurological system, 82
  nutrition for elderly patients, 82–83
  pathophysiology and, 79–86

  renal function, 81–82
  sleep and, 54, 57
Agratroban (Argatroban®), 598
AIDS and HIV, 589–594
  antiretroviral medications, 592–593
  case study, 593
  drug side effects, 592–593
  HIV lab tests, 591
  HIV life-cycle, 590t
  HIV transmission, 589–590
  HIV treatment, 592–593
  immune system and, 590–591
  online resources, 595
  patient outcomes, 593
Airborne transmission, 68
Air embolism, 150
Air leak disease. *See also* Barotrauma
Air quality, 31–32
Airway, breathing, and circulation (ABC) evaluation, 669
Airway adjuncts, 299–301
Airway pressure release ventilation, 311
Albuterol (Proventil®), 329
Aldoctone® (spironolactone), 505
Aldosterone, 503, 504
Aldosterone antagonists, 201–202, 505
Alkalosis, 286–287
Allergic reaction. *See* Anaphylactic shock
Allopurinol, 583
Alpha blockers, 176t
Alprazolam (Xanax®), 688
ALS. *See* Amyotrophic lateralizing sclerosis
Alternative medical systems, 109
Alternative therapy. *See* Complementary and alternative therapy (CAT)
Alveolar cellular composition, 277, 278f
Alveoli, 275, 276–277, 278f
Amantadine hydrochloride (Endantadine®), 322, 696t
Ambient temperature, sleep quality and, 60
Amenorrhea, 514
American Association of Critical-Care Nurses (AACN), 3, 11
Amidate® (etomidate), 653
Amiloride hydrochloride (Midamor®), 505
Aminopan® (somatostatin), 424
Amiodarone hydrochloride (Cordarone®), 202, 220, 233, 732
Ammonia, 696t
Amniotic fluid embolism, 294
Amobarbital (Amytal®), 687
Amphetamines, 686–687, 696t
Amprenavir (Agenerase®), 592
Amyl nitrite, 691
Amyotrophic lateralizing sclerosis (ALS), 297t
Amytal® (amobarbital), 687

Anaphylactic shock, 251
Anaphylactic transfusion reactions. *See* Transfusion reaction
Anastomotic leak, 707–708, 710–711
Anastomotic strictures, 711–712
Anectine® (succinylcholine), 653
Anemia, 500
Anesthesia, 46t, 651–657
  anesthetic agents, with neurologic disorders, 377
  epidural, 654–655
  inhalation agents, 651–652
  intravenous, 653–654
  local, 654, 696t
  moderate sedation/MAC, 656–657
  muscle relaxants, 652–653
  regional, 654–656
  spinal, 655–656
Aneurysm
  left ventricular, 188
  repair, 378
  surgical clipping, 401
Angina, 164, 181. *See also* Chest pain
Angiodysplasia, 444
Angiography, 187, 445
Angiotensin-converting enzyme (ACE) inhibitors, 81, 101, 166, 176t, 189, 199, 200–201, 505
Angiotensin-receptor blockers (ARBs), 176t, 201
Anion gap metabolic acidosis, 691
Annuloplasty, 232
Anorectal disease, 444
Anoscopy, 445
Antacids, 448
Antiarrhythmics, 696t
Antibiotics, 653t, 679, 696t
Anticholinergics, 448, 696t
Anticholinesterase drugs, 652
Anticoagulant therapy, 379, 581, 607
  oral, 656t
Anticonvulsants, 46t
Antidepressants, 46t, 101, 694–695, 696t
Antidiabetic agents, 696t
Antidiuretic hormone (ADH), 511–512
Antifibrinolytic therapy, 189, 611
Antihistamines, 696t
Antihypertensive drugs, 101
Anti-inflammatory agents (NSAIDs), 46t
Anti-ischemic therapy, 189
Antimicrobials. *See* Antibiotics
Antiplatelet medications, 166, 379, 599, 656t
Antipsychotic drugs, 699t
Antiresorptive therapy, 580
Antiretroviral therapy, 592. *See also* AIDS and HIV
Antithrombin III, 610, 611
Antithrombotic therapy. *See* Antifibrolytic therapy
Antizol® (fomepizole), 692

Anxiety, 643
  critical care cardiac patients and, 192
  disturbed sleep and, 57
  medications, 176t
Anxiolytics, 688
Aortic rupture, 668
Aortoenteric fistula, 444
Apnea, 279t, 307
Apneustic, 279t
Appalachians, 99
Apresoline® (hydralazine hydrochloride), 201, 263
ARBs. *See* Angiotensin-receptor blockers
ARDS. *See* Acute respiratory distress syndrome
Aredia® (pamidronate), 580
Argatroban® (agratroban), 598
Aristocort® (triamcinolone), 329
Aromatherapy, 32t, 34–35
Arrhythmias. *See* Dysrhythmias
Arsenic, 697t
Arterial blood gas (ABG)
  analysis, 678
  monitoring, 284–287, 285t, 286f, 286t
Arterial occlusion, 263–265
Arteriovenous malformations (AVM), 395–399
  AVM incidence, 395
  diagnosis, 396
  endovascular treatment, 397–398
  nursing care, 398–399
  pathophysiology, 395–396
  presentation, 396
  radiosurgery, 398
  Spetzler-Martin Surgical Grading Scale, 397t
  treatment, 396–398
Artwork, 33–34
Ascites, 199, 418, 425, 456, 460
  refractory, 425
Asian cultures, 99, 101, 102
Aspiration pneumonia. *See* Pneumonia
Aspirin, 101, 189, 692, 693
Assessment
  AVPU method, 632
  cultural, 97–104
  pain, 43–45, 165
  primary and secondary assessment, 671
  respiratory, 278–281
  sleep assessment in ICU, 61–62
Assisted living, 642
Assurance, family need for, 19
Asthma, 279t, 298–299, 313, 327–330
  factors contributing to attack of, 327t
  pathophysiology, 327–328
  severity, classification of, 328t
  signs and symptoms of, 328
  treatment, 328–329

Atelectasis, 294–295
Atenolol (Tenormin®), 504
Atherosclerosis, as cause of arterial occlusion, 264
Atherosclerotic changes, in the elderly, 80
Atherosclerotic lesions, 159–161, 161f
Ativan® (lorazepan), 311, 653, 687, 690
Atrial ectopy, 81
Atrial fibrillation, 233
Atromid-S® (clofibrate), 514
Atroven® (ipratropium), 329
Auscultation, 134, 280
Autonomic nervous system, 349
Autonomy, 722, 723
Autopsies, cultural approaches to, 102
AVM. *See* Arteriovenous malformations
AVPU assessment method, 632
Axillary block, 654
Axon, 350

Babinski sign, 355
Bacterial endocarditis, 238
Bacterial meningitis, 380–381
Balloon valvuloplasty, 232
Barbiturates, 653, 687–688, 697t
Bariatric patients, 705, 709–713. *See also* Bariatric surgery
    anastomotic leaks, 710–711
    anastomotic strictures, 711–712
    aspiration, 711
    case study, 712
    gastrointestinal bleeding, 711
    hemodynamic instability, 710
    indications for bariatric surgery, 705, 706t
    infection/sepsis, 711
    management of, in ICU, 708–712
    nutrition, 710
    obesity pathophysiology, 708–709
    online resources, 713
    patient outcomes, 712
    pharmacology, 709–710
    sedation and extubation, 710
    surgical complications, 707–708
    venous thromboembolism/pulmonary embolism, 711
Bariatric surgery, 705–707
    biliopancreatic diversion, 706–707
    duodenal switch, 706–707, 707f, 708t
    gastric binding, 708t
    malabsorptive and restrictive surgery, 706–707
    restrictive surgery, 706
    Roux-en-Y gastric bypass (RYGB), 707
Barium studies, 418, 445
Barotrauma, 313, 342–343
Base deficit changes, 80
Base excess, 287–288

Basilar skull fracture, 389
"Beating heart" coronary artery bypass, 231
Beclomethasone (Beclovent®), 329
Beclovent® (beclomethasone), 329
Bedside vigil, 743–744
Behavior (family), 19–20
Behavior (patient), 4, 45
Benadryl® (diphenhydramine), 540
Beneficence, 722, 723
Benign pituitary adenoma, 513
Benzodiazepines, 653–654, 687, 688, 690, 695, 697t
Beta blockers, 166, 176t, 189, 199, 201, 498–499, 697t
Beta stimulants, 697t
Bile, 456
Bilevel positive airway pressure (BiPAP), 302, 311
Biliopancreatic diversion, 706–707
Bilirubin metabolism, 457
Bioethics, elderly patients and, 78
Bioethics, life-and-death decisions, 722
Biologically based therapies, 109
Biological variations, and disease risk, 101
Biorhythms, 58
Biot's respirations, 279t
BiPAP. *See* Bilevel positive airway pressure
Bispectral index monitoring, 367–368
Biventricular pacemakers, 203, 222–223
Blaylock Discharge Planning Risk Assessment Screen, 644–645f
Blenoxane® (bleomycin sulfate), 578
Bleomycin sulfate (Blenoxane®), 578
Blood
    loss, 235, 669
    platelets, 597
    products, 249
    red blood cell production, 538
    supply and demand, 163–165
    transfusions, 248, 249, 679
    types, 250
Blood pressure. *See also* Hypertension
    aging and, 80
    ischemic stroke and, 379
    regulation, 537–538
Blood smear, 610
Bloodstream infections, catheter-related, 69
Blood urea nitrogen (BUN) levels, 82, 538–539
"Blow-by," 316
Blunt trauma, 668, 675, 677
BMI. *See* Body mass index
Body mass index (BMI), 432, 433
"Body stuffing", 687
Bowel evisceration, 674
Bowel motility, 417
Brachial plexus block, 654

Brachial plexus injury, 237
Bradyarrhythmias, 732. *See also* Dysrhythmia interpretation
Bradycardia, postoperative, 233
Brain. *See also* Brain death; Invasive brain monitoring;
        Neurological monitoring
    brain tissue oxygen monitoring, 365–366
    components of, 352, 353f
    injury, 672, 673t, 679
    penumbra, 363
    temperature monitoring, 366
    ventricles within, 364f
Brain death
    clinical criteria for, 382–383
    physiology, 728
Breathing. *See also* Mechanical ventilation; Respiratory
        assessment
    abnormal, 279t, 280t
    negative- *vs.* positive-pressure ventilation, 307
    normal breath sounds, 280t
Brethine® (terbutaline), 329
Brevibloc® (esmolol), 174t, 499
Brevital sodium (Methohexital®), 653
Bronchial glands, 276
Bronchospasm, 298
Bruits, 137, 356, 417
BUN. *See* Blood urea nitrogen levels
Bupivacaine (Marcaine®), 654
Burn(s), 629–639, 668, 669
    acute phase, 635
    assessment, 629–633, 630t
    biological dressings/skin substitutes, 636t
    case study, 638
    chemical, 634–635
    circulatory compromise, 632–633
    electrical, 634–635
    emergent (shock) phase, 630–631
    emotional/psychological/social function and therapy,
        637–638
    eye, 635
    first degree, 629, 630t
    hypovolemic shock and, 246
    Lund and Browder, 630–631t
    management, 630–638
    metabolic and nutrition support, 636–637
    nutrition and, 432, 637
    online resources, 639
    Palmer method of burn assessment, 630
    patient outcomes, 638
    physical/occupational function/therapy, 637
    referral criteria, 637
    rehabilitative/reentry phase, 637
    second degree, 629, 630t
    secondary survey, 634

    third degree, 630t
    wound care, 635–636
Burns Weaning Assessment Program, 315f
Butabarbital (Butisol®), 687
Butalbital (Fiorinal/Fiorcet®), 687
Butisol® (butabarbital), 687
Bypass surgery. *See under* Cardiac surgery

CABG. *See* Coronary artery bypass grafting
CAD. *See* Coronary artery disease
Calan® (verapamel hydrochloride), 405
Calcitonin (Miacalcin®), 580
Calcium antagonists, 166–167, 189, 698t
Calcium channel blockers, 166–167, 189, 199, 405, 505, 698t
Calcium, corrected serum, 579
CAM. *See* Confusion Assessment Method
Cambodians, 100
Cancer. *See also* Oncologic emergencies
    biological risk for, 101
    therapeutic touch and, 111
Candida albicans, 71
Capnography, 288
Carafate® (sulcrafate), 459
Carbamazepine (Tegretol®), 514
Carbocaine® (mepivacaine), 654
Carbon dioxide
    detection, EtCO$_2$ monitoring and, 289
    mainstream and sidestream analysis, 288
    monitoring, 677
Carbon monoxide poisoning, 632, 688–689, 698t
Car crashes, 667, 668
Cardene® (nicordipin), 174t, 234
Cardiac assessment, 132–137
    carotid arteries, 134
    extremities, 137
    general appearance, 133
    health history, 133
    heart, 134–137
    jugular veins, 134
    risk factors, 133
    signs/symptoms of disease, 133
    skin, 134
    vital signs, 133–134, 133t
Cardiac assist devices, 209–226
    case study, 225–226
    implantable cardioverter-defibrillators, 223–224
    implantable hemodynamic monitoring systems, 218
    online resources, 227
    pacemakers, 218–223
    patient outcomes, 224
    ventricular assist device (VAD), 209–216
Cardiac catheterization, 187
Cardiac glycosides, 698t

Cardiac index, 140
Cardiac monitoring, 283
Cardiac output, 140–145
    afterload, 141–142
    cardiac reserve, 144–145
    contractility, 142–143
    heart rate, 144
    measurement, 151, 153
    preload, 140–141
Cardiac resynchronization therapy, 203
Cardiac rhythm irregularities, 198–199
Cardiac surgery, 229–238. *See also* Cardiac transplantation
    beyond immediate postoperative period, 237–238
    case study, 240
    conduit choices, 231–232
    day of, 230
    discharge preparation, 238
    minimally invasive, 229, 232
    off-pump coronary artery bypass, 229, 231
    online resources, 242
    on-pump coronary artery bypass graft, 230–231
    open chest resuscitation, 236
    operating room, 230–232
    patient outcomes, 240
    postoperative assessment and monitoring, 233–236
    preoperative education, 230
    preoperative workup, 229–230
    valve surgery, 232
    weaning from mechanical ventilation, 236–237
Cardiac tamponade, 577–578, 669
Cardiac transplantation, 238–239
    diagnostic evaluation for, 239
    donor criteria, 239
    ventricular assist devices, 239–240
Cardiogenic shock, 187, 244t, 669. *See also* Shock
Cardiolite® (thallium-201), 187
Cardioprotective therapy, 189
Cardiovascular disease, 229. *See also* Cardiac assessment
    cardiac assessment, 132–137
    dysrhythmia interpretation, 125–132
    risk factors, 133
Cardiovascular patients
    elderly, 80–81
    therapeutic touch, 111
Cardiovascular status, in shock, 253
Cardiovascular system, 121–125
    cardiac cycle, 123f
    cardiac output, 123–124
    circulation, 123
    conduction system, 126–127, 126f
    depolarization/repolarization, 124–125, 124f
    electrophysiology, 124–125
    heart, 121

    nervous system innervation, 124
    online resources, 138
    physiology of, 122–123
    refractory/supernormal periods, 125
Carina, 272f, 275
Caring practices, 4, 6
    creating a healing environment in the ICU, 27–39
    family-focused care, 15–25
    infections in the ICU, 67–73
    pain issues in the ICU, 41–49
    sleep disturbances in the ICU, 53
Carotid arteries, 375, 376t
CAT. *See* Complementary and alternative therapy
Catapres® (clonidine), 504, 698t
Catecholamines, 503
Catheter(s)
    catheter-associated urinary tract infection (CAUTI), 70
    catheter knotting, 150
    catheter-related bloodstream infections, 69
    central venous, 147
    fluid-filled intraventricular placement, 361f
    intra-aortic balloon pump, 234
    intra-arterial, 147
    Licox® Catheter, 365
    peritoneal dialysis catheters, 558t
    pulmonary artery, 147–148, 149t, 153–154
CCFAP. *See* Critical Care Family Assistance Program
CCFNI. *See* Critical Care Family Needs Inventory
CD4 count, 591
Cell body, 350
Cellular dehydration, 82t
Central nervous system (CNS), 351–353
Central nervous system drugs, 101
Central venous access, 147
Central venous catheters (CVCs), 69, 69t
Cephulac® (lactulose), 459
Cerebellum dysfunction, 355
Cerebral aneurysm(s), 378, 399–406
    classification by size, 400t
    diagnosis, 400–401
    endovascular stenting prior to aneurysm coiling, 403f
    endovascular techniques, 402–403
    Hunt-Hess Subarachnoid Hemorrhage Classification, 402t
    hyponatremia, 405
    incidence of, 399
    locations of, 400f
    neurogenic pulmonary edema, 405–406
    nursing care, 404
    pathophysiology, 399
    presentation, 399–400
    staged endovascular coiling, 403f
    surgical techniques, 401–402, 403f
    treatment, 401–403

vasospasm, 404–405
Cerebral angiography, 356, 401
Cerebral edema, 364, 379, 455, 458
Cerebral metabolic decompensation, 380
Cerebral perfusion pressure (CPP), 376, 388
Cerebral vasospasm, 404–405
Cerebrovascular accident (CVA), 80, 175
Cerebrovascular complications, 378–379
Cerebrovascular disorders, 395–408
    arteriovenous malformations, 395–399
    cardiac dysfunction and, 406
    case study, 407
    cerebral aneurysms, 399–406
    hydrocephalus, 406
    online resources, 408
    patient outcomes, 406
Chemical burns, 634–635
Chemical tracheobronchitis, 632
Chemotherapy, 580, 581
Chest pain, 164, 181, 189–190, 464. *See also* Angina
Chest palpation, 279–280
Chest radiograph, 186, 677
Chest shape, 278–279
Chest trauma, 671
Cheyne-Stokes, 279t, 741
Chickenpox (varicella-zoster virus), 68
Chief cells, 415
Children, and patient visits, 19
Chinese medicine, 113
Chinese patients, and drug therapy, 101
Chlorpropamide (Diabinese®), 514
Cholesterol, 162
Chromotherapy, 30
Chronic bronchitis, 299t
Chronic heart failure, 200–203, 203–204. *See also* Heart failure
Chronic intrinsic restrictive disease, 296t
Chronic kidney disease, 565–566. *See also* Renal failure
Chronic obstructive pulmonary disease (COPD), 273, 278, 279, 298, 299
    classification of severity of, 331t
    pathophysiology, 330–331
    patient/family education, 332–333
    signs and symptoms of, 331–332
    treatment, 332
Chronic pain, 42, 85. *See also* Pain
Cilia, 276
Cimetidine (Tagamet®), 538
Circadian rhythms, 29–30, 55
Cirrhosis, 424, 425, 454–456
CK. *See* Creatine kinase
Clinical inquiry, 4, 7
Clinical judgment, 4, 6
Clinical trials

abdominal aortic aneurysm management, 262t
    meds for chronic heart failure, 202t
Clofibrate (Atromid-S®), 514
Clonidine (Catapres®), 504, 698t
Clopidogrel (Plavix®), 113, 189, 403, 598
Clostridium difficile, 434
Clot formation, 150
Clotting cascade, 606–607
CNS. *See* Central nervous system
Coagulation, 606–608. *See also* Disseminated intravascular coagulation
    cascade, 607f
    pathways, 606–608
    platelets, 606
Coagulopathies, 460, 678
Cocaine, 689–690, 698t
Codeine, 49t, 101
Code of Ethics for Nurses, 642
Code status, of patients, 721
Cognitive responses, aging and, 82
Cold, application of, 47
Cold caloric test, 357
Collaboration, 4, 6
Colonic varices, 444
Colonoscopy, 418–419, 423, 445
Color, in environment, 30–31, 31t
Colorimetric detector, 289
Coma (myxedema coma), 499–500
Communication
    consistency and, 18
    family-focused care and, 16
    nonverbal, 98–99
    nurse-to-nurse, 5
    pain assessment, 42–45
    principles, for family understanding, 20
    transcultural, 98
Compartment syndrome, 265–266, 678
Compazine® (prochlorperazine), 663
Complementary and alternative therapy (CAT), 109–114
    case study, 114
    categories of, 109
    herbs, 112–113
    music therapy, 111
    online resources, 115
    patient outcomes, 113
    prayer and spirituality, 111–112
    therapeutic touch, 110–111
Complex partial seizures, 380
Compound skull fractures, 389
Computed tomography (CT) scan, 368, 396, 674, 675. *See also* CT scan
Computerized tomographic colonography, 423
Concussion, 388, 672

Concussion (spinal cord), 390
Conducting airways, microanatomy of, 276, 277f
Confusion Assessment Method (CAM), 82
Coning, 728
Conn's disease, 504–505
Contact transmission, 68
Continuous positive airway pressure (CPAP), 302, 310, 709
Continuous renal replacement therapy (CRRT), 559–560
Contractility, 142–143, 144t
Control volume mode, 310
Contusion (cord), 390
Contusions, 388
COPD. *See* Chronic obstructive pulmonary disease
Coping methods, 19
Cordarone® (amiodarone hydrochloride), 202, 220, 233, 732
Corlopam® (fenoldpam), 174t
Coronary arteries, 159–160, 160f
Coronary artery bypass grafting (CABG), 191. *See also*
    Cardiac surgery
Coronary artery disease (CAD), 159–168
    blood supply and demand, 163–165
    case study, 167
    chronic stable angina and, 165–167
    endoscopic atraumatic, 231
    genetic risk for, 101
    markers of inflammation, 163
    online resources, 168
    pathophysiology of, 159–161
    patient outcomes, 167
    pharmacological management, 166
    risk factors, 161–163
Corticosteroids, 581, 584
Corticotrophin, 512
Cortisol, 28, 58, 503
Cortrosyn® (cosyntopin), 506
Cosyntopin (Cortrosyn®), 506
Coughing, 283
Coumadin® (warfarin), 113, 190, 499, 581
COX-1 and -2, 46t
CPAP. *See* Continuous positive airway pressure
CPOT. *See* Critical Care Pain Observation Tool
CPP. *See* Cerebral perfusion pressure
Cranial nerves, 355–356, 356t
Craniopharyngioma, 513
Craniotomy, 401
C-reactive protein, 163
Creatine kinase (CK), 185–186
Creatinine, 538
Creatinine clearance (glomerular filtration rate), 539
Crepitus, 279
Cricoid cartilage, 272f
Critical care environment design, 27–36. *See also* Healing
    environment
Critical Care Family Assistance Program (CCFAP), 20

Critical Care Family Needs Inventory (CCFNI), 17
Critical Care Pain Observation Tool (CPOT), 45
Critical illness myopathies and neuropathies, 314
Cromolyn (NasalCrom®), 329
CRRT. *See* Continuous renal replacement therapy
Cryoprecipitate, 611
C-spine injuries, 632
CT scan. See Computed tomography
Cullen's sign, 476
Cultural issues, in critical illness, 95–106
    biological variations, 101–102
    care planning considerations, 97–100
    case study, 105
    cultural assessment, 97
    cultural concepts, 96–97
    decision making, 101
    disease risk, 101
    drug therapy, 101
    end-of-life issues, 102
    evaluating cultural care, 104
    evidence-based transcultural care, 103t
    key cultural terms, 96t
    online resources, 106
    research summary, 103t
    social organization, 100–101
    target outcomes/sample indicators, 105
    time orientation, 100t
    transcultural care guidelines, 102, 104
Cultural remedies, 99
Curling's ulcer, 633
Cushing's response, 728
Cushing's Syndrome, 492t, 506–507, 513, 514
Cutting balloon angioplasty, 190
CVA. *See* Cerebrovascular accident
CVCs. *See* Central venous catheters
Cyanide poisoning, 690–691, 698t
Cyanosis, 284
Cystic fibrosis, 295
Cystoscopy, 539

Danaparoid sodium (Organan®), 598
Dantrium® (dantrolene sodium), 661
Dantrolene sodium (Dantrium®), 661
Darvon® (propoxyphene), 692
Daylight, 29–30
D-dimer, 609
Deadspace, 289, 293–294
Debridement, 635
Decadron® (dexamethasone), 506
Decision making
    in critical illness, 101
    patient participation in, 4, 5
Declomycin® (demeclocycline hydrochloride), 582
Deep vein thrombosis (DVT), 70, 678, 679

Dehydration, 82t
Delirium, 57, 82, 643
Deltasone® (prednisone), 599, 734t
Demeclocycline hydrochloride (Declomycin®), 582
Demerol® (meperidine), 235, 692, 693
Dendrites, 350
Depakene® (valproic acid), 476
Depressed skull fractures, 389
Depression, 643
Depression medications, 694–695, 696t
Desflurane (Suprane®), 652
Destination therapy, 210t
Dexamethasone (Decadron®), 506, 599
Dexamethasone suppression tests, 507
Dexedrine® (dextroamphetamine), 686
Dextroamphetamine (Dexedrine®), 686
Diabetes/diabetic emergencies, 162, 491, 519–531
    assessment of patient knowledge of, 528
    case study, 529–530
    diabetes insipidus, 514, 733
    diabetic ketoacidosis, 522–523
    etiologies of diabetes, 520t
    flow sheet for DKA/HHS, 527–528
    hyperglycemia, 522–526
    hyperosmolar hyperglycemic states, 523–524
    hypoglycemia, 520–522
    long-term complications, 520t
    online resources, 531
    pathophysiology, 519–520
    patient outcomes, 528
    prevention/lifestyle program, 526
    renal failure risk, 553
    types of diabetes, 520t
Diabinese® (chlorpropamide), 514
Dialysis. See Renal replacement therapies
Diamox® (acetazolamide), 548
Diaphragm, 272
Diarrhea, 438
Diastolic heart failure, 198, 203. See also Heart failure
Diazepam (Valium®), 690, 695
Dibenzyline® (phenoxybenzamine), 504
Dibucaine (Nupercaine®), 654
Didanosine (Videx®), 592
Diffuse axonal injury, 388–389, 672
Digestion, 413–414, 415f
Digoxin (Lanoxin®), 201, 499
Dilantin® (phenytoin), 690, 695, 699t
Diphenhydramine (Benadryl®), 540
Diprivan® (propofol), 311, 433, 653, 679–680, 695
Dipyridamole (Persantine®), 187, 598, 599
Directional atherectomy/rotational atherectomy, 190–191
Direct thrombin inhibitors, 189
Disability (trauma) check, 670
Discharge planning. See Transitional planning

Discomfort, 102
Disease risk, biological variations, 101
Disseminated intravascular coagulation, 605–615
    acute vs. chronic, 605–606
    cardiac care, 612
    case study, 614
    coagulation, 606–608
    conditions associated with, 606t
    detection, 613
    diagnosis, 608–610
    gastrointestinal care, 612–613
    genitourinary care, 613
    neurological care, 612
    online resources, 615
    pain, 612
    pathophysiology, 608
    patient/family support/education, 613
    patient outcomes, 613
    respiratory care, 612
    skin assessment, 611–612
    systemic assessment and support, 611–613
    tests, 609t
    treatment, 610–611
    underlying disorders, 605
Dissociative agents, 653
Distraction technique, 47
Distributive shock states, 244t, 669. See also Shock
Diuretics, 201, 581, 583
Diversity, response to, 4, 7, 21–22
    cultural issues, 95–106
    gerontological issues, 77–91
Diverticulitis, 83
Diverticulosis, 444
DNA damage, 685
Dobutamine (Dobutrex®), 187, 199, 234, 249, 612, 732
Dobutrex® (dobutamine), 187, 199, 234, 249, 612, 732
Documentation systems (patient), 8
Dofetilide (Tikosyn®), 203
Doll's eyes reflex, 357
Do-not-resuscitate orders, 720, 721
Dopamine (Intropin®), 199, 578, 612, 624, 732
"Dowager's hump," 297
Droplet transmission, 68
Drotrecogin Alfa (activated) (Xigris®), 341, 625
Drug elimination, 538
Drug overdose and poisonings, 685–701
    acetaminophen, 685–686
    amphetamine/methamphetamine, 686–687
    barbiturates, 687–688
    benzodiazepines, 688
    carbon monoxide, 688–689
    case study, 700
    cocaine, 689–690
    cyanide, 690–691

Drug overdose and poisonings—*continued*
  initial nursing management, 695
  methanol, 691–692
  online resources, 701
  opiates, 692–693
  patient outcomes, 695
  salicylates, 693–694, 693t
  select poisonings and emergency management, 696–699t
  tricyclic antidepressants, 694–695
Drugs, recreational, 689–690
Drug therapy, ethnicity and, 101
Duodenal switch procedure, 706–707, 707f, 708t
Durable health care power of attorney, 721
DVT. *See* Deep vein thrombosis
Dysfunctional families, 20
Dyslipidemia, 734
Dysrhythmia interpretation, 125–132
  atrial dysrhythmias, 129
  atrioventricular heart blocks, 131–132
  bradycardia, 128
  configuration of normal ECG, 127
  ectopic beats, 127–128
  electrode placement and skin care, 125
  junctional dysrhythmias, 129–130
  sinus disturbances, 128
  tachycardia, 128–130
  ventricular dysrhythmias, 130–131
Dysrhythmias, 188, 732
  postoperative, 660

ECG. *See* Electrocardiogram
Echinacea, 112
Echocardiogram, 186, 577
  stress, 187
  two-dimensional, 286
ECMO. *See* Extracorporeal membrane oxygenation
Edema, 137
EDHs. *See* Epidural hematomas
Education, of patients, 99
EEG. *See* Electroencephalograms
Efferent division, 354
Efferent neuron, 349
EGD. *See* Esophagogastroduodenoscopy
Elderly patients. *See* Aging
Electrical burns, 634–635
Electrocardiogram (ECG), 19
Electroencephalograms (EEG), 54
Electrolyte balance, 500, 538
Electrolyte management, 460
Emergent hypertension, 173–174, 174t. *See also* Hypertension
Emergent (shock) phase, 630–631
Emotion

color and, 30
  expression of, 19
Enalapril (Vasotec®), 174t
Encephalitis, 381–382
Encephalopathy, 455
Endantadine® (amantadine hydrochloride), 322
Endocrine cells, 415
Endocrine function, of pancreas, 415
Endocrine system
  anatomy/physiology, 487–490
  assessment, 490–491
  case study, 493
  disorders, 491
  glands, 488f, 488t
  hypothalamic-pituitary-thyroid feedback loop, 490
  online resources, 495
End-of-life issues, 740
  cultural approaches to, 102
  professional misconceptions in management of, 723–724
  strategies for challenging issues, 723t
  symptoms/management, 741–743
  withdrawal of life support, 724
Endoscopic procedures, 422–424
Endoscopic retrograde cholangiopancreatography (ERCP), 424
Endovascular therapy, 397–398
End stage renal disease, 553, 565–572. *See also* Renal failure; Renal replacement therapies
  acutely ill patient in, 566–568
  chronic kidney disease staging, 565–566
  comorbid conditions with, 567
  nursing interventions, 567
  patient and family teaching, 567–568
  renal transplantation, 568–569
End-tidal carbon dioxide monitoring (ETCO$_2$), 288, 289, 677
Energy therapies, 109
Enflurane (Ethrane®), 652
Enfuvirtide (Fuzeon™), 592
Enoxaparin (Lovenox®), 113, 709
Enteral nutrition, 434–437
  contamination and, 438
  formula selection, 436–437
  gastric feeding, 435
  management/safety issues, 437–438
  rate of delivery, 435–436
  selecting route of, 434–435
  small bowel feeding, 435
  timing of, 435
Enterobacter spp., 69
Enterococci, 69
Enteroscopy, 445
Entrainment, 33

Entry/fusion inhibitors, 592
Environment, healing. *See* Healing environment
Environmental control, cultural factors in, 99–100
Eosinophilic granuloma, 296t
Ephedrine, 686
Eplerenone (Inspra®), 505
Epicardial pacing, 221–222
Epidural anesthesia, 654–655
Epidural hematomas (EDHs), 389, 672
Epiglottis, 272f, 275
Epinephrine (Adrenaline®), 43, 503, 654, 732
Epivir® (lamivudine), 468, 592
Eptifibatide (Integrilin®), 598
Equianalgesia, 47
Equipment, noise and, 29
ERCP. *See* Endoscopic retrograde cholangiopancreatography
Errors, in patient care, 15, 16
Esberitox N, 113
Esmolol (Brevibloc®), 174t, 499
Esophageal varices, 444
Esophagitis, 444
Esophagogastric tamponade tubes, 425, 426t
Esophagogastroduodenoscopy (EGD), 422, 445
Esophagus, 414
Essential oils, 32, 34
Estrogen, 161–162
ETCO$_2$. *See* End-tidal carbon dioxide monitoring
Ethambutol (Myambutol®), 326
Ethrane® (enflurane), 652
Ethanol, 687
Ethical dilemmas, 722–723
    case study, 722–723
    online resources, 725
    withdrawal of life support, 724
Ethnic/ethnicity, defined, 96
Ethnicity, coronary artery disease and, 161
Ethylene glycol, 698t
Etomidate (Amidate®), 653
Europeans, southern, 99
Euthyroid sick syndrome, 500
EVEREST clinical trial, 232
Evisceration of the bowel, 674
External strain gauge, 360–361
Extracorporeal membrane oxygenation (ECMO), 341
Extremities, trauma to, 671
Extrinsic nerves (outside digestive tract), 414
Eye contact, 99
Eye movement assessment, 356–357

Faces Rating Scale, 85
Face trauma, 670–671
Factor II, 610
Factor V, 610

Factor VII, 609–610, 611
Factor VIII, 610, 611
Factor IX, 610
Factor X, 610
Factor XI, 610
Factor XII, 610
"Failure to thrive," elderly patients and, 83t
Family. *See also* Family-focused care
    cultural issues in, 100–101
    defined, 16
    history, coronary artery disease and, 161
    trauma assessment and, 670
Family-focused care, 15–25
    accessible healthcare delivery systems, 21
    assurance, need for, 19
    awareness of family strengths/coping methods, 19
    case studies, 23
    communication principles, 20t
    critical care family needs, 17t
    defined, 15–16
    effect of critical illness on family, 17
    family as constant in patient's life, 17–18
    family assessment/information checklist (example), 21t
    family need for information, 19, 20–21
    family need to be comfortable, 19–20
    family need to be near patient, 18–19
    implementing, 17–22
    invasive procedures/resuscitation, 21, 22t
    key elements of, 16t
    online resources, 24
    patient pain assessment, 45
    support, need for, 21–22
FAST. *See* Focused assessment with sonography for trauma
Fat embolism, 294, 678
Fat metabolism, alterations in, 456
Fat-soluble vitamin deficiency, 456
Femur fracture, 678
Fenoldpam (Corlopam®), 174t
Fentanyl, 49t, 661, 679, 692, 710
Fevers, cultural remedies for, 99–100
FDP. *See* Fibrin degradation products
FFP. *See* Fresh frozen plasma
Fiber-optic monitoring, 362
Fibrin degradation products (FDP), 608–609
Fibrinogen, 609
Fibrinolysis, 608, 621
Fibrosis, 80
Fiorinal/Fiorcet® (butalbital), 687
Fish oils, 112
Flagyl® (metronidazole), 459
Flail chest, 298
Flexible sigmoidoscopy, 418, 422–423
Flonase® (fluticasone proprionate), 329

Florinef® (fludrocortisone), 506
Fludrocortisone (Florinef®), 506
Fluid balance, ARDS and, 340–341
Fluid resuscitation, 255, 633–634
Fluids, monitoring, 283
Flumadine® (rimantadine hydrochloride), 322
Flumazenil (Romazicon®), 688
Flunisolide (AeroBid®), 329
Fluorescent lighting, 30
Fluothane® (halothane), 652
Fluoxetine (Prozac®), 694
Fluticasone proprionate (Flonase®), 329
Focal motor seizures, 380
Focused assessment with sonography for trauma (FAST), 674, 677–678
Foley catheter, 633–634
Folk medicine, 99–100
Follicle-stimulating hormone (FSH), 512
Fomepizole (Antizol®), 692
Foradil Aerolizer® (formoterol fumarate), 329
Forane® (isoflurane), 652
Formoterol fumerate (Foradil Aerolizer®), 329
Fraction of inspired oxygen (FiO$_2$), 310
Fractures, 389, 678
Frank-Starling law of stretch, 143, 245
Fresh frozen plasma (FFP), 610
FSH. *See* Follicle-stimulating hormone
Full code, 721
Full-spectrum light, 29–30
Fulminant hepatic failure, 453. *See also* Hepatic failure
Functional change (patient), 4
Functional residual capacity, 310
Fungal infections, 71
Furosemide (Lasix®), 249, 476, 580
Fuzeon™ (enfuvirtide), 592

Gastroesophageal sphincter, 414
Galactorrhea, 513, 514
Garlic supplements, 112, 113
Gastric feeding, 435
Gastric lavage, 421–422, 447
Gastric secretion, 415
Gastric stress ulcers, 679
Gastric tubes, 633–634
Gastroenteritis, 466
Gastrointestinal anatomy/physiology, 413–416
    basic digestive process, 413–414
    digestive system components, 414–416
    online resources, 419
    regulation of digestive tract, 414
Gastrointestinal bleeding, 443–451, 711
    case study, 450
    diagnostic testing, 444–445

drugs used in, 448–449t
etiology, 444
locations of, 444, 445t
lower, 443
medical management, 445–447
nursing management, 447
online resources, 451
patient education for, 449t
patient outcomes, 447
problem list for, 449t
upper, 443
Gastrointestinal bleeding scan, 445
Gastrointestinal hormones, 414
Gastrointestinal interventions, 421–429
    case study, 427–428
    endoscopic procedures, 422–424
    gastric lavage, 421–422
    liver biopsy, 425–426
    online resources, 429
    paracentesis, 426–427
    patient outcomes, 427
    surgical procedures, 424–425
Gastrointestinal status, in shock, 254
Gastrointestinal system assessment, 416–417, 418t
Gastrointestinal tract malfunctions, 434
G cells, 415
Gender
    coronary artery disease and, 161–162
    transcultural care differences, 102
Generalized tonic-clonic seizures, 380
Gerontological issues, 77–91
    cardiovascular function, 80–81
    case study, 87–90
    functional status assessment, 86
    gastrointestinal tract and nutrition, 82–83
    hormonal function, 83–84
    immunity and infection, 84
    neurological system, 81
    online resources, 91
    oxygenation and ventilation, 79–80
    pain management for critically ill elders, 84–85
    pathophysiology and aging, 79–86
    physical restraints in ICU, 85–86
    predicting outcomes for elders, 78
    renal function, 81–82
GFR. *See* Glomerular filtration rate
Gigantism, 513
Giger and Davidhizar Transcultural Assessment Model, 97, 98
Ginger, 112
Ginkgo biloba, 112, 113
Ginseng, 113
Glasgow Coma Scale, 354–355, 359, 632, 669
Glomerular filtration rate (GFR), 80, 536–537, 539

Glomeruli, 535
GlucaGen® (glucagon hydrochloride), 521
Glucagon hydrochloride (GlucaGen®), 521
Glucocorticoids, 341, 499
Gluconeogenesis, 636
Glucosamine, 112
Glucose-6-phosphate dehydrogenase (G6PD) enzyme deficiency, 101
Glycemic control, with ischemic stroke, 379
Glycols, 698t
Glycoprotein IIb/IIIa inhibitors, 189
Glycopyrrolate (Robinul®), 653
God, belief in, 111–112
"Golden hour" of trauma, 668
Gonadal dysfunction, 513
Gonadotropin deficiency, 513
Graves' disease, 498
Gray-Turner sign, 476
Grief responses, cultural differences in, 102
Growth hormone, 512
Guglielmi detachable coil, 402
Guided imagery, 47
Guillain-Barré syndrome, 297t
Gunshot wounds, 677

HAIs. See Healthcare-associated infections (HAIs)
Halcion® (triazolam), 688
Haldol® (haloperidol), 101, 687, 695
Haloperidol (Haldol®), 101, 687, 695
Halothane (Fluothane®), 652
Hand hygiene, 68–69, 69t, 70t, 71
HCO3, 287
Head injuries, 388–390. See also Head trauma; Neurologic injuries
    concussion, 388
    contusions, 388
    diffuse axonal injury, 388–389
    fractures, 389
    intracranial hemorrhage, 389–390
    nursing management of, 391
Head trauma, 670–671, 672, 673t
Healing environment, 27–39
    air quality, 31–32
    ancient perspective, 27–28
    aromatherapy, 34–35
    artwork, 33–34
    benefits, 35
    case study, 37
    color and, 30–31
    environmental landscape, 31
    environmental noise, 28–29
    light, 29–30
    online resources, 38
    patient control of, 33, 35

    patient/family needs and wants, 32–33
    psychological/physiological connection, 28
    recommendations for creating, 35–36
    therapeutic sounds/music therapy, 33–35
    traditional and healing environment compared, 36t
    visitation, 32
Healing touch, 110–111
Healthcare-associated infections (HAIs), 67–73
    antibiotic-resistant, in critically ill adults, 69
    case study, 72
    catheter-related bloodstream infections, 69
    control and prevention strategies, 71
    fungal infections, 71
    healthcare-associated pneumonia, 70
    online resources, 73
    patient outcomes, 71
    patient risk factors, 67–68, 67t
    surgical site infections, 70
    transmission modes, 68–69, 68t
    urinary tract infections, 70
Healthcare environment/system, 4
Health practices, cultural remedies, 99
Heart. See also Cardiovascular disease; Cardiovascular system; Heart failure
    anatomy, 121, 122f
    auscultation, 135–136, 135f
    examination of, 134–137
    extra heart sounds, 136
    first and second heart sounds, 136
    inspection, 135
    murmurs, 136
    palpation, 135
    pericardial friction rubs, 137
Heart failure, 81t, 187, 197–207. See also Acute coronary syndrome; Cardiovascular disease
    acute decompensated, 199–200, 203
    case study, 205–206
    causes, 198t
    chronic, 200–203, 203–204
    clinical trials, 203
    diagnostic tests, 199, 200t
    diastolic, 203
    drugs to avoid, 202–203
    nonpharmacologic treatment, 203–204
    online resources, 207
    pathophysiology, 197–198
    patient/family education, 204
    patient history/physical exam, 198–199
    patient outcomes, 204
    pharmacologic treatment, 199–203
    possible surgical/interventional procedures for, 204t
HeartMate IP, 214–215
HeartMate XVE, 215, 217
Heart transplant. See Cardiac transplantation

Heat, application of, 47
Heat stroke, 83
Helicobacter pylori, 419, 444
Hemicraniectomy, 364
Hemodialysis, 34, 555–558
Hemodynamic changes, pain assessment and, 85
Hemodynamic instability, 688
Hemodynamic monitoring, 139–157
    accuracy of, 148–51
    cardiac output, 140–145
    case study, 155–156
    clinical inquiry/decision making, 154–155
    factors that alter heart rate, 144f
    implantable hemodynamic monitoring system, 218
    online resources, 157
    oxygen delivery, 145
    physical assessment, 146–151
    physiologic basis of, 140–146
    pulmonary gas exchange, 140
    terms, 145
    troubleshooting systems, 151–154, 152t
Hemodynamics, 243–245, 246t, 247t
Hemoglobin
    hemodynamic monitoring and, 145
    respiratory monitoring and, 283
Hemolysis, 101
Hemolytic transfusion reactions, 249
Hemorrhagic stroke, 378–379
Hemothorax, 676, 677t
Heparin, for DIC, 611
Heparin-induced thrombocytopenia, 598
Hepatic failure, 453–463, 685, 686
    acetaminophen overdoses management, 460
    ascites management, 460
    bilirubin metabolism, alteration in, 457
    case study, 462
    cerebral edema, 455
    clinical findings of, 458t
    collaborative management, 457–459
    encephalopathy management, 459
    etiology, 453–454
    fluid/electrolyte management, 460
    GI bleeding management, 459
    hepatic encephalopathy, 455
    hepatorenal syndrome, 457
    late onset, 453
    liver transplantation and, 460–461
    metabolic alterations, 457
    nutrition management, 459–460
    online resources, 463
    pathophysiology and clinical manifestations, 454–456
    patient outcomes, 461
    portal hypertension, 456
    protein metabolism alterations, 457

Hepatitis, 465–473
    case study, 472
    etiology, 466
    fulminant, 466
    Hepatitis A, 466–467, 466t
    Hepatitis B, 467–468, 467t, 468t
    Hepatitis C, 469–470
    Hepatitis D, 468–469, 469t
    Hepatitis E, 470–471
    Hepatitis F and G, 465
    online resources, 473
    pathophysiology, 465–466
    patient outcomes, 471
    vaccines, 466t, 467
Hepatocellular carcinoma, 470
Hepatomegaly, 199
Hepatorenal syndrome, 457
Hepsera® (adefovir), 468
Herbs, 112–113
Herniation, 376
Heroin, 692
Herpes simplex encephalitis type 1, 382
Herpes simplex virus (HSV), 68
Herpetic whitlow, 68
Hirsuitism, 514
Hispanics, 99, 102
Histamine, 276, 448
HIV. *See* AIDS and HIV
Home health, 642
Hormone metabolism, alterations in, 456
Hormone replacement therapy, in organ donors, 732
Hormones, 487–488, 489–490t. *See also* Endocrine system
    adrenocorticotropic hormone (ACTH), 28, 503
    corticotropin-releasing hormone (CRH), 28, 503
    gastrointestinal, 414
    secreted by the pituitary, 511–513
    thyroid, 497–498
Hormone secretion, 538
Hospice care, 642
HSV. *See* Herpes simplex virus
Human immunodeficiency virus. *See* AIDS and HIV
Hunt and Hess grading scale, 378
Hydralazine hydrochloride (Apresdine®), 201, 263
Hydrocarbon absorption, 635
Hydrocephalus, 401
Hydrocodone, 49t
Hydrocortisone, 499, 500
Hydromorphone, 49t
Hydrostatic pressure, 149
Hydrostatic systems, 360–361
Hyoid bone, 272f
Hyoscine hydrobromide® (scopolamine), 663
Hyperaldosteronism, 505
Hypercalcemia, 578–580

Hypercatabolism, 636
Hyperdynamic response, 636–637
Hyperdynamic therapy, 404
Hyperglycemia, 162, 438, 478, 522–524
    diabetic ketoacidosis, 522–524, 525f, 526
    hyperosmolar hyperglycemic states, 523–526
    osmolarity calculation, 524t
    signs/symptoms, 524
    treatment, 524–526
Hyperkalemia, 81
Hyperlipidemia, 478
Hypermetabolic response, 636
Hypermetabolism, 432
Hyperosmolar hyperglycemic states. See under
        Diabetes/diabetic emergencies
Hyperparathyroidism, 492t
Hyperpituitarism, 513
Hyperresonance, 280
Hypersensitivity pneumonitis, 296t
Hypertension, 101, 171–179
    acute aortic dissection, 175
    after cerebrovascular accident, 175
    blood pressure levels in adults (categories), 178
    case study, 178
    coronary artery disease and, 162
    decision tree for drug treatment, 177f
    end-stage renal disease and, 175
    mechanisms of secondary, 173t
    medications, 176t, 177
    nursing management, 174–177
    online resources, 179
    pathophysiology, 171–173
    patient education, 177–178
    patient outcomes, 178
    pheochromocytoma and, 504
    postoperative, 175, 660
    prior to discharge, 175–177
    renal failure risk, 553
    urgent and emergent, 173–174, 174t
Hypertensive therapy, 404
Hyperthermia, 83
Hyperthyroidism, 498
Hypoadrenalism, 500
Hypoalbuminemia, 477
Hypocalcemia, 478
Hypoglycemia, 500, 520–522, 521t, 522f
Hypogonadism, 513, 514
Hypokalemia, 505
Hypomagnesemia, 680
Hyponatremia, 405, 680
Hypoparathyroidism, 492t
Hypopharynx, 275
Hypopituitarism, 500, 513
Hypotension, 313

    in critically ill trauma patients, 680
    neurogenic shock and, 250–251
    postoperative, 659–660
Hypothalamus, 488f, 488t
Hypothermia, 83, 670, 678
    induced, 377, 379
    postoperative, 660
Hypoventilation, 286, 659, 676
Hypovolemia, 289, 477, 669
    in potential organ donors, 728
Hypovolemic shock, 244t, 246–247, 445–446. See also Shock
Hypoxemia, postoperative, 659
Hypoxia, 387, 676
    severe, 308

IABP. See Intra-aortic balloon pump
IADLs. See Instrumental activities of daily living
ICH. See Intracranial hemorrhage
ICP. See Intracranial pressure
"ICU psychosis," 57
IHD. See Ischemic heart disease
Imaging modalities
    CT scan, 674–675
    FAST, 674, 677–678
Immune system
    elderly patients and, 84
    GI tract and, 83
    therapeutic touch for treatment of disorders in, 110
Immunosuppresive therapies, 733, 734t
Implantable cardioverter-defibrillators, 203, 223–224
Inactivity, health problems and, 163
Indirect calorimetry, 433
Indirect contact transmission, 68
Indocin® (indomethicin), 238, 514
Indomethicin (Indocin®), 238, 514
Inderal® (propranolol), 101, 459, 498–499, 690
Infections. See also Healthcare-associated infections (HAIs);
        Sepsis
    cardiac postoperative, 237
    elderly patients and, 84
    hepatic failure and, 460
    intracranial pressure monitoring and, 360
    multisystem organ failure-associated, 434
    of the nervous system, 380–382
    pulmonary artery catheter monitoring and, 150
    prevention of, 626
    VADs and, 216t
Infectious colitis, 444
Inferior vena cava, 277
Inflammation
    coronary artery disease and, 161, 163
    sepsis and, 620–621
Inflammatory bowel disease, 444
Influenza, 101, 321–322

Information, family need for, 19
Inhalation agents, 651–652
Inhalation injury, 632
Injury stress syndrome, 432
Insomnia, 30, 57
Inspiratory pressure level (IPL), 309
Inspiratory time (Ti) and inspiratory to expiratory ratio (I:E Ratio), 309
Inspra® (eplerenone), 505
Instructive advance directives, 720
Instrumental activities of daily living (IADLs), 642
Integrilin® (eptifibatide), 598
Intercoronary stenting, 191
Intercostal muscles, 273
Intercostal retractions, 273
Interferon alpha (Intron® A), 468
Interneurons, 350
Interpreters, 98
Interstitial edema, 337
Intra-abdominal pressure monitoring, 419
Intra-aortic balloon pump (IABP), 188, 199, 203, 234, 235f
Intra-arterial catheters, 147
Intra-arterial waveform, 154
Intracerebral hematomas, 672
Intracerebral hemorrhage, 396
Intracranial hemorrhage (ICH), 378, 389–390, 390
Intracranial pressure (ICP)
    elevated, 375–377, 379
    monitoring, 360–362
    neurologic injuries and, 388
Intraparenchymal hemorrhage, 396
Intraparenchymal monitor, 363
Intravenous anesthetics. See Anesthesia
Intravenous pyelogram, 539–540
Intraventricular hemorrhage, 396
Intraventricular monitoring, 363–365
Intrinsic nerve plexi, 414
Intron® A (interferon alpha), 468
Intropin® (dopamine), 199, 578, 612, 624, 732
Intubation, 289, 632, 669
Invasive brain monitoring, 365–366
    intracranial pressure monitoring, 360–362
    intraventricular monitoring, 363–365
Invasive devices, infection and, 68
Invasive ventilation. See Mechanical ventilation
INVOS cerebral oximeter system, 366
Ipratropium (Atrovent®), 329
Irritable bowel syndrome, 423
Ischemia, 164, 183, 376
Ischemic colitis, 444
Ischemic heart disease (IHD), 164–165, 165t, 182
Ischemic stroke, 378, 379
Isoflurane (Forane®), 652

Isopropyl alcohol, 698t
Isoproterenol (Isuprel®), 732
Isordil® (isosorbide dinitrate), 201
Isosorbide dinitrate (Isordil®), 201
Isuprel® (isoproterenol), 732

Jehovah Witnesses, 102
Jugular venous oxygen saturation, 365
Justice, 722

Ketalar® (ketamine), 653, 654
Ketamine (Ketalar®), 653, 654
Kidney disease. See Renal failure; Renal replacement therapies
Kidney Disease Outcomes Quality Initiative, 565
Kidney(s). See also Renal failure; Renal system
    ADH and, 512
    hypoperfusion of, 478
    shock and, 254
    size of, and aging, 81
    transplantation, 735
Kinetic therapy, 340
Klebsiella pneumoniae, 69
Kussmaul's respiration, 279t
Kyphosis, 297

Labetalol (Normdyne®, Trandate®), 173, 174t, 263, 687, 690
Lactic acid, 146
Lactogenic hormone, 512
Lactulose (Cephulac®), 459
Lamivudine (Epivir®), 468, 592
Language barriers, 98
Lanoxin® (digoxin), 201, 499
Laparoscopic adjustable gastric banding, 708t
Large intestine, 416
Laryngospasm, postoperative, 659
Larynx, 275
Laser angioplasty, 191
Lasix® (furosemide), 249, 476, 580
Law of stretch, 175, 245
Learning facilitation, 4, 7
Left ventricular aneurysm, 188
Left ventricular assist device (LVAD), 203
Left ventricular end diastolic pressure (LVEDP), 141
Lepirudin (Refludan®), 598
Levalbuterol (Xofenex®), 329
Levophed® (norepinephrine), 234, 612, 711, 732
Levorphanol, 49t
Levothyroxine (Synthroid®), 500
Licox® Catheter, 365
Lidocaine (Xylocaine®), 654, 690, 732
Lifestyle alterations, and coronary artery disease, 165–167
Life support, withdrawal of, 724

Light
   environmental, 29–30
   light therapy, 30
   sleep-wake cycles and, 60
Liothyronine (Thyrolar®), 500
Lipid-lowering medications, 166
Lip necrosis, 314
Lipophilic drugs, 710
Lipoproteins, 162
Liquid chromatography-mass spectroscopy, 507
Liver, 415f, 416
   biopsy, 425–426
   transplantation, 460–461, 734–735
Liver disease/damage, 254, 685, 686. See also Hepatitis
Living wills, 720–721
Long-term acute care, 642
Loop diuretics, 176t
Lorazepam (Ativan®), 311, 653, 687, 690
Lou Gehrig's disease, 297t. See also Amyothrophic
      lateralizing sclerosis
Lower airway injury, 632
Lower respiratory tract, 275–276
Low-molecular-weight heparin, 189, 656t
Lovenox® (enoxaparin), 113, 709
Luminal® (phenobarbital), 687, 690, 695
Lund and Browder chart, 630, 631t
Lung anatomy. See Respiratory anatomy
Lung cancer, 101
Lung collapse, 677t
Luteinizing hormone, 512
LVAD. See Left ventricular assist device
LVEDP. See Left ventricular end diastolic pressure
Lymphangiomyomatosis, 296t

Magnetic resonance imaging (MRI), 187, 356, 368, 396,
      397f, 401
Ma Huang, 686
Malignant disease. See Cancer; Oncologic emergencies
Malignant hyperthermia, 660–661, 662
Mallory-Weiss tear, 444
Malnutrition. See also Nutrition (for critically ill adult)
   in the elderly, 83
   healthcare-associated infections and, 67–68
Malonylurea, 687
Manipulative and body-based therapies, 109
Mannitol (Osmitrol®), 364, 377
MAP. See Mean arterial pressure
Marcaine® (bupivacaine), 654
Massage, 47
Mast cells, 276
Maxair® (pirbuterol), 329
Mean arterial pressure (MAP), 147, 154, 245, 388
Mean pulmonary artery pressure (MPAP), 245

Measles, 68
Mechanical ventilation, 307–319
   acute respiratory distress syndrome and, 339–340
   alarms, 311, 312–313t
   avoiding complications of, 311, 313
   case study, 318
   nursing management of patient on, 311–314
   obese patients, 709
   online resources, 319
   patient outcomes, 316
   positive-pressure ventilation, 307–308
   sepsis and, 621
   sleep disorders and, 58
   ventilator parameters and modes, 308–310
   volume modes, 310–311
   weaning from, 236–237, 314–316, 317f
Mechanism of injury, 668
Mediastinitis, 237
Medications. See also specific medication
   drug dosages eliminated via the kidney, 81
   ethnicity and effects of, 101
   pain, 45–47, 46t
   pupillary response and, 357
   respiratory monitoring and, 283
   sleep impairment and, 59t
Melatonin, 30, 58
Meningioma, 513
Meningitis, 380–381
Meperidine (Demerol®), 49t, 235, 692, 693
Mepivacaine (Carbocaine®), 654
Metabolic cart, 433
Metabolic syndrome, 163
Metaproterenol (Alupent®), 329
Metastic carcinoma, 513
Metformin HCl, 696t
Methadone, 49t
Methamphetamines, 686–687
Methanol, 691–692, 698t
Methicillin-resistant S. aureus (MRSA), 69
Methimazole (Tapazole®), 498
Methohexital® (brevital sodium), 653
Methylene blue, 691
Methylphenidate (Ritalin®), 686
Methylprednisolone (Solu-Medrol®), 673–674
Metoclopramide (Reglan®), 437
Metronidazole (Flagyl®), 459
MDRO. See Multidrug-resistant organisms
Miacalcin® (calcitonin), 580
Microperfusion, 365
Midamor® (amiloride hydrochloride), 505
Midazolan (Versed®), 311, 653, 688
MIDCAB. See Minimally invasive direct coronary artery
      bypass

Milrinone (Primacor®), 199, 234, 249, 299
Mind-body interventions, 109
Mineralocorticoids, 503
Minimally invasive direct coronary artery bypass (MIDCAB), 231, 232
Minnesota tube, 446–447
Minute ventilation (MV), 309
Mitral valve regurgitation, 188
Mitral valve repair techniques, 232
Mixed venous oxygen saturation, 145
MODS. *See* Multiple organ dysfunction syndrome
Mometasone furoate monohydrate (Nasonex®), 329
Monoamine oxidase inhibitors, 698t
Monroe-Kellie doctrine, 364
Montelukast (Singulair®), 329
Mormons, 100
Morphine, 47, 49t, 101, 679, 690, 692
Motility, 413
Motor nerve damage, 355
Motor nerve roots, 377t
Motor vehicle crashes, 667, 668
Mouth, 414
MPAP. *See* Mean pulmonary artery pressure
MRI. *See* Magnetic resonance imaging
Mucomyst® (n-acetylcysteine), 460
Mucosal protective agents, 448
Mucous membranes, respiratory assessment and, 279
Mucous neck cells, 415
MUGA. *See* Multiple gated acquisition scan
Multicenter Automatic Defibrillator Implantation Trial, 203
Multidrug-resistant organisms (MDRO), 69
Multimodal monitoring, 359
Multiple gated acquisition (MUGA) scan, 187
Multiple organ dysfunction syndrome (MODS), 82, 145, 619, 634
Multisystem organ failure-associated infections, 434
Muscle atrophy, 355
Muscle relaxants, 652–653
Muscular dystrophies, 297
Musculoskeletal injuries, 678
Music therapy, 33–35, 47, 111
Muslims, 99
Mustargen® (nitrogen mustard), 578
Mutated viruses, 591
Myambutol® (ethambutol), 326
Myasthenia gravis, 297
Mycobacterium tuberculosis, 68, 325, 326
Myocardial infarction (MI), 159, 181–182, 182f, 183, 187–188. *See also* Acute coronary syndrome
Myocardial perfusion scan, 187
Myxedema coma, 499–500

N-acetylcysteine (Mucomyst®), 460
Naloxone (Narcan®), 650, 692

Narcan® (naloxone), 650, 692
Naropin® (ropivacaine hydrochloride), 654
Nasal cavity, 273–274
NasalCrom® (cromolyn), 329
Nasogastric tube, 675
Nasonex® (mometasone furoate monohydrate), 329
Nasopharyngeal airways, 300
Nasopharynx, 274
National High Blood Pressure Education Program, 177
Native Americans, 99, 101, 102
Natriuretic peptide (nesiritide), 199
"Natural therapies," 112–113
Nausea, 438
Neck trauma, 671
Necrotizing pancreatitis, 475–476, 478. *See also* Pancreatitis (acute pancreatitis)
Nedocromil (Tilade®), 329
Negative-pressure wound therapy, 635
Nelfinavir (Viracept®), 592
Nembutal® (pentobarbital), 687
Neoplasm, 444
Neostigmine (Prostigmin®), 652
Neosynephrine® (phenylephrine), 404
Nephrons, 535, 536t
Nesiritide (natriuretic peptide), 199
Neurogenic pulmonary edema, 405–406
Neurogenic shock, 250–251, 391
Neuroleptics, 687
Neurological anatomy/physiology, 350–354
    brain components, 353f
    central nervous system, 351–353
    peripheral nervous system, 353–354
    synaptic structure/function, 352f
Neurological assessment, 354–357
    cranial nerves and sensory system, 355–356
    Glasgow Coma Scale, 354–355
    online resources, 358
    posturing, 355f
Neurological death, 728
Neurological monitoring, 359–372
    case study, 370
    invasive brain monitoring, 360–366
    noninvasive brain monitoring, 366–368
    online resources, 372
    patient outcomes, 368–369
    physical neurological exam, 359–360
Neurological procedures, 357t
Neurologic disorders, 375–384
    brain death, 382–383
    case study, 383
    elevated intracranial pressure, 375–377
    evidence-based interventions, 377–383
    hemorrhagic stroke, 378–379
    infections of the nervous system, 380–382

ischemic stroke, 378
online resources, 384
patient outcomes, 383
status epilepticus, 379–380, 381
Neurologic injuries, 387–393
case study, 393
drug therapy, 390
head injuries, 388–390
intracranial pressure and cerebral perfusion pressure, 388
neurogenic shock and spinal shock, 391
nursing management of, 391
online resources, 394
pathophysiology, 387–388
patient outcomes, 392
spinal cord injuries, 390
vertebral fractures, 390–392
Neurologic status, in shock, 253
Neuromuscular blocking agents, 652–653, 653t
Neuromuscular disorders, 297
Neuromuscular monitoring, 368
Neurons, 349–350, 350f
Neuropathic pain, 42. *See also* Pain
Neuroscience nursing, 375
Neutropenia, 69
Newborns, and sense of smell, 31–32
Nicardipine (Cardene®), 174t, 234
Nifedipine (Procardia®), 173
Nimodipine (Nimotop®), 404
Nimotop® (nimodipine), 404
Nipride® (nitroprisside), 173, 174t, 188, 690
Nitrates, 166
Nitric oxide, inhaled, 341
Nitrobid® (nitroglycerin), 174t
Nitro-Bid® ointment (nitropaste), 690
Nitrogen mustard (Mustargen®), 578
Nitroglycerin (Tridil®, Nitrobid®, Nitrostat®), 173, 174t, 199, 414, 690
Nitropaste (Nitro-Bid® ointment), 690
Nitroprusside (Nipride®), 173, 174t, 188, 199, 263, 690
Nitrostat® (nitroglycerin), 199, 414
Nitrous oxide, 652
NIV. *See* Noninvasive ventilations
Nociception, 42
Noise
environmental stress and, 28–29
sleep disruption in ICU from, 59
Nonbarbiturates, 653
Noncardiogenic pulmonary edema, postoperative, 659
Nonhemolytic febrile reactions, 249
Noninvasive ventilations (NIV), 303t
Nonmaleficence, 722
Nonopioids, 45, 46t
Nonrapid eye movement (NREM) sleep, 53-55

Nonsteroidal anti-inflammatory drugs (NSAIDs), 46t, 444, 699t
Nonverbal communication, 98–99
Norcuron® (vecuronium), 368
Norepinephrine (Levophed®), 43, 234, 503, 504, 612, 711, 732
Normdyne® (labetalol), 173, 174t, 690
Nosocomial infections, 295. *See also* Infections
Novapressin® (terlipressin), 424
Novocain® (procaine), 654
NREM. *See* Nonrapid eye movement sleep
NRTIs. *See* Nucleoside/nucleotide reverse transcriptase inhibitors
NSAIDs. *See* Nonsteroidal anti-inflammatory drugs
Nuclear imaging studies, 187
Nucleoside/nucleotide reverse transcriptase inhibitors (NRTIs), 592
Nupercaine® (dibucaine), 654
Nurse(s)
competencies, 4t
cultural competence of, 97
dimensions of nursing practice, 4
educating, 9 10
performance standards applied to selected, 9t
Synergy Model, 3–12, 8–10
Nursing homes, 642
Nutrition (for critically ill adult), 431–440
best practices, 432–434
body mass index calculation, 432
case study, 439
delivery method, 433–434
enteral nutrition, 434–437, 436t
estimating caloric needs/nutrient requirements, 433
formula selection, 436–437
online resources, 441
parenteral nutrition, 434
patient outcomes, 438–439
rate of delivery, 435–436
starvation *vs.* stress hypermetabolism, 431–432
timing (early *vs.* late), 435
weight categories based on BMI, 433

Obesity. *See also* Bariatric patients
as cause of death, 705
coronary artery disease and, 163
effect on immune/metabolic reserves, 709
measurement of, 432
morbidly obese defined, 705
pathophysiology, 708–709
Observational sedation assessment, 366–367
Obstructive shock, 244t, 249–250. *See also* Shock
Obstructive sleep apnea, 708–709
Octreotide infusion (Santostatin®), 424, 447, 459, 478
Ocular burns, 635

Oculocephalic reflex, 357
Oculovestibular reflex, 357
Odor, effects of, 31–32
Off-pump coronary artery bypass (OPCAB), 229, 231
Omalizumab (Xolair®), 329
Oncologic emergencies, 577–586
    cardiac tamponade, 577–578
    case studies, 585
    hypercalcemia, 578–580
    online resources, 586
    patient outcomes, 584
    spinal cord compression, 583–584
    superior vena cava syndrome, 580–581
    syndrome of inappropriate antidiuretic hormone
        secretion, 581
    tumor lysis syndrome, 582–583
Ondansetron (Zofran®), 663
OPCAB. *See* Off-pump coronary artery bypass
Open surgical liver biopsy, 426
Opiates, 692–693, 699t
    endogenous, 42
Opioid agonists, 45, 46t, 47, 49t, 699t
Oral cavity, 274
Organ donation, 727–737
    brain death physiology, 728
    cardiac criteria, 239
    care of recipient, 733–735
    case studies, 735, 736–737
    complications associated with specific, 734t
    complications following transplant, 733t
    confirmation of brain death, 382
    consent, 728
    contraindications for, 727–728
    critical pathway for, after cardiac death, 729–730f
    critical pathway for donor, 730–731f
    cultural approaches to, 102
    hemodynamic management of potential donor, 732t
    immunosuppressive therapies, 734t
    kidney evaluation criteria, 568t
    medical management, 728–732
    online resources, 737
    patient outcomes, 735
    rejection signs/symptoms, 733
Organ transplants
    cardiac, 204, 238–239
    kidney, 568–569
    liver, 460–461
Orgaran® (danaparoid sodium), 598
Oropharyngeal airways, 299–300, 300f
Oropharynx, 274
Orthodox Jews, 102
Orthopedic trauma, 678
Orthostatic hypotension, 356
Oseltamivir (Tamiflu®), 322

Osmitrol® (mannitol), 364, 377
Osmotic agents, 364, 377
Ovaries, 488, 488f
Overcrowding, ICU infections and, 71
Oxycodone, 49t
Oxygen
    consumption, 146
    delivery, 145
    saturation, 676
Oxygenation
    critical care cardiac patients and, 192
    elderly patients and, 79–80
Oxygen therapy, 657
Oxyhemoglobin dissociation curve, 286
Oxytoxin, 512

Pacemakers, 218–223, 233
    biventricular, 222–223
    duel chamber, 219
    epicardial, 221–222
    failure to capture/failure to sense, 221f
    ICHD codes, 222t
    100% capture of dual chamber pacer, 220f
    100% capture of ventricular pacer, 219f
    permanent, 222, 223
    temporary, 218–222
    transcutaneous, 218–219
PaCO$_2$, 286–289
PACs. *See* Pulmonary artery catheters
PACU Behavioral Pain Rating Scale (PACUBPRS), 45
PACUBPRS. *See* PACU Behavioral Pain Rating Scale
Pain, 41–49
    acute, 42, 85
    aromatherapy and, 35
    assessment, hemodynamic changes and, 85
    assessment, in nonverbal patients, 42, 44–45
    assessment, PQRSTU, 43, 44, 165
    behavioral/physiological indicators for, 45t
    case study, 48
    clinical practice guidelines for management of, 47
    components of, 41
    critical care cardiac patient and, 191
    definition and types of, 41–42
    end of life symptoms, 741–742
    equianalgesia, 47
    intensity scales, 44f
    mangement of, for critically ill elders, 84–85
    mechanical ventilation weaning, 237
    medication, cultural approaches to, 102
    music therapy and, 33
    nociception, 42
    nociceptive *vs.* neuropathic, 43f
    nonpharmacological methods for management of, 47
    observable indicators for, 44–45

patient outcomes, 47
patient's self-report of, 42, 43–44
pharmacological management of, 45–47, 49t
physiology of, 42–43
postoperative, 662–663
sleep disorders and, 58
steps for complete assessment of, 44
stress response, 42
traumatic brain injury and, 679–680
Pain Assessment and Intervention Notation, 45
Palliative care, 739–747
    advance directives, 741
    barriers to implementing, in ICU, 743
    case study, 745
    communication, 744
    delirium management, 743
    family-focused care, 744
    fever management, 742–743
    goals of, 739–740
    hydration/nutrition, 742
    ICU environment, 740
    nausea/vomiting management, 742
    online resources, 746–747
    pain management, 741–742
    patient outcomes, 744
    shift from curative to comfort care, 743, 744
    shortness of breath/dyspnea management, 742
Palmar method of burn assessment, 630
Palpation, 418
Pamidronate (Aredia®), 580
Pancreas, 83, 415–416, 488t
    exocrine function, 415
Pancreatitis (acute pancreatitis), 424, 475–482, 476f
    case study, 481
    challenges for nursing student/faculty, 478, 480
    classification of, 475–476
    clinical presentation, 476
    etiology and incidence, 475–476
    key research summary, 478
    local complications, 478
    management of, 480t
    metabolic complications, 478
    necrotizing, 475–476, 478
    nursing care guide for patient with, 479t
    online resources, 482
    patient care management, 478
    patient outcomes, 480–481
    predicting severity of, 477
    Ranson's criteria for, 477t
    surgical management, 478
    systemic complications, 477–478
Pancuronium (Pavulon®), 368
PAOP. See Pulmonary artery occlusive pressure
Papaverine (Para-Time® SR), 405

Paracentesis, 426–427
Paralytic agents, with neurologic disorders, 377
Parasympathetic nervous system, 349
Parathyroid gland disorders, 491
Parathyroid gland, 488t
Para-Time® SR (papaverine), 405
Parenchymal hemorrhage, 396
Parenteral nutrition, 434
Parietal cells, 415
Partial lobectomy, 364
Patient acuity, 8
Patient characteristics, 4
Patient participation, in care, 4, 5
Patient Self-Determination Act, 721–722
Pavulon® (pancuronium), 368
PAWP. See Pulmonary artery wedge pressure
PC. See Pressure Control
PC/IRV. See Pressure Control/Inverse Ratio Ventilation
PCIs (percutaneous coronary interventions), 190
PCWP. See Pulmonary capillary wedge pressure
Pectoralis major, 273
Pectus carinatum, 296
Pectus excavatum, 296
PEEP. See positive end expiratory pressure
Pelvic fractures, 678
Pelvis trauma, 671
Penetrating trauma, 668, 674
Pentobarbital (Nembutal®), 687
Pentothal® (thiopental sodium), 653, 687
Penumbra, 363
Peppermint, 34, 112
Peptic ulcers, 444
Perception, of pain. See Pain
Percussion, 280, 417–418
Percutaneous balloon angioplasty, 405
Percutaneous coronary interventions (PCIs), 190
Percutaneous liver biopsy, 426
Percutaneous transjugular intrahepatic portosystemic (TIP) shunt, 424–425
Percutaneous transluminal coronary angioplasty (PTCA), 190
Pericarditis, 188
Perineum, trauma to, 671
Periodic limb movements, during sleep, 57
Peripheral nerve blockade, 654
Peripheral nervous system, 349, 353–354
    afferent division, 353–354
    efferent division, 354
Peripheral parenteral nutrition (PPN), 434
Peristalsis, 413
Peritoneal dialysis, 558–559
Peritoneal inflammation, 418
Peritonitis, 674
Persantine® (dipyridamole), 187, 598

Personal protective equipment (PPE), 68

PET. *See* Positron emission tomography

Petroleum-based ointments, 635t

pH, 286–287

Phantom pain, 42

Pharyngoesophageal sphincter, 414

Pharynx, 274–275, 275f

Phencyclidine, 699t

Phenergan® (promethazine), 663

Phenobarbital (Luminal®), 687, 690, 695

Phenothiazines, 699t

Phenoxybenzamine (Dibenzyline®), 504

Phentolamine (Regitine®), 690

Phenylephrine (Neosyrephrine®), 404

Phenytoin (Dilantin®), 690, 695, 699t

Pheochromocytoma, 504

Phlebostatic axis, 151f

Photodynamic therapy, 30

Physical function, 642–643

Physical restraints, in ICU, 85–86

Pigeon breast, 296

Pineal body, 488

Pirbuterol (Maxair®), 329

Pitressin® (vasopressin), 424, 459, 612, 732

Pituitary gland, 488f, 488t, 491, 511–516
  anatomy and physiology, 511–513
  case study, 515
  disorders of, 513–515
  online resources, 516
  patient outcomes, 515

Pituitary hormones, 449

Plantar reflex test (Babinski's sign), 355

Plaque rupture, 161

Plasma (fresh frozen) therapy for DIC, 610–611

Plasmapheresis, 599

Plasma renin activity (PRA), 172

Platelet count, 608

Platelet disorders, 597–598

Platelets, 606

Platelet transfusions, 610

Pleural effusion, 297–298

Plavix® (clopidogrel), 113, 189, 403, 598

Pneumocystis carinii pneumonia, 324, 339, 589

Pneumonia, 322–325
  acute process, 295
  aspiration pneumonia, 67, 438
  elderly patients and, 79
  healthcare-associated, 67, 70
  pathophysiology, 322–324
  patient/family education, 325
  pneumocystis carinii, 339, 589
  signs and symptoms of, 324–325
  treatment, 325
  ventilator-associated, 69, 70, 313, 679

Pneumothorax, 298

Poiseuille's law, 361

Poisonings. *See* Drug overdose and poisonings

Pollution, noise, 28–29

Pontocaine® (tetracaine), 654

Portal caval shunt, 425

Portal hypertension, 454, 456

Positioning, in OR, and related problems, 661

Positive end-expiratory pressure (PEEP), 289, 296, 310, 340

Positive-pressure ventilation, 307–308

Positron emission tomography (PET), 187

Postanesthesia recovery, 651–665
  anesthetic agents/adjuncts, 651–657
  assessment, 657
  case study, 664
  complications, 659–663
  discharge criteria, 658
  documentation, 658
  extubation criteria, 657
  initial postoperative care, 657–658
  online resources, 665
  oxygen therapy, 657
  pain management, 662–663
  patient outcomes, 663
  postanesthesia recovery score (PARS), 658t
  postoperative nausea/vomiting, 663
  stir-up regime, 657–658
  temperature regulation, 658

Postcardiotomy failure, 210t

Post-pericardiotomy syndrome, 237–238

Posturing, 355f

Potassium ions, 350

PPE. *See* Personal protective equipment

PPN. *See* Peripheral parenteral nutrition

PRA. *See* Plasma renin activity

Prayer, 110, 111–112

Predictability (patient), 4, 5

Prednisone (Deltasone®), 599, 734t

Preload, 140–141, 234, 245

Pressure Control/Inverse Ratio Ventilation (PC/IRV), 310

Pressure Control (PC), 310

Pressure support ventilation (PSV), 310

Primacor® (milrinone), 100, 234, 249

Primaquine, 101

Primary hyperaldosteronism, 504–505

Primary hypertension, 172–173. *See also* Hypertension

Primary pituitary carcinoma, 513

Printzmetal's angina, 181

Procaine (Novocain®), 654

Procardia® (nifedipine), 173

Process S and process C, 55, 57

Prochlorperazine (Compazine®), 663

ProCord study, 392

Prolactin, 512

Promethazine (Phenergan®), 663

Propofol (Diprivan®), 311, 433, 653, 679–680, 695

Propoxyphene (Darvon®), 692

Propranolol (Inderal®), 101, 459, 498–499, 690

Propylthiouracil (PTU), 498

Prostaglandin analogues, 448

Prostigmin® (neostigmine), 652

Protease inhibitors, 592

Prothrombin time, 609–610

Proton pump inhibitors, 448

Proust phenomenon, 31

Proventil® (albuterol), 329

Proxy advance directives, 720

Prozac® (fluoxetine), 694

Pruritus scores, aromatherapy and, 34

Pseudocholinesterase deficiency, 661

Pseudomonas aeruginosa, 69

PSV. *See* Pressure support ventilation

PSV trials, 316

Psychoacoustic therapy, 33

Psychological function, 643

Psychoneuroimmunology, 28

Psychosis, circadian rhythms and, 30

PTCA. *See* Percutaneous transluminal coronary angioplasty

PTU. *See* Propylthiouracil

Pulmonary alveolar proteinosis, 296t

Pulmonary artery catheters (PACs), 139, 147–148, 148f, 149t, 150, 339

Pulmonary artery catheter waveforms, 153–154, 153f

Pulmonary artery occlusive pressure (PAOP), 141, 245

Pulmonary artery rupture, 150

Pulmonary artery wedge pressure (PAWP), 141

Pulmonary capillary wedge pressure (PCWP), 141

Pulmonary contusion, 675, 677t

Pulmonary disease, obesity and, 709

Pulmonary edema, 295–296, 295t

Pulmonary embolism, 80t, 294, 339, 678, 679, 711

Pulmonary emphysema, 299t

Pulmonary fibrosis, 296

Pulmonary secretions, 283

Pulmonary surfactant, 277

Pulmonary system
   circulation and gas exchange, 277
   shock and, 253

Pulmonary vascular resistance (PVR), 141

Pulse assessment, 137

Pulse oximetry, 283, 284, 285

Pupil assessment, 356–357

PVR. *See* Pulmonary vascular resistance

Pyloric sphincter, 414

Pyrazinamide (Tebrazid®), 326

Quality of life, 4

Quantitative plasma HIV RNA, 591

Radiation therapy, 580, 581

Radiographs, 675

Radiography, 368

Radiosurgery, 398

Ramsay Scale, 366–367

Ranson's criteria for acute pancreatitis, 477

Rapid eye movement (REM) sleep, 53

Recombinant human B-type natriuretic peptide, 199

Rectal examination, 675

Rectal ulcer, solitary, 444

Red blood cell production, 538

Red blood cell treatment, of DIC, 610

Refeeding syndrome, 438

Reflexes, 352, 355

Refludan® (lepirudin), 598

Regitine® (phentolamine), 690

Reglan® (metoclopramide), 437

Rehabilitation services, 642

Relaxation, 47

Relenza® (zanamivir), 322

REM. *See* Rapid eye movement sleep

Renal arteriogram, 540

Renal biopsy, 539

Renal failure, 543–550. *See also* End stage renal disease; Renal transplantation
   acute hepatic failure, 457
   case study, 549
   diuretic stage, 548
   initiation stage, 546–547
   intrarenal acute renal failure, 545–546, 545t
   nursing interventions, 544–545, 546, 547, 548
   oliguric stage, 547
   online resources, 551
   patient and family teaching, 545–546, 546
   patient outcomes, 548
   postrenal acute renal failure, 546
   prerenal acute renal failure, 544–545, 544t
   recovery stage, 548
   research, 548
   rhabdomyolysis and, 679

Renal replacement therapies, 553–562
   acute renal failure and, 554
   case study, 561
   chronic kidney disease staging, 554
   circulatory access types, 555t
   continuous arteriovenous hemofiltration (CAVH), 559–560
   continuous arteriovenous hemodiafiltration (CAVHDF), 559
   continuous arteriovenous hemofiltration-dialysis (CAVHD), 559–560
   continuous renal replacement therapy (CRRT), 559–560
   continuous venovenous hemofiltration (CVVH), 559
   continuous venovenous hemodiafiltration (CVVHDF), 559

Renal replacement therapies—*continued*
  continuous venovenous hemofiltration dialysis
    (CVVHD), 559
  dialysis of drugs, 560–561
  diffusion, 554
  hemodialysis, 555–558, 555t
  need for, 553–554
  nursing interventions, 558, 559, 560
  online resources, 563
  osmosis, 555
  patient and family teaching, 558, 559, 560
  patient outcomes, 561
  peritoneal dialysis, 558–559, 558t
  post-dialysis assessment, 557t
  predialysis assessment, 556t
  principles of dialysis, 554–555
  research, 561
  untrafiltration, 555
Renal status, in shock, 254
Renal system. *See also* Renal failure; Renal replacement
  therapies
  anatomy of, 535–536, 536t
  assessment, 538–540
  interventions, 553–562
  online resources, 540
  physiology of, 536–538
  radiological studies, 539–540
  regulation of blood pressure/osmolarity, 537–538
  renin-angiotensin-aldosterone system, 537
Renal transplantation, 568–569
  assessment for, 569t
  case study, 572
  kidney evaluation criteria, 568t
  online resources, 572–573
  patient and family teaching, 569–570
  patient outcomes, 570
  post-transplant nursing interventions, 569
  pre-transplant nursing interventions, 568–569
  research, 570
Renal ultrasound, 539
Reopro® (abciximab), 598
Resiliency (patient), 4, 5
Resonance, 280
Resource availability (patient), 4, 5, 7
Respiratory anatomy, 271–278
  breathing muscles, 271–278, 273f
  diaphragm, 272
  nerve impulses, 274f
  online resources, 281
  respiratory tract, 273–276
  rib cage, 272f
  thoracic cavity, 271, 272f
Respiratory assessment, 278–281, 281t. *See also* Respiratory
  monitoring

  auscultation, 280
  inspection, 278–279
  palpation, 279–280
  percussion, 280
Respiratory bronchioles, 276
Respiratory defense mechanisms, 323
Respiratory disorders. *See also* Respiratory failure; specific
  disorder
  case study, 334
  online resources, 335
  patient outcomes, 333
Respiratory failure
  airway adjuncts, 299–301
  case studies, 303–304, 305
  noninvasive ventilation, 301–302, 301f
  obstructive causes of, 298–299
  online resources, 305
  patient outcomes, 302
  vascular causes of, 293–294
Respiratory monitoring, 283–291
  arterial blood gas monitoring, 284–287, 285t
  base excess, 287–288
  case study, 290
  compensation, 287
  HCO_3, 287
  online resources, 291
  $PaCO_2$, 286–287
  PaO_2, 285t, 286
  patient outcomes, 289
  pH, 286
  pulse oximetry, 284, 285
  terms, 284t
Respiratory muscle fatigue, 308
Respiratory rate (RR) or frequency, 308–309
Respiratory status
  elderly patients and, 79–80
  shock and, 253
  sleep disorders and, 58
Resting potential, 350
Restless legs syndrome, 57
Restoril® (temazepam), 688
Restrictive lung disease, 294–298
Retrovir® (zidovudine), 590
Retroviruses, 590
Rhabdomyolysis, 679, 687
Ribavirin, 470
Rib cage, 271, 272f
Richmond Agitation Sedation Scale, 367
Rifadin® (rifampin), 326
Rifampin (Rifadin®), 326
Rimantadine hydrochloride (Flumadine®), 322
Ritalin® (methylphenidate), 686
RNA virus, 466
Robinul® (glycopyrrolate), 653

Romazicon® (flumazenil), 688
Ropivacaine hydrochloride (Naropin®), 654
Roux-en-Y gastric bypass (RYGB), 707, 708t
Rule of Nines, 630, 631t
RYGB. *See* Roux-en-Y gastric bypass

SAH. *See* Subarachnoid hemorrhage
Salicylates, 693–694, 693t, 699t
Salivary glands, 416
Salmeterol (Serevent®), 329
Sandostatin® (octreotide), 424, 459, 478
Sarcoidosis, 296t
SARS. *See* Severe acute respiratory syndrome
Satisfaction with care (patient), 4
Scalenes, 273
Scar tissue formation, 637
Scleral endoscopic therapy, 423–424
Scoliosis, 297
Scopolamine (Hyoscine hydrobromide®), 663
ScvO₂, 145
SDH. *See* Subdural hematoma
SE. *See* Status epilepticus
Seasonal affective disorder, 30
Secobarbital (Seconal®), 687
Seconal® (secobarbital), 687
Secondary hypertension, 172–173, 173t. *See also*
        Hypertension
Secondary hypothyroidism, 513
Second degree burn, 629, 630t. *See also* Burn(s)
Sedation
    mechanical ventilators and, 311
    monitoring, 366–368
    physiological assessment of, 367–368
Sedative hypnotics, 688, 699t
Sedentary lifestyles, health effects of, 163
Segmented branches, 276
Seizures, 366, 379–380
    focal motor, 380
    tonic-clonic, 380
Sengstaken-Blakemore tube, 447
Sensitivity (breathing and), 309–310
Sensory nerve roots, 377t
Sensory system, 355–356
Sepsis, 84t, 477, 619–628
    cardiovascular assessment/intervention, 621, 623–624
    coagulation, 621
    fibrinolysis, 621
    gastrointestinal assessment/intervention, 622, 625
    hematologic assessment/intervention, 622, 625
    infection prevention, 626
    inflammation, 620–621
    integumentary assessment/intervention, 623, 625
    interventions, 623–626, 624t
    lab values, 625–626, 629

neurological assessment/intervention, 622–623, 625
nursing assessments, 621–623
online resources, 628
pathophysiology, 620
patient/family education/communication, 626
patient outcomes, 626
pulmonary assessment/intervention, 621, 624–625
renal assessment/intervention, 621, 625
signs/symptoms of, 619–620, 622
Septal defect, 188
Serevent® (salmeterol), 329
Serum creatinine, 538
Serum electrolyte monitoring, 538
Serum laboratory tests, 538–539
Serum lactate elevation, 691
Severe acute respiratory syndrome (SARS), 113
Sevoflurane (Ultane®), 652
Sheehan's syndrome, 505, 513
Shivering, postoperative, 235
Shock, 80t, 243–258
    anaphylactic, 251
    blood transfusion steps, 248
    burn shock, 633
    cardiogenic, 187, 247, 249, 669
    case studies, 256–257
    classification/etiology/underlying effects, 244t
    compensated, 251–252
    distributive, 244t, 250–251
    emergent phase, 630–631
    fluid resuscitation, 255, 633–634
    hemodynamics review, 243–245, 246t
    hypovolemic, 246–247, 445–446
    irreversible, 252–253
    neurogenic, 250–251, 391
    nurse management of, 255
    obstructive, 244t, 249–250
    online resources, 258
    patient management, 254–255
    patient outcomes, 255, 256
    progressive, 252
    renal status, 254
    spinal, 391
    stages, 251–253
    syndromes, classified, 245–246
    system progression/management, 253–254
Shunt, 289, 294
SIADH. *See* Syndrome of inappropriate antidiuretic
        hormone secretion
Sigmoidoscopy, 422–423, 445
Sildenafil citrate (Viagra®), 189
Silver nitrate (AgNO3), 635t
Silver sulfadiazine, 635t
Simple pneumothorax, 677t
Simplified predictive formula, 433

Singulair® (montelukast), 329
SIRS response, 636
Skeletal deformities, 296–297
Skin breakdown, 342
Skin grafts, 636
Skin inspection, in respiratory assessment, 279
Skin integrity, with shock, 254–255
Skin substitutes, 636t
Skull fractures, 389, 672
Sleep
    architecture in young *vs.* older adults, 55f
    benefits of uninterrupted, 111
    case study, 62
    deprivation, and delirium, 82
    disturbed, in intensive care unit, 53, 55–60
    function of, 54–55
    history, 57
    improving, in ICU, 60–62
    noise and, 28–29
    nonrapid eye movement (NREM), 53–55
    online resources, 63
    overview of normal, 53–55
    pain perception and, 41
    process s and process c, 55–58
    rapid eye movement (REM), 53–55
    regulation, 55
    slow-wave, 54
    stages, 54f
    therapeutic touch and, 111
Sleep disorders
    chronic illness and, 57–58
    demographics and, 57
    sleep apnea, 57
Small bowel feeding, 435
Small intestine, 416
Smells, effects of, 31–32
Smoking, coronary artery disease and, 162
SNS. *See* Sympathetic nervous system
Social function, 643
Social organization, family, 100–101
Sodium bicarbonate, 583
Sodium ions, 350
Sodium nitrite, 691
Sodium retention, 81t
Sodium thiosulfate, 691
Solu-Medrol® (methylprednisolone), 673–674
Somatic nervous system, 354
Somatostatin (Aminopan®), 424, 478
Somatostatin analogues, 449
Somatotropin, 512
Sound
    absorption, 29
    therapeutic, 33

Soy supplements, 112
Space, cultural preferences for, 99
Space-occupying lesion of the pituitary, 514
Spetzler-Martin Surgical Grading Scale, 397t
Sphincters, 414
Spinal anesthesia, 655–656
Spinal cord compression, 583–584
Spinal cord/spinal cord injuries, 352–353, 375, 390–392
    care of patient with, 391–392
    neurogenic shock and spinal shock, 391
    nursing management of, 392
    research, 392
    spine trauma, 672–674
    steroid use after, 392
    vertebral fractures, 390–392
Spirituality, 111–112
Spiriva® (tiotropium bromide), 329
Spironolactone (Aldoctone®), 505
Square wave testing, 149, 151
St. John's wort, 112
Stability (patient), 4, 5
Stab wounds, 677
Staphylococcus aureus, 69
Statins, 190
Status asthmaticus, 329–330
Status epilepticus (SE), 379–380, 381
Stavudine (Zerit®), 592
Stent-assisted coiling, 403
Stenting, 191
Stereognosis, 355
Sternal abnormalities, 296
Sternomastoids, 273
Steroids, and spinal cord injuries, 392
Stir-up regime, 657–658
Stomach, 414–415
Stool assessment, for gastrointestinal bleeding, 444
Streptase® (streptokinase), 581
Streptokinase (Streptase®), 581
Stress, lack of sleep and, 57
Stress echocardiography, 187
Stressors, 42
Stress perfusion imaging, 187
Stress-related erosive syndrome, 444
Stress response, 42
Stress testing, 186–187
Stress ulcers, 342
Stroke
    hemorrhagic, 378–379
    ischemic, 378, 379
Stroke volume, 140
Strychnine, 699t
Subacute care, 642
Subarachnoid bolt, 362

Subarachnoid hemorrhage (SAH), 378, 380, 389, 395
Subcutaneous emphysema (crepitus), 279
Subdural hematoma (SDH), 389, 672
Subfulminant hepatic failure, 453. *See also* Hepatic failure
Subjective global assessment, 432
Succinylcholine (Anectine®), 653
Sulcrafate (Carafate®), 459
Sulfamylon, 635
Sulfanilamide, 101
Sulfonylurea, 696t
Sumycin® (tetracycline), 476
Superior vena cava (SVC), 277
Superior vena cava syndrome, 580–581
Suprane® (desflurane), 652
Surfactant administration, 341
Surgical resection, AVMs and, 396–397
Surgical site infections, 70
SVC. *See* Superior vena cava
Sympathetic nervous system (SNS), 349
Synapse, 351, 352f
Syndrome of inappropriate antidiuretic hormone secretion (SIADH), 514, 581–582
Synergy Model, 3–12, 4t
    case study (Clarian Health Partners), 11
    healthcare environment/system, 4
    nurse competencies, 6–7t
    online resources, 12
    overview, 3–4
    patient characteristics, 4, 5t, 8
    plan of care development and, 9, 10t, 38
    in transcultural care, 97
Synthroid® (levothyroxine), 500
Systemic inflammatory response syndrome (SIRS), 79, 619, 620f. *See also* Sepsis
Systemic vascular resistance, 142
Systems thinking, 4, 6–7
Systolic heart failure, 198. *See also* Heart failure
Systolic peak, 154

Tactile fremitus, 279, 280
Tagamet® (cimetidine), 538
Tamiflu® (oseltamivir), 322
Tapazole® (methimazole), 498
T-cell count, 591
Tebrazid® (pyrazinamide), 326
TEE. *See* Transesophageal echocardiogram
Tegretol® (carbamazepine), 514
Temazepam (Restoril®), 688
Tenormin® (atenolol), 504
TENS. *See* Transcutaneous electrical nerve stimulator
Tension pneumothorax, 669, 677t
Terbutaline (Brethine®), 329
Terlipressin (Norapressin®), 424

Terminal airways, microanatomy of, 276
Testicles, 488f, 488t
Tetracaine (Pontocaine®), 654
Tetracycline (Sumycin®), 476
Thallium-201 (Cordiolite®), 187
Therapeutic touch (TT), 110–111
Thermoregulation, 83
Thiazide diuretics, 176t
Thiopental sodium (Pentothal®), 653, 687
Thioplex® (thiotepa), 578
Thiotepa (Thioplex®), 578
Third degree burn, 630t. *See also* Burn(s)
Thoracic cavity, 271, 272f
Thoracic trauma, 675–678, 677t, 679
Thoratec HeartMate II Lef Ventricular Assist System, 215
Thoratec HeartMate Implanted Pneumatic Left Ventricular Assist System, 214–215
Thoratec Heartmate XVE Left VAD, 215f
Thoratec Implantable VAD, 214, 217
Throid storm, 498–499
Thrombin time, 610
Thrombocytopenia, 597–603
    case study, 602
    clinical presentation of, 598–599
    evaluation/diagnosis, 599–600
    heparin-induced, 598
    idiopathic thrombocytopenic purpura, 598–599
    mechanisms/associated clinical conditions, 599t
    online resources, 603
    patient outcomes, 601
    platelet disorders, 597–598
    platelets and normal hemostasis, 597
    qualitative platelet disorders, 598
    quantitative platelet disorders, 598
    treatment/management, 600–601
Thrombolytic therapy, 190, 379, 581
Thrombophlebitis, 283
Thromboprophylaxis, 709
Thrombosis, 263
Thrombosis of renal artery/vein, 478
Thrombotic thrombocytopenic purpura (TTP), 599
Thrombus formation, 161
Thymus gland, 488t
Thyroid cartilage, 272f, 275
Thyroid disorders, 491, 497–502
    case study, 501
    euthyroid sick syndrome, 500
    myxedema coma, 499–500
    normal hormone levels, 498t
    normal thyroid function, 497–498
    online resources, 502
    patient outcomes, 500, 501
    thyroid storm, 498–499

Thyroid gland, 488t
Thyroid hormone replacement, 500
Thyroid-stimulating hormone (TSH), 512
Thyroid storm, 498–499
Thyrolar® (liothyronine), 500
Thyrotoxic crisis, 498
Thyrotropin, 512
Thyrotropin deficit, 513
TIA. *See* Transient ischemic attack
Tidal volume, 308
Tikosyn® (dofetilide), 203
Tilde® (nedocromil), 329
Time orientation, 100
Tiotropium bromide (Spiriva®), 329
TIPS. *See* Transvenous intrahepatic portosystemic shunt
Tirofiban hydrochloride (Aggrastat®), 598
Tissue factor pathway inhibitor, 611
Tissue perfusion, 139, 140, 365
Tongue, 416
Tongue obstruction, 669
Total parenteral nutrition (TPN), 434
Touching, 99, 110–111
Toxin elimination, 538
"T-piece," 316
TPN. *See* Total parenteral nutrition
Trachea, 272f, 275
Trandate® (labetalol), 173, 174t, 263, 690
Tranquilizers, 688
Transcranial Doppler studies, 368
Transcultural care
    evidence-based, 103t
    guidelines, 102, 104 (*See also* Cultural issues, in critical illness)
    summary of key research, 103t
    transcultural nursing, defined, 96
Transcutaneous electrical nerve stimulator (TENS), 47
Transducer systems, 148–149
    fluid-filled, 361
Transducer-tipped systems (fiberoptic), 362
Transduction, 42
Transection, 390–391
Transesophageal echocardiogram (TEE), 186
Transfusions
    complications from, 679
    platelet, 601
    reactions, 269
Transient ischemic attack (TIA), 80
Transitional planning, 641–647
    case study, 646
    economic domain, 644
    nursing role in, 642–644
    online resources, 647

    patient outcomes, 646
    physical function, 642–643
    planning as collaborative practice, 642
    post-acute care alternatives, 642
    psychological function, 643
    screening, 644–646
    social function, 643
Transmission, 43
Transthoracic (transcutaneous) temporary pacemaker, 218–220
Transvenous biopsy, 426
Transvenous intrahepatic portosystemic shunt (TIPS), 424–425, 445, 447
Transvenous temporary pacemaker, 220
Trauma, 667–682, 671t
    abdominal trauma, 671, 674–675, 675t, 676t, 679
    assessment, 669–671
    case study, 681
    elderly patients and, 680
    head injury, 670–671, 672, 673t
    ICU considerations, 678–680
    imaging modalities, 674–675
    mechanism of injury, 668
    monitoring adjuncts, 676–677
    monitoring equipment/diagnostic studies, 671t
    online resources, 682
    orthopedic, 678
    patient outcomes, 680
    phases of trauma care, 668
    physiology of trauma/injury, 668–669
    primary/secondary survey, 676t
    spine trauma, 672–674
    "systems approach" to, 667
    thoracic, 675–678, 677t, 679
    trauma systems, 667–668
Trauma centers, 668
Triamcinolone (Aristocort®), 329
Triazolam (Halcion®), 688
Tricyclic antidepressants, 694–695, 699t
Tridal® (nitroglycerin), 174t
Trigger sensitivity, 309
Triglycerides, 161–162
Triple-H therapy, 404–405
Troponin, 185
Trust, 4, 16, 22
TSH. *See* Thyroid-stimulating hormone
TT. *See* Therapeutic touch
TTP. *See* Thrombotic thrombocytopenic purpura
Tube clogging, 437–438
Tube malposition, 437
Tuberculosis, 325–327
    pathophysiology, 325–326

patient/family education, 327
signs/symptoms of, 326
treatment, 326–327
Tumor lysis syndrome, 582–583

Ultane® (sevoflurane), 652
Ultrasound, 419
Understaffing, ICU infections and, 71
Unfractionated heparin, 189, 656t
United Network for Organ Sharing, 239, 728
Unstable angina, 181
Upper airway obstruction/edema, 632
Upper GI endoscopy, 422
Upper GI series, 445
Upper GI tract, bleeding and, 443. *See also* Gastrointestinal bleeding
Upper respiratory tract, 273–275, 274f
Urea breath test, 419
Urgent hypertension, 173. *See also* Hypertension
Urinalysis, 539
Urinary catheter, 675
Urinary tract infections, 70
Urine creatinine, 539
Urine free cortisol level, 507
Urine laboratory tests, 539
Urokinase (Abbokinase®), 581

Vaccinations, 84
Vacuum-assisted closure, 635–636
VADs. *See* Ventricular assist devices (VADs)
Valium® (diazepam), 690, 695
Valproic acid (Depakene®), 476
Valve surgery, 232
Valvuloplasty, 232
Vancomycin-resistant *Enterococcus* (VRE), 68, 295
Variceal banding, 424
Varicella-zoster virus (Chicken pox), 68
VAS. *See* Visual Analogue Scale
Vascular changes, in the elderly, 80
Vascular disorders, 261–267
abdominal aortic aneurysm, 261–263
arterial occlusion/venus occlusion, 263–265
case study, 267
compartment syndrome, 265–266
online resources, 268
patient outcomes, 266
Vascular ectasias, 444
Vascular stenting of the vena cava, 581
Vasoactive drugs, 578
Vasodilation, 732
Vasodilators, 176t
Vasopressin (Pitressin®), 424, 447, 459, 612, 732

Vasospasm, 404–405
Vasotec® (enalapril), 174t
Vecuronium (Norcuron®), 368
Venogram, 581
Venous occlusion, 263–265
Venous thromboembolism, 711
Ventilation, 32. *See also* Mechanical ventilation; Respiratory monitoring
elderly patients and, 79–80
neurologic disorders and, 377
noninvasive, 301–302
Ventilation/perfusion mismatch, 294–298
Ventilator-associated pneumonia (VAP), 69, 70, 313, 342, 679
Ventilator liberation, 314
Ventilatory failure, impending, 308
Ventricular assist devices (VADs), 234, 239–240
basics, 209–216
biventricular assist device, 212
bridge to recovery, 212
bridge to transplant, 212
care of patient with a VAD, 216–218
choosing, 213
compared, 218t
current applications, 212
destination therapy, 210t, 212
discharge teaching, 217t
FDA-approved systems, 213–215
future device therapy, 215
in heart failure patients, 199
infection control guidelines, 216t
left ventricular assist devices, 210–211, 211f
patient selection/timing, 212–213, 213t
physical assessment, 217t
physiology, 210–212
potential postoperative concerns, 215–216
right ventricular assist devices, 211f
terminology, 210t
Ventricular dysrhythmias, 150, 694
Ventricular ectopy, 81
Ventriculogram, 187
Ventriculostomy, 360
Veracity, 722
Verapamil hydrochloride (Calan®), 405
Versed® (midazolam), 311, 653, 688
Vertebral arteries, 375, 376t
Vertical banded gastroplasty, 708t
Viagra® (sildenafil citrate), 189
Videx® (didanosine), 592
Vietnamese families, 102
Viracept® (nelfinavir), 592
Viral encephalitis, 381–382

Viral hepatitis. *See* Hepatitis
Virchow's triad, 264
Virtual colonoscopy, 423
"Virtual window," 31
Visiting policies, 18–19, 32
Visual Analogue Scale (VAS), 85
Vitamin deficiencies, 456t
Vocal chords, 275
Vocal fremitus, 279
Voice box, 275
Volume-guaranteed pressure modes, 311
Volume ventilation, 308
Volu-trauma, 313–314
VRE, *See* Vancomycin-resistant *Enterococcus*
Vulnerability (patient), 4, 5

Warfarin sodium (Coumadin®), 113, 190, 499, 581
Waste elimination, 538
Waveform interpretation, 153–154
Wear-and-tear theory of aging, 79

"Wedge" pressure, 245
Weight-reduction surgery. *See* Bariatric patients; Bariatric surgery
Windows, light/view and, 29–31
Wood alcohol (methanol), 691–692, 698t
Workstation design, 29

Xanax® (alprazolam), 688
Xigris® (drotrecogin alfa (activated)), 341, 624
Xofenex® (levalbuterol), 329
Xolair® (omalizumab), 329
Xylocaine® (lidocaine), 654, 690, 732

Zanamivir (Relenza®), 322
Zerit® (stavudine), 592
Zidovudine (Retrovir®), 590
Zofran® (ondansetron), 663
Zoledronate acid (Zometa®), 580
Zometa® (zoledronate acid), 580
Zovirax® (acyclovir), 382